MEDICAL-SURGICAL NURSING

■ KATHLEEN NEWTON SHAFER, R.N., M.A.
Formerly Associate Professor of Out-Patient Nursing, Cornell University–New York Hospital School of Nursing; formerly Assistant Consultant in Orthopedic Nursing, National League for Nursing Education; formerly Instructor in Medical Nursing and Instructor in Surgical Nursing, Cornell University–New York Hospital School of Nursing, New York, N. Y.

■ JANET R. SAWYER, R.N., Ph.D.
Associate Professor, School of Nursing, University of Vermont, Burlington, Vt.; formerly Instructor, School of Education, Department of Nurse Education, New York University; formerly Instructor in Surgical Nursing, Cornell University–New York Hospital School of Nursing, New York, N. Y.

■ AUDREY M. McCLUSKEY, R.N., M.A., Sc.M.Hyg.
Associate Director, Continuing Education Project, New England Board of Higher Education, Wellesley, Mass.; formerly Associate Professor and Chairman, Public Health Nursing, Yale University School of Nursing, New Haven, Conn.; formerly Associate Professor in Nursing, Cornell University–New York Hospital School of Nursing

■ EDNA LIFGREN BECK, R.N., M.A.
Formerly Associate Director of Nursing Education, Muhlenberg Hospital School of Nursing, Plainfield, N. J.; formerly Assistant Professor in Fundamentals of Nursing and Instructor in Surgical Nursing, Cornell University–New York Hospital School of Nursing; formerly Clinical Instructor in Surgical Nursing, Roosevelt Hospital School of Nursing, New York, N. Y.

■ WILMA J. PHIPPS, R.N., A.M.
Professor and Chairman of Medical-Surgical Nursing, Frances Payne Bolton School of Nursing, Case Western Reserve University, Cleveland, Ohio; Director of Medical-Surgical Nursing, University Hospitals of Cleveland; formerly Associate Professor, Medical-Surgical Nursing, University of Illinois at the Medical Center, Chicago, Ill.; formerly Instructor in Tuberculosis Nursing, Herman Kiefer Hospital, Detroit, Mich.

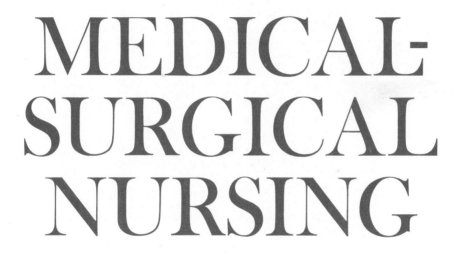

MEDICAL-SURGICAL NURSING

KATHLEEN NEWTON SHAFER

JANET R. SAWYER

AUDREY M. McCLUSKEY

EDNA LIFGREN BECK

WILMA J. PHIPPS

SIXTH EDITION

With 608 Illustrations

THE C. V. MOSBY COMPANY

SAINT LOUIS   1975

■ DEDICATION

To all our students past and present from whom we have gained so much. We trust that this book will assist them to practice nursing at the highest possible level.

Sixth edition

Copyright © 1975 by The C. V. Mosby Company

All rights reserved. No part of this book may be reproduced in any manner without written permission of the publisher.

Previous editions copyrighted 1958, 1961, 1964, 1967, 1971

Printed in the United States of America

Distributed in Great Britain by Henry Kimpton, London

Library of Congress Cataloging in Publication Data

Shafer, Kathleen Newton.
    Medical-surgical nursing.

    Includes bibliographies and index.
    1. Nurses and nursing. I. Title.
[DNLM: 1. Nursing care. WY150 M489]
RT41.S5 1975   610.73   74-20829
ISBN 0-8016-4516-6

TS/U/B 9 8 7 6 5 4 3 2 1

Contributors

■ **RANDALL K. BEEDLE, Ph.D.,** Director of Audiology, Cleveland Speech and Hearing Center; Associate Professor of Audiology, Case Western Reserve University

■ **FRANCES R. BROWN, R.N., M.S.N.,** Assistant Clinical Professor of Nursing, Frances Payne Bolton School of Nursing, Case Western Reserve University; Nurse Clinician, Cardiovascular Nursing, University Hospitals of Cleveland

■ **PATRICIA BUERGIN, R.N., B.S.N.,** Senior Clinical Nurse, University Hospitals of Cleveland

■ **MARY E. BUSHONG, R.N., M.S.N.,** Assistant Professor of Operating and Recovery Room Nursing, Frances Payne Bolton School of Nursing, Case Western Reserve University; Nurse Clinician, Recovery Room Nursing, University Hospitals of Cleveland

■ **DOROTHY A. BUTLER, R.N., Ed.M.,** Clinical Instructor in Medical-Surgical Nursing, Frances Payne Bolton School of Nursing, Case Western Reserve University; Nurse Clinician, Orthopedic Nursing, University Hospitals of Cleveland

■ **ELIZABETH J. BYRNES, R.N., M.S.N.,** Assistant Clinical Professor of Nursing, Frances Payne Bolton School of Nursing, Case Western Reserve University; Assistant Director of Medical-Surgical Nursing, University Hospitals of Cleveland

■ **LYNN W. CHENOWETH, R.N., M.S.N.,** Instructor in Medical-Surgical Nursing, Frances Payne Bolton School of Nursing, Case Western Reserve University; Associate in Nursing, University Hospitals of Cleveland

■ **ELLA A. CINKOTA, R.N., Ed.M.,** Associate Professor of Maternity Nursing, Frances Payne Bolton School of Nursing, Case Western Reserve University; Associate in Nursing, University Hospitals of Cleveland

■ **BARBARA J. DALY, R.N., M.S.N.,** Clinical Instructor in Medical-Surgical Nursing, Frances Payne Bolton School of Nursing, Case Western Reserve University; Administrative Nurse Clinician, Intensive Care Nursing, University Hospitals of Cleveland

■ **BARBARA A. GESSNER, R.N., M.S.N.,** Nursing Specialist, University of Wisconsin Extension, Madison

■ **SISTER PAULA GONZALEZ, Ph.D.,** Associate Professor of Biology, College of Mount Saint Joseph, Cincinnati

■ **C. JOAN GOWIN, R.N., M.A.,** Associate Professor of Operating and Recovery Room Nursing, Frances Payne Bolton School of Nursing, Case Western Reserve University; Director of Operating and Recovery Room Nursing, University Hospitals of Cleveland

■ **JUDITH L. GREIG, R.N., M.S.N.,** Assistant Professor of Operating and Recovery Room Nursing, Frances Payne Bolton School of Nursing, Case Western Reserve University; Nurse Clinician, Operating Room Nursing, University Hospitals of Cleveland

■ **GRACE McCARTHY HARLAN, R.N., M.A.,** Assistant Professor of Medical-Surgical Nursing, Frances Payne Bolton School of Nursing, Case Western Reserve University; Associate in Nursing, University Hospitals of Cleveland

■ **VIRGINIA BURKE KARB, R.N., M.S.N.,** Clinical Instructor in Medical-Surgical Nursing, Frances Payne Bolton School of Nursing, Case Western Reserve University; Nurse Clinician, Neurosurgical Nursing, University Hospitals of Cleveland

■ **MARJORIE A. KINNEY, R.N., M.S.N.,** formerly Assistant Professor of Medical-Surgical Nursing, Frances Payne Bolton School of Nursing, Case Western Reserve University; Nurse Clinician, Rehabilitation Nursing, University Hospitals of Cleveland

Contributors

■ **DONNA J. KUKLO, R.N., M.S.N.,** Assistant Clinical Professor of Medical-Surgical Nursing, Frances Payne Bolton School of Nursing, Case Western Reserve University; Coordinator of Decentralized Staff Development, Medical-Surgical Nursing, University Hospitals of Cleveland

■ **PAULA J. LAMBRECHT, R.N., M.S.,** Assistant Clinical Professor of Medical-Surgical Nursing, Frances Payne Bolton School of Nursing, Case Western Reserve University; Nurse Clinician, Renal Nursing, University Hospitals of Cleveland

■ **BARBARA C. LONG, R.N., M.S.N.,** Associate Professor of Medical-Surgical Nursing, Frances Payne Bolton School of Nursing, Case Western Reserve University; Associate in Nursing, University Hospitals of Cleveland

■ **CAROL J. MITTEN, R.N., M.S.N.,** Assistant Clinical Professor of Medical-Surgical Nursing, Frances Payne Bolton School of Nursing, Case Western Reserve University; Nurse Clinician, Metabolic Nursing, University Hospitals of Cleveland

■ **FRANK E. MUSIEK, M.A.,** Doctoral Candidate in Audiology, Case Western Reserve University

■ **JANICE NEVILLE, D.Sc.,** Associate Professor of Nutrition, Case Western Reserve University

■ **ALICE D. NORMAN, R.N., M.S.N.,** Assistant Clinical Professor of Medical-Surgical Nursing, Frances Payne Bolton School of Nursing, Case Western Reserve University; Nurse Clinician, Pulmonary Nursing, University Hospitals of Cleveland

■ **CATHERINE O'MALLEY, R.N.,** Supervisor of Specialty Units, Cleveland Metropolitan General Hospital

■ **ELIZABETH A. SCHENK, R.N., M.S.N.,** Nurse Clinician, Rehabilitation Nursing, Highland View Hospital, Cleveland

■ **SHIRLEY SLEEKER, R.N., M.S.N.,** Cardiovascular Nurse Clinician, Baptist Memorial Hospital, Kansas City, Missouri

■ **FRANCES WHITE, R.N.,** Senior Clinical Nurse, University Hospitals of Cleveland

■ **MAY WYKLE, R.N., M.S.N.,** Assistant Professor of Psychiatric-Mental Health Nursing, Frances Payne Bolton School of Nursing, Case Western Reserve University; Associate in Nursing, University Hospitals of Cleveland

Preface

Since the previous edition of *Medical-Surgical Nursing* was published, many changes have taken place in society in general, in medical and health care, and in the practice of nursing. This sixth edition seeks to faithfully reflect these changes. Increasing emphasis has been placed on understanding the physiologic basis of deviations from normal, and additional attention has been given to all aspects of the role of assessment in nursing practice. The reader will find that these threads are carried throughout the book. Although the format of the book remains essentially the same, those familiar with past editions will find many changes. For example, a new chapter, Ecology and Health, has been added to accentuate this very important issue, and Chapters 32 and 33 in the fifth edition have been combined to better present the problems of patients with musculoskeletal injuries and disorders. The chapter on neurologic diseases has also been extensively revised and updated.

In order to assist all nurses—both students and those in active practice—to keep abreast of changes in the delivery of health care, many experts contributed to this revision. I am deeply grateful to each of them for the time and energy they contributed to this revision. I am also indebted to the many members of the faculty of the Case Western Reserve University, School of Medicine, who read parts of the manuscript and whose valuable suggestions are incorporated in this edition.

I am especially grateful to Sister Paula Gonzalez, Ph.D., who wrote Chapter 3, Ecology and Health, and to Mrs. Geraldine Mink, Librarian, Health Sciences Library, Case Western Reserve University, for her valuable assistance with research for the book. The new illustrations for this edition are by Barbara M. Rankin and William Holmes. Their expert assistance is gratefully acknowledged. My special thanks go to Janet Mitchell and Sondra Patrizi, who assisted with the typing and editing of the manuscript, and to my cousin, Donna M. Hone, who helped with the many last-minute details. Most of all I am indebted to the original four authors of this book who first conceived the idea of a joint medical-surgical nursing text. I trust that this edition will meet their goal of providing a book that is truly patient centered and assists nurses to provide better health care to all persons with whom they interact.

Wilma J. Phipps

Contents

Contents

Contents

Contents

Contents

32 Neurologic diseases, 847

33 Musculoskeletal injuries and disorders, 933

Trends and problems influencing patient care

1 The patient and the nurse
understanding, interaction, and the nursing process

■ Nurses in all practice settings have as one of their goals the therapeutic use of self as a means by which the patient or client being served is assisted to maintain, restore, or improve health. In order to better understand human behavior and the forces that shape individuals and their responses in time of stress and crisis, the nurse needs to have a broad background in the behavioral sciences. An increased awareness of cultural patterns, normal defense mechanisms, emotional responses to crisis, coping behavior, and interpersonal relationships may be obtained from formal courses, by reading articles or books, or by viewing audiovisual materials and the like. Current social forces demand that all nurses, as health professionals, be continuing learners. Thus no one should be discouraged by what they do not know at a given point in time as long as they are committed to seeking answers to questions and acquiring new knowledge, skills, and increased sensitivity. Because most of nursing is practiced in dynamic, ever-changing settings, it is essential that each nurse understand and accept the need to continue to grow both as a person and as a nurse. Only a few of the basic concepts involved in developing a therapeutic relationship with a patient can be discussed in this chapter, and it is assumed that the reader will be stimulated to seek out additional information from the many references listed at the end of this chapter and throughout the book.

■ UNDERSTANDING AND INTERACTION
The concept of patient

"The patient is a person" and "patients are people" are phrases used frequently in the nurse's education. These or similar phrases serve to remind the nurse that the patient, whoever he may be, is a human being with hopes and desires, likes and dislikes, strengths and weaknesses. The patient may be a man or a woman, a boy or girl, an infant or an elderly person. *Who* he is and *his place* are important. They are of paramount importance to him and they should be a most important consideration in his care.

Being a patient places the person in a unique setting. The number of places where patient care is offered today are numerous and differ greatly. The person who becomes a patient is often described as "one who is under the care of a physician or in a hospital." Patients also receive care in the physician's office, in the outpatient service of a hospital, in their own homes, in nursing homes, in other institutions, and more recently in offices of nurses in private practice. Regardless of where care is given, each experience has special meaning to the patient. Perhaps for most people, institutional care has the greatest significance. The fact that the person is away from his home, family, friends, and usual way of life, even for only a short time, and is faced with threat of disease or illness and unpleasant experiences may tax his resources in understanding and in adaptation.

The individual who becomes a patient in a hospital takes on a different status and is surrounded by circumstances quite unlike his usual ones. His total environment becomes different from the familiar. He is requested to wear clothing he normally wears only for sleep. His living quarters are only a room or cubicle that is little more than a place to rest. He may have private bathing or toilet facilities, but most likely he will share a community-type room. A public lounge may be available to him and his family, or there may be only a bench in the corridor. His family, perhaps some friends, hospital personnel,

■ STUDY QUESTIONS

1 Keep a record for a week of each patient for whom you care. Include the patient's age, his nationality, his place of birth, the language spoken in his home, his education, his place in his family, and his religion. Consider whether or not any of these influenced the nursing care you gave.

2 How has knowledge of the patient's background, as listed above, influenced your teaching of a patient during his preparation for leaving the hospital?

3 What are some of the ways in which anxiety may be expressed? List some questions that patients and members of their families have asked you that indicate anxiety.

and fellow patients complete the group of people who will be his close associates during his hospitalization. The latter two groups of people are determined for him by circumstances rather than by his choice.

A patient in the hospital is the recipient of suggestion, direction, explanation, and treatment. He is observed, tested, exposed to situations over which he may have little or no control and is given a variety of medications and treatments. He may have surgery. As he recovers from illness or completes a diagnostic survey, he usually is given a final checkup, and then he may be declared well enough to resume life at home or he may go to another institution for further care. On the other hand, the hospitalization may be his last life experience.

The patient's response to illness may be quite different from his response to hospitalization. Illness outside a hospital may be accepted and the patient may experience physical and emotional discomfort with little outward expression. With hospitalization, his response to illness may be intensified, or his reaction may be one of relief with a lessening of his reaction to illness. The significance of the hospital or hospital care to each patient needs careful consideration. Hospital surroundings, atmosphere, and ways of doing things are very familiar to personnel and to some patients. Most patients, however, are not familiar with them and need help in adjusting to the experience.

The patient's concept of the nurse

The nurse should be aware that each patient has a mental image of the nurse and that wide variations exist. The same factors influencing his behavioral responses to illness and care will influence his concept and expectations of the nurse.

The image the patient has of nurses may speed or delay his acceptance of them and of what they help him to do. For example, his mental image of the nurse may be that of a woman in a white uniform, cap, shoes, and stockings. Thus the patient may not be quite prepared for the male nurse, and in some instances the male nurse may have to work harder to gain the patient's trust. Public health nurses may also find that the patient questions their identity since they wear colored uniforms and come into his home to give care.

The patient's concept of the nurse is frequently based on the general public's idea, particularly if the patient has had no previous contact with nurses. Nurses are often thought of as persons who are good, immaculately groomed, efficient, and kind. They are thought of as persons who "do for the sick." Therefore when the patient is asked to participate in his own care, he may feel that the nurse does not understand how sick he is and that he is being "picked on." Unfortunately in the past much of the "caring" in nurse-patient relationships has been conveyed through doing *for* the patient rather than *with* the patient.

The public frequently turns to nurses for answers to questions regarding health, but the nurse is seldom considered a teacher. When nurses attempt to teach the patient and family about measures to prevent illness and to maintain health, they may elicit little interest from them. Thus, if continuing nursing care consists primarily of health supervision in the home, the patient and his family may feel that a nurse is not needed. If treatment or physical exercises must be given, the patient may recognize this as concrete evidence of "doing" and accept the need for a nurse. When nurses make arrangements for patient care, particularly in the change from care in the hospital to care in the home, these factors should be borne in mind.

Some patients may have had traumatic experiences that lead them to distrust and reject the nurse. Others may have listened to harrowing experiences of their friends and assume that their association with nurses will not be pleasant. The nurse should try to help the patient correct this distortion by spending time with him and getting to know him as an individual. This is the first step in establishing a therapeutic nurse-patient relationship.

Psychologic factors may affect the patient's response to the nurse. When any person becomes ill and dependent on others, he regresses to some extent. Just having to be in a hospital and having to abide by the regulations places the patient in a dependent position. Some patients unconsciously respond to the nurse as they did to their mothers during childhood. This may be demonstrated by docile obedience, eagerness for approval, or a number of other ways. Their behavioral expressions will depend on what they learned as appropriate responses. Others may identify the nurse with a domineering mother from whom they may be seeking emancipation or with an unwanted mother-in-law. They may respond with stubborn and contradictory behavior that the nurse must try to understand.

The patient may have come from a cultural background in which women are considered inferior to men, one in which women unquestionably wait upon men. For example, a man who had recently come to this country antagonized all the female members of a nursing staff by ordering them about and by refusing to help himself at all. His convalescence was being delayed by his firm conviction that the women about him, the nurses, must "do for him" on all occasions. An alert nurse noticed that he also ordered his wife about during visiting hours and that she accepted this in a satisfied fashion. Only then did the nurses realize the meaning of his behavior. In this particular instance the situation was remedied by working through the physician, whose opinions, suggestions, and judgments were accepted readily by the patient. Thus the nurses learned from this insight into the patient's behavior and no longer needed to feel resentful.

Interpretation of all we see is based on our own experiences and learning. Therefore it is not strange that the nurse is seen in a different light by each patient and his family members. Accepting this, the nurse needs to work toward responding to each patient individually, respecting his differences and placing emphasis on common elements. In this way the most effective care will be given.

The nurse's concept of the patient

The nurse-patient relationship is a term commonly used to identify the complex interaction between the patient and the nurse. Every nurse needs to understand this relationship, for upon it will rest success in helping the patient and in achieving personal satisfaction.

Each of us is uniquely different from any other individual. Nurses need to be aware of their own biases and prejudices. Each nurse needs to work toward meeting each person with an open mind. To be successful in working with patients as individuals, the nurse needs to accept each as he is without attaching conditions to the acceptance. The patient then does not need to be burdened with trying to earn the nurse's approval, and it also is easier for the nurse to work with the patient and his family with genuine sincerity, sensitivity, and understanding. The nurse who attempts to convey outwardly one response when inwardly feeling another way only confuses the patient, and relationships remain superficial.

The nurse may encounter many situations that require acceptance of things that cannot be changed. All nurses at some time will care for patients with incurable illnesses that may result in immediate death or that may become chronic. Some patients may require disfiguring surgery. Others may have deformities or communicable diseases with attendant social stigma. The nurse needs to develop the ability to accept things that cannot be changed and to respect the opinions of others in the determination of what can be or should be changed within reasonable limits.

Nurses need to learn to distinguish between their own goals, values, and standards of conduct and those of the patient. Discovery of what situations mean to the patient is one of the first steps nurses can take to truly help the patient. All nurses should realize that although they attempt to anticipate what the patient may need, the patient may be the best interpreter of what he needs and wants, if only someone will listen. Much can be learned about the patient through observation, collection of information by other health personnel, talking to the patient's family, and talking to other nurses who take part in his care. However, the best source of information is most often the patient, and he should be given every opportunity to express his own feelings about situations. If the meaning of observed patient behavior is not clear, the nurse should not make assumptions. Verifying the meaning with the patient brings the concern into the open, and together the patient and the nurse learn the meaning.

There will be situations that nurses find difficult to understand and that they cannot accept. They may need assistance in resolving conflict and should seek aid from persons who can help them better understand such situations and their part in them. Through this kind of discussion they then may give care to patients with greater awareness of the meaning of their own behavior and the behavior of the patient. Above all, nurses need to understand that value systems differ and that even though they do not agree with the patient's values, they can accept him as an individual with the right of choice. *Acceptance* of the patient is especially difficult when his behavior is considered antisocial or outside accepted patterns of behavior. However, it is a sign of professional and personal maturity when one is able to accept the patient for what he is and not for what he does.

There can be no set rules or techniques to determine the nurse's responses to patients. Each response is made according to the individual and the situation. The following suggestions may help as guidelines:

1. Be yourself, for nothing else draws more genuine response from others.
2. Let others respond in their own way rather than trying to make them respond the way you would.
3. Reflect upon situations that are unsatisfactory or frustrating and ask yourself the following questions: Why do these situations exist? What did the patient do and say, and what did you do and say? Did you really understand what it meant to him, or were you interpreting it by your values?
4. Continue to grow intellectually, emotionally, and socially by developing broad interests both within and outside nursing.

Emotional and cultural responses to illness

In general the patient's behavior is influenced by his previous knowledge and experience, his cultural background, his emotional makeup, and alterations in his physiologic functioning. These influences are so closely tied to each other that it is often very difficult to sift out a single reason for his behavior. However, nurses should bear in mind that whatever the patient's behavior may be, it has a very definite meaning. It may be relatively simple or very complex. The patient may not be able to verbalize the reason for his behavior, or if he does, his interpretation may be quite different from the nurse's interpretation.

To understand his behavior, the patient's age needs to be considered along with other factors. A child will react according to his stage of emotional and physical development in addition to the factors already listed. A discussion of the stages of growth and development cannot be included here, but every nurse should remember that the child's reactions are different from those of the adult and are in keeping with behavioral patterns expected at particular stages of development.

The adult patient is expected to face his problems in an adult fashion. However, his behavior may illustrate that the level of emotional maturation he has attained makes this impossible under the circumstances.

Anxiety and *fear* are part of the natural reaction of every normal human being when threats to his health appear. Anxiety has been defined as a feeling of uncertainty and helplessness in the face of danger. It is caused to some extent by the nature of the human organism but can be intensified by lack of knowledge, lack of trust, and social, cultural, and economic forces bearing directly on the affected individual. Fear of cancer, for instance, is almost universal in our society. This fear can be transferred from one person to another in such a way that it has been defined as one of the most common "communicable diseases" of man. It is imperative that the nurse have some understanding of the anxieties and fears of patients.

Illness may be a new experience for the patient. He may be uncertain of what it will mean for him, of the reactions expected of him by others, and of how others will react to him. His anxiety may be the result of his present situation. He may be fearful of the many activities that directly affect him and that occur around him, such as diagnostic procedures and treatments. His own incidental observations of other patients in the hospital may cause concern.

Illness often separates the patient from those he loves and those who perhaps know him best and can comfort him most. Even a short hospitalization may seem very long to the patient and his family who are accustomed to daily support from each other. Being denied this accustomed source of warmth and security increases the patient's anxiety and fear. Small children, who cannot always be given a satisfactory explanation of what may be done to them, often suffer greatly from anxiety.

The loss of financial security and the economic effects of illness may cause the patient and his family to feel threatened. This may be particularly true of a person who is head of a household. One response may be anger and hostility. If this response occurs,

the patient needs acceptance of this behavior and a good listener. By listening, the nurse may help the patient to release tensions. Sometimes the social worker can help these patients resolve some of their problems. In the hospital it is the social worker who knows the most about such community resources as financial aid, housekeeping services, child-placement facilities, nursing homes, and job-placement agencies.

The signs of anxiety, fear, and tension are variable. An indifference to his symptoms and to the tests being made may mean that the patient has not accepted the possibility that anything may be wrong. He may not be able to face reality and still maintain stability and integrity of his personality. The patient who is noisy and demanding, perhaps declaring that he is not worried, is one who, if closely observed, may reveal what he dares not verbalize. The patient who "forgets" the clinic appointment at which he is to learn the results of a test is probably fearful of these results. Other patients manifest their anxiety, consciously or unconsciously, by repeatedly asking the same question, making many complaints, or being preoccupied with bodily functions. Still others struggle with their fears alone, leaving the nurse unaware of their problems. Insomnia, anorexia, frequent urination, irritability, inability to listen or to concentrate, and detachment are signs of anxiety. Sometimes marked physical signs such as perspiring hands, increased pulse and respiratory rates, and dilated pupils denote anxiety and fear. Perhaps the best way a nurse can estimate helpfulness to the anxious patient is by his progress. If he becomes more tense, the nurse should seek expert assistance.

Cultural background is related so closely to emotional response that it must always be considered in determining the basis for the patient's behavior. This evaluation may be difficult to make and may necessitate careful observation and study. It is important that the nurse try to identify whether the patient's response is a cultural or an emotional one because the nurse's response will depend on this knowledge.

Certain diseases may have implications that are not culturally acceptable to the patient or his family. In some societies it is a disgrace to become ill. Diseases such as epilepsy and mental illness may be carefully guarded secrets within families. Some diseases, such as venereal disease, may be associated with uncleanliness or immorality.

Various parts of the body may have significant meaning in certain cultures. Some patients may refuse to permit amputation of a limb because physical fitness and the "body beautiful" are valued highly. The modern woman in the United States may have an almost intolerable emotional reaction to a mastectomy because of the emphasis placed on women's breasts in our culture. It will be interesting to see if this will change now that the "women's movement" is stressing that women should not be viewed as sexual objects.

The patient may be censured for displaying behavior acceptable in his own cultural group. For instance, in one culture "the picture of health contains a normal amount of disease." For this reason, early medical care or a program of prevention may meet resistance. In another culture the family usually prefers to care for the patient at home, but if hospitalization is necessary, many relatives and friends cluster around lest the patient feel rejected in his time of need. In still another culture it is proper to go to bed with much moaning and groaning if one is ill, so that the relatives may fulfill their rightful role of beneficence. Hospital personnel frequently consider these patients "problems" rather than recognizing that such behavior is culturally determined and trying to work out acceptable adjustments. Explanation to the patient and his family of hospital policies such as visiting hours and isolation requirements may prevent undue anxiety in both the patient and his relatives.

Hospitalization should not deprive the patient of the right to follow his religious convictions (Fig. 1-1). To provide total patient care, the nurse must be aware of and make provision for the patient's participation in his preferred religious activities. A significant part of many religions is the observation of *dietary laws*. While most of the major religions waive such restrictions in time of illness, individuals frequently prefer to follow them. The anxiety produced in the patient who is confronted with food he feels he should not eat can usually be prevented by keeping the dietary department informed about religious persuasions.

In addition to religious restrictions on food, patients may have cultural preferences. For example, Mexican diets contain spicy foods, while Swedish diets are bland and high in fat. Many illnesses necessitate major changes in eating habits and most patients accept dietary changes reluctantly. Good patient and family teaching is necessary if the medical regimen is to be successful. Some patients "just don't like the food." If there are no medical contraindications, families can be encouraged to bring in food for patients. This provides excellent opportunities for health teaching in nutrition.

Complaints about food in hospitals are very common. While sometimes legitimate, they are more often the result of patient dissatisfaction in other areas. Good nurse-patient relationships that provide for open communication may help eliminate these misplaced complaints.

■ THE NURSING PROCESS

In recent years the nursing process has been identified as a means by which nurses can be assisted to give nursing care to patients. Formerly, nurses were considered to be more "doers" than "thinkers" and much of nursing care was based on intuition, common practice, and carrying out the orders prescribed by the physician for the patient's care. Today it is accepted that nurses can and should take a more systematic approach to the care of the patient or client. The question is no longer "How many baths are there to be done?" or "How many treatments are there to be given?" but rather what are the patient's nursing care needs and how may they best be met? In order to answer the latter question the nurse must have an organized method for planning, giving, evaluating, and recording the care the patient receives. This method, which involves a problem-solving approach, has become known as the nursing process.

Components of the process

Although there may be minor variations in the component steps in the process, in general it includes the following: (1) *assessment* of the patient through data collection, data analysis, and identification of patient problems; (2) a *written nursing care plan* that includes objectives or goals for each of the identified problems, a statement of possible

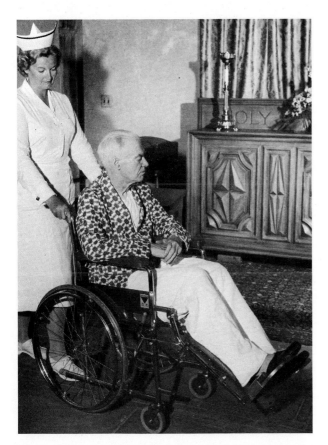

FIG. 1-1. Many patients derive great comfort from a few moments of silent prayer in the chapel.

nursing interventions to meet each problem, and an indication of the priority of each objective in terms of short-term and long-term goals; (3) *implementation* of the written plan by giving direct care to the patient or by directing others in giving the care, teaching the patient and his family in regard to his care, and consulting and collaborating with other health professionals about the patient's care; and (4) *evaluation* of the effectiveness of the nursing intervention and replanning care accordingly. This includes recognizing and planning for new patient care problems and updating the nursing care plan so that it will be readily available to others.

In acquiring the data base necessary to plan nursing care the nurse may seek information from many sources—the patient, his family, the patient's record, and the like. Although data may be collected from the patient in an informal manner, there is much evidence that a systematic approach is the most efficient way to do this. Thus several history and interview forms are presented in nursing literature. Since the forms vary in format and content, most nurses will find it helpful to test them out with actual patients in the setting in which they are working. Sometimes it is helpful to borrow elements from several different forms and combine them into a new form. This eclectic approach is often very useful and assists the nurse or a group of nurses in developing the form that best meets the needs of a given practice situation.

The "Patient Information Guide for the Nurse" is an example of the kind of form that can be used to collect information about the patient. There are many other forms available and several are listed in the references at the end of this chapter.[28,36,52,53,71]

Problem-oriented approach. In using the patient information guide presented or any other history or interview form, the nurse should bear in mind that the nursing care plan will only be as good as the data base. That is, if only three patient care problems are identified when there are really six problems that should be dealt with, the patient will not receive the care he should. In the past few years many physicians and other health professionals have begun to

---

PATIENT INFORMATION GUIDE FOR THE NURSE

I Physical, emotional, and social observations
  A Physical
    1 General appearance
      a. Body build, weight, height, posture, gait
      b. General day-to-day appearance
      c. Changes in appearance
      d. Appearance before illness
    2 Symptoms and signs
      a. Temperature
      b. Pulse
      c. Respiration
      d. Blood pressure
      e. Color
      f. Specific complaints such as pain, nausea, fatigue, dyspnea
      g. Usual pattern of specific complaints; e.g., in cardiac patient, time and nature of chest pain over a period of days in relation to activity
      h. Intake and output
      i. Other physical symptoms and signs that occur in relation to self-care (see II, Self-care activities)
    3 Previous state of health
      a. Number of admissions—present hospital and others
      b. Contact with other health agencies—public health nursing, family service
  B Emotional and social
    1 Behavior
      a. Adjustment—to illness, roommates, staff, therapy
      b. Previous behavior—collection of observations made by patient and by family and/or friends
      c. Usual day-to-day behavior—interest, occupation, general frame of mind or spirits
      d. Changes in behavior—circumstances at time of change and before and after change
      e. Family relationships—at home, reaction to visitors, reaction to lack of visitors, family interest, family members who seem to help
    2 Social activities
      a. Usual way patient likes to spend time
      b. Amount of free time available and how used
      c. Friends or lack of friends
      d. Activities at home or outside home or both
    3 Family
      a. Nationality
      b. Birthplace
      c. Religion
      d. Place in family—mother, father
      e. Siblings
      f. Children
      g. Language spoken in home
    4 Mental ability and education
      a. Vocabulary
      b. Ability to understand explanations
      c. Ability to carry out functions in relation to care needed
      d. Ability to repeat actions such as giving self-medication after a demonstration
      e. Ability to retain knowledge to be used another time
      f. Ability to make suggestions regarding own care
      g. Amount of schooling
      h. Kind of schooling
      i. I.Q.—if psychologic testing has been done
    5 Household
      a. Importance to patient
      b. Importance to family

PATIENT INFORMATION GUIDE FOR THE NURSE—cont'd

c. Patient satisfied or dissatisfied
d. Location of home
e. Physical setup of home

6 Finances
  a. Kind of work patient has done
  b. Kind of work patient is doing
  c. Income of patient and family
  d. Attitude toward job—satisfaction, dissatisfaction
  e. Use of income—values of individual in relation to finances
  f. Use of public assistance or private funds—acceptance of, reaction to
  g. Effect of finances on health habits, purchase of prescribed medications, follow-through on prescribed diagnostic tests

II Self-care activities
Include factors such as patient's interest in doing, specifically how the activity is done, progression in doing activities

A Personal hygiene
  1 Bathing
    a. By patient, nurse, member of family, or combination
    b. Usual method—bed, tub, shower
    c. Frequency
  2 Nails
    Care of, by patient, nurse, member of family, or combination
  3 Hair
    a. Shampoo by patient, nurse, member of family, beautician, or combination
    b. Where shampooed and type of equipment used or needed
    c. Usual method
  4 Shaving
    a. By patient, nurse, member of family, barber, or combination
    b. Usual method and equipment used
    c. Frequency

B Grooming and appearance
  1 General appearance
    a. Neat
    b. Untidy
    c. Interest in
  2 Use of cosmetics
    a. Used by self or with help
    b. Interest in
  3 Combing hair
    a. By self, nurse, member of family, or combination
    b. Special device necessary
  4 Dressing
    a. By self, nurse, member of family, or combination
    b. Special devices used
    c. Difficulties involved, need for practice

C Eating
  1 Type of food
    a. Regular
    b. Special diet
  2 Appetite

3 Likes and dislikes
4 Accomplished by self, nurse, member of family, or combination
5 Special devices or setup necessary

D Elimination
  1 Continent
  2 Incontinent
  3 Constipation
  4 Amount of urinary output
  5 Habit
  6 Need for special training schedule and management—bladder and bowel
  7 Facility used
    a. Bedpan
    b. Commode
    c. Toilet
    d. Special equipment

E Activity
  1 Bed activities
    Ability to turn, lift, pull, balance, attain sitting position
  2 Special devices for bed activity
    a. Bars
    b. Trapeze
    c. Others
  3 Ability to go from bed to chair, from bed to wheelchair, from wheelchair to chair
  4 Ability to return to bed
  5 Ability to stand
  6 Walking and stair climbing
  7 Use of any devices in standing and walking
  8 Tolerance for activity
  9 Amount of activity advised in comparison to that carried out
  10 Activity on unit and activity off unit
  11 Ability to move about in house and how
  12 Ability to go outside house and how
  13 Ability in managing transportation

F Rest
  1 Usual habit
  2 Habit on hospital unit
  3 Habit since illness
  4 Prescribed amount in comparison to amount taken
  5 Problems of maintaining or securing rest—when and how helped

III Special teachings for future
Need for special teaching may be in relation to any of above activities

A Special diet—selection, purchase, and preparation of food
B Administering medication
  1 Purchasing and obtaining medication and necessary equipment
  2 Method
C Household activities
  1 Easier ways of managing
  2 Relocation of articles in home
  3 Scheduling activities
D Care of other members of family by patient
E Care of patient by other members of family
F Provision for follow-up of patient and reevaluation

use problem-oriented medical records, commonly referred to as POMR. One of the objectives of the problem-oriented approach is to provide an organized means for listing all the patient's problems in a problem list and then stating the initial plan for meeting each problem. By numbering each problem and subsequently charting on the progress notes about each problem by number, a more systematic assessment can be made of the handling of each problem and the patient's response to the planned intervention. In this way no problem is forgotten, and the patient may be spared readmission to the hospital for a problem that was not attended to during his hospitalization.

In some hospitals, physicians and nurses work from a joint problem list, while in other settings there is a separate medical and nursing problem list. The method used will depend on a variety of factors that cannot be discussed adequately here. Nevertheless, all nurses will need to keep themselves informed about the problem-oriented approach since it is becoming more and more widely used. Although several excellent references are listed at the end of this chapter,* the nurse will need to be alert to new articles appearing in nursing and medical literature.

Nursing audit. Some nursing service departments in hospitals and other health care agencies are evaluating the effectiveness of the nursing care given to their patients by doing a retrospective chart audit. In a *retrospective* chart audit, charts of discharged patients are audited to learn whether or not each patient received the care deemed necessary for a patient with his particular medical and nursing care problems. Thus, if the patient was recently diagnosed as being diabetic, did the chart indicate that he had been taught how to test his urine for sugar and acetone and take his prescribed medications properly? Did it also indicate that he knew what his diet restrictions were and how he should care for his feet? By examining several charts of patients with the same diagnosis and analyzing the results, an estimation can be made of the quality of care patients are receiving. With society as a whole becoming more and more interested in health care delivery and its cost, all nurses can expect to be involved in nursing audit at some time. The problem-oriented approach to charting on patients' records should simplify the audit process, and therefore many institutions are going to the POMR in preparation for audit.

Peer review. Another aspect of evaluation of nursing care is peer review. In peer review or *ongoing* audit the care that the patient is receiving is reviewed while he is in the hospital. As the name implies, the review is carried out by a nursing peer. Thus the data base, problem list, nursing interventions, and rationale for each are reviewed by a nurse

who is knowledgeable about the care that a certain patient or group of patients should be receiving. In discussion with the nurse or nurses responsible for planning the patient's care, the reviewer may suggest ways in which the care could be improved while the patient is still in the hospital. Although some nurses may look at peer review as a threat, other nurses will welcome it as a means by which they can profit from peer evaluation of the care they give to patients. It would appear that peer review will become much more common in the future.

Standards of care. In order to provide criteria against which the quality of patient care can be measured, many institutions are developing standards of care for patients with specific problems. Most of these standards are written in terms of patient outcomes; that is, what the outcome for the patient should be on discharge from the hospital or other health care setting. For example, an outcome for the newly diagnosed diabetic who is to take insulin daily would be that he can measure and administer his own insulin safely. Thus it can be seen from this outcome that there is a clear statement of what the patient should be able to do and this could be used for both retrospective chart audit and peer review.

As a part of nursing care planning, the nurse must make provision for maintaining the patient's physical capacities, assist in the prevention and release of anxiety, and provide for the patient's return home. These points are discussed next.

Maintaining the patient

Physical capacities. Although the nurse may begin with recognizing the patient's emotional strengths and weaknesses, at the same time his physical strengths and weaknesses should be carefully assessed. The patient should be kept as active as possible within the limitations set by his diagnosis and the physician's prescribed regimen. The nurse should be particularly attentive to the maintenance of activity in the case of patients who are confined to bed or who have severely restricted activity. Patients who have partial restriction of activity and are left without encouragement to move may readily develop limitations in motion or contractures.

Patients confined to bed or allowed only limited activity will have problems of body mechanics. Helping the patient to keep as active as possible within his limitations and to keep good bodily alignment may enable him to resume usual activities sooner. The nurse should have a thorough understanding of joint motion and either should help the patient go through the full range of motion or should move each joint through its range of motion once or twice daily or as often as necessary to preserve the ability to move freely. The daily bath and assistance with self-care activities provide excellent opportunities for helping to preserve mobility. The nurse should

---

*See references 2a, 3a, 4, 23a, 66a, 68, 69, 78, and 83-85.

know the ranges of motion in a systematic fashion and should be familiar with their terminology (Figs. 1-2 to 1-4). As the patient is helped to preserve motion, the importance of these activities is explained to the patient and his family.

If a patient has lost an extremity (amputation) or has loss of function (paralysis), careful attention given to bed posture, changes in position, and follow-through on exercise programs will help prevent development of additional disability. Many patients who require extended periods of bed rest can be helped to maintain muscle tone by use of a footboard, foot exercises, quadriceps setting, self-care

within the limits permitted, correct position, and frequent turning unless contraindicated. If there is doubt about the appropriateness of certain exercises, the physician or a physical therapist should be consulted.

Most patients are placed on progressive activity programs as their condition permits. As new activities are introduced, nurses should give clear explanations of the nature of the activity, what they will do to help, and what the patient must do. Preparation of the patient prior to changes in activity will help to pave the way for better acceptance of the change and will help allay the patient's apprehen-

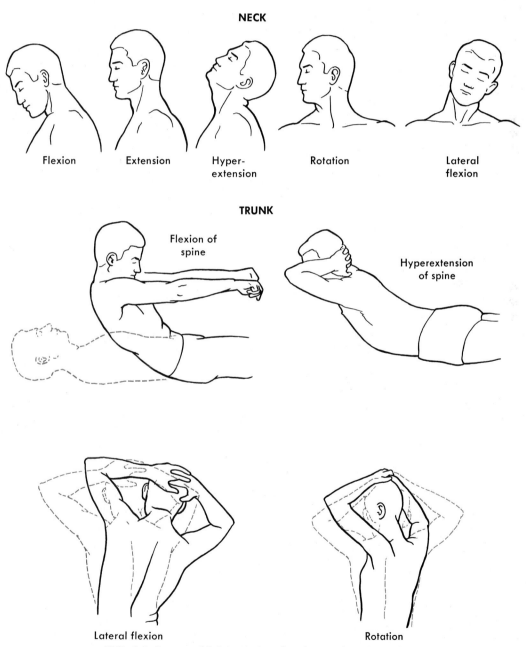

NECK

Flexion   Extension   Hyper-extension   Rotation   Lateral flexion

TRUNK

Flexion of spine

Hyperextension of spine

Lateral flexion   Rotation

FIG. 1-2. Range of joint motion for the neck and trunk.

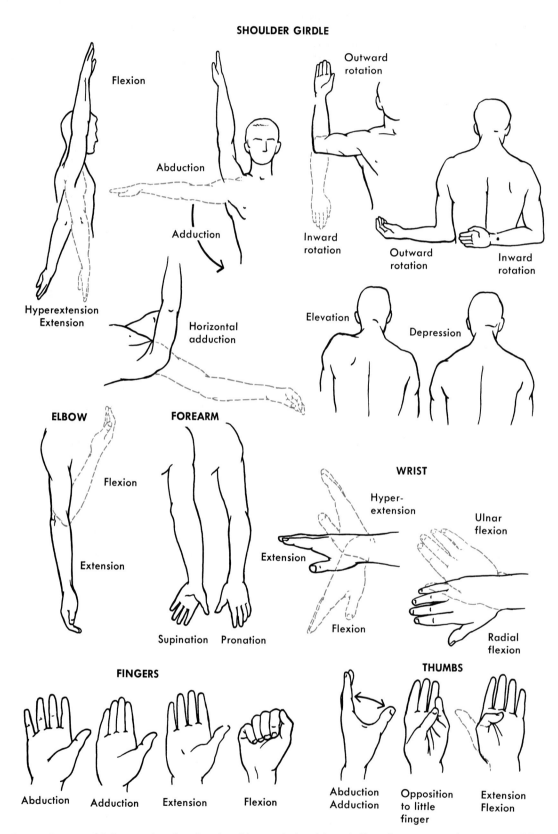

FIG. 1-3. Range of joint motion for the shoulder and shoulder girdle, elbow, wrist, forearm, and hand.

sion. For example, the patient who has pain on moving in bed and has been on bed rest for weeks may become apprehensive and fearful when approached with the idea of being moved out of bed. The nurse can do much to allay fears and apprehension by knowing exactly how the patient can be moved—and with the least effort on his part. The nurse with a

confident but understanding manner can make a new procedure much less traumatic for the patient than can the competent, technically skilled nurse who lacks understanding.

Nurses can and should contribute suggestions for working out activity problems with their patients. One way of finding a method to assist the patient

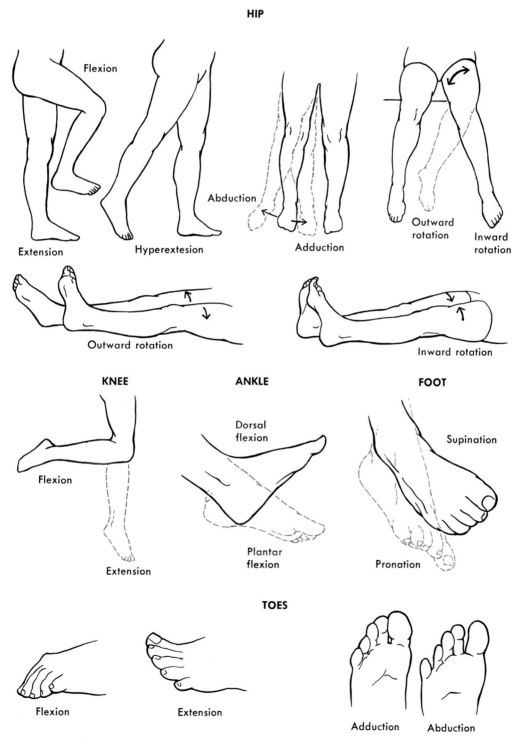

FIG. 1-4. Range of joint motion for the hip, knee, ankle, foot, and toes.

with a particular movement is for the nurse to assume the same limitations as the patient and proceed from there. For example, if the patient has weak upper and lower extremities, it may be difficult for him to assume a sitting position in bed. By experimenting the nurse will find that starting from a back-lying position it will be necessary to place the palms of one's hands close to the hips, push on the elbows, and then raise the head and shoulders from the bed. The next step is to slide one elbow back and then the other until both elbows are under the shoulders. This puts one in a supported position but the hands are not free. By pushing on the right hand and extending the right elbow and then pushing on the left hand and extending the left elbow an unbalanced sitting position can be assumed. To assume a balanced position it will be necessary to move first one hand forward and then the other until a secure sitting position is attained. Whereas this may be an easy procedure for the nurse who is strong and not hindered by weakness, it may be painstaking and slow for the patient who has weak extremities. However, through a step-by-step demonstration the nurse can teach the patient exactly how he can achieve a sitting position in bed. Since almost all rehabilitation is a slow process, it is important not only to have an ultimate goal but also to set intermediate goals that may be obtained in a shorter time. Unless patients experience some success, discouragement usually develops.

The nurse can be a source of encouragement to the patient in finding new ways to manage necessary self-care. However, nurses can learn much about techniques from their patients. Faced with a problem that he knew had to be lived with for the rest of his life, many a patient as well as physicians, nurses, and therapists have been spurred to develop easier ways of managing daily needs as well as meeting occupational needs. A recent article by a nurse who had experienced a stroke gives insight into such a problem and its management.[21]

Extension handles for combs, toothbrushes, and eating utensils are simple to construct and make it possible for many patients to be self-sufficient (see Figs. 33-2 to 33-5). If given a picture or sample drawing with explanations of what is needed, members of the family can often assist in making self-help devices for the patient. In this day of small gadgets one can find numerous useful articles already on the market. However, patient and family may need help in recognizing the needs for such aids, in learning where to find them, and in learning how to use them effectively.

Careful nursing attention to prevention of pressure areas, incontinence, and malnutrition also helps speed the patient's return to his usual activities. Nursing care contributing to prevention of these problems is discussed in detail in subsequent chapters.

Emotional capacities. Although the patient may have serious physical limitations, he may be able emotionally to accept them and either compensate for them or through sheer inner strength manage his own daily care and his life despite them. Discussion of understanding the patient's emotional responses to illness or threat to health was included earlier in this chapter. Nurses cannot possibly know all the factors contributing to anxiety or their particular application for each patient. However, they can do much to help the patient rally the emotional strength necessary to continue with a prescribed medical program.

Nursing intervention to prevent and release anxiety

Orienting the newly admitted patient and his family to the hospital routine tends to minimize anxiety (Fig. 1-5). Each new experience should be explained to the patient and, if possible, related to familiar experiences. It is helpful to inform the patient how he may call the nurse, when he will see his physician, the hours the religious adviser is available, and how he may contact his family. In addition, the family should be told how to obtain information concerning the patient, when they may visit, and any immediate plans for the patient.

If a patient is to have a treatment or test, he must be given some idea of what will be done, the preparation involved, and the reasons why the procedure is necessary. To remove the water pitcher and inform a patient that he cannot have any more water until

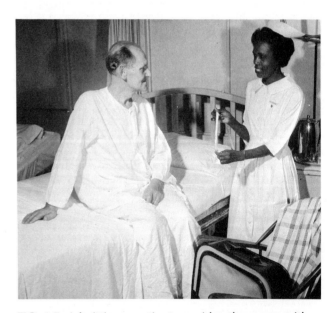

FIG. 1-5. Admitting a patient provides the nurse with the opportunity to allay some of his fears and anxieties by thorough explanation of the environment and expected procedures. It also provides the opportunity to do an admission interview to collect data necessary to planning his care.

after his x-ray examination can leave him with many anxious thoughts: "What x-ray examination?" "I wonder when it is?" "What will it be like?" "It must be something special if I can't have any water." Lack of knowledge as a cause of anxiety reflects the nurse's lack of consideration for the patient's rights as an individual.

Explanations should be given in the patient's own terms at appropriate times and repeated as necessary. If the patient is very anxious, he may need repeated explanation, since extreme anxiety reduces intellectual function. It is useless to give detailed explanations to patients who are overanxious or sedated or to those who have high temperatures or severe pain. Repetition is often required for older persons and children because they may have a short memory span.

Time spent in giving explanations to relatives is not wasted. Not only does it relieve their anxieties, which may be transmitted to the patient, but it also saves having to untangle misinformation. Often the family is helpful in interpreting necessary instructions to the patient in such a manner that he understands and accepts them.

In most instances a large part of the nurse's work is to encourage the patient to express his anxieties, to help him see the universality of fear in his situation, to help him seek outlets for his fears and tensions, and to allay them whenever possible. Nurses should provide opportunities for the patient to talk, but they should not probe. There is a difference between prying into a patient's thoughts and beliefs and eliciting information that will aid in the understanding of his behavior and in planning for his care. Without seeming unduly curious, one can usually find some topic of personal interest to the patient that will provide an opening. A picture on the bedside table may create such an opening. Then, nurses who listen with sincere interest and without making judgments about the patient may begin to gain insight into the patient as a person. And more important, he may begin to speak about his fears.

As soon as the patient begins to talk about his feelings, the nurse should proceed with conversation, taking cues from what the patient offers. The nurse who feels inadequate or anxious may cut off the conversation. For instance, if a patient says, "You know, I don't think I'll ever get to see my little boy again," a common response is "Oh, don't say that, certainly you will; you're going to be all right." The patient may very well not be all right. Would it not be better to respond, "What makes you feel this way?" Such a response helps the patient explore the subject and leaves opportunity for the patient to examine this fear himself. It also gives the nurse a chance to find out what the patient fears. The nurse who is willing to listen to patients, to be guided by their reactions and to work with them rather than

to make decisions for them will give them needed emotional support. Solving patients' problems for them, even if it were possible, is not the aim of nursing. Indeed, it would tend to make patients less healthy psychologically.

The art of meaningful communication involves more than just listening: it includes moving the conversation so that the patient's attempts to communicate are assisted. Observing the patient for facial changes and general body movements provides opportunities for the nurse to discover from the individual the full meaning of his situation. For example, consider the patient who sucks in air as he talks. His mouth becomes drier and drier; his tongue seems to stick in his mouth. He is not at ease and shows his anxiety even though his words may be quite innocuous. A simple statement such as, "Your mouth seems very dry; would a glass of water help?" allows the nurse to clarify observations made. Such an approach gives the patient a chance to tell what he is experiencing, and he may gain understanding by talking about it.

The nurse is prepared only to help the patient look at those problems that he himself is able to bring into awareness. Underlying problems should be handled by people trained in psychotherapy. A nurse needs to be able to recognize normal anxiety reactions and to report exaggerated reactions that may indicate the need for psychiatric referral. Stuttering and blocking of words may indicate increasing tension. Depression and sadness are normal reactions to illness and particularly to changes in body image, but feelings of guilt and worthlessness should make the nurse aware of the possibility of suicide. Apathy may indicate that the patient has given up not only fear but also hope. Fortunately most normal and abnormal anxiety is self-limiting and improves with a cheerful and encouraging attitude on the part of the staff, renewed activity for the patient, and a chance to talk. Independence should be allowed and encouraged as soon as possible, since for most people nothing is so demoralizing as complete dependence on others. Independence cannot be forced, however, because it results from changes within the patient himself. This motivation may sometimes be initiated by first allowing the patient to be dependent. The desired goal is interdependence—the result of collaboration of the health team and the patient to help the patient regain and maintain normal health.

The nurse has a responsibility to the patient for maintaining channels of communication with others who may be better prepared to meet his needs. The patient should feel free to communicate with others such as the physician, his family, spiritual advisers, and social workers. At times the nurse may need to be a "go-between" because some patients are unsure as to whether their questions are appropriate. When accompanying the physician, a statement by the nurse, such as, "Mr. Jones asked about how long he would be hospitalized, and I believe you have some other questions, don't you, Mr. Jones?" may provide the necessary opening.

Providing for the patient's return home

Throughout the patient's illness, nurses should be aware that the patient is a member of a family and community to which he will return. This fact must be considered in planning for home care in order to avoid unnecessary anxiety. It is important for nurses to ascertain with whom the family authority lies, since this person is usually the one who should be brought into planning. They also need to gain insight into reactions to such things as disability, infectious diseases, and care of the aged, which may be culturally determined. A patient may find it difficult for others to accept him. In such a case the nurse should assist him to prepare for this adjustment.

The aged patient is not always readily accepted into the home of his children. In some cultures the older person rarely has this problem, since he is highly respected as the head of the family. In others it may be expected that the aged person who is widowed will go to a home for the aged when he is no longer able to live by himself. Awareness of any such possibilities should make the nurse alert to early planning with the patient and his family for his discharge, whether it be for convalescent, rehabilitative, chronic, or terminal care. Here again, the plans must stem from the patient and his family.

Planning is also necessary in carrying out any patient-teaching program. The nurse's goal is to help the patient and his family toward self-sufficiency and independence by suggesting needed materials, routines, and techniques. The patient, with his family, should be encouraged to work out the details, such as the equipment available, the best time of day, the best place, and the easiest technique. They

must plan, for example, how a special diet can be worked in with the family meals. The nurse should be available to give guidance as needed. In teaching patients, the following suggestions may be helpful:

1. Explain to the patient the desired results, suggesting possible means to these ends.

2. Explore with the patient and his family the possibilities of carrying out instructions. Listen carefully for factors that might interfere with carrying out instructions and try to make adjustments that will make the treatment acceptable and practical to the patient and his family.

3. Have the patient practice the procedure as it is to be carried out in the home.

4. Provide some channel for assistance if the patient should meet with difficulty.

Nurses have a unique opportunity to provide comprehensive care to patients if they use each interaction with the patient to the best advantage. At the same time all nurses need to understand that not every problem will be solved during one or even more patient-nurse interaction. Some problems may never be solved or at least not in the manner that seems, in the nurse's judgment, to be in the best interest of the patient.

In this chapter great stress has been placed on the need for the nurse to understand human behavior, to recognize and accept differing value systems and life-styles, and to use a systematic approach to provide appropriate nursing care to patients. Above all it is hoped that the reader sensed the importance of the nurse's being warm, responsive, and sensitive in interactions with patients. Therapeutic nurse-patient relationships develop from *genuine feelings and appropriate application of techniques*. It is hoped that this chapter and the succeeding ones will assist the nurse to understand more about patients and the problems that they face, and that the patients will benefit from this increased knowledge and understanding.

REFERENCES AND SELECTED READINGS*

1 American Nurses' Association: Standards: nursing practice, Kansas City, Mo., 1973, The Association.

2 Anxiety recognition and intervention, programmed instruction, Am. J. Nurs. **66:**129-152, Sept. 1965.

2a Aradine, C. R., and others: The problem-oriented record in a family health service, Am. J. Nurs. **74:**1108-1112, June 1974.

3 Bernstein, L., and Dana, R. H.: Interviewing and the health professions, New York, 1970, Appleton-Century-Crofts.

3a *Bloom, J., Molbo, D. M., and Pardee, G.: Implementing the problem-oriented process in nursing, Supervisor Nurse **5:**24-38, Aug. 1974.

4 Bonkowsky, M. L.; Adapting the POMR to community child health care, Nurs. Outlook **20:**515-518, Aug. 1972.

5 Bower, F. L.: The process of planning nursing care, St. Louis, 1972, The C. V. Mosby Co.

6 Brown, E. D.: Newer dimensions in patient care, ed. 2, New York, 1965, Russell Sage Foundation.

7 Burkhardt, M.: Response to anxiety, Am. J. Nurs. **69:**2153-2154, Oct. 1969.

8 Burton, G.: Personal, impersonal, and interpersonal relations, ed. 2, New York, 1964, Springer Publishing Co., Inc.

9 Carlson, S.: A practical approach to the nursing process, Am. J. Nurs. **72:**1589-1591, Sept. 1972.

10 *Carrieri, V. K., and Sitzman, J.: Components of the nursing process, Nurs. Clin. North Am. **6:**115-124, March 1971.

11 *Chamings, P. A.: Need a little help . . ., Am. J. Nurs. **69:**1918-1920, Sept. 1969.

12 Clancy, K. M.: Concerning gifts, Perspect. Psychiatr. Nurs. **6:**169-175, 1968.

13 *Clemence, Sister Madeleine: Existentialism: a philosophy of commitment, Am. J. Nurs. **66:**500-505, March 1966.

14 *Connolly, M. G.: What acceptance means to patients, Am. J. Nurs. **60:**1754-1757, Dec. 1960.

*References preceded by an asterisk are particularly well suited for student reading.

15 *Cuthbert, B. L.: Switchoff, tune in, turn on, Am. J. Nurs. **69:**1206-1211, June 1969.

16 *Davis, M. Z.: Cancer dwells here, Nurs. Forum **6**(4):379-381, 1967.

17 *Dicks, R. L.: Who is my patient? New York, 1943, Macmillan Publishing Co., Inc.

18 Duff, R., and Hollingshead, A.: Sickness and society, New York, 1968, Harper & Row, Publishers.

19 Eckelberry, G. K.: Comprehensive nursing care, New York, 1971, Appleton-Century-Crofts.

20 *Eldred, S. H.: Improving nurse-patient communication, Am. J. Nurs. **60:**1600-1602, Nov. 1960.

21 *Ellis, R.: After stroke sitting problems, Am. J. Nurs. **73:**1898-1899, Nov. 1973.

22 *Freund, H.: Listening with any ear at all, Am. J. Nurs. **69:**1650-1653, Aug. 1969.

23 Garrett, A.: Interviewing: its principles and methods, New York, 1942, Family Service Association of America.

23a *Goldfinger, S. E.: The problem-oriented record: a critique from a believer, N. Engl. J. Med. **288:**606-608, March 1973.

24 *Goldsborough, J.: Involvement, Am. J. Nurs. **69:**66-68, Jan. 1969.

25 *Greenhill, M. H.: Interviewing with a purpose, Am. J. Nurs. **56:**1259-1262, Oct. 1956.

26 *Gregg, D. E.: Anxiety—a factor in nursing care, Am. J. Nurs. **52:**1363-1365, Nov. 1952.

27 *Gregg, D.: Reassurance, Am. J. Nurs. **55:**171-174, Feb. 1955.

28 Haferkorn, V.: Assessing individual learning needs as a basis for patient teaching, Nurs. Clin. North Am. **6:**199-209, March 1971.

29 Hagerman, Z. J.: Teaching beginners to cope with extreme behavior, Am. J. Nurs. **68:**1927-1929, Sept. 1968.

30 *Hall, E. T.: The silent language, Greenwich, Conn., 1959, Fawcett Publication, Inc.

31 *Hall, E. T.: The hidden dimension, Garden City, N. Y., 1966, Doubleday & Co., Inc.

31a *Hamdi, M. E., and Hutelmyer, C. M.: A study of the effectiveness of an assessment tool in the identification of nursing care problems, Nurs. Res. **19:**354-358, July-Aug. 1970.

32 *Harrison, C.: Deliberative nursing process versus automatic nurse action, Nurs. Clin. North Am. **1:**387-397, Sept. 1966.

33 Henderson, V.: The nature of nursing: a definition and its implications for practice, research, and education, New York, 1966, Macmillan Publishing Co., Inc.

34 *Ingles, T.: Understanding the nurse-patient relationship, Nurs. Outlook **9:**698-700, 1961.

35 *Jaco, E. G.: Patients, physicians and illness, ed. 2, New York, 1972, The Free Press.

36 Johnson, I.: The art of history taking, J. Neurosurg. Nurs. **2:**5-17, Dec. 1970.

37 *Johnson, J. E., Dumas, R. G., and Johnson, B. A.: The essence of nursing care, Nurs. Forum **6**(3):324-334, 1967.

38 *Jourard, S. M.: How well do you know your patients? Am. J. Nurs. **59:**1568-1571, Nov. 1959.

39 *Jourard, S. M.: The transparent self, New York, 1964, D. Van Nostrand Co.

40 *Jourard, S. M.: Disclosing man to himself, New York, 1968, D. Van Nostrand Co.

41 Kachelski, M. A.: The nurse-patient relationship, Am. J. Nurs. **61:**76-81, May 1961.

42 *Keller, N.: Care without coordination: a true story, Nurs. Forum **6**(3):280-323, 1967.

43 *Kelly, M. M.: Exercises for bedfast patients, Am. J. Nurs. **66:**2209-2213, Oct. 1966.

44 *King, J. M.: Denial, Am. J. Nurs. **66:**1010-1014, May 1966.

45 King, S. H.: Perceptions of illness and medical practice, New York, 1962, Russell Sage Foundation.

46 Kinlein, M. L.: Independent nurse practitioner, Nurs. Outlook **20:**22-23, Jan. 1972.

47 *Levine, M. E.: Four conservation principles of nursing, Nurs. Forum **6**(3):45-57, 1967.

48 *Levine, M. E.: Introduction to clinical nursing, ed. 2, Philadelphia, 1973, F. A. Davis Co.

49 Little, D., and Carnevali, D.: Nursing care plans: let's be practical about them, Nurs. Forum **6**(3):61-67, 1967.

50 Ludemann, R. S.: Empathy—a component of therapeutic nursing, Nurs. Forum **7**(3):275-288, 1968.

51 *Marshall, J. C., and Feeney, S.: Structured versus intuitive intake interview, Nurs. Res. **21:**269-272, May-June 1972.

52 *McCain, R. F.: Nursing by assessment—not intuition, Am. J. Nurs. **65:**82-84, April 1965.

53 *McPhetridge, L. M.: Nursing history: one means to personalize care, Am. J. Nurs. **68:**68-75, Jan. 1968.

54 Menninger, K., Mayman, M., and Pruyser, P.: The vital balance: the life process in mental health and illness, New York, 1963, The Viking Press, Inc.

55 *Monaco, J. T., and Conway, B. L.: Motivation by whom and toward what? Am. J. Nurs. **69:**1719-1722, Aug. 1969.

56 Murphy, J. F.: The patient's plea. In Bergersen, B. S., and others, editors: Current concepts in clinical nursing, vol. 2, St. Louis, 1969, The C. V. Mosby Co.

57 *Neylan, M. P.: The depressed patient, Am. J. Nurs. **61:**77-78, July 1961.

58 *Neylan, M. P.: Anxiety, Am. J. Nurs. **62:**110-111, May 1962.

59 *Orlando, I. J.: The dynamic nurse-patient relationship, New York, 1961, G. P. Putnam's Sons.

60 *Peplau, H. E.: Talking with patients, Am. J. Nurs. **60:**964-966, July 1960.

61 Perry, G. S.: Families of America, New York, 1949, Whittlesey House, McGraw-Hill Book Co.

62 *Pluckhan, M. L.: Space: the silent language, Nurs. Forum **7**(4):386-397, 1968.

63 *Prange, A. J., Jr., and Martin, H. W.: Aids to understanding patients, Am. J. Nurs. **62:**98-100, July 1962.

64 *Quint, J. C.: The threat of death: some consequences for patients and nurses, Nurs. Forum **8**(3):287-300, 1969.

65 *Quint, J., Strauss, A., and Glaser, B.: Improving nursing care of the dying, Nurs. Forum **6**(3):368-378, 1967.

66 Ramphal, M.: Values of routines in nursing, Nurs. Forum **6**(3):335-340, 1967.

66a *Reinstein, L.: The problem of the problem-oriented record, New. Engl. J. Med. **288:**1133-1134, May, 1973.

67 Robinson, L.: Psychological aspects of the care of hospitalized patients, Philadelphia, 1969, F. A. Davis Co.

68 *Ryback, R., and Gardner, J. S.: Problem formulation: the problem oriented record, Am. J. Psychiatry **130:**312-316, March 1973.

69 *Schell, P. L., and Campbell, A. T.: POMR—not just another way to chart, Nurs. Outlook **20:**510-514, Aug. 1972.

70 *Skipper, J. K., and Leonard, R. C., editors: Social interaction and patient care, Philadelphia, 1965, J. B. Lippincott Co.

71 *Smith, D. M.: A clinical nursing tool, Am. J. Nurs. **68:**2384-2388, Nov. 1968.

72 *Smith, D. W.: Patienthood and its threat to privacy, Am. J. Nurs. **69:**278-282, Feb. 1969.

73 Sorensen, G.: Dependency—a factor in nursing care, Am. J. Nurs. **66:**1762-1763, Aug. 1966.

74 Starlie, F.; The world of Mr. Wickersham, Am. J. Nurs. **68:**2389, Nov. 1968.

75 *Stevens, B. J.: Why won't nurses write nursing care plans? J. Nurs. Admin. **2:**6-7, 91-92, Nov.-Dec. 1972.

76 Tarnower, W.: Psychological needs of the hospitalized patient, Nurs. Outlook **65:**28-30, July 1965.

77 *Taylor, C. D.: The hospital patient's social dilemma, Am. J. Nurs. **66:**96-99, Oct. 1965.

78 *Thoma, D., and Pittman, K.: Evaluation of problem-oriented nursing notes, J. Nurs. Admin. **2:**50-58, May-June 1972.

79 Towle, C.: Common human needs, New York, 1965, National Association of Social Workers, Inc.

80 *Travelbee, J.: Interpersonal aspects of nursing, Philadelphia, 1968, F. A. Davis Co.

81 *Velazquez, J. M.: Alienation, Am. J. Nurs. **69:**301-304, Feb. 1969.

82 *Wagner, B. M.: Care plans: right, reasonable, and reachable, Am. J. Nurs. **69:**986-990, May 1969.

83 *Walker, H. K., Hurst, J. W., and Woody, M. F.: Applying the problem-oriented system, New York, 1973, Medcom Books, Inc.

84 Weed, L. L.: Medical records, medical education, and patient care, Cleveland, 1970, The Press of Case Western Reserve University.

85 *Woody, M., and Mallison, M.: The problem-oriented system for patient-centered care, Am. J. Nurs. **73:**1168-1175, July 1973.

86 *Zimmerman, D. S. and Gohrke, C.: The goal-directed nursing approach: it does work, Am. J. Nurs. **70:**306-310, Feb. 1970.

2 Age a factor in care of patients

Diseases and disorders requiring medical or surgical treatment afflict persons of all ages, from newborn infants to octogenarians. The age of the patient influences his nursing needs and must always be considered in planning and providing care for him. Each person, regardless of his age and whether he is sick or well, has needs related to his physical and emotional welfare. These include being fed, clothed, and housed, being safe and comfortable both physically and spiritually, and being important to others. It is not possible or appropriate to discuss each aspect fully in this book. The student should refer to the many excellent books and periodicals related specifically to the various age groups for additional information. Some are listed in the suggested readings at the end of the chapter.

In the United States two age groups in the population have received a great deal of society's attention—children and the elderly. The number of elderly people in the United States has increased steadily over the past 50 years. Approximately 21 million persons are 65 years of age or over.[52,56] By 1980 it is estimated this number will reach or surpass 25 million.[52,56] At present those persons 75 years of age or over are increasing proportionately faster than the total age group who are over 65. The increasing number of elderly persons has come about primarily through the decrease in infant mortality, the prevention and control of communicable disease during childhood, the improved treatment of adult acute and chronic dis-

ease, and improvements in medical care in general. At the same time the birth rate in the United States is declining; in 1973 it was slightly above zero population growth.

Society's youth

Concern first was aroused about infant and child welfare during the latter half of the nineteenth century. There were extremely high morbidity (illness) and mortality (death) rates among this group. The problem was especially serious among the children of the poor and of immigrants living in urban communities. Children often were housed in crowded and unsanitary tenements, played in the streets, and were utilized and exploited by developing industries as their labor force. In addition to being overworked and subjected to disease and accidents, most children received little schooling. Contaminated water and food also caused much illness. In response to public sympathy for these children, the Children's Aid Society of New York was founded in 1853. Shortly thereafter, children's hospitals and clinics began to be established. Interest in child care (pediatrics) has continued since this time. In 1909 the first national effort to conserve children's health was started by the President, who called a White House Conference on Children and Youth. Since then, this group, with nationwide representation from all professional and social groups (both public and private) interested in child care, has convened every 10 years to

STUDY QUESTIONS

1 Outline some of the problems that you feel contribute to the present "generation gap."
2 List the stresses most common to persons in your age group. How do these compare with stresses in your parents' age group?
3 Review the physiologic changes that occur with aging. What are the developmental tasks for the elderly person?
4 Review the normal schedule for physical development in children. What are the developmental tasks of each age group?
5 Review the eating patterns of an elderly person of your acquaintance; compare his food intake with your understanding of an adequate diet.
6 From what you have read in newspapers and heard discussed, what would you select as major problems of elderly people in your community?
7 From what you have learned in fundamentals of nursing, what are some practical measures you can take to prevent accidents involving elderly patients in the hospital environment and in their own homes?
8 What services are available in your community for infants and children? What ones are available for the elderly?

discuss the problems of youth. As a result of the first conference, The United States Children's Bureau was formed. The bureau is now known as the Office of Child Development and is a special office in the U. S. Department of Health, Education and Welfare. This office is an excellent source of literature for parents, and it is active in working with the states to help them provide improved services for children and their families.

Stemming from the aroused interest of our society in children, considerable social legislation improving the welfare of children has been enacted. The education of children is now compulsory in all states, and child-labor laws now prohibit hiring children in industries producing goods sent across state lines. All states have laws limiting child labor within their boundaries.

Through the international activities of the Children's Bureau and through such organizations within the United Nations as the World Health Organization, UNICEF, and UNESCO, as well as Vista and voluntary groups such as churches, assistance is being given to developing countries throughout the world to improve child care. The Fourteenth General Assembly of the United Nations in 1959 approved the Declaration of the Rights of the Child, which is based on the idea that mankind everywhere owes children the best it can give.[34]

In the United States many services are available to children free of cost. Many communities have free well-baby clinics and immunization programs. Public schools may provide free yearly health examinations for children. Financial assistance is available in every state in the country for medical care of crippled children and the blind. Nurses should become familiar with the services available in their communities so that they may guide parents to seek help as needed.

Despite these efforts, there are still many serious problems related to the youth of our society. Because of poor delivery and inequality of health services offered to the underprivileged members of society, the United States is far behind many Western European countries in regard to decreasing its infant mortality rate. Physical abuse of infants and young children by adults seems to be increasing. In addition, many children are neglected. The injuries sustained by an abused child are known as the "battered child syndrome." The physician is now required by law to report any case of abuse that comes to his attention. Appropriate community agencies then provide for the protection of the child and counseling of the parent or parents. Placement of the child in other settings will be carried out when necessary. (See p. 260 for other suggestions.)

Many times the abuse and neglect of infants is related to the problems of teenagers and young adults. Teenage marriages and pregnancies (often of unmarried mothers) have become exceedingly common. Many of these teenagers are emotionally immature and unprepared to accept the responsibilities of marriage and parenthood. The incidence of venereal diseases, even in young teenagers, is increasing at an alarming rate (p. 535). Drug abuse (p. 159), abortions (legal and illegal), and accidents among young people have increased, and many of our youth have serious emotional problems.

Society did not foresee the problems that youth would face today and did not prepare itself to solve them. Although the public now recognizes many problems, there is still a great deal of ignorance about such things as drug (including alcohol) abuse and venereal disease, which are paramount threats to the health of many young people. Facilities for giving help to youth are frequently inadequate. There is growing awareness, however, that society must deal more creatively with the problems of young people. One example of this is the free clinics that have been founded across the country to provide care for adolescents and others who might not otherwise receive care. In many of these, youths can remain anonymous and receive treatment free from the fear of being discovered by parents or teachers. Treatment is often given free or for a minimal charge.

Communities often provide opportunities for recreation and other activities to help young people fill their free time. Also, the federal government has urged business and industry to provide jobs for youths, especially during summer months, and has provided some funds to assist communities with job programs. In addition, special attention has been given to the school dropout in an attempt to prepare him for obtaining work and to help him develop interests with which to fill hours of leisure time.

The elderly person in our society

Unfortunately social adjustments adequate to meet the challenges presented by the increasing number of elderly persons were not made over the years. It was not until 1950 that much social planning for the elderly was instituted. Meanwhile the plight of many elderly people had become almost insufferable. Many, typical of their age group, had one or more chronic illnesses and many had been replaced on the work force by younger people. Consequently, the problems of this group often were overwhelming. As the number of elderly people was increasing, the patterns of living were changing. No longer were homes large enough to accommodate aging relatives. In fact, society seemed to have begun to frown on elderly parents living with their children. This arrangement, therefore, even if possible, frequently was distasteful to both the elderly and their children. Also, the increased mobility of today's society has made it more likely that parents and children may live far from one another. The provision of living facilities for this group of persons, many of whom needed some nursing care or home-making assistance and could barely afford even the basic essentials of life, became a tremendous challenge. Formerly the elderly person could continue to work as long as he wished. Many now being forced to retire had been accustomed to working long hours in their earlier years. Consequently, many of the elderly had not prepared for retirement. Not only did they have little money, but they frequently had no interests or hobbies with which to fill their newfound leisure time.

In 1950 the first National Conference on Aging was held in Washington. Following this, the Committee on Aging and Geriatrics (the care of the elderly) was formed within the federal government. In the same year the National Social Welfare Assembly, a voluntary organization, formed a Committee on Aging. This committee became an independent organization, the National Council on Aging,* in 1961. This group has concerned itself with matters affecting the aged, such as standards for sheltered care, employment of the aged, and retirement regulations. It is a valuable source for literature relating to the elderly. In 1956 the Center for Aging Research in the National Institutes of Health was established. In 1962 the President's Council on Aging was created to coordinate efforts in behalf of the elderly in the various departments of government and to broaden the range of federal activities. The Administration on Aging was created within the Department of Health, Education and Welfare in 1965. This office publishes a monthly newsletter, *Aging*.

Many state and local committees have been formed to work for the aged. In several states, joint legislative committees have been formed to guide lawmaking bodies in passing legislation concerning the welfare of older people. Many church and other local groups have set up special committees to study what their contribution can be to housing, recreation, and other community planning for the aging. Most county medical societies now have geriatric sections, as does the American Nurses' Association. There are two national scientific societies devoted exclusively to the aging and the aged, the Gerontological Society, Inc., and the American Geriatrics Society.[3]

As a result of society's interest in the elderly, the majority of them now have a small income from one or more sources, such as voluntary insurance plans, state and federal government plans, and individual savings. The average income per family unit, however, is still substantially below that of families the heads of which are 45 to 65 years of age, and the elderly as a group have a lower standard of living.

*Headquarters, 1828 L St., N. W., Suite 504, Washington, D. C. 20036.

Persons whose income is largely from pensions, which do not increase or decrease with the cost of living, have the greatest difficulty.

It is impossible to determine exactly how many receive benefits since sources overlap. However, in 1971 about 24 million persons 62 years of age and over received income from Old-Age, Survivors, and Disability Insurance (Social Security) and approximately 7,841,000 wives and other dependents of retired and deceased workers also received income from this source.[52] Although Social Security benefits have been increased periodically in recent years, they often have not kept pace with increases in the cost of living, and many of the recipients have difficulty making ends meet during periods of inflation.

Unfortunately it is still very difficult for the person over the age of 65, even if he is physically able and anxious to work, to find employment. Hopefully, however, society is learning that gainful employment seems to be essential for the happiness of many. It cannot be replaced by provision for economic security. There is presently a genuine effort to encourage job development and employment for the elderly.[3]

There has also been a great deal of concern about suitable housing for the elderly. Many aged persons live in private homes that are too large, in poor neighborhoods, in isolated rural areas, on the top floor of walk-up tenements, and in housing that is otherwise unsuitable. They may live in these dwellings for financial reasons or because they may wish to remain in familiar surroundings. Many still live with children, and disturbing problems have occurred from crowding, economic pressures, and dissimilarity in cultural backgrounds of various members of the family. Some elderly persons live with distant relatives or friends and see their children only occasionally. Still others are able to live alone quite independently and yet maintain close ties with their children who show interest in their welfare.

Progress has been made recently in setting aside a portion of low-cost housing for elderly persons. These facilities are located on ground floors of buildings with special heating and safety features such as electric instead of gas stoves, good lighting, and doorways without sills to minimize the danger to the person with locomotor disability from stumbling and falling.

At first there was a movement to provide communal homes (homes for the aged) and building developments exclusively for the aged. Soon, however, it was learned that a variety of housing facilities was needed. What one older person prefers, another may not. Although homes for the aged and group housing planned specifically for the aged may be acceptable to those who fear to be alone and who need the security and protection of group living, they are not the answer for everyone. Many wish to live where they may associate with all ages (Fig. 2-10), and indeed this may be preferable.

Every effort should be made to enable the aged person to live in his own home and in his customary setting if he so wishes. This is sometimes made possible by providing such services as housekeeping for the frail and visiting nursing for the ailing. Sometimes arrangements for bringing one hot meal each day to the home may be all that is necessary to enable a feeble elderly couple to carry on together. Others can maintain a home if provision can be made for assistance with some relatively simple tasks such as grocery shopping. Provision for a telephone and for daily visits by a neighbor is frequently all that is necessary. Making prior arrangements to enter a home for the aged whenever the need arises has made it possible for many elderly persons to continue on their own with less apprehension. It is important for the elderly to take part in choosing a nursing home or home for the aged if they are able. Adjustment is usually much easier then.

In an effort to help the elderly use their free time in a satisfying manner and to help them maintain social contacts, despite the death of a husband or wife and lifelong friends, many community and voluntary agencies have organized clubs and day care centers for the aged. Here they can make new friends (Fig. 2-1) and participate in activities suitable to their physical stamina (Fig. 2-2). These clubs also provide a way for the elderly to get together to discuss concerns and problems. Many groups bring in outside experts to advise the elderly concerning their special interests such as social security, Medicare, maintaining health, and providing for safety. Visitors, either voluntary or employed, are provided by some community agencies to go into the homes

of elderly shut-ins solely for socialization. They are also being used for lonely hospitalized patients. Often an elderly person can give this service, thus providing him with a useful occupation.

Compared to other age groups, the geriatric age group requires medical, nursing, and other professional services as well as medications and appliances more often, in larger amounts, and for longer periods. They also have more frequent and longer hospital admissions.[53] Previously (as at present) the implications of illness were more important for the aged person than was the illness or disability itself. He often could not afford to be ill, and he was frequently uncertain who would care for him during illness. General hospitals often were reluctant to admit him, and he often found it necessary to enter a chronic illness hospital or nursing home. He frequently put off medical care, delayed the purchase of medications, and refused treatments or home nursing care because he felt he could not afford them. With the amendment to the Social Security Act (Title 18, "Medicare," and Title 19, Medical Assistance), a great step forward has been made to alleviate this problem. Hospital care and nursing home care, for a limited period at least, are now assured by the federal government for all persons over 65 years of age. For $6.70 a month, medical insurance to assist in paying for a doctor's services and other medical items can be obtained. The legislation also includes specific requirements that an institution must fulfill to qualify for Medicare and Medical Assistance funds. This legislation has brought about improvements in many facilities.

The adult in our society

Nonelderly adults in the United States are usually considered to be those persons between 21 and 65

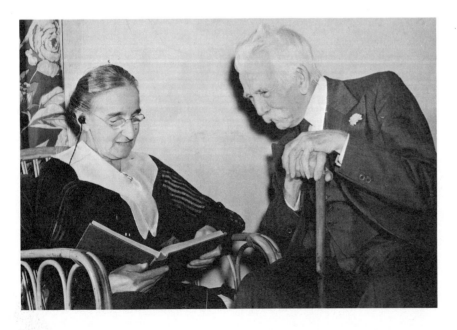

FIG. 2-1. Elderly persons often find that loneliness is relieved when they can share activities and memories with someone in their age group. (Courtesy New York League for the Hard of Hearing, New York, N. Y.)

years of age. This group makes up the majority of the work force and the homemakers. By far the greatest number are married and have children, but there is also a sizable number of single people in this age group.

Most of the community planning and organization is done by the adult age group and, consequently, health teaching related to community needs usually is directed toward them. The younger members of this group often need to be taught about child rearing and homemaking, and they are usually receptive to such teaching.

It is during early adulthood that people should begin to prepare physically, psychologically, and economically for retirement and their later years. Good planning at this time will make the transition to retirement easier and more secure. Maintenance of good health practices related to diet, exercise, and rest may help to prevent many of the chronic ills of the aged. Yearly medical examinations may help to assure that early symptoms of disease are recognized and treatment instituted before conditions become acute or chronic.

Adults should be taught the early signs of cancer, since it frequently occurs in the later adult years. Certainly they need to maintain immunizations (p. 311). People in this age group, especially those having jobs in industry and construction, are frequently

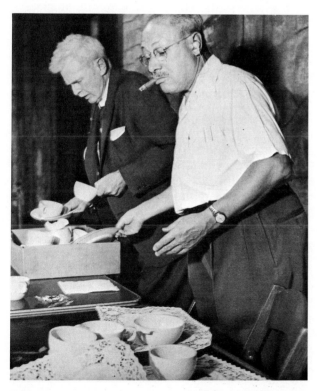

FIG. 2-2. Community recreational programs fill in many empty hours. (Courtesy New York League for the Hard of Hearing, New York, N. Y.)

involved in accidents. Accident prevention programs, the institution of safety devices, and the supervision of their use are important for this group. Teaching working people and homemakers how to prevent stasis of blood in the legs may prevent them from developing peripheral vascular disease (p. 374). Teaching this age group to avoid obesity is certainly essential (p. 144) and may help to prevent serious chronic diseases such as diabetes and atherosclerosis in later years. Teaching avoidance of cigarette smoking also is essential and may prevent diseases such as cancer of the lung, emphysema, and coronary artery disease.

In our society today, people undergo great stresses, both on the job and in life in general. We live in a highly competitive and fast-moving society. The adult is especially affected by the age-graded competition, as it may influence his ability to maintain a job and a home for his family. The resulting stress may contribute to such diseases as peptic ulcers, coronary heart disease, and hypertension. Therefore it is extremely important to encourage adults to relax. Physical activities and diversional recreation of all kinds are essential because they help to reduce tensions. Some of these activities, especially in the later adult years, should be ones that can be continued into retirement.

Labor unions have done more for the welfare of the adult group than any other agency in our society. They have been concerned with wages and working conditions and have instituted pension and insurance plans for many working groups. Insurance companies have also directed their efforts toward adults, urging them to participate in voluntary insurance plans and providing them with a great deal of literature concerning health practices. Industry, of course, focuses a great deal of attention on the adult consumer. Laborsaving devices planned for adults have often been useful. "Do-it-yourself" materials have also been useful in helping many fill their leisure hours, although they have also resulted in an increased number of accidents among persons in this age group.

Recently the United States Government and some businesses have begun to help the adult prepare psychologically for retirement. Programs have been instituted to gradually reduce the working year. It is hoped that this reduction will help people adjust more readily to retirement.

The generation gap

Despite the protestations of some to the contrary, there seems to be little doubt that there is a worldwide generation gap between the young and the old. There is increasing evidence that those born and reared before the atomic age and those born since World War II have a different view of our world. As Margaret Mead[35] and others have pointed out, it is only when both the young and the old accept the existence of the generation gap that communication can be established.

In some respects it seems that both adults and young people as a group have not squarely faced some of the realities that must be looked at and worked on together if the human race is to survive. But first this requires creative listening—the kind of listening that charges and inspires individuals to respond to each other and act toward continuous change and renewal that can lead to social solutions.

■ AGE AS A FACTOR IN DEVELOPMENT AND IN ILLNESS

The nurse whose patient is an infant, child, or adolescent should remember that he is growing physically and developing physically, mentally, and emotionally. Therefore in planning nursing care it is just as important to provide for the patient's growth and development needs as it is to meet needs generated by his illness. The nurse also may need to help parents understand and provide for their children's present and future needs.

To give effective care to patients in this age group, the nurse should know the usual stages of growth and development and the special attention needed by each group for maintaining normal development. The emphasis the nurse should place on the various aspects in giving care will vary, depending on the age of the child, how long he is ill, whether he must be hospitalized, and the nature of his illness.

The infant (birth to 2 years of age)

Care of the infant. Infants have all the basic needs of the person of any age and they may be afflicted with similar ailments. However, the ways in which their needs are expressed, their ability to cope with them even when well, and their response to illness are quite different. In caring for an infant a cardinal rule to remember is *babies are not little adults, physically, physiologically, or emotionally.*

Physical and physiologic characteristics of infants. An infant's physical development is incomplete, and therefore his metabolism is extremely active. His need for calories, fluids, and all the nutrients is proportionately greater than that of persons in any other age group. His reserves of fat, glycogen, and extracellular water are so limited that he cannot withstand loss of fluid or the omission of food or fluids for more than a few hours without developing signs of acidosis (p. 118) and dehydration (p. 111). If dehydration occurs, the baby will go rapidly into shock from subsequent loss of blood volume. Unless immediate treatment is given, death will soon follow. Parents should know of the need to seek immediate medical attention for any baby who has fever,

diarrhea, or vomiting or who fails to take several consecutive feedings. Because of the ease with which they become dehydrated, infants seldom are given cathartics or enemas. Any order for a cathartic or enema should be carefully verified with the physician, and after it is given, the infant should be observed closely for signs of dehydration.

Because his metabolism is so active, the infant generates large amounts of heat. He also loses proportionately larger amounts of fluid than do physically larger persons in dissipating the same amount of heat and therefore becomes quickly dehydrated by fever. The infant also is quickly chilled because his vascular dilation and constriction are poorly controlled, preventing body heat from being retained efficiently. This poor control is probably related to the incomplete development of the nervous system in infants.

Because the nervous system of an infant is incompletely developed at birth, he is not able to do such things as focus his eyes, use his hands to grasp objects, and localize pain. Even after physical development of the nervous system is complete, physical and emotional responses, except for reflex ones (which are part of the body's defense system), must be learned by repetitive practice. Those that produce satisfying results for the person usually are retained. They may or may not be appropriate according to the standards of society. However, responses that are unacceptable to others usually are not satisfying. It is in this way that the family and the community mold behavior according to social and cultural patterns. The child who is given no opportunity to practice appropriate physical and emotional responses will not develop normally even if he has no innate physical or physiologic limitations.

If physical development is incomplete for some reason or if there is a malfunction of some physiologic process, the child may not be able to develop normally in every aspect. For example, the mechanism for seeing or hearing may be incomplete, and as a result the baby will be blind or deaf. A muscle in his leg may be congenitally absent, making it impossible for him to learn to walk. Failure of the anterior lobe of the pituitary gland to secrete the growth hormone may cause him to be a dwarf; oversecretion may cause him to grow excessively. His brain may fail to develop normally for various reasons, making him mentally retarded and, in turn, possibly preventing his learning such activities as walking and talking.

During the first year or two of life the infant's endocrine functions are sluggish. His fluid and electrolyte balance is easily upset and he has little resistance to infection or stressors of any kind. Therefore babies respond quickly and critically to illness. They may be apparently well one moment and an hour later seriously ill. The younger the child, the more pronounced is this response.

Young babies, especially ill ones, are very prone to infections and often die as a result of them. They are more likely than are older children to have generalized systemic involvement even from such seemingly minor conditions as a cut or a cold. Therefore the nurse and others caring for a sick infant should wear an isolation gown to protect the infant against organisms carried on the clothing. Some authorities advise that a mask be worn, and some feel that sterile masks and gowns should be used. No one with an upper respiratory infection or any type of staphylococcal infection should care for a baby. Before giving care to an infant, it is essential to carefully wash one's hands. The baby's room should be kept clean and dust free, and it should be comfortably warm but well ventilated. All treatments should be carried out with the utmost gentleness to prevent traumatizing tissues, and strict surgical aseptic techniques should always be used whenever the treatment involves an opening on the skin or entry into any body cavity.

Since the infant tolerates respiratory embarrassment poorly, special precautions must be taken to prevent accidental suffocation. The importance of these measures should be stressed to parents. Materials such as soft pillows, filmy plastic, or heavy blankets that might smother a baby should not be used around him or left anywhere near him. Pins or small objects that he might put into his mouth and accidentally swallow must never be left within his reach.

Any infant who is "croupy," has a dusky color, shows sternal retraction on respiration, or has irregular respirations (Cheyne-Stokes) needs immediate medical attention. The nurse caring for a sick baby should always know how to give mouth-to-mouth resuscitation (p. 262). Teaching parents to do this might at some time save the life of their child. Parents should also be taught the signs of respiratory embarrassment in an infant and be alerted to the need to seek immediate medical attention should they occur.

A baby with any respiratory embarrassment, no matter how slight, may be given oxygen to make each inspiration more effective and to reduce the work of the heart as it attempts to transport adequate oxygen to all parts of the body. This is usually given by a small oxygen tent or a head tent (Burgess box). Steam tents (croup tents) may be needed to provide humidity to loosen mucous secretions. (Pediatric nursing texts should be consulted for detailed discussions of these procedures.) Mucus in the nose and throat may need to be removed with suction (p. 215). A temporary tracheostomy sometimes must be done (p. 612). All of these procedures may be very upsetting for the child's parents. The considerate nurse will find time to explain to them the reason they are necessary and arrange for the parents to talk with the physician about the child's condition. If oxygen is being used only prophylactically, the parents should be told this fact.

Anticipating the infant's physical needs. Not only is the infant unable to take care of himself in any way, but he is unable to express his needs except by crying. Therefore others must anticipate them. The nurse who cares for an ill baby must observe his appearance and behavior closely and frequently for signs and symptoms of abnormality. Parents also should be taught to recognize these signs and symptoms so that they will know when to seek medical attention for their baby.

A restless, irritable infant may be manifesting pain that he has no other way of expressing. Since pain is difficult to evaluate and localize in babies, any symptoms suggesting it should be reported in detail to the physician.

Failure of the infant to eat properly may be a sign of any one of many serious disorders and should always be discussed with the physician. Apathy to food and loss of appetite may signify an incipient infection. It may have many other causes. Failure to gain weight in spite of taking food is always a serious sign. Unusual fussiness between feedings is often indicative of ill health. A satisfied and healthy baby usually sleeps soon after his feeding and awakens prior to the next one. Persistent vomiting, as contrasted with the normal occasional regurgitation that occurs in many well infants, nearly always is a serious sign and may be the first evidence of infection anywhere in the body or of other disease.

Changes in the character and timing of stools may indicate serious gastrointestinal disease. When an infant is sick, the color and amount of each stool should be noted and recorded. The time of each stool also should be recorded. The color, odor, and amount of urine and the frequency of urination should be recorded (p. 121). Any significant changes in the stool or urine from normal should be brought to the physician's attention at once.

Caring for the infant's needs. Attention must be given to the infant's *general hygiene.* Each day the infant's entire body should be thoroughly inspected. This is usually done during the bath. The eyes, ears, and nostrils should be inspected for discharges and cleaned as necessary. The skin and scalp should be observed for any lesions. Rashes on the back of the head, the buttocks, and the perineum are rather common. They can be minimized by keeping the baby clean and dry. If the baby has any urinary tract infection, special care needs to be taken because the urine is likely to be more acid or alkaline than normal.

If the baby is hospitalized or sick at home for a long period, plans should be made for him to be in the outside air and sun at intervals. Care should be taken, however, not to chill the baby or to overexpose him to the sun.

The infant must be given *food* and *fluids*. If the ill infant can tolerate food and fluid orally, he usually is given his regular formula. Otherwise food and fluids are given parenterally. Occasionally a baby will have to be gavaged (fed through a nasogastric tube) (p. 122).

Well babies, beginning soon after birth, usually receive prescribed formulas equivalent to $2\frac{1}{2}$ ounces and 50 calories/pound of body weight a day.[34] Formulas may be supplemented by orange juice and vitamins A and D. Solids in the form of cereals, strained vegetables, and fruits are usually started at least by the third or fourth month. They should be fed to the baby before he is given his bottle. When the infant begins to get teeth and learns to chew, he is usually advanced to chopped foods (junior foods) and given hard teething biscuits when teething. Most children go to an adult diet sometime between the eighteenth and twenty-fourth month.[34] When the baby no longer takes a formula, his diet should include the basic food groups given as finger foods when possible.

Often a sick infant will need extra fluids, and the doctor should specify the amount and type of fluid. Plans must be made to space this extra fluid between feedings. Medications are usually given by medicine dropper or spoon. Any baby, especially an ill one, should be held for his bottles and medications to prevent aspiration. Holding him will give him the security, love, and tactile stimulation he needs to develop properly; it may also improve his appetite.

If the baby is hospitalized over a period of many months, the nurse should consult the physician about increasing his diet. There usually is no reason why a hospitalized infant's diet should not progress with his age in the same way it would normally. New foods should be started one at a time. If an infant rejects a food, a substitution should be made and the food tried again later. To help the child learn to chew, the nurse may give him crackers or dry toast. Chopped food should never be given before he has learned to chew.

Before the baby is discharged from the hospital, the nurse should be sure that the mother knows the formula or food he is receiving and how to prepare it. Nurses from the nursery for newborn infants may be called on to teach formula preparation, or the nutritionist or dietitian will teach it. The visiting nurse can be asked to go into the home to give the mother additional help as necessary.

Attention needs to be given to the baby's *physical development.* Not all babies develop at the same rate, and the sick baby may be expected to be somewhat retarded in his development. As the infant develops, he soon should begin to look about him. At around 4 months of age he usually begins to clutch at large objects, although he may be 8 months old or more before he can hold small objects. Around 5 months of age he begins to roll over and by 8 months

of age he may be able to crawl. Babies vary greatly in the time they learn to walk and speak. The average age for walking is 12 months. Many children can also say several words by this age.[34] (See pediatric nursing texts for further details.)

Nurses caring for an infant should know the usual schedule of development. They should be alert for any indications of abnormality in the development of infant patients and bring these to the physician's attention. They also should provide care that will in no way impede development. If the infant is ill for a long time, either at home or in the hospital, they should see that provisions are made whenever possible for normal development to continue.

Provisions should be made for the baby to have as much normal movement as possible. A firm mattress helps the sick baby who has poor muscle tone to move about more easily. If possible, the baby should be turned on his abdomen as well as each side several times a day. When any part of the infant's body must be restrained, it is desirable for the restraint to be released for 5 or 10 minutes every 2 to 4 hours day and night. This allows the infant to move the part freely at intervals. The nurse should remain with the infant while he is unrestrained to protect him from injury.

Equipment appropriate for the infant's stage of development should be provided. Bright rattles or mobiles strung over the crib provide exercise in eye movements. When the baby begins to clutch with his hands, a rattle or some similar toy should be provided. If the baby is beginning to crawl and pull himself up, it is often permissible to put him in a playpen or some other safe area where he can move about more freely than in a crib.

Special attention should be paid to the *safety* of a baby. A baby, no matter how young, should never be left alone with the crib side down or in any other place where he might fall (Fig. 2-3). Even young babies are usually quite active with their arms and legs and can accidentally propel themselves over the edge of a bed or table. When the baby begins to move about more actively, a harness restraint often is used to secure him even in the crib. The harness slips over the shoulders and chest, fastens in the back, and is tied to the lower bar at the head of the crib with a square knot that holds securely but is easily untied. Preferably the harness should be made like a vest, and its ties should be short enough to prevent the infant from becoming entangled in them and choking. Any body restraint used for an infant or small child must be approved by the medical staff of the hospital and must be ordered specifically by the physician for each patient.

Occasionally it may be necessary to use restraining measures to prevent a baby from moving about during a procedure, to prevent him from pulling on catheters or dressings, or to keep him from scratch-

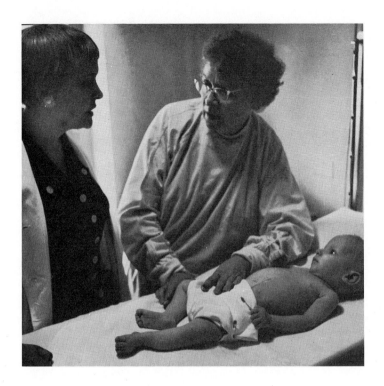

FIG. 2-3. The social worker is visiting while the grandmother helps care for the infant. Note that the grandmother is standing so as to protect the child from rolling out of the bed accidentally. (Courtesy Today's Health, American Medical Association, Chicago, Ill.; photograph by Dorothy Reed.)

ing an itchy rash. Usually holding the baby's arms and legs firmly at the ankles and wrists provides sufficient restraint for a procedure, but sometimes it may be necessary to place him in a blanket restraint ("mummy" him) (Fig. 2-4). To prevent the baby from pulling at dressings and tubes or scratching himself, elbow splints usually are effective. They prevent bending of the elbow but allow movement of the arm as a whole (Fig. 2-5). Since the baby is as agile with his feet as with his hands, a splint may need to be placed behind the knee. Special care must be taken to ensure that any splints are well padded and do not press into soft tissues to prevent ulceration of the tissue. At other times it may be necessary to apply wrist or ankle restraints. These restraints should be well padded and should allow for maintenance of correct body alignment and slight movement of the part. For a tiny baby a long gown that fastens snugly in the back and can be tied below the feet may suffice to keep dressings and catheters out of reach. A gown with mittens also may give adequate restraint. No restraint should impede circulation to the part and, if permitted, it should be removed periodically (see above).

It is normal and necessary for a baby to be fondled and loved. "Mothering" is essential for his *psychologic development.* The plan for care, therefore, should include time for cuddling the infant of any age, and some time should be taken each day to play with him. If a rocking chair is kept at the bedside, the infant can be held comfortably, talked to, and stroked while he is being bathed, dressed, and fed, and even while he is being given certain treatments.

Some babies may have restrictions of movements and cannot be held. The resourceful nurse, however, will still find ways of providing loving care. Even a baby who cannot be held can be talked to and stroked. Wheeling his crib back and forth in a rocking motion often is comforting to a baby. The baby who has apparatus such as catheters attached usually can be held safely provided that the persons caring for him are properly instructed in the necessary precautions.

The nurse can provide some of the "cuddling" needed by the infant as daily care is given. However, the nurse seldom has time to give the infant the amount of attention he needs. Since this is a period of life when the mother and baby are normally together, it is preferable that whenever possible the mother provide the "mothering" and those aspects of care that she can perform. It is probably not essential for the welfare of a young infant that the mother be present 24 hours a day. However, as he approaches the age of 2 years, it becomes more important. (See discussion later in this chapter.) If the mother cannot be with her baby, another family member such as a grandmother, a teenage sister, or the father may wish to assist with the care. Sometimes a volunteer or paid worker may be assigned as "mother" for the infant who must be hospitalized for a long time and whose family is not present.

The infant's *spiritual needs* must not be neglected. The religious or denominational affiliation of the infant's family should be ascertained, and the nurse should be meticulous in assuring that appropriate observances are carried out. In the initial interview

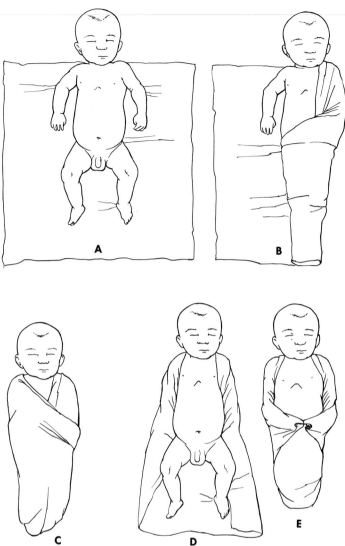

FIG. 2-4. Mummying an infant. **A,** Place infant on sheet or blanket to be used. **B,** Wrap one side of sheet snugly around and under baby so that the arm is at his side and legs are together. **C,** Bring other side of sheet across body, securing the other arm. Pin the sheet securely at the side and bottom. **D** and **E,** A modification that can be used for treatments requiring that the chest and/or abdomen be uncovered.

it should be ascertained whether or not the baby has been baptized and, if not, whether the family wishes to have the baby baptized. The family also should be consulted about their desire to have a priest, minister, or rabbi informed should the baby become critically ill. In discussing the infant's progress with the family members, the nurse should give assurance that their desires in these matters have been complied with.

The infant's family. The baby who is hospitalized usually belongs to a family who will be interested in the course of his illness and his general development. Arrangements should be made for the family to speak with the physician about the infant's medical progress and about plans for his continued treatment. The nurse can tell the family about any new symptoms displayed by the infant, signs of physical or psychologic improvement, and advances in normal development. The family should also receive an explanation of the procedures and tests that the infant is undergoing.

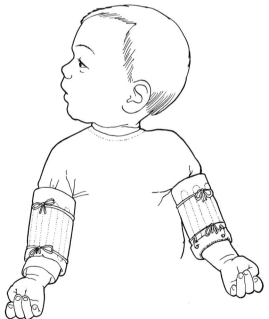

FIG. 2-5. Elbow splints prevent infant from disturbing dressings or scratching, yet permit free movement of the shoulders and arms.

When a family member wishes to assist in the nursing care of the infant, a specific plan should be worked out so that he or she receives the assurance, support, and teaching necessary to give the care. At the same time the nurse must reassure the family member who does not wish to participate in giving care that this is acceptable. Otherwise feelings of guilt about not giving direct care to the infant may develop.

The nurse usually gives the infant his medications and treatments, but if he will need continued treatment at home, the family member who will be responsible should have the opportunity to learn and practice the procedures involved under the guidance of the nurse. Often a baby whose mother has been allowed to assist with his care in the hospital will be able to be discharged from the hospital sooner than otherwise because the family is less fearful and is prepared to provide continuing care in the home.

Home care. It is usually advisable to arrange for a visiting nurse to make a home visit to the family of any baby who has been hospitalized. The visiting nurse is also helpful to parents whose child is ill but does not require hospitalization. If the baby has been hospitalized, an early referral should be made so that the nurse may visit the home before the baby's return to help the family make the necessary preparations. It may be helpful for the visiting nurse, before doing this, to visit the baby in the hospital. In writing the referral, information concerning nutrition, development, medications, details of dressings, and other treatments should be included so that the nurse coming into the home can provide continuity in follow-up care.

The young child

The term "young child" applies to children in two age groups: those 2 to 5 years of age (preschool children) and those in elementary school. Although both groups are growing and developing rapidly, they differ somewhat physically, physiologically, and psychologically. Children in both groups grow rapidly for a time, slow down, and then have another spurt of growth. Their appetite may parallel the growth pattern. Physiologic controls, especially of fluids and electrolyte balance and temperature, are still not fully developed in the preschooler, although they are somewhat more effective than those of an infant. By about the age of 7 years, physiologic controls appear to be fully developed.

The preschool child is still learning basic muscle coordination and speech, is developing the basic behavior patterns necessary for socialization, and is exploring his environment. He does not express himself with complete facility yet and often has not learned to cooperate with spoken instructions. The schoolchild, on the other hand, usually can express himself well, can follow instructions, and has learned to cooperate with others. He often can be reasoned with effectively.

Children in both age groups need love and affection. To be happy, they also need discipline. Knowing the acceptable limits seems to give security to persons of every age.

The ill child. Children, especially those under the age of 5, tolerate any systemic upset, such as may occur with infection, tissue trauma, or anesthesia, poorly. Their ability to withstand fluid and electrolyte loss is still poor, and they still may readily respond with fever. Therefore extensive bowel preparations for diagnostic procedures or surgery are rarely given, and physicians rarely withhold food or fluids for long. The usual plan when food or fluids must be withheld is described on p. 110. If more than one enema is given to a child under 7 years of age, or if food and fluids are withheld for more than 2 to 4 hours, he should be observed closely for signs of dehydration, and the physician must be notified at once if they appear.

There is rarely any reason why children who are not seriously ill or who do not have a fever cannot be dressed during the day. Most hospitals provide playclothes as well as underclothes and nightclothes. Children who are hospitalized should be encouraged to continue activities they have learned to do for themselves at home, such as dressing themselves, washing, and going to the toilet. Bathrooms with low fixtures usually are available or a sturdy step stool can be used. The nurse should ask the mother what her child does for himself and make as few radical changes from the home routine as possible. The child responds best to as much normality as possible. If the child must be kept in bed, the nurse should be sure he understands about the use of the bedpan, bed bathing, and eating from trays.

Many children in the younger age groups are finicky eaters, and feeding the hospitalized child may present special problems. Most children eat better if given small servings and if they are not constantly coaxed. They usually eat better at a table with others, and making mealtime a "party" occasion is often helpful. Snacks between meals may supplement inadequate meals. Food likes and dislikes should be ascertained from the mother in the admission interview.

The older child may have a voracious appetite, especially if he is growing rapidly and is very active. He should be given foods high in protein and carbohydrates. Starches and fats sometimes should be restricted because overweight may become a problem. The mother should be told about diet requirements because they also apply to the child's diet at home.

Play should be provided for children unless they are acutely ill. A variety of amusements should be available, especially for young children. Even when well, the attention span of children is short, and sick children may tire of an activity even more readily. Preschool children often enjoy crayoning, finger painting, and make-believe activities (Fig. 2-6). The school-age child may be interested in reading, listening to records, observing and caring for birds or fish, making such objects as model planes or jewelry, painting, or taking part in competitive activities. Playing with others usually is possible even for the bedridden child, but care should be taken that the child does not overexert himself or become overtired. Educational play activity and play with others are especially important for the child who has a prolonged illness, so that continued mental and social development is assured.

If a child of school age is hospitalized or is sick at home for a long period of time (usually over 2 weeks), most boards of education provide visiting teachers. Parents need to be reminded of this service. Continuing with his schoolwork not only provides diversion for the child but also assures that he will not fall behind his classmates.

Every ill child, whether in the hospital or at home, should receive some special attention from adults. This attention is needed especially by the bedridden child. The form of the attention needed varies with the child. Most children, even those of school age, need to be held and hugged occasionally; others respond better to interest in their activity or just quiet talking. Almost all children like to have stories read to them, and quiet play activities such as games are usually enjoyed. Helping the mother or nurse with such small tasks as picking up toys or cleaning the table may provide the desired attention. A very ill child of any age may want little more than the comfort of a parent's presence, but this is very important to him.

When a child requires treatments or medication, the nurse must adapt the procedures to the age of the child and to his response. Before a procedure is performed, it should be described to the child and his part in it explained. With preschool children, painless but strange procedures can often be accomplished most easily by using play techniques. For example, a rockinghorse seat may be provided for the child while a radiograph of the lungs is taken. A similar arrangement can be made for holding a potty for the collection of urine specimens. The resourceful nurse can devise many techniques of this type. The school-age child usually follows instructions well and is surprisingly cooperative if explanations of procedures are given to him. Often he can assist with his tests. For example, he may watch the clock for the time to collect specimens. The capacity to cooperate will, of course, vary from child to child and depends on the extent of his development.

If the procedure will be uncomfortable, a parent or a nurse who is well liked by the child should be present to comfort and firmly hold him as necessary. A child of any age should be told truthfully what type of sensation he may expect, and it usually is advisable to tell him when he is about to be hurt. Restraining techniques such as "mummying" (Fig. 2-4) occasionally must be used for the safety of a preschool child who is overactive, but usually just talking to the child and holding him firmly is all that is needed. School-age children who have been properly instructed rarely need restraining. Appropriate praise, comfort, and attention should be given to the child at the completion of a painful procedure.

Giving oral medication to children often requires ingenuity. The most successful technique should be recorded on the nursing care plan. It is helpful to ask

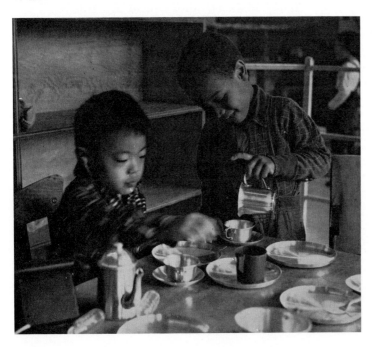

FIG. 2-6. Make-believe play activities amuse many preschool children. These two little boys are playing house. (Jan E. Ott from Monkmeyer Press Photo Service; from Winter, C. C., and Barker, M. R.: Nursing care of patients with urologic diseases, ed. 3, St. Louis, 1972, The C. V. Mosby Co.)

the mother about methods she has found successful with her child. Some children will swallow pills disguised with food, and others will take them dissolved in small amounts of fruit juices, but care should be taken not to develop a food dislike by its use with medications. Children's medications often come in both liquid and pill form and usually are flavored. The child may accept one form better than the other. Usually children accept medicine better when they are among other children who are also receiving it. Therefore it may be helpful to offer medications to children in a group situation. Special care must be taken, if this method is used, not to give the wrong medication to a child. Medication should *never* be given to any child before his identification band is carefully checked.

Medications should not be forced on a child. If difficulty is encountered in getting a child to take a medication, the nurse should wait a few minutes and then try a new approach. There usually is some approach that is effective, but if not, the physician should be consulted.

Special needs of the hospitalized child. If hospitalization is necessary, the child of any age should be prepared for the experience by his parents. The nurse in the physician's office or clinic should be sure the parents know how to prepare him. They should tell the child truthfully about the hospital and why he must go there. He should not be frightened about the experience, but neither should he be led to expect the experience to be completely pleasant. He should be told about the high beds, bedpans, urinals, bed baths, eating in bed, the attire of nurses and physicians, and the play facilities in a matter-of-fact and reassuring way. If possible, the preparation for hospitalization should be done gradually. Well-written storybooks

concerning hospitalization are available in bookstores and may be helpful in introducing the topic (Fig. 2-7).* In addition, many children's hospitals have written their own books for patients.

Children, especially those between 2 and 5 years of age, tend to form attachments to inanimate objects such as well-loved toys or blankets. Such an object, whatever it may be, gives the child comfort and security. Even a sick child of school age may want to bring some favorite object to the hospital. He should be allowed to do so, and no one should worry if it is old or ragged. The object is the child's link with home, and he should be free to take it with him wherever he goes, even to treatment rooms and to the operating room.

It is important, too, for parents to allow children of any age, prior to their departure for the hospital, to help prepare for their return home. This tells the child he is expected home again. Often the child can pack a bag with clothes that he will wear when he is discharged from the hospital, or he may help prepare the room where he will stay while he is recuperating.

Hospitalization and separation from the mother has been found to be especially upsetting for the child between 2 and 4 years of age. He has a tendency to regress to earlier behavior patterns while in the hospital, on his return home, or at both times. This regression may take many forms. Some children return to earlier behavior of bed-wetting or soiling their clothes; others may have bad dreams and cry during

---

*Two helpful publications are Ray, H. A.: Curious George goes to the hospital, Boston, 1966, Houghton-Mifflin Co.; Flandorf, R. S.: Books to help children adjust to hospital situations, Chicago, 1967, American Library Association.

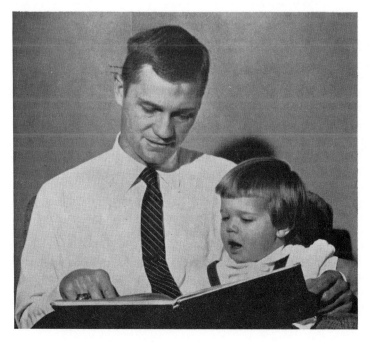

FIG. 2-7. A child's father can help in preparing the child for hospitalization. This one is reading a book about going to the hospital to his daughter. (Bloom from Monkmeyer Press Photo Service; from Winter, C. C., and Barker, M. R.: Nursing care of patients with urologic diseases, ed. 3, St. Louis, 1972, The C. V. Mosby Co.)

sleep. Some refuse to eat; others revert to baby talk and whining or stop talking altogether. The child may be "too good" or he may be unusually naughty. Temper tantrums and clinging to the mother are common. If the child has to be separated from his mother, the regression may be more noticeable and last much longer. Consequently, physicians now seldom hospitalize children in this age group unless it is absolutely necessary. Whenever possible, the child is cared for in his home, in an outpatient department, or in the physician's office.

If the child must be hospitalized, many experts advise the mother to "room in" with the child during the entire hospital stay. Many hospitals have lounging chairs or cots placed at the child's bedside; some of the cots slide under youth beds. The mother's comfort should be considered, and the thoughtful nurse will be sure that she knows the location of rest rooms, dressing and eating facilities, and a telephone booth. The mother should be informed about hospital regulations by which she is expected to abide. For example, it may be customary for her to leave the room during certain treatments or she may be forbidden in other children's rooms or in workrooms of the unit. Often, if the mother stays at the hospital with her child, plans must be made for the care of the rest of the family. The social service department of the hospital or of a public health agency may be helpful in this regard. It is certainly not always possible or practical for a mother to stay with her child constantly, especially if the hospitalization is to be for more than a few days. If she cannot stay, she should not be made to feel that she is a poor mother.

When his mother does not stay with the hospitalized preschool child, he should be cared for by as few nurses as possible. This procedure seems to add to his security. A substitute mother (p. 27) may also be used. Frequent and regular visits from the parents are helpful, even though the child often ignores them during the visit and cries bitterly after they leave. This behavior may be very upsetting to parents, and the nurse should prepare them to expect it. They should be helped to realize that it is a completely normal response and that no amount of reasoning with the child will change his reaction. He is angry at his parents because he thinks he has been deserted. They should be cautioned not to add distrust to anger by failing to visit at appointed times or by deceiving him in any way. For instance, they should tell the child when they are leaving and not slip away without telling him they are leaving. If frequent visits cannot be made, children seem to enjoy receiving some daily momento such as a brightly colored greeting card or a note from the family. Nurses should allow the child to keep the card with him and should be willing to read and reread it for him. Telephone conversations between the older child and his parents also seem to give comfort.

Hospitalization apparently is not too psychologically traumatic for the schoolchild, especially if he has been adequately prepared for it. Unless the child is acutely ill or will be having an operation, he rarely needs the constant attendance of his mother. However, his parents should be urged to visit him regularly or, if frequent visits are not possible, to keep in regular contact with him by telephone or letter.

The parents will want to know about their child's activities, behavior, and progress in the hospital. Although no child should be discussed with his parents when he is present, the nurse is responsible for keeping parents informed and for giving them necessary explanations. Plans also should be made to teach the mother any procedures she will need to know when the child returns home. The parents should be told to expect that a young child on return home may exhibit some form of regressive behavior. He can be managed best by giving him extra "mothering" and resuming former expectations for behavior at once. Arrangements should be made for parents to discuss the medical aspects of the child's care with the physician.

The teenager

The early adolescent (12 to 16 years of age) is neither a child nor an adult, and he may alternately respond and wish to be treated as either a child or an adult. Adequate handling of this group offers a real challenge. One must feel one's way and alter the approach accordingly.

Many boys and girls in their early teens are physically awkward and poorly coordinated because their growth during this period progresses in uneven stages. The young teenager should not be expected to handle any tasks that would put him in the embarrassing position of "falling over" his hands and feet. Great tact is needed to avoid being obvious about avoiding such a situation. He also may drop and spill things but should not be reprimanded.

The teenager, especially the young one who is growing rapidly, consumes large amounts of food. Girls between 13 and 15 and boys between 16 and 19 years of age need more calories than at any other time during their life cycle. Teenagers often need double or even triple servings of food at meals and nourishing snacks between meals. Good food habits should be stressed to ensure an adequate nutritional intake as well as a "filling" one (Chapter 6). Teenagers often tend to maintain a hamburger-and-coke diet. Teenage girls, especially, often omit breakfast.

Young teenagers of both sexes are likely to be subject to disorders involving the skin. Acne vulgaris is a common condition at this age. It is related to the hormonal changes of puberty. Although it cannot be prevented, the symptoms can be minimized and complications prevented by attention to skin care and to diet. This condition is very upsetting to most teenagers, and they usually are willing to follow suggestions for care.

Teenage girls often spend much time languishing and primping. They are flattered by attention by men but also enjoy "woman-to-woman" talk. Teenage boys often try to get a "rise" from young women by acting like a "man-about-town." At other times they may seem quite rude, failing to respond to people who are talking to them or responding curtly. If these reactions are handled matter-of-factly or ignored, they will usually pass.

Teenagers, especially older ones, are often confronted by ambivalence, and they may become quite confused and worried. They feel a need to be the same as others in their group and yet they are beginning to become individuals. They may be the size of an adult and have the sexual drive of an adult but still be emotionally immature. Society, however, may expect them to behave as adults. Teenagers are inherently idealistic, yet the realities of the world are constantly being revealed to them. They have a great amount of energy and enthusiasm. These qualities are all too frequently rejected by adults, perhaps because the realization that their own years of life are passing makes them uncomfortable.

Teenagers need to talk about their problems and feelings. The teenage boy often likes to talk with an older adult, either a man or woman. The teenage girl may confide in a young woman. Both boys and girls may find it easier to talk with someone other than a family member. Priests, ministers, rabbis, club leaders, nurses and physicians, and friends of parents may be useful in this role. The teenager should be allowed to express his feelings freely and should be helped to explore them. Sometimes professional help may be needed.

The ill teenager. When teenagers, especially older ones, require hospitalization, they are often assigned to the adult service. They are usually considered adults as far as physical aspects of preparation for diagnostic tests and therapy are concerned. However, their psychologic needs must be met quite differently from those of an adult.

It is most important that the teenager's relative maturity be acknowledged by nurses. They should talk to him as an adult. He is likely to be flattered by this and usually responds well. The teenager is usually interested in his disease even though he may appear very blasé and even disinterested. Unless nurses make a deliberate effort, this attitude may cause them to be negligent about exploring the true reaction of the patient to his condition and even about explaining procedures to him. Actually the teenager usually is eager for health teaching and is likely to accept it well. He often enjoys discussions of a scientific nature.

Nurses should understand that the teenager has fears. They should anticipate these and by their manner let him know that they do not think less of him for showing them. Teenagers worry most about being different from others in their age group. They worry about their condition, and, surprisingly, many also worry about death, although they rarely mention it. The comfort and consultation of a priest, minister, or rabbi may therefore be desirable. An adolescent boy may become panicky about the effect of disease on his sexual and reproductive capacity. The female nurse, becoming aware of his fear, should refer the problem to a male nurse or physician, who can often give the best reassurance. Girls often worry about having a vaginal examination. The nurse can help reduce their fears greatly by explaining procedures they must undergo factually, telling them who is likely to be present during examinations, anticipating for them questions that may be asked by the physician or others, and seeing that they are kept informed about the probable course of their treatment.

Adolescents, both boys and girls, are likely to be quite modest. Their privacy should be ensured, and any personal teaching or supervision such as that involving physical examination is more acceptable to them from a nurse of the same sex. If a male nurse if not available, a male physician will often give special attention to supervision of a boy. If a female nurse must attend to situations of this kind, an adolescent boy is much more at ease with a mature nurse than with a nursing student or a recent graduate who is near his own age. When the teenage girl is hospitalized, on admission she should be given the necessary supplies and instructions for caring for her menses. In this way she may be saved from embarrassment. She also should be told that her illness may cause her menstrual period to be skipped or to be premature. If a menstrual irregularity occurs without the girl being aware of the possibility, she may be quite concerned and yet not mention it.

Appropriate diversional activities should be provided for teenage patients, who usually find the days very long. Most of them enjoy watching television, and many like to read and do things with their hands. If they can be out of bed, they may enjoy participating in useful activities about the house or hospital unit. Young friends should be encouraged to visit them, and if they have a hobby, they may be encouraged to work on it. If the duration of the illness is longer than 2 weeks, plans should be made with the school to continue schoolwork unless contraindicated.

The teenager should participate in plans for his convalescence since continuing progress will depend on his cooperation. If he has had a serious illness, he should be helped to assess his health situation realistically and to set short-term and long-term goals for himself accordingly. Sometimes his fondest dreams for the future must be given up. Such an occurrence can be so devastating that he may need to be referred for psychiatric help.

The adult

By about the age of 22 years, physical growth is complete, behavior patterns are firmly established, and the personality is molded. There is also some evidence that mental faculties may decline gradually, through lack of use, after the age of 35, although the adult is perhaps better equipped than a younger person to use his knowledge effectively.

Adulthood is often referred to as the time of maturity. However, the nurse must understand that a particular patient may not necessarily have attained what would normally be considered "mature adult behavior." Emotional maturity varies from person to person, as do intellectual ability and physical characteristics. In addition, an adult who appears reasonably mature under usual circumstances, may, when under severe stress, exhibit behavior more typical of a child. He may, for example, demand undivided attention or even have a temper tantrum.

Too often the adult patient is considered to be a person who, without outside assistance, can always handle all his problems except his medical one. Actually the adult often is confronted with the most acute socioeconomic and psychologic problems of any patient, primarily because a spouse, children, or aging parents may all be dependent on the patient for support. Regardless of the level of maturity the patient has attained, these problems may seem almost insurmountable, and indeed they may be. Perhaps it is the complexity of the problems faced by adults that makes nurses reticent about discussing them with patients. Nevertheless, the patient cannot settle down to the business of getting well if his mind is filled with anxieties. Therefore finding out what may trouble the patient and obtaining suitable help to assist with the problem should be one of the primary objectives in giving nursing care to the adult.

The adult patient's major concern often is not about himself. He or she may be the breadwinner of a family. How is the family being supported during the illness? How are the medical bills to be paid? The patient may be a mother with a family of small children. Who will care for the children? If she is hospitalized, she often is concerned about how her family is getting along at home. The patient may have no family. Who will look in on him if he is ill at home? If he had an emergency admission to the hospital, who will take care of his unfinished business? Who will care for him during convalescence? These are only a few of the pressing problems frequently facing the adult patient. Some problems of hospitalized patients may be alleviated by providing the use of a telephone or by arranging a visit with a family member, friend, or business associate. Help needed by the patient may be available through social services in the hospital or through family service or public health agencies. It is helpful if assistance in family care can be arranged prior to the patient's being hospitalized. The nurse in a physician's office or clinic should be alert for patients who need this type of help.

The adult patient is often expected "to act like an adult," and this is especially true if he is a male. Most males reared in the United States and Canada are taught to be brave, not to cry, and to conceal their emotions. Thus, when they are ill, they may become irritable, withdrawn, and depressed because they conceal their true feelings. The nurse needs to be able to convey sincere interest in the patient as a unique human being and acceptance of him even though his behavior is not what one usually expects of an adult.

Teaching of the adult patient is a very important and too often neglected part of patient care. The nurse first needs to ascertain what the patient understands about his illness and the care he is receiving for it and then devise a teaching plan appropriate for the patient. An important part of the patient teaching is timing, and the teaching should begin when the patient's behavior indicates readiness and should progress at a level and rate suited to him. As part of discharge planning, the nurse should be sure that the patient and/or his family will be able to care for his needs at home. When this is not so, the patient needs to be aware of community resources available to assist him in this care. Oftentimes the assumption is made that a well-educated patient with no obvious financial problems will have no difficulty arranging for his own care after discharge. Often this is not true, and all patients need to be aware of options open to them for assistance with health care problems when they are no longer in the acute care setting.

The adult patient quite commonly has been taking medication or following a special diet for a condition other than the one for which he is currently being treated. This information should be sought in the admission nursing history and the patient should be instructed about not taking any medication that is not currently being ordered for him. At the same time the nurse can explain to the patient the need to discuss with the physician any over-the-counter medications such as aspirin taken on a regular basis. Sometimes these medications are antagonistic to the ones currently being used to treat the patient or may potentiate their action. For this reason the patient needs a careful explanation of the need to refrain from taking any medications without discussing it with the physician.

Occasionally a lactating mother is admitted to the hospital. Arrangements need to be made within a few hours to pump her breasts at regular intervals or to dry up the milk supply. Otherwise the breasts will become painfully engorged. Nurses on the maternity service may be consulted for assistance with the procedure. The nurse should always ascertain whether arrangements have been made for the care and feeding of the baby. A visiting nurse may need to be asked to visit the home at once.

Adults who are ill need diversion as much as patients in any other age group. Many relish the opportunity to just relax and read or watch television or listen to the radio. Others are happier keeping actively busy. They may like some occupational therapy (Fig. 2-8), or they may prefer to do useful activities about the hospital unit or for their own homes. Diversional activities should be determined by the patient's interest and his physical limitations. Sometimes it may be possible and desirable for adults to carry on their business from their bedside. Adults are more likely than any other age group to need their social and business contacts restricted at times during illness. Since adults are likely to be active in the community, they may have many visitors. These visits sometimes are more tiring than diversional for the ill patient, and the nurse may have to restrict visitors after discussing the situation with the patient.

The elderly person

Although 65 years of age is usually considered the beginning of late maturity or old age, tremendous individual variation exists. Age is really a sociocultural concept and not wholly physiologic and chronologic. Chronologic age is related to but not identical with the term "aging" because individual and personal variables enter the picture. The U. S. Department of Health, Education and Welfare has defined age in terms of three classes. These classes are biologic age (a person's position in time relative to his potential life span), psychologic age (the individual's capacity for adapting to his environment), and social age (a

person's role in the family, at work, and in his community as well as his interests and activities).[56] Some people may be old at 45 years of age, while others are not old at 80. Persons under 75 are usually considered to be the "young old," and persons 75 years of age and over are the "old old" or "really old." The problems and needs of these two groups may be quite different. The "old old" usually have more physical changes typical of aging and far more social problems such as loss of friends and loss of independence than the "young old." The reverse, of course, may be true. There now exists a tendency to see middle age as the first stage of aging.

Characteristics of aging. Aging is a normal process in which certain *anatomic* and *physiologic changes* take place. The changes are associated with a decline in the effectiveness and functioning of the organism that eventually results in death. The speed with which aging occurs varies and depends on hereditary factors and the stresses of life. The genetic factor in these biologic processes determines the time of onset, the course and direction, and the time sequences of the various aging processes.

Aging is now being explored by many researchers. Many models of aging have been hypothesized. These models are generally divided into three classes. The first concerns models centered around aging due to loss of cellular synthesis. The loss of cellular synthesis can be attributed to genetic damage (DNA), loss of messenger synthesis ability of the cells, or a loss of message-translating ability. A second class of models to explain aging concerns loss of cellular function. The loss of function can occur because of loss of function of cellular organelles, insufficiency of growth factors, or an accumulation of inhibitors. Finally, the third class of models or hy-

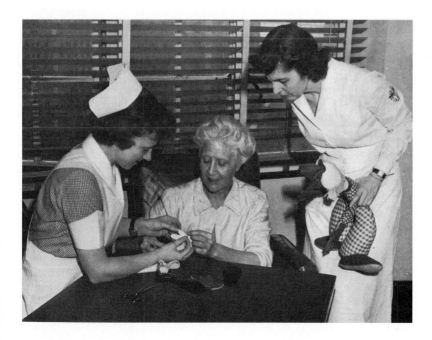

FIG. 2-8. Adult patients also need diversion. (From Anderson, H. C.: Newton's geriatric nursing, ed. 5, St. Louis, 1971, The C. V. Mosby Co.)

potheses centers around loss of intercellular coordination. Reasons hypothesized to explain this include physical alteration, decreased cell responsiveness due to loss of receptor sites or cells, or just cell loss. Total cell loss with age may average 10% to 40% in some parts of the body. This cell loss occurs to the greatest extent in the nervous and endocrine systems. Kidney, liver, heart, and muscle tissue seem affected to a lesser degree.

Biologic aging leads to different responses in the older person. Healing takes place more slowly, and the body's response to infection is less rapid and apparently less effective. Tissues gradually lose their elasticity, leading to a decreased speed of muscle response and decreased strength. Loss of tissue elasticity also causes increased rigidity of such body structures as the rib cage. This rigidity in turn may cause decreased lung expansion and predisposes the aged person to lung congestion. Bones become rarefied in the aging process and fractures occur easily. This is true particularly of the vertebral bodies and the neck of the femur that begin to lose their density while a person is in his thirties.

The elasticity of the blood vessels also lessens, causing circulatory changes. Peripheral resistance increases with age, despite a reduction in cardiac output. Blood pressure also shows a marked increase with age, both in systolic and diastolic readings. A rule of thumb is that normal systolic blood pressure is roughly equal to 100 plus the age. The elderly person does not tolerate radical changes in position such as lowering of the head for postural drainage or elevation of the feet above heart level. Vessels in the head may become engorged, and there is inadequate circulation to the lower extremities. With prolonged standing, blood may accumulate in the lower extremities so that not enough is provided for the brain. Dizziness and accidents may follow.

There is gradual degeneration and atrophy of the nervous system in old age, leading to lessened nerve acuity and impaired sensation. There is a generalized loss of neurons with age and a progressive decrease in the weight of the brain. The older person's gag reflex may be less acute than that of a younger person, and therefore aspiration of mucus or other foreign material such as food may occur easily. He may be unaware of burning himself or of pressure on soft tissues. Mental deterioration, known as senility, may also occur. However, not all old people whose mental processes appear slow and muddled are senile. An inadequate blood supply to the brain may cause this condition. Bed rest causes the elderly person's circulation to slow up; consequently, many elderly people become confused when they must stay in bed. This is noticeable in some even after several hours of sleep. Loss of interest in life may also make an elderly person appear dull mentally. Oftentimes these individuals will become more bright and alert when their stimuli is increased by being in contact with others. Therefore it is often preferable to put the elderly person in a room with others rather than in a single room by himself.

The liver, heart, kidneys, and other vital organs of many elderly people may be working hard to maintain normal function with little margin available for adaptability to stress. Any additional burden may be enough to tip the balance unfavorably unless particular care is given. The physiologic controls of fluid and electrolyte balance and temperature also are less adaptable in the aged. Faintness and shock may follow relatively short periods without food and fluid because of fluid and electrolyte imbalances. Therefore the elderly person should receive medical attention for even apparently slight indispositions.

The basic *psychologic needs* of the elderly are no different from those of adults. In one survey,[26] elderly persons were asked what they considered essential for their happiness. They mentioned good health, a place to live, enough money to live comfortably, recognition by others, participation with others, and opportunity for a variety of experiences. However, the elderly typically have greater difficulty obtaining their desires than do younger adults. Both their desires and the difficulties that must be overcome to obtain them should be considered in planning the nursing care of elderly people. The primary objective in caring for the elderly person is to help him make the adjustments necessary to make life worth living. Each patient has different limitations and frustrations, and each will react to them differently. In general the elderly person will react essentially as he has reacted to other stresses throughout his life.

The elderly person who is ill. Most diseases from which the aged suffer are chronic, and most patients have several chronic ailments. Some of these ailments are not particularly troublesome. Most have developed slowly and usually take time to alleviate. Heart disease, cancer, renal disease, vascular disease such as cerebrovascular accident, chronic obstructive pulmonary disease such as emphysema, and accidents are the most common problems that bring older patients to the hospital. Other chronic ailments such as arthritis, skin disorders, and mild neuromuscular conditions are very common but are usually cared for while the patient is ambulatory. The most prevalent acute illnesses of later life are acute respiratory conditions such as pneumonia and pulmonary edema.

When the elderly person becomes ill, he is particularly apprehensive and worried, probably because his security is more profoundly affected by illness than that of younger persons. He often fears helplessness and physical dependence on others. The elderly patient may face many adjustments that make it difficult and sometimes impossible for his basic emotional needs to be met. In addition to illness and the depleted physical energy almost always accompanying it, he may have no family and few friends, or his spouse may be ill also. He often has an inadequate income and housing problems. Even before his illness, he may have been depressed because of feeling unwanted and useless.

Illness may break down psychologic defenses that have been built up over a lifetime. The aged individual may be overwhelmed with fear of increased dependency needs or other problems to which he may react with extreme irritability. If his self-esteem is low due to years of suffering from economic and/or emotional deprivation, he may use his illness aggressively as a means of revolt. A trivial and purely incidental event may precipitate irritability. Other individuals, even those who had been quite active, may develop excessive lethargy with the onset of illness and may seem to give up all hope and desire to live.

Similarities between childhood and old age should not be assumed, because they are not valid. Even in the matter of helplessness there is no similarity. The child is in ascendance; he is developing new power daily and marking up achievements over his environment. The aged person's helplessness is infinitely more frustrating because it is increasing rather than decreasing.

Providing for the elderly patient's nursing needs. The goal of geriatric medical and nursing care is to keep the patient functioning at the highest possible level for his age. This includes living with chronic ailments and continuing degenerative changes. The nurse who views aging as a normal, inevitable process, one requiring adjustments in living patterns but not a withdrawal from life, is best prepared to work with the aging patient. The nurse's philosophy of aging should be one of ever-changing life that eventually will end in death, not one of approaching death.

Necessary nursing care depends on the physiologic and anatomic changes that have taken place, the disease from which the patient is suffering, and his own emotional makeup and apparent adjustment to his particular situation. In planning nursing care for elderly patients, the nurse should consider each patient's physical, social, economic, and psychologic capacities and limitations. The older patient frequently talks at length about his family and the past to the nurse who is willing to listen. This is his way of remembering the past good times when he may have been happier. His conversation may give clues of interests that should be encouraged and of problems that are confronting him. The nurse should evaluate these clues and make plans to help the patient maintain as much independence as possible despite his limitations. Sometimes plans must first focus on ways of encouraging the elderly patient to regain an interest in living.

When giving nursing care to elderly patients, it is necessary to take special care *to build up and protect their sense of worth and their feelings of adequacy.* Remembering the names of patients and calling them by name instead of using such terms as "grandma" or "grandpa" helps. Giving clear and slow explanations to the patient may spare him the embarrassment of mistakes caused by misunderstanding. Since many elderly patients are deaf, special care must be taken to be sure the patient has heard the explanation. The best method to use to ensure that he hears and understands should be recorded on his nursing care plan. The nurse should always face an elderly patient when speaking and speak distinctly so that he can lip-read inconspicuously if necessary. If hearing is better in one ear than the other, the nurse should talk into the good ear. It usually does no good to shout in an attempt to help the elderly person to hear, since with shouting the voice frequency increases and the elderly have the greatest difficulty hearing sounds in the higher frequency range. If the patient uses a hearing aid, the nurse should be sure that it is working properly. Written instructions are helpful for some elderly patients. The nurse should also be thoughtful about repeating instructions because the short-term memory span decreases with age.

Placing equipment conveniently so that assistance need not be requested also makes the elderly patient feel more adequate. Self-help devices may help him maintain some degree of independence. For example, an overbed trapeze or side rails on the bed may allow him to pull himself about in bed. Handrails along hallways and in the bathroom or a walkerette may make it possible for him to walk alone. Sturdy chairs with arms and wooden seats make it easier for many elderly patients to get into and out of chairs themselves. Hi-Lo beds also allow them to be more independent. If the patient uses a cane, glasses, hearing aid, or dentures, these devices should be readily available. Showers or bathtubs equipped with handrails and with nonskid strips may make it possible for some patients to bathe independently.

Many adjustments can be made to help the patient who is confined to a wheelchair retain some measure of independence. If the patient is able to transfer himself to the toilet, having a bathroom fixed in such a way that this maneuver is possible may be desirable. Some patients, especially if they have urinary frequency or incontinence, appreciate their wheelchair or chair being fixed as a commode (p. 184). Removal of door sills may make it possible for an elderly patient confined to a wheelchair to move about the house. Elderly patients are often unable to propel their chair manually. They may, however, be able to use a motorized wheelchair.

Elderly patients often need help with personal

care such as arranging the hair, applying cosmetics, shaving, and dressing. This help, if necessary, should be given regularly, and special care should be taken to assure that it is given before the patient goes about his daily activities. Personal appearance is important to everyone's morale.

Many elderly patients can give most or all necessary *physical care* to themselves. Some may need encouragement to do so; others resent not being allowed to care for themselves. The nurse or the family member caring for them, however, must be patient and give them adequate time. The older patient often is exceptionally slow in the morning and, in fact, geriatricians instruct their patients to take twice the usual time to shave, to dress slowly, and to avoid hurry of any kind, particularly in the morning hours. Since the elderly patient may tire easily, the nurse should be sure that he is physically able to give his own care.

If the patient is in a general hospital, a slow pace is often hard to assume. For example, many diagnostic procedures must be carried out in the morning, and breakfast must usually be served with that of other patients. However, many hospital routines can be adjusted for the elderly patient. For instance, he may prefer to bathe and shave in the afternoon or early evening. He then will only need minimal personal care during the morning hours and will feel less rushed. The nursing care plan for physical care of each elderly patient should include what self-care he gives, what assistance he needs, the method used, and the schedule the patient follows. Most elderly patients find comfort in familiar things and processes. It is therefore important to maintain routine as much as possible. The elderly are not unable to make changes, but require more time to adjust to new routines. The patient should participate in planning his schedule, and whenever possible it should parallel his pattern of care at home.

Since *physical change* occurs in the aging process, elderly people, especially the "old old," need to use somewhat different hygienic practices than an adult uses to maintain an optimum physical condition. The *skin* of an elderly person is usually thin, delicate, and sensitive to pressure and trauma. The loss of subcutaneous fat and the hardening of the tiny arterioles near the surface cause the skin to be wrinkled, sagging, and sallow. Sweat glands atrophy and the excretory function of the skin is lessened, making the skin dry and flaky and sometimes causing it to itch. Color changes occur in the skin with aging, and seborrheic keratoses, which are lesions resembling darkened, greasy warts, are common (Fig. 28-1). These lesions are nonmalignant but should be inspected frequently for signs of any irritation or change.

Because the skin is likely to be very dry, daily bathing is often contraindicated for the elderly. Usually one or two baths a week are sufficient, although the patient who is incontinent needs local sponging at frequent intervals and perhaps more frequent baths. Because regular soaps can be irritating, mild superfatted soaps are preferred. Bath oils may be used, or lanolin or body lotions can be applied after bathing.

If the patient is confined to bed, an alternating pressure mattress, flotation pad, or flotation mattress may be extremely helpful in maintaining the skin in good condition. Above all, the patient's position should be changed frequently, and bony prominences and weight-bearing areas should be massaged at least every 2 hours. Sheepskin pads placed under bony prominences are also used to relieve pressure and to prevent irritation of the skin. Every effort should be made to get the elderly out of bed as much as possible. This not only helps to redistribute pressure over the body and improve circulation but can also give patients a psychologic boost.

Because of dryness, poor circulation, and low resistance to infection, the skin of elderly persons readily becomes infected. Special care should be taken to prevent fungous infections such as epidermophytosis (athlete's foot) (p. 780). Elderly persons often need assistance in drying their feet after bathing and in cutting and caring for their toenails. Nails are often hard and scaly; soaking the feet in warm water or applying oil to the nails for a day or two prior to cutting softens them and makes cutting easier and safer. A podiatrist should be asked to care for very hard nails and other conditions such as calluses, corns, and bunions.

As the tissues age and circulation becomes sluggish, the *hair* becomes thin, dry, and colorless. Massage of the scalp and daily brushing with a soft-bristled brush help to preserve its beauty. Lanolin cream in small amounts may be used for massage, and oil treatments may be given before shampoos. Frequent shampooing should be avoided. Every 2 to 4 weeks is sufficient for most aged patients, although some people who have washed their hair more frequently throughout their lives may wish to continue to do so. A mild soap dissolved in water or a shampoo with a nonalcoholic base should be used. The older person should not experiment with new shampoos because many preparations contain alcohol and other agents that may have a drying effect.

The distribution and quality of hair change with age. Hair in the axillary and pubic areas becomes finer and scanty, whereas that of the eyebrows becomes coarse and bristly. To many women, hair on the face is a most annoying feature of growing old. If the patient is ill for a long time and is unable to care for herself, the nurse may have to assist in the removal of superfluous hair on the face. Shaving or using a pumice stone, followed by the application of cream to prevent drying, usually suffices. Plucking stray hairs from the face is often necessary. Hairs should not be plucked from moles but may be snipped close to the surface of the skin with small scissors. Stray hairs on the face may be made less conspicuous by bleaching them daily with a weak solution of hydrogen peroxide and ammonia if this can be done without irritating the skin.

Changes occur in the *eyes* with aging. There is a decrease in the conjunctival secretions, and sometimes the lower lid droops (ectropion), causing the moistening fluid of the eye to be lost. Therefore irritation of the conjunctivae and tearing are common complaints of the aged. Smoke also may be more irritating to their eyes than to those of younger persons. Eyedrops are frequently ordered as a comfort measure.

An accumulation of secretions at the inner canthus of the eye may be present, particularly on awakening, and may be uncomfortable and unsightly. A sterile cotton sponge moistened with a physiologic solution of sodium chloride can be used to cleanse the eyes. Care must be taken not to press on the eyeballs or to irritate any exposed conjunctiva.

The lens of the eye loses its ability to accommodate effectively as aging progresses. Most people over 60 years of age need glasses, at least for reading. Care of glasses, making certain that they are not lost or broken, is important in the nursing care of the elderly. It is advisable to label glasses with the patient's name. They should also be kept clean. Smudged glasses rather than failing vision may be the cause of difficulty in seeing. The patient should have his glasses available at all times, since confusion and inability to deal with situations in an adequate fashion may result if they become misplaced.

The eyes of older people also accommodate more slowly to changes in light. Bright lights or sunlight may be almost unbearable to some elderly people, and they will want the window shades pulled and the room lights dim. The nurse should arrange lights so that there is adequate illumination without glare. Many elderly persons see very poorly in the dark. Therefore night-lights should always be used to reduce confusion in patients and to prevent those who get up during the night from having accidents.

Cataracts, failing vision, and actual blindness are common in the aged. (See p. 843 for care of the patient with visual impairment.)

The elderly person should be urged to give special attention to the care of his *mouth* and *teeth*. Free hydrochloric acid in the stomach may be decreased, predisposing the elderly to poor oral health as well as to impaired digestion. The gums become less elastic and less vascular. They may recede from the remaining teeth, exposing areas of a tooth not covered with enamel. These areas are sensitive to injury from brushes and coarse dentifrices. In addition, diseases of the gum that may have been progressing symptom free for years may cause loss of teeth. Many elderly persons have decayed, broken, or missing teeth. This leads them to avoid foods that are difficult to eat but that may be necessary for health. The effect of oral health on nutrition is very real; definite improvement in appetite has followed correction of unhealthy conditions in the mouth.

A recent study has demonstrated that almost 80% of the population over 65 years of age have oral lesions of which they are unaware. Some of these lesions are potentially malignant.[6] Moreover, approximately 80% of all women and 70% of all men have lost their teeth by the time they are 70 years of age and therefore require dentures. Consequently, care of dentures and prevention of their loss are part of the general nursing care of most elderly patients. Patients may be encouraged by their dentists to keep dentures in place while they sleep as well as when they are awake, since this helps to preserve the normal contours of the face. Dentures should be cleansed following each meal. Because dental plates may be conductors of heat, and since the mouths of aged patients are often not too sensitive to excessive heat, they should be urged not to consume very hot food or fluids. Care should be taken that dentures are not lost, as they are costly. Dentures can also be easily mixed up, especially if the patient removes them frequently and then forgets where he puts them. Dentures should be marked, and there is equipment now available to do this.

The feet and legs usually show the results of limitation in peripheral circulation before any other body part. Therefore it is important for the aging person to *exercise the feet and legs regularly,* to avoid constriction or stasis of the circulation to their lower extremities, and to avoid injury and infections of their feet and legs. Precautions similar to those described for the patient who has peripheral vascular disease (p. 374) should be taken by all elderly people.

As the muscles become less active in age, slumped posture may result. The abdomen may sag, the spine becomes rounded, and the chest and shoulders droop forward. Lessened elasticity of tissue tends to make these changes fixed. Attention to preventive posture is therefore essential. Although corrective postural exercises and general exercise must be prescribed carefully by a physician, teaching good posture and encouraging deep breathing are part of the daily nursing care of all elderly patients. Any improvement in posture will enable the elderly person to use his diminishing resources to better advantage. Good body alignment adds to the comfort of the patient confined to bed as well as decreasing the need for corrective exercises later. A firm mattress is usually preferable and helps to make the use of pillows more effective. If greater stability is needed, a fracture board can be placed under the mattress. Bedcovers should be light and warm and should be tucked loosely, giving sufficient room for the patient to move about in bed. A block or board placed at the foot of the bed helps to keep covers off the toes and provides something firm against which the patient may press his feet and thereby get some exercise. A pillow placed lengthwise under the head and shoulders helps to bring the chest forward, thereby permitting good chest expansion. Pillows placed under the arms support the muscles of the shoulder girdle and provide comfort for the patient who must have the head of the bed raised for long periods of time.

Unless there is some particular contraindication, exercises for the arms and legs, exercises to keep abdominal and gluteal muscles in good tone, and exercises to strengthen the extensor muscles of the spine should be performed several times each day by every bed patient. The patient is taught to flex, abduct, adduct, and extend each leg separately and both legs simultaneously. The heel of one foot can be placed on the knee of the opposite leg and then the heel passed slowly down the leg to the ankle. This can then be repeated, alternating the legs. Arm, hand, neck, and shoulder movements can be encouraged by having the patient first raise and lower his head, neck, and shoulders from a flat supine position without a pillow and then by having the patient extend his arms in front of his chest, followed by raising them above his head. Each of these exercises should be done, if possible and if not contraindicated, in time to regular, deep respiration to encourage deep breathing while bedfast.[29] These exercises should be taught to the patient by the nurse, and they should be supervised daily by the nurse or the family member caring for the patient. The regular performance of exercises will help to prevent the loss of muscle tone that occurs in all bed patients, regardless of age, unless activity is continued. If the elderly person is unable to do active range of motion exercises independently, the nurse should assist with them or do passive range of motion exercises.

The elderly person should wear the *clothing* that is comfortable for him. He often feels cold and may wear woolen clothing even when it seems very warm to others. The hospitalized patient often wishes to wear socks, woolen underwear, a bed jacket, a cap, or other items of clothing to which he is accustomed. Some provision must be made for the care of this clothing. Sometimes members of the family are glad to care for special clothing that the patient needs.

Elderly women often appreciate assistance with altering their clothes. They may be unable to afford new ones, but they are often interested in remaining stylish. Wearing a well-fitted brassiere and corset not only improves the elderly woman's appearance, but the support given to sagging tissues may make her more comfortable.

The elderly person should be encouraged to wear firm, well-fitted shoes with good support to prevent damage to the arches of the feet since the muscles are often weak. Hospitalized patients should have their shoes and should wear them when they are up. If an elderly person wears slippers, they should also fit well and be firm, since the person is less likely to slip or stumble and fall.

Fresh air is especially necessary for the elderly person because, with his diminished chest expansion, poorly oxygenated air may not provide him with a sufficient blood level of oxygen. The aged, however, may be susceptible to drafts not even noticed by younger persons; consequently, they may dislike open windows.

Protective adipose tissue under the skin disappears with age, and the volume of circulating blood, particularly to the small outer arteries, may be diminished, thus affecting the ability to withstand chilling without discomfort. Decreased activity also lessens circulatory function, resulting in lowering of skin temperature and susceptibility to chilling. Many elderly people suffer from mild arthritis and fibrositis, which produce vague muscle and joint pains, and these conditions are aggravated by chilling. Measures to provide fresh air but to avoid drafts and chilling are essential. Sometimes windows can be opened wide in adjoining rooms, or perhaps a screen can be placed in front of an open window to prevent drafts and extra covers given to the patient to keep him warm.

Rest is essential for the aged. However, confusion, decubitus ulcers, lung congestion, and general deterioration may result from prolonged bed rest. Circulation to the brain as well as to the body in general is markedly slowed during long periods of inactivity, and therefore rest should be alternated with activity. It is undesirable for an elderly patient to be confined to bed, and even acutely ill elderly people are often gotten up in a chair for most of the day. They may even be encouraged to walk. When the patient is being cared for by his family, the nurse should try to impress on them the great importance of keeping the patient active, since they may be oversolicitous of the patient or it may seem to require too much effort to get him in and out of bed.

Elderly people usually *sleep* lightly and intermittently with frequent waking. At home the aged person may get out of bed, read, wander about the house, and even prepare something to eat at odd hours. Actually this activity is probably good, since it prevents excessive slowing of circulation. Some wakefulness, therefore, can be expected in the elderly patient who is hospitalized. If the patient is allowed out of bed, it probably is best for him to get up as he would at home. However, a low bed, nightlights, and adequate supervision should be employed to avoid accidents, and the nurse should be sure that the patient is not constantly wakeful. Elderly patients, similar to all others, may be unable to sleep.

They are rarely given sedation, however, since many become excited rather than sedated by it.

The time-tested aids such as a warm drink, a back massage, and quiet surroundings may help to get the night of sleep off to a good start. Interesting activities to keep patients awake during the day may result in better sleep at night. Most important, however, are the patient's peace of mind and feeling of well-being, which may be achieved by giving individual attention to the elderly patient, making him feel at home and secure. A kind word and a wish for a good night of sleep or an unobtrusive inquiry into some mentioned fear or uncertainty for which reassurance can be given may alleviate worries and will do much to help the patient sleep (Fig. 2-9).

Noise should be avoided during the hours of sleep because it is particularly disturbing to the elderly ill person, especially if he has a hearing loss. Partial deafness may set the person "on edge" and alert him to catch every sound. Even those persons with inability to hear conversation may be disturbed by the sound of a distant radio, shrill voices, or rattling equipment.

Many elderly people are undernourished, and for this reason a great deal of emphasis is placed on *nutrition* for the aged. Other than acute and chronic illness, possible causes of malnutrition in the elderly are limited financial resources, psychologic factors such as boredom and lack of companionship when eating, edentia, lifelong faulty eating patterns, fads and notions regarding certain foods, lack of energy to prepare foods, and lack of sufficient knowledge of the essentials of a well-balanced diet. Many elderly persons, particularly those living alone, subsist on a diet high in carbohydrates and low in vitamins, minerals, and protein. Often they think that because they are elderly they do not need much food. A diet composed largely of tea and toast may seem sufficient to them.

The nurse should instruct the patient and those responsible for his care in the essentials of a well-balanced diet (Chapter 6). Dietary patterns should not be changed too quickly, and it is useless to attempt to change many established food patterns. Simply prepared and easily digested foods are best, and meals should be distributed throughout the day. Usually elderly persons do not tolerate fried food. Large amounts of roughage should be avoided, but bulk is necessary. Fluid intake is important, yet many do not drink much water. Tea, coffee, and other beverages are usually preferred. Drinks prepared with dry skim milk supply essential protein and are useful in helping to meet the protein and calcium needs of older patients without supplying too many calories.

Some elderly persons are obese even though they may be undernourished. Excess weight burdens the heart, liver, kidneys, and musculoskeletal system and should be avoided. Weight reduction for the aged person, however, should be gradual and must be supervised by a physician. Sudden loss of weight is poorly tolerated by many elderly persons whose vascular system has become adjusted to the excess weight. Sudden weight reduction may lead to serious consequences, including confusion associated with lowered blood pressure, exhaustion, and vasomotor collapse.

Elderly patients may worry about their *bowel function.* They tend to forget that less food and less activity will result in reduced bowel function. Any marked change in bowel habits, however, and any unusual reactions to normal doses of laxatives should be reported, since malignancies of the large bowel and diverticulitis are fairly common among this age group.

Regularity in going to the toilet is important, since it provides stimulus to evacuate the bowel. Motor activity of the intestinal musculature may be decreased with age, and supportive structures in the intestinal walls become weakened. Sense perception is less acute, so that the signal for bowel elimination may be missed. Constipation may occur and in turn lead to impactions. The very elderly and somewhat confused patient should be reminded to go to the bathroom following meals.

Daily attention must be given to elimination, and sometimes small enemas may be needed every 2 or 3 days. Many physicians now order laxative rectal suppositories such as bisacodyl (Dulcolax). Small daily doses of a mild laxative may be ordered. The mild bulk laxatives such as psyllium seed and agar-agar combined with mineral oil are usually preferred to the saline cathartics, which may cause dehydra-

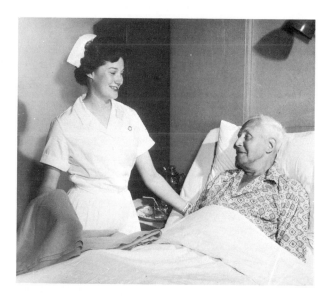

FIG. 2-9. A few minutes of special attention at bedtime often make it easier for the patient to relax and fall asleep.

tion. If the patient is constipated, it may be necessary occasionally to carefully insert a gloved finger into the rectum to be certain impaction has not occurred.

Frequency of *micturition* is common in old age and becomes a problem during illness. The ability of the kidneys to concentrate urine during sleeping hours usually decreases slowly with age. In addition, decreased muscle tone in the bladder with resultant impairment of emptying capacity may result in residual urine in the bladder and subsequent infection. It may be necessary to catheterize the patient to check for residual urine. One of the first signs of diminishing or failing kidney function is frequency of micturition during the night. Frequency and slight burning on urination are symptoms of bladder infection.

Elderly women have relaxation of perineal structures, which may also interfere with complete emptying of the bladder and predispose to bladder infection. Some elderly patients have decreased sensation and do not realize when the bladder must be emptied. Periodic dribbling of urine suggests that the bladder is not being emptied completely. The nurse should observe the very elderly patient for distention of the bladder and consult the physician about it.

Unless there is a definite contraindication to high fluid intake, the elderly patient should be urged to take sufficient fluids to dilute urine and decrease its irritating properties. Fluids may be limited in the evening if nocturia is troublesome and is interfering with sleep. If the patient is quite feeble, it is well to offer a urinal or bedpan during the night.

Involutional changes in the lining of the vagina lead to lessened resistance to invasion of organisms. Mild infections with troublesome discharge are not unusual in elderly women. This condition should be reported to the physician, who may order specific therapy for it. Frequent local bathing may be helpful in allaying itching. Application of cornstarch also relieves itching. Embarrassment may prevent the elderly patient from reporting symptoms. The nurse should be aware of the symptoms of this condition and watch for them.

Almost all elderly men have hypertrophy of the prostate, which makes urination difficult. The nurse must report, or must urge the patient to report, such complaints to his physician because specific treatment is often necessary and can be safely administered even when the patient is far advanced in years.

Incontinence of urine and/or feces has been found to be over three times more prevalent among the hospitalized or institutionalized aged, but about 10% of the aged being cared for at home also have this problem. It is twice as common among women as men.[53] It is a particularly upsetting problem not only to the patient and his family but also to the nursing staff. Every effort should be made to insti-

tute and maintain the patient on a bowel and bladder training regimen. Specific details about bladder and bowel training can be found in Chapter 9.

An important part of nursing care for the elderly is helping to meet their *emotional needs.* Elderly patients are often lonely, and individual attention should be given to them. They often appreciate just talking with others. If possible, the nurse should plan time to visit with them daily. Volunteers may also be used to visit the elderly. Some patients appreciate visits with a clergyman.

When visiting with elderly patients, one should remember that, although they commonly talk about events and activities in their own past, they usually are interested in the activities of young people and of the world about them (Fig. 2-10). These interests often must be satisfied for them through the eyes and ears of others. If the patient is unable to see well enough to read, he may enjoy being read to by others.

Provision should be made for the patient who requires long hospitalization to maintain his family contacts. A grandfather or grandmother often wishes to see a grandchild, and a visit should be arranged, if possible. Sometimes plans can be made for the patient to make a short visit outside the hospital. This is especially important if a wife or husband is physically unable to visit the patient. Arranging for telephone conversations with family members also is desirable.

If the elderly patient likes to read, reading materi-

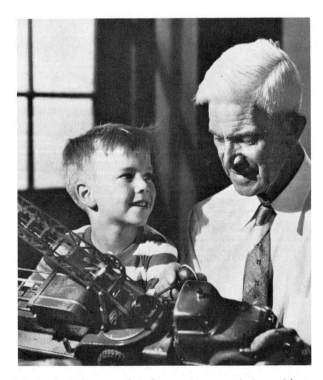

FIG. 2-10. Older people often enjoy association with youngsters. (© 1958, Parke, Davis & Co.)

als should be provided. If he is unable to see to read, talking books, available through public libraries, may be appreciated. It is also possible to get books and magazines with large print for persons with reduced vision. Television and radio also provide desirable diversion.

Elderly people often are interested in doing useful tasks. There are many tasks in which even the elderly person who is ill may be able to participate. Women may enjoy mending or knitting. If they are at home, they may be able to help with dishes or meal preparation. Men may be interested in repairing toys or making useful gadgets for the house. Many elderly persons enjoy painting. The older person may be quite slow in all his activities, and great care must be taken not to show impatience, which may discourage further participation.

Elderly patients are usually aware of death as an imminent possibility and sometimes see it as a welcome event. The nurse should not avoid this issue. If the nurse senses that the patient is genuinely concerned about death, he can be urged to discuss his feelings about it. He may also wish to see a clergyman, a family member, or the physician or perhaps to arrange to transact some unfinished business. The nurse must always be responsive to such requests, since they frequently are more important for the patient's peace of mind than his medical treatment. The feelings of the family of the elderly person must also be considered in dealing with the question of death. They may find it a very uncomfortable subject.

Special precautions related to diagnosis and treatment. Elderly persons usually tolerate *medications* poorly and may have bizarre reactions to them. This occurs for several reasons. Older persons experience a reduction in metabolic turnover so that a lower dosage of a drug produces the desired effect. A second factor to be considered with drug therapy in the elderly is the altered response of medication on the central nervous system. The decreased blood flow to the brain is a contributing factor to this response. Medication that produces sedation in younger adults may cause extreme confusion in the elderly. This is especially true of the barbiturates.

Many elderly persons maintain a delicate balance between normal and abnormal because of impairments of homeostatic mechanisms, especially if disability or impairment is already present. Drugs given may produce toxic effects that occur quickly and may have far-reaching manifestations. One of the most common of these manifestations is drug-induced hypotension, which can lead to ataxia, falls, and possible injuries. Another factor that affects medication therapy in the elderly is the decreased blood flow to the kidneys and liver. This leads to decreased function of both organs, and drugs are not detoxified and eliminated as quickly as in the healthy adult. Toxic concentrations of drugs may occur because of the cumulative effects. One drug that does this easily is digitalis. With any elderly person who is maintained on a medication for a prolonged length of time, frequent checks of blood levels should be made. Another factor is that the delayed effects of drugs may be observed in the elderly weeks or even months after the drug has been discontinued.

Drug treatment in the elderly has its definite place in the therapeutic regimen, but it must be handled carefully. One general principle in treatment of the elderly with medication is that the drug level should be built up gradually. Small doses should be given at first and then increased slowly until the desired effect is observed. The minimal number of medications possible should be given. It is not uncommon to find the elderly taking medication to counteract untoward effects of other medication.[48]

The nurse should carefully check for untoward reactions from medications and report them to the physician. Narcotics and sedatives are tolerated especially poorly, and small doses usually are prescribed. If the patient is emaciated or of very advanced years, the use of full adult doses of drugs should be questioned.

Many elderly patients must administer medicines to themselves. The nurse should carefully determine their ability to do so and should report to the physician if the practice does not seem to be safe, so that other plans can be made. In planning self-administration of drugs with the elderly, it is frequently helpful to determine the easiest time for him to remember to take medication. This time is usually tied in with some incident of daily living such as arising or taking meals. The use of a medication check sheet is helpful in reminding some patients. Plans may also include placement of the medication so that seeing it will be a reminder. Special care needs to be taken, however, to put it where it will not accidentally be taken in place of another drug or where other family members such as small children may take it. Some elderly persons have found it helpful to use something such as an egg carton with the days marked. One dose is put into each hole and it is easy to know if the medication has been taken.

The elderly person should understand the medications they are taking. They should be cautioned against taking extra doses of the medication because some believe that if one tablet or pill helps, two will really be better.

Elderly patients who are undergoing *diagnostic tests* requiring withholding of meals or the use of enemas or cathartics should be attended unless they are in their beds because they often become quite weak and dizzy. The nurse should encourage the physician to prescribe milder laxatives and cathartics than he would in the younger adult. No elderly patient should ever be left unattended on a treatment table, and he should be helped on and off the table. Since he often is quite dizzy, it is advisable for him to arise slowly and sit on the edge of the table for a few moments before standing. The dizziness is caused by the slow compensation of inelastic blood vessels. Older patients with cardiovascular disease may also be orthopneic and cannot tolerate lying flat for examinations.

Because of the rapidity with which they develop pressure ulcers, elderly patients who must lie on x-ray, treatment, or operating room tables for lengthy periods of time need pads placed under the normal curves of their backs and a pad of material such as sponge rubber placed under bony prominences. Skin

over bony prominences should be rubbed occasionally to improve the circulation to the area. On return to the unit the patient's skin should always be checked for pressure areas, and if any signs of pressure are evident, these areas should be massaged frequently until the tissue appears normal in color. If possible, the patient should be kept off these areas until signs of pressure disappear. If the patient is placed in lithotomy position, care must be taken to place both legs in the stirrups at the same time to prevent undue pull on unresilient muscles. The same principle applies when removing the legs from the stirrups. Care must also be taken to prevent hyperextension and hyperflexion of the joints since many elderly patients have arthritis.

REFERENCES AND SELECTED READINGS*

1 *Ambler, M. C.: Disciplining hospitalized toddlers, Am. J. Nurs. 67:572-573, March 1967.

2 Amend, E. L.: A parent education program in a children's hospital, Nurs. Outlook 14:53-56, April 1966.

3 Anderson, H. C.: Newton's geriatric nursing, ed. 5, St. Louis, 1971, The C. V. Mosby Co.

4 *Austin, C. L.: The basic six needs of the aging, Nurs. Outlook 7:138-141, March 1959.

5 *Bailey, T. F.: Puppets teach young patients, Nurs. Outlook 15:36-37, Aug. 1967.

6 Bhaskar, S.: Oral lesions of the aged population, Geriatrics 23:137-149, Oct. 1968.

7 Birren, J. E.: The psychology of aging, Englewood Cliffs, N. J., 1964, Prentiss-Hall, Inc.

8 *Blaesing, S., and Brockhaus, J.: The development of body image in the child, Nurs. Clin. North Am. 7:597-608, Dec. 1972.

9 *Blake, F. G., Wright, F. H., and Waechter, E. H.: Nursing care of children, ed. 8, Philadelphia, 1970, J. B. Lippincott Co.

10 *Brooks, M. M.: Why play in the hospital? Nurs. Clin. North Am. 5:431-441, Sept. 1970.

11 *Bruce, S. J.: What mothers of 6- to 10-year olds want to know, Nurs. Outlook 12:40-43, Sept. 1964.

12 Busse, E.: Behavior and adaption in late life, Boston, 1969, Little, Brown & Co.

13 *Byers, M. L.: The hospitalized adolescent, Nurs. Outlook 15:32-34, Aug. 1967.

14 Caring for the aged—an AJN feature, Am. J. Nurs. 73:2049-2066, Dec. 1973.

15 *Davis, R. W.: Psychologic aspects of geriatric nursing, Am. J. Nurs. 68:802-804, April 1968.

16 *Deakers, L. P.: Continuity of family-centered nursing care between the hospital and the home, Nurs. Clin. North Am. 7:83-93, March 1972.

17 *Dempsey, M. O.: The development of body image in the adolescent, Nurs. Clin. North Am. 7:609-616, Dec. 1972.

18 *Duran, M. T.: Family-centered care and the adolescent's quest for self-identity, Nurs. Clin. North Am. 7:65-74, March 1972.

19 *Eyres, P. J.: The role of the nurse in family-centered nursing care, Nurs. Clin. North Am. 7:27-40, March 1972.

20 *Fujita, M. T.: The impact of illness or surgery on the body image of the child, Nurs. Clin. North Am. 7:641-650, Dec. 1972.

21 *Gimpel, H. S.: Group work with adolescent girls, Nurs. Outlook 16:46-48, April 1968.

22 *Goda, S.: Speech development in children, Am. J. Nurs. 70:276-278, Feb. 1970.

23 *Goldfarb, A. I.: Responsibilities to our aged, Am. J. Nurs. 64:78-82, Nov. 1964.

24 Hammar, S. L., and Eddy, J. A. K.: Nursing care of the adolescent, New York, 1966, Springer Publishing Co., Inc.

25 *Havighurst, R. J.: Developmental tasks in education, ed. 2, New York, 1952, David McKay Co., Inc.

26 Havighurst, R. J., and others: Psychology of aging, Bethesda Conference, Public Health Rep. 70:837-856, Sept. 1955.

27 *Issner, N.: The family of the hospitalized child, Nurs. Clin. North Am. 7:5-12, March 1972.

28 *Jones, L., and Wakeley, C.: Tell me about your picture: insights into children's ideas about the hospital, Imprint 21:20-22, Feb. 1974.

29 Kelly, M.: Exercise for bedfast patients, Am. J. Nurs. 66:2209-2213, Oct. 1966.

30 *Kimball, C. P.: Psychosocial aspects of cardiac disease in children and adolescents, Heart & Lung 2:394-399, May-June 1973.

31 Kosa, J., Antonovesky, A., and Zola, I. K., editors: Poverty and health, Cambridge, 1969, Harvard University Press.

31a *Kunzman, L.: Some factors influencing a young child's mastery of hospitalization, Nurs. Clin. North Am. 7:13-26, March 1972.

32 *Lore, A.: Adolescents: people, not problems, Am. J. Nurs. 73:1232-1234, July 1973.

33 *Luciano, K. B.: Components of planned family-centered care, Nurs. Clin. North Am. 7:41-52, March 1972.

33a *Mann, S. A.: Coping with a child's fatal illness, Nurs. Clin. North Am. 9:81-87, March 1974.

34 Marlow, D. R., and Sellew, G.: Textbook of pediatric nursing, ed. 4, Philadelphia, 1973, W. B. Saunders Co.

35 *Mead, M.: Culture and commitment: a study of the generation gap, Garden City, New York, 1970, Doubleday & Co., Inc.

36 *Mead, M., and others: The right to die, Nurs. Outlook 16:20-28, Oct. 1968.

37 *Meyer, H. L.: Predictable problems of hospitalized adolescents, Am. J. Nurs. 69:525-528, March 1969.

37a *Meyer, V. R.: The psychology of the young adult, Nurs. Clin. North Am. 8:5-14, March 1973.

38 Nelson, W. E., editor: Textbook of pediatrics, ed. 9, Philadelphia, 1964, W. B. Saunders Co.

*References preceded by an asterisk are particularly well-suited for student reading.

39 Neugarten, B. L.: Middle age and aging, Chicago, 1968, University of Chicago Press.

39a *Northrup, F. C.: The dying child, Am. J. Nurs. **74:**1066-1068, June 1974.

40 *Olsen, E. V., and others: The hazards of immobility, Am. J. Nurs. **67:**779-794, April 1967.

41 *Patrick, M. L.: Care of the confused elderly patient, Am. J. Nurs. **67:**2536-2539, Dec. 1967.

42 *Penalver, M.: Helping the child handle his aggression, Am. J. Nurs. **73:**1554-1555, Sept. 1973.

43 *Perlman, H. H.: Persona (the adult), Chicago, 1968, University of Chicago Press.

44 *Petrillo, M.: Preventing hospital trauma in pediatric patients, Am. J. Nurs. **68:**1468-1473, July 1968.

45 *Pittman, R.: The man in the family, Nurs. Outlook **16:**62-64, April 1968.

46 *Redman, R. E.: Black child-white nurse: a nursing challenge and privilege. In Duffey, M., and others: Current concepts in clinical nursing, vol. 3, St. Louis, 1971, The C. V. Mosby Co.

47 *Riddle, I.: Nursing intervention to promote body image integrity in children, Nurs. Clin. North Am. **7:**651-662, Dec. 1972.

48 Rossman, I.: Clinical geriatrics, Philadelphia, 1971, J. B. Lippincott Co.

49 *Rubin, M.: The therapeutic use of separation during hospitalization: an alternative to pediatric rooming-in. In Duffey, M., and others: Current concepts in clinical nursing, vol. 3, St. Louis, 1971, The C. V. Mosby Co.

50 *Schwartz, D.: Problems of self-care and travel among elderly ambulatory patients, Am. J. Nurs. **66:**2678-2681, Dec. 1966.

51 Shock, N. W.: The physiology of aging, Sci. Am. **6:**100-110, Jan. 1962.

52 Statistical abstracts of the United States, 1973, 74th annual edition, Washington, D. C., 1973, U. S. Bureau of the Census.

53 Stosky, B. A.: The elderly patient, New York, 1968, Grune & Stratton, Inc.

54 *Tierney, T. M.: The continuing partnership, Nurs. Outlook **16:**22-24, Jan. 1968 (Medicare).

55 U. S. Department of Health, Education and Welfare: Working with older people, Public Health Service Publication no. 1459, vol. 1, Washington, D. C., March 1969 (revised), U. S. Government Printing Office.

56 U. S. Department of Health, Education and Welfare: Working with older people, Public Health Service Publication no. 1459, vol. 2, Washington, D. C., April 1970, U. S. Government Printing Office.

57 *Waechter, E. H.: Children's awareness of fatal illness, Am. J. Nurs. **71:**1168-1172, June 1971.

58 *Webb, C.: Tactics to reduce a child's fear of pain, Am. J. Nurs. **66:**2698-2701, Dec. 1966.

59 Williams, S. R.: Nutrition and diet therapy, ed. 2, St. Louis, 1973, The C. V. Mosby Co.

60 Wolff, K.: A new conceptualization of the geriatric patient, Geriatrics **23:**157-162, Aug. 1968.

61 *Wu, R.: Explaining treatments to young children, Am. J. Nurs. **65:**71-73, July 1965.

62 Wygant, W. E., Jr.: Dying, but not alone, Am. J. Nurs. **67:**574-577, March 1967.

3 Ecology and health

Homeostasis in the biosphere: the balance of nature
Imbalance—affluence and pollution
Perspectives for human health

■ HOMEOSTASIS IN THE BIOSPHERE: THE BALANCE OF NATURE

Thanks to the marvel of modern communications technology, millions of persons around the globe joined with the Apollo astronauts in gazing at a spectacular sight—the earth! Through this occurrence we have been given the opportunity to go far beyond an intellectual understanding of ecologists' descriptions of our finite planet; we have experienced it. We are becoming increasingly aware of the message in Adlai E. Stevenson's last speech, "We all travel together, passengers on a little spaceship, dependent on its vulnerable supplies of air and soil; all committed for our safety to its security and peace, preserved from annihilation only by the care, the work, and I will say the love we give our fragile craft."*

We must change from the "frontiersman" mentality, which has characterized the growth and progress of industrialized nations, to the "astronaut" outlook through which it will be possible to assure the continuation of life on our finite planet. The need is urgent and it challenges each of us to strive for as complete an understanding as possible of the complex interaction and interdependence within and among the various components of the biosphere.

*Speech before the Economic and Social Council, Geneva, Switzerland, July 9, 1965.

Composition of the biosphere

Environ systems. The biosphere is the thin "layer" of air, water, and soil on the planet Earth within which all living things exist. Fig. 3-1 establishes the components of the biosphere and suggests their interrelationships. John McHale, the eminent futurist, calls the material components of ecosystems "environ systems" to distinguish them from the "human systems," which we will survey later. Note that in each of the biosphere compartments there are both living and nonliving portions and that these interact in energy-dependent interrelationships to form a complex, interconnected web. Urbanization and industrialization place a severe strain on many of the natural cycles in the biosphere, as illustrated by contrasting a typical forest area with a city (Fig. 3-2). Note that in the forest, large amounts of oxygen are being produced as a result of photosynthesis. This maintains the normal ratios of the atmospheric gases. In the urban area, oxygen is consumed in much greater quantities than it is produced. Also, carbon dioxide and other materials are present in concentrations that often can be harmful. This example dramatically points up an important ecologic principle—the cyclic nature of almost all events in the biosphere.

A look at the water cycle (Fig. 3-3) illustrates not only this cycling activity but also the integral interrelatedness of the major biosphere compartments: hydrosphere, atmosphere, and lithosphere. Not only are water molecules being constantly cycled through the soil, air, and water, but many other substances are being transported with the water, thus constantly influencing the chemical composition of all three com-

■ STUDY QUESTIONS

1 Discuss the relationship between chemical wastes and disease. If you were a legislator, where would you begin to attack this problem?
2 Describe the difference between "intentional" and "incidental" food additives and give examples from your own experience.
3 What are the major pollution problems in the area in which you reside?
4 All of us have heard much in recent years about air, water, and soil pollution. Think about the possible interrelatedness of these forms of pollution. What implications might this have in pollution abatement efforts?
5 Explain your current concept of the relationships involving air pollution, smoking, and lung cancer. Do you think the "Smoking is hazardous to your health" warning on cigarette packs should be taken seriously?

partments. Water serves as one of the chief instruments both in the building of soil through weathering of rock and in its breakdown through erosion. We shall see later how even a slight imbalance in one of the compartments affects not only that compartment but the others also.

ATMOSPHERE

Airborne spores, pollen,
and dust
Air, water, radiant
energy, and gas cycles

LITHOSPHERE
(terrestrial)

Plant and animal
organic populations (including man)
Rock, mineral deposits,
and cycles

HYDROSPHERE
(oceans, rivers, lakes, etc.)

Plant and animal
organic populations
Water, mineral deposits,
and cycles

FIG. 3-1. Material components of the biosphere. (Modified from McHale, J.: World facts and trends, ed. 2, New York, 1972, Macmillan Publishing Co., Inc.)

Physical processes such as those involved in the water cycle can cause significant and often dramatic changes in the three biosphere compartments; consider the effects of such events as volcanic eruption, earthquake, and tornado. However, when weather conditions are relatively normal, the chief factors affecting the homeostatic or steady-state condition of any ecosystem are the activities of the living organisms that inhabit the area. All ecosystems—oceans, deserts, grasslands, forests, etc.—have a characteristic structure and organization: (1) a typical combination of abiotic factors such as soil or water composition, temperature, altitude, and humidity and (2) specific populations of living organisms, the variety and number being dependent to a large extent on the combination of abiotic factors characteristic of a given region.

Biotic factors and energy flow. The biotic components of any ecosystem in the biosphere—plants, animals (including man), and microbial organisms—exist in what is fundamentally an energy-dependent interrelationship. Radiant energy in the form of sunlight is the ultimate source of energy for all ecosystems. When sunlight enters the biosphere, it is used in the process of photosynthesis through which carbon dioxide and water are converted into energy-rich carbon compounds such as carbohydrates, proteins, and lipids. Green plants are the organisms that perform this function in each ecosystem; so they are called *producers* and are said to be *autotrophic* (self-feeding). They form the first link in the many and diversified "food chains" that characterize ecosystems. Almost all other organisms are said to be *heterotrophic* (other-feeding), since their nutritional needs are met by feeding on other organisms. There are two groups of heterotrophs, the *consumers* and the *decomposers*.

In the consumer group those that derive their nutrition directly from plants are called *herbivores* (primary consumers); those that obtain nourishment by

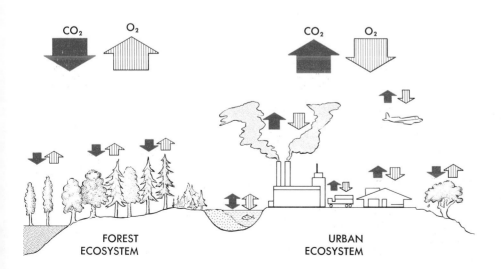

FIG. 3-2. Carbon oxygen cycle. Summary of events in a forest ecosystem and in an urban ecosystem. The atmosphere and bodies of water serve as reservoirs of carbon dioxide and oxygen. Carbon dioxide is produced by animal respiration, burning fuels, and dissolving carbonates and is used by plants in photosynthesis. It is consumed in the process of plant photosynthesis and the combustion of fuels.

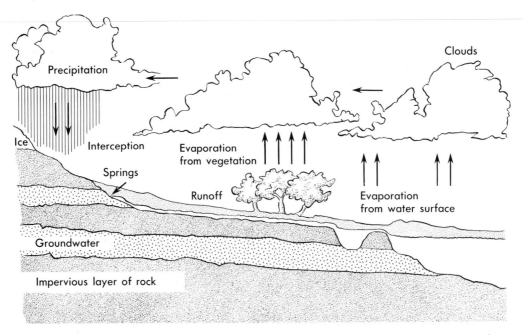

FIG. 3-3. Water cycle activity and its interrelatedness to major biosphere compartments. (Redrawn from Humphrey, C. C., and Evans, R. G.: What's ecology? Northbrook, Ill., 1971, Hubbard Press.)

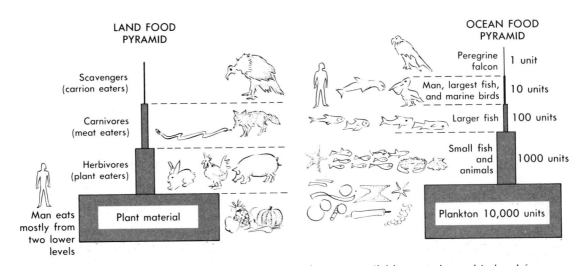

FIG. 3-4. Ecologic pyramids. Left: The relative amounts of matter available at each trophic level for conversion into energy. Right: The 90% reduction in available energy in ascending steps of a food pyramid. (Redrawn from Humphrey, C. C., and Evans, R. G.: What's ecology? Northbrook, Ill., 1971, Hubbard Press.)

consuming herbivores are called *carnivores* (secondary consumers); and in some food chains there may be one or two other levels of carnivores. In Fig. 3-4 these organism-energy interrelationships are illustrated clearly through use of what ecologists call a *pyramid,* in which the amounts of available energy (Fig. 3-4, *A*) or the number of organisms (Fig. 3-4, *B*) at each of the trophic levels are represented by blocks of decreasing width. It should be evident that the reason there are only a few types of food chains

with second- and third-level carnivores and that the number of these is very low is because of the enormous loss of available energy that occurs from one trophic level to the next.

Decomposers are the other type of heterotrophs and include chiefly bacteria and fungi. These organisms do not ingest food as do the consumers; rather, they produce and release enzymes into dead plant and animal material and then absorb some or all of the digested products. Aside from assuring their own survival, these organisms contribute an invaluable service to an ecosystem by releasing to the environment (soil or water) various minerals found in protoplasm, thereby making them available for reuse by producers. Thus in all ecosystems two processes are always proceeding simultaneously, the noncyclic flow of energy with much of it lost as heat and the cycling of nutrient elements such as carbon dioxide, water, and minerals. Thoughtful study of Fig. 3-5 should help in the realization not only of the complexity of the interrelationships in the "web of nature" but also of the fact that the slightest change at any point will necessarily produce some effect in the entire system. Keep this in mind later as we begin to investigate a few of the changes that man's technology makes on the energy flow and the materials' cycling of the biosphere.

Figs. 3-4 and 3-5 should also suggest the fact that a wide variety of factors can influence the number of organisms that can survive simultaneously at each trophic level. Any decrease in availability of energy to the producers (through the influence of clouds, smog, changes in temperature, etc.) will automatically influence the number of herbivores and in turn the carnivore population. Other great influences on the populations at each level are factors such as predation, parasitism, competition for nutrients, mates, and space, and other factors. Fig. 3-6 shows the effects of some of these factors on population growth. Fig. 3-6, *A*, shows a generalized growth curve. Fig. 3-6, *B*, shows typical S-shaped growth

curves and illustrates the difference in rate of growth as well as the final number within populations as influenced by an abiotic factor, temperature. The enormous influence of nutrient availability is shown in Fig. 3-6, *C*; if these curves were shown for a longer time, one would expect the "equilibrium" (lag phase) population of the typical S-shaped curve to become established (as in Fig. 3-6, *B*) due to lack of space and accumulation of toxic metabolic wastes. The combination of factors that exists during the "equilibrium" portion of the curve is called the *carrying capacity* of the particular system.

In animals with longer life cycles this equilibrium actually represents a series of seasonal fluctuations as seen in Fig. 3-7, *A*. If the carrying capacity deteriorates permanently, the equilibrium-level population will decrease as shown in Fig. 3-7, *B*; the implications of this figure for the subsequent brief study of pollution effects should be obvious. There are many other aspects of population dynamics that would better enable us to understand the interrelationships among living organisms, but they are beyond the scope of this brief survey. You may wish to consult some of the readings suggested at the end of this chapter to gain more information.

Human systems

Man, as we have just seen, is an integral part of the particular ecosystem in which he lives. However, it is vital to human survival that more and more of us recognize that man alone is in a position both to

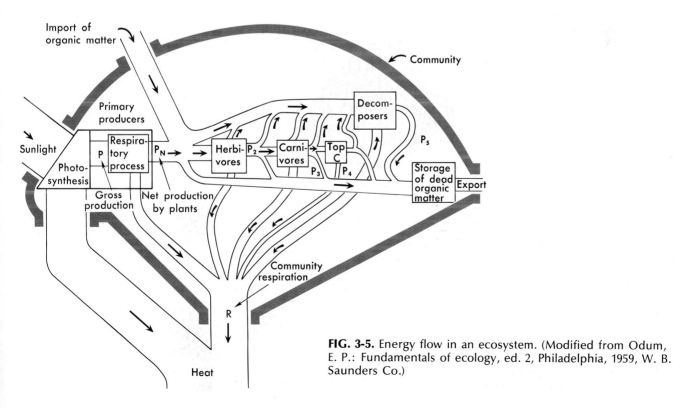

FIG. 3-5. Energy flow in an ecosystem. (Modified from Odum, E. P.: Fundamentals of ecology, ed. 2, Philadelphia, 1959, W. B. Saunders Co.)

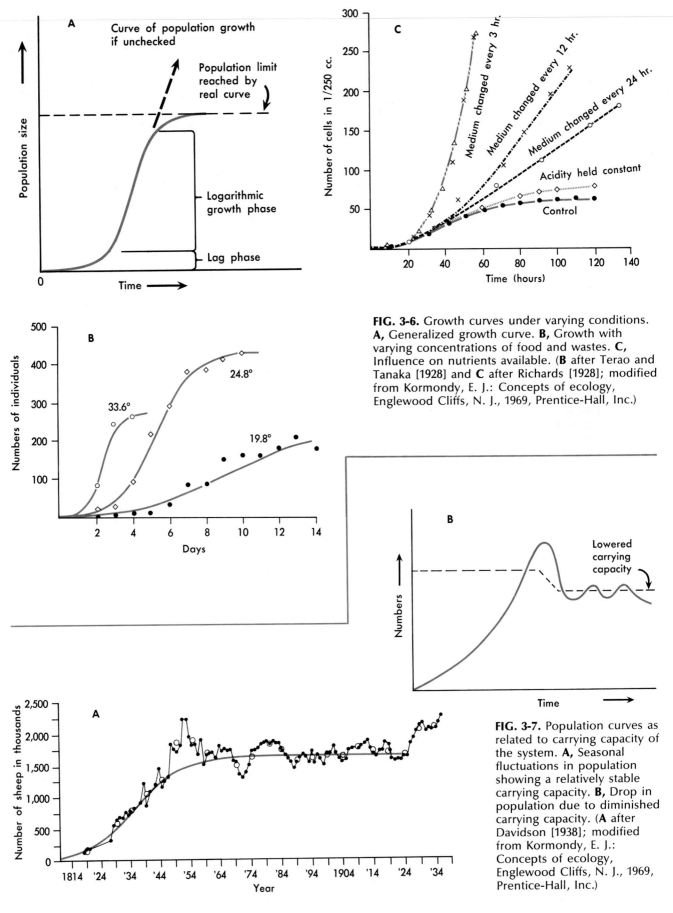

FIG. 3-6. Growth curves under varying conditions. **A,** Generalized growth curve. **B,** Growth with varying concentrations of food and wastes. **C,** Influence on nutrients available. (**B** after Terao and Tanaka [1928] and **C** after Richards [1928]; modified from Kormondy, E. J.: Concepts of ecology, Englewood Cliffs, N. J., 1969, Prentice-Hall, Inc.)

FIG. 3-7. Population curves as related to carrying capacity of the system. **A,** Seasonal fluctuations in population showing a relatively stable carrying capacity. **B,** Drop in population due to diminished carrying capacity. (**A** after Davidson [1938]; modified from Kormondy, E. J.: Concepts of ecology, Englewood Cliffs, N. J., 1969, Prentice-Hall, Inc.)

realize his role in the biosphere and to plan and control his influence on it. Fig. 3-8 shows a simple scheme that might be used as we proceed to look at the interrelationships between man and nature. A thoughtful look at each component of this "human ecology" cycle suggests the many ways in which man, especially in industrialized nations, will have to change his life-style in order to restore homeostasis in the biosphere.

In Fig. 3-9 we can see some of the various aspects of man's complexity and the interrelationships involved; these are aptly described as "internal and external human metabolism." Man's basic biophysical functions are similar to those of many other organisms in the ecosystems he inhabits. "Ecologically" considered, he is basically a heterotroph who can consume food from any and all levels of the food pyramid and can survive only within very narrow ranges of temperature, pressure, and other factors of the abiotic environment. But man is "human" and finds personal meaning largely in the psychosocial sphere, more by his sense of belonging to the larger human society and to a particular cultural heritage than by his understanding that he is an organism of a particular species within an ecologic population. Even when he attempts objectivity, man perceives

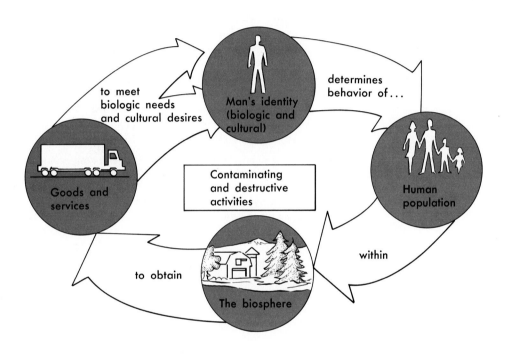

FIG. 3-8. A human ecology cycle. A simple scheme showing interrelationships between man and nature. (From Humphrey, C. C., and Evans, R. G.: What's ecology? Northbrook, Ill., 1971, Hubbard Press.)

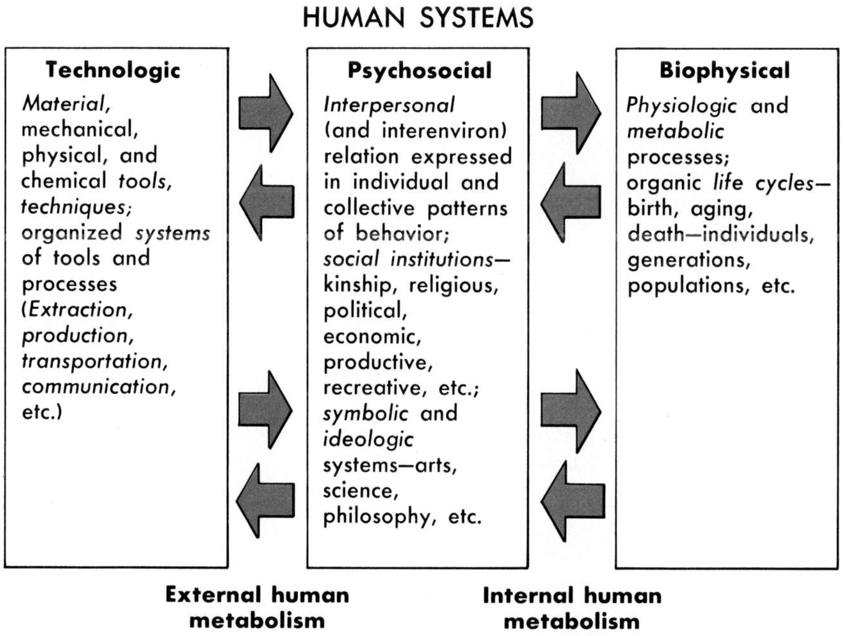

HUMAN SYSTEMS

Technologic	**Psychosocial**	**Biophysical**
Material, mechanical, physical, and chemical *tools, techniques;* organized *systems* of tools and processes (*Extraction, production, transportation, communication,* etc.)	*Interpersonal* (and *interenviron*) relation expressed in individual and collective patterns of behavior; *social institutions*—kinship, religious, political, economic, productive, recreative, etc.; *symbolic* and *ideologic* systems—arts, science, philosophy, etc.	*Physiologic* and *metabolic* processes; organic *life cycles*—birth, aging, death—individuals, generations, populations, etc.

External human metabolism   **Internal human metabolism**

FIG. 3-9. Unique interactions of the human populations in the biosphere. (Modified from McHale, J.: World facts and trends, ed. 2, New York, 1972, Macmillan Publishing Co., Inc.)

the environment from a uniquely human perspective; man's uniqueness is evidenced in the use of language to interpret and communicate the reality of what he experiences.

Through technology man has learned to transcend his physical limitations by controlling his environment so well that for brief periods he can live in considerable comfort even in outer space. Since the nineteenth century, medical advances have significantly lowered mortality rates in infants and in those

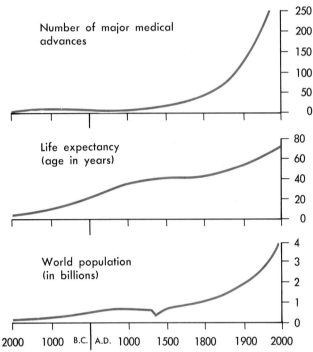

FIG. 3-10. Medical advances and effect on life expectancies and population. (Modified from McHale, J.: The future of the future, New York, 1969, George Braziller, Inc.)

with infectious diseases (Fig. 3-10). The result has been an unprecedented rise in the rate of human population growth during a very brief period.

Fig. 3-11 shows that it took hundreds of thousands of years for the human population to reach the current level of 3.6 billion; yet United Nations' projections, even at a "medium" rate, suggest that the global population will exceed 6 billion by the year 2000—a doubling in less than 40 years!

This is more clearly seen in Fig. 3-12, and this can alert us to an important implication—the projected growth will not be evenly distributed. Rather, the populations of the underdeveloped regions, with their much higher birth rates, will increase much more rapidly than those of the industrialized areas, where the birth rate has become more stabilized. As the underdeveloped nations make agricultural and medical advances, the total world population may grow for generations at a rate even greater than the present one before the establishment in these areas of industrialized societies in which lowered birth rates are characteristic.

A brief review of Fig. 3-7, *B,* should clearly point out the importance of understanding that the increasing deterioration of the Earth's carrying capacity by pollution, mining, deforestation, urbanization, etc., along with the current rate of population increase, cannot be tolerated if human life as we have known it is to continue. At present our prospect can be reasonably optimistic, but it will call for greater personal and social discipline. Technology and proper management of resources can eliminate many of the current insults to the environment, but this will require a commitment to the restoration and maintenance of environmental quality that can only result if major changes in personal values are accepted. These assume major adjustments in consumption patterns, income, and life-styles, especially

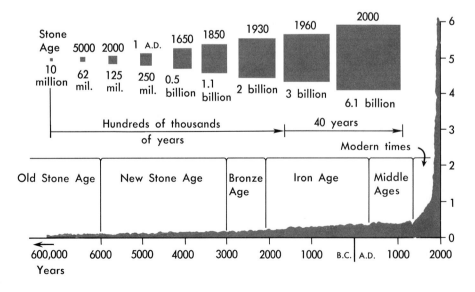

FIG. 3-11. The growth of human numbers. (Modified from Desmond, A.: Pop. Bull. **18:**5, Feb. 1962.)

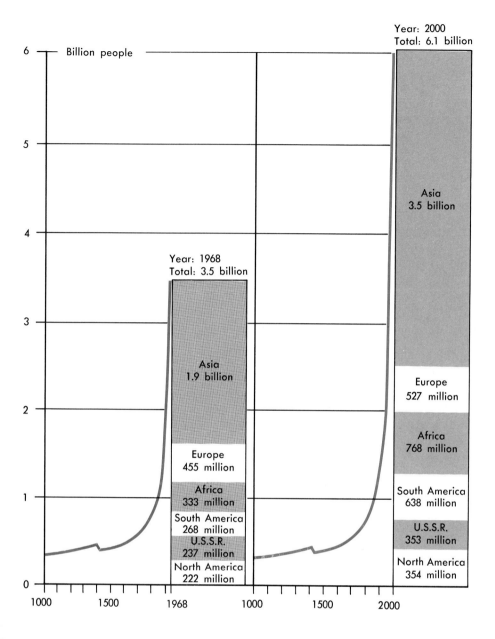

FIG. 3-12. Growth of the human population from 1000 A.D. to 2000 A.D. showing population distribution. (Modified from McHale, J.: World facts and trends, ed. 2, New York, 1972, Macmillan Publishing Co., Inc.)

for us in the United States; for though we make up only 6% of the world's population, we consume 30% to 60% of its various resources. In the context of the ecologic crisis in which the global populations of the next few decades will live, Fig. 3-13 summarizes simply the unique position of man in the biosphere; it is political man, economic man, and social man who will determine whether or not our planet will regain homeostasis. The situation does not yet call for despair, but there is urgent need for sustained concern and action on the part of every citizen of the world community.

■ **IMBALANCE—AFFLUENCE AND POLLUTION**

An ecosystem can be studied in much the same way as an organism. In the preceding section we have

looked briefly at the "anatomy and physiology" of that collectivity of ecosystems called the biosphere and we have found it to be an amazingly complex steady-state system. In it, homeostasis can be maintained only if energy supplies are adequate and if the cyclic feedback processes that regulate the system are all operating properly. Before reading further, stop for a moment and try to list some of the strains and imbalances on the various compartments of the biosphere that result from (1) urbanization, (2) industry, (3) modern agricultural methods, and (4) affluence in general. Study Fig. 3-14 carefully until you begin to gain some realization of the fact that twentieth-century man in industrial societies is affected far more by technologic and psychosocial factors than by those that unite him to the more fundamental cycles of the particular ecosystems in which

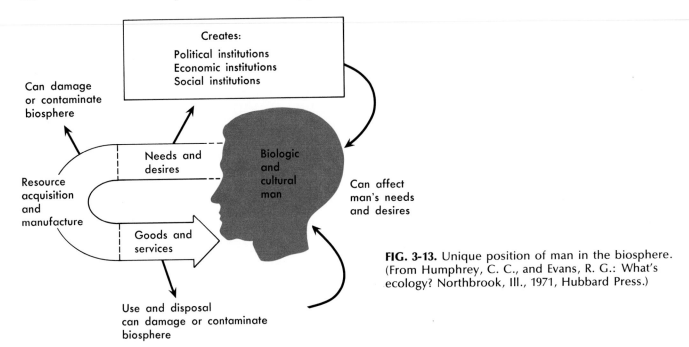

FIG. 3-13. Unique position of man in the biosphere. (From Humphrey, C. C., and Evans, R. G.: What's ecology? Northbrook, Ill., 1971, Hubbard Press.)

he lives. Affluence has been defined as "that state of societies or of individuals in which materials and facilities are available in excess of those necessary for the maintenance of physical and psychological health."[62] Increasingly we are beginning to see that the unbridled production and consumption associated with affluence are not only damaging the physical compartments of the biosphere but are endangering man's interrelationships in the psychosocial sphere through serious imbalances in the distribution of global resources. Let us prepare for a consideration of how these imbalances affect man's physical health by looking briefly at how human activities, especially during the past century, have altered the atmosphere, hydrosphere, and lithosphere.

The damaged atmosphere

When we look for the weather report in newspapers or on television, we have learned to take for granted that a "pollution index" will be one of the items. Yet how many of us know what air pollution really is and how serious a problem it presents? The air we breathe is part of the tropospheric layer of the atmosphere that extends outward about 6 to 10 miles. It functions as a great reservoir within which move all the great wind systems, carrying water, gas, and particulate materials that are constantly circulated from one part of the globe to another. Air in its natural state is very pure; it is essentially a mixture of approximately 79% nitrogen and 20% oxygen with small amounts of carbon dioxide and argon and traces of other gases, including water vapor. However, since the time when he discovered fire, man began to contaminate the air with smoke, the volume of which continually increased as he

moved into cooler latitudes where combustion of fuel was necessary to provide heat. Urbanization and the industrial revolution have resulted in the addition of many foreign substances to the atmosphere. Industrial growth, internal combustion, jet engines, and incineration of refuse have only served to multiply these effluents through the ever-increasing combustion processes required to serve man's desires for warmth, power, and material goods. The enormous magnitude of the problem, if current trends continue, is dramatically illustrated in a recent projection (Fig. 3-15). In spite of governmental efforts to prevent and control pollution through such measures as the Clean Air Act of 1963 with its several amendments, it is unlikely that the degree of improvement in air quality that is urgently needed will be achieved unless there is a considerable change in the life-style of many individuals.

The types and quantities of pollutants and the sources of these materials in the air are shown in Fig. 3-16. It is interesting to note that the total tonnage of pollutants in the air exceeds our annual steel production. Soot, hydrocarbons, oxides of nitrogen and sulfur, carbon dioxide, and carbon monoxide all result from fossil-fuel combustion; the latter two are relatively stable, but the other substances are unstable and can react with one another, making air both toxic and corrosive. For example, hydrocarbons and oxides of nitrogen are relatively harmless, but when combined in sunlight, they can generate large volumes of ozone. Other substances that can accumulate to potentially toxic levels are sulfuric acid mists, lead aerosols from gasoline and paints, asbestos fibers, pesticide sprays, and radioactive emissions. The effects of these toxic agents are often intensified

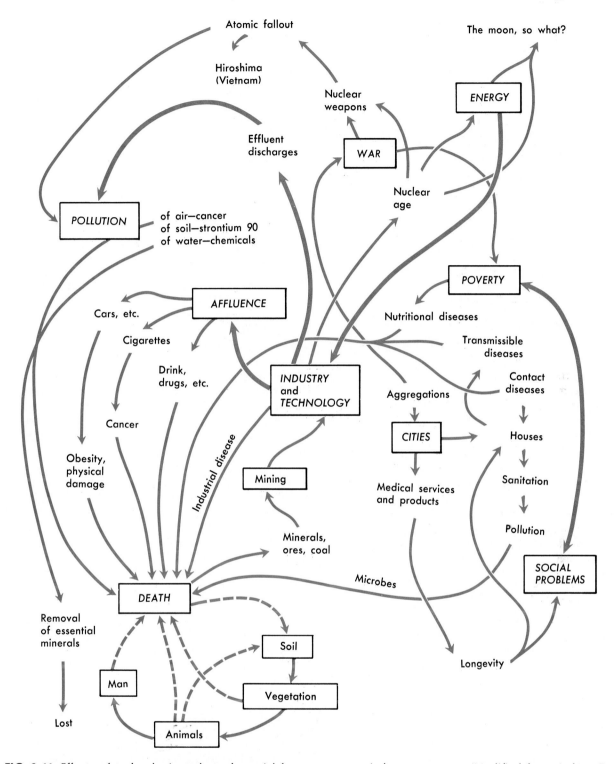

FIG. 3-14. Effects of technologic and psychosocial factors on twentieth-century man. (Modified from Arthur, D. R.: Man and his environment, London, 1969, The English Universities Press.)

by atmospheric turbidity, both sulfur-based smog such as that found over New York and London and the photochemical smog typical of areas such as Los Angeles that results largely from the action of sunlight on auto emissions such as hydrocarbons and oxides of nitrogen.

We can see, then, that most of the pollutants originate in metropolitan areas. In the past we have relied on wind movement to disperse and dilute the contaminants, a rather efficient process where air temperatures decrease rapidly with altitude. Commonly, however, temperatures may decrease only slightly with height or be even warmer above than near the surface, a condition known as inversion. This situation is frequent at night, especially over large urban areas, and because it is often coupled with very weak winds, it may last several days and become very dangerous to health. It has not yet been

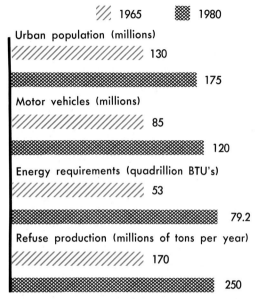

FIG. 3-15. Current trends affecting air pollution in the United States. (Modified from Middleton, J.: Pop. Bull. **24**:117, Dec. 1968.)

fully established to what extent pollutants interfere with global and local climates, but careful study of the effects of increasing accumulations of carbon dioxide and particulates is important lest these result in major global temperature changes or marked rises in sea level. With regard to effects on human health, the establishment of specific causes and effects is difficult because poor air quality is primarily a characteristic of urban areas, where there are so many other factors that contribute to physiologic stress. However, there seems to be little doubt that air pollution increases both the incidence and seriousness of many respiratory disorders, and more and more evidence suggests a high incidence of carcinogenic factors in the total environmental complex of airborne chemicals to which man is exposed.

The recovery and maintenance of clean air will be increasingly expensive, as pollution can be effectively controlled only by decreasing pollutant levels at their source; most of this economic burden will be borne by the consumer of goods and services. Because dispersion of air depends on wind movements, control measures must be undertaken at least on a regional basis and should eventually become international in scope. Early efforts toward global management of the problem have resulted from the United Nations Conference on the Human Environment that has begun an "Earthwatch" program in which various nations are monitoring several aspects of global air quality. How vital such efforts will become should be evident if we consider not only the direct effects of air pollution on a global scale but also the influences of the many foreign chemicals, particulates, and radioactive products as precipitation washes them into the lithosphere and hydrosphere.

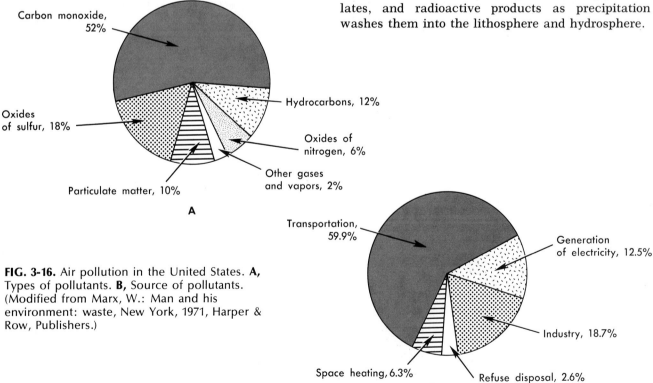

FIG. 3-16. Air pollution in the United States. **A,** Types of pollutants. **B,** Source of pollutants. (Modified from Marx, W.: Man and his environment: waste, New York, 1971, Harper & Row, Publishers.)

Degraded waters

Everyone has discussed water pollution at one time or another, each person having his own concept of what it is. The term may have meanings ranging all the way from occasional litter in a body of water to bacteriologic content so high as to make the water seriously dangerous to living organisms, including man. As seen in Table 3-1, even natural waters are never pure and they range in quality from tasty, safe water to poisonous drinking water and from fresh rainwater to ocean water. Because of the enormous quantity of water in the hydrosphere, the ability of bodies of water to rid themselves of wastes through natural processes such as dilution, water movement, and bacterial decomposition has been too heavily relied on in many areas. Fig. 3-17 will make us aware that much of the domestic and industrial sewage and the agricultural runoff that constitute "water pollution" are received primarily by the surface waters; these make up only about 0.02% of the total water in the world! Most of the organic wastes from cities are highly concentrated and enter rivers and lakes through pipes so large that they produce concentrations of materials that can completely exhaust the dissolved oxygen content of the waterway. Once a body of water's capacity to meet the biologic oxygen demand (BOD) is exceeded, most of the living organisms die and are decomposed by anaerobic bacteria, producing a septic condition often accompanied by very foul odors. Undecomposed wastes can settle to the bottom and build up sludge bands. Natural re-aeration occurs downriver, but the number of outfall discharges along major waterways, particularly in our highly industrial regions, often makes impossible the recovery of conditions suitable for maintaining most living organisms. Some of our rivers and lakes have enormous populations of the very few species of organisms that can survive in polluted conditions instead of the rich diversity of living things characteristic of freshwater ecosystems; some have virtually no living organisms at all.

Domestic and industrial sewage can be treated to lower its biologic oxygen demand level and still release large quantities of waste products such as the plant nutrients from artificial fertilizers and detergents. An idea of the scope of the problem can be gained from Fig. 3-18. Lakes are particularly prone to excessive enrichment or "eutrophication" because re-aeration cannot occur as rapidly as it does in rivers and streams. A body of water may be overwhelmed not only by organic wastes but also by enormous loads of inorganic and nonbiodegradable materials. Many human activities such as strip mining and bulldozing for highways and subdivisions greatly increase sediment loads to a point where they cannot be diluted effectively. The increased water turbidity can interfere with algal photosynthesis with resultant effects all the way up the food chains. It can also produce amounts of silt that are very injurious to gill-breathing organisms and eventually form sediments capable of completely burying such forms as clams and oysters. In addition, such sediments

Table 3-1 Impurities in natural waters: source and classification*

Particle size classification

Source	Suspended	Colloidal	Dissolved		
			Molecules	Positive ions	Negative ions
Atmosphere Mineral, soil, and rock	⟵ Dusts ⟶ ⟵ Sand ⟶ ⟵ Clays ⟶ ⟵ Mineral soil particles ⟶		CO_2, SO_2, O_2, N_2 CO_2	H^+ Na^+, K^+, Ca^{++}, Mg^{++}, Fe^{++}, Mn^{++}	HCO_3^-, $SO_4^=$ Cl^-, F^-, $SO_4^=$, $CO_3^=$, HCO_3^-, NO_3^-, various phosphates
Living organisms and their decomposition products	Algae Diatoms Bacteria ⟵ Organic soil (topsoil) ⟶ Fish and other organisms	 Viruses Organic coloring matter	CO_2, O_2, N_2, H_2S, CH_4, various organic wastes, some of which produce odor and color	H^+, Na^+, NH_4^+	Cl^-, HCO_3^-, NO_3^-

*Modified from Turk, A., and others: Ecology, pollution, environment, Philadelphia, 1972, W. B. Saunders Co.

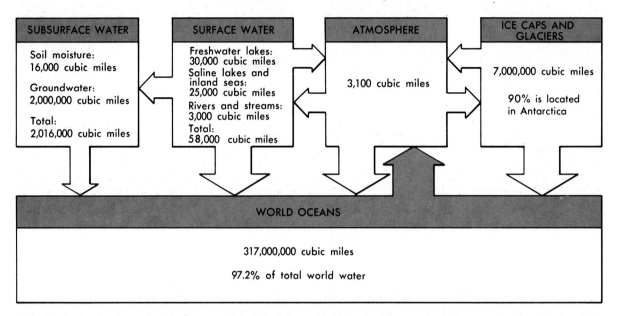

THE HYDROSPHERE
Total world water = 326 million cubic miles
(cubic mile contains 1,101,117,143,000 gallons)

FIG. 3-17. Distribution of global water. (Modified from McHale, J.: The ecological context, New York, 1970, George Braziller, Inc.)

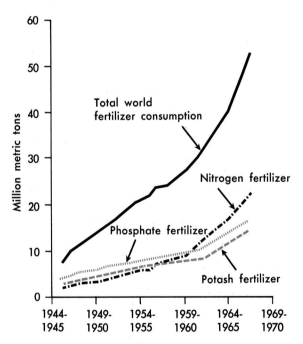

FIG. 3-18. Increase in fertilizer consumption. (From Brown, L. R.: Sci. Am. **223:**161, Sept. 1970;)

can carry tremendous loads of toxic wastes such as DDT and other pesticides, herbicides, acid drainage from mines, heavy metal residues, radioactive wastes, and a host of highly toxic organic compounds from industrial processes. Many of these ma-terials, even if present only in trace quantities, can become severely toxic by being taken up in the food web and concentrated through the process of *biologic magnification* (Fig. 3-19). Toxic concentrations sufficient to interfere with reproductive processes and that may even be lethal to creatures at the top of the food pyramid have been recorded.

Waterways that can handle the organic and inorganic waste loads may still not be safe from pollution, for thermal pollution can be as disruptive of aquatic ecosystems as the chemical types. Power plants and industries remove millions of gallons of water to cool electric-generating processes and then return the water 20° to 30° F. warmer. This problem is likely to be greatly aggravated by the increase in nuclear power plants projected for the very near future.

Although the oceans are enormous, pollution conditions similar to those in fresh water are becoming increasingly present at ocean outflow sites, causing considerable damage to coastal ecosystems and even to marine life at enormous depths through dispersion of nonbiodegradable chemicals such as pesticides and radioactive wastes. Despite their magnitude, even the oceans can become ecologic "disaster areas" if man is as careless with them as he has been with surface waters.

The marred face of the land

The surface of the lithosphere is being influenced constantly by the action of wind and water; so many of the pollutants we have just discussed are trans-

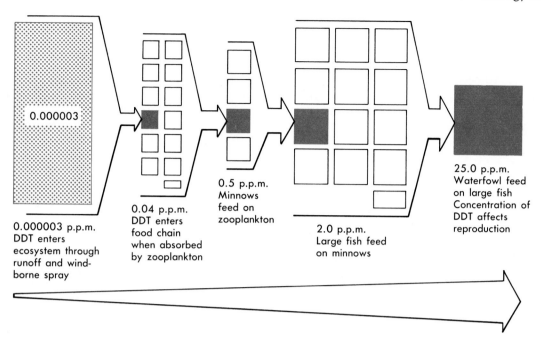

FIG. 3-19. Biologic magnification of DDT. Concentration of DDT and effect on reproduction through the food chain. (Reprinted by permission from TIME, The Weekly Newsmagazine; Copyright Time Inc.)

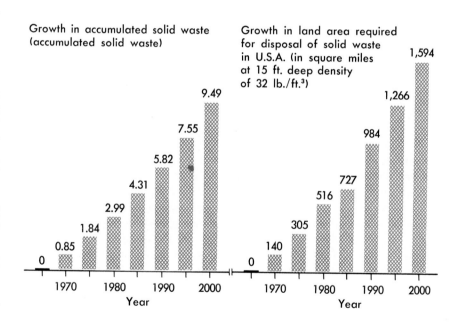

Growth in accumulated solid waste (accumulated solid waste)

Growth in land area required for disposal of solid waste in U.S.A. (in square miles at 15 ft. deep density of 32 lb./ft.³)

FIG. 3-20. Projected scope of the solid waste disposal problem in the United States. Accumulated solid waste shown in billion tons. (Modified from Closing the cycle from use to reuse. The fusion torch, May, 1969, Washington, D. C., U. S. Atomic Energy Commission.)

ferred to the land and then percolate into the groundwater through the soil. Groundwater and soil also can be contaminated by acid or radioactive wastes from surface mining of metals and uranium, pesticide residues, synthetic chemicals, heavy metal salts, and other soluble materials. Marked effects of biologic magnification on the soil's ability to support plant life have not been reported as yet, and we cannot predict the results of a long-term buildup of potentially toxic materials.

Historically, man has used the surface of the land in its natural condition as rangeland or forest; with an increasing population, more and more of these regions have been converted into croplands. Table 3-2 shows some international projections for land use that make the finiteness of land surface on the planet readily apparent. Increasingly the loads of wastes resulting from the production characteristic of affluent societies produce solid waste disposal problems that are critical, especially in densely populated areas. The rate at which the problem is growing is evident from Fig. 3-20, a projection resulting from a 1969 Atomic Energy Commission study.

Solid wastes fall into five major categories:

Table 3-2 Present and potential uses of land surface of planet (percent of total area)*

Use	Present	Potential
Croplands	11	24
Rangelands	20	28
Managed forests	10	15
Reserves (80% forest)	26	0
Not usable	33	33
Total	**100**	**100**

*From Matthews, W. H., and others, editors: Man's impact on terrestrial and oceanic ecosytems, Cambridge, Mass., 1971, The M.I.T. Press.

urban, which includes domestic, commercial, and municipal; industrial; agricultural; mineral; and those from federal establishments. The mountains of urban wastes—garbage, paper, furniture, abandoned cars, ashes, dead pets, street sweepings, materials resulting from construction and demolition, and the many nonbiodegradable, "disposable" products—not only utilize enormous amounts of land surface but they also tend to be esthetically offensive because of the appearance and odor, to enhance the multiplication of disease-producing organisms, and to create fire and explosion hazards. Improvements in management are beginning to be evident in a few cities through use of sanitary landfills, composting, metal reclamation, and other recycling efforts, but open dumping still remains by far the most widely used means of urban waste disposal. Industrial concerns are struggling to cope with up to 115 million tons of waste yearly: waste plastics, scrap metals, paper wastes, and large inventories of off-grade products, sludges, slags, etc. Most of these materials cannot be processed and reintroduced into use.

Wastes from agriculture and forestry include animal manures and residues from such activities as crop harvesting, pruning, fertilizing, and spraying. Domestic animals produce close to 2 billion tons of animal wastes annually, as much as 50% of which is generated in concentrated growing and feeding operations close to urban areas.

Mountains of mineral wastes, such as submarginal grade ores, coal waste piles, tailings, slag, and wastes from chemical processing are produced by about 80 mineral industries, with the copper, iron, steel, phosphate rock, bituminous coal, lead, zinc, and anthracite industries generating the most wastes. Dredging and strip mining also produce large-scale pollution and destruction of the land; by 1980 it is estimated that more than 5 million acres will have been defaced by strip-mining operations alone. Research in solid waste disposal will increase as an urgent need, and it is to be hoped that a unified, comprehensive approach to solid waste management will be sought if the enormous cost of effective management is to be reduced. Some idea of the projected cost of solid waste control can be gained from a recent study by the National Academy of Sciences (Fig. 3-21, A.) The projected figure probably includes support of the new technologies that will be required to ensure that recycling techniques are made effective enough to reduce significantly the pollution of all compartments of the biosphere. Fig. 3-21, B, indicates, however, that recent trends have shown nearly a doubling of refuse production per person; so much of the economic burden projected is due to the increasing "throwaway" mentality of an affluent society.

It is becoming more and more apparent that the environmental crisis confronting us today has a cultural basis. It is industrial man's affluence, technology, urbanization, increasing individual wealth, and exploitive attitude toward nature that are wrecking

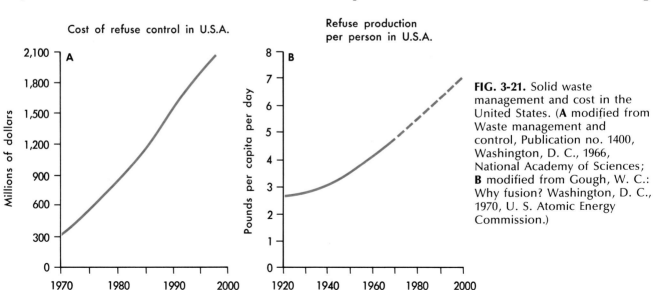

FIG. 3-21. Solid waste management and cost in the United States. (**A** modified from Waste management and control, Publication no. 1400, Washington, D. C., 1966, National Academy of Sciences; **B** modified from Gough, W. C.: Why fusion? Washington, D. C., 1970, U. S. Atomic Energy Commission.)

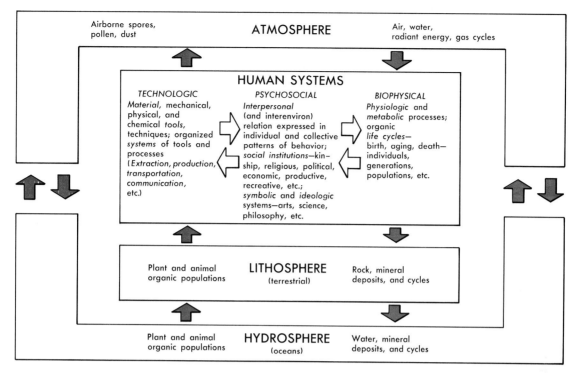

FIG. 3-22. Integral interrelatedness of environ systems and human systems in the biosphere. (Modified from McHale, J.: World facts and trends, ed. 2, New York, 1972, Macmillan Publishing Co., Inc.)

the environment. If man is concerned about his own physical, mental, and social health as well as the welfare of generations yet unborn, his attitudes toward nature must change enough to result in new individual behavior and new institutions; both of these must be enlightened by the global perspective that social justice demands. Man must come to a recognition of the interdependence of all creatures and a respect not only for life in all its forms but also for the nonliving components of the biosphere (Fig. 3-22). He must learn to live as part of the community of life—as the steward of the planet, not its master.

■ PERSPECTIVES FOR HUMAN HEALTH
Metabolic homeostasis and health

Health is often thought of as freedom from disease, weakness, or malfunction. Viewed positively, however, it is quite appropriate to equate it with homeostasis or steady-state functioning. In many ways the human body can be likened to an ecosystem with the metabolic systems accomplishing the producer-decomposer roles, the musculoskeletal complex and (on a less consistent basis) the reproductive system being the consumers of the energy produced by the metabolic systems, and the entire interacting "ecosystem" under exquisite neuroendocrine control. Such an analogy is shown schematically in Fig. 3-23.

Just as in an ecosystem, an imbalance or malfunction in part of this steady-state complex is re-

flected throughout the organism; this we know as disease or illness. Historically, man has suffered primarily from the infectious diseases caused by invading microorganisms, and to a large extent this is still true in many of the underdeveloped regions. In the developed nations, however, especially since the discovery of antibiotics (Fig. 3-24), infectious disease has been all but eradicated, yet simultaneously, the incidence of chronic metabolic and degenerative disease continues to rise in the more affluent areas of the world (Table 3-3). Data such as these reflect a complex interaction of factors characteristic of affluent, highly industrialized urban regions. Many persons in such regions show high cholesterol levels and obesity resulting from overconsumption of food coupled with decreased activity. Heavy cigarette smoking seems to be more prevalent in sophisticated, urban cultures, and the deleterious effects of smoking are significantly aggravated by intake of polluted air characteristic of these densely populated regions. Noise tends to produce psychologic trauma of varying seriousness by limiting efficiency, interfering with sleep, and generally adding to the many other stressful conditions from which industrial man suffers. Thus it is difficult to implicate individual environmental factors directly as causative of specific disease conditions.

The task of studying the environment as it relates to human health is enormous because it requires simultaneous handling of a multitude of variables that

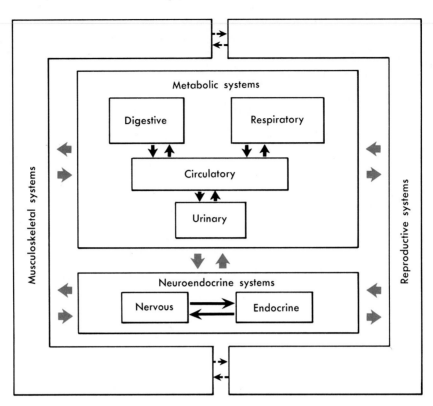

FIG. 3-23. Human body viewed as an "ecosystem."

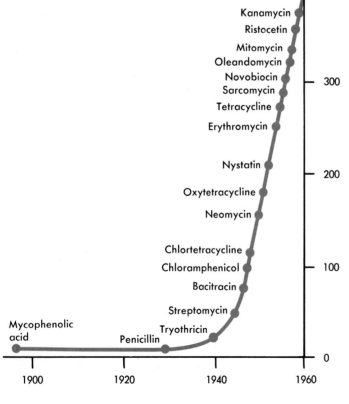

FIG. 3-24. Years in which antibiotics were developed and the number in use. (Modified from McHale, J.: The future of the future, New York, 1969, George Braziller, Inc.)

Table 3-3 International mortality statistics: comparison of death rates from arteriosclerotic and degenerative heart diseases per 100,000 population in developed and underdeveloped countries—1966*

Developed countries		Underdeveloped countries	
Scotland	366.5	Venezuela	47.8
Denmark	327.7	Mauritius	46.5
Eire	326.1	Costa Rica	45.8
United States	320.0	Singapore	35.9
England and Wales	317.0	Mexico	16.9
Australia	290.0	Philippines	14.5
Canada	240.1		
Switzerland	218.6		
Netherlands	184.5		
France	81.4		

*From Smith, G., and Smyth, J. C., editors: The biology of affluence, Edinburgh, 1972, Oliver & Boyd, Ltd.

can be understood only as a whole system rather than as separate parts. This is a staggering realization to researchers, since historically medical research investigations have been those of individual scientists testing effect of one variable at a time on test animals and sometimes on humans. Only through the use of integrated team efforts, aided by systems analysis and projection possible through computer use, is there any hope that man will arrive at an understanding of the many cause-effect relationships between himself and his environment. Institutional response has begun to be evident in the new departments of community medicine and environmental health being formed in some medical schools and schools of public health. Such programs evidence the growing realization that today's health personnel should not simply restore patients to health but should be instrumental in helping to educate them concerning the many environmental factors that can influence their health directly or indirectly.

Pollution and physiologic imbalance

Because of the complexity of the interacting body-environment system that must be studied, there is very little solid evidence to date of cause-effect relationships between specific pollutants and particular disease processes. In order to clarify the effects of chronic, low-level exposure to pollutants, fundamental research must include (1) basic studies on the physiologic effects of pollutants on various body tissues and organs; (2) animal experimentation on the effects of these substances on susceptibility to infectious diseases; (3) industrial and urban/rural morbid-ity studies in relation to known exposures; and (4) controlled epidemiologic studies. To date the only concerted research efforts that fulfill these criteria have been made in two areas: the relationship of smoking to health and the somatic and genetic effects of radioactivity. We shall study these in greater detail later in an effort to comprehend how difficult it will be to marshal sufficient interest and financial backing to make the necessary investigations for the enormous number of compounds that would have to be tested. But first let us survey briefly a few of the pollutant-disease relationships that have come under suspicion, usually through a dramatic incident such as a localized air-pollution episode or an industrial or research accident that exposed victims to unexpected quantities of a hazardous material.

The entry site for disease-producing pollutants is always one of the body surfaces that is exposed to the environment—the digestive and respiratory tracts and the skin. A general indication of how easily any of the wastes that we surveyed earlier can enter the body is seen in Fig. 3-25. Note that because of the integral interrelationships among the biosphere compartments any waste from any source can eventually influence the food and water ingested and the air taken in by the respiratory tract and be potentially disease producing.

Two groups of substances that enter the mouth are "intentional" and "incidental" food additives. In our affluent society, man has come to expect enormous variety in his diet, regardless of seasonal availability and location of production. To make this possible as well as to aid the homemaker, often employed full time outside the home, processors add a large variety of materials to color, flavor, sweeten, ripen, add firmness, thicken, soften, moisten, dry, emulsify, enrich, hasten chemical reactions, or retard oxidation and rancidity in foods. In many cases such additives have enhanced nutritional health. For example, addition of potassium iodide to table salt has all but eliminated simple goiter, and the enrichment of bread with B vitamins has greatly cut down the incidence of pellagra in the United States.

Just before Thanksgiving in 1959 all cranberries and cranberry products were removed from the market because it was feared that they might contain residual aminotriazole, a herbicide that had been found to induce cancerous growths in the thyroid glands of rats. This is a dramatic example of the "incidental" additives that find their way into food. Among these are (1) insecticides and herbicides, (2) substances that might diffuse from packaging materials, (3) heavy metals, and (4) radioactive materials from fallout. Warnings similar to those for cranberries were made abroad relative to the black dye in jelly beans and the diethylstilbestrol used in chickens to produce caponettes. The death rate from pesticides is estimated at 150 persons a year, 50% to 75%

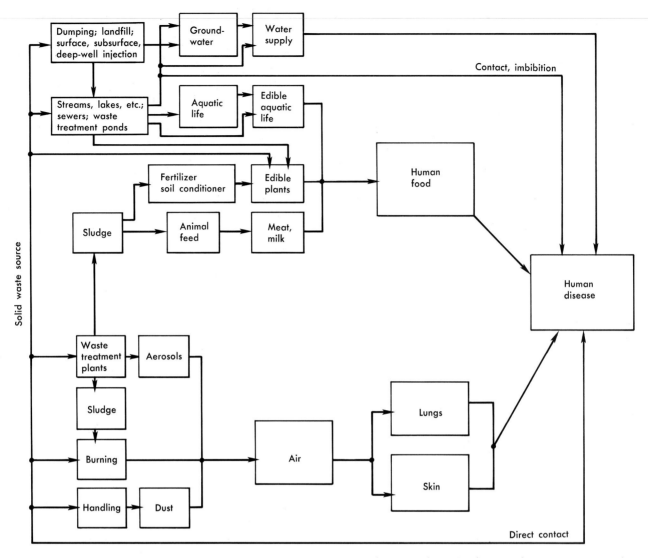

FIG. 3-25. Relationship between chemical waste and disease. Schematic drawing showing how any source of waste can contaminate air, food, or water. (Modified from Marx, W.: Man and his environment: waste, New York, 1971, Harper & Row, Publishers.)

IMPACT OF CONTROL PROGRAMS

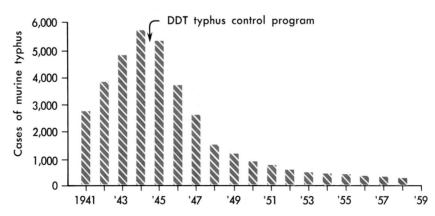

FIG. 3-26. Effect of DDT on the incidence of typhus. (Redrawn from Benarde, M. A.: Our precarious habitat, New York, 1970, W. W. Norton & Co., Inc.)

being children who have accidentally eaten lethal doses. There is some danger for spray pilots, insecticide producers, and greenhouse personnel. Recently the migrant workers who pick the crops have been agitating for improved working conditions, among them more protection from insecticides and herbicides. The dangers from these substances, both with regard to acute exposure and to low-level effects over a long period, must be weighed against the benefits to health as illustrated in Fig. 3-26 and the enormous rise in global food productivity that have been made possible. Such increases in food production are essential if we are to achieve the projected increases in total food supply needed just to maintain present diet levels—a 50% increase by 1985 and a 75% increase by the year 2000. This is just one more example of the complexity of every problem that involves some trade-off between adverse effects to environment and health and the increased productivity necessitated by rising population numbers.

Exposure to lead and mercury poisoning has attracted much attention. Incidences of lead poisoning from paints ingested by children begin to rise in spring and peak in July and August. It is thought to show this seasonal pattern because increased temperature and ultraviolet light are thought to act on old paint chips and result in increased intestinal absorption of lead. Evidence of severe damage to the nervous system has been seen among many employees of an industrial complex in Japan where industrial wastes loaded with mercury were discharged into the water and underwent magnification via the food chain. No amount of financial settlement by the industry involved can ever reverse the misery of the weakened, grotesquely deformed victims of Minamata disease. It has been suggested that several other metals such as cadmium, vanadium, and beryllium might be implicated in disease, and although the extent and effects of exposure of these and many other suspected materials may not be known for sometime, there is certainly reason for caution.

Chemicals added by those wishing to market nearly spoiled goods are called "malicious" additives; these may be dangerous particularly because of the concentrations in which they are often used. In 1958 the Food Additives Amendment was enacted containing the "Delaney clause": "No additive shall be deemed safe if it is found, after tests which are appropriate for the evaluation of safety of food additives, to induce cancer in man or animal." Within the past few years many Americans saw the speed with which cyclamate-sweetened products were removed from distribution because of the possible danger of cancer and/or chromosome damage. However, it is difficult to see how the Food and Drug Administration will ever keep up with the enormous number of new substances that are introduced through new production and packaging processes.

Man can survive for weeks without food and for about 5 days without water, but he cannot survive even 5 minutes without air. Perhaps this is why the adverse effects of air pollution on health, comfort, and property have consistently generated more public concern and research activity than other types of pollutants that produce more subtle effects. A major piece of evidence of the health implications of air pollution came in 1930, when the Meuse Valley in Belgium was blanketed by a heavy smog and 63 persons died as a result of the dense layer of fog and smog that hung low and bottled up contaminants for nearly 4 days. Similar weather conditions occurred in 1948 in Donora, Pennsylvania, where almost half of the city's 14,000 residents were seized by fits of coughing and vomiting; 19 persons died, 17 more than the average number of deaths a week in this small town. Several other acute episodes of this type (Table 3-4) have made public health officials very aware that though it is usually impossible to implicate a particular component of polluted air as causative, there is no doubt that air pollution can kill and disable people and that the effects could easily become a great deal more widespread. To date there have been no acute air pollution episodes resulting from the ozone-rich Los Angeles type of smog that have resulted in recorded fatalities. However, the irritating effects on mucous membranes, the reduced visibility and increased ozone concentrations, which are constant experiences of inhabitants of these re-

Table 3-4 Deaths during acute episodes of air pollution*

Date	Place	Sulfur dioxide value— peak (p.p.m.)	Mortality
Feb. 1880	London	—	1,000
Dec. 1930	Meuse Valley	9.6-38.4†	63
Oct. 1948	Donora	2.0	17‡
Dec. 1952	London	1.47	4,000
Jan. 1956	London	—	1,000
Dec. 1957	London	—	700-800
Dec. 1962	London	Same as 1952	700
Nov. 1953	New York	0.86	200
Jan.-Feb. 1963	New York	0.40-1.50	200-400
Nov. 1966	New York	0.69-0.97-1.02	168

*From Battigelli, M. C.: Sulfur dioxide and acute effects of air pollution, Paper presented at the Air quality criteria symposium, New York, June 4-5, 1968.

†Assumed retrospectively.

‡These deaths are usually counted in the literature as 20. Actually only 19 occurred during the week and two deaths were the usual expected per week.

gions, along with the damage to plants and to residential and industrial properties make a strong economic case for air pollution abatement before a deadly disaster occurs.

It is not simply a case of mustering the scientific and medical manpower needed to analyze the potential health effects of each component of polluted air; even if this nearly impossible task could be accomplished, it would not provide a solution. The constituents of polluted air are very complex and are constantly varying in concentration. They have the potential for additive, synergistic action among themselves, and in addition their effects may be related to many other factors such as climate, age, occupation, state of health of those exposed, and whether they are habitual smokers. It is important to realize that acute exposures such as those indicated in Table 3-4 may be a much less serious health threat than continuous exposure to low-level but cumulative contaminants that may produce or aggravate chronic disease conditions. These possibly hasten the degenerative conditions that are characteristic of aging in various organs and tissues.

In the *Proceedings of the U. S. Technical Conference on Air Pollution* published in 1952 each and every paper on health aspects indicated that although there seemed to be a relationship between polluted air and incidence of bronchitis and lung cancer, there had been no clear causal relation demonstrated between any specific air pollutant and chronic disease. By 1961, in a symposium at the University of California School of Medicine, the following was recognized:

Most of the major medical problems today are not episodic, at least etiologically. Cancer, heart disease and of course the host of degenerative diseases of old age have their roots far back in the life history of the patient. In order to understand these diseases we are learning, slowly, to think of medicine not in terms of organs and diseases, but in terms of interactions in time. We are approaching an ecologic conception of medicine, a conception which emphasizes environment and interaction, to understand the processes of life as processes. . . .*

By 1973 air pollution was assumed to be damaging to health, in spite of the lack of hard scientific data that would implicate specific pollutants, with a few exceptions such as those determined as causative factors in lung cancer in smokers. The extent of the effects observed are evident in the report of the Council on Environmental Quality, which projected damage, avoidance, transaction, and abatement costs for environmental pollutants. That damage to health is one of the most significant components of estimated damage costs is illustrated in Table 3-5.

Table 3-5 Estimated national air pollution damage costs with no pollution control, 1968 and 1977 (in billions of dollars)*

Damage class	1968†	1977‡
Health	6.1	9.3
Residential property	5.2	8.0
Materials and vegetation	4.9	7.6
Total	16.2	24.9

*From The economics of clean air, Senate Document No. 92-67, Washington D. C., 1972, U. S. Government Printing Office.
†In 1968 dollars.
‡In 1970 dollars.

The costs, which cannot be projected in dollars, suggest the magnitude and complexity of the problem as indicated in the report:

Many types of environmental damage will create both tangible and intangible costs. By damaging health, air pollution affects tangible resources by causing lost production and by consuming equipment, supplies, and the time of highly skilled manpower required to restore good health. The illness, as well as the threatened loss of income security, may also arouse anxiety and fear in the individual and his family and friends. These are some of the psychic costs of air pollution—costs that are rarely included in damage estimates.

Although probably comprising a significant portion of total damage costs, psychic costs, unfortunately, cannot be accurately quantified. Further, they change over time. Opinion surveys indicate that the degree of concern about such problems as air and water pollution has increased substantially in less than a decade. . . . In the past, people were less aware of the extent and dangers of environmental degradation and had less interest in the amenities offered by a clean environment. Even as we improve our environment, the psychic costs may be higher than before because of this heightened concern.*

Even a partial cataloging of substances suggested to be associated with various diseases is not possible in this brief chapter, for we would have to consider many types of materials, both chemicals and particulates: nitrogen and sulfur-containing chemicals; particulates such as soot, asphalt, rubber, and asbestos; gases such as hydrogen sulfide, chlorine, and fluorine; heavy metals such as cadmium, vanadium, and lead; and many others. Instead, we will look at some of the data from the Surgeon General's report on the health effects of smoking and leave the reader to wonder about and hopefully to maintain a concerned vigilance as more and more studies come out

---

*From Farber, M., and Wilson, R. H. L., editors: The air we breathe, Springfield, Ill., 1961, Charles C Thomas, Publisher.

*From Council on Environmental Quality: Fourth annual report on environmental quality, Washington, D. C., 1973, U. S. Government Printing Office.

that implicate specific substances in the causation or aggravation of disease.

It is interesting—and somewhat alarming—to note that what is perhaps the most definitive report of cause-effect relationships between pollutants and specific diseases, the Surgeon General's report *Smoking and Health* has not produced any lasting reduction in smoking in the United States. This indication of attitude is particularly significant if we consider that it has been estimated in a report to the Muskie Subcommittee on Air and Water Pollution in 1968 that a person breathing the air of the average large city probably receives at least as much carcinogens as if he smoked one pack of cigarettes a day. In heavily polluted areas the risk of simply breathing may produce an accumulation of known carcinogens equal to that of inhaling two packs of cigarettes daily. The gravity of the situation for the urban smoker should be obvious.

Reports, even in the late 1950's, indicated that epidemiologic studies revealed a worldwide increase in the prevalence of lung cancer, with a greater incidence in males and urban residents and especially in those with a history of prolonged or excessive cigarette smoking. Thus urban air alone was associated early with an increased risk of developing lung cancer. This rise in lung cancer was described to the Muskie Subcommittee as "a dramatic increase . . . now approaching epidemic proportions." The dra-

matic nature of the increase is evident in Fig. 3-27, which clearly illustrates the summary of the report: "Cigarette smoking is causally related to lung cancer in men; the magnitude of the effect of cigarette smoking far outweighs all other factors. The data for women, though less extensive, point in the same direction".[68] Among the other findings summarized were the establishment that "cigarette smoking is the most important of the causes of chronic bronchitis in the United States and increases the risk of dying from chronic bronchitis." A correlation was definitely found between pulmonary emphysema and cigarette smoking, but the facts did not definitively implicate smoking as causal. That cigarette smoking is a "significant factor in the causation of laryngeal cancer in the male" and "associated with" cancer of the esophagus and urinary bladder can be seen in Fig. 3-28. No relationship was established between cigarette smoking and stomach cancer.

Among the other conditions thought to be aggravated are ulcers, the association being greater for gastric than for duodenal ulcer, and pulmonary emphysema. For all of these conditions, as well as for cirrhosis of the liver, increased mortality of smokers has been shown in the seven prospective studies that were carried out on 1,123,000 men during the study. In Table 3-6 the accumulated and combined data are summarized on 14 disease categories for which the mortality ratio of cigarette smokers to nonsmokers

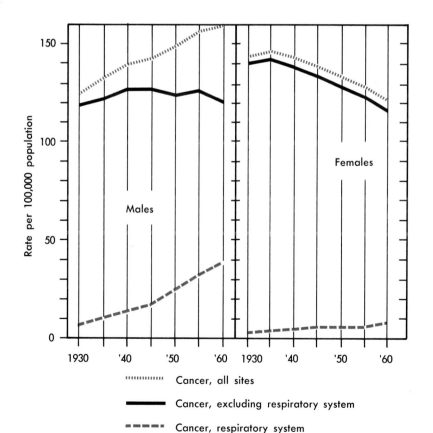

FIG. 3-27. Trends in age-adjusted mortality rates for cancer by sex. All sites and respiratory system in the United States, 1930-1960. (From U. S. Department of Health, Education and Welfare, Public Health Service: Smoking and health, Washington, D. C., 1964, U. S. Government Printing Office.)

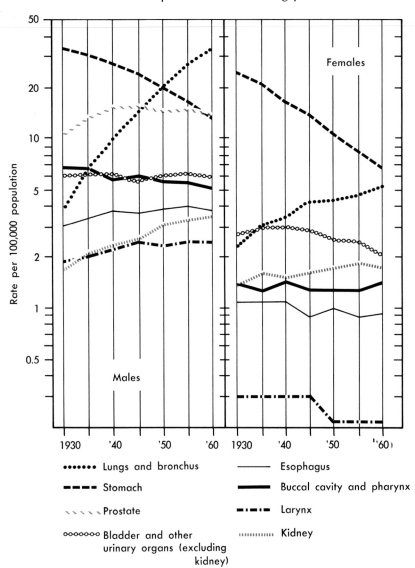

FIG. 3-28. Trends in age-adjusted mortality rates for selected cancer sites by sex in the United States, 1930-1960. (Data from U. S. Department of Health, Education and Welfare, Public Health Service: Smoking and health, Washington, D. C., 1964, U. S. Government Printing Office.)

•••••• Lungs and bronchus — Esophagus

–––– Stomach —— Buccal cavity and pharynx

╲╲╲╲╲ Prostate –•–•– Larynx

ooooooo Bladder and other urinary organs (excluding kidney) ⋯⋯⋯⋯ Kidney

was 1:5 or greater (that is, in which the death rate for cigarette smokers is at least 50% higher than for nonsmokers). It is significant to note that cigarette smoking, besides causing lung cancer and chronic bronchitis, at least predisposes to or aggravates a large number of the degenerative conditions that are the major causes of death in industrialized, economically affluent regions.

One of the most potent of all the carcinogens now known is benzopyrene. It has been shown to be one of the two most potent of the seven carcinogens detected in tobacco smoke, and it is present in much larger quantity than any of the other carcinogens listed. Since 1933, it was known to be the coal tar constituent that evoked skin cancer when applied to the skin of mice. The particular significance of this single finding is that benzopyrene is one of the gaseous hydrocarbons found in automobile emissions and thus reaches high concentrations in urban air. The concentration in cities such as New York, Chicago, and Los Angeles has been reported to be as much

as 50 million times that of Grand Canyon National Park.

A recent report by the genetic study section of the National Institutes of Health suggests that the danger of birth defects from airborne chemicals may dwarf even the well-documented dangers of radiation. Since the effects of air contaminants may be much less acute than those of radiation, the danger may be even greater because the increased mutation rates might spread over many generations and include ill-defined abnormalities such as subtly increasing aging and susceptibility to diseases such as leukemia and cancer. It is significant to note in this regard that benzopyrene has been shown to produce many malformations in mice. Although knowledge of chemical mutagenesis and teratogenesis in man is much less certain than that of radiation, a number of chemicals have been discovered already that are known to induce genetic or teratogenic effects in some organisms.

It is outside the scope of this brief chapter to con-

Table 3-6 Expected and observed deaths for smokers of cigarettes only and mortality ratios in seven prospective studies*

Underlying cause of death	Expected deaths	Observed deaths	Mortality ratio
Cancer of lung	170.3	1,833	10:8
Bronchitis and emphysema	89.5	546	6:1
Cancer of larynx	14.0	75	5:4
Oral cancer	37.0	152	4:1
Cancer of esophagus	33.7	113	3:4
Stomach and duodenal ulcers	105.1	294	2:8
Other circulatory diseases	254.0	649	2:6
Cirrhosis of liver	169.2	379	2:2
Cancer of bladder	111.6	216	1:9
Coronary artery disease	6,430.7	11,177	1:7
Other heart diseases	526.0	868	1:7
Hypertensive heart	409.2	631	1:5
General arteriosclerosis	210.7	310	1:5
Cancer of kidney	79.0	120	1:5
All causes	15,653.9	23,223	1:68

*From U. S. Department of Health, Education and Welfare, Public Health Service: Smoking and health, Washington, D. C., 1964, U. S. Government Printing Office.

sider in any detail the well-documented genetic and somatic hazards of long-term exposure to low-level ionizing radiation. Somatic effects involve mostly the induction of cancer. Whether there is a threshold below which exposure to radioactivity has no somatic effects has been a major uncertainty. If the relationship between exposure and cancer induction can be extrapolated back to the very light exposure to which the general population could be subjected under current radiation standards, an impressive number of deaths would be attributable to man-made radiation if the maximum permissible levels were reached for everyone. It is not likely that we will reach such levels from reactor operation, but the problem of disposing of the enormous increases of radioactive wastes for thousands of years presents hazards of a social and political nature.

The fundamental causes of environmental problems, as we have seen, are in the psychosocial and technologic spheres. In the final analysis it is political, economic, and social man who will determine whether to pay the price required to restore the biosphere to homeostasis. The choice is in our hands.

REFERENCES AND SELECTED READINGS*

1 American Chemical Society: Cleaning our environment: the chemical basis for action, Washington, D. C. 1969, The Society.
2 *Arthur, D. K.: Man and his environment, New York, 1969, American Elsevier Publishing Co., Inc.
3 *Barbour, I. G., editor: Western man and environmental ethics, Reading, Mass., 1973, Addison-Wesley Publishing Co., Inc.
4 Bates, M.: Man in nature, ed. 2, New York, 1964, Prentice-Hall, Inc.
5 *Benarde, M. A.: Our precarious habitat, New York, 1970, W. W. Norton & Co., Inc.
6 Beranek, L.: Noise, Sci. Am. 215:66-76, Dec. 1966.
7 *Blau, S. D., and Rodenbeck, J. von B.: The house we live in, New York, 1971, Macmillan Publishing Co., Inc.
8 Borgstrom, G.: The hungry planet, New York, 1967, Collier-Macmillan International, Inc.
9 Boughey, A. S.: Ecology of populations, New York, 1968, Macmillan Publishing Co., Inc.
10 Boughey, A. S.: Man and the environment, New York, 1971, Macmillan Publishing Co., Inc.
11 Brubaker, S.: To live on earth, Baltimore, 1972, The Johns Hopkins University Press.
12 Cailliet, G., and others: Everyman's guide to ecological living, New York, 1971, Macmillan Publishing Co., Inc.
13 Carson, R.: Silent spring, Boston, 1962, Houghton Mifflin Co.
14 Chute, R. M.: Environmental insight, New York, 1971, Harper & Row, Publishers.
15 *Clark, J.: Thermal pollution, Sci. Am. 220:18-27, March 1969.
16 Colinvaux, P. A.: Introduction to ecology, New York, 1973, John Wiley & Sons, Inc.
17 Commoner, B.: Science and survival, New York, 1966, The Viking Press, Inc.
18 *Commoner, B.: The closing circle: nature, man and technology, New York, 1971, Alfred A. Knopf, Inc.
19 Council on Environmental Quality: Fourth annual report on environmental quality, Washington, D. C., 1973, U. S. Government Printing Office.

*References preceded by an asterisk are particularly well suited for student reading.

20 *Curtis, R. and Hogan, E.: Perils of the peaceful atom, New York, 1970, Doubleday & Co., Inc.

21 Dansereau, P.: Challenge for survival: land, air, and water for man in megalopolis, New York, 1970, Columbia University Press.

22 Dasmann, R. F.: Man and the biosphere—a challenge for UNESCO in a new international program, Washington, D. C., 1970, The Conservation Foundation.

23 DeBell, G., editor: The environmental handbook, New York, 1970, Ballantine Books, Inc.

24 *Deevey, E. S.: The human population, Sci. Am. **203**:194-204, Sept. 1960.

25 Detwyler, T. R.: Man's impact on environment: McGraw-Hill series in geography, New York, 1971, McGraw-Hill Book Co.

26 Dubos, R.: The mirage of health, New York, 1961, Doubleday & Co., Inc.

27 Dubos, R.: So human an animal, New York, 1968, Charles Scribner's Sons.

28 Ehrlich, R. P., and Ehrlich, A. H.: Population, resources and environment: issues in human ecology, San Francisco, 1970, W. H. Freeman & Co., Publishers.

29 Fabun, D.: The dynamics of change, Englewood Cliffs, N. J., 1970, Prentice-Hall, Inc.

30 Farber, M., and Wilson, R. H. L., editors: The air we breathe, Springfield, Ill., 1961, Charles C Thomas, Publisher.

31 Fowler, J. M., editor: Fallout, New York, 1960, Basic Books, Inc., Publishers.

32 Frakes, G. E., and Salberg, S. B.: Pollution papers, New York, 1971, Appleton-Century-Crofts.

33 Galbraith, J. K.: The affluent society, Boston, 1958, Houghton Mifflin Co.

34 *Handler, P., editor: Biology and the future of man, London, 1970, Oxford University Press, Inc.

35 Hanks, T. G.: Solid waste-disease relationships, Washington, D. C., 1967, U. S. Department of Health, Education and Welfare.

36 Helfrich, H. W., Jr., editor: The environmental crisis, New Haven, Conn., 1970, Yale University Press.

37 *Holt, S. J.: The food resources of the world, Sci. Am. **221**:180-194, Sept. 1969.

38 *Hulett, H. R.: Optimum world population, Bioscience **20**:160-161, 1970.

39 Humphrey, C. C., and Evans, R. G.: What's ecology, Northbrook, Ill., 1971, Hubbard Press.

40 *Hutchinson, G. E.: The biosphere, Sci. Am. **223**:44-58, Sept. 1970.

41 *Johnson, H. D.: No deposit—no return, Reading, Mass., 1970, Addison-Wesley Publishing Co., Inc.

42 Kahn, H., and others: The year 2000, New York, 1967, Macmillan Publishing Co., Inc.

43 Kormondy, E. J.: Concepts of ecology, Englewood Cliffs, N. J., 1969, Prentice-Hall, Inc.

44 Marquis, R. W., editor: Environmental improvement (air, water and soil), Washington, D. C., 1966, U. S. Department of Agriculture.

45 Marx, W.: Man and his environment: waste, New York, 1971, Harper & Row, Publishers.

46 Matthews, W. H., and others, editors: Man's impact on terrestrial and oceanic ecosystems, Cambridge, Mass., 1971, The M.I.T. Press.

47 McCabe, L. C., chairman: Air pollution: proceedings of the U. S. Technical Conference on air pollution, New York, 1952, McGraw-Hill Book Co.

48 *McDermott, W.: Air pollution and public health, Sci. Am. **205**:49-57, Oct. 1961.

49 *McHale, J.: World facts and trends, ed. 2, New York, 1972, Macmillan Publishing Co., Inc.

50 McHarg, I.: Design with nature, New York, 1969, Natural History Press.

51 Means, R. L.: The ethical imperative, New York, 1969, Doubleday & Co., Inc.

52 Mumford, L.: The myth of the machine, New York, 1967, Harcourt Brace Jovanovich, Inc.

53 Murphy, E. F.: Man and his environment: law, New York, 1971, Harper & Row, Publishers.

54 National Association of Science—National Research Council: Research needs in environmental health: a symposium, NAS-NRC Publication no. 1419, Washington, D. C., 1966, U. S. Government Printing Office.

55 National Association of Science—National Research Council: Resources and man: a study and recommendation, San Francisco, 1969, W. H. Freeman & Co., Publishers.

56 National Association of Science—National Research Council: Rapid population growth, Baltimore, 1971, The Johns Hopkins University Press.

57 Novick, S.: The careless atom, Boston, 1969, Houghton Mifflin Co.

58 *Odum, E. P.: Fundamentals of ecology, ed. 2, Philadelphia, 1959, W. B. Saunders Co.

59 Odum, E. P.: Ecology, New York, 1963, Holt, Rinehart & Winston, Inc.

60 Packard, V.: The waste makers, New York, 1964, Pocket Books.

61 Shepard, P., and McKinley, D., editors: The subversive science, Boston, 1968, Houghton Mifflin Co.

62 Smith, G., and Smyth, J. C., editors: The biology of affluence, Edinburgh, 1972, Oliver & Boyd, Ltd.

63 Teilhard de Chardin, P.: The future of man, New York, 1964, Harper & Row, Publishers.

64 Thomas, W. L., Jr., editor: Man's role in changing the face of the earth, Chicago, 1956, University of Chicago Press.

65 Toynbee, A.: Surviving the future, New York, 1971, Oxford University Press, Inc.

66 *Turk, A., and others: Ecology, pollution, environment, Philadelphia, 1972, W. B. Saunders Co.

67 Udall, S. L.: The quiet crisis, New York, 1963, Holt, Rinehart & Winston, Inc.

68 U. S. Department of Health, Education and Welfare, Public Health Service: Smoking and health, Washington, D. C., 1964, U. S. Government Printing Office.

69 *U. S. Department of Health, Education and Welfare, Environmental Health Service/Public Health Service: Environmental health problems, Washington, D. C., 1970, U. S. Government Printing Office.

70 *U. S. Department of Interior: Man . . . an endangered species? Conservation yearbook no. 4, Washington, D. C., 1968, U. S. Government Printing Office.

71 U. S. Public Health Service: Today and tomorrow in air pollution, Publication no. 1555, Washington, D. C., 1966, U. S. Government Printing Office.

72 *Woodwell, G. N.: Toxic substances and ecological cycles, Sci. Am. **216**:24-31, March 1967.

73 World Health Organization: World health statistics report, **22**:448-476, 1969.

74 World Health Organization: Global environmental health monitoring, Geneva, 1970, The Organization.

4 Maintaining the body's defenses against harmful factors in the external environment

External defenses
Internal defenses against invasion by pathogens
Internal defenses against foreign proteins
Internal defenses against stressors in the environment
Internal defenses against inadequate food, water, and
  oxygen supplies
Internal defenses against temperature changes in the external
  environment

■ Since the turn of the century, great strides have been made in the prevention and treatment of disease and disability. This progress has been made possible by application of the results of epidemiologic investigations. *Epidemiology* is the study of the patterns of health and disease in man. The factors that influence the occurrence and distribution of health, disease, defects, disabilities, and deaths among groups are sought and analyzed. Attempts are made to discover which population groups and which individuals in the group are affected, what the causative agent is, and under what environmental circumstances the disease or disability becomes prevalent. Although epidemiology started as the study of infectious disease, epidemiologists are now studying many noninfectious conditions such as cancer, heart disease, accidents, and the effects of environmental pollution. With increased knowledge about the causative agents of disease, how they act on the host (person afflicted), and how the host responds (body reaction), much medical

■ STUDY QUESTIONS

1 What is a normal white blood count? Distinguish between the various types of white blood cells. What is the normal proportion of each? What are the main functions of the polymorphonuclear leukocytes?

2 In disease, what is the significance of leukocytosis? Of leukopenia? Study the laboratory findings of a patient who is or has been acutely ill; compare repeated white blood count reports. What treatments or circumstances appear to have contributed to these changes?

3 What is the therapeutic action of aspirin? What untoward side effects does it have? When is it contraindicated?

4 Review the procedure for an alcohol sponge bath, a sterile dressing, and a blood transfusion.

5 Where are the sympathetic and parasympathetic nervous systems located in relation to the central nervous system, and how are they linked to it? What functions are controlled by the autonomic nervous system?

6 Describe the appearance and actions of a frightened person. Describe your own physical and emotional state when you have been frightened or anxious.

7 Distinguish between epinephrine and norepinephrine. Where in the body are these hormones produced? What is the effect of each? Review the commonly used drugs containing these hormones.

8 How is oxygen transported in the blood? What is the mechanism that comes into action when the blood oxygen level is low?

9 What is the normal oxygen concentration of the air? What is the normal atmospheric pressure? As the atmospheric pressure decreases, what happens to the oxygen availability? Review the physical laws relating to the pressure of gases (Dalton's law, Boyle's law, and the law of solubility of gases).

10 What nutrients are essential for life? Which ones are stored by the body? What essential body functions require expenditure of water?

treatment has changed from palliative to curative.

Increased knowledge of the effect of environment on the host, as well as on biologic agents that attack the host, has made possible the discovery and institution of many measures for prevention and control. At the same time increased world population, urbanization, increased mobility of people, decreased levels of acquired immunity, and increased resistance to antibiotics and insecticides have created new epidemiologic problems. These problems are presently being studied in an attempt to plan appropriate control measures.[43]

Since it usually is easier and more economical to prevent a disease or disability than to cure or correct it, the nurse should become familiar with current epidemiologic knowledge about the cause and prevention of disease and disability. This knowledge should be applied in all aspects of nursing practice, including the teaching of others. Because of the rapidly expanding knowledge in this field, the nurse needs to be constantly alert to new insights into the relationship between agent-host and environment. The nurse also should be able to identify areas in need of further research.

Disease or disability may be caused by *external* or *internal* agents. The external agents may be classified as *biologic* (living matter such as bacteria, viruses, fungi, worms, or insects), *chemical* (poisons), *nutritional* (excesses or deficiencies in diet), *mechanical* (surgery, accidents), or *physical* (exposure to excess heat, cold, or radiation). The internal agents may be classified as *genetic* (anomalies or hormonal, metabolic, or glandular deficiencies), *physiologic* (structural changes due to aging or the body's response to other disease processes), or *psychologic* (structural or physiologic changes due to psychosomatic response). In studying each disease process the nurse should try to classify the causative agents. An ability to identify the causative agents will enable the nurse to incorporate preventive measures in nursing practice.

Much preventive nursing care is concerned with maintenance of the body's defenses against harmful factors in the external environment. The body has built-in mechanisms to protect it from the constantly changing and frequently hazardous external environment. Although some of the defenses are structural parts of the body, many are adaptive processes. To exist, all living matter must constantly adapt to its environment, which consists not only of inanimate matter (air, water, soil, cars, houses) but of living matter (people, other animals, insects, plants, microorganisms). This adaptation is a purposeful adjustment and is necessary to maintain the integrity of the organism. The remainder of this chapter will deal with the body's defense mechanisms against environmental factors that attack it physically, the results of failure to adapt to the attack, and the treatment then instituted to modify or to supplement them. Chapter 7 deals with the psychologic defense system. Maintenance of the internal environment in a homeostatic state also involves body defense against changes in its equilibrium. These changes usually are brought about originally by factors in the external environment. This aspect will be discussed in the following chapter.

■ EXTERNAL DEFENSES
Skin

The skin is the first line of defense against injury and disease. If the skin is intact and its glands secrete normally, pathogenic bacteria cannot enter the body through it. The skin also protects the delicate tissues of the body from injury by such external forces as heat, cold, and trauma.

The normal acid secretion of the skin (pH 5.5) tends to inhibit the growth of disease-producing microorganisms (pathogens). Bacteria that are normally present on the skin (resident bacteria) are usually nonpathogenic. Staphylococci are the exception. Of the transient organisms, only the bacilli causing anthrax and tularemia are able to live or multiply in the acid flora of the skin.

Resident bacteria, including staphylococci, however, are present on the skin in great numbers. They penetrate the hair follicles and the glands of the skin, and perspiration continuously brings them to the surface. Scrubbing with soap and water removes only the surface bacteria. The skin, therefore, can never be considered sterile (free from all organisms). For this reason, in addition to thoroughly scrubbing the hands, sterile gloves are worn and sterile instruments are used to prevent contamination during surgical aseptic procedures.

Thorough hand washing, by its mechanical action, is effective in decreasing the number of bacteria on the skin. Shaving the hair to which bacteria cling also tends to reduce their numbers. The use of bacteriostatic soaps containing hexachlorophene such as hexachlorophene liquid soap (pHisoHex) and of disinfectants such as 70% isopropyl alcohol and povidone-iodine (Betadine) to cleanse the skin prevents rapid multiplication of bacteria remaining on the skin. Recent evidence regarding the toxic effects of hexachlorophene on the nervous system has altered its use. The Federal Drug Administration (FDA) has recommended restrictions in its use in certain areas with the exception of practices involving its use for routine hand washing. These agents are all effective supplements to the body's defenses because a few pathogens gaining entrance to the body are more likely to be destroyed by the body's internal defenses than are large numbers of them.

Sensory receptors (touch, pain, pressure, heat, cold) are located in the skin. These receptors are protective mechanisms against injury because they warn the person against continued contact with dangerous external forces. The responses to the sensations, however, are learned, and their effectiveness depends on mental maturation and consciousness. They are ineffectual in infants and young children and in the unconscious patient. For this defense mechanism to operate, neural pathways, along which the sensations are carried to the spinal column and the brain, must be functioning. Consequently, persons with diseased or absent nerve pathways will not be protected. The acuity of these sensations also decreases with aging. In the absence of fully functioning sensory receptors in the skin, compensatory measures to avoid contact with dangerous external forces must be taken by the person or by others for him.

Melanin (skin pigment) screens out some of the burning rays of the sun and thus acts as a protective agent. However, since people have varying amounts of melanin in the skin, it is not a universally protective mechanism, and it needs to be supplemented as necessary with the use of protective lotions and with the use of caution in exposure to sunshine.

Mucous membranes

Mucous membranes protect the eyes and line all parts of the body that have external openings. When intact, the mucous membranes, like the skin, are impervious to bacteria. They also contain some sensory receptors. In addition, their secretions may deter the growth of bacteria, and the cilia along the membranes of the nose and respiratory tract tend to sweep bacteria and other foreign material out of the body. Mucous membranes also are highly vascular, so that internal defenses are readily available to destroy bacteria gaining entrance through them. The danger of bacterial invasion through the mucous membranes is greatest when they are dry and the person is chilled, because dryness causes cracking and chilling causes the superficial blood vessels to constrict.

The eyes

The eyes, including the conjunctivae, are protected from the entrance of bacteria and particles of dirt by the lids and eyelashes. Foreign material that gains entrance tends to be washed out by tears. The blinking reflex also protects the eyes against damage by shutting out foreign material and bright light. In the absence of these protective devices, special care must be instituted to protect the eyes (p. 189).

Nose, mouth, throat, and respiratory system

The nose and mouth normally contain many pathogens such as streptococci and pneumococci. Usually these organisms are not harmful since most pathogens that enter through the mouth are washed back into the throat by saliva, swallowed, and destroyed by the gastric secretions. Bacteria and other foreign material that are inhaled into the nose are usually blocked by the cilia in the anterior nasal passages. If they succeed in passing through this barrier, the mucous secretions of the nose move the bacteria into the nasopharynx, where they are swallowed and destroyed by gastric secretions. Pathogenic organisms are unlikely to gain entrance to the body through the nose, mouth, or throat unless there is a break in the mucous membrane. Although mouthwashes, gargles, and irrigations with antiseptic solutions decrease the number of organisms in the mouth and throat slightly for a limited time, their effectiveness is very minimal.

Occasionally bacteria and other minute particles of foreign material from the nose and throat are aspirated into the lungs instead of being swallowed. If this happens, the movement of the cilia and mucous secretions normally propels them forward into the pharynx, where they are expectorated or swallowed. The cough reflex prevents aspiration of large particles of foreign material into the lungs. The person must be conscious for this mechanism to be effective. It also is less effective in the very young, the very old, and the debilitated. In these circumstances, special care must be taken (p. 187).

The greatest threat of pathogens in the nose, mouth, throat, and respiratory system is the spread of the organisms of one person to others who are susceptible because of age, wounds, or debility. To prevent the spread of bacteria from the nose and throat, people are taught to cover the nose and mouth when sneezing or coughing and to blow the nose and expectorate into disposable handkerchiefs. A dry mask worn over the nose and mouth helps to decrease the spread of bacteria to others. Acceptable types of masks are described on p. 315. Masks are worn during surgical aseptic procedures and while caring for burned patients to decrease the possibility of introducing organisms from the nose and throat into the wounds. A damp mask incubates bacteria and increases their numbers and their spread. When there is known respiratory disease, a mask worn by the patient may prevent spread of infectious organisms to others.

When the gastric acidity is low, special precautions need to be taken to avoid introducing organisms through the nose and mouth because they may not be destroyed in the stomach. Since infants have a low gastric acidity, bottles and nipples used for feeding them and equipment used to prepare their formulas are sterilized. Hands should be washed thoroughly before feeding or handling a baby. Sometimes masks are worn by persons caring for an infant to prevent pathogens from their nose and throat from passing to him. This latter precaution is not necessary for the mother or family members to take unless they have an upper respiratory infection. The baby has antibodies that were passed to him from his mother through the placenta. They usually protect him against organisms normally found in the nose and throat of persons in his family. Because of these antibodies, unless the mother has a communicable disease, breast-feeding probably exposes the infant to fewer organisms to which he has no resistance than other means of feeding him. Special precautions to avoid ingestion of large numbers of organisms orally should also be observed by adults who for any reason have low gastric acidity.

Gastrointestinal tract, urinary tract, and vagina

If pathogens get through the stomach into the upper gastrointestinal tract, many of them are destroyed by the proteolytic enzymes or the alkaline bile. However, pathogens such as typhoid and paratyphoid bacilli, the virus that causes infectious hepatitis, and *Entamoeba histolytica,* which causes amebic dysentery, enter through the mouth and are unaffected by the gastric or intestinal secretions. In fact, they set up infection in the bowel and use it as their portal of exit from the body. The bowel is the natural habitat of some pathogens such as *Escherichia coli* and *Clostridium perfringens.* Although these organisms do not produce disease in the bowel, they may be transported in the feces to areas of the body that are favorable for their growth and multiplication and set up infection there. *Clostridium perfringens,* the causative agent of gas gangrene, produces disease only when it reaches sites with little oxygen such as deep wounds. *Escherichia coli* frequently causes infections of the urethra and bladder in women, and it may cause vaginal infections. Therefore after a bowel movement the anus should be cleansed away from the vagina and urethra.

Some pathogens also are normally present in the anterior urethra and some may leave the body through the kidneys. Unless they are very virulent, are massive in number, or are left in an obstructed kidney, ureter, or bladder, they rarely cause difficulty. The mucous lining of the urinary tract prevents their invasion of tissue, and normal urine flow from the upper urinary tracts and normal voiding washes them out. Trauma such as may occur in catheterization, however, may predispose to infection by these organisms, especially if the patient is not emptying his bladder completely when he voids. Practices that reduce the danger of infection from catheterization are described on p. 178.

Vaginal secretions contain acid, which usually destroys most pathogens entering the vagina. The spirochete and the gonococcus are notable exceptions. Vaginal secretions, however, are not present before puberty and they decrease in amount after the menopause. Young girls and older women, therefore, should be especially careful not to introduce organisms into the vagina (p. 510). Frequent use of vaginal douches tends to wash away the protective secretions.

If the hands are not washed after using the toilet, bacteria that exist in or pass through the bowel, urethra, or vagina may be transmitted via eating utensils or food to others. All employees of food establishments are required to have laboratory examinations of the stools before employment to determine whether they are carrying infectious organisms in the intestinal tract. The employer is responsible for providing approved toilet and hand-washing facilities and for insisting upon their proper use. All eating and drinking facilities and meat-handling establishments are inspected regularly by a health department sanitarian in an attempt to decrease the spread of infectious diseases by inadequate methods of cleansing utensils and other poor practices. The practice of hand washing after handling excreta, of course, also applies to the nurse. Patients should be taught this practice and provided with opportunities to carry it out during hospitalization.

Sheltered areas

All parts of the body without openings to the outside are considered "sheltered areas" and are normally free of any organisms. Internal defenses seem to be less effective in these parts. Therefore extreme caution needs to be used to prevent the introduction into or growth of organisms in areas such as the bloodstream, the spinal canal, the peritoneal cavity, and the bones.

■ INTERNAL DEFENSES AGAINST INVASION BY PATHOGENS

When the external defenses fail to prevent the injury of body tissues or their invasion by biologic agents, the internal defense mechanisms come into action. Pathogens may enter the body to cause primary disease or they may enter in the wake of other conditions. Staphylococci and streptococci frequently invade cells already damaged by other organisms, disease, or injury. *Clostridium perfringens* and *Clostridium tetani* always enter through traumatized tissues. Regardless of whether the invasion by pathogenic organisms is a primary or secondary condition, the body's defensive response is the same.

Inflammatory response

When cells are damaged by any kind of agent, there is an active local reaction of tissue to injury. This is called *inflammation.* The suffix *itis* is added to a combining word to indicate inflammation; for example, phlebitis means inflammation of a vein (phlebo). The inflammatory response is an attempt by the body to localize the effects of the injury and to overcome any invading bacteria. It is the first line of internal defense against invasion. The agent can be physical (heat or cold, radiant or radioactive rays, trauma), chemical (acids, bases, digestive juices), or biologic (microorganisms).

There are three major physiologic responses that occur during the inflammatory process: vascular response, fluid exudation, and cellular exudation. The *vascular response* consists of a transitory vasoconstriction (stress response) followed immediately by vasodilatation. This is thought to occur as a result of chemical substances such as histamine or kinins released at the site of injury or invasion. The amount of blood flow to the area is thus increased *(hyperemia),* causing redness and heat. As the capillaries dilate, there is increased permeability of the capillary walls facilitating fluid and cellular exudation. *Fluid exudation* from the capillaries into the interstitial spaces begins immediately and is most active during the first 24 hours after injury or invasion. Initially the fluid exudate is primarily serous fluid, but as the capillary wall becomes more permeable, protein (albumin) is lost into the interstitial spaces. This increases the colloid osmotic pressure in the interstitial spaces, which encourages more fluid exudation. The swelling of the tissue from the fluid in the interstitial spaces is called *edema* (p. 353). *Cellular exudation* refers to the migration of white blood cells (leukocytes) through the capillary walls into the affected tissue. An increased number of white blood cells are attracted to the vessels in the affected area, adhere to the capillary wall, and then pass ameboid fashion through the widened endothelial junctions of the capillary wall. Neutrophils (polymorphonuclear leukocytes), which comprise about 60% of the circulating white blood cells, are the first leukocytes to respond, usually within the first few hours. The neutrophils ingest the bacteria and dead tissue cells *(phagocytosis);* then they die, releasing proteolytic enzymes that liquefy the dead neutrophils, dead bacteria, and other dead cells (pus). Monocytes and lymphocytes appear later. The monocytes continue the phagocytosis and the lymphocytes play a role in the antigen-antibody response (p. 77).

The five cardinal symptoms of inflammation were identified many centuries ago. These are redness *(rubor)* and heat *(calor)* due to the hyperemia, swelling *(tumor)* due to the fluid exudate, pain *(dolor)* due to the pressure of the fluid exudate and to chemical (bradykinin) irritation of the nerve endings, and loss of function of the affected part due to the swelling and pain.

The inflammatory response serves to prepare the tissue for healing or to contain the spread of bacterial invasion. To prevent the spread of bacteria, fibroblasts are attracted to the area and secrete fibrin, a threadlike substance that encircles the affected area to wall it off from healthy tissue. If there is interference with this walling-off process, bacteria can spread into the surrounding tissue. This explains why an abscess should not be incised and drained until it has "come to a head" or until the walling-off process is completed.

Bacteria may fail to be contained locally and spread to other parts of the body by means of the lymph system or bloodstream. If picked up by the lymph stream, the bacteria will be carried to the nearest lymph node. These nodes are located along the course of all lymph channels, and here, too, bacteria can be ingested and destroyed. If the bacteria are virulent enough to resist the action in the lymph nodes, leukocytes are brought in by the bloodstream to attack and engulf the bacteria in the node. The node then becomes swollen and tender because of the accumulation of phagocytes, bacteria, and destroyed lymphoid tissue. This is known as *lymphadenitis.* Swollen lymph nodes can be palpated primarily in the neck, axilla, and groin.

If bacteria spread from the local site into the bloodstream *(bacteremia),* they can be ingested by tissue macrophages (large phagocytic cells) that are located along the course of the blood vessels in the spleen, liver, lungs, bone marrow, and adrenal glands. These cells function similarly to lymph nodes and will engulf and digest bacteria, dead cells, and foreign particles in the bloodstream. When bacteria are present, growing and producing toxins in the bloodstream, the infection is called *septicemia.* Bacteria circulating in the bloodstream may lodge at points distant to the original site of infection and cause a *secondary infection.* This is the process by which infections such as bacterial endocarditis and pyelonephritis occur.

Certain pathogenic bacteria can produce chemical substances called *toxins* that can be disseminated by the bloodstream to other parts of the body, producing a toxic effect on distant cells. Toxins destroy cells by interfering with enzyme activity. The toxins of hemolytic streptococci, producing symptoms of a "strep throat," may cause complications such as rheumatic fever or glomerulonephritis. The heart can be damaged by the toxin produced by the bacteria that cause diphtheria. The systemic reaction caused by the absorption of toxins in the bloodstream is called *toxemia.*

Moderate to severe inflammatory responses can produce generalized systemic effects. Products from the breakdown of bacteria can affect the temperature-regulating center in the hypothalamus and produce fever. A severe infection without an accompanying fever may suggest a poor prognosis. Loss of appetite (anorexia) and fatigue may be due to conservation of body energy needed to resist the infection. The body increases the production of white blood cells to help fight the infection and *leukocytosis* (serum white blood cell levels greater than 10,000/mm.³) may occur. With infection there is also an increased blood sedimentation rate; that is, when an anticoagulant is added to the blood in the laboratory, the red blood cells settle to the bottom of a test tube more rapidly than normal. This increase in the sedimentation rate is believed to be caused by an increase in fibrinogen (a blood protein essential to the healing process). The sedimentation rate is elevated during the acute inflammatory stage of infection. Its elevation is an indication that the body's defense mechanism for the repair of damaged tissue is operating. Because the sedimentation rate gradually returns to normal as tissues heal, it also is used to determine when physical activity can be safely resumed following an acute infection.

Inflammations can be classified as *acute* or *chronic.* Acute inflammations are characterized by a sudden onset and an increase in the fluid exudative response. Chronic inflammations have a slower more insidious onset and are characterized by increased cellular exudation.

Knowledge of the physiologic changes that occur during the inflammatory process helps the nurse to understand the changes that occur in a wide variety of diseases. For example, whenever cells die as a result of injury or disease *(necrosis)* such as during a myocardial infarction (p. 343), the inflammatory process will occur. Fat deposits (atheromas) on blood vessel walls cause injury to the lining of the vessel wall and initiate an inflammatory response. Irritation of the peritoneum by trauma or bacterial invasion can cause inflammation of the peritoneum *(peritonitis)*. Bacteria that can cause disease *(pathogenic)* may resist the body's defense mechanisms, multiply, and spread from the portal of entry to produce a continued stimulus for an inflammatory response in susceptible tissue. Infectious diseases are those caused by pathogenic bacteria (p. 308).

There are several factors relating to the agent per se, the invasiveness of the agent, or the host that determine the severity or extent of an inflammatory response. If the agent is a pathogenic microorganism, the degree of each factor determines the *infectivity potential.* Factors relating to the agent per se are strength *(virulence),* number, and nature of the agent. Different pathogenic microorganisms produce different effects on the host. Pyogenic bacteria usually produce fever and leukocytosis. Virus infections are characterized by increased fluid exudation. Certain diseases such as German measles (rubella) are usually mild, while measles (rubeola) can produce severe reactions. Factors relating to the invasiveness of the agent are the duration of the exposure or the ability of the agent to reach the host and the portal of entry or ability of the agent to enter the host. Some bacteria such as streptococci can produce inflammation through any portal of entry to the body; other bacteria such as gonococci produce inflammation only when entry is at a specific site such as the genitourinary tract or eyes of the newborn.

Several factors determine the ability of the host to respond to injury or invasion:

1. *Age.* Both extremes of age (the infant and the aged) are the groups most susceptible to infection. Infants have not yet built up immunity factors. The elderly have decreased lymphoid tissue and decreased antibody formation. The young adult or middle-aged person has increased resistance to infection but may have an increased reaction when infection does occur.

2. *Nutrition.* Individuals who are malnourished do not have reserve stores for energy consumption. Excess energy is expended during fevers (p. 135). When cells break down (catabolism), nitrogen is lost. Nitrogen loss that exceeds nitrogen intake is called *negative nitrogen balance.* White blood cells and fibroblasts are composed primarily of protein, the basis of which is nitrogen. For the body to produce sufficient quantities of these cells to resist infection, additional protein is needed. Nitrogen is also needed in wound healing; therefore a malnourished individual will have decreased resistance to infection.

3. *Adequacy of blood supply.* Tissue affected during inflammation needs sufficient blood to supply the fluid exudate to dilute the toxins, white blood cells and fibroblasts to fight infection, and oxygen and nutrients to promote healing. If the blood supply is decreased through vascular disease (p. 385) or shock, the inflammatory process is impeded.

4. *Availability of white blood cells.* If the number of leukocytes is below normal *(leukopenia)* or if there is an increased number of immature cells such as occurs in leukemia, the ability of phagocytes to ingest offending organisms is lessened.

5. *Antigen-antibody response.* The ability of the host to resist foreign protein depends on the autoimmune mechanism of the host (p. 234). The presence of specific antibodies or antitoxins will decrease the inflammatory response.

6. *Hormonal influences.* The hormones of the adrenal cortex have an anti-inflammatory effect. Individuals who have increased production of the corticosteroids (p. 762) or who are receiving corticosteroid therapy (p. 82) are more susceptible to infection.

Symptoms of infectious disease caused by biologic agents do not appear until enough cells have been damaged to cause a generalized systemic reaction. The period between entry of the pathogens into the body and the appearance of symptoms is called the *incubation period.* Pathogens that localize at the site of entry have short incubation periods, while those that must be transported for a distance from the portal of entry to the site of tissue invasion usually have longer incubation periods.

Signs and symptoms vary according to the portal

of entry and the specific tissues finally invaded by the pathogen. Often symptoms appear in two stages. The symptoms related to involvement of tissues at the portal of entry appear and then subside, only to be followed several days later by symptoms produced by damage of cells in the specific tissues invaded. Localized invasion of skin or soft tissues produces symptoms of local inflammation (p. 74). Invasion of the respiratory tract produces symptoms of an upper respiratory infection, with increased mucous secretions (catarrhal exudate) and congestion. Invasion of the gastrointestinal tract produces nausea, vomiting, and diarrhea. Invasion of the central nervous system produces severe headache and stiff neck. Invasion of muscle may cause muscle pain, weakness, or spasms. Microorganisms producing toxins frequently cause skin rash, high fever, and chills. Symptoms of general malaise, anorexia, dull headache, and generalized aching usually occur when there is widespread tissue involvement, as in viral infections such as influenza.

Antigen-antibody response

Pathogens and their toxins are foreign proteins, and the body has a mechanism for dealing with any foreign protein (antigen) that invades it. This mechanism is a very effective second line of defense against pathogenic organisms.

As the cells of the body come into contact with sufficient amounts of any specific foreign protein, they become sensitized to it and produce a chemical substance that tends to reject the protein by repelling or damaging it in some way. The chemical substances that are formed in response to pathogens are called antibodies; those formed in response to toxins are called antitoxins. The antibody or antitoxin for each type of pathogen is specific. The antibodies enable the phagocytes to engulf organisms. The antibody may cause the organisms to stick together in clumps (agglutinate), or to break up (lyse), or it may coat the organisms or prevent their reproduction. The antitoxin neutralizes the toxin released by the pathogen. The process is known as the antigen-antibody response, and it occurs in the lymphoid tissue. It is by this mechanism that infecting organisms finally are overcome by the body.

Antigens gain access to the body and are processed by the reticuloendothelial system. The principal cells involved in the formation of antibodies and antitoxins are the macrophages, lymphocytes, and plasma cells. On the surface of the antigens are specific patterns of atoms designated as antigenic determinants. It is postulated that these natural patterns of atoms direct the reactions of the antigen with the macrophages, lymphocytes, and plasma cells causing changes in the molecular structure and resulting in the synthesis of antibodies and antigens. The resulting changes from this process may be temporary or permanent

and provide resistance to the specific pathogen, which is known as active immunity.

Antibodies and antitoxins remain in the blood for varying periods of time, and as long as they are present they provide protection for the person against a repeated attack from the specific organism. When the antibodies form in response to disease, the process is called natural active acquired immunity. If the molecular structure or the pattern of the cells remains permanently changed, the patient remains immune. This condition is called permanent active immunity. Even when a permanent change in molecular structure does occur in the cell, periodic contact with small numbers of the organism seems to be needed to maintain continued effectiveness of antibodies. A permanent immunity against diseases that cause antibody production and appear endemically (some of the population having the disease every few years) is usually maintained in this manner. Immunity acquired for common childhood diseases is an example.

Methods have been developed to artificially inject certain pathogens or their toxins into the body to stimulate active antibody production without disease. This is called artificially acquired active immunity. It is used to enhance the body defenses against disease-producing organisms. The use of this method is discussed on p. 311.

The young child seems to be best equipped to acquire natural active immunity. He is old enough to withstand infection, and the level of his histamine response, although high enough to stimulate the internal defenses against infection, is also low enough so that symptoms are rarely severe. Consequently, it is considered a good practice to begin to expose the preschool child to the usual environment in which he will live. He should not be intentionally exposed to known disease, but isolation of the child in his home environment should be avoided. Artificially immunizing the child against diseases that might cause serious complications, as well as seeing that he receives natural acquired immunity, is recommended (p. 312).

Studies show that people who have grown up in crowded and unhygienic conditions seem to be less prone to attack by many of the more common infecting organisms than are those whose living conditions have been better.[9] For example, draftees to the armed services who have lived in rural areas are more prone to develop influenzal diseases soon after induction than are their city compatriots. Before the advent of vaccine against poliomyelitis, many children living under slum conditions were less susceptible to the virus that causes poliomyelitis than were rural or suburban children living in more hygienic surroundings.

Natural active immunity sometimes is inherited and does not require actual contact by the body with a pathogen. This is known as *natural immunity* and is thought to be genetically determined. It probably accounts for the resistance of certain species, races, or individuals to specific diseases. In the study of many diseases, absence of this resistance factor is of more concern than its presence. For example, its absence apparently influences the increased susceptibility or tendency of certain persons to such diseases as tuberculosis. Susceptibility to such noninfectious diseases as cancer, coronary artery disease, and diabetes mellitus apparently is also genetically determined.

In *passive immunity,* antibodies against specific pathogens are present in the bloodstream, but the person has not produced them himself. Therefore their effectiveness is *temporary.* In infants this kind of immunity is accomplished by a natural mechanism. Antibodies pass through the placental membrane into the infant's bloodstream prior to birth and protect the infant from many of the common infections and communicable diseases (provided that the mother has an active immunity to them) up to the age of approximately 6 months. Other types of passive immunity are acquired by injecting human or other animal serum containing antibodies against specific pathogens into the bloodstream of a person who has been exposed to the disease. This is an emergency measure to supplement the body's defense mechanism, and the effects are temporary. The use of passive immunization is discussed further on p. 312.

The healing process

No healing will occur until infection has subsided and pus and dead tissue have been removed. Pus is a local accumulation of dead phagocytes, dead bacteria, and dead tissue. The bacteria most commonly causing this reaction are the staphylococci, streptococci, and *Pseudomonas aeruginosa (pyocyanea).* A collection of pus that is localized by a zone of inflamed tissue is called an *abscess* (Fig. 4-1). An inflammation that involves cellular or connective tissue is called *cellulitis,* whereas an inflammation in which pus collects in a preexisting cavity such as the pleura or gallbladder is called *empyema.* When infection forms an abscess within the body, develops a suppurating channel, and ruptures onto the surface or into a body cavity, it is called a *sinus.* If the infection forms a tubelike passage from an epithelium-lined organ or normal body cavity to the surface or to another organ or cavity, it is called a *fistula* (Fig. 4-1).

After the infected area is clean, new cells are produced to fill in the space left by the injury. They may be the normal structural cells or they may be fibrotic tissue cells known as *scar tissue.* If they are fibrotic cells, they will not function as formerly but only serve to fill in the injured area. Some body cells

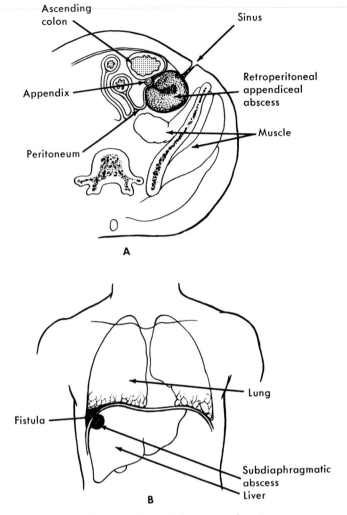

FIG. 4-1. A, Cross section of the torso showing an appendiceal abscess with a sinus that has developed through the abdominal wall. **B,** Subdiaphragmatic abscess that has developed a fistula opening into the pleural cavity.

readily regenerate; for instance, after the bowel has healed, it is almost impossible to find the injured area. The respiratory tract also regenerates its tissues readily. Liver tissue has the capacity to regenerate its tissue, but over a longer period of time. Some nerve cells are always replaced with fibrous tissue. If a large amount of tissue is destroyed, structural cells may not be replaced, regardless of the type of tissue.

When little scar tissue is produced, the process is called *healing by first intention.* This type of healing usually occurs in a clean, incised wound that is sutured. The edges of the injured tissue become connected by shreds of fibrin, a thin layer of blood clot, and a crust of dry, protective plasma. Within 3 days, fibroblasts multiply and grow across the gap while leukocytes, blood, and lymph continue to remove the debris. Collagen fibrils are then formed to replace the fibrin, and the injured area is quickly filled with granulation tissue composed of new capillaries, fibroblasts, and collagen fibers. Meanwhile, cells typical of the tissue bridge the gap from each side of the wound. As the fibrous connective tissue increases in amount, shrinkage of this tissue occurs and the scar increases in strength. The rapidity with which healing occurs is influenced by the maintenance of a good blood supply, adequate lymph drainage, a high-protein diet, and a continuous supply of vitamin C.

When there is excessive loss of tissue and the skin edges cannot be brought together, healing by granulation must occur. This process is called *healing by second intention.* It is similar to healing by first intention, but it takes longer because a large area must be filled with granulation tissue. The scar from healing by second intention is usually large and appears uneven. If it involves skin or any other tissue that normally contains nerve endings, it will be numb. As the healing progresses and the scar tissue shrinks, contraction of surrounding tissue may occur and lead to malfunction and deformity.

Some people, especially those with brown or black skin, are prone to excessive scar formation. Such tissue formation, known as a *keloid,* is hard and shiny in appearance and may enlarge to a surprising degree. It may cause disfigurement or undergo malignant degeneration and for this reason is usually excised surgically. Serous membranes sometimes become adherent during inflammatory and healing processes, and as the inflammation subsides, fibrous tissue forms, holding the membranes together. This fibrous tissue is called an *adhesion.* Adhesions may occur in the pleura, the pericardium, about the pelvic organs, and in many other parts of the body. They often occur in and about the intestinal tract, where they may cause an obstruction.

Instead of healing, there may be necrosis, or death of the tissue. Bacteria, both pathogens and nonpathogens, often invade the necrotic tissue and cause putrefaction (decomposition), which is called *gangrene.* The body defenses are useless in preventing or curing gangrene because no blood can get to the area. Gangrenous tissue must be completely removed before healing can occur.

Principles basic to invasion by pathogens

The nurse needs to understand the principles that make invasion of human beings by pathogens possible. The following principles are basic to the prevention of both local and generalized infections and to their spread. They underlie medical asepsis (isolation and reverse precautions) and surgical asepsis.

1. The greater the number of microorganisms (both pathogenic and nonpathogenic), the greater the possibility of infection.
2. By genetic mutation a microorganism can change from a nonpathogen to a pathogen, or

a pathogenic organism may become more viable or more virulent. (Since microorganisms multiply at an exceedingly rapid rate, mutations frequently occur.)
3. Desirable conditions for growth (available food supply, warmth, moisture, and an appropriate supply of oxygen and light) increase the number of pathogens.
4. The number of susceptible hosts and the passage of time tend to increase the virulence of organisms because their numbers increase.
5. The more virulent the pathogen, the more serious the disease is likely to be.
6. Resistance of a host to a pathogen usually increases with contact with it, because antibodies against the pathogen are produced.
7. A pathogen with which the host is unfamiliar is likely to produce disease.
8. A host with lowered body defenses against infectious organisms is more likely to contract infection.

Surgical asepsis. The purpose of surgical asepsis is to prevent as many organisms as possible from entering the body during procedures that require perforation or incision through the skin or mucous membranes that usually protect these areas. All materials that are used in these procedures are sterilized (made free of all organisms). The patient is further protected from infection by the following practices. In the operating room, caps and masks must be worn by everyone, since the hair, nose, and throat are sources of airborne pathogens. Shoe covers should also be worn. The surgeon, his assistants, and the scrub nurse take special precautions to ensure the safety of the patient by scrubbing their hands and forearms for a prescribed period of time. The routine for this scrub is variable but essentially involves the use of a sterile brush and one of the antiseptic detergent preparations (p. 72) containing hexachlorophene (pHisoHex) or one of the organic iodine detergents (Betadine). On completion of the scrub the hands and forearms are blotted dry with a sterile towel and the individual dons sterile gown and gloves. Usually the patient's skin has been scrubbed and shaved (p. 199) the day before surgery. After the patient has been anesthetized and positioned on the operating table, the operative site is cleansed to eliminate bacterial flora from the site. Preparations used for this procedure vary with each hospital and with the preference of the surgeon. They include antiseptic detergents that contain hexachlorophene or those that contain an iodine complex. Some surgeons prefer using antiseptic solutions without a detergent scrub. Antiseptic solutions in common use are tincture of Zephiran, Merthiolate, and IoPrep.

The field of operation is then draped with sterile towels, or one of many available adherent plastic films is applied directly to the skin. Large sterile cloths or disposable paper drapes are placed so as to provide a wide sterile area around the proposed field of operation. Sterile supplies that may be needed during the surgical procedure are brought to the scrub nurse or technician by the circulating nurse. The circulating nurse wears appropriate surgical attire but is not scrubbed, and therefore is free to procure sterile supplies, instruments, special equipment, and medications for the scrubbed members of the surgical team. Nurses in the operating room have a unique opportunity to provide the unconscious patient with expert nursing care at a most critical time.

Excessive talking and movement in the operating room should be discouraged because they increase spread of airborne pathogens. Obviously the environment of the entire operating room must be kept scrupulously clean. This involves thorough cleaning at the end of each operation. All linen, instruments, and supplies used during the procedure are removed and all movable equipment (operating table, buckets, instrument table, overhanging surgical lights, etc.) is washed with a germicidal detergent; the floor is "flooded" or mopped and then vacuumed dry. Periodically, operating rooms are cleaned thoroughly with a germicidal detergent. Fogging machines have replaced the manual scrubbing of walls and floors in the surgical suite. Germicidal detergents with a phenolic base such as Matar, Turgisol, and Ves-phene are commonly used.

The isolated patient. Medical asepsis (isolation of a patient) has one of two purposes—either to prevent spread of a pathogen from the infected patient to others or to protect the susceptible patient from pathogens carried by others or present in the environment. The principles basic to preventing spread of a pathogen from an infected patient are discussed on p. 314.

Reverse isolation precautions (also referred to as protective isolation) are used to protect the highly susceptible patient from pathogens. The patient is placed in a single room that should be thoroughly cleaned and aired prior to his admission. It often is fumigated with a bacteriostatic spray and left to air for 24 hours. This process may be repeated at 1- or 2-week intervals, but the repetition means moving the patient from room to room. Anyone entering the room wears a face mask and sometimes the hair is covered. The door to the room usually is kept closed, and traffic in and out of the room is kept at a minimum. No one with a known infection of any kind (local or generalized) should be allowed in the room. Anyone giving direct care to the patient should wash his hands thoroughly first and wear a freshly laundered (sometimes sterile) gown. In some instances only sterile bed linen is used. If possible, the patient is not transported to other areas of the hospital, but should this be necessary, he usually is asked to wear a face mask, and any open wounds are covered with a sealed dressing. His room should be kept free from dust. However, only damp dusting and mopping or vacuuming should be permitted.

Sometimes even stricter precautions are desired, and the patient may be placed in an *isolator* (Life Island)—a plastic tent that completely shields him from the environment (Fig. 4-2). The inside of the tent is rendered nearly microbe free, and the patient

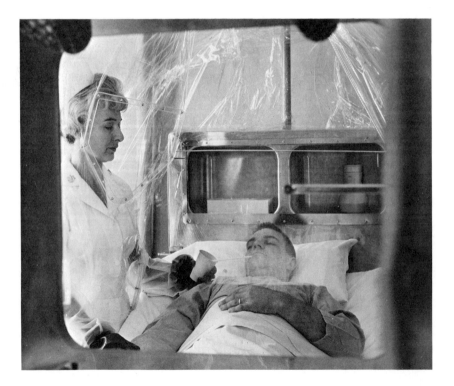

FIG. 4-2. The patient may be placed in an isolator (Life Island), or plastic tent, to completely shield him from the environment. (Courtesy Walter Reed Army Institute of Research; reprinted, with permission, from Ginsberg, M. K., and LaConte, M. L.: Am. J. Nurs. **64:**88-90, Sept. 1964.)

is bathed and his hair shampooed with soap containing hexachlorophene before he is placed in it. Only sterile materials are used in the tent, and they are passed through portholes (Fig. 4-3). Even the food is sterilized. The nursing and medical personnel work through gauntlets that protect the patient from their hands. This procedure has been completely described by Seidler.[60]

Social isolation is a form of sensory deprivation and anyone who is medically isolated is also socially isolated. Therefore the nurse must make plans to minimize social isolation. The patient and his family and friends need to understand why isolation is necessary. See the discussion of ways to overcome this problem on p. 298. Unless special care is taken, the patient of any age may undergo personality changes. The young child fails to develop at a normal rate, whereas the older child may revert to earlier patterns of social behavior that often persist after he returns home. Adolescent and adult patients sometimes become paranoid and may even have hallucinations or become delirious.*

If the patient is isolated from his physical environment for any length of time, he must be reintroduced to it carefully. He should be warned to avoid contact with persons who have a known infectious disease and to notify his physician if he develops any infection. Probably it is best if he does not have to

---

*For further information see Chodil, J. and Williams, B.: The concept of sensory deprivation, Nurs. Clin. North Am. 5:453-465, Sept. 1970.

be around school-age children, because they frequently are carriers of pathogens.

Management of the patient with an inflammation

Application of heat. Heat, applied locally, increases vasodilation in an inflamed area and thus augments the natural defense mechanism. Dry heat in the form of heat lamps or diathermy may be ordered, or moist heat in the form of warm compresses or soaks may be used. Many physicians prefer massive warm, moist packs because they insulate the part, preventing loss of body heat from the physiologically dilated vessels. Warm packs, however, may cause reflex vasoconstriction and decrease, instead of increase, the blood supply to the affected part. Hot applications are used rarely and with great caution for infants because their tender skin is easily burned. The temperature of the solution used for soaks should not be over 37.8° C. (100° F.). If moist compresses are used for long intervals on an extensive area such as an extremity in an infant or small child, the body temperature should be checked at least every 2 hours because a large percentage of the body area is exposed to extra heat and deprived of dissipation of heat. If the temperature rises, the compresses should be discontinued and the physician notified. Sterile procedures are not necessary unless there is an open lesion. These procedures are described in texts on fundamentals of nursing.

Application of cold. Vasoconstriction occurs when cold is applied to an area, thus decreasing the blood supply. In those instances when the inflammatory response is not desired, that is, when further tissue

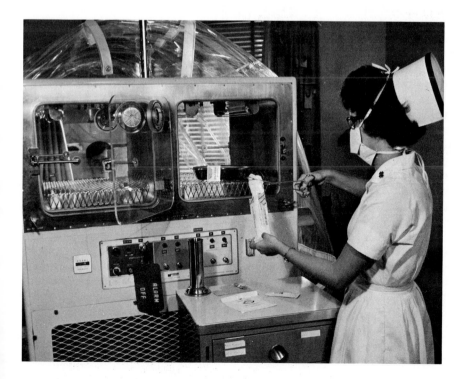

FIG. 4-3. Only sterile materials are used in the isolator. Here the nurse is passing sterile equipment through a porthole. (Courtesy National Institutes of Health, Bethesda, Md.; reprinted, with permission, from Seidler, F. M.: Am. J. Nurs. **65:**108-111, June 1965.)

damage or increased pain can occur because of the effect of the fluid exudate, application of cold rather than heat may be more effective. Examples of these situations are following trauma such as a sprained ankle or in acute bursitis in the initial phase when the increased fluid exudate creates pressure in the joint capsule. In some instances it is desirable to slow down the inflammatory process to prevent complications. Thus, if appendicitis is suspected, cold is applied to the lower abdomen to try to prevent rupture of the appendix with subsequent peritonitis and to aid in decreasing pain.

Corticosteroids. Because hormones produced by the adrenal cortex (corticosteroids) are anti-inflammatory agents, they are widely used to treat inflammation. The exact mechanism of action of the corticosteroids is unknown and investigators are constantly searching for new knowledge about them. The corticosteroids are not curative, but they do suppress the adaptive phenomena of the body to inflammation; therefore they are used to treat severe inflammatory conditions that are not self-limiting.

Corticosteroids may be administered systemically or topically and sometimes are injected into involved joints or into body cavities. The adrenocorticotropic hormone (corticotropin or ACTH) or one of the corticosteroids may be used. ACTH is used less commonly since it must be given parenterally and is only effective for those patients whose adrenal glands are capable of producing the adrenocortical steroids. The corticosteroids used to treat inflammation include cortisone and hydrocortisone and their many derivatives. Some of the more commonly used ones are prednisone (Meticorten), prednisolone (Meticortelone), methylprednisolone (Medrol), triamcinolone (Aristocort), paramethasone acetate (Haldrone), dexamethasone (Decadron), and betamethasone (Celestone). Paramethasone acetate is twice as potent as triamcinolone but is essentially devoid of mineralocorticoid activity. Dexamethasone and bethamethasone are 16 to 30 times more potent than cortisone itself and are often used to treat patients with a severe inflammatory reaction.[6] Because knowledge about the corticosteroids is increasing rapidly, new preparations are constantly becoming available to supplement or replace older ones. The nurse should keep informed about the latest developments by reading current literature from drug companies and by regular perusal of medical, nursing, and other scientific periodicals.

Because corticosteroids affect a wide variety of body functions (p. 761), their therapeutic uses are numerous, but their effects also make them potentially dangerous. They should be used only with the utmost care and discretion.

The nurse working with a patient receiving corticosteroids should know the functions of the body that are controlled by these hormones and be prepared to recognize and deal with untoward reactions and to prevent the disastrous effects of rapid withdrawal of the drugs. The preparation used may have the total effect of the adrenocortical hormones or it may have only a partial effect. Deoxycorticosterone (DOCA) is a mineralocorticoid primarily affecting the fluid and electrolyte (sodium and potassium) balance. Cortisone and hydrocortisone preparations are glucocorticoids exerting effects on glucose metabolism, electrolyte balance, lymphoid tissue, eosinophils, and fibroblasts and producing anti-inflammatory and antistress effects. Adrenocortical extract or corticotropin preparations produce full adrenocortical hormone effects—that is, the effects of deoxycorticosterone and cortisone plus gonadal hormone effects. The adrenogenic hormone, which is secreted by the adrenal cortex as well as by the testicles (testosterone), stimulates protein anabolism and has masculinizing effects. The estrogenic hormone, secreted by the adrenal cortex as well as by the ovary, exerts its effects on tissues reflecting secondary sex characteristics. Corticosteroids applied topically do not produce systemic effects unless they are used in large amounts in areas where they can be absorbed readily.

The nurse should watch all patients on corticosteroid therapy for side effects and untoward reactions and immediately report any early signs of these responses. If a patient is being cared for at home, he and/or his family should be taught to watch for the signs. Many of the side effects of this therapy, while unsightly and annoying, do not contraindicate therapy unless more severe untoward reactions occur. Some patients find they become quite "jittery" and may have difficulty sleeping; others feel euphoric. Usually these effects are self-limiting, but some patients may develop psychotic reactions. Therefore personality changes should be recorded carefully and reported. Some patients become very depressed. The typical "moon face" so often described in patients who are on corticosteroid therapy often changes the person's appearance noticeably. Since this change in appearance is related to fluid and electrolyte changes, it forewarns of the need for careful measurement of the serum sodium and potassium levels, but it rarely necessitates stopping treatment. Hirsutism in women and engorgement of mammary tissue in men are common but not serious side effects of adrenocortical extract, or ACTH.

To avoid his undue concern, any patient receiving systemic treatment with corticosteroids should be forewarned that at first he may feel nervous and overalert and may have difficulty sleeping. If this condition continues beyond 3 or 4 days or becomes worse, he should contact his physician. The patient on long-term therapy needs to be told about the "moon face," the hirsutism, and mammary gland changes. The patient often needs help in making an emotional adjustment to changes in physical appearance. He should be observed carefully for any signs of withdrawal from personal contacts or other personality changes that suggest difficulty. A woman who is at the climacteric and receiving ACTH should be told that the hormone may cause menstrual bleeding. Any change in the menses should be reported.

Serious untoward effects that require immediate attention may result from long-term treatment with corticosteroids. They can follow the use of either cortisone or ACTH. The patient may develop hypokalemia (low potassium content of the blood) and hypernatremia (excessive amount of sodium in the blood). Muscle weakness, cardiac arrhythmias, hypertension, edema (dependent and pulmonary), and neurologic symptoms suggest these conditions. He may develop diabetes mellitus due to interference with the body's use of insulin (see p. 745 for the symptoms). He also may show signs of tissue wasting due to increased protein catabolism. Wounds may fail to heal well, and old healed lesions such as peptic ulcer craters and the tubercle of primary tuberculosis (Ghon tubercle) may break down. New peptic ulcers may develop (see p. 665 for the symptoms). Eosinopenia and lymphopenia may develop. Because of these side effects, corticosteroids are rarely given for a long period to patients with histories of healed peptic ulcer, tuberculosis, heart failure, hypertension, cardiac arrhythmias, or blood dyscrasias. They are not used after surgery or for traumatic injury unless the patient has been on the drug previously and must be maintained on it postoperatively. If the nurse is aware of any circumstances that make the use of these drugs dangerous for the patient, the physician should be informed.

Today many people take drugs prescribed by various specialists, and the physician ordering the most recent drug may not be aware of other drugs being taken. Before the patient starts taking corticosteroids, the nurse should find out what other drugs he is taking and have him discuss them with his physician. The patient should also be instructed to inform any other physician who may be prescribing for him that he is taking corticosteroids. Adrenergic drugs (such as amphetamine) and psychic stimulants are definitely contraindicated because they increase the possibility of hypertension and manic states. Tranquilizers also may be undesirable due to their psychic effects. Corticosteroids may counteract the effects of antihypertensive drugs, and the two types of drugs should not be taken simultaneously without medical advice. Patients who are receiving estrogens or androgens may need the dosage of these drugs adjusted.

Because corticosteroids depress the inflammatory process and the production of lymphocytes, the body's first line of defense against invading pathogens, the patient on corticosteroid therapy must be carefully protected against infection. Frequently during hospitalization reverse isolation techniques are used. The patient should be told that reverse isolation protects him from exposure to others who may be carrying infectious organisms and why this protection is important. He should be advised that when he returns home he should minimize his exposure to crowds and his contact with persons who have colds and other infectious disorders. He also should avoid chilling and fatigue. If he sustains even slight cuts or injuries or develops any sign of infection, he should contact his physician at once. If infection does occur, antibiotics may be used. Several of the antibiotics, however, are contraindicated because of the side effects they may cause. For example, chloramphenicol (Chloromycetin) sometimes causes agranulocytosis (a depression of white blood cells), and monilial infections may result from chlortetracycline (Aureomycin). These side effects may produce serious consequences in a patient on corticosteroids because the hormone makes him more susceptible to infections.

When adrenocorticosteroids are being taken, sodium tends to be retained and to increase the retention of water in the body. Salt intake, therefore, is almost always restricted. The nurse should ask the physician about the patient who does not have an order for a low-sodium diet. Even if the patient is not to be on a special diet, the nurse should suggest that he avoid salty foods and use less salt than usual in food preparation. A diet high in potassium also may be ordered, and additional potassium may be given. The hospitalized patient on corticosteroids usually is on recorded intake and output. Daily weight and blood pressure may be taken, and usually a urinalysis is done at least once a week.

Systemic administration of adrenocorticosteroids suppresses the secretion of ACTH by the pituitary gland. Sudden withdrawal of the drug or a marked decrease in dosage may cause an acute adrenocortical hormone deficiency due to the failure of the inactivated pituitary hormone to take over effectively at once. This may precipitate addisonian crisis, which, if not treated immediately, can cause death from hypotension and vasomotor collapse. This condition and its management are described fully on p. 763. Hypoglycemia also may develop (p. 761). Adrenocortical hormones usually are discontinued gradually. The drug should not be discontinued for diagnostic tests without a specific order.

Every patient receiving systemic adrenocorticosteroids on an ambulatory basis should be warned of the serious consequences of omitting the drug and the need to take it at the prescribed intervals. The patient and his family should know the symptoms that may occur if the blood levels of the hormones are inadequate, and they should understand the need to seek immediate medical attention if these symptoms occur. The patient should carry an identification card giving his name and address, the drug he is taking, the name and address of his physician, and instructions as to what should be done in event of sudden injury or unconsciousness. Some patients on steroids wear Medic Alert bracelets.*

Because many corticosteroids are ulcerogenic, the patient should be instructed to take his medication after meals or with milk. Some patients will also be placed on antacid therapy.

Errors in giving corticosteroids to hospitalized patients and cancellation of orders when patients are transferred from one unit to another or when diagnostic tests or operations are scheduled can lead to serious consequences. Since one of the signs of adrenocortical deficiency is hypotension, it is apparent that this deficiency may affect adversely the postoperative course of a patient whose blood pressure may also be lowered by the operation. When patients are receiving the corticosteroids intravenously, the nurse must know what flow rate is necessary to maintain the desired blood level of the drug. If for any reason this flow rate cannot be maintained, the physician should be notified at once.

Corticosteroids rarely are given to infants and young children. If they are, special precautions should be taken. The infant and young child are likely to tolerate these medications poorly and should be watched carefully for untoward reactions. The younger the child, the shorter the time he can tolerate an untoward reaction. Therefore any signs of reaction should be noted promptly and treatment instituted at once.

Management of the patient with generalized infection

A generalized infection is one that causes widespread tissue sensitization and therefore a generalized histamine response. The patient usually has an elevation of temperature accompanied by hot, dry skin, coated tongue, rapid pulse, general malaise, anorexia, and chills. Profuse diaphoresis may occur. In severe infections with high fever, delirium also may develop. (See p. 156 for management of the delirious patient.) Because the central nervous system is less fully developed and less stable than in adulthood, convulsions are not uncommon in infants and young children who have an infection with a high fever. (See p. 878 for management of the patient who has convulsions.)

Symptoms of generalized infection are seen in many disorders. Symptomatic treatment, however, is similar regardless of the cause and will be discussed here. Management of specific infections with their specific symptoms are discussed in the appropriate chapters in Section 2 of this book.

*For further information see Fish, S. A.: Medic Alert, Nurs. Forum 8:428-431, 1969.

The patient with fever. Fever is an elevation of body temperature above normal. Fever that occurs as a result of infection may be intermittent or continue over several days. The chemical agents that give rise to a fever are classified as pyrogens. The fever is apparently due to the action of pyrogens on the thermoregulatory mechanisms in the hypothalamus. The result is that these regulatory mechanisms behave as if they were adjusted to maintain body temperature at a higher than normal level. Body dehydration also leads to an elevated temperature characterized as fever. The reverse is also true; fever causes dehydration because of the activity of the body defenses.

Certain nursing interventions should be taken to help the patient with a fever. A sponge bath helps dissipate body heat by increasing evaporation from the skin surface. To prevent or treat dehydration, every effort should be made to assist the patient to increase his fluid intake. Acetylsalicylic acid also helps to dissipate heat.

Although fever is an essential part of the defense mechanism, most physicians advise that a patient with a temperature over 38° C (100.4° F.) stay in bed, since his respiratory and pulse rates are increased. Usually he is permitted to get up to go to the bathroom. Because headache and irritability often accompany severe systemic infection with a high fever, the room should be kept quiet and lights dimmed. The patient should be encouraged to sleep. A warm sponge bath, a back rub, and a smooth bed may help to induce sleep. Frequent baths may be needed since more body wastes may be excreted through increased perspiration. Bathing also helps to dissipate body heat by increasing evaporation from the skin surface. To prevent drying of the mucous membranes of the mouth and nose, the patient should be provided with a lubricant such as cold cream with which to lubricate the anterior nasal passages and his lips. He should also be encouraged to brush his teeth several times a day and be urged to take a generous amount of fluids.

In an infection with an accompanying fever, toxins are often excreted through the kidneys, more fluid than usual is lost by evaporation from the skin and by the rapid respiration, and more fluids are needed for accelerated metabolic processes. The adult patient, therefore, usually is urged to take 2,500 to 3,000 ml. of fluid a day. Infants and children should be given smaller amounts. (See p. 123 for a detailed discussion of limitations and precautions to be observed in administering fluids to children and to certain adults.) In addition to water, fluids high in calories and containing vitamin C, protein, salt, and potassium, if not contraindicated by the disease, should be taken by the patient because they help to supply the body's metabolic and electrolyte needs. Solid foods usually are not palatable to the patient with a fever but may be eaten if desired.

Since kidney damage can occur, the nurse should determine whether or not the urine excreted is normal in appearance and adequate in amount. Often there is an order to measure it. If, despite forcing fluids, the urine becomes concentrated or less than 1,000 ml. is voided daily by an adult, less then 500 ml. by a child, or less than 300 ml. by an infant, the physician should be notified.

Sudden rises (spikes) in temperature are not unusual in infants and young children who have acute infections because their temperature control mechanism is labile. They do not, however, tolerate fever well. Infants and young children are easily dehydrated because their body surface is proportionately greater than that of an adult. Consequently, they rapidly develop fluid and electrolyte imbalance.

Temperatures that are considered too high to be permitted to continue without heart or other tissue damage (usually over 40° C. [104° F.] in an older child or adult and over 39° C. [102° F.] in an infant or young child) and prolonged elevations that tend to debilitate the patient by increasing his metabolic needs may be lowered to safer levels by the administration of acetylsalicylic acid orally or rectally. The physiologic action of the salicylates in reducing temperature is not completely understood, but in most persons vasodilatation and diaphoresis occur and heat is dissipated by this mechanism. Even in the absence of diaphoresis, the salicylates are usually effective in lowering temperature. It is felt that these antipyretic effects are either due to protection of the heat-regulating center against pyrogens or interference with the peripheral release or production of endogenous pyrogenic factors.[33]

Sponge baths with tepid water or alcohol (half alcohol and half water) may be given (Fig. 4-4). Ice bags are sometimes applied to the head, groin, and axillae. Care should be taken not to initiate shivering by the excessive use of cold applications. (For details of the procedure see fundamentals of nursing texts.)

If chills accompany a fever, the patient should be lightly covered to prevent further dissipation of surface heat until the fever can be lowered. Shivering is the body's physiologic response to excessive loss of heat from its surface and acts to raise the body temperature. The mechanism comes into play regardless of fever. The use of warm covering only serves to raise the temperature higher and to produce excessive sweating, which can cause a serious loss of sodium and water in the infant and small child.

A high fever increases metabolism, which in turn increases heart action and subsequently the rate of the pulse. It also causes nitrogen wastage and weight loss and increases loss of fluid and sodium through perspiration. For these reasons, hypothermia may be used to treat serious generalized infections, especially in patients who tolerate high fever poorly, such as infants, debilitated patients, and patients who have

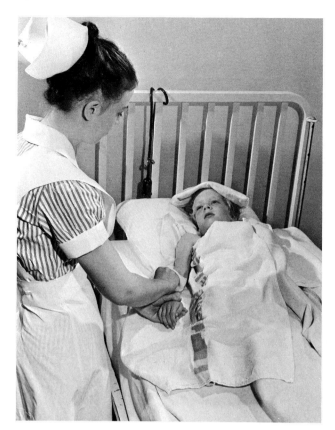

FIG. 4-4. Elevated temperatures may be lowered to safer levels by sponging the patient with alcohol solution.

cardiac or renal disease. Hypothermia decreases the body's metabolic needs. The lowered body temperature also inhibits multiplication of the infecting organism, making it easier for the body's defenses and the prescribed treatment to control the infection producing the fever. (See p. 209 for management of a patient being treated with hypothermia.)

After a high fever the patient usually stays in bed until his temperature has been normal for 24 hours. After a high or prolonged fever most adults feel weak, perspire on physical exertion, and become tired easily. For several days (or even weeks after a prolonged fever) the patient of any age should have extra rest and should eat foods high in protein and calories. Children and young adults usually recover much more rapidly than elderly persons, even when the infection has been severe. During recovery the patient of any age needs visitors and quiet activities such as reading to help pass the time.

Management of local symptoms. Nausea and vomiting often accompany a generalized infection. If they occur, food and fluids should be withheld for a time. Dimenhydrinate (Dramamine), prochlorperazine (Compazine), chlorpromazine (Thorazine), or trimethobenzamide (Tigan) are often helpful in relieving nausea. If the fever is very high and/or the fluid loss from vomiting is large, fluids may be given parenterally. Infants need fluid replacement much sooner than adults. Carbonated beverages, tea, broth, and soda crackers and dry toast are usually retained best as nausea subsides.

Symptoms of an upper respiratory infection also frequently accompany generalized infections. An antihistaminic drug is often prescribed to relieve these symptoms. Otherwise they are treated similarly to those of the common cold (p. 553). Muscle aches and pains, which often occur with an elevation of temperature, are usually relieved by giving aspirin. Urticaria may also occur and present a difficult nursing problem (p. 784). Antihistaminic drugs sometimes give relief.

Management of the patient with local infection following injury

Wounds. The nurse may be called on to care for persons with wounds sustained through injury. Therefore the nurse needs to determine the seriousness of the wound, know what emergency care to give, and when to advise the patient to seek medical attention.

All wounds sustained accidentally may be infected. If they do not bleed, bleeding should be encouraged to help wash away bacteria. They should be washed well with running water, soap and water, or an antiseptic such as hydrogen peroxide (an oxidizing agent), which effervesces and helps to debride the wound. Excessive bleeding should be controlled. For even minor wounds caused by bites or by dirty or rusty material, the person should seek medical attention. The wound may need to be incised surgically and drained. If there is any danger of its being infected with *Clostridium tetani,* tetanus toxoid or antitoxin is given (p. 87). Medical attention also should be sought for large or deep wounds because sutures may be needed to prevent unsightly scarring. If any appendage such as a fingertip has been amputated, the patient and the amputated part should be brought to the physician at once, since he may be able to suture it in place so that union may occur.

An *incised wound* is one caused by a sharp, cutting object such as a knife, glass, or razor blade. Several layers of tissue are cut and the wound gapes apart. A *laceration* is similar to an incised wound except that it has jagged, rough edges. It may be caused by such things as animal bites, wire, or machinery. Both of these wounds usually bleed profusely, and bleeding may have to be controlled by pressure over the wound or at pressure points (p. 264).

A *puncture wound* is caused by a sharp, pointed, narrow object such as a nail, pin, bullet, or splinter of wood. As the tissues are penetrated by the object, pathogenic organisms may be introduced. Since the skin quickly seals over, the wound rarely bleeds enough to wash out organisms. Bacteria such as

Clostridium tetani that thrive without air may infect these wounds. Because anaerobic bacterial infections are extremely serious, a physician should be consulted if the puncture was made by a dirty object. Puncture wounds received from objects such as contaminated needles used for any parenteral treatment also should be reported to a physician. Viral hepatitis may be contracted from this type of injury. Immune serum globulin may be given as prophylaxis. Any puncture wound should be made to bleed, and it should be watched carefully for signs of developing infection.

A *stab wound* is caused by a sharp, pointed, cutting instrument such as a knife. Deep tissues are usually penetrated, and the instrument may be plunged into a body cavity or into an organ. In the case of a stab wound of the chest, the instrument should never be removed unless a "sealing" dressing such as petroleum jelly gauze is available for immediate application. Otherwise air may be drawn into the pleural cavity, breaking the normal vacuum and causing a *pneumothorax* (collapse of the lung) (pp. 265 and 582). All stab wounds require medical attention since they are deep and should be well debrided. If the injury has been on the trunk, the patient should be examined carefully and observed to determine whether an organ has been perforated.

A wound caused by a blunt instrument that breaks the skin and bruises the surrounding tissues is known as a *contusion.* There is hemorrhage into the tissue with a resultant *hematoma* (swelling caused by leakage of blood into the tissues). The immediate application of ice to the area and elevation of the injured part may reduce swelling due to bleeding of superficial tissues.

Complications from contaminated wounds. If the tissue around any wound becomes swollen, reddened, or painful, medical attention should be sought at once because these signs indicate infection. Wounds are most often infected by staphylococci. Both the pathogenic strain *(Staphylococcus aureus A)* and the nonpathogenic strain *(Staphylococcus aureus B)* are found normally in the nose, throat, hair follicles, and sweat glands of man. Most people have a high tolerance for these microorganisms, but the very old, the very young, and those with metabolic disease, acute infections, wounds, or abrasions are very susceptible to them. Although staphylococci are responsible for most suppurative infections of the skin, streptococci and enteric organisms also may infect wounds. Open wounds that are exposed frequently to the air may become infected with the airborne bacteria *Pseudomonas aeruginosa.* Their presence may be detected by the appearance of a blue-green watery discharge.

Staphylococcal infections. The incidence of serious coagulase-positive *Staphylococcus aureus* infections in hospitals is a continuing problem and poses one of the most difficult aspects of caring for hospitalized patients today. In recent years staphylococcal organisms have become increasingly resistant to one or more antibiotics. Staphylococci can be isolated from patients and from staff members. One third of the general population are nasal carriers of *Staphylococcus aureus*.[2] In hospitals the most important mode of transmission is the hands of personnel, with air and fomites being much less important sources of infection.[2] The nurse is primarily responsible for teaching other staff members and supervising good aseptic technique in matters such as washing hands and the prevention of transmission from open suppurative lesions. In current practice, patients with open lesions are isolated, and strict medical asepsis is observed. All or most hospital personnel may be required to have nose and throat cultures. Those who are carriers of staphylococci usually are treated with antibiotics and are not permitted to be in contact with susceptible patients until subsequent cultures are negative.

If, when the staphylococci are implanted in susceptible tissues, body defenses do not overcome them quickly, they produce coagulase and toxins that destroy cells and phagocytes and cause a dense, hard, fibrinous wall to surround the infected area. This wall protects staphylococci from the body defenses, allowing the bacteria to multiply and extend the infection. Necrosis of tissue develops, and the subsequent degeneration and liquefaction of cells results in abscess formation. If the infection is allowed to progress without adequate treatment, necrosis of soft tissues may occur, underlying bone may become infected, the lymph nodes may become involved, and generalized bacteremia may occur and cause death.

Local infections caused by pathogenic staphylococci usually are treated by hot soaks, incision and drainage of the abscess, and penicillinase-resistant penicillin or other effective antibiotics. Surgical incision of the abscess is necessary because the drugs are less effective in the presence of pus.

Pseudomonal infections. *Pseudomonas aeruginosa,* a gram-negative bacillus often found in necrotic tissue in wounds and burns, is the cause of some urinary tract infections and can cause meningitis following a lumbar puncture. It is a relatively new "opportunist" and has been frequently cultured from IPPB tubing. Removal of necrotic tissue may be sufficient treatment but in certain situations, especially in debilitated patients, severe infection may be produced by this organism.[5] *Pseudomonas aeruginosa* is generally resistant to most antimicrobial therapy. Because of this resistance, it tends to emerge as the dominant infecting organism following the eradication of other bacteria and may be responsible for a suprainfection as occurs in bronchopulmonary infections.

Pseudomonas aeruginosa is the most frequently encountered organism in a burn wound infection, and if it cannot be controlled, septicemia results

with the systemic invasion causing vasogenic (endotoxic) shock and death. Many efforts have been made to develop methods to prevent "burn wound sepsis." A *Pseudomonas* vaccine is being tested clinically with favorable results, and the use of hyperimmune gamma globulin and hyperimmune plasma is also being evaluated; but because the *Pseudomonas* organism is airborne and can also be transmitted by water, it is very difficult to control its spread. Reverse isolation precautions have been somewhat successful in protecting the patient, but his body defenses may be overwhelmed by an autoinfection from his own bacterial flora, which are not controlled by environmental contaminants.[75]

Wounds infected with *Pseudomonas aeruginosa* are irrigated with Dakin's solution or acetic acid (0.25% to 1%) to aid debridement. No special care of the surrounding skin is needed when acetic acid is used, but precautions must be taken with Dakin's solution (p. 89). A bactericidal antibiotic of the aminoglycoride group, gentamicin sulfate (Garamycin), is effective against a wide variety of pathogenic gram-negative and gram-positive bacteria. It can be injected intravenously or used as an ointment on the infected wound.

Tetanus.* Tetanus, or lockjaw, is an infectious disease caused by the gram-positive, anaerobic, spore-forming bacteria *Clostridium tetani,* which are normal inhabitants of the intestinal tracts of men and other animals and can survive for years in soil and dirt. They enter the bloodstream of human beings through wounds and travel to the central nervous system.[5] They produce a powerful toxin that acts at the myoneural junction, causing prolonged muscular contractions. The symptoms of tetanus appear from 3 days to 3 weeks after the introduction of the bacteria into a wound. The patient first notices stiffness of the jaws and then develops difficulty in opening his mouth. He complains of rigidity of the facial and sternocleidomastoid muscles. They become hypertonic and cause stiffness of the neck and spasm of the facial muscles, which produces the characteristic sardonic smile *(risus sardonicus).* The abdominal and lumbar muscles also become rigid, and opisthotonos (arching of the back) occurs. Painful muscle spasms may occur on the slightest stimulation (a draft, jarring the bed, touching the bedclothes).

Even with rigorous treatment, about 25% of patients with tetanus die. Prophylaxis is the only sure treatment (p. 311). Once tetanus has developed, treatment is directed toward neutralizing the toxin with tetanus immune globulin (human)—TIG—ad-

---

*Since tetanus is rarely seen today, details of nursing care will not be discussed in this text. For further information see Burton, M. R.: When tetanus struck, Am. J. Nurs. **65:**107-110, Oct. 1965; and Cirksena, W. J.: Tetanus, Am. J. Nurs. **62:**65-69, April 1962.

ministered intramuscularly, with part of the dose infiltrated around the wound.[2] Tetanus antitoxin (TAT) of equine origin is only used when TIG is not available. Anyone who is to receive tetanus antitoxin must be tested for hypersensitivity to horse serum and desensitized if hypersensitivity is present. Penicillin G or tetracycline is often administered to reduce the number of vegetative forms and to control secondary infection.[2]

Other therapy includes constant care in a quiet, semidark room, sedation, and muscle relaxants to reduce the severity and frequency of muscle spasms. The treatment of choice in severe disease is d-tubocurarine (curare) to produce paralysis, tracheostomy, and artificial ventilation.[2] Concomitant sedation with diazepam (Valium) is also essential.

Gas gangrene. Gas gangrene (clostridial myositis) is a much feared infection that usually occurs following traumatic wounds in which there is damage to muscles. It is caused by *Clostridium perfringens,* which is found in the intestinal tract of human beings and domestic animals. These bacteria are able to survive for indefinite periods of time in dust, dirt, and woolen clothing.

Gas gangrene is characterized by the onset of pain and swelling in the infected area within 1 to 5 days after the introduction of the bacilli. The patient becomes prostrated with extreme weakness and exhaustion and is very pale. The pulse and respirations become rapid, and the blood pressure falls. The temperature may be only slightly elevated. The infected area is extremely tender, and there may be gas bubbles within the wound and under the skin. A thin, brownish, odorous, watery discharge comes from the wound. This drainage contains large numbers of the bacteria. The involved area is swollen, brick red, and necrotic. The surrounding area may be blanched at first and later a mottled purple. Because not all wounds containing gas bubbles are infected with gas gangrene, the diagnosis can be made only by culture of wound discharge.

Gas gangrene can be spread to others and therefore precautions must be taken. The patient should be isolated, his soiled dressings burned, and any instruments used for wound care washed and sterilized immediately after use. Gas gangrene, fortunately, is less prevalent and less serious since the advent of antibiotic therapy. However, an occasional patient may still develop the disease. Specific treatment includes early surgery with meticulous cleansing and debridement. Large doses of penicillin and tetracycline or chloramphenicol are given. Tetanus toxoid and/or antitoxin should also be given.[2] Usually the patient is quite alert and requires constant supportive nursing care to keep him comfortable and as free from pain and apprehension as possible.

Hyperbaric oxygen has been used successfully to treat some patients with gas gangrene. The use of hyperbaric oxygen increases the oxygen level in the blood and aids in the destruction of the anaerobic *Clostridium perfringens.* *

Polyvalent gas gangrene antitoxin prepared from the blood of hyperimmunized horses is now available for passive immunization.[2]

Wound irrigation and packing. The nurse is often asked to irrigate or pack infected or gaping wounds. It is important that these wounds heal from the bottom since, if the skin and superficial layers of tissue heal first, a collection of pus may form in the unhealed space. When irrigating deep wounds or sinus tracts, a catheter usually is placed as deep into the wound as possible. Then, with an Asepto syringe, the irrigating fluid is instilled until the returns are clear (Fig. 4-5). The physician should be consulted as to the direction in which the catheter should be inserted and the depth to which it should go. This information should be recorded on the nursing care plan. In irrigating fistulas the fluid instilled in one opening should return from the other. The patient should turn so that all the irrigating solution drains back, or the solution should be aspirated from the wound with an Asepto syringe, since fluid that is left in a deep wound becomes a culture medium for bacterial growth.

If the wound is to be packed, the packing also should be placed into the bottom of the wound cavity

---

*For further information see Gunter, V.: Gas gangrene treated by hyperbaric oxygen, Nurs. Times **65:**526, April 1969.

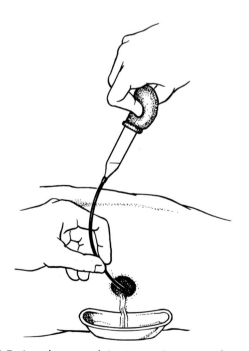

FIG. 4-5. A catheter and Asepto syringe are often used to irrigate an infected wound that may have a deep abscess or a sinus tract to the exterior.

to prevent surface healing. Packs should be kept moist. If they become dry, they should be moistened with normal saline solution before being removed to prevent damage to the newly formed granulation tissue. This tissue will ooze readily, and it should be handled gently. The physician often trims it with scissors to stimulate further healing. The patient feels no pain from this procedure since there are no nerve endings in the new tissue.

Diluted sodium hypochlorite solution, 0.5% (modified Dakin's solution), often is used to irrigate or pack infected wounds. It is a powerful germicide and deodorant and dissolves necrotic tissue, preparing the area for granulation. It also interferes with formation of thrombin and delays clotting of blood and usually is not used if there are catgut sutures, since it may dissolve them. Dakin's solution is irritating to normal skin, and a protective ointment such as petroleum jelly gauze should be applied before it is used. Since Dakin's solution is unstable, it should be made freshly every 48 hours. Hydrogen peroxide solution also is ordered for the irrigation of infected wounds and is the solution most often used for home care. It acts as a cleansing agent, by removing organic debris, but its bactericidal action is limited in the presence of blood or pus.

The antiseptic povidone-iodine (Betadine), in 0.5% dilutions, may also be used. Antibiotic solutions and solutions containing proteolytic enzymes such as *streptokinase* and *trypsin,* which digest the necrotic tissue, may be instilled into the wound. No special care of the skin is needed when using hydrogen peroxide, povidone-iodine, acetic acid, or antibiotic solutions. If solutions containing enzymes are used, however, care should be taken to keep them off the normal skin, where they will cause irritation. If, in caring for the wound, the nurse notices any increased inflammation or any increased suppuration or necrosis, this change should be recorded and the physician notified.

Common local infections

Patients often ask the nurse for advice on minor infections involving the superficial tissues. Therefore the nurse must be able to recognize the most common infections, know when medical attention is indicated, and teach measures for preventing these infections.

Infections of the hand. Infections of the hand occur frequently because the hands are functionally involved in most activities and thus are likely to be injured or exposed to infection. These injuries and infections usually are painful, and rest is essential to healing. Therefore, although the patient rarely is hospitalized, he may be partially incapacitated.

An infection involving the soft tissues around and underneath the nail is called a *paronychia* (Fig. 4-6, *A*). It usually results from the infection of a hang-

nail. The involved finger is very painful, and the patient complains of a continuous throbbing sensation. The pain is relieved immediately by lifting the soft tissues away from the nail with a scalpel and draining the pus. The patient then may be given an antibiotic and instructed to soak his finger in warm, sterile saline solution for 15 to 20 minutes several times a day and to refrain from using his hand.

An infection that involves the soft tissue of the fingertip is called a *felon* (Fig. 4-6, *B*). It often is caused when staphylococci are introduced into the finger by a pinprick and sometimes can be prevented by making pinpricks bleed. In the early stages the infection responds to warm soaks, and sometimes an antibiotic is given. If it is allowed to progress untreated, the swelling may cause obstruction of the arterial blood supply to the soft tissues of the finger, and necrosis of the tissue and underlying bone may occur. The infected area will then have to be surgically incised and drained and the necrotic tissue excised. A pricked finger should be watched carefully, and if swelling or pain develops, medical treatment should be obtained.

Infection of the tendon sheath (Fig. 4-6, *C*), particularly on the palmar surface, often follows puncture wounds of the fingers or hand. Streptococci are most often the infecting organisms. The hand becomes red and swollen along the tendon, and movement is very painful. This kind of infection usually responds to early treatment with antibiotics and hot soaks, but surgical incision and drainage may be necessary. Untreated infections of the tendon sheath lead to destruction of the tendon with resulting finger and hand deformities. If the tendon has been damaged, a tendon graft to correct deformities may be necessary after healing has occurred.

Lymphangitis and lymphadenitis. Lymphangitis is an inflammation of the lymphatic vessels. It is usually of streptococcal origin and is a sequela of infections of the feet, legs, hands, or arms. The first symptom to appear is a red, tender streak under the skin of

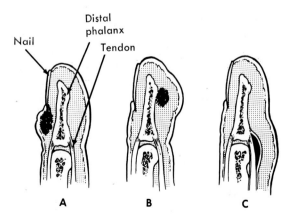

FIG. 4-6. Common infections of the finger. **A,** Paronychia. **B,** Felon. **C,** Tendon sheath infection.

the leg or forearm, indicating the spread of the infection to the lymphatic vessels. The lymph nodes above the infection (in the knee, groin, elbow, or axilla) become swollen and tender as the infectious organisms invade them. This condition is known as lymphadenitis. If the infection continues uncontrolled and bacteria reach the bloodstream, septicemia with fever, chills, malaise, and increase in the pulse rate may develop. Infections of the lymph channels are treated by drainage of the original infection, antibiotics, hot wet dressings, and elevation of the affected extremity.

Furuncles and carbuncles. Furuncles (boils) and carbuncles (multiple boils) are common local infections. They are discussed on p. 781.

Ulcerations. An ulcer is a superficial loss of skin due to the death of cells. It may be caused by infection, second-degree burns, or inadequate blood supply and nutrients to the part. Debilitated persons are prone to develop pressure sores or decubitus ulcers from prolonged pressure over bony prominences. Ulcers of the lower legs and feet are rather common in persons with poor arterial or venous circulation in the lower extremities. If the ulcer does not become secondarily infected, it will heal by second intention. Because of their location, however, ulcers of the skin usually become infected with staphylococci, streptococci, or enteric bacteria and require extensive treatment with antibiotics both systemically and locally.

Warm saline soaks usually are prescribed to cleanse the ulcer and stimulate granulation. If the ulcer is infected, irrigations and packings similar to those described on p. 88 may be ordered. Pressure on the part should be relieved and circulation to it stimulated. Patients with large ulcers on the trunk may be placed in CircOlectric beds or on Stryker frames and turned from the abdomen to the back at 1- to 2-hour intervals. Patients with ulcers on the legs or feet may be placed on CircOlectric beds and the bed tilted up or down at regular intervals. An oscillating bed may also be used. There may be an order to keep the part elevated, with intermittent exercise prescribed. Alternating air-pressure mattresses or flotation pads should be used. Padding bony prominences with lamb's wool also reduces pressure. There is some evidence that topical hyperbaric oxygen treatment may be a promising approach in the therapy of certain superficial skin ulcers. If the ulcer does not heal, as often occurs in arteriosclerotic diseases, a skin graft may be necessary to close the wound.

An ulcer of the skin usually is easier to prevent than to cure. The measures just discussed for relief of pressure over bony prominences and for improvement of circulation should be used prophylactically for debilitated patients, patients who must be confined to bed for long periods, and patients with any disease that tends to impair circulation.

Home care of local infections

Many patients with local infections are not hospitalized. Therefore the nurse will often be asked to instruct patients in how to apply warm dressings, soak hands or feet, provide rest for the part by splinting,

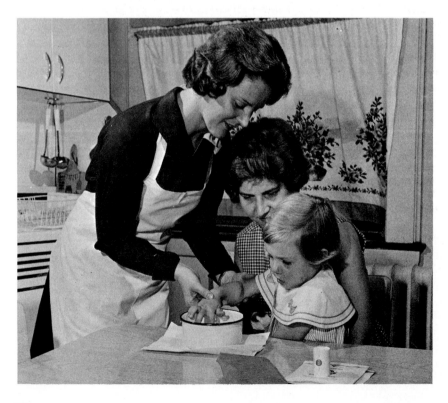

FIG. 4-7. The nurse in the patient's home is teaching the mother how to carry out the prescribed procedure of warm soaks for her child's infected finger.

or elevate the part with a sling or pillows (Fig. 4-7).

Sterile normal saline solution is most often used for warm dressings and soaks to open wounds. The patient can make this solution in the home by adding 8 ml. (2 tsp.) of table salt to each quart of water and boiling the solution for 10 minutes. The solution must be allowed to cool until it can be used without danger of causing a burn (from 90° to 100° F.). Magnesium sulfate (Epsom salts) may be ordered. It should be prepared according to the physician's orders.

If warm moist dressings are to be applied, the area covered by the dressing should be lubricated with petroleum jelly to prevent burns. Sterile dressings are placed in the solution and wrung out with forceps, eyebrow tweezers, or two sticks. These instruments should be boiled for 10 minutes before the initial use. They then can be stored in a sterilized jar containing 70% alcohol or benzalkonium chloride or be boiled before each use. If sterile dressings are not available, the dressing material can be boiled with the solution. Unsterile warm dressings can be prepared by immersing a bath towel in hot water and wringing it out. Heat will be maintained for longer periods if the wet dressing is covered with a piece of plastic and flannel. A hot-water bottle may also be placed over the dressing to maintain the heat. The length of time warm dressings are to be kept in place will be determined by the physician, but 20 minutes to half an hour, four times a day, is the usual time.

If warm soaks are being used, a basin large enough to immerse the part completely should be obtained. If an open wound is being soaked, the basin and solution should be sterile. Sterilization can be accomplished by filling the basin with the solution and boiling it for 10 minutes. After it has cooled sufficiently for the soak (90° to 100° F.), the excess solution can be poured off. Soaking is usually ordered for 15 to 20 minutes, three or four times a day. Soaks are often done with the dressing left in place. However, outside layers of the dressing should be removed. The wound usually is completely redressed after the soak.

Rest for a finger is often accomplished by wrapping it in a bulky dressing. This prevents bending of the joints. A *splint* may sometimes be made by placing a tongue blade under the finger before applying the dressing. If the wound is on the fingertip, a splint of this type is helpful in preventing accidental trauma. Unless contraindicated, the joints should be moved each time the dressing is removed to prevent stiffening.

Slings are frequently used to provide elevation and rest for an infected finger or hand. A scarf or a triangle of muslin will serve as a sling. The sling should be applied so that the hand is supported with only the tip of the little finger showing, and it should be tied so that the hand is elevated above the elbow.

In order to prevent pressure sores, care must be taken to avoid knotting the sling over the spinous processes. To prevent "frozen" joints, a sling should be removed several times a day and the joints put through their range of motion. The sling should be removed at bedtime and the part elevated on a pillow.

Elevation of arms or legs on pillows should be done according to the principles of good body mechanics, making sure that the part is in proper body alignment and is supported along the entire length of the limb. Care should also be taken to assure that the part is in a position that will enhance rather than impede drainage of blood vessels.

If the infection involves the leg or foot, the patient may not be able to be up and about to care for himself, and a family member may need to be taught to prepare the dressings or soaks. However, if no such assistance is available, the patient may be admitted to the hospital. The nurse should discuss plans for home care with the patient and consult the physician if home nursing care seems inadvisable.

■ INTERNAL DEFENSES AGAINST FOREIGN PROTEINS

The body's mechanism for dealing with foreign proteins (the antigen-antibody response, p. 77) is not reserved only for pathogenic organisms. It also comes into action against other foreign substances such as pollens, food, animal serum, and dander as well as a variety of other material such as house dust, cosmetics, synthetic products, and drugs. Some people also develop allergic response (hypersensitivity) to bacteria.

Allergy

Antigenic substances that produce hypersensitivity are known as *allergens,* and the hypersensitivity is called an allergy. About 20% of the population will react to allergens that are not antigens for the remainder of the population. These individuals are referred to as being "atopic." This tendency to become hypersensitive is inherited genetically. What these individuals become hypersensitive to, however, will be determined by the allergens to which they are exposed. The most common allergens are (1) *food,* which is primarily a problem from infancy to 2 years of age; (2) *environmental inhalants* such as house dust and animal dander, which most commonly cause allergic response between the ages of 2 and 6; and (3) the *seasonal inhalants* such as tree and grass pollens and fungus spores, which cause allergy in those over the age of 6.

When a person who has a tendency to become allergic first comes into contact with the specific allergen to which he is sensitive, antibodies are formed. When he comes in contact with this allergen again, an antigen-antibody reaction occurs, which results in the release of histamine or a histamine-like substance. Histamine has three main effects: (1) it constricts smooth muscle such as that found in the bronchi; (2) it increases vascular permeability; and (3) it increases mucous gland secretions. Allergies most commonly affect the nose, chest, or skin. The symptoms seen in the patient will be determined by the organ affected. The patient who has hay fever will have sneezing, tearing of the eyes, and watery discharge from the nose. The individual who has asthma will wheeze when his bronchial muscles are constricted, and the person with a skin allergy will have hives, urticaria, and skin rash. Nausea, vomiting, and diarrhea may also be allergic reactions (Fig. 4-8). Infants and children who develop eczema are highly sensitive individuals and about 80% of them will develop hay fever or asthma before the age of 6. Environmental and seasonal inhalants are about equally important in causing allergies in atopic persons. Environmental inhalants are easier to control, however, and with proper precautions these individuals can often remain symptom free.

Epinephrine (Adrenalin) and antihistaminic drugs such as tripelennamine (Pyribenzamine), diphenhydramine (Benadryl), and chlorpheniramine (Chlor-Trimeton) may provide temporary symptomatic relief. Newer antihistamines include triprolidine (Actifed), dexbromphen (Drixoral), and carbinoxamine (Rondec). These recent additions use pseudoephedrine hydrochloride as the drying agent, which causes little, if any, "rebound" congestion. Antihistamines have a tendency to produce drowsiness, and epinephrine may cause nervousness. Persons who must drive motor vehicles or work around machinery should schedule their doses of these drugs so that they are not understimulated or overstimulated during times when alertness is essential. If drowsiness is a serious problem, they should consult the physician who prescribed the drug. A newer drug, cromolyn sodium (Aarane), has been found to be effective in the treatment of patients with chronic asthma. It works by partially or completely preventing the immediate allergic response to the offending allergen. It should not be used to treat an acute asthmatic attack.

It usually is possible to determine the specific allergens to which a person is hypersensitive by taking a detailed history and then testing for sensitivity. *Skin tests* are often used to determine whether a person has a sensitivity to certain substances in his external environment. Several methods of testing are used. Small amounts of extracts of various allergenic substances to which the patient is suspected to have a sensitivity may be injected intradermally at spaced intervals, usually on the outer surface of the upper arm, on the forearm, or in the scapular region. The extract also may be placed on the skin and the skin scratched lightly *(scratch test)*. These two methods are used most often to test for sensitivity to pollen, feathers, dander, and dust. They also may be used to test for sensitivity to foods, but the results are often inaccurate. When clothing or other material is the suspected allergen, a small piece of it may be put against the skin under an airtight patch for 48 to 72 hours *(patch test)*. Sensitivity to soaps and other cleaning agents such as detergents is often tested in this way. An infant may be tested indirectly by injecting his blood serum at spaced intervals under the skin of a nonallergic person. Twenty-four

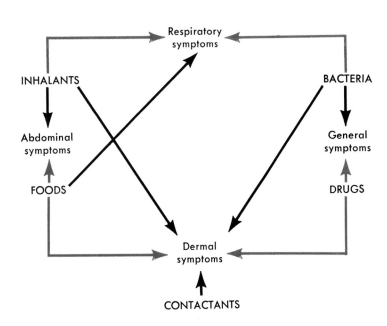

ALLERGY

FIG. 4-8. Illustrating the causes of allergic responses and their relative severity. (Courtesy Dr. Paul F. deGara, New York, N. Y.)

hours later the extract of the suspected allergenic substance is injected at these sites. Tests for allergenic substances usually are done in series; for example, pollens from trees are tested first, then pollens from grasses, and so on. Positive reactions to allergens are indicated by the appearance of a *wheal* or redness at the test site. Occasionally one drop of a test extract is instilled into the eye to test for sensitivity *(conjunctival test)*. Redness of the conjunctiva and tearing will appear within 5 to 15 minutes in an allergic person.

A person with a food allergy usually is asked to keep a food diary for at least a week. On the basis of this diary, suspect foods such as milk, wheat products, and eggs may be removed from the diet *(elimination diet)* until symptoms subside and then added one at a time in an attempt to identify the offending foods. Babies on this diet often must be given a special nonmilk formula made of products such as soybeans or barley. The mothers need instructions in preparing this formula. A similar elimination process may be used to test for allergy to other substances such as cosmetics or fabrics.

Some hospitals now have environmentally controlled rooms, which may be used to remove a highly allergic person from his usual environment and thus facilitate the search for the substances to which he is sensitive. The rooms also may be used for treatment. When the symptoms have subsided, various articles used at home may be introduced one at a time. Only a limited number of staff members are allowed to enter the room, and they may be requested to avoid the use of cosmetics and to wear a special gown.

The nurse may be helpful to the allergic patient during the period of testing by encouraging him to continue the program, which often takes weeks and months. By suggesting common allergenic substances to him, the nurse may help the patient give the physician a more complete history. Nurses are often called on to help the patient plan for elimination testing.

The best treatment for an allergy is to prevent the patient from coming in contact with the allergen or allergens to which he is sensitive. If the allergen is a *food,* it should be eliminated from the diet. Often infants who have food allergies will outgrow them by 2 years of age. Infants who could not tolerate cow's milk can often drink it as they grow older. Persons who are sensitive to environmental or seasonal inhalants should be taught how to control exposure to these allergens. This is most often accomplished by having a controlled room (usually the bedroom) in which the individual can spend much of his time when at home. A properly prepared room is especially important for the atopic child, since he is apt to be hypersensitive to a variety of allergens.

Persons whose allergies are due to *environ-* *mental* inhalants will need a room free of house dust, animal dander, fungus spores, and other allergens. Because 90% of the airborne particles in the house (such as house dust) are 5 microns or less in size, an electrostatic filter will be necessary. An electrostatic filter attracts particles by means of highly charged metal plates, which can be removed for cleaning. These filters come in portable models for room use or can be attached to the central heating system.

The room should also have wooden floors or be covered with linoleum or plastic tile. No rugs other than cotton throw rugs that can be washed frequently should be used, since carpets trap material that will produce house dust. Closet doors should be rendered "airtight" by applying weather stripping around the door. It also may be helpful to place clothes in plastic bags. The closet should be cleaned frequently to prevent the accumulation of house dust. Atopic children and adults are often allergic to animal dander, and most allergists will not allow them to have any fur-bearing pet. Goldfish may be a suitable substitute pet. Persons who are allergic to animal dander must also avoid feather pillows and other inanimate articles that may contain animal dander. Only cotton curtains that are smooth and can be easily washed should be used. The bed should have a mattress made from an allergen-free material such as foam rubber or be completely encased in an allergen-proof cover. Pillows should be made of a nonallergenic substance such as foam, Dacron, or Acrilan. A room air conditioner may add to the comfort of the individual and is often prescribed by the physician. Daily damp dusting of the room should be done to lessen the amount of dust in the air.

The person who is sensitive to *seasonal* inhalants (tree and grass pollens and fungus spores) will benefit from eliminating all outside air from his bedroom. This can be achieved by sealing the windows and installing an air conditioner or an electrostatic window filter. The cost of electrostatic filters and air conditioners that are prescribed by the physician is income tax deductible medical expenses.

In addition, some patients with allergies such as that caused by ragweed may be advised to vacation outside of the ragweed area during the peak of the pollinating season. This is quite possible for many persons and prevents them from having seasonal attacks of hay fever or asthma.

Usually the individual with hay fever will find relief from symptoms after only a brief time in an environmentally controlled room. However, the symptoms of the individual with asthma may not be relieved for days or weeks. Experience has shown that individuals who understand what they are hypersensitive to can remain symptom free for years as long as they avoid these allergens. Since the antibodies to the allergens are always present in the body, the individual will have symptoms should he come in contact with the offending allergen. This is especially true of animal dander, and parents should understand that atopic children can probably never have a fur-bearing pet.

Sometimes an attempt is made to slowly desensitize a patient by injecting small but increasingly larger doses of the allergen at regular intervals (usually 1 to 4 weeks) over a long period of time. This treatment may take years, or it may have to be continued indefinitely. It is about 80% effective in hay fever, but less effective in asthma and dermatitis.[1]

When a patient has been desensitized to a particular food, he may resume eating the food, but only small amounts should be taken at first. If any symptoms develop, the food should be stopped and the physician notified.

Specific care of the patient with asthma is discussed on p. 571, and care for the patient with allergic dermatitis is discussed on p. 783.

Anaphylactic shock

The patient may be so sensitive to an allergen that its subcutaneous injection will cause an acute, severe allergic reaction known as anaphylactic shock. The initial symptoms of anaphylactic shock are edema and itching about the site of the infection, apprehension, and sneezing. These mild reactions are rapidly followed, sometimes in a matter of seconds or minutes, by edema of the face, hands, and other parts of the body, wheezing respirations, cyanosis and dyspnea, dilation of the pupils, rapid weak pulse, and falling blood pressure. Death may follow in a few minutes. The respiratory and circulatory symptoms are caused by constriction of smooth muscle by histamine or a histamine-like substance.

Parenteral injections of penicillin are the most frequent cause of anaphylactic shock. Animal serum used in the preparation of antitoxins and extracts of allergenic substances used for testing or desensitization of an allergic patient also frequently cause it. Sudden death resulting from a bee sting is due to anaphylactic shock. Contrast media containing iodide, such as those used for intravenous pyelograms and angiograms, may produce this serious allergic response. Persons also have been known to develop anaphylactic reactions to acetylsalicylic acid as it is absorbed into the bloodstream. Therefore this drug is not as innocuous as many people believe.

Since people with a history of allergies are more likely to develop anaphylactic reactions to drugs than are those without such a history, all patients should be questioned about allergies and sensitivity to drugs before drugs are initiated. If there is any positive history, the physician should be consulted before a new drug is started, and if it is given, the patient should be watched closely for allergic response. In hospitals it is now common practice to have the fact that the patient is sensitive to certain substances posted conspicuously on the outside of his chart where it cannot be overlooked by anyone responsible for the care of the patient. In addition, many hospitals use a special color identification bracelet for the patient who is sensitive to certain substances. This alerts personnel throughout the hospital to the patient's hypersensitivity.

People who are known to be allergic or who have received a specific type of animal serum and who must receive antiserum should be given another type if it is available in order to lessen the possibility of an allergic response. When it is necessary to use animal serum, the individual should first be tested for sensitivity to the substance. An intradermal skin test, preceded by a scratch or eye test, is recommended.[2] A scratch test is performed by applying a drop of 1:100 saline dilution of serum to a superficial scratch and observing it for 20 minutes. A positive reaction consists of *erythema* or *wheal* formation. An eye test consists of instilling a drop of 1:10 saline dilution of serum in one eye and a drop of normal saline solution in the other eye to serve as a control. A positive reaction consists of tearing and conjunctivitis (redness) appearing in 10 to 30 minutes.[2]

If the scratch test or eye test is negative, an intradermal test is performed. This consists of injecting 0.1 ml. of a 1:100 saline dilution intradermally. A positive test is a wheal appearing in 10 to 30 minutes. In persons with a history of allergy, it is recommended that the intradermal dose be reduced to 0.05 ml. of a 1:1,000 dilution.[2] In persons who have a positive reaction to any of the above tests, desensitization may be undertaken.[2]

Any time animal sera, allergenic extracts, or contrast media containing iodide are given, a syringe containing 1:1,000 epinephrine hydrochloride (Adrenalin) should be at hand. An antihistamine such as tripelennamine (Pyribenzamine) or diphenhydramine (Benadryl), aminophylline, and isoproterenol (Isuprel) also should be available, and the patient should be kept under surveillance for at least 20 minutes. Any reaction that occurs within a few minutes forewarns of an impending emergency. At the first sign of untoward symptoms (redness and itching about the injection site, itching of the eyes, nasal symptoms, tightness in the chest) epinephrine, 1:1,000 (0.01 ml./kg.), is administered subcutaneously or intramuscularly. In case of a more severe reaction an antihistamine is given parenterally, a tourniquet is applied above the injection site, and epinephrine is injected into the site. Additional epinephrine may be given at intervals until the reaction subsides or tachycardia develops. Aminophylline may have to be given to relax the bronchial spasm and a vasopressor to raise the blood pressure. ACTH or corticosteroids may also be administered. Sometimes, to counteract shock, the patient's lower limbs are elevated, oxygen may be given by positive pressure mask, and an infusion is started. If there is tracheal edema, an endotracheal tube may be inserted or a tracheostomy may be done.

Transfusion reactions

Blood from another person is in itself a foreign protein. It may contain allergens to which the patient is sensitive, antibodies, and pathogens. Consequently, blood is a dangerous therapeutic agent that must be used only with the greatest care.

If the blood contains allergens to which the patient is sensitive, he may have an allergic response. Urticaria usually is the first symptom. It may be followed by dyspnea and cyanosis. If any of these symptoms appear, the blood should be discontinued at once, but the vein should be kept open with the physiologic saline solution until the physician has been contacted for further orders. Sometimes, if the blood is absolutely essential and the reaction is not severe, an antihistaminic drug is given and the transfusion continued. Epinephrine hydrochloride, 1:1,000, will cause prompt disappearance of the symptoms. Diphenhydramine and tripelennamine also may be ordered to relieve an allergic reaction.

With the exception of anaphylactic shock the most serious reaction to a blood transfusion is caused by giving the patient incompatible blood—that is, blood with which antibodies in the recipient's blood react. When this is done, the red blood cells of the donor's blood are agglutinated and dissolved (lysis) by the recipient's serum, and the product of this hemolysis is circulated throughout the bloodstream.

After he receives about 50 ml. of incompatible blood, the patient usually complains of fullness in the head, severe pain in the back, and a sensation of constriction in the chest. Nausea and vomiting may occur, and the patient's pulse usually becomes rapid and his blood pressure drops. If the transfusion is discontinued at this point, these symptoms will disappear, but a few hours later the urine becomes red (port-wine urine) and the urinary output is diminished. The urine contains red blood cells and albumin. This reaction is thought to be caused by the release of a toxic substance from the hemolyzed blood that causes a temporary vascular spasm in the kidneys, resulting in renal damage and blockage of the renal tubules by the hemoglobin precipitated out in the acid urine (hemoglobinuria). If the patient receives more than 100 ml. of the incompatible blood, irreversible shock with complete renal failure may occur, and death may follow. This renal failure is similar to the renal damage that sometimes results from ingestion of poisons and highly toxic drugs (p. 468).

At the first sign of a reaction the blood transfusion should be discontinued and the physician notified.

Epinephrine hydrochloride, 1:1,000, is given at once, and the urine is rapidly alkalized by an intravenous injection of sterile $\frac{1}{6}$M sodium lactate solution. This procedure reduces the precipitation of hemoglobin in the kidneys.

As blood cells disintegrate (lyse), large amounts of potassium are released into the bloodstream, and if the renal function is impaired, hyperkalemia (excessive amount of potassium in the blood) will develop (p. 116). If this condition occurs, the patient may be treated with an artificial kidney machine (p. 475).

Pyrogenic reactions can occur with the administration of any intravenous fluid, including blood. Pyrogens are toxic products of bacterial growth, and if tubing, needles, and solutions such as sodium citrate are improperly processed, pyrogens may be present despite sterilization that has killed any viable bacteria. The symptoms of a pyrogenic reaction differ little from early symptoms of reaction to incompatible blood. They include fever, headache, nausea and vomiting, weakness, and lumbar pain. However, they subside shortly and require no definitive treatment.

The most common pathogens transmitted to other persons through blood are the viruses causing hepatitis (both serum and infectious). (See p. 712 for the symptoms and treatment.) In order to prevent transmission of the hepatitis virus via blood transfusion, the following precautions are indicated: routine testing of all donor blood for HB-Ag, rejection of blood donors who have received transfusions or who have been exposed to hepatitis within a 6-month period, and rejection of donors with a previous history of hepatitis.[2] Other pathogens such as gram-negative coliform bacilli, diphtheroids, and staphylococci can also be introduced into the body with blood, and the resulting bacteremia may cause death.

Precautions in administering blood. Before blood is given to the patient, a sample of his blood is drawn for typing and crossmatching. His blood is then matched with the blood of possible donors to see if there is compatibility between the patient's serum and a donor's red cells. If they are compatible, the red blood cells do not clump together or agglutinate when the serum of the donor and the red cells of the recipient are mixed, and vice versa. The blood also is tested for the Rh factor. Approximately 85% of the population are Rh positive, which means that their blood contains agglutinins that will sensitize and later cause agglutination of the red cells of those persons (15% of the population) who are Rh negative (do not have these agglutinins). Several other tests are now done to determine the presence of unusual antibodies, many of which seem to be racial or geographic in origin.[12] With more sensitive testing, blood is less likely to produce untoward reactions, but it becomes increasingly difficult to find appropriate donors. A central clearinghouse for blood, the American Association of Blood Banks,* has been organized to help locate donors with unusual factors in the blood. The donor's blood also is tested for syphilis, and if the test is positive, the blood is not used.

The administration of the blood transfusion is the responsibility of the physician, but the nurse gathers the equipment and prepares the patient. (For the procedure see a fundamentals of nursing text.) The blood should not be obtained from the blood bank until the physician is ready to start the transfusion, and only one unit at a time should be brought to the unit. Refrigeration on the unit usually is not suitable for storage of blood, and without adequate refrigeration the blood cells may release potassium that may be detrimental when given to some patients (p. 116). Just before the transfusion is started, the label should be checked against the accompanying card by both the nurse and the physician for the patient's name, donor type and number, the Rh and other factors, the expiration date, and for abnormal cloudiness or color. The nurse should take the patient's temperature to establish a baseline. If the physician is assured that the blood is intended for the patient, he starts the transfusion.

If possible, the patient should be attended constantly by a nurse until the first 100 ml. of blood has been received, since any serious reactions usually occur by this time. If he cannot be given special attention, the nurse should check the flow of the blood frequently and observe the patient for signs of any reaction. An infant, young child, or acutely ill person should be attended constantly by someone on the nursing team throughout the procedure. A child's attention can often be distracted from the procedure by reading to him. When the adult patient is not attended constantly, his call bell must be placed within reach of his free hand, and he should be advised to call the nurse if he experiences any unusual sensation such as chilliness, dizziness, or any aches or pains.†

Rejection of tissue and organ transplants

One of the most serious problems surgeons face in trying to transplant any tissue from one person to another is tissue rejection. It is felt that the antigen-antibody response is responsible for this rejection. Tissue from another person is a foreign protein, and the body proceeds to destroy it. Patients who are to receive tissue transplants will be treated with agents that suppress the antigen-antibody response both before and after the implant. The agents most commonly used are the corticosteriods, Imuran, and total body irradiation with cobalt. Specific organ transplants are discussed on pp. 369, 480, and 726.

---

*Located at the Chelsea Navy Hospital in Massachusetts.
†For further information see Child, J., and others: Blood transfusions, Am. J. Nurs. **72:**1602-1605, Sept. 1972.

■ INTERNAL DEFENSES AGAINST STRESSORS IN THE ENVIRONMENT

The body has a self-preserving mechanism that automatically and immediately comes into action in times of stress or danger. The stressors can be physical, as in injury or disease, or psychologic, as in fear, anger, or frustration. Although stress often arises from changes in the external environment that threaten survival, it also may result from changes in the internal environment of the body. It has been suggested that the body responds to stress beginning with stimulation of the hypothalamus, which then activates two different mechanisms, the *sympathetic-adrenal medullary* mechanism and the *anterior pituitary–adrenocortical* mechanism. Impulses are conducted from the hypothalamus to the sympathetic centers in the thoracolumbar segments of the autonomic nervous system. Impulses then go from these ganglia to various effectors to prepare the body for "fight or flight" (or the responses may be that of immobility). This first mechanism, the sympathetic-adrenal mechanism, suppresses functions that are nonessential for life and augments those that facilitate overcoming or escaping the stressful situation. An adequate blood supply to the brain and heart is maintained and that to the skeletal muscles is increased. Provision is made to maintain the body's water, electrolyte, and temperature balances and to supply extra energy. To achieve these responses, the adrenergic fibers (sympathetic) of the autonomic nervous system are stimulated to produce a chemical norepinephrine, and the adrenal *medulla* secretes norepinephrine and epinephrine.

The second mechanism, the anterior pituitary–adrenocortical mechanism, is not activated by nerve impulses but by a neurosecretion, *corticotropin-releasing factor* (CRF). This chemical is produced in the hypothalamus and released into the pituitary portal veins. CRF causes the "master" gland to augment the amount of *adrenocorticotropic hormone* (ACTH) released, which in turn causes an outpouring of adrenocorticosteroid hormones (glucocorticoids). The action of these hormones provides emergency fuel by stimulating the release of glucose from liver and muscle glycogen. They also help to maintain the fluid and chemical balance that is usually upset by initial stress responses. The glucocorticoids will later help to provide the body with materials for repair of any damage incurred.

Norepinephrine acts as a vasoconstrictor (increases the peripheral resistance to blood flow) and consequently causes an elevation in blood pressure. *Epinephrine* stimulates the central nervous system; causes increased cardiac output; dilates the bronchioles of the lungs, which aids in the exchange of oxygen for carbon dioxide; and enhances metabolic activity so that more energy is available. Perspiration is increased, allowing for dissipation of excess body heat. Gastrointestinal peristalsis is decreased, and the blood vessels in the kidney constrict. The pupils dilate, making vision for darkness and distance more acute. Clotting of blood is enhanced. There is some evidence that epinephrine also causes the spleen to contract and discharge blood into the general circulation.

The protective mechanism used in response to stress is called into action frequently in everyday life, but the response usually is minimal and too short-lived to produce symptoms. In times of severe stress or danger, however, the person appears pale, his skin is cool and moist, his pupils are dilated, his muscles are tense, and he is keenly alert. His pulse is full and rapid, his systolic blood pressure is elevated, and his respirations are deep but usually show little increase in rate. The person having a pronounced reaction to stress may have abdominal distention, and he usually becomes nauseated. After the immediate threat has been removed, he may vomit or have diarrhea. If the stress is not severe enough to cause vasoconstriction of the renal vessels, the person usually has a full bladder and a desire to void as soon as the stress is relieved. If the stress continues as it does after severe trauma or during serious illness, the urine may be concentrated and the output reduced.

If moderate to severe responses to stress occur frequently, permanent damage to the body may result. For example, constant exposure to emotional stress is thought to be the cause of gastric ulcers and of coronary heart disease and hypertension in some people. It also appears to play a part in the response of some people to allergenic substances.

The body's response to stress may be detrimental to a patient with heart disease, generalized arteriosclerosis, or aneurysms because he may be unable to tolerate the increased stress on the cardiac muscle or blood vessel walls. The epinephrine output accompanying the alarm response may cause the patient with diabetes mellitus to go into insulin reaction (p. 756) because epinephrine (as well as insulin) facilitates the metabolism of glucose and the insulin in the blood may not be used. Later, however, when the adrenocortical hormones come into action and release glycogen from the liver, and when the epinephrine response is lessened, the patient may have an elevated blood glucose level unless extra insulin is administered. Patients with inadequate adrenocortical hormones and those with a diseased liver often withstand stress poorly because necessary energy supplies may not be available and the homeostatic regulation of body fluid and electrolytes is inadequate. Under all these circumstances the nurse may need to help the patient and his family plan their life so as to avoid unnecessary stress. Some special precautions are discussed in the chapters dealing with each disease condition.

Recently it has been learned that persons do not tolerate stress equally well at all times of the day. For example, the adrenocorticosteroid output seems to be lessened during the night hours. Probably urine specimens will be tested for 17-ketosteroids more frequently in the future because this test done on specimens voided at various hours may give clues as to when an individual should withstand stress best. It is quite likely that in the future, operations and stress-producing treatments will be scheduled with the individual's optimum period for withstanding stress in mind, so that shock, which is caused by poor accommodation to stress, can be minimized.

The intensity of the response to physical stressors seems to be related to the extent of the injury or the severity of the illness. For example, the more tissue removed in an operation, the greater the stress response will be. The sudden appearance or an increase in symptoms of stress and their failure to respond to treatment may be the first sign that the patient's condition is getting worse. Unless measures are instituted to relieve the primary condition causing the stress, the body's mechanism for dealing with it may soon be overtaxed. Transitory signs and symptoms of stress such as a temporary rise in the systolic blood pressure and the pulse rate and periodic deep breathing probably signify an increase in emotional stress or that the patient is overexerting physically.

The original stressor may be so damaging to the body that it is impossible for the defense mechanism to be effective. Examples of extreme stress situations are arterial bleeding, pressure on the hypothalamus, overwhelming infection, and blockage of a major branch of the coronary artery. In these situations, unless the primary condition can be controlled promptly, death will occur.

Every nurse should understand the body's mechanism for handling stressors. Otherwise nursing actions may impede rather than complement and supplement the defense mechanism. It should be remembered that the purpose of the initial response to stressors is to help the person escape the stress-producing situation or mobilize all his defenses to resist it. Severe and continuing stress, however, may overtax the body's mechanism for self-preservation.

Although physical activity may be useful in reducing anxiety, it is contraindicated in severe stress caused by trauma or illness because it will impede maintenance of body functions essential for life. Thus a patient showing signs and symptoms of severe stress usually is kept in bed and sometimes is given sedation. Although he should be kept warm, he should never be too warm, because overheating causes vasodilation, counteracting arteriolar constriction, which assures an adequate blood supply to the vital organs.

Although the patient may be able to cope with one stress-producing situation, his body may not be able to adapt to further stressors. Therefore it is always extremely important to prevent additional physical or emotional stress. Special care needs to be taken to prevent further trauma or superimposed infection. Anxiety and fear both produce stress reactions, and special care should be taken to alleviate them in any patient who has suffered a serious injury, is undergoing surgery, or is seriously ill. Extraordinary thoughtfulness may be required since the patient is likely to be very alert. Anxiety-producing conversations with the patient or in his vicinity should be avoided, and noise, bright lights, and movement should be kept at a minimum. Pain should be alleviated because it increases the stress reaction.

Even a minor stress reaction causes annoying symptoms, which the nurse should attempt to relieve. The backache, general muscle tension, and headache that commonly accompany illness are often stressors. Comfort measures such as back rubs, frequent position changes, and maintenance of proper body alignment and support help to relax the muscles. After a severe stress reaction, food and fluids should be withheld until nausea subsides and gastrointestinal activity returns to normal.

■ INTERNAL DEFENSES AGAINST INADEQUATE FOOD, WATER, AND OXYGEN SUPPLIES

The body, even under normal circumstances of health, has a very limited ability to withstand inadequate replacement of nutrients, water, and oxygen from the environment. Some oxygen in the external environment must always be available, and a complete absence of water can be tolerated by an adult only for several days. A baby or child can tolerate it for no more than 1 day because he has proportionately less fluid reserve and uses more than an adult. A well-nourished young adult can exist without food for several weeks if necessary, but he will develop electrolyte imbalances. The baby and young child must have daily replacement of nutrients because their needs are great and their reserves minimal. Elderly people need a constant supply of nutrients because they may have impaired circulation, which makes the distribution of nutrients to cells inefficient. In addition, vital organs such as the heart and kidneys may be functioning near maximum capacity and be less able to withstand inadequate cellular nutrition and the resultant additional strain caused by the electrolyte imbalance. Elderly persons tolerate starvation no better than children but for different reasons.

Food and water

If adequate food is not available, the body burns its own tissues to supply its energy needs. It cannot do this for any length of time, however, without the development of ketosis with resultant fluid and electrolyte imbalance. Many vitamins and minerals essential for body processes that help to maintain the homeostatic state are not stored in the body and must be supplied daily in food.

To maintain its energy requirements without adequate food, the body first burns its glycogen stores. Fats are then oxidized, and finally body proteins are mobilized and burned for energy. Burning of body fats produces ketones, and as proteins are burned, nitrogen and potassium accumulate in the blood. If lack of food is associated with an inadequate fluid intake, these end products of metabolism may be retained by the body and electrolyte imbalance rapidly ensues. Symptoms of metabolic acidosis (p. 117) appear, the blood urea nitrogen (p. 427) rises, and symptoms of hyperkalemia (p. 116) develop. Lack of adequate food and water is a stressor, and the resultant outpouring of adrenocortical hormones causes sodium to be retained to help maintain the blood volume by holding water in the bloodstream. Hypernatremia (p. 116) can result from this retention of sodium. Despite adequate intake of water, electrolyte imbalance will occur eventually because of inadequate mineral replacements.

To maintain essential body functions, an adult uses at least 1,700 ml. of water a day, an infant about 300 ml., and a child about 500 ml. Water produced from the burning of tissues (oxidation) and water pulled from the interstitial spaces can be used to maintain the body's needs for a short time. The kidneys, too, will conserve water as much as possible. However, since only 150 ml. a day is produced by oxidation (proportionately less in infants and children despite their higher metabolic rate), the available supply is rapidly depleted and the patient becomes seriously dehydrated (p. 111). This sequence of events may be speeded up by illness.

Although it is possible to live for short periods without food and fluid, the results are likely to be very serious for the person who is ill. Therefore seeing that food and fluid intake is maintained is of primary importance in caring for any patient. The nurse should remember that lack of adequate food and water is a stress situation. In stress, energy requirements increase, which quickly compounds the problems.

Oxygen

Although the body must always have a supply of oxygen, it normally can make some adjustments to decreased amounts of available oxygen. For example, people who live at high elevations, where less oxygen is available to the body, gradually develop an increased number of red blood cells. This compensatory mechanism provides for greater oxygen transport in the blood, and although each blood cell may carry less oxygen than normally, the increased number of carriers may provide for adequate oxygenation of tissues.

Since travel has become so rapid and widespread,

it is important to teach the public the implications of this adjustment, which normally is slow. Because extreme or unusual exercise or stressful situations always require extra oxygen supplies, care should be taken to avoid these situations for several days after arriving in a place where the altitude is higher than that to which a person is accustomed. In high altitudes the atmospheric pressure is low, and at low atmospheric pressures less oxygen diffuses across the alveoli into the blood, while carbon dioxide diffuses more rapidly than usual from the blood, causing respiratory alkalosis. This reaction is an application of Dalton's law of gases. If precautions are not taken until the body has had an opportunity to compensate by increasing the number of red blood cells, the tissues may not receive enough oxygen. Men whose work takes them to places where the altitude is high are likely to have serious difficulty if they contract respiratory illness. They also need to avoid strenuous physical activity for several days after arrival.

Because of the dangers accompanying atmospheric pressure changes, most planes now have pressurized cabins as well as additional oxygen supplies. It is unwise for anyone who would be susceptible to the development of problems due to a low concentration of oxygen to fly in a plane without these protections. Elderly persons and those persons who have circulatory or respiratory diseases often tolerate atmospheric pressure changes poorly. They should be advised to consult their physician before planning a trip that entails going to mountainous regions.

A precipitous change from an area of high pressure to one of low pressure can cause rupture of the alveoli because of the expansion of the gases in them. This is an application of Boyle's law. This type of pressure change also causes a decrease in the solubility of the nitrogen in the blood, causing the nitrogen to form bubbles that obstruct blood flow. This is an application of the law of the solubility of gases. The latter condition is commonly known as "the bends" (*decompression sickness* or *caisson disease*) and may be a problem for pilots, divers, and others such as "sand hogs" who work underwater for long periods of time. Unless pressurized cabins or tanks are used, descent from planes or ascent from diving should be gradual enough to allow time for accommodation to pressure changes. Informing the public about this reaction is very important because many people today engage in flying and diving for recreation.

When extra oxygen is needed, respirations increase in rate and may become gasping, allowing more air to be inspired. This response is brought about by the low oxygen level in the blood with increased carbon dioxide and the stimulating effect of carbon dioxide on the respiratory center. The bronchioles in the lungs also dilate to enhance the gaseous exchange unless disease prevents dilation. This dila-

tion is a stress response that helps to assure an adequate supply of oxygen to vital organs. Therefore the person suffering from an inadequate supply of oxygen should be protected from any additional physical exertion or emotional stress that might overtax and consequently decrease the body's stress response. Additional stress also increases the need for oxygen.

If the body is unable to accommodate to an inadequate oxygen supply in the external environment, or if, even though oxygen is available, the blood is unable to carry adequate amounts of it because of a low hemoglobin level (anemia), 100% oxygen may be administered. Usually adequate amounts can be provided by face mask, nasal catheter, or cannula. Occasionally oxygen must be administered under positive pressure, and hyperbaric oxygen chambers also may be used.

■ INTERNAL DEFENSES AGAINST TEMPERATURE CHANGES IN THE EXTERNAL ENVIRONMENT

Life cannot exist unless the temperature of the body is maintained within a relatively narrow range. For normal body function this temperature is about 37° C. (98.6° F.). However, various parts of the body have different temperatures. The extremities are generally cooler than the rest of the body. The magnitude of the temperature differences between body parts varies with the environmental temperature. The rectal temperature is representative of the temperature at the core of the body and varies least with the environmental temperature.

There is a clear circadian rhythm in temperature. The normal human core temperature undergoes a regular diurnal fluctuation, being the lowest during sleep and highest during the waking state. In the female the temperature pattern follows the menstrual cycle, with a rather sharp rise in temperature occurring at the time of ovulation.

Since the external environment is often much cooler or warmer than body temperature and because heat tends to radiate from a warm area to a cooler one, the body must constantly adjust in order to release or retain heat. The body is able to produce heat as a result of a variety of basic chemical reactions that include metabolic processes and the ingestion and metabolism of food. The major source of heat, however, is the contraction of skeletal muscles, which occurs with activity or with shivering. Heat production also is influenced by endocrine mechanisms. *Epinephrine* and *norepinephrine* produce rapid but transient increases in heat production; *thyroxine* causes a slowly developing but prolonged increase in heat production.

Body heat is lost, on the other hand, by various processes such as radiation and conduction, vaporization from perspiration, respiration, urination, and defecation. Tissue conductance, or the rate at which heat is transferred from deep tissue to the skin, is dependent on the blood flow to the skin. Local temperatures also affect blood flow and thus body cooling and heating.

The primary neural integrating area for temperature regulation is located in the hypothalamus. There appear to be two main neural pathways to it. First, there are the skin receptors, and second, there is the thermaceptine property of the hypothalamus itself. The hypothalamus also operates functionally as the source for releasing factors for the tropic hormones for the endocrine glands such as the thyroid and as the source of sympathetic drive for adrenal medullary secretion of epinephrine and norepinephrine. The neurochemical effects of epinephrine and norepinephrine regulate blood flow, causing vasoconstriction or vasodilatation resulting in heat losses by radiation and conduction. Thus there is a system of neural-controlled mechanisms that regulate body temperature. Through the responses of these processes the body is able to adjust to the constantly changing environmental temperatures.

When the environment is hot, the body temperature begins to rise. The blood vessels in the skin then dilate so that heat can be released. The person perspires, and as the moisture evaporates, the air enveloping the skin is cooled so that body heat can radiate to the environment. Respirations also increase and this process, too, releases heat as well as moisture. Usually the person who is too warm instinctively stays somewhat inactive, thus avoiding the burning of additional body fuel with the production of heat.

When the external environment is cold, the superficial blood vessels constrict so that the body radiates less heat. If too much heat is still being lost, shivering occurs. Shivering is a form of muscle contraction that causes additional body fuel to be burned. In the same way, exercise also helps to warm the body.

The ability to regulate body temperature undergoes some changes with age. Infants have no difficulty with the production of heat, but do have difficulty regulating heat loss. This difficulty is due to their scanty layer of insulating fat, smaller size, and greater surface–to–body weight ratio as compared to adults. Under conditions of favorable environmental temperatures the elderly are capable of maintaining constancy of their internal temperature. Their responses to extreme environmental temperatures, however, are less efficient than in younger adults. The reasons for this are believed to be a slowing of the circulation and structural and functional changes that occur in the skin as the result of aging. There are a variety of diseases that affect temperature regulation secondary to pathologic changes in blood flow. These include congestive heart failure (p. 352), Raynaud's disease (p. 387), and Buerger's disease (p. 387). Recent studies have shown that environmental temperatures have an influence on the incidence of myocardial infarction and cerebrovascular accidents.

Even the normal person may be unable to compensate for extremely high or extremely low environmental temperatures. If he cannot compensate, heat syncope, heat exhaustion, sunstroke, or freezing may occur (p. 271). Heat syncope results from the extensive peripheral vasodilatation that may combine with orthostatic hypotension to produce cerebral ischemia. Drugs that cause vasodilatation, such as those used to lower blood pressure, may predispose an individual to heat syncope. In addition, sedative and tranquilizing drugs suppress or interfere with temperature regulation. All persons, especially those on medications that predispose them to these states, should be warned against unnecessary exposure to temperature extremes.

In giving nursing care to patients it is important to avoid measures that counteract the natural defenses for heat control. For example, providing too much warmth for a patient who has a fever, yet feels chilly, may cause the temperature to rise higher. However, if he is not protected enough to prevent shivering, the temperature also will be increased. Sudden warming of a person whose body temperature has been markedly lowered may actually cause it to drop further because, unless the environment is very warm, the heat is lost through the dilated vessels.

Nursing measures may be taken to help the body regulate its temperature. Recently consideration has been given to the role prostaglandins may play in temperature regulation. This is a new area of research about which the nurse will need to keep informed. Patients such as the elderly who have a poor arteriolar constrictive mechanism, persons with arteriosclerotic disease, and persons whose autonomic nervous system is blocked by drugs, surgery, or injury have a tendency to lose body heat. It is important for them to be protected against the cold by the use of light, yet warm clothing and bed coverings. Patients with disease of the hypothalamus or medulla, those who have just been treated with hypothermia or hyperthermia, and infants, whose nervous system still is not fully developed, need to have their body temperatures carefully checked at frequent intervals because their body mechanism for temperature control may be ineffective. The temperature control mechanism is especially ineffective when there is a wide swing in environmental temperature or if a person has a disease that is causing fever. Therefore the temperature of the external environment should be carefully controlled when giving care in these situations, and treatment to reduce fever needs to be instituted promptly.

REFERENCES AND SELECTED READINGS*

1 Allergy and hypersensitivity, a programed review for physicians, ed. 3, New York, 1966, Charles Pfizer & Co., Inc.

2 American Academy of Pediatrics: Report of the Committee on Infectious Disease, ed. 17, Evanston, Ill., 1974, The Academy.

3 Anthony, C. M., and Kolthoff, N.: Textbook of anatomy and physiology, ed. 8, St. Louis, 1971, The C. V. Mosby Co.

4 Axelrod, J.: Neurotransmitters, Sci. Am. 230:58-71, June 1974.

5 Beeson, P. B., and McDermott, W.: Cecil-Loeb textbook of medicine, ed. 13, Philadelphia, 1971, W. B. Saunders Co.

6 Bergersen, B. S.: Pharmacology in nursing, ed. 12, St. Louis, 1973, The C. V. Mosby Co.

7 *Bruton, M. R.: When tetanus struck, Am. J. Nurs. 65:107-110, Oct. 1965.

8 *Bunting, F. W.: Immunity against the infectious disease, Nurs. Times 67:634-636, May 1971.

9 Burnet, Sir Macfarlane: The natural history of infectious disease, ed. 4, London, 1972, Cambridge University Press.

10 Burrows, W.: Textbook of microbiology, ed. 12, Philadelphia, 1973, W. B. Saunders Co.

11 Carlson, L. D., and Hsieh, A. C. L.: Control of energy exchange, New York, 1970, Macmillan Publishing Co., Inc.

12 Child, J., and others: Blood transfusions, Am. J. Nurs. 72:1602-1605, Sept. 1972.

13 *Chodil, J., and Williams, B.: The concept of sensory deprivation, Nurs. Clin. North Am. 5:453-465, Sept. 1970.

14 *Cirksena, W. J.: Tetanus, Am. J. Nurs. 62:65-69, April 1962.

15 *Cleland, V., and others: Prevention of bacteriuria in female patients with indwelling catheters, Nurs. Res. 20:318-320, July-Aug. 1971.

16 Cox, J. S. G.: Disodium cromoglycate: mode of action and its possible relevance to the clinical use of the drug, Br. J. Dis. Chest 65:189-204, May 1971.

17 *Craven, R. F.: Anaphylactic shock, Am. J. Nurs. 72:718-721, April 1972.

18 Davis, B. G., and others: Microbiology, ed. 2, New York, 1973, Harper & Row, Publishers.

19 DeCoursey, R. M.: The human organism, ed. 4, New York, 1974, McGraw-Hill Book Co.

20 *Devney, A. M., and Kingsbury, B. A.: Hyperthermia: in fact and fantasy, Am. J. Nurs. 72:1424-1425, Aug. 1972.

21 Eckstein, G.: The body has a head, New York, 1970, Harper & Row, Publishers.

22 *Fish, S. A.: Medic Alert, Nurs. Forum 8(4):428-431, 1969.

23 Fisher, B.: Topical hyperbaric oxygen treatment of pressure sores and certain skin ulcerations, Nurs. Times 66:613-616, May 1970.

24 *Francis, B. J.: Current concepts in immunization, Am. J. Nurs. 73:646-649, April 1973.

25 Frieden, E., and Lipner, H.: Biochemical endocrinology of the vertebrates, Englewood Cliffs, N. J., 1971, Prentice-Hall, Inc.

26 Frobisher, M.: Microbiology in health and disease, ed. 13, Philadelphia, 1973, W. B. Saunders Co.

27 Frohman, I. P.: The adrenocorticosteroids, Am. J. Nurs. 64:120-123, Nov. 1964.

28 Fuerst, E. V., and Wolff, L. V.: Fundamentals of nursing, ed. 5, Philadelphia, 1974, J. B. Lippincott Co.

29 *Garner, J. S., and Kaiser, A. B.: How often is isolation needed? Am. J. Nurs. 72:733-737, April 1972.

30 Gaul, A. L., and others: Hyperbaric oxygen therapy, Am. J. Nurs. 72:92-96, May 1972.

31 *Ginsberg, M. K., and LaConte, M. L.: Reverse isolation, Am. J. Nurs. 64:88-90, Sept. 1964.

32 *Gluck, L.: A perspective on hexachlorophene, Pediatrics 51:400-406, Feb. 1973.

33 Goth, A.: Medical pharmacology, ed. 7, St. Louis, 1974, The C. V. Mosby Co.

34 Gunter, V.: Gas gangrene treated by hyperbaric oxygen, Nurs. Times 64:526, April 1969.

35 Ham, A. W.: Histology, ed. 6, Philadelphia, 1969, J. B. Lippincott Co.

36 Hanawalt, P. C., and Haynes, R. H.: The chemical basis of life: an introduction to molecular and cell biology, San Francisco, 1973, W. H. Freeman & Co.

37 *Hardy, C. S.: Infection control, what can one nurse do? Nursing '73 3:18-21, Aug. 1973.

38 *Hargiss, C. O.: Epidemiology, a new area for nurses, A.O.R.N. J. 18:210-214, July 1973.

39 Horrobin, D. F.: An introduction to human physiology, Philadelphia, 1973, F. A. Davis Co.

40 Hyde, J. S.: Short and long-term prophylaxis with cromolyn sodium in chronic asthma, Chest 63:647-649, June 1973.

41 Infection control in the hospital, Publication no. 2010, Chicago, 1968, American Hospital Association.

42 Jacoby, F.: Care of the burned patient, Nurs. Clin. North Am. 5:563-575, Dec. 1970.

43 Jekel, J. F.: Communicable disease control and public policy in the 1970's—hot war, cold war or peaceful coexistence, Am. J. Public Health 62:1578-1585, Dec. 1972.

44 *Johnson, K. J.: Allergen injections, Am. J. Nurs. 65:121-122, July 1965.

45 Kinbrough, R.: Review of recent evidence of toxic effects of hexachlorophene, Pediatrics 51:391-394, Feb. 1973.

46 Langley, L. L., and others: Dynamic anatomy and physiology, ed. 4, New York, 1974, McGraw-Hill Book Co.

47 MacBryde, C. M.: Signs and symptoms: applied pathologic physiology and clinical interpretation, ed. 5, Philadelphia, 1970, J. B. Lippincott Co.

48 *Mangon, H. M.: Care, coordination and communication in the Life Island setting, Nurs. Outlook 17:40-44, Jan. 1969.

49 Marlow, D. R.: Textbook of pediatric nursing, ed. 4, Philadelphia, 1973, W. B. Saunders Co.

50 McCallum, H. P.: The nurse and the isolator, Nurs. Clin. North Am. 1:587-596, Dec. 1966.

51 *McDermott, N. K.: The nursing role in specialized infection control unit, Nurs. Clin. North Am. 5:113-121, March 1970.

52 McQueen, E. G.: Hexachlorophene, Drugs 5:154-156, 1973.

53 *Morse, L. J., and Schonbeck, L.: Hand-lotions—a potential nosocomial hazard, N. Engl. J. Med. 287:376-378, Feb. 1968.

54 Mountcastle, V. B.: Medical physiology, ed. 13, St. Louis, 1974, The C. V. Mosby Co.

55 *Nichols, T., and others: Diurnal variations in suppression of adrenal function by glucocorticoids, J. Clin. Endocrinol. Metab. 25:343-349, March 1965.

56 Pai, A. C.: Foundations of genetics: a science for society, New York, 1974, McGraw-Hill Book Co.

57 Riley, R. L.: Air-borne infections, Am. J. Nurs. 60:1246-1248, Sept. 1960.

58 Rosenthal, A. M., and others: Hyperbaric treatment of pressure sores, Arch. Phys. Med. Rehabil. 52:413-415, Sept. 1971.

59 Schottelius, B. A., and Schottelius, D. B.: Textbook of physiology, ed. 17, St. Louis, 1973, The C. V. Mosby Co.

60 *Seidler, F. M.: Adapting nursing procedures for reverse isolation, Am. J. Nurs. 65:108-111, June 1965.

61 *Selye, H.: The stress of life, New York, 1956, McGraw-Hill Book Co.

62 Shiff, P.: Modern trends in immunization, Med. J. Aust. 1:551-557, March 1973.

*References preceded by an asterisk are particularly well suited for student reading.

63 Smith, A. L.: Microbiology and pathology, ed. 10, St. Louis, 1972, The C. V. Mosby Co.

64 Smith, A. L.: Principles of microbiology, ed. 7, St. Louis, 1973, The C. V. Mosby Co.

65 *Some psychological effects of medical and surgical advances, Frontiers Hosp. Psychiatry **3**:1, June 1966.

66 Sotaniemi, E.: Environmental temperature and the incidence of myocardial infarction, Am. Heart J. **82**:723-724, Dec. 1971.

67 Sotaniemi, E., and others: Effects of environmental temperature on hospital admissions for cerebrovascular accident, Ann. Clin. Res. **4**:233-235, Aug. 1972.

68 *Streeter, S., and others: Hospital infection—a necessary risk? Am. J. Nurs. **67**:526-533, March 1967.

69 Tarnawski, A., and Balko, B.: Antibiotics and immune processes, Lancet **1**:674-675, March 1973.

70 Vasile, J., and others: Prognostic factors in decubitus ulcers of the aged, Geriatrics **27**:126-129, April 1972.

71 Van Cleave, C. D.: Late somatic effects of ionizing radiation, Washington, 1969, United States Atomic Energy Commission.

72 Vander, A. J., and others: Human physiology: the mechanisms of body function, New York, 1970, McGraw-Hill Book Co.

73 Williams, A.: A study of factors contributing to skin breakdown, Nurs. Res. **21**:328-343, May-June 1972.

74 Williams, S. R.: Nutrition and diet therapy, ed. 2, St. Louis, 1973, The C. V. Mosby Co.

75 Wilson, M. E., and Mizer, H. E.: Microbiology in nursing practice, New York, 1969, Macmillan Publishing Co., Inc.

5 Maintaining the body in dynamic equilibrium

Maintaining respiration
Maintaining the energy supply and intact body tissues
Maintaining the circulation of blood
Maintaining fluid and electrolyte balance
Management of patients with fluid and electrolyte imbalance

■ We live in two environments—an external one of heat and cold, noise, dirt, and physical force and a much more constant internal one of fluid, electrolyte, and temperature balance. The human machinery, carefully steered by the hormones and the central nervous system, is constantly adapting to changes in body requirements and to variations in the availability of essential elements. This human machinery operates on a cellular level. Each cell is capable of growing and functioning as long as it is provided with the required amount of oxygen, nutrients, and electrolytes. Body cells are bathed in the extracellular fluid, which comprises about one third of the total body fluid. This extracellular fluid, also called internal environment, must be kept at a relatively constant condition to provide the cells with their requirements of oxygen, nutrients, and electrolytes. The process of maintaining this condition in the internal environment is the process of dynamic equilibrium. While each cell is dependent on the internal environment, each cell contributes to maintaining the internal environment. The respiratory system provides oxygen and removes carbon dioxide; the kidneys remove wastes and maintain a relatively constant electrolyte concentration; the digestive system provides glucose, fats, and amino acids needed by the cells. The nurse must know how essential body functioning is maintained in order to help people maintain health and to give supportive nursing care when disease or injury upsets the body's ability to maintain its checks and balances.

■ MAINTAINING RESPIRATION

Oxygen is essential for the metabolic processes of the body. Chemical reactions in the cell that release adenosine triphosphate (ATP), which is one of the

■ STUDY QUESTIONS

1 What is oxidation? What is the action of a catalyst? What are some common catalysts in the body?
2 What is the normal blood hemoglobin level? Check the hemoglobin level of the patients on your unit who have oxygen deficits and relate it to their diagnosis.
3 Differentiate between anabolism and catabolism. List several body processes other than anabolism requiring expenditure of energy. What is the caloric value of a gram of carbohydrate, fat, and protein?
4 What are the sources of aldosterone and antidiuretic hormone (ADH)? Describe the main action of each.
5 Review the process of diffusion. How does it differ from osmosis? What happens when a 5% solution of salt is placed in a container in which it is separated by a semipermeable membrane from a 1% solution of salt? What would happen if a solution of sugar or protein, such as gelatin, were separated by a semipermeable membrane from water?
6 What happens to the extra salt and water you consume when ham is served for dinner?
7 Review these procedures: hypodermoclysis, venoclysis, blood transfusion, nasogastric intubation, Murphy drip. What are the special details for the nurse to remember when these procedures are ordered?
8 If you (or a close friend or member of your family) have recently had severe diarrhea, vomiting, or elevation of temperature, what symptoms did you observe that might indicate change in fluid or electrolyte balance?

most important energy compounds in cellular work, require oxygen. When oxygen is present in sufficient amounts, 38 molecules of ATP are formed from one glucose molecule, as compared to only two molecules of ATP being formed during anaerobic glycolysis. Refer to physiology and biochemistry texts for further information.

For the oxygen to be used by the body, it must reach the bloodstream and be carried to the cellular level. It does so through the process of respiration.

Ventilation is a mechanical process by which air is brought to the alveoli and carbon dioxide is brought back for expiration. Impulses from the inspiratory center in the medulla cause contraction of the external intercostal muscles and the diaphragm. The net result enlarges the thoracic cavity and the pressure in the lungs decreases. Air enters the lungs to equalize the pressure and inspiration occurs. Expiration is largely a passive process secondary to the elastic recoil of the alveoli. A rise in the carbon dioxide or hydrogen ion concentration in the blood stimulates the respiratory center and increases the respiratory rate. Any disease that inhibits expansion of the thorax or the lungs, including the bronchioles and alveoli, or that decreases the elastic recoil of the alveoli may lead to an oxygen deficit.

When the levels of carbon dioxide and hydrogen ions in the blood are low *(alkalosis)*, respirations are slow and shallow. As the levels rise *(acidosis)* respirations become deep and rapid. If the serum level of carbon dioxide becomes very high, the medullary centers will become depressed *(carbon dioxide narcosis)*, and the aortic and carotid chemoreceptors that respond to low oxygen levels will assume the stimulus for respiration. If oxygen is administered to these patients in sufficient quantity to increase the arterial oxygen concentration, the stimulus for respiration will be removed and breathing will stop. Ventilation may need to be mechanically sustained until the body mechanism is reinstated. Every nurse should know how to perform mouth-to-mouth resuscitation (p. 262).

When the oxygen reaches the lung, it must *diffuse* through the alveolar membrane, the interstitial space, and into the capillary, where it is picked up primarily by the hemoglobin of the red blood cells and transported to cells throughout the body. Interference with diffusion can occur in the following situations: certain lung diseases, due to decreased alveolar surface area, thickened membranes, or secretions in the alveoli; pulmonary edema, due to fluid in the interstitial spaces between the alveoli and capillaries as well as fluid within the alveoli; or circulatory problems that interfere with the *perfusion* of blood through the pulmonary capillaries. Failure of the exchange of adequate oxygen and carbon dioxide at this level leads to low oxygen tension in the blood and acid-base imbalance. The nurse should be alert to signs of inadequate oxygenation (restlessness, dyspnea, tachycardia) and carry out measures to enhance optimum oxygenation such as positioning to facilitate breathing and assisting the patient to clear and maintain his airway and to perform appropriate breathing exercises. When these measures are not effective, suctioning and ventilatory support may be necessary. The use of mechanical ventilators is discussed on p. 594.

■ MAINTAINING THE ENERGY SUPPLY AND INTACT BODY TISSUES
The energy supply

All body functions require energy, and physiologic oxidation-reduction reactions (the burning of foodstuffs and/or body tissues) are the only source of this energy. Energy production is so vital that if nutrients are unavailable from other sources the body has a protective mechanism by which it can burn its own tissues.

Oxygen and carbohydrates, fats, or proteins, and usually enzymes (biologic catalysts) are essential ingredients for producing energy. Enzymes are special proteins built under genetic control, and some work only when specific minerals and vitamins (coenzymes) are available. Thus for adequate energy production all nutrients must be available.

The healthy adult man of average size who lives in a moderate climate needs 1,500 calories a day just to maintain the basic functions essential to life (those functions that go on even while the person is at rest). However, basic caloric needs vary with age, sex, body size, climate (p. 133), and body temperature (see the discussion of fever, p. 84, and of hypothermia, p. 209). Extra calories are required to sustain additional activity.

The body always meets its energy requirements before nutrients are used for any other purpose. Extra caloric intake, therefore is essential to prevent the burning of body tissues in any situation in which extra energy is being used, whether in normal life or in illness.

Whenever food cannot be ingested, digested, assimilated, and metabolized normally by the body, some body tissues must be burned. For example, patients with untreated or uncontrolled diabetes mellitus (a condition in which carbohydrates are not metabolized effectively) burn excessive amounts of fat for energy. Because they often are unable to dispose of the acid end products of fat metabolism, acidosis may develop (p. 117). People who are starving also develop this problem as soon as the body's carbohydrate stores are depleted and body fat must be used.

The normal body stores whatever excess nutrients are taken in. Excess fat can be converted into glycogen or stored in adipose tissue. Similarly, excess carbohydrate can be stored as glycogen or converted into neutral fats and stored in adipose tissue. Whenever fats cannot be assimilated or stored, as in some diseases of the liver, additional glucose should be given so that the body proteins are not burned for energy. The burning of body proteins is undesirable because it results in tissue breakdown. Burning body proteins and fats for energy causes weight loss.

Some body proteins are almost always used for energy under conditions of severe stress. When there is extensive tissue damage, however, this metabolic process seems to be accelerated and usually continues for 7 to 10 days despite adequate intake of food. This acceleration is thought to be due to the action of the adrenocortical hormones. The burning of body proteins often causes serious chemical imbalances in the body because large amounts of nitrogen and potassium are lost in the urine. Fluid intake should be increased when large amounts of urea, the end product of protein catabolism, are excreted by the kidneys. Potassium and solutions containing amino acids may be given intravenously to patients after surgery, burns, or injuries that have resulted in extensive tissue damage. This measure may be contraindicated, however, if coexistent renal damage causes the nitrogen and potassium to be retained in the blood.

It is not possible to meet even the basic energy requirements of a person by the administration of intravenous glucose solution alone. For example, 1,000 ml. of 5% dextrose in water contains only 50 Gm. of dextrose, or the equivalent of 200 calories. For this reason, parenteral hyperalimentation is becoming more widely used in some situations since it is possible by this method to supply approximately 1,000 calories/L. of fluid. Hyperalimentation is discussed in detail later in this chapter (p. 125).

Despite the ability to deliver more calories parenterally, it is important for gastrointestinal function that the patient be fed by the alimentary route (either orally or through nasogastric intubation) as soon as possible. When it is expected that a person will be unable to eat for several days, as after certain surgical procedures, special emphasis will be placed on improving his nutritional status beforehand.

In the stress situations in which intravenous fluids are often needed there is an increase in the production of adrenocortical hormones that tend to cause retention of sodium and water. Therefore the danger of overloading the circulatory system is even greater than normal and the nurse should monitor the patient closely so as to detect any signs of overload immediately.

Tissue building and repair

The metabolic process by which proteins are synthesized by the body is called *anabolism.* All body cells are basically protein, and anabolism makes possible the development of new cells for tissue growth and replacement. It is also by this process that blood is replaced and enzymes and hormones produced. Anabolism, however, cannot take place until after the body's energy requirements are met.

Since catabolism of protein is unavoidable in conditions of severe stress such as serious infectious disease or extensive tissue damage, patients with these conditions must be provided with the complete proteins essential for synthesis of body protein as soon as possible. The amino acids that are given intravenously are not complete proteins. Therefore they are only useful to supplement other food or to be burned as energy to conserve body proteins. A nutritious diet should be given as soon as the patient is able to tolerate it. The diet needs to be relatively high in calories (2,000 to 3,000 calories a day) despite the limited physical activity of the patient, since extra energy is being expended because of the increased metabolism, resulting at first from the stress and later from tissue repair. The diet should also be high in protein. If the patient is at home or is returning home after an illness, he should be instructed to continue this diet until he regains his normal weight. Caloric and protein intake should then be reduced to normal.

The pituitary, adrenal, thyroid, and parathyroid glands all affect metabolic processes in various ways. A disturbance of the function of any one of these glands may cause a disruption in anabolic processes.

■ MAINTAINING THE CIRCULATION OF BLOOD

To maintain life, nutrients and oxygen must be transported throughout the body to cells and the waste products of metabolism must be removed from each cell. This process is accomplished by the circulatory system. Maintenance of this system, therefore, is essential to life.

Shock

The circulatory system is made up of three components: fluid to circulate (blood), a pump (heart), and channels (blood vessels). A failure in any one of these components results in a disruption of circulation. When this disruption is severe, blood flow through tissues is inadequate, and cellular hypoxia and shock occur. Shock may be caused by a variety of unrelated conditions such as severe infection, toxemia, anaphylaxis, severe dehydration, hyperinsulinism, severe physical or psychic trauma, massive hemorrhage, loss of blood plasma such as occurs in burns, or severe cardiac disease. A simple classification of shock based on the three components of the circulatory system is as follows:

1. Shock caused by blood or fluid loss is classified as hypovolemic.

2. Shock caused by failure of the heart to perform as a pump is classified as cardiogenic.
3. Shock caused by vasodilation in the vascular tree is classified as neurogenic when caused by nervous control of blood vessels or vasogenic when caused by humoral factors such as histamine.

In *hypovolemic shock* there is a decrease in circulating blood volume to a level that is inadequate to meet the body's needs for tissue oxygenation. Common causes of hypovolemic shock are excessive bleeding such as seen in massive gastrointestinal hemorrhage; blood loss secondary to surgical procedures or trauma; fluid loss that accompanies extensive burns or loss from the gastrointestinal tract as seen in severe vomiting or diarrhea; or loss from fistulas.

Cardiogenic shock is caused by failure of the heart to pump an adequate amount of blood to the vital organs. This reduction in cardiac output means that the amount of blood that reaches the vital organs is not adequate for tissue perfusion. Left ventricular failure secondary to congestive heart failure or acute myocardial infarction can cause cardiogenic shock. It can also occur when there is cardiac tamponade that interfers with cardiac output.

Neurogenic shock is a fleeting type caused by spinal anesthesia, surgery and drugs that inhibit the sympathetic nervous system, and psychic trauma such as fear, worry, and emotional tension. Fainting is the commonest form. Symptoms are caused by sudden vasodilation of the peripheral blood vessels into which much of the circulating blood rushes. There is no actual loss of blood volume. Vasodilation caused by psychic trauma is considered an important contributory factor in other types of shock.

In *vasogenic shock,* vasodilation by drugs such as histamine and alcohol or histamine released in the body in response to foreign proteins or toxins from infectious organisms causes leakage of plasma into the tissues. This *bacteremic* or *endotoxic* shock is seen most commonly as a complication of gram-negative infections, especially with the coliform bacilli, meningococci, *Proteus,* and *Salmonella* organisms. Anaphylactic shock, discussed on p. 94, is also a type of vasogenic shock.

Very young patients, elderly patients, and patients with cardiovascular diseases and metabolic disorders such as diabetes are more likely to develop shock following trauma, disease, or surgery than is a young, healthy adult. A patient who is receiving cortisone therapy or who has had it discontinued recently may have a rapid onset of shock because the adrenal glands may be unable to compensate by secreting additional hormones as they normally would. These patients may be given corticosteroids intravenously.

To prevent the occurrence of shock following elective surgery, the patient is prepared preoperatively so that he is in the best physical and emotional state possible. Typing and cross matching of blood are done before surgery so that if blood is needed to combat shock, it will be available. An infusion usually is started in the operating room so that if the patient needs blood, it can be given easily.

In shock, regardless of the cause, there is a drop in the systolic blood pressure. The significance of the drop must be evaluated in terms of the patient's blood pressure prior to the shock condition. With the drop in systolic blood pressure the pulse increases in rate and becomes weak and thready, the patient becomes extremely weak, and the skin is pale, cold, and covered with perspiration. As shock progresses, the respirations become rapid and shallow and the temperature becomes subnormal. The earliest signs of shock often are apprehension and restlessness and an often unexplained feeling that something is wrong. The patient may also become apathetic, indifferent, and finally unconscious. Symptoms of neurogenic shock often appear rapidly, but those of other types of shock usually do not appear until the condition is well established. It is only by careful observation and assessment of the vital signs and of the general physical appearance of the patient that shock may be recognized and treated early. Restlessness, apprehension, coldness, and pallor may be the first noticeable symptoms. The blood pressure and pulse usually are within relatively normal limits in the early stages. Since blood flow through the kidneys becomes inadequate during shock and the glomerular filtration rate is reduced, incipient shock can often be detected before other symptoms appear by observing hourly urine output in postoperative patients with indwelling catheters.

When there has been loss of fluid from the circulating blood, the venous return to the heart is slowed and the cardiac output is decreased. A compensatory vasoconstriction due to the excretion of epinephrine and norepinephrine maintains the blood pressure at a normal level for a short period of time. However, as fluid losses increase, the vasoconstriction becomes ineffectual and the blood pressure drops markedly, decreasing the blood supply to vital body tissues. This decrease leads to tissue anoxia (*ischemia*), and if it is allowed to persist, the shock becomes irreversible; that is, no amount of treatment will restore tissue function. The liver, kidneys, and nervous tissues tolerate a lack of oxygen and nutrients for only a very short time before permanent tissue damage occurs. If the systolic pressure remains below 50 mm. Hg for long, the patient usually dies.

Treatment. The primary aim in the treatment of all types of shock is to increase tissue perfusion.[8] Therefore treatment will be directed toward correcting the factors responsible for the hypotension. The symptoms of neurogenic shock readily disappear when the patient is placed in a recumbent position. One of the best ways to treat shock caused by fluid loss is to replace the fluid. If the loss is due to internal or external loss of blood or plasma, whole blood usually is given. Concentrated albumin, dextran, Ringer's lactate solution, or 5% dextrose in water may also be used to increase blood volume. Normal human plasma may be used, but many physicians prefer other blood expanders because the risk of transmitting viral hepatitis in pooled plasma is so great. Oxygen is usually given by mask to increase the oxygen available to the blood. If the shock is due to electrolyte imbalance, appropriate fluids and electrolytes are given either intravenously or orally to restore the normal balance. When shock is caused by vasodilation from substances within the body, vasoconstricting drugs such as phenylephrine (Neo-Synephrine) or metaraminol bitartrate (Aramine bitartrate) may be given, but they are not used in hypovolemic shock. Patients in hypovolemic shock are not treated with vasopressor drugs, since it is now recognized that the patient in hypovolemic shock is already in a state of peripheral vasoconstriction as his body attempts to overcome the decrease in blood volume. Therefore any increase in vasoconstriction is undesirable, since it will further limit the perfusion of vital organs. When it is felt that peripheral vasoconstriction is already present, vasodilators such as phentolamine (Regitine) or phenoxybenzamine hydrochloride (Dibenzyline) are usually given. The purpose for giving vasodilators is to overcome peripheral vasoconstriction and increase tissue perfusion. Some physicians give chlorpromazine (Thorazine) for this purpose. When vasodilators are given, provision must also be made for adequate and rapid fluid replacement.

Treatment of cardiogenic shock centers on increasing the efficiency of the heart as a pump. This is usually accomplished with rapid digitalization. In addition, isoproterenol (Isuprel) may be given by microdrip. This drug can cause ventricular arrhythmias and patients receiving it must have constant ECG monitoring.[8] (See p. 345 for a further discussion of cardiac monitors.)

Nursing intervention. Any patient suspected of incipient shock should be observed closely by the nurse for early signs and symptoms. The patient in shock should be kept quiet and warm, but he should have only enough covering to maintain his body temperature. If he perspires, he is too warmly covered and the peripheral blood vessels have become dilated, dissipating the available blood to the surface vessels. Any movement of the patient in shock is contraindicated. All physical care, except for essentials such as using the bedpan and comfort measures such as washing the face and hands, should be omitted until the blood pressure stabilizes.

In the past the patient was often placed in the Trendelenburg position (head-low position) to increase the flow of blood to the brain. However, this position has been found to inhibit cardiac output and respiration through pressure of the visceral organs against the diaphragm. Many physicians now prefer that the lower extremities be elevated at a 45-degree angle from the hip, with the knees straight and the head level with or slightly higher than the chest. This position promotes increased venous return from the legs without interfering with the cardiac output. The nurse should assess each patient's situation to determine the position of maximum physiologic effect and comfort. In some settings in which the nurse is functioning there may be policies concerning positioning of the patient in shock. Nevertheless, the nurse should assess the patient's response to such positioning and take appropriate action as necessary.

After the patient is positioned properly, other measures to prevent further stress should be instituted at once. The patient's questions should be answered and all procedures explained in an attempt to decrease his anxiety. Barbiturates may be prescribed for their sedative effect. Relief of pain also decreases shock, and morphine sulfate is often ordered for this purpose. Usually it is given by the physician intravenously since subcutaneous injections may be too slowly absorbed because of decreased circulation to the tissues. Repeated injections of any drug given subcutaneously or intramuscularly during shock may cause symptoms of overdosage on the return of normal circulation. If the patient is receiving a vasopressor drug such as levarterenol bitartrate or metaraminol by infusion, the blood pressure must be checked frequently (every 5 to 15 minutes) so that the rate of flow can be adjusted according to the rise and fall of the blood pressure. The aim is to maintain a mean blood pressure of 70 to 80 mm. Hg.[8]

$$\text{Mean blood pressure} = \frac{\text{Systolic} + \text{Diastolic}}{2}$$

Levarterenol is now used less frequently because it causes necrosis and sloughing if it infiltrates tissues.

The nurse should keep very accurate records of intake and output for patients in shock. An indwelling catheter is often inserted to facilitate collection of hourly urine specimens. Monitoring of the *central venous pressure* is commonly done to determine the adequacy of the fluid replacement. (See p. 326 for more details of this procedure.)

Hemorrhage

Hemorrhage is the loss of a large amount of blood from the bloodstream due to rupture or injury of a blood vessel, slipping of a ligature from a blood vessel postoperatively, erosion of a vessel by a drainage tube, tumor, or infection, or some interference with the clotting mechanism of the blood such as occurs in hemophilia. The patient may lose small amounts of blood over a long period of time, or he may lose a large amount of blood in a short period of time. The bleeding may be arterial (bright red and spurting), venous (continuous flow of dark red blood), or capillary (oozing). The blood may be expelled from any body orifice, from an incision, or from the site of an injury, or it may collect under the subcutaneous tissues as a tumor mass *(hematoma)* or in a body cavity such as the peritoneal cavity.

Symptoms of massive hemorrhage, both internal and external, are apprehension, restlessness, thirst, pallor, a cold, moist skin, drop in blood pressure, increased pulse rate, subnormal temperature, and rapid respirations. As hemorrhage continues, the lips and conjunctivae become pale and the patient may complain of spots before the eyes, ringing in the ears, and extreme weakness. If the hemorrhage is not controlled, unconsciousness and finally death will occur.

Management. The treatment of hemorrhage is directed toward stopping the bleeding, if possible, and replacing blood loss. When bleeding occurs, the vessel walls constrict, narrowing the lumen of the vessels, and a clot forms over the end of the bleeding vessel. Clotting usually occurs much earlier in the child and very young person than in older patients because the blood vessels of children and young persons are more elastic. In arterial bleeding the clotting phenomenon is not possible until there has been enough blood loss to decrease the pressure of the blood circulating through the bleeding vessel. However, pressure against the artery proximal to the bleeding point decreases the flow of blood through it and permits clotting to take place. Elevation of the part also may decrease arterial bleeding. *Direct pressure* at the site of the bleeding also decreases the blood flow and encourages clotting. This method is frequently used in superficial wounds, and a gelatin sponge (Gelfoam) also may be applied to help form a clot. The principle of direct pressure may also be used to control hemorrhage from esophageal varices. An esophageal balloon is inserted and then inflated until it compresses the bleeding vessels. In a similar way bleeding from the prostate gland, such as may occur following prostatectomy, is controlled by direct pressure. A Foley catheter is inserted and the balloon inflated to compress bleeding vessels.

Cold applications are often used to control bleeding into tissues or into body cavities, since the cold causes the small vessels to constrict. In uterine hemorrhage an ice bag may be applied to the abdomen over the uterus. In gastric hemorrhage, cold can be applied by irrigating the stomach with iced solution through a gastric tube. (See p. 666 for additional information.)

Very *hot applications* cause reflex vasoconstriction and control bleeding temporarily. This method is often used during surgery in which there is considerable vascular oozing. To control the bleeding permanently, large vessels usually have to be ligated, and smaller ones may be electrically cauterized. A ruptured organ such as the spleen may have to be removed to control bleeding. Removal of the spleen also may be necessary to control bleeding due to a blood dyscrasia such as idiopathic thrombocytopenic purpura.

When the bleeding is caused by a prothrombin deficiency, such as occurs in liver diseases in which hepatic ducts are obstructed or in biliary duct obstruction, *vitamin K_1* is given parenterally. Vitamin K_1 is helpful in controlling hemorrhage following overdoses of bishydroxycoumarin (Dicumarol). Protamine sulfate is given after overdoses of heparin.

If possible, the blood loss should be measured so that the physician can prescribe replacement more accurately. Dressings saturated with blood can be weighed, and bloody vomitus, which may be bright red or coffee-ground color, and drainage from gastric tubes should be measured. Whenever possible, tarry stools and bright blood discharged from the rectum should be measured. If this is not feasible, the amount should be estimated. The physician often will want to see evidence of bleeding, such as bloody stools or urine, vaginal clots, and bloody vomitus.

Blood replacement usually is started before complete hemostasis has been accomplished, since the restoration of blood volume is imperative in preventing the occurrence of irreversible shock. Blood plasma or a plasma expander may be given until whole blood is available. The physician's determination of the amount of blood to be given depends on the amount of blood loss, the central venous pressure, and the condition of the patient. When large amounts of blood must be given rapidly, the blood should be warmed to body temperature, since cold blood can act as a hypothermic agent. A decrease in the body temperature may cause cardiac slowing, with decreased cardiac output or the development of ventricular fibrillation.[8] The speed at which blood is given depends on the patient's condition. If the blood pressure is very low, the blood may be given very rapidly and may even be pumped in under pressure by the physician. (See p. 95 for additional information about transfusions.)

The patient is usually very apprehensive because of the hemorrhage and because of the emergency measures that follow it. Every attempt should be made to keep him quiet, reassured, and comfortable. He should never, under any circumstances, be left alone while a hemorrhage is occurring. Morphine sulfate is often ordered as a sedative. Evidences of bleeding should be removed from the bedside, and stained linen and clothing should be replaced. Noise and excitement should be kept to a minimum, and all treatments and procedures, such as frequent blood pressure readings, transfusions, the use of unusual positions, and, if necessary, restriction of food and fluids, should be explained to the patient and his family. The patient with a massive hemorrhage usually is given nothing to eat or drink until the hemorrhage is controlled, since he may have to be taken to the operating room. Food and fluid also are often withheld when the bleeding is from the gastrointestinal tract.

■ MAINTAINING FLUID AND ELECTROLYTE BALANCE

In order to survive the cells must be bathed in the extracellular fluid, which not only provides oxygen and nutrients to the cell but also maintains a certain concentration of electrolytes and fluids. Alterations in the normal concentration of these substances impairs cell functioning, which is the basis of life. Without proper fluid and electrolyte concentration in the extracellular fluid, the cell cannot maintain its intracellular electrolyte concentration.

Body fluid component

Fluid is found in the body either within the cell (*intracellular*) or outside the cell (*extracellular*). The extracellular fluid is contained in two subcompartments, the *interstitial* fluid between the cells and the *intravascular* fluid in the blood vessels. The volume and distribution of body water varies with age and sex. In the average young adult male, about 60% of his body weight is water; two thirds of this fluid is intracellular. In the newborn infant, almost three fourths of his body is water, with the greatest percentage in the extracellular fluid. By 1 year of age almost half of the total body water is extracellular

(Fig. 5-1). The intravascular fluid comprises only about 5% of body weight at any age.

Normal exchange of body fluids. Body fluid is constantly being lost and, for normal processes to continue, must be replaced. With an average daily intake of food and liquids, the healthy body easily maintains compartmental balance (Table 5-1).

Loss. Fluid normally leaves the body through the kidneys, lungs, and skin, with very small amounts being lost through the gastrointestinal tract and negligible amounts being lost in saliva and tears. Two vital processes demand continual expenditure of water—the removal of body heat by vaporization of water and the excretion of urea and other metabolic wastes. The volume of water used in these processes varies greatly with external influences such as temperature and humidity.

The daily loss of fluids in babies and growing children is proportionately greater than that of an adult. Their extremely active metabolism generates large amounts of heat that must be dissipated. The baby loses large amounts of fluid through the skin because the skin surface is larger proportionately than that of an adult. In addition, the kidneys of infants do not conserve water as effectively as the kidneys of adults. In the older child and adult, if the body needs water, the pituitary antidiuretic hormone promotes its reabsorption from the renal tubules, and fluid ingested in excess of need is eliminated through the kidneys.

Approximately 120 ml. of fluid, which is essentially plasma minus the protein content, is filtered

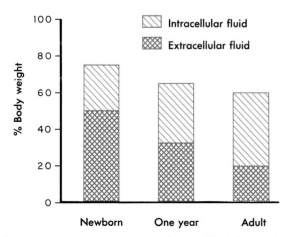

FIG. 5-1. In the newborn more than half of the total body fluid is extracellular. As the child grows, the proportions gradually approximate adult levels.

Table 5-1   Normal fluid intake and loss in an adult eating 2,500 calories/day (approximate figures)*

Intake		Output	
Route	Amount of gain (ml.)	Route	Amount of loss (ml.)
Water in food	1,000	Skin and lungs	1,000
Water from oxidation	300	Kidneys	1,500
Water as liquid	1,200	Total	2,500
Total	2,500		

*Adapted from Fluids and electrolytes, North Chicago, Ill., 1968, Abbott Laboratories.

Note that the intake of water in solid food is almost equal to that taken as liquid. Two-thirds as much water is lost from the skin and lungs as from the kidneys. This is significant in the care of patients with severe burns, who have lessened ability to perspire, and in the care of those who have poor pulmonary function.

through the glomeruli every minute. Normally, however, only 1 ml./minute is excreted as urine. The remainder is reabsorbed by the kidney tubules into the bloodstream. The baby's urinary output is similar to that of an adult, or one half of his total intake. His total water "turnover," however, is much larger in that he takes in and excretes proportionately much more water.[38]

Replacement. The body receives water from ingested food and fluids and through metabolism of both foodstuffs and body tissues. Solid foods such as meat and vegetables contain 60% to 90% water. Metabolic processes release about 12 ml. of water for each 100 calories of fat, carbohydrate, or protein oxidized.[24] Table 5-1 shows the approximate daily intake for an average adult. Note that the normal daily replacement of water equals the normal daily loss. Easily measurable intake (liquid) and easily measurable output (urine) are also approximately equal. These figures, therefore, serve as guides for determining normal fluid balance and emphasize the great need for recording intake and output accurately.

An infant's reserves of extracellular fluid are much more limited than are those of older children and adults. Since his daily turnover of water is more than half of his extracellular fluid volume, it is essential that his fluid losses be replaced at once. He cannot live even as long as an adult without fluids.

Body electrolyte component

All body fluids contain chemical compounds. Chemical compounds in solution may be classified as electrolytes or nonelectrolytes based on their ability to conduct an electric current in solution. Electrolytes in solution break up into charged particles called *ions*. Sodium chloride in solution exists as positively charged sodium ions, Na^+, and negatively charged chloride ions, Cl^-. Positively charged ions are called *cations*. Negatively charged ions are called *anions*. Proteins are special types of charged molecules. They have a charge that is dependent on the pH of the body fluids. At normal plasma pH (7.4) the proteins exist with a net negative charge (Table 5-2). Nonelectrolytes such as urea, dextrose, and creatinine remain molecularly intact and are essentially uncharged.

Electrolytes account for most of the osmotic pressure of the body fluids, are important in the maintenance of acid-base balance, and help to control body water volume. The three fluid compartments contain similar electrolytes, but the concentration of the various electrolytes in each compartment varies markedly (Table 5-2).

Differences in individual ion concentrations occur in various extracellular fluids. For instance, the gastric secretion is acid; hence the concentration of hydrogen ions is high. Pancreatic secretion, on the other hand, is more alkaline than plasma and contains a high concentration of bicarbonate. Gastric, pancreatic, and intestinal juices and bile all contain high concentrations of sodium ions.

In health the ratio of cations to anions in each of the body fluids and the concentration of the various ions in these fluids is relatively constant. Knowing the common electrolytes found in various body fluids is helpful for nurses in planning to prevent depletion

Table 5-2 Normal electrolyte content of body fluids and normal daily loss of ions in urine*

	Maintenance levels of fluid compartments			
	Extracellular			
Electrolytes (anions and cations)	Intravascular (mEq./L.)	Interstitial (mEq./L.)	Intracellular (mEq./L.)	Daily loss in urine (mEq./L.)
Sodium (Na^+)	142	146	15	200
Potassium (K^+)	5	5	150	90
Calcium (Ca^{++})	5	3	2	90
Magnesium (Mg^{++})	2	1	27	20
Chloride (Cl^-)	102	114	1	200
Bicarbonate (HCO_3^-)	27	30	10	17
Protein (Prot$^-$)	16	1	63	0
Phosphate ($HPO_4^=$)	2	2	100	26
Sulfate ($SO_4^=$)	1	1	20	22
Organic acids	5	8	0	50

*Adapted from Fluid and electrolytes, North Chicago, Ill., 1968, Abbott Laboratories.

Note that the electrolyte level of the intravascular and interstitial fluids (extracellular) is approximately the same and that sodium and chloride contents are markedly higher in these fluids, whereas potassium, phosphate, and protein contents are markedly higher in intracellular fluid. Normally most loss of electrolytes occurs through the kidneys, but with high fever or excessive perspiration an additional 25 to 50 mEq./L. of both sodium and chloride may be lost through the skin and lungs.

of necessary substances and in noting early signs of imbalance.

Normal exchange of electrolytes. Electrolytes move more readily between interstitial (surrounding the cells) and intravascular (within the blood vessels) fluids than between intracellular and interstitial fluids. Therefore normally most of the electrolyte exchange occurs between interstitial and intravascular fluids.

Loss. Electrolyte loss is mainly through the kidneys, with smaller losses through the skin and lungs and relatively minimal losses through the bowel. The kidneys selectively excrete certain electrolytes, retaining those needed for normal body fluid composition. Hormonal influences affect the kidneys' selective function. For example, the adrenocortical hormones favor sodium reabsorption and the excretion of potassium. Because of their rapid loss of water through the skin, infants normally lose more sodium than adults. They also tend to lose more potassium because more is freed by their rapid metabolism for growth, and its loss through the kidneys appears to be less finely controlled by hormonal action.[24]

Cells are very sensitive to changes in the pH (hydrogen ion concentration) of body fluids. The maintenance of a stable pH of body fluids is essential to life. The normal body fluid is slightly alkaline (pH 7.35 to 7.45) and is maintained in a relatively stable condition by "buffer systems" in the body. A buffer is a substance that can act as a chemical sponge, either soaking up or releasing hydrogen ions so that pH remains relatively stable. The main buffer systems of the extracellular fluid are hemoglobin, protein, and the carbonic acid-bicarbonate system. The latter is one of the most important clinically. Two types of carbonate are present in body fluids: carbonic acid

(H_2CO_3) and bicarbonate (HCO_3^-). The ability of the body to keep pH of body fluids within normal limits relies essentially on maintenance of the normal ratio of 1 part of carbonic acid to 20 parts of bicarbonate (Fig. 5-2).

The carbonic acid concentration is controlled by the lungs and the amount of carbon dioxide expelled is varied by the depth and rate of respiration. The bicarbonate concentration is controlled by the kidneys, which selectively retain or excrete bicarbonate depending on body needs. Refer to a physiology text for a more detailed description of the mechanism by which the normal ratio is maintained.

Replacement. A healthy person eating a well-balanced diet will easily ingest all the substances needed to maintain electrolyte balance. Any excess of electrolytes ingested will be excreted by the kidneys.

Fluid and electrolyte imbalance

Almost all medical and surgical conditions threaten fluid and electrolyte balance. Excessive amounts of body fluid and the electrolytes contained therein may be lost through the skin due to diaphoresis or to oozing from severe wounds or burns. They are lost from the gastrointestinal tract when profuse salivation, vomiting, or diarrhea occurs and when the gastrointestinal tract is drained by intubation or purged with cathartics or enemas. In hemorrhage, body fluids and electrolytes are always lost. Fluids with their electrolyte constituents may be trapped in the body by conditions such as wound swelling, edema, ascites, and intestinal obstruction and therefore may not be available for normal processes. Any person under stress (emotional or physical) loses additional amounts of potassium through the kidneys because production of adrenocortical hormones increases. Potassium depletion, therefore, is common in all disease, injury, and surgery. When the respiratory system does not provide an adequate exchange of oxygen and carbon dioxide, serious electrolyte imbalance usually results.

For clarity of discussion, imbalance of each ion and of body fluid will be considered separately. Actually, several imbalances occur simultaneously because of the interrelationship of body fluids and their electrolytes.

Fluid loss. When too much fluid is lost from the body, *dehydration* occurs. In the normal individual, increased thirst is the first symptom of fluid loss. If, for some reason, the individual is unable to maintain an adequate fluid intake and there is need to conserve body water, the antidiuretic hormone (ADH) will be secreted. ADH regulates osmotic pressure of the extracellular water by controlling the reabsorption of water in the distal tubules of the kidney. When these homeostatic mechanisms are not sufficient to overcome fluid loss, dehydration occurs. Fluid moves from the interstitial spaces into the intravascular compartment to help maintain adequate blood vol-

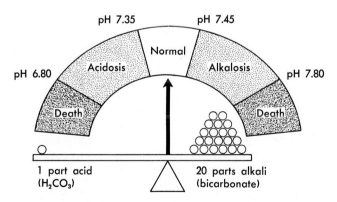

pH 7.35   pH 7.45

Normal

pH 6.80   Acidosis   Alkalosis   pH 7.80

Death   Death

1 part acid   20 parts alkali
(H_2CO_3)   (bicarbonate)

Carbonic acid-base bicarbonate balance

FIG. 5-2. Note that a relationship of 1 part carbonic acid to 20 parts of bicarbonate will maintain the hydrogen ion concentration (pH) within normal limits. An increase in H_2CO_3 or decrease in HCO_3 will cause acidosis; similarly, a decrease in H_2CO_3 or increase in HCO_3 will cause alkalosis. (Redrawn from Fluid and electrolytes, North Chicago, Ill., 1970, Abbott Laboratories.)

ume. The mechanism may occur either because there is increased plasma colloid osmotic pressure (due to protein concentration) or because there is decreased capillary fluid pressure. Both pressures serve to pull the fluid into the capillary, while the loss of water from the interstitial spaces causes fluid to move out of the cells, resulting in cellular dehydration.

The symptoms of dehydration are flushed, dry skin with poor turgor; dry lips; a dry, coated tongue; abnormal thirst; sunken, soft eyeballs; and atonic muscles. If the cause of dehydration continues unchecked and treatment is not given, anorexia, dyspepsia, and constipation develop as a result of inadequate fluids for gastrointestinal fuctioning. Normally about 8 L. of fluid are used daily for gastrointestinal fluids (Table 5-3), most of which is reabsorbed. As both intracellular and interstitial fluids decrease, cell function is impaired because food, oxygen, and waste products are diffused inadequately. The cells then release potassium, upsetting not only the potassium levels but the sodium levels of the body fluids and causing electrolyte imbalance with all its symptoms.

When there is a low serum sodium level, high serum potassium level, or dehydration, aldosterone is secreted by the adrenal cortex. Aldosterone promotes the *retention of sodium and water* by the kidney and increases the *excretion of potassium.* The sodium, which is retained, increases the retention of water because of osmolarity, and the urinary excretion of water is decreased. If an adequate blood volume cannot be maintained by these measures, cardiac output will be decreased and the blood pressure will drop. Renal function and vaporization then decrease, causing body wastes to be retained in the blood, which disturbs the potassium-sodium and acid-base balances still further. The heat-regulating mechanism also is upset. Unless fluid and electrolyte

replacement is begun at once, the patient may die. Because of his smaller water reserve, the baby quickly goes into shock from loss of blood volume.

In treating dehydrated patients, glucose and water often are given first to replace the water losses and to increase urinary flow. The urinary output must be normal for those electrolytes in excess of body needs to be excreted. Therefore solutions containing electrolytes needed by the body are not given until the urinary output is adequate to regulate the amount to be retained. When the renal function is adequate, normal saline solution or one-half strength normal saline solution is often given. In the treatment of dehydration, saline solutions usually constitute about one half of the 24-hour intake of parenteral fluids. Many experts now feel it is better to give a more dilute solution of sodium chloride (one-half strength saline solution) since this puts less of a load on the kidneys. Therefore the patient may receive all of his parenteral fluids as 5% glucose in 0.45% sodium chloride solution rather than half of his fluid replacement as 0.9% sodium chloride solution and the remainder as 5% glucose in water.[21] Additional electrolytes such as potassium chloride and sodium bicarbonate may be added to replace shortages of potassium and bicarbonate ions. If the patient can retain fluid given orally, fluids high in potassium content such as fruit juices and salty fluids high in sodium may be ordered.

If plasma proteins are lost from the body, as occurs in hemorrhage, or if they are shifted from the blood to the interstitial fluid, as occurs in burns, the blood volume drops rapidly because fluid from interstitial spaces cannot be mobilized to maintain it and shock follows. Whole blood, plasma, or plasma expanders usually must be given to these patients to replace the protein loss before extensive fluid therapy is effective.

Fluid excess. Fluid that is retained in the body in excess of normal is termed *overhydration.* If there is an excess of water without an increase in sodium or protein, water will enter the cells through osmosis, causing them to swell. This is referred to as *water intoxication* (dilution syndrome). If the excess fluid is isotonic, the fluid will remain in the extracellular compartments and *edema* will occur.

Water intoxication. This form of overhydration can occur when the water intake is greater than the kidneys' ability to excrete it. Water excess can occur in the following situations:

1. Excess secretion of ADH as seen in acute stress such as trauma or surgery, pain, fear, acute infections, administration of anesthetics or analgesics such as morphine or meperidine (Demerol), and cerebral lesions
2. Low renal blood flows as seen in congestive heart failure, cirrhosis of the liver, acute renal insufficiency, or Addison's disease
3. Large amounts of water given rectally as occurs

Table 5-3 Fluid composition of total internal secretions*

	Approximate ml. of fluid (daily)
Saliva	1,500
Gastric juice	2,500
Intestinal juice	3,000
Pancreatic juice	700
Bile	500
Total	8,200 ml./24 hr.

*Adapted from Fluid and electrolytes, North Chicago, Ill., 1968, Abbott Laboratories.
Note that approximately 8 L. of fluid is used daily for digestive purposes. Normally most of this fluid is reabsorbed. Some of each of the ions found in blood plasma is present in each of the fluids listed, but the individual concentration varies with each fluid.

with repeated enemas or x-ray studies of the bowel

4. Frequent and continuous amounts of water taken orally, especially the seriously ill patient who drinks sodium-free liquids rather than eating solid foods

5. Absorption of irrigating fluids during transurethral resection of the prostate[27]

The signs and symptoms of acute water intoxication are due to swelling of the cells and may develop rapidly and dramatically. These include changes in behavior, confusion, incoordination, convulsions, hyperventilation, sudden weight gain, and warm, moist skin. If the condition develops gradually, there may be apathy, sleepiness, anorexia, nausea, and vomiting. The patient will usually recover with careful water restriction unless convulsions and coma are present.

Edema. If there is an excess of body water with a concomitant increase in sodium (isotonic fluid), the excess fluid will be retained in the *extracellular* compartments and lead to the formation of edema. Edema is the accumulation of fluid in the interstitial spaces. In the normal tissue there is a negative interstitial fluid pressure and cells are held in close approximation to facilitate the exchange of gases, nutrients, and waste products between the cells and capillaries. If fluid accumulates in the interstitial space and is not removed either by direct return to the blood vessel or through the lymph system, a positive interstitial fluid pressure develops and cells are pushed farther apart. If a finger is pressed over an edematous area, the indentation made by the finger may remain briefly as the fluid is pushed to another area; this is called *pitting edema.* Fluid refills the interstitial space in the "pit" area within a few seconds. In the healthy individual, edema does not develop immediately with the initial inflow of fluid into the interstitial spaces due to the body's compensatory mechanisms, that is, the existing negative interstitial fluid pressure and the removal by the lymph system of excess fluids and proteins.

A review of normal capillary dynamics will help to understand the various factors that can cause edema to develop. There are two different types of pressures that influence the flow of fluid across a capillary membrane: fluid pressure (pressure resulting from the hydrostatic force of fluid) and colloid osmotic pressure, or *oncotic* pressure (pressure resulting from the presence of the proteins that do not diffuse across the membrane wall). Fluid pressure within the capillary is much greater than fluid pressure in the interstitial space; therefore this force *filters* fluid out of the capillary. Since there are a larger number of proteins in plasma than in interstitial fluid, the oncotic pressure within the capillary serves as a force to *absorb* fluid back into the capillary. According to Starling's "law of the capillaries,"

there is an equilibrium between the forces filtering fluid out of the capillary and forces absorbing fluid back into the capillary. The fluid hydrostatic pressure gradient (the difference between the fluid pressures inside and outside the capillary) should equal the oncotic pressure gradient (Fig. 5-3). If there is a change in the oncotic pressure in or out of the capillary or in the capillary fluid pressure, there will be a rapid fluid flow across the capillary membrane, creating a change in the interstitial fluid pressure until an equilibrium is reached again.*

Edema was defined earlier as an accumulation of fluid in the interstitial spaces creating a positive fluid pressure. Thus edema can be produced by the following: increase in capillary fluid pressure, decrease in capillary oncotic pressure, or increase in interstitial oncotic pressure (Table 5-4).

The same mechanisms that create edema in the interstitial spaces can create fluid collection in potential fluid spaces. These are spaces between two membranes that normally contain only traces of fluid. The main potential fluid spaces are intrapleural (lung and chest wall), pericardial (heart and pericardial sac), peritoneal (intestines and abdominal wall),

---

*For example, a decrease in capillary oncotic pressure to 16 mm. could produce the following (see Fig. 5-3).

$$17 - (x) = 16 - 4$$
$$17 - x = 12$$
$$x = 5 \text{ mm. of interstitial fluid pressure}$$

Fluid would filter rapidly into the interstitial space until a pressure of 5 mm. is reached. This would then effect a balance of 12 mm. of fluid pressure gradient and 12 mm. of oncotic pressure gradient.

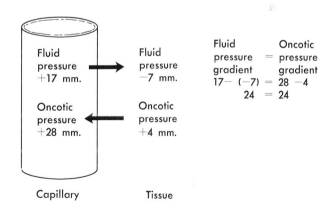

Diagram of Starling's law of capillaries

FIG. 5-3. An equilibrium exists between forces filtering fluid out of the capillary and forces absorbing fluid back into the capillary. Note that the fluid pressure within the capillary is greater than the fluid pressure in the tissue. This differential (fluid pressure gradient) serves as a filtering force. Note also that the oncotic pressure (colloid osmotic pressure) is greater within the capillary. This serves as an absorbing force.

Table 5-4 Etiology of edema with clinical example

FLUID PRESSURE	ONCOTIC PRESSURE

Increased (↑) capillary fluid pressure
Increased venous pressure
  Vein obstruction
    Varicose veins
    Thrombophlebitis
    Pressure on veins from casts, tight
      bandages, or garters
  Increased total blood volume with
    decreased cardiac output or decreased
    ADH
    Congestive heart failure
    Fluid overloading
Sodium retention: increased aldosterone
  due to
  Decreased renal blood flow
    Congestive heart failure
    Renal failure
  Increased production of aldosterone
    Cushing's syndrome
  Aldosterone added to system
    Corticosteroid therapy
  Inability to destroy excess aldosterone
    Cirrhosis of liver
	Decreased (↓) capillary oncotic pressure
	Loss of serum protein
	  Burns
	  Hemorrhage
	  Nephrotic syndrome
	  Chronic diarrhea
	Decreased production of protein
	  Malnutrition
	  Liver damage
	Increased (↑) interstitial oncotic pressure
	Increased capillary permeability to protein
	  Burns
	  Inflammatory reactions
	    Trauma
	    Infections
	  Allergic reactions
	Blocked lymphatics: decreased removal of
	  proteins
	  Malignant diseases
	  Surgical removal of lymph nodes
	  Elephantiasis

and joint spaces. The symptoms of fluid collection in these spaces are usually caused by the pressure of the collected fluid against adjoining organs or walls. Large amounts of fluid may collect in the peritoneal space *(ascites)*. This fluid is high in protein and electrolytes (p. 720). Accumulation of large amounts of fluid in all body tissue is called *anasarca*.

Overloading of the vascular system with fluid results in an increase in the hydrostatic pressure of the blood resulting in generalized tissue edema. More important, if the increase in hydrostatic pressure is great enough to push large amounts of fluid into the alveoli of the lungs, it rapidly leads to death from "drowning" in one's own fluids *(pulmonary edema)*. The hydrostatic pressure in the pulmonary vessels normally is much lower than that in the general circulation and therefore any increase in it is reflected rapidly in the lungs.

Overloading of the vascular system may be caused by giving too much fluid within a short period of time to a person who, because of circulatory or renal disease, cannot dispose of the surplus. Infants and young children can also be overloaded easily because they normally have little extravascular fluid reserve. Elderly people tolerate increases in blood volume very poorly since, with inelastic vessels, only relatively small increases in volume are needed to markedly increase the hydrostatic pressure. Monitoring the central venous pressure is the best way to determine if overloading is occurring.

Overloading of the vascular system also may be caused by increasing the oncotic (pull) pressure of the intravascular fluid by giving proteins so rapidly that the body cannot dispose of those that are in excess of its need. This overloading causes fluids to be pulled into the intravascular compartment from other body fluid compartments. The blood volume increases rapidly, neutralizing the oncotic pressure but increasing the hydrostatic pressure of the vascular system and the oncotic pressure of the interstitial fluid compartment. Fluid is then pushed into the tissues. Overloading the vascular system is a danger when fluids such as plasma, plasma expanders, albumin, or blood are given to any patient regardless of age or state of health.

Edema often is treated with diuretics, the action of which is on the kidneys. Some, such as the mercurial diuretics, block sodium reabsorption and consequently water reabsorption by the renal tubules. Other diuretic agents are partially or completely unabsorbable by the renal tubules and tend to carry sodium and water with them into the urine. When diuretics are given, a large amount of fluid is lost from the vascular compartment, increasing its oncotic pressure and causing fluid to be pulled back into it from the tissues. Potassium is usually lost along with the sodium and the water.

Reducing the salt intake also may reduce edema because the remaining supply of sodium seems to be needed to maintain the isotonicity of the blood and therefore is not available for holding water. If the edema is caused by venous stasis, elevating dependent body parts and applying supportive stockings promote venous return.

Overloading of the circulation is most often treated by phlebotomy (withdrawal of blood), and rotating tourniquets may be applied. If severe pulmonary symptoms are present, the administration of oxygen under positive pressure is started at once. (See treatment of acute pulmonary edema, p. 361.)

Blood volume determination. Since maintenance of normal blood volume is essential to electrolyte balance and the prevention of shock, a blood volume determination may be made. This procedure often is done preoperatively so that normal blood volume can be restored if necessary. It also may be done to monitor the effectiveness of fluid or blood therapy. A hematocrit reading usually is taken too because it gives an index of the ratio of plasma to cells and thus indicates the need for whole blood, plasma, or fluid replacement only.

In making blood volume determinations, one of several substances may be used such as a blue dye (Evans blue), radioactive iodinated blood albumin (RISA), or red blood cells tagged with a radioactive substance such as radioactive phosphorus. A known quantity of one of these substances is injected intravenously, and blood samples are taken from the opposite arm at a specified time and are examined to determine how much the injected substances have been diluted. Either Evans blue or RISA is used to determine the plasma volume. Tagged red cells are used to determine the red cell mass. By using appropriate formulas, the entire fluid content of the intravascular compartment (red cell mass plus plasma) can be calculated from either the red cell mass determination or the plasma volume determination.

When Evans blue dye is used, the patient should be informed that his urine will be a bluish green color and his skin may have a blue tinge for several days until all the dye is excreted. Since only trace doses of radioactive substances are given, no radiation precautions are necessary.

Electrolyte imbalance. No single electrolyte can be out of balance without causing some others to be out of balance also. This fact should be kept in mind while reading this section.

Imbalance of cations. Sodium, potassium, and calcium are all essential for the passage of nerve impulses. Whenever the concentrations of any of these cations are increased or decreased in body fluids, the increase or decrease is reflected in the stimulation of muscles by nerves. The muscles may become weak and atonic because of inadequate stimulation, or they may become somewhat spastic because of excess stimulation. A decrease in calcium concentrations in body fluids may cause the stimulus to be irregular, and muscle spasms may result. Gastrointes-

tinal and cardiac symptoms, so often produced by electrolyte imbalances, result in part from changes in neural stimulation of the muscles of these systems.

With cation imbalances, the distribution of body fluids frequently is upset. Abnormal collections of fluid probably cause some of the gastrointestinal symptoms such as nausea, vomiting, and diarrhea. Decreased amounts may cause anorexia, dyspepsia, and constipation. It is thought that edema of cerebral tissues may be responsible for headache, convulsions, and coma.

Sodium deficit. Whenever sodium is lost from the body fluids, they become hypotonic. Sodium loss from the intravascular compartment, therefore, causes fluid from the blood to diffuse into the interstitial spaces. As a result, the sodium in the interstitial fluid is diluted. In response to this reduction of the sodium concentration in the extracellular fluid, potassium moves out of the intracellular fluid. Therefore the patient with sodium imbalance is also likely to have potassium imbalance.

Sodium depletion results most often from the loss of gastrointestinal secretions. This can occur through vomiting, diarrhea, gastrointestinal or biliary drainage, or fistulas. Symptoms of sodium depletion appear rapidly in patients with profuse ileostomy drainage. Diarrhea in infants is extremely dangerous. Infants normally have large sodium losses through the skin; therefore, when large amounts of sodium are lost through the bowel as well, their sodium supply quickly becomes depleted. Sodium depletion can also occur in the shifting of body fluids so that the sodium is not accessible for use. This can occur in massive edema, ascites, burns, or small bowel obstruction.

Anyone who is perspiring profusely because of climate, exercise, or fever is losing large amounts of both sodium and water. If salt is not replaced with water such as by drinking, water intoxication will occur (p. 112). Salt can be replaced orally by drinking salty fluids, by taking salt tablets (0.5 Gm.), or by drinking a 0.1% solution (one 0.5 Gm. salt tablet in 500 ml. water).[27]

The normal concentration of sodium in the blood is 138 to 145 mEq./L. A low sodium level in the blood (*hyponatremia*) can indicate either a deficit of sodium or an excess of water. The usual symptoms of sodium deficit are headache, muscle weakness, fatigue, apathy, postural hypotension, anorexia, nausea and vomiting, and abdominal cramps. As the sodium loss becomes more severe, the increase in intracellular fluid and decrease in circulating blood volume produce symptoms of mental confusion, delirium, coma, and shock.

Sodium excess. If fluids are markedly limited or if extra salt is retained due to poor renal function or hormonal influences, sodium may be concentrated in the body fluids *(hypernatremia)*. Excess intravascular sodium causes fluid to be withdrawn from the tissues, resulting in dehydration. If fluids are not given to dilute the sodium and if excretion of sodium is not increased, extensive fluid and electrolyte imbalances will occur, causing manic excitement, tachycardia, and eventual death.

Potassium depletion. Potassium is the major cation of the cells. During the formation of new tissues *(anabolism)* or when glucose is converted to glycogen, potassium enters the cell. With tissue breakdown *(catabolism)*, potassium leaves the cell. This occurs with trauma, dehydration, or starvation. The body's mechanism for conserving potassium is not as effective as that for conserving sodium, and the kidneys may excrete potassium even when the body needs it. Whenever sodium is being retained in the body through reabsorption by the kidney tubules, potassium is excreted. Thus, whenever aldosterone secretion is increased such as in stress, potassium will be excreted. Potassium may also be lost through the urine as a result of certain diuretics such as the thiazide derivatives.

The patient who has a balanced diet withheld for several days, is dehydrated, or is given large amounts of parenteral fluids with no replacement of potassium develops potassium depletion. The parenteral administration of 5% dextrose in water without the addition of potassium tends to dilute the potassium in the extracellular tissues. This dilution, in addition to the lack of a balanced diet and to potassium loss due to catabolism of body proteins, accounts for many problems of electrolyte imbalance in the postoperative patient. Patients who eat a nutritionally inadequate diet or take no food for an extended period of time or who are losing large amounts of fluid from the gastrointestinal tract usually are given intravenous fluids containing electrolytes as well as glucose.

The practice of giving multiple enemas is becoming less common because it is now known that some of the enema fluid is absorbed and dilutes the potassium in the interstitial compartment, upsetting the balance between compartments. Solutions for hypertonic enemas may damage cells in the bowel mucosa, causing potassium loss.

The normal concentration of potassium in the blood is between 4 and 5 mEq./L. Potassium has a direct effect on cardiac and skeletal muscle function. The patient with potassium deficit *(hypokalemia)* will show characteristic electrocardiographic changes of flattened or inverted T waves with a prolonged Q-T interval. (See p. 324 for further discussion of a normal ECG.) The most striking symptom of hypokalemia is muscle weakness. Other symptoms are apathy, abdominal distention, and paralytic ileus (p. 229). Digitalis toxicity can occur in patients taking digitalis if they develop hypokalemia (p. 359).

In any of these situations the patient may die unless potassium is administered promptly. The safest way to administer potassium is orally. Fresh fruits (especially oranges and bananas) or foods high in protein are good sources of potassium. When potassium is given intravenously, the rate of flow must be monitored closely so as not to cause hyperkalemia and atrial arrest. The usual rate of infusion should not exceed 20 mEq. of potassium/hour.[27]

Potassium excess. As already stated, whenever there is severe tissue damage, potassium is released from the cells into the extracellular fluids. Since shock usually accompanies this damage, renal function is reduced and a high blood potassium level results *(hyperkalemia)*. There is great danger in giving extra potassium to any patient with poor renal function. If the patient is dehydrated or has lost vascular fluid, glucose and water or plasma expanders usually are given until renal function returns. Untreated adrenal insufficiency also is a contraindication for giving potassium. If the patient who has potassium intoxication needs a blood transfusion, fresh blood must be used. Cells in blood that has been kept for several days tend to release potassium during storage. If it is given, it may increase the patient's blood potassium level still further.

The patient with potassium intoxication develops spasticity of muscles due to their overstimulation by nerve impulses. He complains of nausea, colic, diarrhea, and skeletal muscle spasms. The muscles later become weak because overstimulation produces an accumulation of lactic acid and because potassium is lost from the muscle cells.

If the condition is not controlled, overstimulation of the cardiac muscle will cause the heartbeat to become irregular and eventually stop. ECG evidence of potassium elevation includes tall, peaked, symmetric, or tented T-waves with a short Q-T interval. As the blood potassium level increases further, the QRS spreads and atrial arrest occurs.[2] (See p. 324 for a discussion of ECG readings.)

When potassium intoxication occurs, the patient is allowed nothing orally, and an infusion of 10% glucose with 50 units of insulin is often given to induce transfer of potassium from the serum to the intracellular fluid. If the patient is in a state of acidosis, correction of the acidosis will result in movement of potassium back into the cell (p. 759). Cation exchange resins such as Kayexalate may also be given. If the patient is in acute renal failure, hemodialysis may be necessary. The patient should be on absolute bed rest and should receive complete nursing care until the potassium blood level is returned to normal.

Calcium deficit. Patients with pancreatic disease or disease of the small intestine may fail to absorb calcium from the gastrointestinal tract normally, and they may excrete abnormally large amounts of calcium in the feces, thus reducing the blood level of calcium. Patients who have draining intestinal fistulas also lose calcium. In renal failure and when the parathyroid glands are removed, the level of calcium in the blood is reduced. The normal serum calcium level is 4.5 to 5.8 mEq./L. The patient who has calcium deficiency usually first complains of numbness and tingling of the nose, ears, fingertips, or toes. If he is not given calcium at this time, painful muscular spasms, especially of the feet and hands (carpopedal spasm), muscle twitching, and convulsions may follow (tetany). There are two tests used to elicit signs of calcium deficiency. *Trousseau's sign* is elicited by grasping the patient's wrist to constrict the circulation for a few minutes. If his hand goes into a position of palmar flexion (carpopedal spasm), he probably has a serious calcium deficit. *Chvostek's sign* is elicited by tapping the patient's face lightly over the facial nerve (just below the temple). A calcium deficit is probably present if the facial muscles twitch.

The specific treatment for a low blood level of calcium is the administration of calcium gluconate or calcium chloride intravenously or orally. (See p. 744 for treatment of hypoparathyroidism and p. 470 for treatment of tetany in renal failure.)

Calcium excess. A marked increase in the calcium level of the blood *(hypercalcemia)* may be seen in diseases with extensive bone involvement such as metastatic carcinoma and hyperparathyroidism. One of the most serious consequences of hypercalcemia is the formation of renal stones. Therefore any patient with this condition, regardless of its cause, should always be given generous amounts of fluid. Immobilization is a common cause of hypercalcemia, and the condition is seen frequently in patients with fractures and skeletal muscle paralysis. It can be prevented by helping the patient to exercise muscles in uninvolved parts of the body. This condition is an important reason for encouraging patients who are immobilized in a back-lying position to use a trapeze bar. It is also one reason for encouraging all patients who are able to move about as much as possible and, with the use of side rails and other means, to engage in activities that require muscle action.

Because patients with marked hypercalcemia often are losing calcium from their bones, special care should be taken to prevent pathologic fractures. Even the pressure used in giving a back rub must sometimes be avoided. The patient with hypercalcemia commonly complains of severe thirst and has polyuria. Gastrointestinal symptoms, including anorexia, nausea, vomiting, and constipation, may also develop. Without treatment the patient may become lethargic and confused, and he may become comatose. The only definitive treatment is removal of the cause.

Acid-base imbalance. When the buffer systems are unable to maintain the hydrogen ion concentration (pH) of the blood within the normal range (7.35 to 7.45), the blood will become more acid *(acidosis)* or more basic *(alkalosis).* If the pH of the blood drops below 6.8 or rises above 8.0, death will usually ensue (Fig. 5-2). Carbonic acid excess or deficit is referred to as *respiratory* acidosis or alkalosis, whereas base bicarbonate change is called *metabolic* alkalosis or acidosis.

When acidosis or alkalosis does occur, two compensatory mechanisms are utilized by the body other than the buffer systems. The first is action of hydrogen ions on the respiratory center in the medulla to increase or decrease the rate and depth of breathing. As a result, carbon dioxide is removed rapidly or retained to a greater extent in the blood. This will decrease or increase the carbonic acid content. The second mechanism is the excretion by the kidneys of an acid or alkaline urine. In acidosis the kidney will reabsorb bicarbonate and excrete hydrogen ions with nonbicarbonate ions or as ammonia (NH_4). The reverse occurs with alkalosis. (Refer to a physiology text for a more detailed explanation of these mechanisms.)

The major effect of acidosis is depression of the central nervous system as evidenced by disorientation followed by coma. Alkalosis is characterized by overexcitability of the nervous system and the muscles may go into a state of tetany and convulsions.[30] Acid-base imbalances always produce an imbalance of the body's other cations as well, therefore symptoms of these imbalances will also occur.

Bicarbonate deficit. In some conditions such as uncontrolled diabetes mellitus and starvation, glucose either cannot be utilized or is not available for oxidation. The body compensates for this by using body fat for energy, producing abnormal amounts of ketone bodies. In an effort to neutralize the ketones (fatty acids) and maintain the acid-base balance of the body, plasma bicarbonate is exhausted. The resultant acid-base imbalance is known as *metabolic acidosis,* or *ketoacidosis.* This condition can develop whenever the person does not eat a balanced diet and his body fat must be burned for energy. It is the reason why extremely low-carbohydrate or high-protein/zero-carbohydrate reduction diets are criticized by nutrition experts.

Ketoacidosis rapidly develops in infants because they have minimal glycogen reserves. It also can develop whenever excessive amounts of lactic acid are produced because of strenuous muscle exercise or when oxidation takes place in cells without adequate oxygen such as occurs in shock.[45] Loss of large amounts of alkaline intestinal secretions such as in severe diarrhea or through fistulas can also create a bicarbonate deficit. The patient in acidosis becomes hyperpneic and has deep, periodic breathing. The hyperventilation represents an attempt to blow off carbon dioxide, thus compensating for the acidosis. If the condition is untreated, disorientation, stupor, coma, and death will occur.

Metabolic acidosis is controlled by giving intravenous solutions of sodium bicarbonate or sodium lactate. Sodium bicarbonate sometimes is given orally if it can be retained. Treatment of the condition precipitating the acidosis is then instituted.

Bicarbonate excess. When abnormally large amounts of hydrochloric acid and sodium chloride are lost through vomiting or drainage of the stomach, or when fluids high in potassium chloride are lost abnormally through biliary drainage, intestinal fistulas, or diarrhea, the result is an electrolyte imbalance in which there is an excess of base elements. This type of acid-base imbalance, which is known as *metabolic alkalosis,* is also caused by rapid ingestion of large amounts of sodium bicarbonate or carbonated drinks or the ingestion of these substances when renal function is impaired.

In metabolic alkalosis, breathing becomes depressed in an effort to conserve carbon dioxide for combination with hydrogen ions in the blood to raise the blood level of carbonic acid. Sodium chloride or ammonium chloride may be given to relieve metabolic alkalosis. If the condition is associated with loss of sodium chloride, potassium must be restored because it is lost with the sodium.

Carbonic acid deficit. Excessive pulmonary ventilation will decrease hydrogen ion concentration and thus cause *respiratory alkalosis.*[30] A common cause of respiratory alkalosis is *hyperventilation.* When the patient hyperventilates, he blows off large amounts of carbon dioxide. At the same time there are too many free cations in the blood, and they may be excreted through the kidney, leaving a deficiency. The patient may complain of lightheadedness and numbness or tingling of the fingers and toes. If the alkalosis becomes more severe, tetany and convulsions may be present. Hyperventilation often occurs in persons who are anxious or hysterical. If the patient has fainted, he can be aroused by administering a few whiffs of carbon dioxide or by having the patient breathe into a paper bag and then rebreathe his own exhaled carbon dioxide. If tetany is present, calcium gluconate is given intravenously.

Carbonic acid excess. Any factor that decreases the rate of pulmonary ventilation increases the concentration of dissolved carbon dioxide, carbonic acid, and hydrogen ions and results in *respiratory acidosis.*[30] An excess of carbon dioxide can cause carbon dioxide narcosis. In this condition (as the name implies), carbon dioxide levels are so high that they no longer stimulate respirations but depress them. Associated with the decreased respiratory rate is oxygen lack and hypoxia. During respiratory acidosis, potassium moves out of the cells, producing hyperkalemia. Ventricular fibrillation may occur if the blood

potassium levels are greatly increased. Treatment is aimed at increasing the excursion of the lungs in order to improve the exchange of carbon dioxide and oxygen. This objective is accomplished by using an intermittent positive pressure breathing (IPPB) machine to assist the patient to exhale carbon dioxide. Because the respiratory center is narcotized by increased amounts of carbon dioxide, the lowered oxygen tension of the blood is maintaining respirations. For this reason, oxygen is never given to patients with carbon dioxide narcosis unless they are receiving IPPB, and even then it must be administered in low, controlled concentrations (p. 574).

■ MANAGEMENT OF PATIENTS WITH FLUID AND ELECTROLYTE IMBALANCE

Important nursing functions include prevention of fluid and electrolyte imbalances, assessment of patients in order to recognize and report early signs of imbalances, and planning and carrying out actions related to replacement therapy and relief of symptoms.

Prevention of fluid and electrolyte imbalance

There are many ways in which the nurse can help to prevent fluid and electrolyte imbalance in both the healthy and the ill patient. Teaching patients the principles of good nutrition and encouraging them to eat nutritionally adequate diets promotes maintenance of fluid and electrolyte balance.

Unless preventive measures are employed, many medical and surgical conditions and techniques used to treat them may lead to fluid and electrolyte imbalance. There are some rather frequently encountered situations in which the nurse's attention to preventive aspects may lessen the possibility of the development of serious imbalance.

Inadequate fluid intake. Any patient who is unable to ask for fluids, to identify his own need for fluid, or to swallow easily may develop a fluid deficit. Thus a patient with a cerebral vascular accident and aphasia may not be able to communicate his desire for fluids or may have difficulty swallowing fluids that are offered to him. A confused or disoriented patient may not be aware that he is thirsty. Patients who are comatose, weak, or catatonic may also develop fluid deficits. The nurse should recognize those patients who may not be receiving adequate fluid intake, monitor their intake and output and plan scheduled fluid offerings for them.

Patients receiving tube feedings may also experience fluid deficits since the content of most tube feedings is high in solutes such as dextrose, protein, and salt. These solutes given in high concentrations may act as osmotic diuretics and be excreted by the kidney along with large amounts of water. This can result in a sodium loss as well as a fluid deficit.

Fluid loss from the gastrointestinal tract. Vomiting and diarrhea are common symptoms of many illnesses, and most people suffer from them from time to time. Sodium and some potassium are lost in vomiting and diarrhea, while chloride is lost only in vomitus. As soon as fluids are tolerated, the patient who has vomiting or diarrhea should be served salty broth and tea or another fluid high in potassium in order to replace the losses. This measure often keeps the patient from feeling so weak and exhausted. Dry soda crackers often are tolerated when fluids are not and can be used to replace sodium. Prompt replacement of both water and electrolytes is essential in infants since they have limited reserves. If vomiting or diarrhea persist for even a few hours and oral foods are not tolerated, infants should have medical attention since they may need intravenous replacement of losses.

A patient with a draining fistula from any portion of the gastrointestinal tract loses sodium, calcium, and some potassium. It is important that his diet be supplemented. Extra milk will replace all the losses, and the patient should be instructed to increase his milk intake somewhat above normal levels. For the body to use the calcium, vitamin D also must be available, but most milk is now fortified with vitamin D. People with a permanent fistulous opening such as an ileostomy need to be especially careful to supplement sodium and potassium when vomiting, diarrhea, or fever adds to their already unusually large loss of electrolytes.

Many patients in the course of treatment have a nasogastric tube inserted and attached to suction drainage. Routine intravenous replacement usually is adequate to compensate for losses through this drainage unless the patient has been allowed to take fluids orally or has had the tube irrigated frequently with water. Both of these practices, although they seem to be harmless because the fluid is removed immediately through the aspiration apparatus, stimulate the secretion of gastric juices. Aspiration of gastric juices and other normal secretions of the stomach at rest may lead to electrolyte and sometimes even fluid imbalances. If irrigation of the tube is necessary, physiologic saline solution should be used. Thirst is a problem for these patients, and measures must be taken to relieve it, but special precautions should be taken to be certain that the patient does not consume the fluid from ice chips or mouth rinses.

If there is an order for enemas until the returns are clear, the nurse should not give more than three enemas to the patient without consulting the physician, since this treatment may result in water intoxication or potassium loss (p. 116). The practice of some people, especially those who are older, of taking daily enemas should be discouraged, especially if hypertonic solutions (detergents, for example) are used. If an elderly person living at home complains of pronounced weakness without apparent cause, the nurse should ask whether he has been taking cathartics or enemas. If so, stopping this procedure, eating foods with high sodium and potassium content, and increasing the fluid intake may relieve the symptoms. Methods to combat constipation without purging should be taught.

Abnormal fluid loss through the skin, lungs, and kidneys. Any person who is perspiring profusely is losing sodium, and anyone who is hyperventilating because of fever, strenuous exercise, exposure to excessive heat, or other causes (such as acidosis, difficulty with oxygenation, or stress) is losing abnormally large amounts of carbon dioxide. In all these situations more fluid than usual is lost.

Even the healthy person who is perspiring profusely needs extra salt in his diet and should drink extra fluids, and some salty fluids should be given to any patient with a fever. Patients on salt-restricted diets and those with draining gastrointestinal fistulas are especially likely to suffer from sodium depletion. They should always be taught to increase their salt intake slightly whenever they perspire profusely. Patients who have hot packs applied to large areas of the body also lose sodium and water, although the loss may not be readily noticeable as perspiration. If they are able to take fluids orally, salty broths should be served to them several times a day. Attention to ingesting more salt and water than usual whenever a person is in situations of excessive heat, climatic or otherwise, may prevent heat exhaustion.

Patients who are hyperventilating for long periods of time, regardless of the reason, should have their fluid intake increased somewhat because they are losing more fluid than usual through the lungs. Although this may not actually upset the fluid balance of the body in people with adequate renal function, it does cause the urine to become concentrated, which may allow waste products of metabolism, toxins, and minerals to pass through the kidneys without sufficient dilution. If this process continues for long, renal damage may occur. Infants and adults whose kidneys cannot conserve water because of disease will become dehydrated rapidly whenever more fluid than usual is lost by other routes.

Because an infant loses so much fluid through his skin, there normally may be some discrepancy between his liquid intake and his urine output. Patients who are dehydrated and those who are losing large amounts of body fluids through perspiration, wounds, or the gastrointestinal tract also can be expected to have less urine output in relation to intake. Urinary output in the adult should not fall below 900 ml. a day, and the total fluid lost from all routes should equal the fluid intake.

All diuretics (except Aldactone A) are adminis-

119

tered to encourage excretion of sodium and water that are in excess of body needs. However, potassium, which may not be in excess, is lost also. Therefore the nurse should encourage the patient who is receiving diuretics to eat foods that are high in potassium but low in sodium. Tea, coffee, and fruit juices are good sources of potassium, but the patient usually must limit fluids. Therefore he should be advised to select most of his fluids from liquids containing potassium. Bananas and other fresh fruits also provide good sources of potassium without increasing the sodium or fluid intake. Diuretics such as the thiazides eventually may cause sodium depletion; therefore the patient who is receiving extensive diuretic treatment should be observed for symptoms indicating sodium depletion (p. 115). Since many patients receiving diuretics are at home, they should be taught to report symptoms of sodium depletion to the physician.

Changes in the urinary output may forewarn of fluid and electrolyte imbalance. Therefore persons with a urine output that greatly exceeds fluid intake and persons with oliguria should see a physician.

Renal or circulatory impairment. Any patient with renal or circulatory impairment as may occur in shock, cardiac decompensation, or constriction of blood vessels because of disease, may develop electrolyte imbalance. Sodium and water may be held in the tissues, the potassium level of the blood may rise, acidosis may develop from inadequate tissue oxygenation, or the kidneys may be unable to excrete waste products properly. The nurse should instruct patients with cardiac and renal impairment to avoid taking too much food containing sodium, potassium, or bicarbonate. They should not drink carbonated beverages. Since many people take bicarbonate of soda or similar proprietary products, they should be told about the undesirability of this practice also.

Patients with renal or circulatory impairment can easily be overhydrated. The nurse should be especially aware of overhydration whenever intravenous fluids are being given and should consider it in planning "forced fluid" regimens for these patients.

Respiratory impairment. Any change from the normal pattern of gaseous exchange or any impairment of cell oxygenation can cause acid-base imbalances. Hyperventilation is a common cause of carbonic acid deficit in the blood. Because anyone has a tendency toward alkalosis following strenuous exercise, carbonated drinks, which also contribute to alkalosis, should be omitted until the body has had time to regulate its acidity. Special attention should be paid to patients in respirators and to those who are receiving IPPB to avoid respiratory alkalosis. If a patient complains of dizziness or shows any signs of muscle irritability, it is likely that the depth of respiration is too great, and the respiratory rate of the machine should be decreased. Nursing measures to reduce high body temperatures and anxiety also help to prevent hyperventilation.

Patients with diseases such as emphysema that limit lung excursion and therefore limit gaseous exchange should not take carbonated beverages or bicarbonate of soda. These substances tend to make the blood more alkaline than normal, and respirations are depressed in an effort to correct this imbalance. Depression of respirations is highly undesirable for these patients.

Any patient with symptoms of inadequate oxygenation or carbon dioxide retention requires medical treatment. Early recognition and treatment of the primary condition often prevents its becoming complicated by acid-base imbalance. Therefore any person with symptoms suggestive of anemia, cardiac insufficiency, emphysema, asthma, or other obstructive diseases of the bronchioles should receive medical attention.

Effect of stressors. Any stressful situation (physical or emotional) may precipitate a condition that leads to electrolyte and acid-base imbalance. Therefore alleviation of anxiety, building up the patient's nutritional status preoperatively to increase his glycogen stores, and helping to restore nutrients to patients who are ill or who have had surgery are important aspects of nursing intervention and may be vital in preventing serious complications from fluid and electrolyte imbalance.

A well-hydrated person who is not losing fluids abnormally will excrete amounts of urine approximately equal to his liquid intake. Postoperatively, however, a person not only has decreased urine production due to increased production of ADH, but he also tends to lose slightly larger amounts of fluid than normal as insensible water loss. Although he may have a fluid intake of 2,000 to 3,000 ml./day, he may have a urinary output of only 1,000 to 1,500 ml./day and he should be observed for signs of overloading.

Assessment of fluid and electrolyte balance

The nurse should be familiar with the symptoms of fluid and electrolyte imbalance and make ongoing physical assessments (Table 5-5) of those patients who have a potential for fluid and electrolyte imbalances. For subjective data such as headache, thirst, nausea, or dyspnea, the nurse should ascertain time of origin and extent of the symptoms. Objective data can be compared to baseline assessments obtained at the time of the patient's entry into the health system.

Additional data to be considered in assessing fluid and electrolyte balance are comparison of fluid intake to output and changes in the patient's weight. Acutely ill medical patients and patients undergoing major surgery should have their fluid intake and output and daily weight closely monitored. All those giv-

Table 5-5   Assessment of fluid and electrolyte balance

	Fluid excess	Fluid loss/electrolyte imbalance
Behavior	Change in behavior, confusion, apathy	Change in behavior, confusion, apathy
Head, neck	Facial edema, distended neck veins	Headache, thirst, dry mucous membranes
Upper gastrointestinal	Anorexia, nausea, vomiting	Anorexia, nausea, vomiting
Skin	Warm, moist, taut, cool feeling where edematous	Dry, decreased turgor
Respiration	Dyspnea, orthopnea, productive cough, moist breath sounds	Changes in rate and depth of breathing
Circulation	Tire easily, loss of sensation in edematous areas, pallor*	Pulse rate changes, arrhythmias
Abdomen	Increased girth, fluid wave	Distention, abdominal cramps
Elimination	Oliguria, constipation, scrotal edema	Oliguria, diarrhea, constipation
Extremities	Dependent edema "pitting," discomfort from weight of bedclothes	Muscle weakness, tingling, tetany

*Pallor-edema decreases the intensity of skin color by decreasing the distance between the skin surface and the pigmented or vascular areas. In the dark-skinned individual, pallor is observed by absence of underlying red tones that give brown and black skin "glow." The brown skin appears more yellow-brown and the black skin appears more ashen gray.[42]

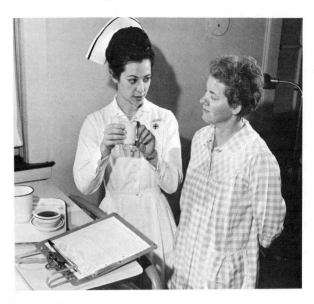

FIG. 5-4. Often the patient needs to be taught to measure and record fluid intake and output accurately.

ing nursing care should understand the need for recording intake and output of selected patients and the importance of accuracy. Patients should know that their intake and output is being recorded so that accuracy can be maintained. If patients are given explanations, their participation can be obtained, when appropriate, in measuring and recording their own intake and output (Fig. 5-4). Totaling the fluid intake and output every shift or every 24 hours gives the nurse and physician additional data for determining if the patient may have a fluid imbalance.

The intake record. The intake record should show the type and amount of all fluids the patient has received and the route by which these were administered. This includes fluids given orally, parenterally, rectally, or fluids administered by tubes and retained by the patient. A record of solid food intake is some-

times necessary, especially with very young children. Foods that are eaten in a semisolid state but which are basically liquid, such as gelatin or ice cream, are recorded as fluids. Ice chips are recorded by dividing the amount of chips by one-half (60 ml. of chips would equal 30 ml. of water). Patients may receive a considerable amount of fluid intake through the frequent sucking of ice chips.

Urinary output. Urinary output should be recorded as to time and amount of each voiding. This record helps to evaluate renal function more accurately. If renal function is a major concern, as in a severely burned patient, an indwelling catheter is used so that the amount of urinary drainage can be recorded every hour and fluid intake regulated accordingly. It has been said that nothing is more difficult to obtain in a modern hospital than an accurate record of urine output, and unfortunately this statement is often true. Conspicuous signs posted on the patient's chart and in the utility room and bathrooms will help to prevent the discarding of urine before it is measured.

Wound drainage. All drainage from body or artificial openings should be measured. This would include such drainage as that from an ileostomy, from a T tube following exploration of the common bile duct, or from any catheter draining a surgical area. If there is excessive drainage from a wound, it may be necessary to weigh the dressings. Fluid loss is the difference between wet weight and dry weight of the dressing.

Other output. Electrolytes are lost in large amounts with vomiting, diarrhea, and gastric drainage. The amount and kind vary according to what type of gastrointestinal fluid is lost. For the physician to determine the amount and type of fluid replacement needed, vomitus, gastrointestinal drainage, and liquid stools should be measured as accurately as possible and should be described as to color, contents, and odor. Gastric secretions are watery, a pale yellowish green, and usually have a sour odor. However, if the acid-base balance has been upset, gastric secretions may have a fruity odor because of the presence of acetone. Bile is somewhat thicker than gastric juice and may vary from bright yellow to dark green in color. It has a bitter taste and acrid odor. Intestinal contents vary from dark green to brown in color, are likely to be quite thick, and have a fecal odor. Fluid used to irrigate nasogastric tubes should be subtracted from total drainage before it is recorded.

It is difficult to determine accurately the amount of water lost in the stools, but a description of their consistency and a record of the number of stools passed give the physician an estimate. The color of stools should be recorded too. Because infants are likely to lose large amounts of water in their stools, daily records usually are kept for any baby who is ill.

Fluid aspirated from any body cavity such as the abdomen or pleural spaces must be measured. This fluid contains not only electrolytes and water but also proteins. Blood loss from any part of the body should be measured carefully.

Diaphoresis is difficult to measure without special laboratory equipment. However, it may be important to estimate the loss of fluid by this route in some patients. Careful note of "excessive" perspiration and its duration should be made. If the clothing and linen become saturated, dry and wet weights may be taken. Accurate recording of body temperature helps the physician to determine how much fluid the patient needs, since fluid loss through the skin and lungs increases as the temperature rises.

Daily weight. The daily weight record is often the best way to determine the onset of dehydration or of the accumulation of fluid either as generalized edema or as "hidden" fluid in body cavities. An increase of 1 pound in weight is equal to the retention of 1 pint (500 ml.) of fluid in the edematous patient. If the weight record is to be useful, the patient must be weighed on the same scale and at the same hour each day, and he must be wearing the same amount of clothing. Circumstances that may affect the weight should be kept as nearly identical as possible from day to day. Usually weights are taken in the early morning before the patient has eaten or defecated, but after he has voided. When extremely accurate measurements are needed, all clothing and even wound dressings are removed from the patient before he is weighed.

Laboratory values. Laboratory determinations of serum levels of the specific electrolytes help in making decisions concerning electrolyte excesses or deficits. Serum pH, pCO_2 (indicator of carbonic acid concentration), and carbon dioxide content (sum of all carbon dioxide dissolved in plasma as carbonic acid or bicarbonate) help in identifying acid-base imbalances. When there is water excess, hemodilution will occur and the hemoglobin and hematocrit levels will be decreased. With excessive fluid loss, there will be hemoconcentration and the hematocrit will be increased.

Replacement therapy

The best way to restore water, electrolytes, and nutrients to the body is to give them orally (Fig. 5-5). When fluids can be tolerated by the stomach but cannot be swallowed, a nasogastric tube may be passed, and fluids containing all the essentials of a balanced diet may be given through it. Normal saline solution or plain water also may be given by slow drip through the tube to replace fluid loss.

If it is not possible for a patient to take food or fluid through the alimentary tract, the most common method of replacement is by intravenous infusion *(venoclysis)*. A vein in the leg or arm commonly is used for a venoclysis, but in infants a vein in the scalp or the femoral or jugular vein may be used. An intravenous infusion may be given by introducing a needle into a vein and taping the needle in place or

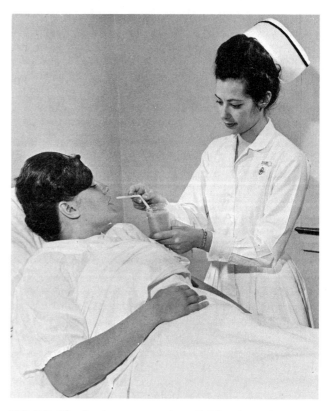

FIG. 5-5. The best way to replace fluids, electrolytes, and nutrients is to give them by mouth.

by making an incision *(cutdown)* and threading a polyethylene catheter *(intracatheter)* into the vein. The intracatheter is the method of choice for parenteral hyperalimentation (p. 125) or for the monitoring of central venous pressure (p. 326).

Physiologic solutions of sodium chloride or solutions containing other electrolytes may be given into subcutaneous tissues *(hypodermoclysis)*. Infants and young children often are given fluids by this method. In adults the fluid usually is injected beneath the skin of the thigh. In babies the thighs, scapular region, or abdomen frequently is used. Infants and young children also may be given fluid intraperitoneally. Normal saline solution or plain water sometimes is given by slow drip *(Murphy drip)* into the rectum, where it is absorbed quickly in most instances.

Fluids given by any route should be spaced throughout the 24-hour period. Not only does this practice help to maintain normal body fluid levels, but it also provides for better regulation of the electrolyte balance by the kidneys and prevents the end products of metabolism and toxic materials from being excreted in concentrated form. In this way the danger of renal damage, formation of calculi, and irritation of the lower urinary tract is reduced. In addition, fluid spacing prevents overloading of the circulation, which may result in dilution of body fluids, with resultant fluid and electrolyte shifts, the most serious of which causes pulmonary edema.

Concentrated solutions of sugar or protein should always be given slowly in small amounts at a time because they will require fluids from the body for dilution. Hypertonic saline solution may cause fluid to diffuse from the tissues to equalize the concentrations of salt in the fluid compartments. Therefore it, too, should be given slowly and in small amounts. The superior vena cava is the preferred site for infusions of hypertonic solutions given by parenteral hyperalimentation methods because of the rapid dilution by the larger amount of blood at this site. If any of these concentrated solutions flow too rapidly into the vascular system, pulmonary edema can develop.

Giving concentrated solutions rapidly and in large amounts into the alimentary tract causes the blood volume to drop, and if large amounts of fluid are needed to dilute the substance, irreversible shock can result. The "dumping syndrome," which sometimes occurs after a gastric resection (p. 671), is caused by this abnormal shift of fluid. Concentrated solutions sometimes are given intentionally to reduce cerebral edema (p. 124). Giving large amounts of fluid either orally or parenterally is potentially dangerous even in a healthy person and therefore fluids of any kind should never be replaced faster than they are lost.

The size of the patient should be considered in

Table 5-6 Approximate division of total body fluid into compartments

Body fluid compartments	Liters of fluid	
	Lean adult weighing 100 pounds	Lean adult weighing 150 pounds
Intravascular (plasma)	2.8	4.2
Interstitial	8.4	12.5
Intracellular	22.3	33.3
Total	33.5	50.0

Note that the smaller the individual, the less fluid he has in each compartment and that plasma is reduced most markedly with decrease in size. The normal size and body type of the individual are considered when fluid replacement is ordered.

giving fluids. The small person normally has less fluid in each body compartment, especially in the intravascular system (Table 5-6). He therefore becomes seriously dehydrated more quickly than a larger person and needs his fluid losses replaced more promptly. Prompt replacement is even more important in infants and young children. Because so much of their body fluid normally is extracellular, they have proportionately less reserve fluid in the cells from which to pull than has a small adult. People with small or inelastic vascular systems also become overhydrated easily. It is important to remember that the vascular system of a person who has had a large portion of his body such as a limb removed either by surgery or trauma is not the same size as previously.

Parenteral fluids. The nurse needs to know the common solutions used parenterally. Dextrose, 5%, in distilled water is often used to maintain fluid intake or to reestablish blood volume. Ascorbic acid and vitamin B (Solu-B) are frequently added. Dextrose, 5%, in saline solution may be given depending on the serum levels of sodium, and potassium chloride may be added to maintain normal intake needs of potassium and to replace losses. A physiologic solution of sodium chloride is given primarily when sodium chloride has been lost in large amounts such as in loss of gastrointestinal fluids or in burns. One-sixth molar lactate solution may be ordered when sodium, but not chloride, needs replacement; ammonium chloride solution may be used to replace chlorides without adding sodium. Balanced solutions containing several electrolytes may be used. Ringer's solution, Hartmann's solution (lactated Ringer's solution), and Darrow's solution are examples.

Body needs for carbohydrates may be partially

met by giving fructose or 10% or 20% glucose in distilled water. Since these solutions are hypertonic, they will require more water for excretion.

Amino acid preparations (Aminosol) are seldom given by standard intravenous methods. Whole blood, plasma, concentrated albumin, or plasma volume expanders can be given to substitute for blood protein loss and are used to reestablish normal blood volume and prevent shock (p. 107). Dextran is the most generally accepted plasma volume expander. It increases the oncotic pressure of the blood, thus increasing the reabsorption of fluid from interstitial spaces. This creates an increase in plasma volume. Low molecular weight dextran decreases the viscosity of the blood, allowing greater flow of blood through the capillaries; thus it is useful in treating cardiogenic, hemorrhagic, or septic shock. It may cause a prolonged bleeding time and should not be used if renal disease with severe oliguria or anuria is present or during pregnancy.[27] The nurse should be alert for signs of anaphylactic reaction (apprehension, dyspnea, wheezing respirations, tightness of chest, itching, hypotension) when dextran is being given.

Intravenous fluids containing electrolytes should be run slowly to allow the body to regulate their use. The patient should be watched carefully for signs of intoxication (excess of fluids or electrolytes). Increased serum potassium (hyperkalemia) can be particularly dangerous, since it may cause cardiac arrest. When solutions containing electrolytes are given, the nurse should monitor the urinary output carefully and report any decrease in the amount to the physician. Since the kidneys select the ions needed and excrete surplus ones, a normal output is significant. If the nurse is planning the sequence of intravenous fluids, hydrating fluids such as one-half strength physiologic solution of sodium chloride or glucose in water solution should be given first. Renal failure and untreated adrenal insufficiency are contraindications for the use of potassium. If these conditions are known or suspected to exist, the nurse should verify orders for its administration. Many physicians do not start intravenous therapy for the day until chemical analyses of the blood have been reported.

The rate of administration of fluids usually is ordered by the physician and will depend on the patient's illness, the kind of fluid given, and the patient's age. An infusion is rarely run at a rate faster than 4 ml./minute. If it is given continuously or if it is given when there is impaired renal function or impaired cardiac function, it is rarely run faster than 2 ml./minute. The usual rate for replacement of fluid loss is 3 ml./minute. This rate allows time for the fluid to diffuse into the extracellular fluid compartments and avoids overloading the circulation or raising the blood volume high enough to produce a diuret-

ic effect. (For precautions as to the rate for concentrated solutions, blood, and blood products, see p. 123.) The nurse should realize that the various equipment for fluid administration may have varying numbers of milliliters per drop. This number must always be checked, since it is not the drops per minute but the milliliters per minute that are important.

Nurses should question the advisability of the rather common practice of speeding up the rate of flow of solutions given intravenously primarily to complete the treatment at a specified time. Every nurse should recognize the initial signs of pulmonary edema (bounding pulse, engorged peripheral veins, hoarseness, dyspnea, cough, or pulmonary rales) and should observe closely for them in patients who are receiving concentrated solutions, those who must be given any intravenous solution rapidly, and those whose age or physical condition makes them special risks. At the first signs of increased blood volume the rate of flow of the infusion should be greatly reduced and the physician notified. Special care needs to be taken in giving fluids to infants, elderly patients with circulatory impairment, patients whose hearts are decompensated, those with renal impairment, and those who have had plasma shifts such as burned patients and those with extensive tissue trauma from other causes. Patients whose plasma has shifted need to be watched especially carefully after a few days because the plasma tends to shift back suddenly from the interstitial tissue to the blood, producing an increase in blood volume with resulting pulmonary edema (p. 361).

It is imperative that the nurse check fluid bottles carefully for correctness of content and record accurately the fluids given. Too much fluid or too much of any of the electrolyte substances can be disastrous for the patient. The greatest care also should be taken to see that any needle that enters a vein has been sterilized by autoclaving to avoid its being contaminated by organisms (p. 714). (For details of equipment and nursing techniques needed in parenteral fluid administration refer to a textbook on fundamentals of nursing.)

Patients who are receiving fluids intravenously should be observed frequently to check the rate of flow so that symptoms indicating the need to slow down, speed up, or stop the infusion may be noted. Signs of developing pulmonary edema should be watched for especially. The tissue at the site of the inserted needle should be checked at intervals for signs of infiltration or inflammatory reaction. If infiltration occurs, the infusion should be stopped at once and plans made to restart it. Solutions such as those containing potassium, are very irritating and may cause tissue necrosis. When checking to see why an infusion is not running properly, the nurse should be extremely careful not to accidentally introduce air or a clot from the needle into the tubing.

Either may act as an embolus when it reaches the bloodstream and cause death.

Parenteral hyperalimentation. Parenteral hyperalimentation is a method of giving highly concentrated solutions intravenously to maintain the nutritional needs of an individual over a period of time for the purpose of protein synthesis (Fig. 5-6). Indications for this therapy are patients having major gastrointestinal diseases, fistulas, or inflammatory disease; patients who develop extensive negative nitrogen balance such as occurs with major body burns, extensive wounds, or starvation; and patients with cancer who are experiencing gastrointestinal side effects from radiation therapy.

The physician initiates the infusion by inserting an intracatheter either into the brachial artery and into the subclavian vein or directly into the subclavian vein and threading it through the innominate vein into the superior vena cava. The large amount of blood in the superior vena cava helps to dilute the highly concentrated solution rapidly and thus prevent phlebitis or vein occlusion. The jugular vein is preferred in infants for ease of insertion but is too close to hair-growing areas in adults (possibility of sepsis) and is more restraining of neck movements. The insertion of the intracatheter is not painful, but the patient may experience a feeling of pressure. The intracatheter is sutured with one suture and covered by an air-occlusive dressing. The infusion is started with a standard intravenous fluid until an x-ray film confirms the location of the catheter tip in the superior vena cava.

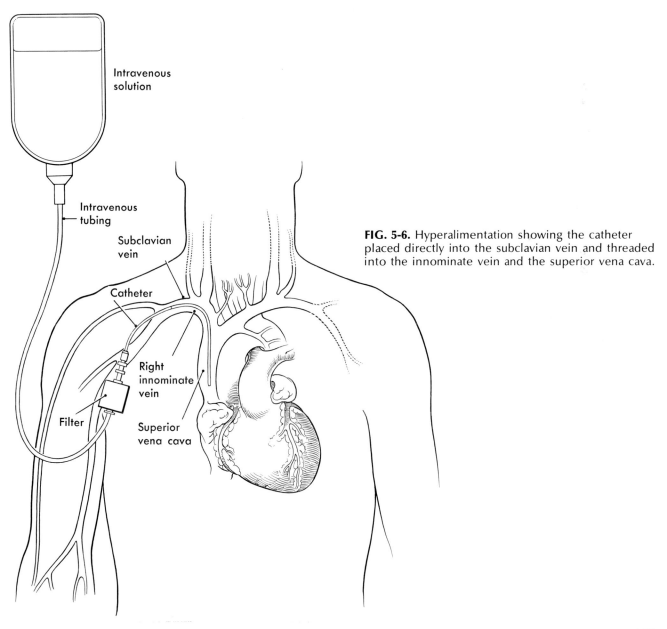

Intravenous solution

Intravenous tubing

Subclavian vein

Catheter

Right innominate vein

Filter

Superior vena cava

FIG. 5-6. Hyperalimentation showing the catheter placed directly into the subclavian vein and threaded into the innominate vein and the superior vena cava.

Solutions for parenteral hyperalimentation are good culture media and should be prepared under strict aseptic conditions, preferably in the pharmacy under a laminar air-flow hood. The physician orders the solution contents based on the patient's nutritional needs. A sufficient amount of glucose to meet energy needs is necessary so that the amino acids are used for protein synthesis rather than for energy. The basic nutrient solution usually contains 20% to 25% glucose to which protein hydrolysate, minerals, and vitamins are added. The commercial preparations of the protein hydrolysate are relatively trouble-free, but some patients do demonstrate sensitivity reactions (headache, fever, myalgia, chills, nausea and vomiting, rash, vasodilation, abdominal pain, convulsions).[12] Medication should *not* be added to the solutions, and any piggyback intravenous setups, central venous pressure monitoring, or drawing of blood for laboratory analyses should not be done through the parenteral hyperalimentation setup in order to maintain scrupulous aseptic conditions. Prepared solutions that are kept refrigerated should be warmed to room temperature before infusion.[12] Solutions should not be hung for longer than a 12-hour period.

Nursing responsibilities during parenteral hyperalimentation therapy. The following are nursing responsibilities during parenteral hyperalimentation therapy.

PREVENTION OF INFECTION. Strict aseptic technique is mandatory during changing of bottles, tubings, or dressings. The nurse should be knowledgeable concerning the frequency and method of dressing changes being utilized. Wet dressings are changed immediately to prevent transmission of bacteria by capillary action. The dressing should be air occlusive. Presence of an elevated temperature should be reported immediately to the physician, and cultures should be taken of the insertion site, tubing, and solutions for fungal as well as bacterial studies. Patients who experience itching under the dressing are cautioned not to scratch or disturb the dressing.

PREVENTION OF AIR EMBOLISM. The possibility of air embolism is greater with use of the superior vena cava than with a peripheral vein because of the decreased venous pressure as the blood approaches the heart. All connections in the parenteral hyperalimentation setup should be taped to prevent accidental separation. Tubing changes should be made quickly with the patient lying flat in bed. The patient may be asked to perform the Valsalva maneuver, forced expiration against a closed glottis, while the tube is disconnected.[12] Filters are useful for trapping air as well as bacteria.

MAINTENANCE OF FLUID AND ELECTROLYTE BALANCE. The goal of parenteral hyperalimentation is a continued and uniform infusion rate of the hypertonic solution. Frequent checking (every 30 to 60 minutes) of the established drip rate and patency of the infusion are important. A decreased flow rate may be due to a plugged filter. Changes in body position will also alter the flow rate. If the rate becomes too slow, hypoglycemia may develop. The flow rate should be maintained as ordered, and never "speeded up" since overload of the hypertonic solution can cause massive dehydration of body cells. Daily weights and recording of intake and output help in monitoring fluid balance. The patient should be observed for signs of fluid overload (p. 112). Sugar overload can be identified by urine analysis. Serum electrolytes, glucose, and BUN levels are usually monitored daily initially and then at longer intervals.

PROMOTION OF HEALTH. The patient should be encouraged to assume activities of daily living. If he is not allowed food or fluids orally, good mouth care is essential, as initially he is likely to be in a catabolic state, which increases the susceptibility to infections of the mouth and respiratory tract. Ambulation should be encouraged, if possible, as inactivity promotes catabolism.

EMOTIONAL SUPPORT. The patient may have many fears and concerns about being fed by intravenous fluids over a long period of time. He should have an understanding of what is occurring and the reason for the frequent dressing changes. If he is not permitted food orally, he may need aid in coping with stress incurred by the smell of food or watching others eat. If he is receiving parenteral hyperalimentation over an extended period of time, he may be concerned about regaining his appetite, taste, or normal eating patterns.[12] Being fed only by tube, even though temporary, may create stress from a change in body image.

Food by mouth. The nurse needs to know which foods contain large and small amounts of various essential nutrients, minerals, and vitamins. When losses must be restored, the patient needs more than is required in the usual adequate diet. It is especially important to know which foods and fluids are high or low in potassium and sodium and which foods are complete proteins. Bananas, citrus fruits, all fruit juices, many fresh vegetables, coffee, and tea are relatively high in potassium and low in sodium content. Salty broths and tomato juice provide extra sodium but have a high potassium content. Meat, milk, and eggs are all complete protein foods and contain relatively large quantities of both sodium and potassium.[53] Current nutrition literature and the dietitian or nutritionist should be consulted as necessary.

The nurse frequently has an order to "force fluids." Since the amount required depends on the size of the patient, the amount of fluid loss, and the patient's circulatory and renal status, no standard amount can be given. Therefore the nurse must make a judgment as to the desirable amount and inform members of the nursing team or family members who may be caring for the patient. If there is any question, the physician should be consulted. Adults who have no circulatory or renal malfunction usually are given between 2,500 and 3,000 ml./day. Suggested amounts for infants and children are given on p. 98. Precautions should be taken so that the overzealous patient does not drink too much fluid in a day or that he does not take too much (3 to 4 glasses) at one time. Excessive water intake may cause water intoxication (sodium depletion).

When many persons are ill, they find it difficult to eat or drink even though they are allowed to do so. There are many ways that the nurse can help the patient take adequate food and fluids orally and thus avoid the need for parenteral fluids. Fruit ades, tea, coffee, and ginger ale or other soft drinks may be substituted for part of the water. Soup, boullion, milk, eggnog, and cocoa provide both fluid and nutrients. Juicy fruits and other semisolid foods with a high fluid and nutrient content such as custard, ice cream, or gelatin may be more palatable than regular meals and plain water. Care must be taken, of course, that any substitutions are acceptable on the diet prescribed for the patient. If a fluid record is needed, the amount of fluid given in semisolid form should be estimated and recorded. A juicy orange, for example, contains about 50 ml. of fluid.

The methods used in presenting food and fluids to patients may influence their consumption of them. Often a small amount of either food or fluid offered at frequent intervals is more acceptable than is a large amount presented less often. Giving some thought to serving foods that the patient likes may improve his appetite. For example, carbonated beverages may be better tolerated by patients who are nauseated, and consideration should always be given to the cultural and aesthetic aspects of eating.

Gavage (feeding by tube). Water, a physiologic solution of sodium chloride, high-protein liquid foods such as Lonalac, or a regular diet that has been passed through a blender and diluted is often given by gavage to older children and adults. These fluids may be given as a slow, continuous drip, or 250 to 500 ml. may be given at spaced intervals. Infants and small children usually are given a prescribed formula equivalent in amount to their usual formula. The tube is left in place in older children and adults, but for infants and small children it usually is removed and passed for each feeding. (See p. 653 for the technique of passing the tube.)

Some special precautions need to be taken when food is given by gavage (Fig. 5-7). For example, nothing should be introduced into the gastric tube until it has been ascertained that the other end of the tube is in the stomach. (Consult a text in fundamentals of nursing for methods.) If gastric contents are aspirated as a means of testing placement of the tube in the stomach, the gastric contents should be

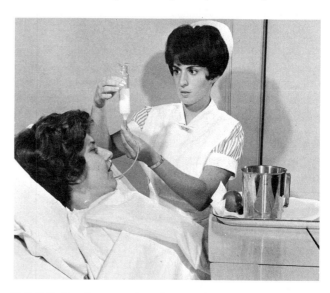

FIG. 5-7. Feeding a patient by gavage is a procedure requiring careful nursing attention.

returned to the stomach to prevent loss of electrolytes. The nurse should be alert for aspiration of the feeding into the lungs. Coughing, choking, and cyanosis indicate aspiration, and if these symptoms occur, the procedure should be discontinued immediately. If the patient is unable to clear his airway on his own, suctioning is indicated.

A small amount of water should always be given before the liquid food because if the tube is displaced, aspirated water is less likely to cause serious trouble than the liquid food. Following the feeding, a small amount of water should be given to flush out the tube. Special care must be taken that high-protein liquid foods are not given in too large quantities at once. Limiting protein intake prevents the movement of excessive quantities of fluids from the bloodstream, which would lower the volume of circulating blood. A patient with a cuffed endotracheal or tracheostomy tube in place is never left alone while fluids are being given by gavage.

Relief of symptoms

Patients with fluid and electrolyte imbalance often have extreme thirst, nausea, and vomiting. These symptoms are distressing, and the nurse should know measures that can be used to give the patient relief.

Thirst. Thirst, the first and most insistent sign of dehydration, sometimes causes the patient more misery than surgery or the symptoms of a disease. It may develop even when fluids have been withheld only for a number of hours. If fluid is being withheld intentionally, thirst often is made more bearable by explaining to the patient why fluid is withheld and when he can expect to receive some.

Thirst usually is relieved rather readily by taking

fluids. If fluids cannot be taken orally, the administration of fluids parenterally usually gives relief. It is often helpful to explain to the patient who is receiving an infusion that the procedure will soon give him some relief from his thirst.

Mouth care will allay some of the discomfort from thirst. This care should include cleansing the tongue and the use of cold mouthwashes. It may be necessary to repeat these procedures every hour. If the patient can be trusted not to swallow, he may be given water or ice chips to be held in the mouth and then expelled. Hard lemon candies (sour balls) often give relief even though they must be expelled. The chewing of gum helps some patients.

When fluids are not permitted, the temptation of a water pitcher at the bedside should be removed, and if the patient cannot be relied on not to get up and drink at a water tap, special provisions such as constant attendance or insistence on bed rest may be necessary. Thirst sometimes compels the patient to obtain water if he can possibly do so.

Pronounced and continued thirst, despite the administration of fluids, is not normal and should be reported. In the patient recently returned from surgery, this kind of thirst should make the nurse suspect internal hemorrhage, elevation of temperature, or some other untoward development. In the chronically ill patient it may indicate the onset of disease such as diabetes mellitus in which extra water is used by the kidneys to eliminate glucose in the urine. It also is a symptom of hypercalcemia.

Nausea and vomiting. Nausea and vomiting often are part of the body's response to insults to its integrity. They usually occur together, but occasionally, if the mechanism for vomiting is touched off by local pressure in the medulla, vomiting may be sudden and not preceded by nausea or any other warning sensation.

It is now known that there are two centers in the medulla involved with vomiting—the chemoreceptor emetic trigger zone and the vomiting center.[17] The vomiting center may be stimulated directly through the vagal or sympathetic nerves. Gastrointestinal irritants, distention or injury of any of the viscera, pain, and psychic trauma cause nausea and vomiting in this manner. Increased intracranial pressure may stimulate vomiting by direct local pressure. The vomiting center also may be stimulated indirectly through the chemoreceptor emetic trigger zone. Emetic agents such as morphine sulfate, meperidine hydrochloride (Demerol), ergot derivatives, digitalis preparations and metabolic emetic substances resulting from uremia, infection, and radiation produce vomiting by stimulation of the chemoreceptor center. Labyrinthine stimulation, the primary factor in the nausea and vomiting of motion sickness, which can occur in healthy people under unusual circumstances involving motion (as in seasickness,

for example), is believed to pass through the trigger center too. It still is not clear by what route irritating gases such as those used in anesthesia affect the vomiting center or what specifically causes vomiting during the first trimester of pregnancy. Toxic substances with an emetic effect probably account for vomiting later in pregnancy.

Nausea and vomiting always are distressing symptoms for the patient, but vomiting also can be a serious symptom. Prolonged and severe vomiting may interfere with nutrition, and it not only is a rather common symptom of electrolyte imbalance, but it may also be a cause of fluid and electrolyte imbalance. The act of vomiting produces a strain on the abdominal muscles, and in the postoperative patient it may cause wound separation, wound dehiscence, or bleeding. Vomiting is especially dangerous for anesthetized patients, persons in coma, and infants because they are likely to aspirate the vomitus into the lungs. Aspiration may cause asphyxia, atelectasis, or pneumonitis. It happens easily, too, in the elderly patient whose nasopharyngeal reflexes are less acute than those of a younger person.

Treatment of nausea and vomiting depends on their cause. Medications or other substances known to cause the trouble are usually stopped or eliminated, and fluid and electrolyte imbalances are treated. Most patients will have less vomiting if the emotional components of its cause are removed. Therefore the nurse should try to relieve the patient's anxiety. Sedation may help to quiet the patient. Nausea and gagging sometimes are relieved by taking deep breaths through the mouth. Ginger ale and other effervescent drinks seem to have a remarkable effect in controlling postoperative vomiting and often can be taken and retained long before other fluids are tolerated. Effervescent fluids also may be effective in controlling vomiting from other causes such as seasickness.

Antihistaminic drugs such as dimenhydrinate (Dramamine), meclizine hydrochloride (Bonine), and trimethobenzamide hydrochloride (Tigan) are used widely in control of motion sickness such as is encountered in air and sea travel. These medications are effective prophylactically when taken about 30 minutes before the initial motion and then continued at regular intervals. They also are ordered with varying success in the nausea and vomiting associated with illness. Tigan in large doses has been quite effective in controlling nausea and vomiting postoperatively. All these drugs are available as rectal suppositories as well as for oral administration. Any of the antihistaminic drugs may cause drowsiness and dizziness, and the possibility of these reactions should be pointed out to persons who are taking them when traveling. They are especially dangerous to use when driving. When antihistaminic drugs are being used in the hospital, the patient must be watched carefully to prevent accidents such as falling out of bed.

The phenothiazine drugs given in relatively small doses are specific antiemetics, blocking the action of emetic agents at the trigger zone and thus preventing activation of the vomiting center.[17] They now are used frequently for postoperative patients and others with prolonged and severe vomiting not of vestibular origin. Many drugs in this category are on the market, and many of them are available for intramuscular injection. Some common ones used are prochlorperazine (Compazine), promethazine hydrochloride (Phenergan), and perphenazine (Trilafon). All of them have side effects of oversedation and hypotension and therefore the hospitalized patient should be protected from accidents, and persons who are taking them at home should be warned about the danger. They should be given cautiously to patients whose blood pressure is already low.

Nausea and vomiting are profoundly affected by sights, sounds, and smells, and the nurse should try to protect the patient from such stimuli whenever possible. Some equipment used in caring for the sick, such as emesis basins, may be psychologically disturbing to patients. Even empty emesis basins may be suggestive of vomiting and should be kept out of a patient's sight unless he actually is vomiting, and then it may be a comfort to have one conveniently placed. Emesis basins should be removed and emptied immediately after use. Relatives learning to care for a patient at home often need help in improvising equipment that will be psychologically acceptable. For example, they may be using a baby's potty as an emesis basin when an empty coffee can lined with paper might be less offensive. Some patients may become nauseated from seeing their dressings changed. If so, the nurse should try to distract their attention while this procedure is done. The sound of retching frequently makes even well people nauseated. Therefore, whenever possible, patients should be protected from others who are vomiting. Food odors and other odors that are part of a hospital setting also may contribute to nausea in the person who is ill. Even perfumes and strongly scented soaps may cause nausea. Rooms should be ventilated carefully during both the day and the night. Smoking should not be permitted in the patient's room since it often causes nausea.

REFERENCES AND SELECTED READINGS*

1 *Abbey, J. C.: Nursing observations of fluid imbalances, Nurs. Clin. North Am. 3:77-86, March 1968.

2 Andreoli, K. G., and others: Comprehensive cardiac care: a handbook for nurses and other paramedical personnel, ed. 2, St. Louis, 1971, The C. V. Mosby Co.

3 Beeson, P. B., and McDermott, W., editors: Cecil-Loeb textbook of medicine, ed. 13, Philadelphia, 1971, W. B. Saunders Co.

4 *Bergersen, B. S.: Pharmacology in nursing, ed. 12, St. Louis, 1973, The C. V. Mosby Co.

5 *Betson, C.: Blood gases, Am. J. Nurs. 68:1010-1012, May 1968.

6 Bland, J. H., and others: Clinical metabolism of body water and electrolytes, Philadelphia, 1963, W. B. Saunders Co.

7 *Bordicks, K. J.: Patterns of shock: implications for nursing care, New York, 1965, Macmillan Publishing Co., Inc.

8 Brand, L., and Thral, A. P.: Shock. In Meltzer, L. E., Abdellah, F. G., and Kitchell, J. R., editors: Concepts and practices of intensive care for nurse specialists, Philadelphia, 1969, The Charles Press Publishers.

9 *Brooks, S. M.: Basic facts of body water and ions, ed. 3, New York, 1973, Springer Publishing Co., Inc.

10 *Burgess, R. E.: Fluids and electrolytes, Am. J. Nurs. 65: 90-95, Oct. 1965.

11 *Cohn, H. D.: Hemostasis and blood coagulation, Am. J. Nurs. 65:116-119, Feb. 1965.

12 *Colley, R., and Phillips, K.: Helping with hyperalimentation, Nursing '73 3:6-17, July 1973.

13 Davenport, R. R.: Tube feeding for long-term patients, Am. J. Nurs. 64:121-123, Jan. 1964.

14 Davis, L., editor: Christopher's textbook of surgery, ed. 10, Philadelphia, 1972, W. B. Saunders Co.

15 *Deitel, M.: Intravenous hyperalimentation, Can. Nurse 69:38-43, Jan. 1973

16 Dicken, M. L.: Fluid and electrolyte balance: a programmed text, ed. 2, Philadelphia, 1970, F. A. Davis Co.

17 *Downs, H. S.: The control of vomiting, Am. J. Nurs. 66: 76-82, Jan. 1966.

18 *Dudrick, S. J., and Rhoads, J. E.: Total intravenous feeding, Sci. Am. 226:73-80, May 1972.

19 Dunning, M. F., and Plum, F.: Potassium depletion by enemas, Am. J. Med. 20:789-792, May 1956.

20 Dutcher, I. E., and Fielo, S. B.: Water and electrolytes: implications for nursing practice, New York, 1967, Macmillan Publishing Co., Inc.

21 Dutcher, I. E., and Hardenburg, H. C., Jr.: Water electrolyte imbalances. In Meltzer, L. E., Abdellah, F. G., and Kitchell, J. R., editors: Concepts and practices of intensive care for nurse specialists, Philadelphia, 1969, The Charles Press Publishers.

22 Eckstein, G.: The body has a head, New York, 1970, Harper & Row, Publishers.

23 *Fenton, M.: What to do about thirst, Am. J. Nurs. 69: 1014-1017, May 1969.

24 Fluid and electrolytes, North Chicago, Ill., 1968, Abbott Laboratories.

25 Gamble, J. L.: Extracellular fluids, Cambridge, Mass., 1954, Harvard University Press.

26 Garb, S. G.: Laboratory tests in common use, ed. 5, New York, 1971, Springer Publishing Co., Inc.

27 *Goldberger, E.: A primer of water, electrolyte and acid-base syndromes, ed. 4, Philadelphia, 1970, Lea & Febiger.

28 *Grant, J. A.: The nurse's role in parenteral hyperalimentation, RN 36:29-33, July 1973.

29 *Grant, J. A. N.: Patient care in parenteral hyperalimentation, Nurs. Clin. North Am. 8:165-181, March 1973.

30 Guyton, A. C.: Textbook of medical physiology, ed. 4, Philadelphia, 1971, W. B. Saunders Co.

*References preceded by an asterisk are particularly well suited for student reading.

31 *Kee, J. L.: Fluids and electrolytes with clinical applications, a programmed approach, New York, 1971, John Wiley & Sons, Inc.

32 *Kee, J. L.: The critically ill patient and possible fluid and electrolyte imbalances, Nursing '72 **2**:6-11, March 1972.

33 *Kee, J. L.: Fluid imbalances in elderly patients, Nursing II '73 **3**:40-43, April 1973.

34 *Levenson, S. M.: Current status of some aspects of parenteral nutrition, Am. J. Surg. **103**:330-341, March 1962.

35 *Metheny, N., and Snively, W. D., Jr.: Nurses' handbook of fluid balance, Philadelphia, 1967, J. B. Lippincott Co.

36 Moore, F. D.: Regulation of the serum sodium concentration, Am. J. Surg. **103**:302-308, March 1962.

37 Mountcastle, V. B.: Medical physiology, ed. 13, St. Louis, 1974, The C. V. Mosby Co.

38 Nelson, W. E., and others: Textbook of pediatrics, ed. 9, Philadelphia, 1969, W. B. Saunders Co.

39 *Plumber, A. L.: Principles and practice of intravenous therapy, Boston, 1970, Little, Brown & Co.

40 *Potassium imbalance: programmed instruction, Am. J. Nurs. **67**:343-366, Feb. 1967.

41 Preston, F. W., and Henegar, G. C.: Use of intravenous fat emulsions in surgical patients, Surg. Clin. North Am. **39**:145-159, Feb. 1959.

42 *Roach, F. B.: Color changes in dark skin, Nursing '72 **2**:20-22, Nov. 1972.

43 *Sargis, N. M.: Cardiogenic shock, N. Y. State J. Nurs. Assoc. **3**:22-28, Oct. 1972.

44 Seal, A. L., and others: Symposium on injection therapy, Nurs. Clin. North Am. **1**:257-307, June 1966.

45 *Simeone, F. A.: Shock: its nature and treatment, Am. J. Nurs. **66**:1286-1294, June 1966.

46 Snively, W. D.: Sea within, Philadelphia, 1960, J. B. Lippincott Co.

47 *Snively, W., and Roberts, K. T.: The clinical picture as an aid to understanding body fluid disturbances, Nurs. Forum, **12**:132-159, 1973.

48 Statland, H.: Fluid and electrolytes in practice, ed. 3, Philadelphia, 1963, J. B. Lippincott Co.

49 Taylor, W. H.: Fluid therapy and disorders of electrolyte balance, ed. 2, Philadelphia, 1970, F. A. Davis Co.

50 Trainex: Fluids and electrolytes:clinical application, film strips, Trainex Corp. PC261-PC264, 1970.

51 U. S. Department of Agriculture: Food for us all; Yearbook of Agriculture, 1969, Washington, D. C., 1969, U. S. Government Printing Office.

52 *Voda, A. M.: Body water dynamics, a clinical application, Am. J. Nurs. **70**:2594-2601, Dec. 1970.

53 Wayler, T. J., and Klein, R. S.: Applied nutrition, New York, 1965, Macmillan Publishing Co., Inc.

54 Weisberg, H. F.: Water, electrolyte and acid-base balance, ed. 2, Baltimore, 1962, The Williams & Wilkins Co.

55 Williams, J. A., and Frank, H. A.: Transfusion therapy guided by blood volume determinations, Am. J. Surg. **103**:325-329, March 1962.

6 Nutrition a dynamic factor in nursing care

■ In 1969 a White House Conference on Food, Nutrition, and Health was called to focus national attention on the problems of hunger, malnutrition, and improving the nutritional health of all Americans.

Many recommendations for action were made, among them: "That nutritional care be an integral part of total medical service based upon the needs of the individual patient."[67]

Good nursing care has always included attention to the patient's food needs. Florence Nightingale established the first diet kitchen in order to provide such care. At that time the major goal was to provide foods that the patient could chew and swallow easily in portions large enough to satisfy him. The nurse no longer prepares the patient's meals, but maintenance of good nutrition is still one of the major objectives in nursing management. This includes both seeing that the patient in the hospital receives and eats the

■ STUDY QUESTIONS

1 Before you read this chapter, write your own definitions of a good diet and good food. After reading the text, check your definitions. What changes, if any, would you make? Do you agree or disagree with the text? Why?

2 Imagine that for one special day you could have anything and everything you wanted to eat. What foods would you choose? Why? Ask a classmate or friend to do the same thing and compare notes. Can you trace the origins of your food likes and dislikes? If you were told to omit a food you like or to eat a food you dislike in order to improve your health, would you do it?

3 Compare your special menu to the food pattern recommended in this chapter. Does your menu meet the recommendations? What changes, if any, would you make?

4 Talk to some patients about their food likes and dislikes. Try to identify the reasons they have for eating or refusing certain foods. How do different family members influence the choice of foods served at home? How might family patterns of eating and living affect a patient's ability to change his food intake?

5 Choose one of the nutrition texts from the reading list at the end of this chapter and turn to the table of food values in the appendix. Compare the values for baked, boiled, French fried, and mashed potatoes and potato chips. How do they differ? Why? How much of each type would you eat at one time? How does your choice of portion size change the number of calories and nutrients you would obtain?

6 In the table of food values consulted for question 5, check the nutrient values for some of the foods often recommended such as liver, spinach, turnip greens, enriched bread, and milk and for some of your favorite foods. What contributions do these foods make?

7 Check the recommended dietary allowances (Table 6-3) for a person of your sex, age, and size. Make a list of the amounts of each nutrient recommended. Take this list with you to the pharmacy or drugstore and compare the ingredients listed on the labels of vitamin and mineral bottles to your list. What differences are there? What might these differences mean in meeting the needs of patients?

8 Glance through the references and selected readings listed at the end of this chapter. Choose one or two that interest you and look them up in the library.

foods he needs and seeing that he learns how to feed himself properly at home. To meet these goals nurses use their own knowledge and skills and those of other members of the health care team, particularly the physician and the dietitian.

Several years ago a book for the general public was published entitled *Food Becomes You*.[35] The title is succinct and easy to remember. Yet in these three words the importance of nutrition to physical, emotional, and social well-being is implied. Nutrition has been defined as the relationship between man and his food. Food supplies raw materials for body structure and function. Food may be used to reward, punish, or gratify; food and its uses are determined by geography, economics, ethnic or religious considerations, habit, and experience.

Nutrition has also been defined as the sum of the processes by which a living organism ingests, digests, absorbs, transports, uses, and excretes nutrients and their metabolites. Given the proper nutrients or raw materials in adequate amounts, the organism can grow, function, and reproduce. Should a needed material be denied or supplied in inadequate amounts, growth, function, or reproduction may be impaired. The science of nutrition is concerned with identifying the materials each organism requires, determining the quantities needed for optimum growth and functioning and discovering the effects of environment, metabolism, disease, and activity on needs. Every living organism—plant, microbe, animal, man—has nutrient needs and is a subject for nutrition research.

Nutrition research has benefited man in many ways. Identification of the nutrient requirements of plants and animals has been applied in agriculture to produce more and better food supplies. Treatments for certain conditions are actually planned interruptions in the nutritive processes of pathogenic organisms so that growth and reproduction are limited. The most direct benefit has been the identification of those substances man must have and the means to supply them. Much of the research effort in nutrition and medicine is now directed toward defining the relationship between disease, diet, nutrition processes, and man.

The nurse in accepting the responsibility of providing care for the patient as an individual, accepts the responsibility for applying the principles of nutrition. In addition, the nurse serves as liaison between the patient and other professional people in interpreting the patient's nutritional and dietary problems. The perceptive nurse identifies problems, seeks answers, and incorporates the solutions in the nursing care plan. This requires knowledge of the principles of nutrition, appreciation of food composition, understanding of the role of food in the individual patient's life, and appreciation of modifications of diet and food behavior as part of the total thera-

peutic regimen. These topics will be discussed in this chapter and examples of the application of nutrition knowledge will be given. Throughout the text the nurse will find nutrition included in the discussion of medical and surgical nursing problems.

■ BASIC NUTRIENT NEEDS

At the present time there are over 35 nutrients known to be required by the human body for normal growth and function (Table 6-1). They are grouped as carbohydrates (starches and sugars), proteins (amino acids), fats, minerals, vitamins, and water. Good nutrition exists when these are supplied in the right amounts and are appropriately used by the body.

All persons need the same nutrients throughout life, but the amounts required vary. These variations occur in predictable patterns in relation to the life cycle. Growth, basal metabolic functioning, and physical activity are the major factors responsible for changes in nutrient needs. In addition, needs can be altered by disease, trauma, normal and abnormal variations in metabolism, treatment or medications, and the accumulated experiences of a lifetime.

Recognition of these patterns has made it possible to predict the amounts of the different nutrients required by people to maintain health and to provide a basis for planning nutritionally adequate diets. Since 1940, the Food and Nutrition Board of the National Academy of Sciences has met periodically to review the existing knowledge of nutrition and to formulate recommendations. Revisions are made as more knowledge of nutritional needs is obtained.[51]

Table 6-1 Nutrients required by the human body

Water	Minerals	Vitamins
Protein	Calcium	Ascorbic
Total nitrogen	Chromium	acid
Isoleucine	Phosphorus	Biotin
Leucine	Copper	Folacin
Lysine	Fluorine	Niacin
Methionine	Iron	Pantothenic
(cystine)	Iodine	acid
Phenylalanine	Magnesium	Riboflavin
(tyrosine)	Manganese	Thiamine
Threonine	Molybdenum	Vitamin B_6
Tryptophan	Selenium	Vitamin B_{12}
Valine	Zinc	Vitamin A
Histidine	Sodium	(carotene)
(infant)	Potassium	Vitamin D
Carbohydrate	Chloride	Vitamin E
Fat		Vitamin K
Linoleate		
(arachidonate)		

The Recommended Dietary Allowances are the levels of intake of essential nutrients considered, in the judgment of the Food and Nutrition Board on the basis of available scientific knowledge, to be adequate to meet the nutritional needs of practically all healthy persons.*

The recommended daily dietary allowances (RDA) for protein and the growth curve for the reference woman and man are illustrated in Fig. 6-1. Note the similar patterns of the curves. Protein is required throughout life but the amount needed changes. Protein needs vary with growth. This is most easily seen by comparing the protein allowance and height curves for boys and girls between 9 and 15 years of age. Protein needs also vary with body size. For both men and women the RDA is 0.8 Gm. protein/kg. body weight, which means that the average male needs more protein per day than the average female because of his larger body size. The pregnant woman should be supplied with extra protein (RDA + 30 Gm.) for fetal growth. For both sexes at all ages, the recommended allowances for protein include an allowance for individual variability and an allowance to compensate for less than 100% efficiency in utilization. The recommendations exceed actual protein requirements for most persons; the protein not needed for synthesis is used as energy or converted to body fat. Variations in body requirements for structure materials such as calcium and phosphorus follow this pattern as well.

Severe limitations in protein supply (50% or less RDA) can stunt growth and reduce body protein content. Generous supplies of protein, however, will not result in increased body protein or muscle mass without exercise or physical activity. Both body protein and calcium may be lost despite generous dietary supplies in the absence of physical activity. Early ambulation of patients, bed exercises, and the exercise regimen for astronauts in space are used to improve nutritional status.

Calorie needs vary with growth and body size as do protein needs, but other factors must be considered as well (Fig. 6-2). There is a constant need for energy to maintain circulation, respiration, muscle tone, and body temperature. This basal energy requirement is related to the amount of muscle tissue and can be predicted from body weight. It is expressed as the number of calories needed per day. Adult basal needs may be quickly estimated by multiplying pounds of normal or ideal body weight times 10 calories/pound for women and 11 calories/pound for men. Ideal or normal weight for height is used since weight above these levels is usually adipose tissue, which requires very little energy for maintenance. People of similar size have similar basal energy requirements. However, the total energy requirement may vary widely among individuals and for the same person day after day, because the total energy requirement is dependent on physical activity. Energy expenditure increases with the vigor with which muscles are used and total body mass is moved (Table 6-2). Since the average adult American spends a great deal of his time sitting, lying, or standing, the recommended calorie allowances are based on this sedentary life pattern. Recommendations for boys and girls are the same for the first decade of life because growth and activity are similar. After this age, calorie recommendations for the average male and female diverge. Basal energy needs differ, since body composition and size differ. The female has less muscle and more adipose tissue per unit of weight than the male and thus needs fewer calories per unit of body weight than the male. In addition, boys grow to a larger size and generally engage in more vigorous physical activity. Energy

---

*From Recommended dietary allowances, ed. 8, Washington, D. C., 1974, National Academy of Sciences–National Research Council.

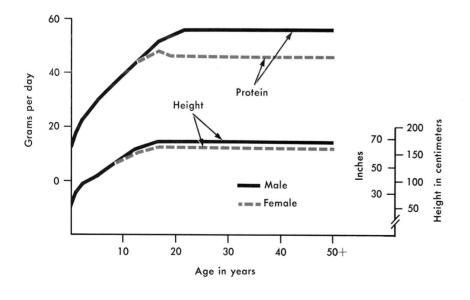

FIG. 6-1. Recommended daily dietary allowances for protein over the life cycle.

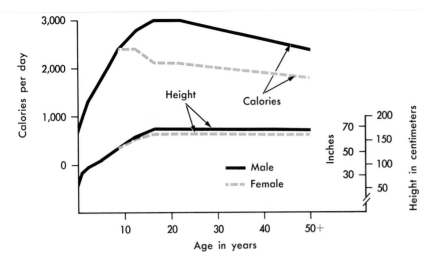

FIG. 6-2. Recommended daily dietary allowances for calories over the life cycle.

Table 6-2 Comparison of calories used in 1 hour for different types of physical activity by a woman weighing 121 pounds and a man weighing 143 pounds (exclusive of basal energy needs)

Activity	Calories expended per hour	
	Woman	Man
Lying quietly	6	7
Sitting	22	26
Standing	28	32
Ironing, dishwashing, driving car	55	65
Office work, painting furniture	82	98
Walking, waltzing, bicycling	138	162
More active walking, skating, foxtrot	220	260
Running, climbing stairs, sawing wood	358	422
High-speed walking, swimming	468	552

needs for fetal growth are met in part by decreased physical activity by the mother.

Energy needs can be predicted from patterns of growth and body size and physical activity. Since physical activity exerts a marked effect on energy needs (Table 6-2) and varies widely from person to person, adjustments must be made for individuals. An inactive teenage boy may become obese when consuming a diet providing the calories recommended, while an active boy would not maintain weight. This principle of energy balance is the basis of a time-honored medical prescription—bed rest. Confining the patient to bed should restrict his physical activity. The energy not used for activity would then be available for growth or rehabilitation. This prescription, however, is effective for some patients but not others. Some patients restrict activity but others amuse themselves by kicking the sheets, wiggling, and developing their skills in calisthenics.

Mineral and vitamin needs also vary with growth. Relatively larger quantities are required of those nutrients that are major structural components of body tissue, such as calcium, phosphorus, and iron, than of those nutrients such as trace elements and vitamins, which function as regulators of metabolic processes. Since males grow to a larger size, their nutrient needs are greater, overall, than those of females. On the other hand, girls, because of menstruation, have a relatively greater need for iron and related nutrients to replace periodic losses. In a recent study of menstruating women, no evidence for an iron requirement much above 11 to 12 mg./day was found.[6]

The RDA for people in the United States are presented in Table 6-3. Note that the table does not include all the substances listed in Table 6-1. If a diet using ordinary foods is consumed in sufficient quantities to meet the RDA, the diet should supply the other nutrients as well. The level of iron intake recommended for women in the reproductive years is high (18 mg.) because many women have not included iron-rich foods in the diet and have poor iron stores. This level of dietary iron is difficult to achieve at the calorie levels recommended.

Currently, many changes are being made in food labeling practices and regulations governing the use of certain terms describing foods.[19] These changes are designed to improve the nutrition information given on food labels and to provide meaningful information to the public. The new nutrition labeling program is voluntary for most foods; however, if a nutrient is added to any product or if a nutritional claim is made either on the label or in advertising, the product label must have full nutrition labeling. On food labels the levels of vitamins and minerals will be listed as a percentage of the US-RDA. To meet the regulations the label must include size of serving, number of servings per container, calories, protein, carbohydrate, fat, and the percentage of the US-RDA for vitamin A, vitamin C, thiamine, riboflavin, niacin, calcium, and iron. Another 12 vitamins and minerals may be listed at the option of the food producer. The US-RDA is based on the standard RDA but is condensed to four categories: infants, children under 4 years of age, adults and children over 4 years of age, and pregnant or lactating women. Consumer memos describing the new regulations are available from the Food and Drug Administration.[65] The regulation allows for a statement of cholesterol, total fat, and polyunsaturated and saturated fat on the label. This will be helpful for patients on fat-modified diets.

A standard of identity has also been established for dietary supplements to distinguish ordinary foods from special dietary foods intended for use as supplements and drugs intended to treat disease.[22] If a product contains less than 50% of the US-RDA, it is considered a food and therefore nutrition labeling is used. If a product contains 50% to 150% of the US-RDA, it is considered a dietary supplement and must meet the standard. If a product contains more than 150% of the US-RDA, it must be labeled and marketed as a drug. This last provision protects the consumer, since the manufacturer must provide information about the proper use of drugs and their adverse effects. The producer must also have evidence to support the claims made for his product. There has been confusion about this regulation. Some people believe that it means no vitamin or mineral preparations will be available without a prescription from a physician. This is not true—the preparations will still be sold over the counter without prescription, but the labeling must conform to the new standards. Prescriptions will be required, however, when an oral preparation of vitamin A contains more than 10,000 I.U./dose or one of vitamin D contains more than 400 I.U./dose.[20] These exceptions were made to protect the public health because of the toxic effects of these vitamins when ingested daily in large amounts. Folic acid may be added to foods and dietary supplements in amounts not to exceed an excess of 0.4 mg. total intake in 1 day for adults.[21] Levels of folic acid permitted in over-the-counter drugs will be determined by the OTC Drug Panel. Daily intake of large amounts of folic acid masks symptoms of pernicious anemia and constitutes a danger to the public health.

General knowledge of nutrient needs must be combined with specific knowledge of the patient to provide good care; for example, fever accompanies many diseases. Energy is required to maintain body temperature, and basal energy requirements increase approximately 7% for each 1° C. rise. Should the patient be fed a high-calorie diet? At one time the answer to this question was yes—"Feed a fever." Now the answer requires careful consideration of the patient. How high is the fever? How long will it last? Does decreased physical activity compensate for increased basal expenditures? Does the patient have sufficient energy reserves in the form of body fat to meet demands not met by diet? The answers to these questions will determine whether a high-calorie intake is or is not an appropriate objective of the nursing care plan for this patient.

■ BASIC FOOD NEEDS

Good *nutrition* exists when protein, fat, carbohydrate, minerals, vitamins, and water are consumed in sufficient amounts and are used appropriately to meet body needs regardless of age, sex, life-style, or

DAILY FOOD GUIDE

Food group	Servings recommended
A Milk	
Fluid milk—whole, skim, cultured, evaporated; milk solids may be in beverage or mixtures fortified with vitamin D	Children: 3 to 4 glasses Teenagers: 4 glasses Adults: 2 or more glasses Pregnant women: 4 glasses
B Vegetables and fruit	
Dark green or deep yellow (broccoli, kale, carrots, squash, turnip, mustard greens, etc.)	1 serving at least every other day ($\frac{1}{2}$ cup)
Citrus fruits and juices, cantaloupe, tomato, broccoli, cabbage, pepper, strawberries, etc.	1 serving ($\frac{1}{2}$ cup or usual portion)
Other fruits and vegetables including potatoes	2 or more servings ($\frac{1}{2}$ cup or usual portion, i.e., medium potato or apple)
C Meat	
Meat, fish, poultry, eggs, dried beans and peas, nuts	2 or more servings (2 to 3 oz. meat, fish, poultry, liver; 2 eggs; 1 cup beans, peas, lentils; 4 tablespoons peanut butter)
D Bread and cereal	4 or more servings (1 slice bread; 1 oz. dry cereal; $\frac{1}{2}$ to $\frac{3}{4}$ cup cooked cereal, rice, macaroni, noodles, spaghetti)

Amounts recommended for a preschool child are 1 pint of milk, $\frac{1}{2}$ cup fruits or juices, $\frac{1}{2}$ cup vegetables, 3 oz. meat and eggs, and 2 servings of bread and cereal.

Table 6-3 Recommended daily dietary allowances[1]* (designed for maintenance of good nutrition of practically all

	Age (yr.)	Weight (kg.)	Weight (lb.)	Height (cm.)	Height (in.)	Energy (kcal.)[2]	Protein (Gm.)	Fat-soluble vitamins			
								Vitamin A activity (RE)[3]	(IU)	Vitamin D (IU)	Vitamin E activity[5] (IU)
Infants	0-½	6	14	60	24	kg. × 117	kg. × 2.2	420[4]	1,400	400	4
	½-1	9	20	71	28	kg. × 108	kg. × 2.0	400	2,000	400	5
Children	1-3	13	28	86	34	1,300	23	400	2,000	400	7
	4-6	20	44	110	44	1,800	30	500	2,500	400	9
	7-10	30	66	135	54	2,400	36	700	3,300	400	10
Males	11-14	44	97	158	63	2,800	44	1,000	5,000	400	12
	15-18	61	134	172	69	3,000	54	1,000	5,000	400	15
	19-22	67	147	172	69	3,000	54	1,000	5,000	400	15
	23-50	70	154	172	69	2,700	56	1,000	5,000		15
	51+	70	154	172	69	2,400	56	1,000	5,000		15
Females	11-14	44	97	155	62	2,400	44	800	4,000	400	10
	15-18	54	119	162	65	2,100	48	800	4,000	400	11
	19-22	58	128	162	65	2,100	46	800	4,000	400	12
	23-50	58	128	162	65	2,000	46	800	4,000		12
	51+	58	128	162	65	1,800	46	800	4,000		12
Pregnancy						+300	+30	1,000	5,000	400	15
Lactation						+500	+20	1,200	6,000	400	15

*From Recommended dietary allowance, ed. 7 (revised 1973), Publication no. 1694, Washington, D. C., 1968, National Academy of Sciences–National Research

[1]The allowances are intended to provide for individual variations among most normal persons as they live in the United States under usual environmental stresses.

[2]Kilojoules (KJ) = 4.2 × kcal.

[3]Retinol equivalents.

[4]Assumed to be all as retinol in milk during the first 6 months of life. All subsequent intakes are assumed to be one-half as retinol and one-half as β-carotene

[5]Total vitamin E activity, estimated to be 80% as α-tocopherol and 20% other tocopherols.

[6]The folacin allowances refer to dietary sources as determined by *Lactobacillus casei* assay. Pure forms of folacin may be effective in doses less than one fourth

[7]Although allowances are expressed as niacin, it is recognized that on the average 1 mg. of niacin is derived from each 60 mg. of dietary tryptophan.

[8]This increased requirement cannot be met by ordinary diets; therefore the use of supplemental iron is recommended.

health of the individual. Logically, then, a good (or balanced) diet consists of any combination of foodstuffs that yields needed nutrients in sufficient amounts to promote growth and metabolism. In common practice, however, the term often refers to any food or combination of foods that are tasty, filling, refreshing, or desirable in the estimation of the person eating or talking about them. As a result, confusion abounds. Similar ambiguities make the terms "normal," "usual," or "average" diet useless unless carefully defined.

Food guides have been developed to help people choose the kinds and amounts of foods needed for health from the abundant and bewildering supplies in the North American market. Such guides, to be effective, are devised for a specific country or culture and feature foods readily available and acceptable to the people. Ordinary staple foods of reasonable cost are emphasized. This same approach is used in diet manuals, which are collections of food guides for persons requiring dietary modifications.

A guide suitable for many patients and families

is shown on p. 135. It groups foods rich in protein, minerals, and vitamins into four main classes according to their major nutrient contributions. Recommendations are made for the number and size of servings to be selected from each food group.[63]

Protein, mineral, and vitamin requirements are substantially met when daily intake of foods includes the recommended servings from each food group. The calorie level of the basic diet is low in comparison with recommended calorie allowances (Fig. 6-2) but is approximately sufficient for adult basal metabolism. Fats, oils, and sweets or additional servings from the food groups may be used to meet energy and growth needs. Cheese may be substituted for some of the milk or meat. Girls and women should be encouraged to choose foods rich in iron during the years of menstruation and child bearing. Liver, meats, egg yolk, whole and enriched grains and cereals, seafood, green leafy vegetables, nuts, and legumes are good sources. New standards for the amount of vitamins and iron to be added to enriched flour and bread are being discussed. They

healthy people in U. S. A.)

			Water-soluble vitamins						Minerals			
Ascorbic acid (mg.)	Folacin[6] (µg)	Niacin[7] (B₁) (mg.)	Riboflavin (B₂) (mg.)	Thiamine (mg.)	Vitamin B₆ (mg.)	Vitamin B₁₂ (µg)	Calcium (mg.)	Phosphorus (mg.)	Iodine (µg)	Iron (mg.)	Magnesium (mg.)	Zinc (mg.)
35	50	5	0.4	0.3	0.3	0.3	360	240	35	10	60	3
35	50	8	0.6	0.5	0.4	0.3	540	400	45	15	70	5
40	100	9	0.8	0.7	0.6	1.0	800	800	60	15	150	10
40	200	12	1.1	0.9	0.9	1.5	800	800	80	10	200	10
40	300	16	1.2	1.2	1.2	2.0	800	800	110	10	250	10
45	400	18	1.5	1.4	1.6	3.0	1,200	1,200	130	18	350	15
45	400	20	1.8	1.5	1.8	3.0	1,200	1,200	150	18	400	15
45	400	20	1.8	1.5	2.0	3.0	800	800	140	10	350	15
45	400	18	1.6	1.4	2.0	3.0	800	800	130	10	350	15
45	400	16	1.5	1.2	2.0	3.0	800	800	110	10	350	15
45	400	16	1.3	1.2	1.6	3.0	1,200	1,200	115	18	300	15
45	400	14	1.4	1.1	2.0	3.0	1,200	1,200	115	18	300	15
45	400	14	1.4	1.1	2.0	3.0	800	800	100	18	300	15
45	400	13	1.2	1.0	2.0	3.0	800	800	100	18	300	15
45	400	12	1.1	1.0	2.0	3.0	800	800	80	10	300	15
60	800	+2	+0.3	+0.3	2.5	4.0	1,200	1,200	125	18[+8]	450	20
60	600	+4	+0.5	+0.3	2.5	4.0	1,200	1,200	150	18	450	25

Council.

Diets should be based on a variety of common foods in order to provide other nutrients for which human requirements have been less well defined.

when calculated from international units. As retinol equivalents, three-fourths are as retinol and one-fourth as β-carotene.

of the RDA.

would increase the levels of iron to 40 mg./pound of flour and 25 mg./pound of bread.[23,50] Many of these foods, especially liver and green leafy vegetables, provide folic acid, which is also needed for erythrogenesis.

This food guide is useful for planning vegetarian diets also.[38] Many people in this country are vegetarians. The reasons vary—religion, food cost, philosophy, etc.[16] Diets vary also; some eliminate only red meat such as beef, veal, lamb, and pork, and others eliminate fish. Still others use only animal products such as milk, cheese, and eggs. Complete elimination of all foods of animal origin from the diet should not be encouraged. Although adequate protein of good quality can be provided by careful attention to planning mixtures of vegetables, grains, and fruits, these foods do not provide vitamin B₁₂.[17,52]

The contribution of food groups to the total diet may be seen in Table 6-4. The daily food guide emphasizes foods readily available and acceptable to most Americans. It provides a simple pattern to ensure dietary adequacy without laborious and time-consuming calculations. When used as the basis for menu planning and patient education, it provides a mechanism for meeting individual needs within a family or an institution. Failure of an individual to adhere to a recommended pattern does not mean that he is failing to meet his nutrient needs. It does mean that the evaluation of his diet may be arduous.

Many combinations of foods may be used. A basic food pattern developed for use in Puerto Rico[53] features five food groups: (1) foods that practically everyone eats; (2) milk (goat's milk, dried milk solids); (3) meat, fish, fowl, and eggs; (4) yellows and greens (local varieties of squash, yellow sweet potatoes, and greens); (5) fresh native fruits. Most Puerto Rican families use rice, beans, viandas (starchy vegetables and fruits such as plantain and green bananas), codfish, lard, and sugar. These are good foods but are not enough in themselves—supplementation with the four other types of food helps ensure adequacy.

The approach used in the Puerto Rican food plan can be used with patients as well. Find out what the patient is doing now, reinforce those practices that

Table 6-4 Contribution of food groups to nutritive value of diets—percentage of total diet in United States

Nutrient	Milk, cream, ice cream, cheese (%)	Meat, poultry, fish, eggs, dry beans (%)	Vegetables, fruits (%)	Grain products (%)	Total (%)
Calories	13	28	10	26	77
Protein	20	52	7	20	99
Calcium	60	7	9	17	93
Iron	1	41	18	31	91
Vitamin A	12	24	50	1	87
Thiamine	10	29	19	40	98
Riboflavin	38	30	9	19	96
Vitamin C	5	1	88	1	95

From Percentage division of money value of food and contribution of home foods to nutritive value. Food consumption in the United States, Report 6, Washington D. C., 1965, United States Department of Agriculture.

are good, make changes only where necessary, and fit the changes wherever possible into patterns already familiar and acceptable to the patient.

For another group of Americans a different food guide is needed. In Alaska, different kinds of foods are readily available or are familiar and acceptable. The principle of grouping foods according to composition and recommending portions from each group is the same, but the foods suggested differ.[1] Foods are grouped as (1) fruits and vegetables (cloudberries, salmonberries, cranberries, canned orange juice, canned tomatoes or tomato juice; willow greens, wild spinach, sourdock); (2) meat, fish, birds, eggs, and dry beans (moose, caribou, bear, muskrat, salmon, herring, blackfish, etc.); (3) milk, bony fish, and shellfish; (4) homemade breads, flour, and cereals (mush, farina, bannock, yeast breads, rice); (5) fats and oils (seal oil, whale blubber, moose fat, fish oils).

All human beings need the same nutrients, but each can obtain his needs from many different combinations of foods. Any combination of foods that supplies the nutrients is a good one. Food plans provide a framework for nutritionally sound food practices, and yet are flexible enough to permit adjustment for individual and family food preferences and economic status. Some people find the plans or guides difficult to use since they specify staple food items. Mixtures such as pizza, spinach souffle, or Spanish rice are not named; however, the ingredients are staples—bread, tomato, cheese, spinach eggs, rice—and are in the guide. Food plans, including those for special dietary modifications, outline recommendations for total daily intake. Menu plans help ensure that all of the recommended foods are included sometime during the day. Menu plans also incorporate food mixtures and help patients under-

stand the proper use of the food guide. For many patients, suggestions for daily food intake are unintelligible and useless unless accompanied by specific help in meal planning.

The convention of three meals a day is just that—a convention and a convenience. Most people eat more often. Snacks have become a part of the eating pattern[61]; life-styles have changed.[25,31] There may be some advantage to eating smaller meals at shorter intervals as long as total nutrient needs are met. Although physiologic reasons do not support a rigid pattern of three feedings a day, there is evidence that skipping breakfast impairs physiologic and mental efficiency.* Each feeding, whether called a meal or a snack, should include a mixture of nutrients.

The nurse, when attempting to teach a patient about diet, is frequently challenged about food cost. Vague generalities such as "use cheaper cuts of meat" are not particularly helpful. Suggestions should be specific, based on the patient's diet and income. They should provide enough information to serve as a basis of action. The price of an envelope of flavored sugar used by many low-income families to make a beverage is equivalent to the price of enough dried skim milk solids for 1 quart of milk. Which is the better buy? Where and how can a person get food stamps? The nurse with personal experience in managing food budgets, purchasing, cookery, etc. is in a position to offer constructive advice. There are many useful materials available on food purchasing, storage, and preparation. The dietitian will be able to help select the materials that are best for the patient.

---

*Hence the Child Nutrition Act of 1966 authorizing pilot breakfast programs in schools.

In most cases, money spent for food can be reduced and the nutritive value of the diet improved by (1) planning the menu at home, (2) listing kinds and amounts of food to be bought, (3) purchasing items on this list, (4) controlling waste due to preparing more food than is needed or due to foods spoiling before use. There are books available that are useful for the nurse working with patients whose food budgets are marginal.[12,64]

Food additives

Recently the public has become more interested in food and nutrition.[7,30,71] The consumer movement has, among other things, focused attention on food processing and food additives.[29] Additives may be foods, derived from foods, or products created in the laboratory. The most widely used food additive is sucrose, ordinary table sugar. Sodium chloride, table salt, is the second. Monosodium glutamate, mustard, and black pepper are food additives used in large quantities also. Most of the current concern about food additives relates to safety. Excessive intake of sugar has been related to obesity, tooth decay, and coronary artery disease; excessive intake of salt has been related to hypertension. Questions have been raised about the safety of nonnutritive sweeteners, nitrates used in curing meats, and antioxidants such as BHT used to keep fat from turning rancid. The food industry's use of additives is regulated by the Food and Drug Administration. In 1958 the food additives amendment to the Food, Drug, and Cosmetic Act of 1938 was passed; it requires proof of safety before a substance may be added to food. In 1960 the color additive amendment was enacted to control all color additives, natural and synthetic.

Generally recognized as safe (GRAS) substances have been classified by technical effect, and each group is being reviewed for use and safety. One such group is Technical Effect Code 16, leavening agents that include yeast and baking powder. The review for each group will be published when completed.

Concern with pesticide residues (as well as food additives) has caused some people to turn to a "natural" or "organic" diet. Some believe that the body can use only nutrients from a natural source despite evidence to the contrary.[69] Others want food that has been grown without the use of chemical fertilizers or pesticides and processed without additives. Foods labeled "organic" or "natural" usually cost more. The terms are not defined by law, and values are being claimed for products without evidence to support them. Current concern with food additives and pesticides has obscured other issues of food safety. It is just as important to be sure that food is free of microbiologic and insect contamination. Foods themselves contain natural substances that can be harmful.[46] Legislation cannot protect the individual from poor food choices nor ensure good food handling practices in the home.

■ OTHER CONSIDERATIONS

There is a constant temptation to isolate one nutrient and label it *the most important*. Resist the temptation, for every nutrient must be supplied in order for life to exist. By definition, a nutrient is an element or compound essential to life and must be supplied to the body from the environment. A nutrient is an element or compound that may be used for fuel, for building and maintaining body structure, and for regulating body processes. All nutrients are of equal importance even though not all are required in equal amounts.

Daily energy requirements are large and are measured in hundreds and thousands of calories. In the United States, from 10% to 12% of the caloric (or fuel) value is obtained from protein, about 44% from fat, and about 46% from carbohydrate. These figures reflect the variety of foods available. In areas where cereal grains are the major food staple, as much as 80% of dietary calories may be supplied by carbohydrate. The relative contributions of protein, fat, and carbohydrate to the fuel value of the diet can be varied within wide limits without harm. Another source of fuel value in many diets is alcohol. Alcoholic beverages have been used by man for centuries to provide pleasure and satisfaction. This is acceptable in moderation, but when alcohol is used to provide a significant proportion of calories, nutrition and health status may be seriously impaired.[47]

The dry weight of energy-yielding nutrients (protein, fat, carbohydrate) in a diet providing 2,500 calories is about 480 Gm. or approximately 1 pound. Some of this is used to provide the nitrogen, amino acids, fatty acids, and saccharides incorporated into the body structure. Fuel supplies are not wasted. Protein, fat, and carbohydrate not required for fuel or growth are converted to body fat and stored in fat depots. In contrast, the dry weights of the nutrients in that 2,500-calorie diet used for body structure are small and are measured in grams and milligrams. Vitamins are needed in minute amounts measured in milligrams and micrograms. If the vitamins in the 2,500-calorie diet were isolated, their total weight would be less than 1 Gm. At least 1.5 L. of water (from food and beverages) is needed as well. This concept of difference in the order of magnitude of body requirements for various nutrients is also demonstrated by body composition. Water is the most abundant body constituent and accounts for one half to three fourths of body weight, depending on age and amount of body fat. The body of a healthy man weighing about 160 pounds might contain about 100 pounds of water, 29 pounds of protein, 25 pounds of fat, 5 pounds of minerals, 1 pound of carbohydrate, and $1/4$ ounce of vitamins.[64]

The body exists in a state of *dynamic equilibrium.* Anabolism and catabolism are continuous. Bone, muscle, fat, organs, and blood participate in the constant exchange of materials. Some tissues are more active than others. There is always some loss, and therefore replacement from food is necessary. When intake exceeds need, a nonfunctioning surplus may accumulate as stores or reserves. Nitrogen and carbohydrate are stored in limited amounts. Reserves of water-soluble vitamins are small; those of fat-soluble vitamins and minerals may be large. Storage of excess fuel as fat has no apparent limit.

In practice, the goal of dietary management is to provide levels of nutrients to maintain top concentrations of nitrogen and water-soluble vitamins and reasonable stores of fat (fuel), minerals, and fat-soluble vitamins. The ability to have reserves is no guarantee of reserves. On the other hand, too generous intakes of fuel or micronutrients such as vitamin A or minerals may gradually increase body concentrations to a point that is harmful.[46]

When a nutrient is eliminated from the diet or if the amounts provided are insufficient to meet needs, there is a long period of gradual depletion before damage becomes severe enough to be recognized. If dietary management has been good, there will be reserves available for use to minimize the effects of illness or truama. Food is the usual source of nutrients; however, there are other means available to nourish patients with special needs. Vitamins and minerals are available in concentrated forms and in a variety of mixtures. Excessively high intakes of one or more nutrients can produce toxic reactions or interfere with proper use of other nutrients. The quantities of vitamins and minerals required are small even for a patient with no reserves. Reports in the literature of persons with toxicity invariably identify excessive use of concentrated medicinal sources of vitamins. Trace minerals are also involved. Generally, continued intake of vitamins and minerals at levels from 10 to 100 times the RDA is associated with symptoms of chronic toxicity. Higher levels are associated with acute toxicity. When supplements are prescribed for the patient, nurses handle them with the same care as they do any other medication. Amino acids, protein, carbohydrate, and fat are available in isolated forms also. These may be mixed with ordinary foods or blended in special formulations. As with vitamins and minerals, care should be taken to meet the patient's needs and to avoid excessively high levels that may provoke undesirable side effects. A recent report in the literature documents the severe effects of administering a tube feeding too high in protein.[26]

Advances in the techniques of administering therapy have made it possible to correct fluid and electrolyte deficits and maintain basal metabolism by infusion of calculated amounts of solutions. Glucose (5%), saline solutions, protein hydrolysates, fat emulsions, and blood have been used to nourish patients. In 1968 a clinical study of the growth and development of an infant with short bowel syndrome, who received all nutrients exclusively intravenously for 44 days, was reported.[69] Success was in part due to increasing the concentration of nonprotein calories or of glucose and to continuous 24-hour delivery of the fluid. The technique requires close and knowledgeable cooperation of physician, nurse, and pharmacist as well as good and frequent laboratory workups. There is an intuitive feeling that supplementation with various nutrients is essential for patients subjected to illness or surgery. The advantages conferred by good nutrition status prior to illness or surgery promotes good response, which is not affected by supplementation.[56,57] Response to such supplements occurs when patients have been relatively deficient, eating diets marginal in nutrient value. There is a point beyond which supplementation does not help and may harm.[45]

■ NUTRITIONAL STATUS

Nutritional evaluation is an important part of total patient evaluation and provides essential information for differential diagnosis. An awareness of nutritional deficits, excesses, or imbalances that may exist can be of particular importance in determining the management and therapy of a patient and in returning him to health as quickly as possible. The basic principles are the same as those used in general evaluation: (1) observing the patient's general appearance and (2) obtaining careful medical and dietary histories, a thorough physical examination, and selected laboratory measurements. A detailed list of the kinds of information useful for nutritional evaluation is presented in the outline below.

I Dietary
  A Usual food patterns
    1 How long followed
    2 Kinds of food eaten
    3 Amounts of food eaten
    4 Items used regularly in large amounts (condiments, beverages, etc.)
  B Use of diet supplements or drugs (type, dose, time, reason)
  C Previous experience with modified diets
  D Food likes, dislikes, intolerances
  E Responses to food
  F Resources for food (money, etc.)
  G Facilities for purchasing, storage, preparation
II Health
  A History of current illness
  B History of previous illness
  C History of previous surgery
  D History of pregnancy and outcome
  E History of blood loss or donation
  F Medications used (dose, time)
  G Proprietary drugs used (dose, time)

III Physical
  A Height, weight, skinfold thickness
  B Muscular development
  C Neurologic
  D Skin, eyes, lips, tongue, mouth
  E Dental status
IV Laboratory
  A Urinalysis
  B Stool (blood, fat, parasites)
  C CBC, blood indices
  D Serum proteins, serum lipids
  E Serum electrolytes, blood pH
  F Liver function studies
  G Blood sugar, BUN, creatinine
  H Nutrient absorption studies
  I Special
    1 Excretion of a nutrient or its metabolite after fasting and/or test dose
    2 Concentration of nutrient in blood, plasma, RBC, WBC, or other tissue
    3 Changes in enzyme activity
    4 Excretion of abnormal metabolites

Evaluation requires the knowledge and skills of the physician, nurse, dietitian, and laboratory staff. Time must also be considered. Homeostatic mechanisms tend to protect the body against minor or temporary changes in nutrient status as nutrient reserves are mobilized and meet the need. When stresses are prolonged or nutrient reserves are depleted, gradual tissue desaturation of the nutrients occurs. Reductions in enzyme activity and altered levels of metabolites develop. If this process is permitted to continue long enough, anatomic lesions become manifest.

The classic picture of malnutrition is one of nutrient deficiency; however, nutrient excesses can also produce malnutrition. When nutrients are supplied in excess of need, mechanisms tend to protect the body by accumulating nutrient reserves or by increasing the rate of excretion from the body. When the excesses are large or prolonged over time, increased concentration of nutrients and alterations in enzyme activities and levels of metabolites develop. If this process is permitted to continue long enough, anatomic lesions occur. The time elapsing before inadequacies or excesses result in anatomic lesions or overt disease varies. For example, if a normal adult is deprived of all dietary ascorbic acid, clinical lesions of scurvy begin to appear in 3 to 6 months. If dietary ascorbic acid supplies are marginal, the onset of overt disease is delayed. If reserves are marginal, onset is faster. If this normal adult is deprived of all vitamin A, clinical lesions might not appear for a year or more. Excesses of vitamin A of 10 or 100 times the RDA may be consumed for months before complaints bring patients to their doctors, but larger doses may precipitate acute toxic reactions. Just as long periods of time may elapse before malnutrition becomes clinically obvious, complete responses to full therapy are correspondingly slow.

The historic deficiency diseases such as scurvy, beriberi, and pellagra can and do occur, although they are rare. The National Nutrition Survey uncovered only a few cases of frank nutritional deficiency disease; however, a significant proportion of those interviewed were malnourished or at high risk of developing nutrition problems.[11] Adolescents had the highest prevalence of unsatisfactory status. People over 60 years of age also gave evidence of poor nutrition. Obesity was also identified as a problem, particularly in adult women; men were less frequently obese. Obesity is a major health problem in the United States regardless of income level and is present in large proportions of the population at all age levels, thus increasing risk of degenerative disease and shortened life span.

Low-level intakes of body nutrients were associated with limited income, cultural and geographic differences, presence of other health problems, and poor food choices.

The prevalence of malnutrition in the general population is disturbing because it need not exist. Food resources are available as is the knowledge of the proper use of foods for health. Income is related to quality of diet as shown in Fig. 6-3, and yet increased income does not necessarily ensure good nutrition. Food habits rather than inadequate income may be causal. Within each income level there are persons who either do not know which foods to select in order to have a good diet or may not choose to do so. Prevention or alleviation of malnutrition in the general population or in the patient requires identification both of its degree and etiology so that appropriate remedies may be instituted to fit the need be it economic, cultural, or educational.

An example of this approach is a study of the nutritional status of children in New York City.[5] The study included information about the food intake of children, physical examinations, and laboratory studies selected to measure the protein, vitamin, and mineral status of their bodies. Six hundred and forty-two children (80% of the fifth and sixth grades in six public schools on the lower east side of Manhattan) were studied. The youngsters were Chinese, Puerto Rican, Negro, and Caucasian. Distinct patterns of vitamin and lipid nutriture were found for each group as were distinct patterns of food intake. Thiamine and ascorbic acid levels in the body were all markedly below the mean values for the total group when protein intake was inadequate. Fortification with multivitamins did not alter these results.

The Chinese youngsters, 15% of the group, consumed diets high in fish, fruits, vegetables, and rice but low in milk and cheese. These children had good levels of thiamine and ascorbic acid in their bodies, but low levels of riboflavin. Puerto Rican youngsters, 65% of the group, reported diets high in fats, milk, and cheese but low in citrus fruits and meat. They

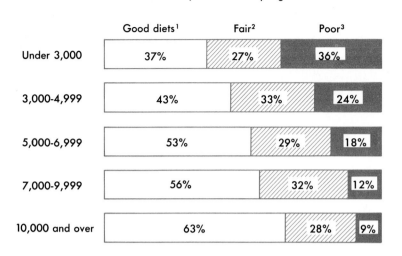

U. S. households, one week in spring

	Good diets[1]	Fair[2]	Poor[3]
Under 3,000	37%	27%	36%
3,000-4,999	43%	33%	24%
5,000-6,999	53%	29%	18%
7,000-9,999	56%	32%	12%
10,000 and over	63%	28%	9%

FIG. 6-3. Diets at three levels of quality, by income. (From U. S. Department of Agriculture: Food for all. Yearbook of agriculture 1969, Washington, D. C., 1969, U. S. Government Printing Office.)

[1]Met recommended dietary allowances (1963) for 7 nutrients.

[2]Met at least ⅔ RDA for 7 nutrients but less than RDA for 1 to 7.

[3]Met less than ⅔ RDA for 1 to 7 nutrients; is not synonymous with serious hunger and malnutrition.

had low body levels of thiamine and niacin, and many were small both in height and weight for their age. Negro youngsters, 10% of the group, reported diets high in meat but low in milk and cheese. Their body levels of thiamine were low. The Caucasian group, 8% of the sample, reported diets high in fats, fruits, and starch-containing vegetables but low in green and yellow vegetables. Their levels of riboflavin and carotene were low. These findings identify both the problems and courses of action to solve them.

The dietary history of a patient can serve as a useful screening device. The adequacy of the diet, in terms of quality and quantity, can be quickly estimated by comparing it to recommended patterns of food intake. If it varies widely from the RDA, a more detailed evaluation should be made. It may also provide information about unusual or bizarre uses of food, which in turn may be a key factor in the health problem. Examples are hypokalemia associated with excessive intake of licorice or cathartics and fever associated with consumption of a gallon of coffee. These imbalances are rare. Identification of factors affecting nutrition status (such as faulty dietary habits, inadequate intake, poor absorption, decreased utilization, increased excretion, increased destruction, increased requirements) permits designing an effective treatment program. Treatment may require dietary modifications, medications, and changes in living patterns.

■ DIET MODIFICATIONS

A diet prescription is based on the determination of each patient's nutrient needs. When no constraints

have been imposed by temporary or permanent alterations in nutritional processes (such as digestion or absorption) or body functioning by illness or trauma, the "normal" ("house") diet is prescribed. This is not considered a "modified diet," since "modified" is used to describe diets different in some way from normal. The nurse will find, however, that meeting the prescription for a "normal" diet does require modification of usual food behavior for patients whose food practices are poor. The diet prescription for a patient may consist of one or many modifications to be followed for varying lengths of time— from 1 day to a lifetime. The patient with chronic disease is often faced with the necessity for permanent changes in food habits. In some instances, dietary modification does not necessitate change in food behavior, since the patient's usual diet actually meets the prescribed modification. A brief discussion of diet modifications and possible applications is included here to illustrate the scope of diet therapy. Consult this text and suggested reading lists for details.

Protein may be increased to levels twice those usually recommended (Table 6-3) for patients with protein losses from tissue catabolism, bleeding, and exudates. On the other hand, protein may be decreased to levels one-half to one-third those recommended. In chronic renal failure, diet management involves providing sufficient protein to prevent tissue protein catabolism and yet avoiding accumulations of urea. In hepatic coma, dietary protein is adjusted to individual tolerance. In some instances, control of the amino acid content of the diet may be required. The child with phenylketonuria needs the same nutrients for growth as the healthy child. His diet must be modified, however, because he cannot convert phenylalanine to tryosine and subsequent normal metabolites. The diet should provide sufficient phenylalanine for growth, but not enough to raise serum levels to those causing central nervous system damage. Phenylalanine cannot be eliminated from the diet as it is an essential amino acid. Tyrosine becomes an essential amino acid for this child as his body cannot convert phenylalanine to tyrosine as normal children do. Specific proteins may be eliminated with gluten-induced enteropathy or allergies.

Fat modifications include increasing or decreasing total fat intake, altering the proportion of dietary calories obtained from fat, and altering the fatty acid composition of the diet. Total fat may be increased to provide essential calories in a concentrated form. Total fat may be decreased for patients with gallbladder disease to reduce pain and contraction of the gallbladder. Alterations in the proportion of dietary calories from fat may be used for patients with primary or secondary disorders of lipid metabolism or to induce ketosis. The prescription should specify the proportions desired for the patient: 10% to 15% of total calories ("low"); 25% to 30% of total calories ("moderate"); 40% to 45% of total calories ("usual"); 60% to 80% of total calories ("ketogenic"). Modifications may also be made in the kind of fat in the diet: short-chain, medium-chain, or long-chain triglycerides or saturated, monounsaturated, and polyunsaturated fatty acids. Modifications in chain length may be prescribed for patients with disorders of digestion and absorption. Modifications in saturated and unsaturated fatty acids may be prescribed to alter serum lipid levels.

Carbohydrate modifications include increasing or decreasing total carbohydrate intake, altering the proportion of dietary calories obtained from carbohydrate, controlling the type of carbohydrate, and eliminating or reducing specific carbohydrate, components. The dietary prescription for a patient with diabetes mellitus might include a decrease in total carbohydrates, a change in the ratio of simple to complex carbohydrates, and substitution of carbohydrate derivatives such as hexitols or dextrins for sucrose. Lactose may be eliminated from the diet of patients with lactase insufficiency and sucrose from the diet of patients with invertase insufficiency. Fructose and sucrose are excluded from the diet of persons with hereditary fructose intolerance and galactose and lactose from the diet of patients with galactosemia.

Modifications in *vitamin* concentrations are generally limited to increasing dosage or providing the vitamin in an alternate form to enhance absorption or utilization. Medicinal sources are frequently used. A diet low in vitamin A and carotene is prescribed for patients with vitamin A toxicity.

Often the *mineral* content of a diet must be controlled. Sodium restriction is one of the most common dietary modifications prescribed and is frequently combined with modifications in calories, sources of carbohydrate, and other minerals. Persons with hypertension, fluid retention, or kidney disease are usually expected to control the amount of sodium they eat. The term "control" is used here deliberately since the goal is to balance sodium intake with sodium need, with the body's ability to handle sodium, and with the physiologic effects of drugs or medications. The level of sodium recommended may vary from 250 mg. to 2 Gm. or more per day. Elimination of sodium from the diet can precipitate dehydration.

Potassium levels may be specified for patients with kidney disease and for those with disorders of electrolyte imbalance. *Other mineral* modifications include diets low or high in calcium and diets low in copper. Medicinal sources of minerals are frequently prescribed.

Liquid (clear and full), *puréed,* and *soft* diets represent modifications in consistency. They may be used when the patient has difficulties in chewing or swallowing[49] or when the patient has lesions of the gastrointestinal tract. They may be used serially for the postoperative patient. Modifications in fiber or residue content of the diet are often prescribed.

Meal size and *frequency* may be modified for treatment of appetite disorders, diabetes mellitus, dumping syndrome, hypoglycemia, peptic ulcer, and other disorders. Modifications in the *method of feeding* include tube feeding, parenteral or intravenous infusions, and sterile food service.[66]

In some cases the prescription may specify elimination of specific foods or beverages from the diet. This approach is used in food allergy. Food elimination may lead to rather bizarre and unusual dietary patterns that should be checked closely for adequacy. Sometimes the diet order specifies foods that may be served to the patient. This is usually a list of bland items such as gelatin, soft-cooked egg, farina, and mashed potato. The nurse may alleviate patient distress and boredom by asking the physician to change the order to "diet as tolerated."

Any diet modification, when imposed, should be justified. Theories of the appropriate nutritional therapy in some diseases vary depending on the interpretation of indirect evidence. Carefully controlled studies are needed to determine the efficacy of modifications, including some that have been used for years (such as the elimination of "gas-forming" or strong-flavored foods). At times it appears as though folklore rather than scientific method fathered some diet and food restrictions.[2] In recent years there has been a trend toward liberal interpretation of dietary therapy. This has been due, in part, to a recognition that many restrictions were without basis in fact and that life lived according to these restrictions was so onerous that emotional well-being was lost without a compensating increase in physical well-being.

Various drugs and medications that a patient is

taking may affect body functions in such a way that diet modification is needed. The obvious illustration of this phenomenon is the treatment regimen for patients with diabetes mellitus: diet, exercise, insulin activity, and hypoglycemic drugs. Moderate to severe elevations in blood pressure may be experienced by patients taking monoamine oxidase inhibitors when they consume large quantities of foods such as aged cheddar cheese, herring, or wines.[42] These foods are rich in tyramine, and metabolism of tyramine is dependent on monoamine oxidase. Some patients on penicillamine therapy may experience a subjective loss of taste for salt and sweet.[34] The diarrhea commonly associated with high-dosage neomycin therapy reflects an induced malabsorption syndrome.[18] Some persons being maintained on barbiturates or anticonvulsants may develop folic acid deficiency, and some taking large doses of isoniazid may show signs of vitamin B_6 deficiency. Thiazide diuretic therapy may deplete cellular potassium. Some medications or products used by a patient may yield so much sodium as to negate any benefit from a sodium-controlled diet; some products contain lactose as a filler. Since new and more powerful drugs are constantly being developed,[10] this list is certain to grow.

■ WEIGHT CONTROL

Despite current emphasis in both the popular press and professional journals, weight reduction is not the goal of nutrition care or diet therapy; weight control is. It is essential that patients, therapists, and the public recognize this fundamental concept.

Weight control involves evaluation of gross body size and proportions of body fat, lean body mass, and body water. The goal of therapy is to promote optimal gross body size and distribution of weight in proper proportions as fat, lean body mass, and body water throughout the life cycle. Obesity, excessive body fat, is the most frequently encountered evidence of malnutrition. Obesity is associated with certain health hazards such as increased risk of developing certain diseases, changes in normal body functions, adverse psychologic reactions, and detrimental effects on established diseases. Relative benefits and risks of any weight reduction regimen must be considered. There are situations in which weight reduction is not indicated (gout, tuberculosis). Drastic weight reduction may be accompanied by cessation of growth in the fetus, the child, or adolescent to the detriment of health.

Since height and weight are measurements that can be made without major investments in equipment and facilities and without discomfort to the patient, body weight for height is used to estimate obesity. Body weight alone is a poor index of maturity, growth, or body composition; height alone is somewhat better (for children), but relative weight for height is a better index than either measure alone. In practice, the patient's weight is compared to a standard table of weight for height to determine degree of overweight or underweight. Skinfold measurements provide a direct estimate of fat. Therapy goals are then stated in terms of the number of pounds of body weight to be lost. This oversimplification is unfortunate. In actuality some patients may be normal in body weight but overfat; others may be overweight but not overfat because of muscular development. In the first group, reduction of body fat but not necessarily reduction of body weight is indicated. In the second group, weight is not a problem.

Therapy for the obese patient should have three objectives: (1) reduction of the body fat compartment, (2) reduction of total body weight when indicated, and (3) maintenance of desirable body size and composition. Far too often both patient and therapist look only at the pounds of weight lost or the rate of loss.[24,62] No differentiation is made as to whether the pounds represent water, muscle, or fat. Very rapid weight loss is satisfying to both patient and therapist, whether the loss is in body fat or water and whether or not the loss is permanent. Fasting regimens are popular because they induce rapid weight loss in a relatively easy way and are immensely satisfying to "scale-watchers." Yet these regimens result in marked protein catabolism with losses of nitrogen, phosphorus, calcium, potassium sodium, and water[60] and may precipitate undesirable effects such as gout or orthostatic hypotension. The questions remain to be answered about the long-term effect of such losses on the health of the individual.

Weight reduction is not achieved simply by lowering the fuel value of the patient's diet. A deficit must be produced between energy expenditure and fuel intake so that body stores of fuel will be mobilized. The

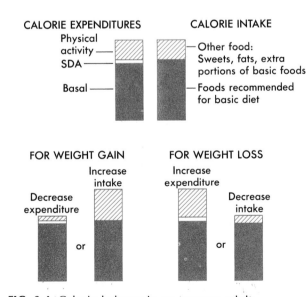

FIG. 6-4. Calorie balance in an average adult.

deficit may be achieved by increasing energy expenditures and/or decreasing calorie intake as illustrated in Fig. 6-4. A pound of adipose tissue has an energy potential of 3,500 calories.[70] To lose 1 pound of adipose tissue/week, a calorie deficit of 500 calories/day must be induced. If a patient requires only 1,500 calories to maintain his current weight, he should not be expected to lose more than 1 pound of body fat/week when adhering to a 1,000-calorie diet. Weight loss is more rapid when lean body tissue is catabolized, since lean tissue has an energy potential of about 1,850 calories. If a deficit of 500 calories/day were met by catabolizing lean tissue, the rate of loss would be about 2 pounds/week. Dehydration produces very rapid loss. Water has no calorie value per se, but 1 pint of water weighs approximately 1 pound.

Patients consuming high levels of calories prior to weight reduction therapy are likely to be successful in achieving rapid weight loss because the calorie deficit between need and the recommended diet is large. Men have a reputation for being more cooperative than women because they lose weight more rapidly. If both a man and a woman are instructed to adhere to a 1,000-calorie intake, the man should lose at a faster rate. This is not because he is more cooperative, but because his calorie deficit is larger (Table 6-2). Although the average adult woman may need 2,000 calories to maintain weight (Table 6-3), the patient may not. It is not inconceivable that a particular patient needs only 1,400 calories to maintain excessive body weight. If she is told to consume a 1,500-calorie diet and she cooperates, she will gain weight despite the fact that an average woman on this regimen would be expected to lose weight. This patient has a right to be upset or indignant when accused of "cheating" on the diet. (Terms such as cheating serve no useful purpose and may lead to silence when communication is essential.) In one study, evaluation of food intakes of a large group of obese adults revealed that half of the women maintained obesity with intakes of 1,500 calories or less and half of the men with intakes of 2,200 calories or less.* An obese patient is not necessarily a glutton. Obesity is not a condition that develops suddenly. Body fat may accumulate slowly over years. A positive calorie balance of 100 calories/day could, in a year's time, result in 10 pounds of adipose tissue. A positive balance of only 10 calories/day could result in 1 pound of adipose tissue in 1 year, or 10 pounds in 10 years. A negative balance of 100 calories/day could result in a loss of 10 pounds in a year's time. Sudden weight changes, gain or loss, should alert the nurse to possible edema, diuresis, or dehydration.

A weight control regimen for female patients who are sedentary, obese, and edematous might include a restriction in dietary calories, an increase in physical activity, control of sodium content in the diet, a diuretic, and other drugs. It should also include teaching the principles of good nutrition so that weight loss, when achieved, is maintained. The weight control regimen should be designed to meet the individual's nutritional, physical, and social needs. Many highly publicized dietary regimens for weight loss emphasize rapid loss at the expense of health. As you can see in Table 6-5, the food guide discussed earlier actually provides a good pattern for weight control as well as for needed nutrients. Obese individuals have large fuel reserves but not necessarily large reserves of vitamins and minerals.

Weight loss is often the first sign of ill health. Loss may be mild or severe, insignificant or serious. It may be caused by inadequate calorie intake, by problems in digestion or absorption, by abnormalities in metabolism, or by excretion of nutrients before they can be utilized. Sometimes weight loss is a result of failure to increase calorie intake when physical activity is increased. Calorie levels sufficient for inpatient activities may not be enough for outpatient activities. Management will vary depending on the basic cause of weight loss.

In every instance, however, the goal is to restore normal body composition, not just weight. A patient will derive no advantage from becoming obese. Restoration of muscle mass occurs slowly. Providing excessive amounts of dietary protein will not hasten this process. Since growth requires energy, calorie intake should exceed calorie expenditures for basal

---

*From Neville, J. N.: Unpublished data, 1965.

Table 6-5 Protein and calorie values of basic diet selected to meet recommendations outlined in food guide for an adult

Group and food chosen	Protein (Gm.)	Calories
Milk, 1 pint Whole (skim)	18	330 (180)
Vegetable-fruit, 4 servings Broccoli, 1/2 cup Potato, 1 medium Lettuce, 1/6 head Apple, 2 1/2-inch diameter	6	190
Meat, 2 or more servings Cheese, 1 oz. Beef, 2 1/2 oz. Poultry, 2 1/2 oz.	56	341
Bread-cereal, 4 servings Cornflakes, 1 oz. Bread, 3 slices	8	290
	88	1,151 (1,001)

and physical activity. There are strong physiologic arguments for preventing obesity and debilitation rather than waiting to treat it after it occurs. Every child, ill or healthy, should be provided with the essentials for attaining his growth potential. As a result, weight control is a component of the health care program for any patient and includes ensuring that the patient knows the principles of weight control and food choice.

■ FOOD FOR THE PATIENT

A diet prescription must be translated into a diet plan or food pattern that will meet the patient's physical needs, and yet provide enough flexibility that the patient will enjoy his food. If a modification is required for only a short period of time, it may not be difficult to plan. However, if the modification is one to be followed at home after the patient is discharged from the hospital, cost, availability, ease of preparation, relationship to family food requirements, etc. must be taken into account.

An unwritten but essential part of each diet order is that the diet should provide all nutrients as generously as its special characteristics permit. If the modification is so restrictive that the food plan will not provide adequate supplies, the physician should be notified so that appropriate adjustments in diet or medication can be made. Clear liquid diets, for example, supply important fluids, some calories, and some sodium and chloride, but they have little other nutrient value. When milk must be eliminated from the diet, it is necessary to identify and eliminate all food items containing milk and replace the calcium, phosphorus, riboflavin, and protein value of milk by incorporating other foods into the food plan. Alterations in the diet—changes in the proportions of calories from protein, fat, and carbohydrate—may in themselves change nutrient requirement. For example, increased polyunsaturated fat should be accompanied by increased dietary levels of vitamin E and increased protein accompanied by increased vitamin B$_6$. This is accomplished by including foods rich in the desired components in the patient's diet. For example, the polyunsaturated fat may be provided by corn oil or safflower oil, which contain both the desired fat and vitamin E.

The value of the nurse's focus on total care of a person, identification of his personal health needs, and coordination of aspects of care, together with the special knowledge gained in day-to-day contact with that person cannot be overemphasized. Constant awareness of the entire spectrum of the patient's needs provides the best safeguard for the patient against iatrogenic disease.

Vigorous therapeutic measures aimed at treating one condition may precipitate others when care is disease focused. For example, the traditional regimen for peptic ulcer emphasized maintaining the patient on a diet of milk, cream, and foods high in calories and fat for months or years. Gain in weight and particularly in body fat was not unusual. Ulcers are most prevalent in middle-aged males, the group most at risk from coronary artery disease.

Foods contain a variety of nutrients in varying proportions. The diet plan should guide selection of the kinds of foods in the amounts dictated by the diet prescription. Calorie, protein, fat, and carbohydrate concentrations of some common foods are shown in Fig. 6-5. Notice how many of the foods contain protein. Intake of all these foods would have to be limited if protein is restricted. Calorie needs would have

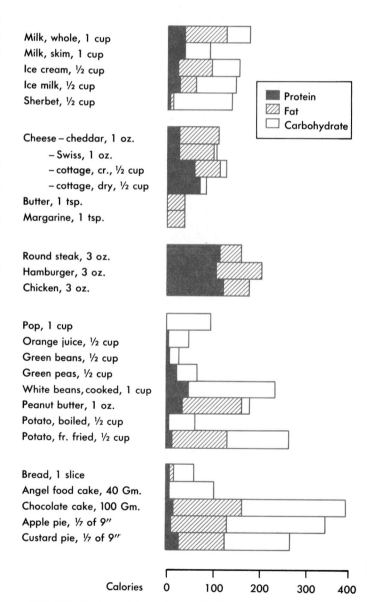

FIG. 6-5. Protein, fat, and carbohydrate concentrations in some common foods presented as calories contributed by each and total calories, in ordinary portions.

to be supplied by foods consisting primarily of carbohydrate or fat.

Some dietary prescriptions can be met only by using different or unusual food items such as casein hydrolysate (low in phenylalanine or starches) made from wheat or corn or other plant sources. These cannot be handled in the same way as the foods they replace. New techniques and recipes must be developed. The final products differ in appearance, texture, and taste from those they replace. Patients whose diets require such products should have help in learning how to cook the products and use them in the diet.

As can be inferred from the discussion of diet modification, detailed and accurate information about food composition is essential. This is a challenge. New food products appear on the market daily. Botanists are busy developing new strains and varieties of food plants. Agricultural experts are applying new techniques of feeding and breeding in animal husbandry to produce animals with more muscle and less fat. Supermarkets stock over 8,000 types of items. Often the only information available is a list of ingredients in the product. Complete information on the concentration of every nutrient (as listed in Table 6-1) in staple food items is not and will not be available until better methods of laboratory analysis are developed. Since information about staple food items is the best available, food plans for diet modifications tend to emphasize staple foods and do not include many new and convenient items on the food market.

Many new products are specifically designed by intent and advertising to replace staple items. There are several breakfast drinks being marketed that look and taste like orange juice and that have been enriched with ascorbic acid so that they may have as much, or more, ascorbic acid as orange juice. But the breakfast drinks are high in sodium and low in potassium, whereas orange juice is low in sodium and high in potassium. A wide variety of substitutes for coffee cream, sour cream, and whipped cream are on the market. They are convenient to use, easy to store, and acceptable in flavor to most people. Can they be used by patients? Many of these products are made from coconut oil, which is a highly saturated fat. Such products cannot be recommended as a source of polyunsaturated fat. They are excellent calorie sources, however.

Notice the difference in protein, fat, and carbohydrate in ice cream, ice milk, and sherbet in Fig. 6-5. The fat of ice cream is butterfat; that of ice milk, is vegetable fat. Sherbet is essentially fat free. All contain sucrose. "Diabetic" ice creams substitute other carbohydrates for sucrose and usually have a high-fat level to provide good texture. As a result, the calorie content of "diabetic" ice creams is often higher than that of conventional ice cream.

The definition of "good" food is very personal and is a product of all the experiences associated with food over a lifetime. The major challenge in diet therapy can be summarized as providing "good" food for the patient within the limits imposed by his health and nutrient needs. One basic principle of learning is that the student learns by building on what he already knows. The patient knows what he is eating now. The patient is much more likely to learn when he is taught how to make changes in his current pattern to meet the diet prescription. Too often a diet is imposed on the patient as though he had no previous experience with food. Instructions for diet modifications should begin with the patient's current food habits and should stress the necessary changes to be made.

■ NURSING RESPONSIBILITIES

Nutrition is a component of nursing care for all patients whatever the medical or surgical problem and whether or not a "special" diet has been prescribed. To use the simplest possible terms, the objectives in nutritional care are to see that the individual patient receives and consumes the foods (nutrients) he needs in the hospital and to see that the individual patient has the knowledge and skills needed to feed himself properly wherever he may be. The nurse may meet these objectives by direct service to the patient. If the patient cannot lift a spoon to his mouth, the nurse may do so for him. If he needs information, the nurse may supply it. On the other hand, the nurse may meet these responsibilities indirectly. If

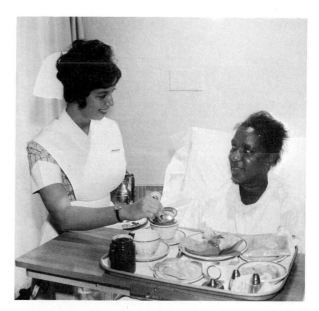

FIG. 6-6. The nurse is responsible for seeing that the patient does not just receive but that he consumes the foods he needs.

the patient cannot lift a spoon to his mouth, the nurse may make arrangements for someone else to feed him or may suggest that the diet be supplied as a liquid that can be drunk through a straw. If the patient needs information, the nurse may secure consultation for him with a dietitian or provide a suitable pamphlet or book. The nurse's responsibility for seeing that the objectives are realized for each patient cannot be delegated (Fig. 6-6).

The nurse's role is that of observer, interpreter, coordinator, and teacher as well as provider of care. The nurse-patient relationship places the nurse in a unique position to observe the patient and define care needs. The nurse serves as an interpreter to the patient by providing brief and easily understood explanations about his diet, any modifications in it, and the food selections on his tray. The nurse also serves as an interpreter by providing pertinent information about the patient to the physician, dietitian, or food service unit so that the diet prescription or food on the tray provides not only nutrients but also conforms insofar as possible to ethnic, religious, or personal preferences and provides eating pleasure. The nurse coordinates the special services the patient requires so that schedule conflicts are avoided. For example, some laboratory studies require that the patient fast; others require that he eat a special type of test meal. Coordination of laboratory, dietary, and nursing care schedules in such situations is essential

to the accuracy of the results and to the patient's comfort. Quite often need for consultation can be identified by the nurse early in the patient's hospital stay. The consultation can then be scheduled and provided before the day of discharge. The so-called discharge diet instruction is often omitted or rendered useless because it is left to the last minute when the patient's major interest is to get home as quickly as possible.

The nurse fulfills a significant role as teacher; by caring for the patient, he is taught to care for himself. The teaching may be informally given during daily nursing care. There may be planned conversations about nutrition or unplanned question and answer sessions. The nurse may integrate principles of therapeutic diet with general health teaching about the patient's disease. The nurse also teaches the patient by actions and attitudes.

In this age of expanding knowledge, major advances in technology and sweeping changes in social structure and patterns of living, it is unrealistic to expect that the few hours spent in a classroom or the few years spent in school will provide all the information and skills that a professional nurse will need for the next 30 to 50 years. The nurse must constantly look for better ideas and procedures and new information in nutrition, for nutrition is a vital part of person-centered nursing care for every patient.

REFERENCES AND SELECTED READINGS*

1 Alaska Basic Five Food Groups. Daily food guide, Public Health Service, Alaska Native Health Program, Nutrition and Dietetics Branch, Anchorage, Alaska, ND-63-30.
2 *American Dietetic Association: Position paper on bland diet in the treatment of chronic duodenal ulcer disease, J. Am. Diet. Assoc. 59:244-245, Sept. 1971.
3 Anderson, L., and Browe, J. H.: Nutrition and family health services, Philadelphia, 1960, W. B. Saunders Co.
4 Anonymous: Food additives: what they are, how they are used, Washington, D. C., 1971, Manufacturing Chemists' Association, Inc.
5 Baker, H., and others: Vitamins, total cholesterol, and triglycerides in 642 New York City school children, Am. J. Clin. Nutr. 20:850-857, Aug. 1967.
6 *Beaton, H. A., and others: Iron requirements of menstruating women, Am. J. Clin. Nutr. 23:275-283, March 1970.
7 *Bernarde, M. A., and Jerome, N. W.: Food quality and the consumer: a decalog, Am. J. Public Health 62:1199-1201, Sept. 1972.
8 Bogert, L. J., Briggs, G. M., and Calloway, D. H.: Nutrition and physical fitness, ed. 9, Philadelphia, 1973, W. B. Saunders Co.
9 Brennan, R.: Nutrition: a book of readings, Dubuque, Iowa, 1967, William C. Brown Co., Publishers.
10 *Butterworth, C. E., Jr.: Interactions of nutrients with oral

contraceptives and other drugs, J. Am. Diet. Assoc. 62:510-514, May 1973.
11 *Center for Disease Control (Health Services and Mental Health Administration): Ten-state nutrition survey 1968-1970. Department of Health, Education and Welfare Publication nos. (HSM) 72-8130, 72-8131, 72-8132, 72-8133, and 72-8134, Washington, D. C., 1972, U. S. Government Printing Office.
12 Cofer, E., Grossman, E., and Clark, F.: Family food plans and food costs, Home Economics Research Report no. 20, Washington, D. C., 1962, U. S. Department of Agriculture.
13 Council on Foods and Nutrition: Improvement of the nutritive quality of foods. General policies, J.A.M.A. 225:1116-1118, Aug. 1973.
14 Cuthbertson, D. P., and Tilstone, W. J.: Nutrition of the injured, Am. J. Clin. Nutr. 21:911-922, Sept. 1968.
15 *Darby, W. J.: The rational use of vitamins in medical practice, Med. Clin. North Am. 48:1203-1216, Sept. 1964.
16 *Dwyer, J. T., and others: The new vegetarians. Who are they? J. Am. Diet. Assoc. 62:503-509, May 1973.
17 *Erhard, D.: The new vegetarians. I. Vegetarianism and its medical consequences, Nutr. Today 8:4-12, Nov.-Dec. 1973.
18 Faloon, W. W.: Metabolic effects of nonabsorbable antibacterial agents, Am. J. Clin. Nutr. 23:645-651, May 1970.
19 *Federal Register 38:2138, Jan. 19, 1973.
20 *Federal Register 38:20737, Aug. 2, 1973.
21 *Federal Register 38:20323, Aug. 2, 1973.
22 *Federal Register 38:20725, Aug. 2, 1973.
23 *Federal Register 38:28558, Oct. 15, 1973.

*References preceded by an asterisk are particularly well suited for student reading.

24 *Fineberg, S. K.: The realities of obesity and fad diets, Nutr. Today 7:23-26, July-Aug. 1972.

25 *Frankle, R. T., and others: Nutrition and life style. I. The Door, a center of alternatives—the nutritionist in a free clinic for adolescents, J. Am. Diet. Assoc. 63:269-273, Sept. 1973.

26 *Gault, M. H., and others: Hypernatremia, azotemia, and dehydration due to high protein tube feeding, Ann. Intern. Med. 68:778-791, April 1968.

27 Goldsmith, G. A.: Nutritional diagnosis, American Lecture Series, Publication no. 356, Springfield, Ill., 1959, Charles C Thomas, Publisher.

28 Griffith, W. H.: Food as a regulator of metabolism, Am. J. Clin. Nutr. 17:391-398, Dec. 1965.

29 *Hall, R. L.: Food additives, Nutr. Today 8:20-28, July-Aug. 1973.

30 *Hegsted, D. M., and Ausman, L. M.: Sole foods and some not so scientific experiments, Nutr. Today 8:22-25, Nov.-Dec. 1973.

31 *Johnston, C. M.: Nutrition and life style. III. Nutrition and contemporary communal living, J. Am. Diet. Assoc. 63:275-276, Sept. 1973.

32 Joint FAO/WHO Expert Committee on Food Additives: Evaluation of food additives, Rome, 1971, FAO.

33 Krause, M. V., and Hunscher, M. A.: Food, nutrition and diet therapy, ed. 5, Philadelphia, 1972, W. B. Saunders Co.

34 Kreiser, H. R., and others: Loss of taste during therapy with penicillamine, J.A.M.A. 203:381-383, Feb. 1968.

35 Leverton, R. M.: Food becomes you, ed. 3, Ames, 1965, Iowa State University Press.

36 Leverton, R. M.: Facts and fallacies about nutrition and learning, J. Nutr. Educ. 1:7-9, Fall 1969.

37 Lowenberg, M. E., and others: Food and man, ed. 2, New York, 1973, John Wiley & Sons, Inc.

38 *Marsh, A. G., and others: About nutrition, Nashville, Tenn., 1971, Southern Publishers Association.

39 Mayer, J.: Overweight: causes, cost, and control (special edition for Consumer Reports), Englewood Cliffs, N. J., 1968, Prentice-Hall, Inc.

40 Mayer, J.: U. S. nutrition policies in the seventies, San Francisco, 1973, W. H. Freeman & Co.

41 Mead, M.: Food habits research: problems of the 1960's, Publication no. 1225, Washington, D. C., 1964, National Academy of Sciences–National Research Council.

42 Meyler, L., and Herxheimer, A.: Side effects of drugs: a survey of unwanted effects of drugs reported in 1965-1967, Baltimore, 1968, The Williams & Wilkins Co.

43 Mitchell, H. S., and others: Cooper's nutrition in health and disease, ed. 15, Philadelphia, 1968, J. B. Lippincott Co.

44 *Morris, E.: How does a nurse teach nutrition to patients? Am. J. Nurs. 60:67-70, Jan. 1960.

45 Murphy, J. V.: Intoxication following ingestion of elemental zinc, J.A.M.A. 212:2119-2120, June 1970.

46 National Research Council, Committee on Food Protection, Food and Nutrition Board: Toxicants occurring naturally in foods, ed. 2, Washington, D. C., 1973, National Academy of Sciences.

47 Neville, J. N., and others: Nutritional status of alcoholics, Am. J. Clin. Nutr. 21:1329-1340, Nov. 1968.

48 *Newton, M. E., Beal, M. E., and Strauss, A. L.: Nutritional aspects of nursing care, Nurs. Res. 16:46-49, Winter 1967.

49 Nizel, A. E.: Nutrition in preventive dentistry: science and practice, Philadelphia, 1972, W. B. Saunders Co.

50 *Norma, C.: Iron enrichment, Nutr. Today 8:16-17, Nov.-Dec. 1973.

51 Recommended dietary allowances, ed. 8, Washington, D. C., 1974, National Academy of Sciences–National Research Council.

52 *Register, U. D., and Sonnenberg, L. M.: The vegetarian diet. Scientific and practical considerations, J. Am. Diet. Assoc. 62:253-261, March 1973.

53 Roberts, L. J.: A basic food pattern for Puerto Rico, J. Am. Diet. Assoc. 30:1097-1100, Nov. 1954.

54 Robinson, C. H.: Normal and therapeutic nutrition, ed. 14, New York, 1972, Macmillan Publishing Co., Inc.

55 *Rubin, R.: Food and feeding: a matrix of relationships, Nurs. Forum 6(2):195-205, 1967.

56 *Sandstead, H. H., and others: Zinc and wound healing: effects of zinc deficiency and zinc supplementation, Am. J. Clin. Nutr. 23:514-519, May 1970.

57 *Schwartz, P. L.: Ascorbic acid in wound healing—a review, J. Am. Diet. Assoc. 56:497-503, June 1970.

58 *Scrimshaw, N. S.: Synergism of malnutrition and infection: evidence from field studies in Guatemala, J.A.M.A. 212:1685-1692, June 1970.

59 Sebrell, W. H., Jr.: Chemical aspects of updating diet quality, J. Agric. Food Chem. 20:518-522, March 1972.

60 *Spencer, H., and others: Changes in metabolism in obese persons during starvation, Am. J. Med. 40:27-37, Jan. 1966.

61 *Thomas, J. A., and Call, D. L.: Eating between meals—a nutrition problem among teenagers, Nutr. Rev. 31:137-139, May 1973.

62 Tullis, I. F.: Rational diet construction for mild and grand obesity, J.A.M.A. 226:70-71, Oct. 1973.

63 U. S. Department of Agriculture: Food for fitness: a daily food guide, Leaflet 424, Washington, D. C., 1964, U. S. Government Printing Office.

64 U. S. Department of Agriculture: Food for us all. Yearbook of Agriculture 1969, Washington, D. C., 1969, U. S. Government Printing Office.

65 *U. S. Department of Health, Education and Welfare, Public Health Service: FDA Consumer memo, nutrition labeling—terms you should know, DHEW Publication no. (FDA) 74-2010. The new look in food labels, DHEW Publication no. (FDA) 74-2036, Washington, D. C., 1974, U. S. Government Printing Office.

66 Watson, P., and Bodey, G. P.: Sterile food service for patients in protected environments, J. Am. Diet. Assoc. 56:515-520, June 1970.

67 White House Conference on Food Nutrition and Health, Final Report, Panel 11-5, Washington, D. C., 1970, U. S. Government Printing Office.

68 Williams, S. R.: Nutrition and diet therapy, ed. 2, St. Louis, 1973, The C. V. Mosby Co.

69 *Wilmore, D. W., and Dudrick, S.: Growth and development of an infant receiving all nutrients by vein, J.A.M.A. 203:860-864, March 1968.

70 Wishnofsky, M.: Caloric equivalents of gained or lost weight, Am. J. Clin. Nutr. 6:542-546, Sept.-Oct. 1958.

71 *Wolff, R. J.: Who eats for health? Am. J. Clin. Nutr. 26:438-445, April 1973.

7 Maladaptive behavior

The patient's behavior
General principles of management
Disorders not related to maladjusted personality
Specific disorders related to maladjusted personality

■ Personality refers to all that a person is, feels, and does, either consciously or unconsciously, as manifested in interaction with his environment.[38] Man is a social being, and one of his basic needs is to feel secure and accepted by others in his social group. His entire life from birth to death consists of a series of adjustments to meet his biologic and emotional needs in socially acceptable ways. The person with a well-integrated personality has learned to live in relative harmony with his environment. Poor adjustment leads to difficulty in interpersonal relationships. Maladjustments vary in degree from occasional withdrawal to overt psychosis. Many people with such emotional problems have, nevertheless, made marginal adjustments within a particular environment. The additional stress accompanying illness may threaten their security enough to disrupt their personalities, causing personality disorganization and disintegration. This disintegration is referred to as a "nervous breakdown" by most people and is classified medically as mental illness.

It is important to remember that the well-integrated person has normal emotional responses to illness. The main difference is that these reactions are usually reversible, while the mentally ill person has an underlying problem that has been "opened up" by stress. Removal of the stress may stop the specific difficulty but it will seldom, if ever, change the basic maladaptive behavior pattern.

At least 55% of the hospital beds in the United States are filled with patients whose primary diagnosis is mental illness. Another 25% are taken by patients with psychophysiologic diseases such as peptic ulcer, colitis, and asthma. Some experts include essential hypertension, arthritis, and other somatic complaints in this classification.

Drug abuse and alcoholism are often seen in persons with maladaptive behaviors. These conditions frequently cause physical illness severe enough to require hospitalization.

It is often difficult to differentiate mental illness from physical illness because of the intimate relationship of the mind and body. Illness of the one always affects the other. Physical illness is often called *organic,* while mental illness is termed *functional.* These terms are used when one is trying to determine the cause of behavior. For example, there may be similarity in the behavior of a patient with an adrenal tumor and the patient with schizophrenia, as can be seen in the following case history.

A 19-year-old high school student had been in a general hospital for diagnosis and treatment of "black out spells." No organic basis for these spells was found. He was transferred to a private psychiatric hospital with a diagnosis of schizophrenic reaction, catatonic type. He appeared somewhat shy, especially with his peer group. Occasionally he was difficult to rouse in the morning and he took frequent naps. One morning the nurses decided to try some TLC while attempting to waken him. He was brought a glass of chocolate milk and fed with a spoon, being assured that people cared about him and wanted to help him face the day. His response was much more rapid than usual and the nurses felt they had hit on a solution to his problem. The psychiatrist was impressed with their reports but questioned if the response to the milk was psychologic or physiologic and ordered blood to be drawn for blood sugar levels the next time he was "catatonic." This was done. The sugar level was 37 mg./100 ml. serum (normal 75 to 105 mg./100

■ **STUDY QUESTIONS**

1 Study the behavior of several selected patients on your ward. What impression do you receive of their mental health from observing their posture and facial appearance, their grooming, their bedside unit, and their relationships with other patients?

2 What provisions does your ward have for the safety of a patient who develops symptoms of mental illness? What is the policy of your hospital regarding care of such patients?

3 How prevalent is drug use among teenagers in your community? How can they be helped to see the dangers of taking drugs?

ml. serum). The patient was transferred to a general hospital for further diagnostic workup. It was determined that he had a left adrenal tumor. This was surgically removed and he took up life again as a relatively normal, healthy young man.

This case history demonstrates that careful observation, laboratory studies, and even surgery may be necessary to determine the cause of a disease.

Naturally the mentally ill are subject to injury and physical illness and when they are sick they may need treatment in a general hospital. Many general hospitals have set aside a few rooms with special safety provisions to meet the particular needs of patients who are emotionally disturbed.

Basic courses in personality development help the nurse understand normal behavior of patients, but specialized help may be necessary when caring for persons with mental illness. If the hospital has a psychiatric division, it may be possible for the psychiatric nurses to consult with the medical and surgical nurses regarding the care of patients who are mentally ill. Many hospitals do not have such experts available, however, and nurses must depend largely on their own knowledge and resources. When the nurse is assigned to care for patients with severe emotional problems, the many good textbooks and other references on psychiatric nursing should be consulted. The following pages contain only a brief discussion of a few important principles or guides to follow in caring for patients with mental illness.

■ THE PATIENT'S BEHAVIOR

Behavior is an expression of personality. Actually the behavior of the maladjusted person does not differ in kind from that of a so-called normal person. It differs only in degree.[38] Many patients with mental illness appear quite normal on casual observation and conversation, and it is only on more prolonged contact that abnormalities of personality may be evident. Consequently, the nurse needs to take time to know the patient. On the other hand, the patient's interactions with others and his self-control may have deteriorated to a point where he is conspicuous. This type of behavior is often manifested during an acute psychotic episode.

The nurse who for the first time encounters a patient in an acute psychotic episode may be truly unprepared for the behavior demonstrated. Most nurses have been accustomed, in their daily living and in their dealings with patients, to meeting persons who are able to face challenges to their security with a normal amount of assurance, thus keeping themselves in harmonious association with others. In the hospital the patient is often expected to repress his fears, irritations, and aggressive impulses to a socially acceptable degree and to be a "good patient." Because the "normal" patient has a reasonably well-integrated personality, and because he anticipates a short stay in the hospital, he usually is able to live up to these expectations. The patient who has a severe emotional disturbance may be unable to control his emotional responses and may react freely and impulsively. He may be out of contact with reality at times, expressing bizarre ideas *(delusions),* and he may have false sensory perceptions *(hallucinations).* Hallucinations are usually auditory or visual, but they may be tactile, olfactory, or gustatory. The patient may also feel pain for no apparent physical reason. Regardless of the unreality of these sensations, they are real to the patient. Hearing voices is very common, and patients often answer the voices or respond to the directions given by them. Tactile sensations usually are of crawling objects, and patients may try to flick them away or to run from them.

It is quite common for an emotionally disturbed person to be *severely depressed.* This depression is much deeper than that experienced in varying degree by normal people. It is described as a feeling of utter hopelessness or as a living death. The patient feels exhausted and is dejected in his posture, facial expression, gait, and verbal reactions. He loses interest in his physical surroundings and his personal appearance. His appetite is poor, and constipation may develop. Although he may be quiet and lie for hours with eyes closed, the severely depressed patient seldom sleeps well. At times a depressed patient may become quite tense and restless, showing signs of agitation such as pacing the floor and wringing his hands. He may be tearful and express feelings of inadequacy, unworthiness, and guilt. A depressed patient may mention and often contemplate suicide. Any severely depressed person who suddenly seems much better should be watched carefully, since this improvement often means only that he has decided on a means of escape that may be suicide.

Studies have shown that the person contemplating suicide almost always shows warning symptoms in a desperate plea for help. He may talk about death or dying; get his affairs in order; ask to see business associates, family members, or friends; and if hospitalized, often make a point of saying good-bye to the nurse who is going off duty or preparing him for sleep. Suicide claimed 10.7 deaths/100,000 population in the United States in 1968 (21,290 reported lives).[62] In 1967 suicide ranked as the tenth leading cause of death in this country.[2] The actual number of suicides is probably much higher than figures indicate, since many experts consider some automobile accidents and other "accidental" deaths as possible suicides.

The emotionally disturbed patient may be *hyperactive* (manic) or aggressive in his behavior. He may flit from one activity or one subject of conversation to another, and it may be impossible to hold his attention for more than an instant. Profanity and vulgarity are common, and the patient may be critical of the hospital and the personnel as well as sarcastic and domineering. He has the exaggerated behavior of the noisy, demanding patient and may become irritated easily and express his irritation in assaultive behavior. Hyperactivity may become so pronounced as to cause exhaustion.

Suspicion (paranoid reactions) may be exhibited by some maladjusted patients. They may appear suspicious, critical, and watchful of every move others make, and they may question activities and refuse medications, treatment, and even food. At the same time they may feel persecuted and neglected if left out of any activity.

Some people with mental illness show *obsessive compulsive behavior.* They are compelled to follow certain rituals or behavior patterns that are far beyond the normal but that in some ways serve to relieve inner tensions. For example, it is normal for many persons to count fence posts as they walk down the road. However, a compulsion neurosis is evident when a person cannot ever walk down a road without counting and touching each post. Ritualistic compulsions in such matters as bathing, washing hands, and dressing in certain sequence are common and, even when carried to great extremes, may sometimes be successfully concealed from the outside world.

The maladjusted person may become overconcerned and preoccupied with body function. This type of behavior is known as *hypochondriasis.*

Hysteria is an abnormal behavior pattern that has been recognized for centuries. Despite the lack of physical cause, the person may not be able to do such things as void or move a particular limb. He may have areas of numbness, lack of one of the special senses, or a variety of other physical complaints. He may have apparent convulsive seizures, although unlike the patient with a true convulsive disorder, he is not likely to injure himself during an attack.

Anxiety states are common among emotionally disturbed patients. The patient may have an abnormal fear of impending disaster, and this fear may be expressed in bodily signs such as flushing, tachycardia, and excessive perspiration. Although there may be no rational basis for his fear, it is very real to the patient and it cannot be dissipated by rational explanation. A word or two picked out of a statement by his physician may serve as a basis for worries and fears. If anxiety becomes too great, *panic*—complete disorganization of behavior in the face of overwhelming terror—may result. The patient then loses complete control of himself and is unable to perceive, communicate, or control motor actions. The environment is often misinterpreted, and the patient may try to escape from what he imagines is acute

danger around him. This behavior may lead to physical injury such as may be sustained from falling out of bed, removing drainage tubes, or falling from an open window. The patient may not be intent on suicide but may destroy himself as he attempts to flee from imagined danger unless special precautions for his safety are taken. The patient in a panic may attack hospital personnel in the belief that they are endangering his life. He acts quickly and impulsively and therefore should be watched most carefully.

■ GENERAL PRINCIPLES OF MANAGEMENT

Basically the care needed by the mentally ill patient on a medical or surgical unit is no different from that needed by any other patient. He needs acceptance as a person, provision for physical needs, and provision for his safety. Bizarre, socially unacceptable behavior can often be handled by a clear statement of recognition of the behavior and its importance to the patient. This will not necessarily change the behavior, but it will often help prevent further disintegration. It is important that the patient not lose self-esteem; therefore he should be protected from the curious eyes of staff and other patients. There are many drugs available that can help the disturbed patient be more comfortable, and when he is more comfortable, he can be more cooperative. The nurse who approaches the disturbed patient with an objective, nonjudgmental attitude communicates acceptance and concern. A positive, expectant manner will shore up the patient's self-respect and help him to be less afraid in a frightening, foreign environment.

Emotional care

It is impossible to tell anyone exactly how to respond to a mentally ill patient. Indeed, no written words could ever transmit this skill, which can be mastered only through practice. Certainly calmness and matter-of-factness combined with a genuine interest in the patient and in trying to help him are positive qualities for the nurse to develop. The nurse's position is that of one who is interested and willing to listen and to help. The nurse cannot take the place of the patient's family and should realize this fact. The patient may hope that the nurse can replace his emotional attachments to his family as he gropes for relationships that are satisfying and yet not too demanding. Inexperienced nurses may encounter serious difficulties if they do not seek help from persons with more experience when patients become too dependent on them.

The patient with mental illness benefits from calmness, consistency, and uniformity in his environment. Procedures should be explained to him calmly, and sometimes repeatedly, even though he may not appear attentive or concerned. Even the smallest details of necessary medical or surgical treatment should be explained before they are undertaken. The equipment used for procedures should be reduced to a minimum, but basic principles such as aseptic technique used in changing dressings should not differ from those used in safe nursing anywhere. The patient must also be prepared for routine nursing measures; for example, when lights are to be turned out, a meal is to be presented, or a visit to the bathroom is to be made, the patient should be told what is going to occur.

Anything that increases the patient's anxiety may be harmful to him. The use of technical language and discussion of disease and technical procedures should be avoided. Subjects that appear to increase the patient's anxiety should be noted carefully, and mention of them should be made in the nurse's notes. Religion is commonly associated with anxiety or feeling of guilt. Sexual maladjustment is common in persons who are mentally ill. Mention of close members of the family may produce anxiety. Often the final failure in interpersonal relationships occurs in the family setting, among those whose acceptance is most valued by the patient. It is safest to let the patient volunteer the information he wishes. If he shares personal information, the nurse must let him know that his confidences will be kept and that his disclosures, regardless of their nature, do not lessen the nurse's opinion of him.

The nurse should be alert for changes in behavior indicating that anxiety is increasing and panic may develop. These may include failure to hear people speaking, muscular tension, perspiring for no observable reason, failure to make connections between details in conversation or conduct, headache, nausea, trembling, and weakness.[45] At this time action should be taken to help the patient release tension. Someone should stay with him, and if possible, he should be removed from the situation that induces the increased anxiety. Activities such as walking, talking, counting, describing something, or playing a simple game reduce anxiety. It also helps to increase the patient's awareness of his surroundings.[45] If panic does occur, the patient can often be handled best by two people calmly approaching him, firmly but slowly addressing him, and leading him away from the situation. A number of people should not suddenly approach a greatly disturbed or active patient unless emergency measures are needed to protect him or others. The patient then should be placed in an environment as free from stimuli as possible, and someone should remain near him until he becomes calmer. When he is left alone again, he should be assured of immediate response if he should need help.

It is useless to argue with the mentally ill person or to attempt to talk him out of his delusions by reasoning with him. He has lost the ability to understand the psychotic nature of his ideas or to see the fallacies in them. No attempt should be made to explain his behavior to him. Many patients become confused and disoriented and may be terrified by their delusions or hallucinations. The nurse can best support the patient by confirming what is real to her. For example, the most bizarre ideation usually has some element of reality in it. Careful listening and reflection of the "real" parts of the patient's experience will help him with his reality testing. It is foolish to ask a confused person such questions as time and place. It is better to tell him in a general, conversant manner, "It's 3:00 P.M., Mr. Smith. I'll be leaving at 3:30 and I wanted to see if you would like to sit up for a while before I go."

Reassurance, in the general sense, should be avoided. Simply telling the patient that he is not going to die or that he is worthy of his family may do more harm than good, since it may destroy a picture of himself that it is necessary for him to have at the moment. However, reassurance in the sense of producing a calm, quiet, accepting environment is always of value. The patient should feel that he will not be censured or rejected because of his behavior. He should be given security by assurance of consistency of routine, of the conduct of others toward him, and of the limitations that are placed on him. He may gain reassurance from consistency in the way in which he is encouraged to express negative feelings. He may show such feelings by disliking the nurse, for example. He may dislike the nurse without the fear of retaliation that would be present if he disliked his wife or any other close member of the family. Thus hostility toward personnel may be a healthy sign and should be accepted as such by the nurse. Effort should be made to have the patient feel that his behavior is understood even though it may not be approved. The right of the patient to want to behave as he does is acknowledged. For example, the patient may have the right to want to hurl his water pitcher but he should know that the staff will continue to prevent him from harming himself or others.

Adequate control of behavior can usually be maintained by the use of drugs such as chlorpromazine (Thorazine), thioridazine (Mellaril), fluphenazine (Prolixin), promazine (Sparine), trifluoperazine (Stelazine), or prochlorperazine (Compazine). These drugs are in the phenothiazine group and have side effects that may be uncomfortable to the patient such as dry mouth, blurred vision, and photophobia. It is especially important to observe him for extrapyramidal reactions that include tremors, shuffling gait, masklike face, drooling, and restlessness. Severe reactions may cause extreme muscle spasm, particularly of the upper body and frequently limited to one side. This reaction can be quickly alleviated by the use of intramuscular or intravenous antiparkinsonian drugs such as benztropine mesylate (Cogentin), biperiden (Akineton), or trihexyphenidyl (Artane). In psychiatric facilities, patients receiving phenothiazines often receive anticholinergic drugs prophylactically. The appearance of side effects may necessitate changing the dosage or even the drug. Intolerance to one drug does not necessarily indicate intolerance to other tranquilizers. Tranquilizers derived from compounds other than phenothiazines and used for mild to moderate anxiety states include chlordiazepoxide (Librium), diazepam (Valium), and meprobamate (Equanil, Miltown).

Antidepressant drugs, often referred to as psychic energizers, produce feelings of well-being in depressed persons. Amitriptyline (Elavil), imipramine (Tofranil), and phenelzine (Nardil) are some of the common ones prescribed. Antidepressant drugs may produce any of the more severe as well as the less severe side effects that are observed in patients taking tranquilizers. Since all of these drugs can produce serious side effects, the nurse is cautioned to be aware of average doses and individual tolerance to the drugs.

The confused or psychotic patient may be unable to comprehend medical orders such as bed rest or intravenous feedings. Repeated clear explanation of treatments and, most importantly, frequent short contact with the patient will do much to gain his cooperation. If the patient is unable to comply with medical orders, it may be necessary to restrain him. For instance, if he has a catheter in place and repeatedly pulls it out, there is danger of injury to the bladder and urethra. In this instance, soft restraints may be enough of a reminder to prevent the catheter from being removed.

Severe restriction of motion such as by leather restraints should be avoided unless there is real danger to the patient or others. Restraining patients often causes increased anxiety, and increased anxiety decreases the patient's ability to deal rationally with his environment. A family member, friend, or staff member who can stay with the patient provides the best way to help the agitated patient adjust to the hospital.

Physical care

When a patient in a general hospital becomes mentally ill, there is a tendency to become overconcerned with his behavior and to neglect his physical needs. It must be remembered that the patient needs good general nursing care, including mouth care, attention to cleanliness, and good grooming. Even if he is physically able to carry out these tasks for himself, he is likely to need help since he may be too preoccupied with his thoughts or with other activities to care for himself completely or safely. Patients have been known to lean against a hot radiator and sustain a severe burn or to step into a tubful of very hot water without flinching. Dressings must be changed and

medications given. Often patients will not even ask for a bedpan or urinal or for medication for pain, and the nurse must be responsible for providing for these needs.

For some time before hospitalization the depressed patient may have eaten too little or improperly. He may refuse to eat, or he may hide his food to give the impression that he has eaten. The hyperactive patient may be too busy, frightened, or preoccupied to eat, and yet he may require more than the usual amount of food. A careful record of *food* and *fluid intake* should be kept on all patients with mental illness. A record of *urinary* and *bowel elimination* is also necessary. The patient who is depressed often suffers from constipation, and the hyperactive patient may delay going to the bathroom because of his many preoccupations.

Medications are often refused by the mentally ill patient, who may be exceedingly clever at concealing drugs not swallowed. When staff have reason to believe the patient is not taking his medication, pills may be crushed and dissolved unless their bitter taste precludes this measure. Serious problems in giving medications orally must be reported to the physician so that he may order another method of administration.

Sleep is necessary for the mentally ill patient but is sometimes hard to achieve. Adequate sleep and good general physical health make it easier for him to face his problems and attempt to solve them. Patients with acute mental illness may require large doses of sedatives or tranquilizers to control daytime behavior, but recent research has shown that such drugs may actually interfere with sleep, particularly dream (REM or rapid eye movement) sleep.[14,34] Exercise outdoors, a quiet environment, a back rub or warm bath, and warm drinks are often surprisingly helpful.

Special needs of the depressed patient

The deeply depressed patient may require almost complete physical care to sustain him, and he may be almost totally unresponsive to any attempts to communicate with him. Nevertheless, the patient needs human contact both physically and interpersonally, even though he may seem oblivious to it. Observant nurses usually will be able to determine to some extent what type of activity or conversation seems to help a particular patient, and they must try to provide it. Overcheerfulness, overt solicitude, abruptness, or a dictatorial manner on the part of personnel is particularly upsetting to depressed patients. A deeply depressed patient may be depressing to the nurse or other personnel caring for him. If so, personnel should plan their contacts with the patient so that they can provide continuity of care, prevent evident avoidance of the patient, and still retain reasonable emotional comfort themselves.

If there is just one person who consistently shows he or she cares for the patient, this fact may be enough to prevent him from coming to the point where he considers that *suicide* is the only means of escape from his untenable situation. Even though he is unable to ask for help openly, the depressed patient wants someone to be concerned about his welfare. He wishes to be protected from himself and his possible impulsive behavior. In contemplating suicide, he does not necessarily really want to die but to express the urgency of escape from an unbearable situation.

It is not true that persons who talk about suicide rarely attempt it. At least a third of those committing suicide talk about it or give some indirect indication of their intent. Mention of suicide intent by the patient should be taken calmly by the nurse but should be reported to the physician at once and recorded in the patient's record. The patient should immediately be given increased attention, with sympathetic and serious concern. By showing more concern for the patient, the nurse indicates to him that he really matters. It is exceedingly important that the nurse not answer the patient in a way that appears to dare him to carry out his threat. Such a comment as "I know you don't mean that" leaves the patient with little choice but to carry out his threat to prove the seriousness of his statement.

Prevention of suicide or other injury requires alert attention on the part of the nurse. Pocketknives and objects such as nail files, razor blades, belts, drugs, and any pieces of equipment that might be used either impulsively or with premeditation should be removed. If the patient is known to be suffering from mental illness, such belongings should be removed on admission, as is done in mental hospitals. If windows can be raised enough so that the patient could crawl through them, they must be equipped with "stop" devices to prevent complete opening, and occasionally protection over the glass is necessary. Doors must be fitted with locks that cannot be turned from the inside. Electrical fixtures must be out of reach of the patient who might attempt to electrocute himself by tampering with the socket or who might injure himself with glass from bulbs.

The physician is responsible for ordering constant observation if it is necessary because of the danger of suicide or injury to others. The order, if issued, must be carried out to the letter. The newspapers bear testimony to many instances of patients leaping from windows or otherwise destroying themselves in the few brief moments when the nurse's back was turned. A decrease in the patient's tension should not cause a relaxation of vigilance, since decision on a plan of action may be its cause.

The nurse must find a way to observe the suicidal patient carefully and sympathetically without making him feel that he is guarded or under constant scrutiny. The patient may resent constant observation, believing that he is being spied on or that he is in danger from the observer. The least conspicuous way to observe a patient is by observing him in a group, but such an arrangement may not be feasible on the medical and surgical unit because of the patient's other illness. The nurse may appear to be busy with a patient in an adjoining room while watching the mentally ill patient. Sometimes locating the observer outside the patient's room may cause the least annoyance. Efforts should be made to convey to the patient that he is being given special attention because the nurse cares about him and feels he needs this attention. When nurses consistently make a genuine and serious effort to find the best way to help a patient, their interest and concern may be crucial in keeping him alive.

Persons who have made unsuccessful suicide attempts are often admitted to general hospitals for emergency care. The immediate care depends on the attempt made. Patients are frequently treated for drug overdoses and other poisoning, severed arteries, and gunshot wounds. They must now face not only the original problem that precipitated the suicide attempt but the consequences of their act. Special care needs to be taken to avoid a repeated attempt, and psychotherapy usually is instituted. Family members, too, often need help in understanding and accepting the patient's problem. Sometimes they need the help of the physician, mental hygiene consultant, social worker, or member of the clergy in planning for the role they will take in the future in helping the patient.

Special needs of the patient with aggressive behavior

A patient with aggressive behavior is often overactive, and he fares best in a nonchallenging and nonstimulating environment. Noise should be kept at a minimum, and distraction and irritations of all kinds should be avoided.

The aggressive patient needs to be allowed to express his feelings in a calm, accepting atmosphere. Although he may be most annoying, he must not be allowed to feel that he is a nuisance or is unliked. He should not be prevented from verbalizing his annoyances, and no attempt should be made to talk him out of his attack or to defend the person or situation being verbally attacked. The patient should never be compared to other patients or to himself on previous occasions, as the comparison may make him feel rejected. Answers to questions should be simple and direct. The nurse should avoid encouraging stimulating conversation while still conferring a feeling of warmth and interest.

The aggressive patient may not respond favorably to direct requests. He usually is happier associating with quiet patients since his aggressiveness often calls forth aggression in others. Attempts should be made to channel the aggressive patient's energy into constructive activity, but he must be observed carefully to detect signs of approaching exhaustion and to prevent upsetting situations from arising because of the possibility of injury to the patient or others. A warm bath in a darkened, quiet room may be helpful for the overactive, aggressive patient, and sedation may also be given.

Special needs of the patient who focuses on physical symptoms

The patient with a psychoneurosis concerning physical symptoms requires infinite patience and understanding. He also needs careful, firm, and thoughtful management. Usually he has told his physical symptoms endless times to numerous people and has worn out his welcome with all. The nurse should listen attentively for a reasonable time and should then try to direct the patient's conversation away from discussion about himself. The nurse should not be trapped into implying that there is nothing wrong with the patient, and it is well to avoid discussion of any medical subject. Activity therapy that can be undertaken at the bedside often helps divert conversation away from the patient and also may result in creativity that earns recognition for him.

The nurse should watch for any attempts the patient may make to aggravate his physical ailment or to produce symptoms. So great may be his need to maintain an acceptable outlet for his problems through illness that he may go to surprising lengths to delay a cure. Patients have been known to hold their thermometers against light bulbs, add water to urine collection bottles, tamper with their wounds to cause infection, and even subject themselves to needless surgery. When the nurse has reason to believe that a patient is attempting to falsify his clinical picture, she has the responsibility to report her suspicions to the physician. An example of such behavior is seen in the following case history.

A 39-year-old unmarried woman who resided with her mother was admitted to the medical service for severe diarrhea and blood loss through her ileostomy. Initially, the staff was concerned about fluid loss and dehydration although there was no clinical evidence such as weight loss, poor skin turgor, or changes in laboratory findings. The patient kept her own intake and output record. In one 24-hour period she recorded 450 ml. intake and 4,700 ml. output, including 28 loose stools, none of which was observed by a staff member. The ileostomy site was reddened and bleeding. The patient in the next bed reported seeing her using a rat-tail comb to irritate the site.

In an attempt to provide more healthy attention-getting activities a very active occupational therapy program was initiated. The patient was quite talented artistically and received many honest compliments on her work. She accepted an invitation to work as a volunteer in the children's ward. Since the intake-output record served no purpose, it was discontinued. No questions were asked about loose stools. She was weighed routinely and without comment about her weight. The patient was most responsive to this regimen and after discharge returned to the hospital weekly for occupational and group therapy. She also entered therapy with a psychologist. The improvement was maintained for 3 months, at which time her mother had a serious fall. The patient was admitted to a surgical floor with an acute exacerbation of symptoms. (The patient had had 27 prior surgical procedures in over 40 hospital admissions.)

To assure reasonable success of this type of approach, each staff member must be well informed about what is being done and why. This prevents the patient from "using" one staff member against another to defeat the program and thus himself.

Observations and recording

The nurse's notes are very important in the care of the mentally ill patient. The nurse is around the patient longer than any other professional person and may be the only one who observes him during evening and night hours. Recorded observations can be of great help to the psychiatrist in his management of the patient. These notes should be remarkable for their quality rather than their length, but it is best to err on the side of length rather than of brevity. They should contain actual expressions of the patient, using quotation marks and taking care that the words recorded are exactly those of the patient. Notes should be recorded immediately after significant conversation or behavior has been noted so that details will be fresh in mind. Although the specialty of psychiatry has a complete vocabulary of its own, rather than place labels such as delusions or hallucinations on the symptoms of the patient, it is better to write factual statements such as "States over and over, 'I see men at the window, they are wearing red, they have come to kill me.'" The nurse's notes should also contain detailed accounts of what the patient does, such as "Sat at the window grimacing and smiling for $2\frac{1}{2}$ hours this P.M.; keeps saying as he smiles, 'I'll be dead tomorrow.'"

■ DISORDERS NOT RELATED TO MALADJUSTED PERSONALITY

Organic and toxic psychoses

Organic psychoses are due to disease processes that have produced physical changes. Among the common causes of organic psychoses are neurologic syphilis, arteriosclerosis, and epilepsy with deterioration. Brain tumors, brain trauma, Huntington's chorea, and encephalitis are other examples of organic origins of mental illness.

Toxic reactions or *toxic delirium* may occur when high temperature is present or when toxins have accumulated in the body from disease (for example, uremia). When such factors are the cause, the toxic reaction is *endogenous.* When psychosis results from a reaction to drugs such as bromides, anesthetics, and alcohol, the reaction is *exogenous.*

Toxic reactions are the most common of the psychoses seen in general hospitals. They usually come on suddenly and may disappear as quickly, particularly if the cause can be found and eliminated. Patients with toxic reactions almost always suffer from confusion, hallucinations, and delusions that usually cause fear and sometimes panic.

■ SPECIFIC DISORDERS RELATED TO MALADJUSTED PERSONALITY

Functional psychoses

Functional psychoses have no demonstrable organic cause, although it is suspected that eventually one may be found. The emotional disorders that are commonly classified as functional psychoses include involutional psychotic reaction (involutional melancholia), manic-depressive reaction, schizophrenia (dementia praecox), and paranoia. Functional psychoses are rarely classified as distinct entities, since most patients have a mixture of reactions. Both schizophrenia and paranoia are serious mental illnesses for which the patient often needs long-term care in a special psychiatric facility. Patients with involutional melancholia and manic-depressive reactions have a fairly good prognosis for recovery from an attack, but attacks tend to recur. If it is known that a patient has suffered from a functional psychosis, the nurse should be alert for early signs of recurring emotional illness since mental health is taxed by physical illness.

Psychoneuroses

Patients with psychoneuroses are seen most often in general hospitals. This is because their behavior, although exasperating to the physician and to all who must help them solve their health problems, is seldom such that care in a mental hospital is necessary. The patient suffering from a psychoneurosis conforms to social standards and is able to appreciate the rights of others in a general sense. He is oriented as to time and place. However, in compromising his desires with social demands he has failed to make a satisfactory emotional adjustment and has escaped from the untenable demands of living by developing psychoneurotic behavior. This behavior may take the form of hypochondriasis, anxiety states, hysteria, or obsessive compulsive behavior. Although the patient may have a physical disease that may or may not be related to his basic emotional disturbance, the emotional problem is predominant and is the one that is really important to the patient. He is less upset by his symptoms than would be expected, and even when extensive diagnostic procedures and surgery are performed, he usually is surprisingly philosophic about the whole experience.

The nurse or anyone else caring for psychoneurotic patients should not assume that these patients are willfully sick. Unfortunately they are too often considered problems by members of the staff who lack the insight to recognize their need to be ill. The patient does feel real pain and discomfort even though no physical cause may be found. Psychoneurotic patients are large consumers of medical care and all related services. It is probable that the economic cost to society of this group of patients is greater than the cost for all the psychoses combined.

Alcoholism

Alcoholism in the United States is on the increase. Conservative estimates are that 80 million people use alcohol and about $6\frac{1}{2}$ million people are afflicted with alcoholism. Alcoholism is defined as "a continuing problem (with alcohol) that affects the person's life; such as his family, his work and/or his social activities." Also, an alcoholic "cannot predict with 100% accuracy what his behavior will be after his first drink."[37] The second definition has to do with the individual's control of the amount he drinks. The nonalcoholic can say he will have one or two drinks and stick to his plan, whereas the alcoholic may not be able to do so.

Industries lose at least 4 billion dollars yearly because of alcoholism.[26] This figure includes the cost of time lost, misjudgments, spoiled materials, broken machines, and other factors. Many companies have special programs for the treatment and rehabilitation of employees with alcoholism. Referrals to the program are made by supervisors and managers on the basis of decreased productivity, thus eliminating the need for them to make a diagnosis.

Habitual drunkenness is the main symptom of the disease of alcoholism. Recent court rulings have declared the drunken person is sick and entitled to medical treatment, not imprisonment. Unfortunately there are not enough facilities to treat the alcoholic; treatment is long, expensive, and often unsuccessful.

The alcoholic as a hospital patient. The nurse in a general hospital is likely to be assigned the care of the alcoholic patient following a drinking bout during which he has sustained an injury or at a time when his physical ailments caused by alcoholism become so severe that treatment is necessary. Alcoholism is so common, however, that the patient may be admitted for a medical or surgical illness completely unrelated to his alcoholism, which may be unknown even to his physician. Or he may be admitted in coma and near death from acute alcohol poisoning. This discussion will consider only a few aspects of care related to general care and information about referring for treatment of alcoholism the patient whom the nurse may encounter either in the general hospital or outside the hospital.

Any patient in the hospital who is not known to

be an alcoholic but who does not respond normally to preoperative medication, to anesthetics, or to sedatives should be observed carefully for signs of alcoholism. The alcoholic patient usually requires large doses of sedatives and anesthesia for effect, and he is likely to be overly excited and active as he reacts from anesthesia. The most apparent signs of chronic alcoholism that may be noted by the nurse are a tremor that is worse in the morning and morning nausea. The patient feels "jittery," and were alcohol available, he would probably have a drink or two to "steady his nerves" before eating.

Alcohol may be prescribed for alcoholic patients during their hospitalization, particularly during an acute illness when reaction to deprivation is severe. However, close observation is necessary because even the patient receiving alcohol as prescribed may be extremely resourceful in obtaining an additional supply. If a patient appears to be obtaining unauthorized alcohol, the physician should be notified. Any alcoholic patient admitted to the general hospital for an acute medical or surgical condition should be observed closely for signs of impending delirium tremens. Early treatment may prevent the development of an acute psychosis.

Regardless of the circumstances surrounding his hospitalization, the alcoholic patient often feels hopeless, guilty, and apprehensive. If his physical ailment is related directly to alcoholism, he is usually quite ill before he consents to be hospitalized. Often he wishes to talk to someone, but the person must be someone who seems to accept him as he is and to understand his problem. The nurses caring for him need to be patient and willing to listen. They should not appear critical of the patient or offer him specific advice but must try to make him feel that he is ill and that help is available. The patient is more likely to be able to accept help if he feels that he still has his self-respect.

Cause of alcoholism. There is no one cause of alcoholism, but alcoholics have been classified empirically into three groups: those whose alcoholism is a symptom of mental disease, those for whom alcohol is a physiologic poison, and those who develop from social drinkers. Persons in the latter group may appear well adjusted until some trouble arises to cause excessive drinking, or they may drift slowly and unknowingly into alcoholism. The alcoholic is likely to be basically insecure and to face realities with difficulty. Alcohol may become a means of escaping the demands of life. The person who is becoming an alcoholic tends to be untruthful about his drinking and to defend himself by rationalizations and pretenses. Alcoholism, like mental illness, is in no way related to social or economic class. It is equally common among the rich and the poor, the intelligent and the mentally limited, the successful and the unsuccessful. Usually alcoholism develops slowly, over a

period of 10 to 15 years, until the person reaches a point where he "drinks to live and lives to drink." At this point he tends to be irritable and unreasonable. He may lack judgment and develop physical as well as mental ailments.

Effects of alcohol. Alcohol contains calories but no vitamins, proteins, or minerals. It is absorbed rapidly from the stomach wall into the bloodstream. However, there is a limited rate at which body cells can use alcohol as food. Any taken in excess of the limit remains in the bloodstream, where it acts as a depressant and an anesthetic, which in turn slows down cellular metabolism. The anesthetic action of alcohol can have serious consequences. The margin of safety for the person anesthetized by alcohol is very small.[25] Unless stimulants are given, alcohol is removed from the stomach, and attention is paid to respiratory function, death may occur. Suctioning, oxygen, and constant nursing attention and observation may be needed.

The true alcoholic is more interested in alcohol than he is in food. The person who drinks a great deal may get as much as a third of his daily intake of calories from alcohol, and the alcoholic may get more calories from alcohol than from any other source. When he obtains the alcohol he wishes, he may become too intoxicated to eat or he may have no appetite for normal food. Alcohol is also the most common cause of acute gastritis that results in severe vomiting, which contributes to poor nutrition. Malnutrition may, therefore, contribute greatly to the alcoholic's physical and mental decline. The alcoholic may be in a general state of poor health with vitamin deficiency, anemia, liver changes, and debility. His resistance to infectious disease is low, and contact with infection is likely during severe bouts of drinking. Consequently, he is often admitted to the hospital with infectious disease such as pneumonia or tuberculosis. Many alcoholics have neurologic symptoms (polyneuropathy) that may include severe pain in the legs and arms and burning of the soles of the feet. Foot drop and wrist drop may develop, and walking and use of the hands may be seriously limited or made impossible. Many alcoholics develop pellagra with its characteristic skin changes of redness, dryness, scaling, and edema. Both pellagra and polyneuropathy are due to vitamin deficiency and are treated with massive doses of vitamin B complex. Weakening of the heart muscle and resultant heart enlargement ("beer heart") is believed to be caused largely by vitamin deficiency. Symptoms of acute heart failure may bring the patient to the hospital. Cirrhosis of the liver occurs often in persons who are alcoholic, and it is believed that the cause is primarily malnutrition—a lack of protein and perhaps other food constituents that are not contained in alcohol.

Chronic alcoholics often exhibit personality

changes and general deterioration of thinking processes. They may be emotionally unstable, suspicious, quick to take offense, and unpredictable in social and related situations. Serious impairment of memory may occur. Severe tremor, visual hallucinations, and loss of memory may develop even if nutrition has been adequate.[25]

Delirium tremens, an acute alcoholic psychosis, can occur when the confirmed alcoholic is denied a regular supply of alcohol, or it may develop when the patient is taking alcohol regularly. It may follow injury, infectious disease, anesthesia, or surgery and may develop in the patient who has not revealed his alcoholic status to his doctor. Delirium tremens is a serious mental illness and may cause the death of the patient. Signs of acute alcoholic psychosis include severe uncontrollable shaking and hallucinations. The patient often says that he sees insects on the wall and that rats or mice are on his bed and sometimes that they are biting him. He becomes extremely restless and apprehensive and perspires freely; sometimes true panic occurs. The treatment consists of tranquilizing drugs such as chlordiazepoxide, sedatives such as paraldehyde given rectally, intramuscularly, or orally, and a high-caloric and high-vitamin diet that may sometimes have to be given by nasogastric tube. The patient must be protected from physical injury and observed carefully for signs of cardiac failure. ACTH and cortisone may be given. Recovery usually takes from 1 to 2 weeks.

Treatment. It is only when the patient truly desires and seeks help with his alcohol problem that treatment is useful. The nurse frequently is the person present at the time the patient is most ready for help —when he has "reached the bottom" and is suffering from the embarrassment and discomfort of a physical misfortune brought on by his drinking. It may be at this time that he is a little more ready to face reality than he has been for some time in his recent past. Nurses' attitudes toward the patient and their knowledge of facilities for treatment of alcoholism may be crucial in the life of the patient and for his family.

The objective of all treatment is to induce the patient to stop drinking alcohol. When the alcoholic does stop drinking, he can *never take one single drink* on any occasion without serious danger of relapsing. He is never considered cured, and abstinence is his only course. Sedatives and tranquilizers may be administered until he recovers from the nervous agitation and insomnia caused by the withdrawal of alcohol. Vitamins and a diet high in calories, proteins, and carbohydrates may be prescribed to improve nutrition and to help overcome weakness and fatigue. Psychotherapy may be helpful to the patient in overcoming the desire to drink.

Because alcoholism is a major health concern, nurses need to be aware of community efforts and resources for its treatment. Most facilities do not require a physician's referral; the patient simply presents himself. If the nurse encounters an alcoholic person in the community who is seeking help, he should be directed to sources of help. If the patient is hospitalized, the nurse would, of course, work through the physician in charge and often through the social worker. Alcoholics Anonymous (AA) is a group of self-acknowledged alcoholics whose aim is to stay sober and to help other alcoholics gain sobriety. There are AA groups in most communities, and usually regular meetings are held. These groups are open to anyone who has a problem with alcohol, and there are no charges involved. Local groups are listed in the telephone directory for each community. A phone call at any hour of the day or night will bring an AA member to see any alcoholic desiring help. Some communities have subgroups of AA that also hold regular meetings. They include Al-Anon for relatives and friends of alcoholics and Al-Ateen for children of alcoholics. Many communities have alcoholic clinics where medical and psychiatric help are available, and many industries now have medical and rehabilitation programs for alcoholics. Information on alcoholism and programs for alcoholics and others are available for interested individuals and groups.*

Drug abuse and narcotic addiction

In recent years drug abuse has risen sharply. There are no reliable statistics on drug abusers and experts disagree as to what actually constitutes drug abuse. Some would include repeated use of any drug, while others limit it to those drugs that, used repeatedly, lead to habituation or addiction.[43]

Drug traffic has particularly increased among teenagers and young adults, and drugs are readily available on most high school and college campuses. The use of marijuana is widespread. There is much controversy as to whether or not it is addicting. Many experts say that it is not. The real danger is that users often go on to LSD (lysergic acid diethylamide) or other hallucinogenic drugs such as peyote or mescaline. There have been many reports of actual psychotic episodes following the use of these drugs. It must be remembered that the person using drugs may have an underlying personality problem that is aggravated by the drug, not necessarily caused by it. Drugs commonly taken in an attempt to "get high" include barbiturates and sedatives, amphetamines, synthetic analgesics, and cough syrups.

---

*National Council on Alcoholism, 2 Park Ave., New York, N. Y. 10016; North American Association of Alcoholism Programs, 1130 17th St. S. W., Washington, D. C. 20036; Alcoholics Anonymous World Service, Inc., Box 459, Grand Central Station, New York, N. Y. 10017; Al-Anon Family Group Headquarters, Box 182, Madison Square Station, New York, N. Y. 10010.

While there is no general agreement on a definition for drug addiction, the World Health Organization has suggested the following:

Drug addiction is a state of periodic or chronic intoxication produced by the repeated consumption of a drug (natural or synthetic). Its characteristics include an overpowering desire or need (compulsion) to continue taking the drug or to obtain it by any means; a tendency to increase the dose; a psychological and gradually a physical dependence on the effects of the drug; and a detrimental effect on the individual and on society.*

Heroin, an opium derivative that quickly produces addiction, is the drug used most often by American addicts today. There is uncertainty as to the extent of the narcotic problem because many narcotic users are not known. In New York City alone it is believed there are over 25,000 heroin addicts. Federal agents estimate that heroin addiction in persons below age 25 years rose by 40% from 1968 to 1969 in the United States.[31] There are many reported cases of children age 14 years and under who admit to heroin addiction.

The use of drugs is not limited to any socioeconomic group. The problem has long existed in the ghetto, and today it has spread to the affluent suburbs and homes of middle-class Americans. Increased social pressures, stresses of puberty and the search for self, frustration, and even boredom can lead adolescents to try drugs as they seek something to ease the pain of growing up.

One of the obstacles to early detection and treatment of addiction is the reluctance of parents to admit that their son or daughter is a drug user. Even members of the health professions "overlook" the often obvious symptoms of drug addiction or, having confronted the user, fail to report their findings to the parents or authorities. The incidence of drug addiction is high also among doctors and nurses, probably because the drugs are more available to them than to other groups of people. Occasionally a patient who must be given narcotics to control pain over a long period of time becomes an addict. It is rare, however, that addiction develops in those given narcotics for real pain, and the nurse should not let fear of the development of addiction keep her from administering prescribed narcotics to patients hospitalized and in severe pain.

Symptoms. Early indications of drug use vary with the individual but frequently include (1) abrupt changes in behavior, mood swings; (2) loss of interest in school, sports, dates, other activities; (3) frequent talking and reading about drugs; and (4) loss of appetite, increased thirst, and constipation. When the drug is actually present in the body, the user may seem drowsy or inebriated and be unconcerned about painful stimuli; the pupils of his eyes may be constricted to pinpoints.

After the individual has developed a tolerance, he may appear quite normal, converse easily, and be able to work. Constipation and appetite loss persist and he may look undernourished. If the person has been "mainlining" (injecting the drug directly into the vein), needle marks, scars, or small scabs can be seen on the hands and forearms or the instep. Addicts often wear long sleeves to hide such marks.

When the addict goes without the drug for a period longer than he can tolerate, he displays *withdrawal symptoms.* These include (1) restlessness, twitching, excessive yawning, sweating, and running eyes and nose; (2) severe abdominal cramps, diarrhea, and vomiting; and (3) dilation of pupils. Complete withdrawal of the drug without the substitution of another drug is called "cold turkey" and is a very uncomfortable physical and psychologic condition that may last up to 3 days.

Because of the expense involved, users often sell their belongings or steal to get the money to buy a "fix." Many addicts spend over $100.00 a day to maintain their habit. The disappearance of such items as transistor radios, watches, jewelry, and other similar objects from the home should arouse the suspicion of parents and friends.

Treatment. In the United States the addiction to narcotics has been considered a crime ever since the passage of the Harrison Narcotic Act in 1914. The general feeling of the Council on Mental Health of the American Medical Association is that narcotic addiction should be considered and treated as an illness. The present methods of treating narcotic addicts are not satisfactory, and the incidence of relapse is high.

One approach to the treatment of narcotic addiction is the methadone maintenance program. Methadone is a synthetic drug, and the average narcotic user's daily dose is inexpensive. The drug is given legally as a part of a rehabilitation program that includes group and/or individual therapy. The drug reduces the severity of the heroin withdrawal and the user can often maintain employment while undergoing treatment. Methadone itself is addictive and must be tapered off or the user may continue the habit the rest of his life. Because this drug is easily available through legal channels and permits the person to work, methadone advocates feel its use is essentially the same as that of the diabetic taking insulin or that of persons on maintenance doses of other drugs such as steroids or digitalis. There is a newer drug, acetylmethadol, which may prove to be superior to methadone.

One of the most effective means of treatment to evolve recently is the use of residential communities, usually run by ex-addicts, with or without profes-

*From Expert Committee on Addiction-Producing Drugs: Seventh report, Technical report series no. 116, Geneva, 1957, World Health Organization.

sionals. Synanon is such a community. It was found-ed in California in 1958 and there are now several chapters across the country. In New York there are the Phoenix and Horizon Houses. Marathon House serves the Rhode Island–Massachusetts area. In Chicago the program is available under the name of Gateway Houses. Such services are usually listed in local telephone directories and the organizations often have literature for distribution and will provide speakers for groups.* The treatment in such communities consists of helping the person through the withdrawal state, and then attempting to help him to increase his self-understanding and to change his life pattern. Therapy is provided by the group. Rules of the community are strict and breaking them results in severe consequences. The programs range in length from 18 to 36 months. Many addicts stay in the community after they no longer use the drug and help to rehabilitate other addicts. This provides support and a good number of former users can "stay clean." Of those who leave the community, there are many who return to drug use.

*Additional information on drugs and drug abuse can be obtained from the National Institute of Mental Health, Box 1080, Washington, D. C. 20013.

There are two federal narcotics hospitals, one in Lexington, Kentucky, and the other in Fort Worth, Texas. Most of the patients in these institutions are there by court order and have little motivation for giving up drugs. Treatment is conservative. More than 90% of these patients return to heroin use. There is much controversy as to the merits of the various programs. Financial problems are serious and there is much competition for the limited available funds.

Although patients receiving treatment for drug addiction usually are housed in special units of psychiatric facilities, the nurse on a medical or surgical unit may have patients who are drug addicts. The drug addict may develop any of the medical and surgical ailments that any other person may have. Because of their poor nutritional state, many addicts have lowered resistance to disease and infection. The use of contaminated syringes and needles often causes hepatitis. In addition, the drug addict, in an attempt to get drugs, may seek admission to a general hospital. He may complain of severe pain such as that from renal colic or back strain, since these are disorders for which narcotics often are given even before a specific diagnosis is made.

REFERENCES AND SELECTED READINGS*

1 A pot primer for parents: Time **95**:56, Feb. 23, 1970.
2 American Cancer Society: 1970 cancer facts and figures, New York, 1969, American Cancer Society, Inc.
3 Anonymous: End of the line and the nurse and the alcoholic patient, Am. J. Nurs. **62**:72-75, Dec. 1962.
4 *Ayd, F. J., Jr.: The chemical assault on mental illness, the major tranquilizers, Am. J. Nurs. **65**:70-78, April 1965; The minor tranquilizers, Am. J. Nurs. **65**:89-94, May 1965; The antidepressants, Am. J. Nurs. **65**:78-84, June 1965.
5 Beck, A. T.: The diagnosis and management of depression, Philadelphia, 1973, University of Pennsylvania Press.
6 *Bowles, C.: Children of alcoholic parents, Am. J. Nurs. **68**:1062-1064, May 1968.
7 *Brooks, B. R.: Aggression, Am. J. Nurs. **67**:2519-2522, Dec. 1967.
8 *Burd, S. F., and Marshall, M. A.: Some clinical approaches to psychiatric nursing, New York, 1963, Macmillan Publishing Co., Inc.
9 *Byrne, M.: Resocialization of the chronic alcoholic, Am. J. Nurs. **68**:99-100, Jan. 1968.
10 Christoffers, C. A.: An existential encounter, Perspect. Psychiatr. Care **5**(4):174-181, 1967.
11 *Clarke, A. R., editor: Conference on hostility in the nurse-patient interaction, Perspect. Psychiatr. Care **7**(4):150-187, 1969.
12 Committee on Alcoholism and Addiction and Council on Mental Health, American Medical Association: Dependence on barbiturates and other sedative drugs, J.A.M.A. **193**:673-677, Aug. 1965.
13 Council on Mental Health, American Medical Association: Narcotics and medical practice, J.A.M.A. **185**:976-982, Sept. 1963.
14 *Current research on sleep and dreams, U. S. Department of Health, Education and Welfare, Public Health Service, Bethesda, Md., 1966, National Institute of Health.
15 *Davis, A. J.: The skills of communication, Am. J. Nurs. **63**:66-70, Jan. 1963.
16 Dixson, B. K.: Dealing with passive-aggressive behavior, Nurs. Forum **3**(3):277-285, 1969.
17 Dulcher, I. E., and Hakerem, H. M.: Mother-child interaction in psychosomatic illness, Nurs. Forum **7**(2):173-189, 1968.
18 *Eiseman, B., Lam, R. C., and Rush, B.: Surgery on the narcotic addict, Ann. Surg. **159**:748-757, May 1964.
19 *Farberow, N., and Shneidman, E. S.: The cry for help, New York, 1961, McGraw-Hill Book Co.
20 *Field, W. E., Jr.: When a patient hallucinates, Am. J. Nurs. **63**:80-82, Feb. 1963.
21 *Fowler, G. R.: Understanding the patient who uses alcohol to solve his problems, Nurs. Forum **4**(4):6-15, 1965.
22 *Freed, E. X.: The crucial factor in alcoholism, Am. J. Nurs. **68**:2614-2616, Dec. 1968.
23 *Gelber, I., and others: Drug addiction—a series of articles, Am. J. Nurs. **63**:53-71, July 1963.
24 *Gerdes, L.: The confused or delirious patient, Am. J. Nurs. **68**:1228-1233, June 1968.
25 Harrison, T. R., and others, editors: Principles of internal medicine, ed. 6, New York, 1970, McGraw-Hill Book Co.
26 Industrial Service Department of National Council on Alcoholism: Prevalence of alcoholism among employees, New York, March 19, 1968, National Council on Alcoholism.
27 Johnson, M. W.: Nurses speak out on alcoholism, Nurs. Forum **4**(4):16-22, 1965.

*References preceded by an asterisk are particularly well suited for student reading.

28 *Jourard, S. M.: Living and dying, suicide: the invitation to die, Am. J. Nurs. **70:**273-275, Feb. 1970.

29 *Kalkman, M. E.: Recognizing emotional problems, Am. J. Nurs. **68:**536-539, March 1968.

30 Kaufman, R., and Levy, S. B.: Overdose treatment, J.A.M.A. **227:**411-413, Jan. 1974.

31 *Kids and heroin: the adolescent epidemic, Time **95:**16-25, March 16, 1970.

32 Klimenko, A.: Multifamily therapy in the rehabilitation of drug addicts, Perspect. Psychiatr. Nurs. **6**(5):220-223, 1968.

33 *Kline, N., and Davis, J. M.: Psychotropic drugs, Am. J. Nurs. **73:**54-62, Jan. 1973.

34 *Long, B.: Sleep, Am. J. Nurs. **69:**1896-1899, Sept. 1969.

35 Ludwig, A. M., and Levine, J.: Patterns of hallucinogenic drug abuse, J.A.M.A. **191:**92-96, Jan. 1965.

36 Manfreda, M. L.: Psychiatric nursing, ed. 9, Philadelphia, 1973, F. A. Davis Co.

37 Mann, M.: New primer on alcoholism, ed. 9, New York, 1968, Holt, Rinehart & Winston, Inc.

38 *Matheney, R. V., and Topalis, M.: Psychiatric nursing, ed. 6, St. Louis, 1974, The C. V. Mosby Co.

39 *McCown, P. P., and Wurm, E.: Orienting the disoriented, Am. J. Nurs. **65:**118-119, April 1965.

40 Mereness, D., and Taylor, C.: Essentials of psychiatric nursing, ed. 9, St. Louis, 1974, The C. V. Mosby Co.

41 *Mertz, H.: How the nurse helps the patient in his experience with psychiatric care, Perspect. Psychiatr. Nurs. **6:**260-263, 1968.

42 *Mueller, J. F.: Treatment for the alcoholic-cursing or nursing, Am. J. Nurs. **74:**245-247, Feb. 1974.

43 *Muhlenkamp, A. F.: Personality characteristics of drug addicts, Perspect. Psychiatr. Nurs. **6:**213-219, 1968.

44 *Nelson, K.: The nurse in a methadone maintenance program, Am. J. Nurs. **73:**870-874, May 1973.

45 *Newson, B., and Oden, G.: Nursing intervention in panic, emergency intervention by the nurse, No. 1, New York, 1962, American Nurses' Association.

46 *Neylan, M. P.: The depressed patient, Am. J. Nurs. **61:**77-78, July 1961.

47 *Neylan, M. P.: Anxiety, Am. J. Nurs. **62:**110-111, May 1962.

48 *Nowlis, H. H.: Why students use drugs, Am. J. Nurs. **68:**1680-1685, Aug. 1968.

49 Parley, K.: Supporting the patient on LSD day, Am. J. Nurs. **64:**80-82, Feb. 1964.

50 *Parry, A. A., McNatt, J., and Sahler, S.: Alcoholism and caring for the alcoholic, Am. J. Nurs. **65:**111-116, March 1965.

51 *Price, G. M.: Alcoholism—a family, community and nursing problem, Am. J. Nurs. **67:**1022-1025, May 1967.

52 Roberts, S. L.: Territoriality: space and the schizophrenic patient, Perspect. Psychiatr. Nurs. **7**(1):29-33, 1969.

53 Scarpitti, F. R., and others: Public health nurses in a community care program for the mentally ill, Am. J. Nurs. **65:**89-95, June 1965.

54 Shneidman, E. S.: Preventing suicide, Am. J. Nurs. **65:**111-116, May 1965.

55 Tallent, N., Kennedy, G. F., Jr. and Hurley, W. T.: A program for suicidal patients, Am. J. Nurs. **66:**2014-2016, Sept. 1966.

56 *Thomas, B. J.: Clues to patients' behavior, Am. J. Nurs. **63:**100-102, July 1963.

57 Ujhely, G.: The nurse and her problem patients, New York, 1963, Springer Publishing Co., Inc.

58 *Ujhely, G.: Nursing intervention with the acutely ill psychiatric patient, Nurs. Forum **3**(3):311-325, 1969.

59 *Umscheid, Sister Theophane: With suicidal patients caring for is caring about, Am. J. Nurs. **67:**1230-1232, June 1967.

60 *Vaillot, Sister Madeleine Clemence: Living and dying, hope: the restoration of being, Am. J. Nurs. **70:**268, 270-273, Feb. 1970.

61 *Wilner, D. M., and Kassebaum, G. G., editors: Narcotics, New York, 1965, McGraw-Hill Book Co.

62 World almanac and book of facts, 1973 edition, New York, 1974, Newspaper Enterprise Association, Inc.

8 The patient in pain

Theories of pain transmission
Physiologic responses to pain
Management of the patient in pain

■ Pain is a two-edged sword. On the one hand, it warns us to move away from heat, cold, and sharp objects before injury occurs and makes us aware of the presence of disease and tissue damage; thus it usually influences us to seek medical attention. On the other hand, fear of pain may cause us to delay medical treatment, and if its cause cannot be located and relieved, its presence serves no useful purpose and it becomes harmful. Continuous, severe pain eventually causes physical and mental exhaustion and prevents the individual from functioning productively. Pain accompanies almost all illnesses, and perhaps no sensation is more dreaded by patients undergoing medical treatment or surgery.

Pain has never been satisfactorily defined or understood. It is an unpleasant feeling, entirely subjective, which only the person experiencing it can describe. It can be evoked by a multiplicity of stimuli (chemical, thermal, electrical, mechanical), but the reaction to it cannot be measured objectively. Pain is a learned experience that is influenced by the entire life situation of each person. What is perceived as pain and the reaction to that pain differ among people and sometimes differ in the same person from one time to another.

Care of patients suffering pain demands skill in both the science and the art of nursing. The nurse's responsibility is to make the patient as comfortable as possible physically and emotionally and to observe and report findings so that they may help the physician make a correct diagnosis and prescribe appropriate treatment.

■ THEORIES OF PAIN TRANSMISSION

There are three theories of pain transmission: the specificity theory, the pattern theory, and the gate control theory. None of these provides all the answers to explain pain transmission, but many recent experiments in pain therapy have been based on the gate control theory.

The *specificity theory* holds that there are certain specific nerve receptors that respond to noxious stimuli and that these noxious stimuli are always interpreted as pain. In addition, this theory states that pain impulses are carried by pain fibers, fast, myelinated A-delta fibers, and more slowly conducting unmyelinated C fibers to the lateral spinothalamic tract in the spinal cord to a pain center in the thalamus. Impulses are then sent to the cerebral cortex via the corticothalamic tract, where the actual perception of pain takes place (Fig. 8-1). Opponents of this theory point out that specific pain receptors have not been identified, nor does the body always interpret certain stimuli as noxious.[29]

The *pattern theory* suggests that pain is produced by intense stimulation of nonspecific fiber receptors. In other words, any stimulus could be perceived as painful if the stimulation were intense enough. This model does not explain, for example, the functioning of the spinal cord in pain transmission and thus does not explain the pain relief provided by many neurosurgical therapies.

In 1965 Melzack and Wall[29] proposed the *gate control theory*. This theory proposes that pain and its perception depend on the interaction of three systems: the substantia gelantinosa in the spinal cord, which modulates impulses entering the spinal cord; a central control trigger, which influences the impulses reaching the brain; and the neural system associated with the perception of pain. This theory

■ STUDY QUESTIONS

1 Review your notes on the nervous system. How are impulses carried to and from the brain? What are the anatomic terms used to describe nerve pathways?

2 Consult your notes on fundamentals of nursing and review the descriptive terms commonly used to describe various kinds of pain.

3 Review the analgesic drugs. What are the main classifications? Review the therapeutic benefit and potential hazard of each.

4 Study a patient in pain on your ward. Describe his physical and emotional reaction to pain. What are the physical causes of the patient's pain? Do any other factors seem to be involved?

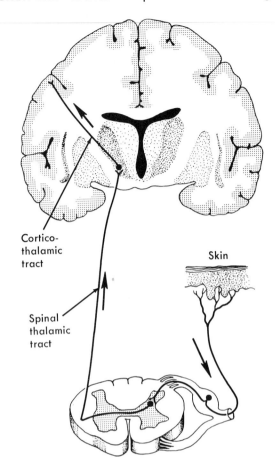

FIG. 8-1. Pathways of pain transmission according to the specificity theory.

holds that at the lower level, nerve impulses from large fibers initially activate transmission in the spinal cord, but later the effect is reduced by a negative feedback mechanism, thus "closing the gate." Small-fiber transmission, however, stimulates a positive feedback mechanism in the spinal cord, "opening the gate." According to this theory, the input of impulses to the brain is thus mediated by the substantia gelantinosa, which in turn is influenced by the number and frequency of nerves stimulated and the balance of activity between large and small fibers.

Not all scientists accept the gate control theory, but it is, at present, the best explanation for the success associated with acupuncture and other more experimental forms of pain relief (p. 170).

■ PHYSIOLOGIC RESPONSES TO PAIN

The simplest response to painful stimuli is the *withdrawal reflex,* in which impulses are conducted over the shortest nerve pathways from the place of injury to the spinal cord, where they synapse and travel back to local muscles as motor impulses. This reflex occurs when one accidentally touches a finger to a

hot object and immediately withdraws the hand. *Visceral responses,* involving the vital organs and the glands of internal secretion, prepare one for "fight or flight." These responses account for the increased pulse and respiratory rates, dilated pupils, and muscle tension that often occur in sudden severe pain. The body is prepared for the possible need to flee from the cause of pain. Because the blood supply is suddenly withdrawn from the viscera, nausea may also occur.

The sensation of pain

Cutaneous or surface injuries usually are more painful than injuries of deeper tissues, since the skin is richly supplied with sensory nerve endings. In surface injuries the intensity of the pain is usually proportional to the extent of injured tissue, but this is not always so, as is exemplified by the severe pain caused by herpes zoster (shingles).

Pain receptors in the visceral organs are fewer in number than those on surface areas and they respond only to marked changes in pressure and chemical irritants. It is also believed that in diseased visceral organs, pain results from traction, pressure, and tension on the parietal peritoneum or on mesenteric attachments. The impulses from pain receptors in the visceral organs are conducted to the spinal cord primarily by sympathetic fibers. The cerebrum frequently misinterprets the source of pain as coming from skin surface areas innervated by sensory fibers, which enter the same segment of the cord as the fibers from the deep structure actually involved. This is the phenomenon of "referred pain." Pain transmitted in this way is usually not well localized, and in diseases affecting the viscera, other symptoms often precede pain. The appearance of pain in visceral disease may indicate far-advanced disease and extensive tissue damage.

The pain caused by a tension or pressure on the viscera may be described as aching, dragging, or boring. Muscle contractions may cause sensations described as cramping or spasm. Muscles that have peristaltic action frequently cause the pain to be stabbing. A sudden, sharp, popping sensation is characteristic of rupture of a visceral organ.

Deep pain does not produce a body defense reaction (visceral response) similar to that which occurs when surface pain is experienced. Severe visceral pain, therefore, can cause shock. The patient becomes weak and prostrate. Blood pressure may drop, the skin may become cold and clammy, and nausea and vomiting may occur. Cardiac and kidney damage can follow, and if the vital organs are already impaired by disease, even death may result.

Perception of pain

The perception of pain or the actual feeling of pain takes place in the cerebral cortex. It is known that a functioning frontal lobe of the brain is required to experience the full suffering and worry that result from pain. The reaction to the same stimuli differs widely among people and in the same person from one time to another because the final perception of pain depends more on the interpretation in the cerebral cortex than on the characteristics of the original stimuli. What the cerebral cortex interprets as pain will depend on childhood training, previous experience, cultural values, religious beliefs, physical and mental health, knowledge and understanding, attention and distraction, fatigue, anxiety, tension, fear, state of consciousness, and the frequency and the intensity of pain impulses.

Atrophy of nerve endings, degenerative changes in the pain-bearing pathways, and decreased alertness may reduce the perception of pain in the elderly, and more stimulation may be required to evoke a response. Elderly persons, therefore, may fail to perceive tissue damage that normally would cause pain and thus alert a younger person.

The perception of a pain stimulus may be altered at many points by both normal and abnormal conditions. A pleasant environment, an enjoyable book, stimulating conversation, or other distracting activity of a pleasing nature may serve to lessen the sensation of pain. Tissue damage or inflammatory conditions at the site where the stimuli originate may increase or decrease the impulse. For example, slapping a person who has a sunburn may set off a far greater impulse than if the person were not sunburned. On the other hand, if the local nerve endings have been damaged by a severe burn, the patient may not respond at all to what would ordinarily be painful stimuli. Abnormal conditions within the spinal cord such as inflammatory diseases, tumors, or injuries may prevent transmission of nerve impulses. This may occur at either the spinal or the thalamic relay stations. The impulse may also be altered at either of these two relay stations by other activity going on simultaneously within the spinal cord. This probably accounts for the fact that sometimes bruises and cuts sustained during absorbing activities go unnoticed until the activity is over. Perception in the cortex may be influenced by abnormal conditions such as inflammatory processes, degenerative changes, and depression of brain function, which may alter the original signal pattern. Anesthesia and analgesia also cause depression of sensory perceptions.

Pain threshold. The point at which a person first feels pain is called the pain threshold. It varies from person to person and may not be constant in the same individual from one time to the next because experience and physical and mental health also enter into its determination. Some authorities believe that the pain threshold and the threshold for tissue damage are the same. The sensation of pain

often appears only a short time before actual damage to the tissue occurs.

The pain threshold or tolerance for pain may be raised by alcohol, drugs, hypnosis, warmth, rubbing, or distracting activities. Strong beliefs and faith seem to increase tolerance for pain, and it is sometimes difficult to judge how much pain a patient with deep faith is actually experiencing. Fatigue, anger, boredom, and apprehension may decrease one's ability to tolerate pain. The pain threshold also is lowered by persistent pain such as that which is sometimes experienced by patients with far-advanced carcinoma. A weak, debilitated patient usually tolerates pain less well than a stronger one, although increasing debility will eventually cause mental dulling, with a resultant decrease in pain perception.

Reaction to pain

Perception of pain is accompanied by reaction to pain. Reaction to pain is influenced also by such factors as past experience, conditioning, cultural values, and physical and mental health. Consequently, people will respond differently to the same stimuli. Some may accept the pain and be patient and resigned; others may become depressed and withdrawn. Some may be fearful, apprehensive, and anxious, while others are tolerant and optimistic. Some weep, moan, scream, beg for relief or help, threaten to destroy themselves, thrash about in bed, or move about aimlessly when they are in severe pain. Others lie quietly in bed and may only close their eyes, grit their teeth, bite their lips, clench their hand, or perspire profusely when experiencing pain.

Some people, by training and example, are taught to endure severe pain without reacting outwardly. American Indian men have rites in which they show their strength by the amount of pain they can endure. Such individuals probably would tolerate pain from disease or injury better than those from a culture in which free expression of feelings is encouraged. Persons from cultures in which health teaching and disease prevention are emphasized tend to accept pain as a warning to seek help and expect the cause of pain will be found and cured.

Parents' attitudes toward pain may determine their children's lifelong reaction to pain. In the American culture, parents usually begin to teach their children what is expected of them in regard to courage and self-control at about the age of 2 or 3 years. They try not to appear too concerned about minor injuries and usually encourage their children not to cry when they are hurt. Children try very hard to be brave, especially in the presence of other children. Boys particularly are expected not to cry when hurt, and girls who cry too easily are ridiculed.

The setting in which injury occurs may influence the external response to pain. Boys may feel, for example, that pain suffered from injury during a football game should be borne quietly, whereas pain resulting from an automobile accident may be expressed freely.

Influence of fear. Morbid fear of a disease may intensify pain caused by it, or it may lead the individual to deny pain in his eagerness to believe that nothing is wrong. Anticipation of pain based on past experience often intensifies pain. For example, the child who enters the hospital for the last of several operations may react more vigorously to postoperative pain than he did on his first encounter with the sensation.

One's personality also influences reaction to pain. A person who reacts hysterically to trying situations may find even a small amount of pain intolerable. People may sometimes use moderate pain as an escape from unacceptable life situations, or they may try to use it to control situations around them. This latter reaction is often demonstrated both in the hospital and in the home.

There is more reaction to pain in the night and early morning hours when the person's physiologic processes are at low ebb and there is little distracting activity. The patient's thoughts may easily turn to concern for himself and his loved ones, and his worrying may increase his reaction to pain.

Age affects the reaction to pain. The young fear it because it may represent an unfamiliar experience and frequently respond to it by crying. The older person may know what to expect and accept it, or he may be withdrawn and quiet while experiencing it because of emotional exhaustion.

■ MANAGEMENT OF THE PATIENT IN PAIN

Assessment

Patience, tolerance, gentleness, technical skill, and keen powers of observation are needed in giving care to the patient in pain. The nurse and the physician are the two professional team members to whom the patient turns when pain is one of his major problems. Every report of pain should be responded to, and the patient should be observed carefully. Making judgments about the real cause of pain or ignoring the patient's and family's observations about the pain can result in emergency situations. In observing a patient in pain the nurse should assess the pain and the patient suffering from pain carefully. It is important that the nurse listen to the patient's interpretation of the pain he has. It is he alone who is experiencing the pain, and only he knows where it is located and how intense it is. His statements should be considered carefully and should not be minimized. In assessing pain the nurse should determine the exact location, type, when it occurred and duration, circumstances preceding it, whether this is the first occurrence, if it is constant

or intermittent, and if it is relieved or increased by medication, food, rest, change in position, or other activity such as application of heat or cold.

Close observation of the patient often gives clues to the intensity of his pain. Pinched facies, drawn and wrinkled brows, clenched teeth, and tightened fists may indicate severe pain. Diaphoresis and a rapid pulse also are valuable clues. The patient who lies very still, who is curled up in bed, or who tosses about is often in pain or at least uncomfortable.

Observing the behavior of the young child who cannot yet talk is the only way to determine whether he has pain and where it is located. The child who tugs at his ear, doubles his body over and clasps his abdomen, or refuses to move a certain area of his body or permit it to be touched may be having pain in the area. Irritability and continuous crying that is unrelieved by the usual comfort measures may mean that the child is in pain. Parents may be asked about activities they have observed that appear to cause discomfort. When signs of pain are apparent, a close examination of the child's body should be made to rule out an injury or other obvious causes of his distress.

The nurse must be able to assess the patient's pain and his emotional response to it without being judgmental about his reaction to pain. How the patient perceives and reacts to pain has been influenced by his whole life, and he cannot voluntarily modify this response very much. Regardless of the cause of pain or his behavior, his immediate need is for relief from pain. Knowing how the patient feels about pain helps the nurse initiate measures to make him more comfortable.

Relief of pain

After the nurse has assessed the patient's pain, nursing intervention is planned. If the pain is the usual type experienced by the patient, the previous methods of relief are indicated. If the pain is different or does not respond to nursing intervention, the physician should be notified.

Even though the nurse can determine no physical cause for the pain, it is important to remember that the patient *feels* the pain regardless of its cause. Recognition of this fact should guide the nurse in care of the patient and thus prevent labeling patients and their families as complainers. The patient whose pain is largely based on emotional reactions needs as much interest and support from the nurse as the one whose pain is largely caused by a physical ailment. At no time should the patient in pain feel that the nursing staff is lacking in sympathy and understanding of his problem, or that the time and effort spent in attempting to alleviate his pain are not worthwhile.

Every member of the nursing team who gives any kind of care to the patient in severe pain should have access to the patient's nursing care plan. The plan should indicate why the patient is in pain, what aggravates it, how he responds to it, and the nursing measures that have been found effective in alleviating or reducing the pain. In addition, the plan should indicate how the patient responds to certain visitors, to his spiritual adviser, to food, and to other patients.

Nursing intervention

Raising the pain threshold. Anything that helps the patient relax raises his pain threshold. Reducing physical tension, unpleasant environmental stimuli, and emotional demands helps people relax. Activities that are pleasantly diversional to them also are relaxing.

Alleviating the family's concern. It is understandable that the family will be upset when the patient is in pain. Not only may he appear uncomfortable, but he may not respond in his usual manner to those about him or relate appropriately emotionally and socially with people because his psychic energy is absorbed by the pain. Prompt attention to the patient's needs helps reduce the family's concern, and the patient's behavior should be interpreted as necessary to his family and friends with simple, clear explanations. Regardless of explanations, persons who are emotionally close to the patient may need extra time to accept his behavior, and they may need repeated explanations. However, reassurance of family members is an essential part of the patient's care because they communicate their concern to him. This tends to make the patient increasingly tense, which in turn lowers his pain threshold. Helping the family understand the patient's behavior often reduces their demands on the patient to try to relate as usual to them and may make the patient feel less guilty when he cannot respond acceptably.

Alleviating apprehension. The patient in pain is often afraid. Fear may be allayed in part by the nurse's calm, quiet manner and particularly by her demonstration of competence. Confidence in the persons who care for him is a tremendous help to the patient. It is a great comfort to the patient to know, for example, that the nurse will not hurry while giving nursing care and increase his pain or be so "busy" that his pain medication is not given at the prescribed intervals.

Sometimes preparation for pain helps to increase acceptance of it and in turn produces relaxation, which will decrease pain. An example is the benefit derived from special preparation for childbirth. Fear and irritability can sometimes be allayed by explaining to the patient why he has pain. This knowledge may let him relax somewhat and thereby lessen his discomfort. If he can be honestly told that the pain is probably of short duration, this should be done. Postoperative pain is often aggravated by movement. Therefore, when certain activities such as

turning and coughing are necessary to prevent complications, the nurse should explain this to the patient. The nurse may be able to comfort a child who is frightened by his pain by holding him, rocking him, or talking to him. Older patients also may be comforted by having someone sit quietly with them, and some patients benefit from the personal contact of holding another's hand.

Reducing emotional demands. Overtalkativeness and overoptimism are often annoying to the patient who has pain. This is particularly true when the patient knows or suspects that his prognosis is poor. Florence Nightingale gave the following advice on this subject:

But the long chronic case, who knows too well himself, and who has been told by his physician that he will never enter active life again, who feels that every month he has to give up something he could do the month before—oh! spare such sufferers your chattering hopes. You do not know how you worry and weary them. Such real sufferers cannot bear to talk of themselves, still less to hope for what they cannot at all expect.*

Every effort should be made to place the patient with pain in a quiet location and reduce activity about him to a minimum. Plans should be made for a minimum number of persons to enter the room of the patient in severe pain. The patient cannot possibly learn to know and trust all the individuals who pop in and out of the average hospital room in the average hospital day. Unless some effort is made to control traffic in and out of his room, the patient may be unable to relax and rest. The same principle applies to care of the patient in his own home, where the problem of visitors is frequently a real one. The nurse, of all members of the health team, is in the best position to give attention to this real need of the patient. Some patients in pain welcome interruptions and distractions, whereas others prefer privacy and seclusion. The nurse should see that the patient's wishes are respected.

Reducing noise. Noise is troublesome to the patient in pain. Even the usual sounds accompanying normal living activities may become almost unbearable to the patient, and sudden unexpected sounds may be quite upsetting. The patient who, after continued effort, has been able to fall asleep often is very irritated when awakened by noise. The irritation and the fact that he has not slept long enough to relax often make it difficult for him to fall asleep again.[30]

Providing spiritual assistance. If no estimate can be made as to the duration of pain, the patient should be given encouragement that the problem will not become too great for him to accept with the assistance that is available. Many patients who have pro-

---

*From Nightingale, Florence: Notes on nursing: what it is, and what it is not, London, 1859, Harrison. (Reprinted by J. B. Lippincott Co., Philadelphia, 1957.)

longed pain with no hope of relief can and do derive benefit from religious faith. This may help them to consider pain in a more positive way and thus make it more endurable for them. The nurse should help to make the appropriate religious adviser's service available to the patient who desires it.

Reducing painful stimuli. Care and treatment should be planned so that the patient in pain is moved about as little as possible and that rest periods between necessary activity are not interrupted. With careful planning it is usually possible to give an analgesic medication and allow time for it to take effect before procedures are performed and to have sufficient help available so that such procedures as the removal of wound packing, an enema, a bed bath, and a change of bed linen can be done in definite sequence. It is distressing to the patient in pain to be moved, bathed, and have his bed linen changed only to find that an enema must be given or that he must be moved for a radiograph to be taken. The nurse cannot control all activity around the patient but can help a great deal by thoughtful planning with him.

With skill and adequate help, the nurse usually can move the patient without causing too much pain. Proper technique when handling the patient with generalized pain or a painful limb or part of the body is important. Support to painful parts of the body is essential. Supporting the trunk and limbs in good body alignment will prevent increasing the pain by unnatural pulling on muscles, joints, and ligaments. A "turning sheet" is often useful in preventing uneven lifting or pull on patients with severe neck, back, or general trunk pain. Painful joints may be moved with less discomfort if they are placed on a pillow or otherwise supported rather than being lifted directly (Fig. 33-1). If there is tenderness or pain in the shaft of the bone, in muscles, or in large skin areas, the limb should be supported at the joints when the patient moves to prevent additional pain.

Binders, surgical belts, and girdles give support to the abdomen. Body casts, corsets, and braces are used to immobilize the vertebral column and thus decrease pain. A firm bed gives support and thereby lessens pain both when the patient is at rest and when he is moving. Traction, splints, casts, and braces are used to immobilize a painful part of the body such as an ankle. Special beds (such as the Stryker frame, Foster bed, CircOlectric bed, and Bradford frame) allow movement with minimal handling of the body and thereby help lessen pain. If the nurse in caring for a patient in pain feels that any of these mechanical devices would benefit him, the problem can be discussed with the physician.

Counterirritation. For some patients a change in the type of stimulation at the site of pain may result in pain relief. For example, lightly rubbing the affected area may cause significant pain reduction. The gate control theory would support changing the amount and type of sensory receptor stimulation, and the nurse with the help of the patient may be able to find a satisfactory and relatively simple stimulus modification to ease the patient's discomfort. Some commonly used counterirritants are discussed later in the chapter.

Psychologic modification of pain. Recent work with patients in pain has also been focused on the perception of pain. In certain settings, hypnosis has met with some success for some patients in reducing pain perception. Other experimenters have tried forms of distraction, suggestion, or operant conditioning with varied success. In some of the operant conditioning trials the patient is connected to an electroencephalogram. When the patient increases his alpha brain wave activity, usually associated with a pain-free state of relaxation, a light is turned on. The patient "trains" himself to turn on the light more frequently and regularly and thus reduces his pain. This mechanism is known as biofeedback.

Medication for pain. The nurse needs to know the precise effect on the body of drugs used in the treatment of pain. The time curve of their beginning effect, the height of their effectiveness, and their declining effect must be understood. In addition, the nurse must also be aware of the possibility that the effects of the drug may vary according to the time of day they are administered and the physiologic status of the individual.

Narcotics. The opiates are drugs most widely recognized and used for the control of pain. Morphine and codeine are usually ordered. Synthetic narcotic drugs such as meperidine hydrochloride (Demerol) and methadone hydrochloride are also widely used. When given in therapeutic doses, narcotics act by depressing brain cells involved in pain perception without seriously impairing other sensory perceptions. They also affect to some extent the patient's feeling about pain and thus affect both physical pain and the reaction to it. In addition, the synthetic narcotic drugs have some antispasmodic action and thereby encourage relaxation.

The effects of narcotics vary with the physiologic state of the patient. The very young and the very old are quite sensitive to the effects of narcotics and require smaller doses to obtain relief from pain. A person of any age may be more depressed physically and emotionally by narcotics during the early morning hours (1 to 6 A.M.) than at any other time of the day and therefore should be watched carefully for untoward effects.

Narcotics cause lowering of the blood pressure and general depression of vital functions. This reaction can be an advantage in treating a condition such as hemorrhage, in which some lowering of blood pressure may be desirable. It may be a disadvantage in treating the debilitated patient, who may go into shock from an excessive dosage of a drug. The narcotic drugs are less likely to cause shock if the patient is up and moving about and taking food and fluids, since these activities tend to maintain the blood pressure at a safe level.

Ataractic drugs. Ataractic drugs, or so-called tranquilizers, which affect the mood of the patient, have been found helpful in the treatment of pain, particularly when given in combination with narcotics. This combination of drugs tends to separate the perception of pain from the reaction to pain. The sensation of pain appears less acute and therefore the reaction to it becomes less severe. When fear and apprehension appear to be the most striking features of the patient's reaction, the tranquilizers alone may be sufficient to help him relax. Prochlorperazine (Compazine) and chlordiazepoxide hydrochloride (Librium) are examples of commonly used tranquilizers. If these drugs cause lethargy and failure of normal response, this reaction should be reported to the physician at once. The physiologic state of the person may cause a variance in response to these drugs similar to that seen with narcotics.

Analgesic drugs. One of the most widely used analgesic drugs is acetylsalicylic acid (aspirin). This is the safest of the coal-tar products; it usually relieves headache, muscle ache, and arthritic pain. The specific action of aspirin on pain is not known, but it does not cause clouding of the sensorium. Aspirin is highly effective when given with codeine, the combined effect being much superior to the use of either drug alone. The nurse needs to be constantly aware that some persons are allergic to aspirin. Death can occur when aspirin is given to such individuals. Other common side effects of acetylsalicylic acid are irritation of the gastric mucosa, ulceration of the gastric mucosa, and reactivation of peptic ulcers. "Salicylism" can occur in persons who take large doses of aspirin over long periods of time. Nausea, vomiting, ringing in the ears, deafness, and severe headache are common manifestations. A decreased prothrombin level with hemorrhagic manifestations can also occur. Hemorrhage is uncommon when the dose is less than 1 Gm./day.[2] Other coal-tar analgesics such as phenacetin and acetanilid may produce toxic effects after prolonged use. They should be used only under the direction of a physician despite the fact that they can be purchased without medical prescription.

Another analgesic widely used is propoxyphene (Darvon). It is said to be as potent as codeine, but some trials have indicated that it has little more than a placebo effect. Propoxyphene is considered nonaddictive, but dependence may occur after repeated use of high dosages. Side effects include dizziness, headache, gastrointestinal disturbances, and rashes. The effectiveness of the drug may be enhanced by use of combination preparations containing propoxyphene.

A commonly used synthetic, nonnarcotic analgesic is pentazocine (Talwin). It is being used to re-place morphine and meperidine for the relief of moderate to severe pain. It is given orally and parenterally. The most commonly occurring reactions are vertigo, nausea, and euphoria. Since sedation and dizziness have been noted in some instances, ambulatory patients receiving pentazocine should be warned not to operate machinery, drive cars, or unnecessarily expose themselves to hazards. Pentazocine is contraindicated in persons with increased intracranial pressure, head injury, or pathologic brain conditions in which clouding of the sensorium is particularly undesirable.

Sedatives. Sometimes the patient needs a sedative drug instead of additional analgesics. This type of drug may permit him to become drowsy and relaxed enough for the analgesic to be effective. Phenobarbital, for example, often enables the patient to be comfortable with less narcotic drug than might otherwise be necessary. The patient with a severe emotional reaction to his illness will often get relief when analgesic drugs are interspersed with sedative drugs. This arrangement has been found useful when the narcotic or other analgesic drug does not seem to quite "hold" the patient for the desired interval. Small doses of phenobarbital appear to relieve most of the discomfort experienced by infants and small children when they have pain. The effect of sedative drugs, similar to narcotics, may be increased by the slowing down of physiologic response. In the presence of fever they sometimes produce excitement rather than relaxation. This effect may occur in older patients as well. Because barbiturates may make the patient less aware of his surroundings, side rails and constant nursing supervision may be necessary to protect him from injuries such as falls.

Drugs to relieve the cause of pain. Pain may be treated by drugs that help to relieve the cause of pain. For example, the belladonna group of drugs (atropine) or synthetic substitutes such as propantheline (Pro-Banthine), which cause relaxation of smooth muscle, may diminish the pain caused by spasm of the smooth muscles. If pain is due to impairment of circulation, drugs that dilate the blood vessels such as papaverine, nitroglycerin, and tolazoline (Priscoline) may do more good than analgesic drugs.

Local application of drugs. Ointments, emollients, and liniments such as ethyl aminobenzoate and methyl salicylate (oil of wintergreen) are counterirritants that may be applied locally to alleviate pain. Oil of clove, used for toothaches, is another example.

Placebos.* Placebos are sometimes used for their psychogenic effect in relieving pain, but they should

---

*For more information on placebos see Jourard, S. M.: The transparent self, ed. 2, New York, 1971, D. Van Nostrand Co.

never be given without a physician's order. Although the most usual response to a placebo is positive, some persons have negative reactions and may report intensified pain or other symptoms. Therefore, when a placebo is being used, the nurse should observe the patient carefully and share with the physician any information that will help determine the best treatment for the patient. Favorable response to a placebo should not lead the nurse to ignore complaints of pain, for the individual who responds to placebos is in great need of the nurse's interest and support. Furthermore, the patient may have a new physical pain that needs to be evaluated.

Treatment

Local. Local applications of heat and cold are examples of counterirritants that often bring relief of pain. Hot sitz baths or a heating pad applied to the abdomen may relieve pain such as that caused by menstrual cramps. Hot gargles may relieve the pain of a sore throat, and an ice cap may be more effective than medication in relief of a headache. If pain in the abdomen is due to gaseous distention, removal of flatus by means of gastric and intestinal drainage, carminative enemas, or a rectal tube often gives more relief than the administration of analgesic drugs. In fact, drugs that cause slowing of peristalsis such as Meperidine may indirectly increase gas pain by allowing larger quantities to collect in the bowel. Pain caused by an overdistended bladder is relieved by catheterization.

Neurosurgical. Constant, relentless pain that cannot be controlled by analgesics (*intractable pain*) may be reduced or abolished by surgery. Interrupting sensory routes just before they enter the spinal canal (rhizotomy) relieves severe pain in the upper trunk. Severing the sensory nerve pathways within the spinal canal (spinothalamic cordotomy) relieves constant pain below the level of the lesion.

For selected patients in whom other methods of pain relief have proved unsuccessful, the creation of a lesion in the midbrain or thalamus may be indicated. These lesions are frequently made by carefully placing long, needlelike electrodes in the desired area and electrically destroying a minute area of brain tissue. Obviously the cause of the pain is not eliminated, but the perception of the pain is altered. These procedures require a skillful neurosurgeon and are not used indiscriminately.

Surgical destruction of the white matter of the frontal lobe or the cingulum can also modify a patient's response to pain, although the actual pain threshold is not changed. These surgeries may have complications, particularly changes in the personality of the patient. Although the assistance of a psychiatrist is helpful in managing all patients with chronic pain, it is highly recommended for any surgery that may change the patient's personality.

Finally, some recent work on pain has been focused on changing the sensory input to the brain rather than reducing it. One type of sensory input modification is provided by *dorsal column stimulators* that can be surgically implanted in the spinal column through laminectomy. Also available is a transcutaneous nerve stimulator, a battery-powered stimulator worn externally that can be controlled by the patient. Both of these stimulators attempt to modify the sensory input by blocking or changing the painful stimulation with stimulation perceived as less painful or nonpainful. The success of this therapy is explained by the gate control theory of pain transmission (p. 163).

Acupuncture. More and more attention is being focused on acupuncture for pain relief. Small acupuncture needles are skillfully inserted and manipulated at specific body points, depending on the type and location of pain, producing often immediate and continued relief of pain. The gate control theory provides the best explanation for the success of acupuncture; the local stimulation of large-diameter fibers by the needles "closes the gate" to pain. It is not known how much part the psyche and the power of suggestion play in this therapy.

Nursing application of medical treatment for pain

Nursing measures to lessen pain or to remove its cause should be considered before medications and treatments for pain are given. Medical treatment, however, should not be withheld when nursing measures alone are ineffectual.

Before giving medication for pain, the nurse should find out whether the patient is really in pain and in need of medication or whether his real need is for company, information, counsel, or acceptance. He also may need a treatment such as hot applications, gastric intubation, or catheterization more than medication. Knowing the patient as an individual as well as understanding what disease condition he has and what treatment he has received, will help the nurse to give the appropriate medications or to seek new orders if they are needed.

So much emphasis has been placed on the danger of drug addiction (and to be sure, the danger is very real) that nurses sometimes withhold narcotic drugs and allow patients to suffer more than is advisable. The patient in severe pain will not become addicted to narcotic drugs if they are given at frequent intervals for several days. Provided there are no physical contraindications, narcotics, when prescribed by the physician, should be given to the patient with intractable pain as often as every 3 or 4 hours regardless of the possibility of addiction. However, before giving any patient an analgesic drug, the nurse should always determine whether the patient's pain is the same as that for which the drug was ordered. If it should be a "new" pain, analgesics may mask symptoms of disease that is undiagnosed.

Providing for independence, physical needs, and decision making

Decision making. Sometimes if the patient helps to make decisions regarding his care, he tolerates pain better. The nurse needs good judgment, however, in deciding when to encourage the patient to make decisions. The patient may feel less helpless by making some decisions, or he may be too uncomfortable to want to be bothered. Pain may alter rational judgment so that the patient may not be able to make sensible decisions. If the nurse knows the patient's usual needs and anticipates necessary action, his care can proceed without burdening him with decisions. However, if he desires, such matters as whether the bed should be changed before or after the nap or whether friends should be encouraged to visit can be decided by the patient. The patient may try to delay necessary moving and treatments. The nurse should know just how long moving should be delayed in the interest of comfort, rest, and benefit to the patient and how much damage will be done to the skin, the circulation, and other vital functions by not moving the patient or by not having him move enough.

Nutrition. Appetite is affected by pain. When one is in continuous pain, nothing, including meals, seems quite right. Care should be taken that foods the patient likes are prepared in a way that he likes. His appetite may be improved by small, attractive servings and by a sincere interest in his reactions to food. Foods that the patient does not like or that he believes disagree with him should not be offered to him. Very gratifying improvement in appetite has followed the control of intractable pain by surgical procedures that interrupt sensory pathways that transmit the painful sensation.

Mental outlook. When caring for the patient who is experiencing severe, continuous, or intractable pain, the nurse must keep in mind the possibility of suicide. Pain is wearing and demoralizing, especially when it is difficult to control with drugs and when the patient knows or suspects that no permanent relief will be forthcoming. The patient may dread the danger of a growing dependence on drugs, he may fear that drugs will no longer help, and he may be depressed by thoughts of being a burden and an expense to his family. He may appear to tolerate pain quite well but at the same time may be planning his own destruction. Plans for protection should be individually made for each patient and will depend on such factors as whether or not he is confined to bed. (For further discussion on patients who contemplate suicide see p. 154.)

REFERENCES AND SELECTED READINGS*

1 Bellville, J. W., and others: Influence of age on pain relief from analgesics, J.A.M.A. **217:**1835-1841, Sept. 1971.

2 Bergersen, B. S.: Pharmacology in nursing, ed. 12, St. Louis, 1973, The C. V. Mosby Co.

3 *Billars, K. S.: You have pain? I think this will help, Am. J. Nurs. **70:**2143-2145, Oct. 1970.

4 Blaylock, J.: The psychological and cultural influences on the reaction to pain: a review of the literature, Nurs. Forum **7**(3):262-274, 1968.

5 Botton, J. E.: Neurosurgical procedures for the management of intractable pain, Clin. Orthop. **73:**101-108, Nov.-Dec. 1970.

6 Breckenridge, M. E., and Vincent, E. L.: Child development, ed. 5, Philadelphia, 1965, W. B. Saunders Co.

7 Brobeck, J. R.: Best and Taylor's physiological basis of medical practice, ed. 9, Baltimore, 1973, The Williams & Wilkins Co.

8 Casey, K. L.: The neurophysiologic basis of pain, Postgrad. Med. **53:**58-63, May 1973.

9 *Cashatt, B.: Pain: a patient's view, Am. J. Nurs. **72:**281, Feb. 1972.

10 Chambers, W. G., and Price, G. G.: Influence of nurse upon effects of analgesics administered, Nurs. Res. **16:**228-233, Summer 1967.

11 *Copp, L. A.: The spectrum of suffering, Am. J. Nurs. **74:** 491-495, March 1974.

12 Davis, L., editor: Christopher's textbook of surgery, ed. 10, Philadelphia, 1972, W. B. Saunders Co.

13 Davitz, L. J., and others: Nurses' inferences of suffering, Nurs. Res. **18:**100-107, March-April 1969.

14 *Drakontides, A. B.: Drugs to treat pain, Am. J. Nurs. **74:** 508-513, March 1974.

15 *Gaumer, W. R.: Electrical stimulation in chronic pain, Am. J. Nurs. **74:**504-505, March 1974.

16 *Goloskov, J., and LeRoy, P.: Use of the dorsal column stimulator, Am. J. Nurs. **74:**506-507, March 1974.

17 *Hanken, A. F.: Pain and systems analysis, Nurs. Res. **15:** 139-143, Spring 1966.

18 *Jourard, S. M.: The transparent self, ed. 2, New York, 1971, D. Van Nostrand Co.

19 Lewis, C. S.: The problem of pain, New York, 1962, Macmillan Publishing Co., Inc.

20 *MacBryde, C. M., editor: Signs and symptoms, ed. 5, Philadelphia, 1970, J. B. Lippincott Co.

21 *Mastrovito, R. C.: Psychogenic pain, Am. J. Nurs. **74:** 514-519, March 1974.

22 McBride, M. A. B.: "Pain" and effective nursing practice, Clinical Sessions ANA (1966), New York, 1966, Appleton-Century-Crofts, pp. 72-82.

23 McBride, M. A. B.: Nursing approach, pain, and relief: an exploratory experiment, Nurs. Res. **16:**337-341, Fall 1967.

24 *McBride, M. A. B.: The additive to the analgesic, Am. J. Nurs. **69:**974-976, May, 1969.

25 McCaffery, M.: Nursing management of the patient with pain, Philadelphia, 1972, J. B. Lippincott Co.

*References preceded by an asterisk are particularly well suited for student reading.

26 McCaffery, M.: Brief episodes of pain in children. In Anderson, E. H., and others, editors: Current concepts in clinical nursing, vol. 4, St. Louis, 1973, The C. V. Mosby Co.

27 *McCaffery, M., and Moss, F.: Nursing intervention for bodily pain, Am. J. Nurs. **67**:1224-1227, June 1967.

28 *McLachlan, E.: Recognizing pain, Am. J. Nurs. **74**:496-497, March 1974.

29 *Melzack, R., and Wall, P. D.: Pain mechanisms: a new theory, Science **150**:971-979, Nov. 1965.

30 Minckley, B. B.: A study of noise and its relationship to patient discomfort in the recovery room, Nurs. Res. **17**: 247-250, May-June 1968.

31 Modell, W.: Relief of symptoms, ed. 2, St. Louis, 1961, The C. V. Mosby Co.

32 Moss, F. T., and Meyer, B.: The effects of nursing interaction upon pain relief in patients, Nurs. Res. **15**:303-306, Fall 1966.

33 *Nightingale, Florence: Notes on nursing: what it is, and what it is not, London, 1859, Harrison. Reprinted by J. B. Lippincott Co., Philadelphia, 1957.

34 *Programmed Instruction: Pain: basic concepts and assessment. I. Am. J. Nurs. **66**:1085-1108, May 1966.

35 *Programmed Instruction: Pain: rationale for intervention, Am. J. Nurs. **66**:1345-1368, June 1966.

36 *Siegele, D. S.: The gate control theory, Am. J. Nurs. **74**: 498-502, March 1974.

37 Walike, B. C., and Meyer, B.: Relation between placebo reactivity and selected personality factors, Nurs. Res. **15**:119-123, Spring 1966.

38 Wang, R. I. H.: Control of pain, Am. J. Med. Sci. **112**:590-609, Nov. 1963.

39 *Zborowski, M.: People in pain, San Francisco, 1969, Jossey-Bass Inc., Publishers.

9 The incontinent patient

Urinary continence
Urinary incontinence
Fecal continence
Fecal incontinence
Uncontrolled urinary and fecal incontinence

■ Incontinence, or involuntary expulsion of feces or urine, is probably one of the most distressing experiences patients can have. Many patients will find incontinence of any amount or frequency intolerable. The associations of thought and past experiences with excreta are very likely to be that excretory products are dirty and that incontinence is childlike and its occurrence is disgraceful. Recollection of childhood mishaps in learning control of elimination may be distressing and may cause an exaggerated reaction in adulthood. Acceptance of loss of control of excretory function will also depend a good deal on the patient's regular habits of personal hygiene. If he is a very fastidious person, his distress usually will be greater. Most people demonstrate uneasiness both physically and emotionally when bladder and/or bowel control is lost even when they are very ill, and even if loss of control happens only once or very occasionally.

Urinary and fecal incontinence accompany many kinds of illness. In giving nursing care, be it in a hospital, a skilled nursing care facility, a nursing home, or in the patient's own home, the nurse will fre-quently be confronted with the problem of incontinence. Some persons who have a long-standing problem of incontinence but are otherwise in relatively good health manage well and can continue working and carrying on a normal life. For others, it may be a relatively new or poorly managed problem. The nurse who has an understanding of normal bowel and bladder physiology and the causes of incontinence will be aided in determining whether functional rehabilitation of the bladder and bowel is possible, or if attempts should be made to make the patient as comfortable and safe as possible, calling on ingenuity in improvising equipment and in using the commercial appliances available.

Patients with incontinence present baffling problems, and to solve them the nurse needs to know the physiologic causes of incontinence.

Incontinence, which may be urinary, fecal, or both, may result from surgery performed to drain the urine or feces temporarily or permanently through an opening that cannot always be controlled. Examples of such surgical procedures are nephrostomy, ureterostomy, ileal conduit, cystostomy, ileostomy, cecostomy, and colostomy. Each of these procedures will be discussed in the chapter dealing with the diseases for which it is performed. Ureterostomy is not performed as frequently as it once was, but the nurse may still encounter patients who have had the procedure. Other causes of incontinence may be (1) disorders involving the central nerve pathways, re-

■ STUDY QUESTIONS

1 Review the anatomy of the bladder, urethra, and lower bowel.
2 Review the physiology of micturition and defecation.
3 What products are formed when urine undergoes decomposition? How does this decomposition affect the skin? List some chemical substances that inhibit or prevent this action.
4 What is constipation? How may it be prevented and/or treated by diet? Review the mild cathartics and laxatives. Study the indications and contraindications for each. What is the therapeutic effect of glycerin suppositories? How should they be stored? How are they administered?
5 What is fecal impaction? How may it be prevented? How is it treated?
6 What foods are omitted or specially prepared in a low-residue diet?
7 What are the common drugs ordered for diarrhea? What is the therapeutic action of each?
8 How can decubiti be prevented? If they occur, what are accepted methods of treating them?

sulting in loss of conscious control of bladder and bowel functions; (2) spinal cord damage, resulting in loss of bladder and bowel reflex mechanisms; and (3) actual tissue damage of the bowel or bladder sphincters or of surrounding supportive tissue.

■ URINARY CONTINENCE

A person must have bladder sphincter control in order to have urinary continence. Such control requires normal voluntary and involuntary muscle action coordinated by a normal urethrobladder reflex. Understanding this coordinated sequence of nerve stimuli and muscle action will help the nurse to understand how continence is maintained.

As bladder filling occurs, the pressure within the bladder gradually increases. The detrusor muscle (the three-layered bladder wall) responds by relaxing to accommodate the greater volume. When a certain point of filling is reached, usually 150 to 200 ml. of urine, the parasympathetic stretch receptors located in the bladder wall are stimulated. The stimuli are transmitted through the afferent fibers of the reflex arc to the reflex center for micturition. This reflex center is located in the S2 to S4 segments of the spinal cord. Impulses are then carried through the efferent fibers of the reflex arc to the bladder, causing reflex contraction of the detrusor muscle. The internal sphincter, which is normally closed, reciprocally opens; and urine enters the posterior urethra. Relaxation of the external sphincter and perineal muscles follows and the bladder content is released. Completion of this reflex act can be interrupted and voiding postponed through release of inhibitory impulses from the cortical center, which results in voluntary contraction of the external sphincter (Fig. 9-1). If any part of this complex function is upset, the patient is likely to be incontinent of urine.

■ URINARY INCONTINENCE
Etiology

The five main causes of urinary incontinence are cerebral clouding, infections in the urinary tract, dis-

FIG. 9-1. Normal nerve pathways involved in bladder function. (From Cordonnier, J. J.: Clinical urology for general practice, St. Louis, 1956, The C. V. Mosby Co.)

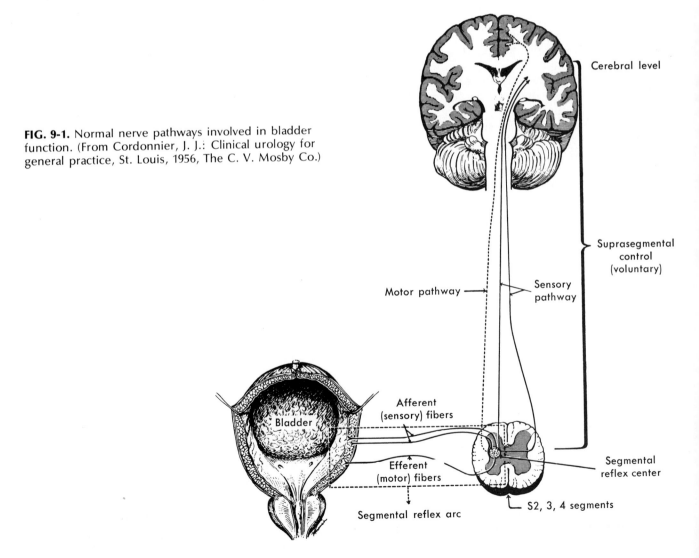

turbance of central nervous system pathways, disturbance of the urethrobladder reflex, and tissue damage resulting from local anatomic and physiologic changes due to age, disease, or trauma. The five major causes of urinary incontinence and the nature of the incontinence they cause are outlined in Table 9-1.

Cerebral clouding. Cerebral clouding is most common in the aged. In many instances the very elderly patient is incontinent of both urine and feces because of a lack of awareness of the need to empty the bladder or bowel. This type of incontinence is often not associated with any definite pathology such as a cerebrovascular lesion. Cerebral clouding also occurs in the acutely ill patient, who may be so ill and so toxic that cerebration is dulled. He may not be able to think, or he may not have the energy to excercise voluntary control. Likewise, a patient who is comatose is incontinent because he has lost the ability to control voluntarily the opening of the external sphincter. As soon as urine is released into the posterior urethra, the bladder contracts and empties. For this reason, patients sometimes void under anesthesia.

Infection. Infection anywhere in the urinary tract may lead to incontinence since bacteria in the urine cause irritation of the mucosa of the bladder and stimulate the urethrobladder reflex abnormally. This condition is quite common in elderly women who have relaxed perineal structures and subsequently poor emptying of the bladder.

Disturbance of the central nervous system pathways. Disease such as cerebral embolus, cerebral hemorrhage, brain tumor, meningitis, or traumatic injury of the brain may prevent adequate voluntary (cortical or cerebral) control of bladder function. Urgency incontinence may be present as a result of an inability to inhibit completion of the urethrobladder reflex by the higher centers.

Disturbance of the urethrobladder reflex. Lesions of the spinal cord or damage to peripheral nerves of the bladder result in disturbance of the urethrobladder reflex and cause incontinence. This form of incontinence may be seen in patients with cord injuries, cord tumors, tabes dorsalis, and compression of the cord from fractures of the vertebrae, herniated disc, metastatic tumor in a vertebra, or postoperative edema of the spinal cord. This type of difficulty can

Table 9-1 Causes of urinary incontinence and factors involved in each

| Cause of urinary incontinence | Factors involved | | | | |
	Awareness of need to void	Cortical ability to inhibit voiding	Reflex arc	Bladder response to filling	Result
Cerebral clouding	Impaired	Impaired	Intact	Normal	Uncontrolled voiding due to reflex response
Infection	Intact	Intact, but overcome by strong reflex response	Abnormally stimulated	Heightened	Voiding due to strong reflex response (urgency)
Disturbance of CNS pathways (cortical lesions)	Diminished	Impaired	Intact	Heightened	Voiding due to reflex response
Disturbance of urethro-bladder reflex					
Upper motor neuron lesion	Destroyed	Destroyed	Intact but deranged	Heightened	Voiding due to reflex response
Lower motor neuron lesion	Destroyed	Destroyed	Destroyed or impaired	Diminished to absent	Distension or incomplete emptying
Tissue damage	Intact	Intact, but not functional due to poor muscle response	Intact	Normal	Loss of control of voiding due to muscular impairment

result in two types of responses known as "neurogenic bladder." The patient with a neurogenic bladder has no way of knowing when he is going to void.

Lesions above the S2 level of the spinal cord or impairment of the cerebrocortical centers do not destroy the reflex arc for voiding, although they may derange it. Such lesions do destroy the potential for cortical control to inhibit the reflex. The result is an "upper motor neuron" or "automatic" bladder. The bladder is hypertonic and has a small capacity (less than 150 ml.). The increased detrusor tone and increased sensitivity to small amounts of urine present in the bladder result in precipitous voiding and the potential for vesicoureteral reflux.

Damage to nerves in the cauda equina or sacral segments of the spinal cord may cause destruction of the reflex arc by interruption of its afferent, efferent, or central components. The result is a "lower motor neuron" or "flaccid" bladder. The bladder is hypotonic with capacities of 500 ml. or more. Overflow incontinence, retention of residual urine, and the potential for vesicoureteral reflux are problems imposed by a hypotonic bladder.

Overflow incontinence is considered to be caused by pressure exerted on the distended bladder by the abdominal muscles. Residual urine, urine remaining in the bladder after incomplete emptying, provides a medium for the growth of bacteria and can be the focus for overwhelming infection. Vesicoureteral reflux is the backflow of urine into the ureters caused by pressure within the bladder.

Tissue damage. Damage to the sphincters of the bladder from instrumentation, surgery, or accidents, scarring following urethral infections, lesions involving the sphincters, or relaxation of the perineal structures may cause urinary incontinence. The latter cause of incontinence is seen occasionally following childbirth. The problem is local in nature and does not involve the nervous system.

Nursing assessment

Until the cause of a patient's urinary incontinence is understood the question of whether functional rehabilitation of the bladder is possible or not cannot be answered. The nurse plays an important role in the assessment of such a patient. This includes records that are as accurate as possible concerning the patient's intake and output, the amount and frequency of his voiding, any symptoms of urgency, indications of his lack of awareness of the need to void, and the appearance of his urine. The nurse may be called on by the physician to assist with tests that will further define the problem such as obtaining midstream or catheterized urine samples for culture to delineate the presence of infection; catheterizing the patient to determine the presence and amount of residual urine; and preparing the patient for and/or helping to perform cystoscopy,

cystometrics, or other tests to demonstrate the status of the patient's bladder, its capacity, and its response to filling.[20]

In the assessment the nurse must also include data concerning the patient's general condition, his ability to follow directions, and certainly any other factors that predispose to or directly cause urinary incontinence.

After all available data concerning the patient's incontinence have been collected and a reasonable cause for his incontinence determined, a program of retraining or management may be attempted.

If the patient's incontinence has been a long-standing problem well managed by him or his family, it would be unwise for the nurse to attempt to change the method of management. In these instances, particularly in a hospital or other institutional setting, the nurse should ascertain the method used by the patient and provide whatever assistance or equipment is needed for its implementation during the patient's stay in the institution.

The nurse should also remember that no program of bladder control or retraining can be accomplished without the patient's cooperation. He needs to be informed of the probable outcomes of such a program and included in the planning for implementing the program. Consequently, the patient's emotional readiness to undertake such a program must also be assessed.

MANAGEMENT OF THE PATIENT WITH URINARY INCONTINENCE

Control of urinary incontinence is largely dependent on the cause of the incontinence. If the cause is cerebral clouding due to acute illness or toxicity or imposed conditions such as anesthesia, the incontinence will clear with effective treatment of the acute illness or removal of the imposed condition. If the cause is urinary tract infection, the incontinence should clear with effective treatment of the infection. When the cause of incontinence is a disturbance of the central nervous system pathways or the urethrobladder reflex, either a program of bladder retraining or the use of internal or external drainage devices is indicated. In instances where the cause is tissue damage, repair of the tissues and retraining of muscles may be effective in reestablishing continence.

Urinary incontinence caused by cerebral clouding. When urinary incontinence is due to dulled cerebration in the elderly, the confused, the acutely ill, or the comatose patient, control can usually be established if a persistent *retraining program* is carried out. A voiding schedule is set up and strictly adhered to until gradually the patient again learns to recognize and react appropriately to the feeling of having to void. A successful program of this type, leading to complete rehabilitation, or *continence,* requires a mentally competent patient. Otherwise someone else must always remind the patient to follow the schedule.

In *toilet training* children, one takes them to the toilet at regular intervals to void. This same plan can be employed with an incontinent adult. People ordinarily void on awakening, before retiring, and before or after meals. If a diuretic such as coffee has been taken, it is usually necessary to void about half an hour later. Using this knowledge, the nurse can begin to set up a schedule for placing the patient on a bedpan or taking him to the toilet. Then, if a record is kept for a few days of the times that the patient voids involuntarily, it is usually possible to determine the individual's normal voiding pattern. If the schedule based on the pattern of incontinence is not successful, toileting every 1 to 2 hours should be carried out on a 24-hour basis.

When it is possible, toileting should be carried out in surroundings that will remind the patient of the voiding function; that is, the patient should be taken to a bathroom where he can use a toilet. If this is not realistic, a bedside commode can be an adequate substitute. Many male patients can void into a urinal more easily if allowed to stand at the bedside. The use of a bedpan is unfamiliar and distasteful to most patients, but in instances where female patients must remain in bed, voiding into a bedpan can be facilitated if the patient's head is rolled up as high as allowed. This kind of positioning is more consistent with the position normally assumed for voiding and facilitates complete emptying of the bladder. Few patients can void adequately in the supine position.

Providing adequate amounts of fluids, a minimum of 3,000 ml./day, is necessary to ensure that there will be adequate amounts of urine produced and present in the bladder to stimulate the voiding reflex at the proper times. Fluids may be given at scheduled times, the largest portion of the 3,000 ml. being given during the day and restrictions being imposed after the evening meal. This type of scheduling may decrease the frequency of voiding through the night.

During the retraining program, mobilization of the patient, attention to the position the patient assumes for voiding, and adequate fluid intake also contribute to reduction of the possibility of infection. Complete emptying of the bladder eliminates the possibility of residual urine acting as a medium for bacterial growth, while a high-fluid intake provides for internal bladder irrigation.

Elderly patients isolated from their families and familiar surroundings, confused by institutionalization, or suffering feelings of loss of self-esteem frequently respond well to mobilization in bladder retraining programs. Their circulation is enhanced by the imposed mobility, their awareness is increased, and they respond to the attention that is given them. In instances where nurses believe that it is easier to change linen than it is to establish an appropriate bladder retraining program, a disservice is done to the patient and more work is actually created for the nurse. The patient becomes subject to skin breakdown or urinary tract infection, and his feelings of worthlessness are increased. For those who can be continent, incontinence is an indignity.

Urinary incontinence caused by infection. The physician who is treating urinary incontinence determines whether or not there is infection of the urinary system before seeking other causes. Infection may be treated systemically with antibiotics. Specific causes of infection such as obstruction must be found and corrected (p. 435). In addition to the specific treatment of the infection, there must be management of the patient's incontinence. This management is largely a nursing measure.

Again, provision must be made for a minimum intake of 3,000 ml./day. Mobilization and positioning for voiding must be attended to. Further, because of heightened bladder sensitivity to even small amounts of urine, urgency to void demands rapid response to the patient's request to void. Patients who are aware of the need to void, but who experience urgency, become quite irritable and embarrassed if their calls for assistance are not answered quickly enough to prevent incontinence.

Urinary incontinence caused by disturbances of the central nervous system pathway or urethrobladder reflex. The patient who has a brain tumor, meningitis, or traumatic injury to the brain that prevents adequate voluntary control of bladder function and causes urgency incontinence by inhibiting cortical control over the urethrobladder reflex may also respond to a bladder retraining program. However, if the patient's condition or response prohibits such a program, an internal or external drainage device may be used.

Patients with injuries of the spinal cord require an indwelling catheter during the acute stage of injury. At this time the catheter is essential in preventing urinary infection and overdistention of the bladder. The physician may order a scheduled clamping of the catheter to prevent contracture of the bladder.[20] Following removal of the catheter, the cooperation of the patient is important in working out a schedule of intake and voiding.

Patients with a lesion above the sacral segments, who have an intact urethrobladder reflex, may initiate voiding by pinching or stroking trigger areas on the thighs or suprapubic area. In a hypotonic bladder the use of the Credé method, which consists of exerting manual pressure over the bladder, will not only help to initiate voiding, but will also provide for more complete emptying. Sometimes special positions such as the patient leaning forward will help. Catheterization is usually done to determine the amount of residual urine. Fluids are spaced in such a way that the bladder is filled and ready to be emptied at designated times. The schedule can be planned for the convenience of the patient and adapted to his living pattern. For instance, if he wishes to go out, the patient will limit fluids for several hours. Most patients limit fluids in the evening so that the bladder will be less likely to empty during the night. However, they should plan to force fluids to 3,000 ml. within the 24-hour period. This measure is necessary because neurogenic bladders seldom empty completely, and infection and stone formation may occur. Since alcohol, the caffeine in tea and coffee, and the theobromine in tea and cocoa tend to stimulate the kidneys and upset the voiding pattern, it is wise to avoid them.

Patients may learn to recognize a full bladder by such systemic reactions as restlessness, sweaty or chilly sensations, or great abdominal discomfort. (Restlessness may also serve as a guide to the nurse in knowing when an unconscious patient should be placed on the bedpan.)

It is important for both the patient and the nurse to know that rehabilitation of the patient with urinary incontinence may take weeks and even months to accomplish. The patient often becomes discouraged by recurring accidental voiding and needs a great deal of encouragement. It is helpful if the patient is taught the physiology of voiding so that he can better understand and help in his rehabilitation. The rehabilitation of the patient with a neurogenic bladder is a complex undertaking. For a more detailed discussion of this subject consult specialized textbooks.[12,20]

Since internal and external catheters do play an important part in the management of incontinent patients, the nurse needs to have a full understanding of what they are, how they are managed, and how they may complicate the patient's condition.

Internal catheters

An *indwelling* urethral catheter may be inserted into the bladder when there is urinary incontinence. However, there are many disadvantages to the use of a urethral catheter, especially if it remains in place for a long time. As a foreign body, it causes irritation of the urethral and bladder mucosa, which in turn predisposes the patient to urethritis and cystitis. Indwelling catheters not attached to a closed drainage system have proved to be a source of infection in the urinary tract.[6] When a urethral catheter is used, men may develop epididymitis because the ejaculatory ducts open into the prostatic urethra, and organisms easily enter at this point and proceed along the vas deferens to the epididymis. Since epididymitis is a painful and serious infection and frequently is complicated by vasoepididymal strictures

that cause sterility, it is always best, if possible, to find means other than a urethral catheter to drain the bladder of a male patient. Penile-scrotal fistulas may also occur from pressure on the urethra. Taping the catheter to the abdomen when the patient is reclining aids in relieving pressure. The nurse must check the drainage system when this is done, as it may interfere with gravity drainage.

If a catheter must be used for a prolonged period, a *cystostomy* is frequently done. A cystostomy is a small suprapubic incision into the bladder through which a catheter is inserted. Because the peritoneum is not entered, the operation is a relatively simple one. Indwelling urethral catheters are somewhat less dangerous for women because, having a shorter and straighter urethra, they are less susceptible to infection originating from traumatic catheterization. Prolonged use of a catheter in either sex may lead to the formation of bladder stones because the urine, instead of maintaining its usual acidity, becomes alkaline as a result of urinary tract infection. This alkalinity encourages inorganic materials found in the urine, especially calcium and phosphate crystals, to settle out and eventually form stones. A bladder that is drained continuously will eventually lose its muscle tone and its normal capacity. For this reason, when a urethral catheter or cystostomy tube is being used for a period of weeks to control incontinence in a patient who is expected to regain normal bladder function, it often is clamped and opened for drainage at regular intervals. Two to four hours is the usual interval. (Catheters should not be clamped in the presence of urinary tract infection.) Sometimes a *tidal drainage apparatus* such as the McKenna irrigator is used to provide automatic filling and emptying. A disadvantage of this type of apparatus is that the patient must remain in bed.

If an indwelling catheter is being used, a minimum of 3,000 ml. of fluid should be taken daily. This amount provides for internal bladder irrigation and assures that waste products are well diluted for excretion, thus lessening the chance of stone formation. A retention catheter should be changed about every 10 days, since mineral deposits collect both within its lumen and at the point where it comes in contact with the bladder and urethra. However, some of the newer specially coated catheters are designed to reduce the formation of mineral deposits. The nurse should be aware of the manufacturer's recommendations for the frequency of changing a particular catheter.

In catheterizing a patient some organisms from the urethra are always introduced into the bladder, where the mucosa, if it is already irritated, is a fertile field for bacterial growth. Therefore prophylactic doses of sulfisoxazole (Gantrisin) are usually ordered for most patients who have indwelling catheters. It is important that the catheter not be permitted to slip out accidentally. The more often a person must have a catheter inserted, the more likely he is to develop a urinary tract infection. To prevent a catheter from becoming displaced, the nurse should anchor it securely and attach the drainage tubing to the bed in such a way that the excess tubing is coiled on the mattress and does not pull on the catheter. If the patient is disoriented, he should be closely observed since he may seriously injure the bladder sphincters and urethra by pulling on the catheter. It may be necessary to obtain an order for the use of mittens that make it difficult for the patient to grasp the catheter firmly.

Care must be taken that drainage is not inadvertently interrupted. Whenever a straight drainage system is being used, one should remember that it functions on the principle of gravity, so that the drainage collection receptacle must be placed at a level lower than the cavity being drained. Tubing should run straight from the mattress to the drainage bottle, and there should be no loops in the tubing. If the patient is out of bed, a plastic leg bag can be used for urinary drainage. This eliminates the necessity of using the long drainage tubing used in bed, which is not only cumbersome but also does not allow adequate drainage when the patient is up. Leg bags are now manufactured with flutter valves to prevent backflow of urine. However, for some patients they may not provide adequate drainage in the recumbent position. In this situation the patient can be taught to change from one drainage system to the other. The connecting tube not in use must be kept sterile, and the tip of the catheter and connectors should be cleansed with benzalkonium chloride (1:750) or 70% alcohol when changing the drainage systems.[20]

The patient who will be discharged with an indwelling catheter must be taught how to care for the catheter at home. He should be supervised in carrying out the necessary techniques while in the hospital. In addition, referral to a public health nurse for supervision in the home is often necessary. Many patients and families are anxious about the details involved. A written referral is sent to the public health agency, explaining what the patient or his family can do and clarifying how much help is needed. The treatment and any nursing problems and approaches already used should be described. Both patient and family attitudes about the patient's incontinence are also described, along with an account of the patient's response to care.

It is not sufficient to give verbal instructions to the patient and his family. They must be given written directions about how to care for the catheter and the equipment being used. Sterilization techniques, complete instructions for all procedures, and equipment resources should be given to them. Suggestions for a home care routine can be found in specialized nursing texts.[20]

Because of the contraindications to the use of indwelling catheters, the resourceful nurse will usually try to control incontinence due to lack of voluntary control by other means.

External catheters

For the incontinent male patient, external drainage can be accomplished since a watertight apparatus can easily be applied to the penis. The following is a satisfactory method. Select a condom of the correct size for the patient. Puncture a hole in the closed end of the condom with an applicator stick. Attach the punctured end of the condom to a firm rubber or plastic drainage tube with either a $1/8$-inch piece of rubber tubing or a strip of adhesive tape (Fig. 9-2). Before applying the condom, clean and dry the penis thoroughly and check it for edema, skin breaks, or discoloration. Invert the condom and roll in onto the penis. There should be no roll at the top that could cause constriction. At least 1 inch of the condom should remain between the meatus and drainage tube to allow for penile erection. There should not be so much slack as to cause twisting and consequent interference with drainage. Elastoplast is then applied over the condom and around the penis (never touching the skin). Under no circumstances should adhesive tape be used. The Elastoplast must not be constricting.

External catheters are also available commercially. Many of these, however, are manufactured of a stiff material that cannot be made to conform to the patient's penis as do the catheters that the nurse can make from the softer condoms.

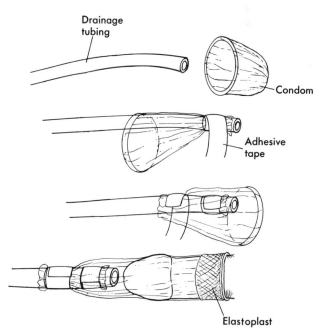

Drainage tubing

Condom

Adhesive tape

Elastoplast

FIG. 9-2. One method of making an external drainage apparatus.

The external catheter must be removed daily and the skin washed and checked. Frequent checking is necessary to determine whether edema or irritation is present and to ensure proper drainage. This is especially important in patients lacking sensation. The external device is attached to straight drainage or to a leg bag.

Since it may be embarrassing and upsetting to a man to have a young female nurse apply an external drainage apparatus, someone else may need to perform this procedure. If there is no male member of the nursing team, an older, more mature female nurse may be called on or the patient's wife, brother, or son may be taught to care for this personal need. At other times the doctor may be willing to do this, or the patient may be able to do it himself. For patients such as paraplegics who need external catheter drainage indefinitely, a rubber urinary appliance (sometimes called an incontinence urinal) may be prescribed. There are several models available, and the one best suited to the patient's need should be selected. The appliance may cause skin irritation, however, since the rubber sheath fits snugly. It is necessary for the patient to have two appliances to allow for cleaning and drying. They must be washed in mild soap, turned inside out, and thoroughly dried before application (Fig. 9-3).

To improvise protection for the incontinent male patient, a shower cap can be used. Cut a hole near the elasticized edge large enough to fit around the penis. Bind the opening with adhesive tape to prevent tearing of the cap and skin irritation. Fill the inside of the cap with absorbent material placed in a doughnut fashion. Then, slipping the penis inside, pin the edges of the cap together. If more support is needed, the cap may be pinned to a belt. This improvisation may be used if skin irritation has resulted from the use of other external devices to collect urine. It may also be used following a perineal prostatectomy when every effort is being made to have the patient void normally. Methods that give more protection may decrease his efforts to achieve continence.

Protection for women with incontinence presents an extremely difficult problem. At present the most satisfactory method is the use of perineal pads and plastic-lined pants (Fig. 9-4).

Urinary incontinence caused by tissue damage. It is practically impossible to repair a sphincter that has been cut. If only the external sphincter has been damaged, the patient will be incontinent on urgency. A voiding schedule can be set up so that he will always void before the bladder is full enough to exert sufficient pressure to open the internal sphincter involuntarily. If only the internal sphincter is damaged, the patient may have no acute feeling of the need to void. Here, the problem is not one of incontinence but of retention. To assure the regular emp-

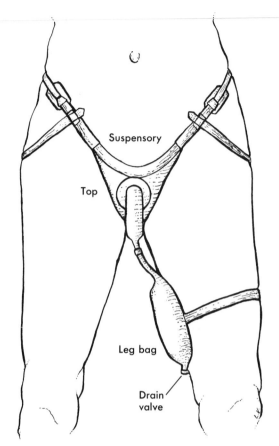

FIG. 9-3. Rubber urinary appliance. Note that it is supported by a strap around the waist and under buttock and is connected to a drainage bag strapped to the leg. The drain valve at the bottom of the bag is removed for emptying.

tying of the bladder, he, too, should use a voiding schedule. If both sphincters are damaged, the patient will be totally incontinent and will require permanent catheter drainage or the use of external protection.

Some conditions respond to treatment. For example, a levator ani muscle that is shortened by scar tissue, thus holding the bladder outlet at a downward angle and allowing a continuous dribbling or causing frequency of urination, may be treated surgically. Sometimes lesions may be surgically removed or improvements effected by plastic surgical procedures.

Incontinence due to relaxation of the sphincters and the perineum presents serious problems. In men this condition may follow prostatic surgery or prolonged use of an indwelling catheter. In women it may follow childbirth, although some women who have had no children have relaxation of the perineum. In both sexes, old age may cause relaxation of the muscles and consequent incontinence. The patient with this type of problem is taught *perineal exercises,* which consist of contracting the abdominal,

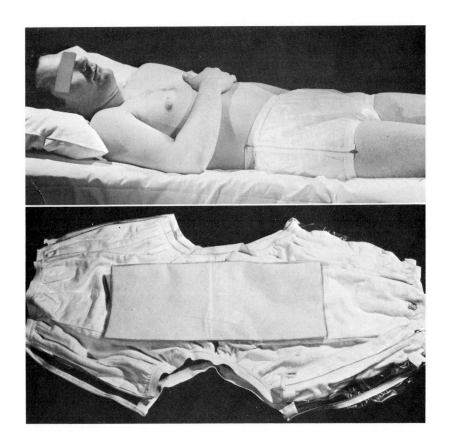

FIG. 9-4. Protective pants for the incontinent patient. The protective pads may be disposable or washable. A cotton jersey liner must be worn under the plastic pants to prevent excoriation of the skin, which must have special care. (Courtesy Ferguson Manufacturing Co., Grand Rapids, Mich.)

gluteal, and perineal muscles while breathing normally. These exercises can be explained by asking the patient to hold himself as he would if he needed to void very badly and there were no available facilities. Sometimes gluteal muscle tone can be increased by having the patient hold a pencil in the fold between the buttock and the thigh. Stopping and starting the urinary stream during voiding will give additional exercise. The patient should strive eventually to maintain a constant muscle tone. Although operations designed to tighten the muscles are sometimes attempted, the results are not always predictable. Much of the problem of incontinence due to a relaxed perineum in women can be prevented if perineal exercises are taught before and following childbirth. These exercises also may be included as part of the health teaching of any woman.

Another serious problem of incontinence occurs in women who have vesicovaginal fistulas. They may result from childbirth injuries or surgical injuries of the vagina or uterus. They also may occur after x-ray therapy for carcinoma of the cervix (p. 526).

Care of the skin of incontinent patients

Care of the skin is very important in the treatment of incontinent patients regardless of the method of management being used. Indwelling catheters cause irritation of the urethral mucosa at the point of insertion. As a result, a mucous discharge may collect around the catheter. The presence of urine on the skin may be irritating and cause a disturbing odor. External catheters of themselves are irritating to the skin and prevent air from reaching the skin to dry it.

The perineal and genital areas should be thoroughly washed several times a day. Tub baths are preferable to showers. Washing the skin with soap and water will help prevent irritation and odor. Exposure to the air is beneficial. Since the acid or alkali in the urine will penetrate any ointment, ointments are useless in protecting the skin. A zinc oxide powder such as one used for babies can be applied and may be helpful in reducing irritation. Cornstarch is often helpful in preventing itching.

Incontinence in children

If incontinence presents baffling problems in the care of adult patients, enuresis, failure of children to gain and maintain urinary control, can sometimes be even more complex for parents to understand and manage. Overcoming this problem may be delayed until the child is in school, and then parents become anxious because teachers and others constantly bring it to their attention. Nurses can be particularly helpful to parents by understanding their emotional distress and by helping them to examine the circumstances in which the problem seems to have developed.

The infant is born with an automatic bladder that

empties reflexly when filled to a certain point. When the nervous system is more fully developed, the child begins to learn voluntary control. Children between the ages of 1 and 2 years usually recognize imminence of micturition and can prevent voiding for a period of time. Day control is usually achieved more readily than night control. Children vary in the rate at which they develop voluntary urinary control just as they vary in other development but by $4\frac{1}{2}$ years of age, approximately 87.8% of all children have complete control.[10] At about 5 years of age most children have the ability to start the urinary stream at will and to stop midstream.[10]

It often is difficult to determine whether the child with enuresis has a psychologic or a purely physical problem. The nurse who is helping the parents can often establish a description of the circumstances for a pediatrician's evaluation. Review of the development of normal bladder control for infants and children may help parents to remember details of events as they occurred for their child. The nurse also should learn about the child's total growth and developmental pattern from birth, including details of bowel control. If the problem developed after urinary control had been established, the nurse should try to elicit the events in the child's family life and relationships preceding the onset of the problem. Questions regarding other children in the family and their development may also give clues.

If the problem seems to be a behavioral one, the parents can be helped to understand the problem and to work through a solution with the child. Bed-wetting may have been a problem for one or both parents, and their acceptance of this or their reaction to it may be quite different from the reaction of those persons who have not experienced it. In some instances the problem may be very complex, and the pediatrician may recommend psychiatric help for the family.

The child's problem, however, may be one of physiologic underdevelopment or actual pathology. Small bladder capacity is one of the most common causes of enuresis. The child may learn to compensate by drinking small amounts of fluid and emptying his bladder voluntarily at short intervals both in the daytime and during the night, but a training program with the objective of increasing the bladder capacity usually is more successful. A record of intake and output is kept for a few days to establish the usual pattern. The child is then encouraged to drink an increased amount of fluid during the day and to postpone voiding for as long as possible. If the child is old enough, it may be helpful to have him help keep the measurements since this participation may encourage him to try for larger capacities. The program should continue until the child has a bladder capacity of at least 250 ml. but preferably 400 ml., and this may take 3 to 6 months.

Uninhibited bladder contraction, urinary tract infection, or other pathologic conditions may cause enuresis. The pediatrician will determine if a urologic examination is necessary.

■ FECAL CONTINENCE

As with urinary incontinence, the problem of fecal incontinence may be better understood if there is first an understanding of fecal continence. Normally the contents of the bowel are moved by peristalsis to the rectum. The rectum then stores this material until defecation occurs. Defecation may occur reflexly because of distention of the rectal musculature, or it may be inhibited voluntarily. Voluntary emptying of the rectum occurs when the anal sphincter (under voluntary control) is relaxed and the abdominal and pelvic muscles contract.[4]

Fecal continence is not so subject to neurologic impairment as is urinary continence. The musculature of the bowel contains its own nerve centers within the wall of the intestine and is not greatly affected by upper or lower motor neuron lesions. Peristalsis persists or can be stimulated even when there is somatic paralysis.[4]

■ FECAL INCONTINENCE

Fecal incontinence is as disturbing as urinary incontinence. It is, however, more readily managed.

Etiology

There are several causes of fecal incontinence. The anal sphincter may be relaxed, the voluntary control of defecation may be interrupted in the central nervous system, or messages may not be transmitted to the brain because of a lesion within the cord or external pressure on the cord. The disorders causing breakdown of conscious control are identical to those affecting the bladder. Perineal relaxation and actual damage of the anal sphincter are often caused by injury during childbirth or during perineal operations. Relaxation usually increases with the general loss of muscle tone in aging. Perineal exercises similar to those used in urinary incontinence may help some patients.

Nursing assessment

The nurse is involved in assessing patients who have fecal incontinence. Records are kept concerning the patient's normal bowel habits, the frequency of his defecations, the nature of his stool, his awareness of the need to defecate, the degree of his sphincter control, and his ability to produce intra-abdominal pressure to aid in expelling the feces. His general condition is also considered, as is his willingness to be involved in a bowel control program. In establishing a bowel control program the nurse must bear in mind that feces may be expelled from the rectum by peristalsis so long as the stool is kept soft.

MANAGEMENT OF THE PATIENT WITH FECAL INCONTINENCE

If fecal incontinence is to be prevented, bowel training or a regular routine of stimulation of peristalsis and of going to the toilet should be carried out. Ordinarily the bowel is trained to empty at regular intervals. Once a day or every other day after breakfast is common. Food and fluids increase peristalsis, which may stimulate defecation. The taking of certain food or fluids may be associated with the accustomed time for defecation. For example, coffee or orange juice may provide the stimulus for some people. Most patients will be more relaxed and thus more likely to have a bowel movement if placed in as near the normal position as possible and if they have privacy. Glycerin suppositories (usually two are needed) help stimulate evacuation of the bowel; they should be inserted about 2 hours before the usual time of defecation. They should be lubricated with petrolatum and pushed well into the rectum against the mucosa with a gloved finger. If the patient is unconscious or has disease of the spinal cord, it may be necessary to use the laxative suppository bisacodyl (Dulcolax). Suppositories are most effective if given following a meal because the gastrocolic reflex will provide additional stimulus. Routine enemas and laxatives are to be avoided since they result in dependence and become less effective with prolonged use. At times, enemas may be necessary for the patient with spinal cord injury. If so, no more than 500 ml. of a nonirritant fluid such as tap water should be used. Usually 200 ml. of fluid is sufficient. Fluid is more easily retained if the patient is on his side. It may be necessary to pinch the buttocks together securely around the rectal tube to retain the fluid in the bowel. Patients may not get full results for 1 to 2 hours or longer following enemas, so they should be provided with protective padding.

Results from bisacodyl usually occur within a half hour. Care must be taken not to insert the suppository into a bolus of stool since it is then ineffective.

It is possible for patients with cord lesions to develop *automatic* defecation. Suppositories are given every day at the same time. If these patients are able to sit up, they should sit on the toilet. In addition to using suppositories, they may have to take stool softeners to keep the stool from becoming hard and causing an impaction. A diet that provides adequate bulk and a minimum of 3,000 ml. of fluids daily is a necessary part of the program. Massaging the abdomen toward the sigmoid area and digital rectal stimulation are additional measures that may be necessary to aid in evacuation. In order to have an effective bowel program it must be consistent, and

it requires cooperation and diligence on the part of the staff as well as the patient. It is necessary to keep a daily record to determine whether the program is producing the desired results. If results are obtained within an hour and impaction and incontinence do not occur, the program can be changed to every other day. When establishing a bowel program, the nurse should include the patient in planning. He can help determine whether a morning or evening program is best. His former habits and current and future activities should be considered in the planning. The general welfare of the patient is benefited so much by automatic defecation that the time and energy expended to accomplish it are well spent.

Incontinent patients may have *diarrhea,* which may be a symptom of *fecal impaction.* The physician usually makes a rectal examination, breaking up the impaction if necessary, and then an oil enema followed by a cleansing enema is given. (Fecal impaction may also cause urinary incontinence by creating pressure on the bladder. Such urinary incontinence will cease when the fecal impaction is removed.) Impaction is frequently a problem of the elderly, and the public health nurse often receives orders to loosen or break up the impaction. The nurse should use lubricating jelly or cream on a gloved finger and gently remove feces from the lower rectum only. If the leakage continues despite enemas and is liquid in consistency, a rectal tube (28 or 30 Fr.) may be inserted into the rectum and anchored in the fold under the buttock with adhesive tape and attached to straight drainage. (See p. 456 for method of anchoring tubes.) If the diarrhea is not due to an impaction, one should look for other causes. A patient may find that certain foods cause him to have diarrhea. The nurse can help him analyze his diet and avoid foods that cause trouble. Emotional stress may also cause diarrhea; so it is important that it be reduced in any way possible. Diarrhea is a rather common reaction to medications, especially antibiotics. Camphorated tincture of opium, bismuth subcarbonate, or kaolin may be given in an attempt to control the diarrhea. Camphorated tincture of opium slows down peristalsis, and the other two medications have a soothing effect in the intestinal mucosa because of their coating property. They are usually given after meals and after each loose bowel movement.

■ UNCONTROLLED URINARY AND FECAL INCONTINENCE

Some patients will have urinary and fecal incontinence despite all efforts. The nurse must see that they are kept clean, odorless, and free from decubiti. Linen must be changed as soon as it is soiled. Newspaper pads covered with a piece of cloth can be used to protect bedding and furniture. Oilcloth and plastic materials also can be used. Many commercial products of soft, absorbent cellucotton backed with light plastic are available. They come in a variety of sizes to be placed just under the buttock area or to cover approximately a square yard. Large rolls of absorbent cellucotton of several thickness can be purchased and then cut to the size desired.

Linen may be protected from soiling and the patient made more comfortable if pants made of some absorbent material backed with plastic are used (Fig. 9-4). A resourceful person may be able to improvise equipment that will be more comfortable and less costly than commercially manufactured pants. Zippers, snap tape and ties, elastic, and a variety of fabrics and waterproof materials may be used. Cellucotton for padding is less expensive if purchased in large rather than small rolls. Commercial diaper service for adult patients is now becoming more available. It ensures a steady supply of dry, soft materials and spares the family from constantly searching for and making up improvised supplies.

Any padding used must be changed often, and the skin must be thoroughly washed and dried at each changing. If possible, the patient should be bathed in a tub of warm water at least once a day. Commercial preparations such as methylbenzethonium chloride (Diaparene) that control urine odor and to some extent lessen its irritating properties are available. Zinc oxide powders also are beneficial to these patients. Deodorant sprays for use on dressings and linen are available, as are deodorants for deodorizing room air.

Elderly incontinent patients, particularly, may be helped to establish a definite time for defecation by using bisacodyl suppositories. By following such a regimen, the patient can be saved the emotional stress of unpredictable movements and can have better opportunities for socialization. In addition, the family members are saved time and linen usage is reduced.

Special bed arrangements are helpful for patients who are confined to bed for long periods of time. A *Bradford frame* with an opening under which a pan or urinal can be placed is helpful for a patient who is incontinent. A similar arrangement can be improvised by building the bed up with padding so that there is a depressed area in which a receptacle for drainage can be placed. This arrangement should be made so that the receptacle does not come in contact with the patient's skin. Sometimes, if the problem is expected to go on for years, a circular hole can be cut in the patient's mattress, the edges padded, and a funnel and collection bottle placed beneath the opening. A *Stryker frame, Foster bed,* or *CircOlectric bed* also can be modified to accommodate the incontinent patient.

If the patient can be up, his favorite chair can be equipped with a commode seat. Special commode wheelchairs are also available, making it possible for the patient to be more comfortable and enabling him to mingle socially with others. Thus he will probably be a happier individual and one with whom it is more pleasant to live.

REFERENCES AND SELECTED READINGS*

1 *Birum, L., and Zimmerman, D: Catheter plugs as a source of infection, Am. J. Nurs. **71:**2150-2152, Nov. 1971.

2 *Buchwald, E., McCormack, M., and Raby, E.: A bladder and bowel training program for patients with spinal cord disease, Rehabilitation Monograph III, New York, 1952, The Institute for Physical Medicine and Rehabilitation, New York University, Bellevue Medical Center.

3 *Delehanty, L., and Stravino, V.: Achieving bladder control, Am. J. Nurs. **70:**312-316, Feb. 1970.

4 Hirschberg, G. G., and others: Rehabilitation: a manual for the care of the disabled and elderly, Philadelphia, 1964, J. B. Lippincott Co.

5 Holliday, J.: Bowel programs of patients with spinal cord injury: a clinical study, Nurs. Res. **67:**4-15, Winter 1967.

6 *Langford, T.: Nursing problem: bacteriuria and the indwelling catheter, Am. J. Nurs. **72:**113-115, Jan. 1972.

7 Lapides, J.: Stress incontinence, J. Urol. **85:**291-294, March 1961.

8 Licht, S., editor: Rehabilitation and medicine, New Haven, Conn., 1968, Elizabeth Licht Publishing Co.

9 *Lindan, R., and Bellomy, V.: The use of intermittent catheterization in a bladder retraining program: preliminary report, J. Chronic Dis. **24:**727-735, Dec. 1971.

10 Muellner, S. R.: Development of urinary control in children, J.A.M.A. **172:**1256-1261, March 1960.

11 *Robertson, C. A.: Manual expression of urine, Am. J. Nurs. **59:**840-841, June 1959.

12 Rusk, H. A.: Rehabilitation medicine, a textbook on physical medicine and rehabilitation, ed. 3, St. Louis, 1971, The C. V. Mosby Co.

13 Saxon, J.: Techniques for bowel and bladder training, Am. J. Nurs. **62:**69-71, Sept. 1962.

14 *Sister Regina Elizabeth: Sensory stimulation techniques, Am. J. Nurs. **66:**281-286, Feb. 1966.

15 *Stafford, N. H.: Bowel hygiene of aged patients, Am. J. Nurs. **63:**102-103, Sept. 1963.

16 Stolov, W.: Rehabilitation of bladder in injuries of spinal cord, Arch. Phys. Med. Rehabil. **40:**467-473, Nov. 1959.

17 Swezey, R., and Hallin, R.: Technics for chronic drainage of bladder, Arch. Phys. Med. Rehabil. **48:**201-208, April 1967.

18 Williams, S. R.: Nutrition and diet therapy, ed. 2, St. Louis, 1973, The C. V. Mosby Co.

19 Winter, C. C.: Practical urology, St. Louis, 1969, The C. V. Mosby Co.

20 Winter, C. C., and Barker, M. R.: Nursing care of patients with urologic diseases, ed. 3, St. Louis, 1972, The C. V. Mosby Co.

*References preceded by asterisk are particularly well suited for student reading.

10 The unconscious patient

Observation and assessment
The environment and the family
Management of the unconscious patient
Convalescence
Death of the patient

■ Disturbances in consciousness may be associated with a variety of conditions. Whatever the cause, the individual has a disturbance in sensory perception to the extent that his awareness and responsiveness to stimuli are altered or lost. The degree and duration of unconsciousness may vary greatly among individuals. For example, periods of unconsciousness may be momentary (the common faint or syncope) or may last for months (as after a serious motor vehicle accident in which extensive brain damage has been sustained).

The term "unconsciousness" is relative since there are many degrees or levels of unconsciousness or awareness, from one of general alertness and responsiveness to the environment to one of complete loss of response to any stimuli. In the past certain terms such as "excitatory," "somnolent," "stuporous," and "comatose" were used to describe an individual's level of consciousness. Although these terms are still used, it is important for the nurse to recognize that these, too, are relative and that there is no unanimity of opinion about their precise meaning.

In *excitatory unconsciousness* the patient does not respond coherently but is easily disturbed by sensory stimuli such as bright lights, noise, or sudden movement. He may become excited and agitated at the slightest disturbance. This stage of responsiveness is commonly seen in the elderly and in patients who are going under anesthesia or who are partially reacted from anesthesia. In caring for such a patient the room should be kept dimly lighted, the environment should be quiet, and any necessary moving of the patient or activity about him should be slow and gentle. Safety and protective measures should always be observed with these patients.

The *somnolent* patient is extremely drowsy and will respond only if spoken to directly and perhaps touched. He may perceive his environment inaccurately; he may be confused and may misinterpret stimuli. Jerky body movements are commonly seen during this state. The *stuporous* patient responds to noxious and painful stimuli (such as pricking or pinching of the skin) by reflex withdrawal, grimacing, or unintelligible sounds. In deep stupor he may respond only to supraorbital or substernal pressure. This response may be a reflex withdrawal from the painful stimulus.

The patient in *deep coma* does not respond to any type of stimulus, and his reflexes are gone. He has no gag or corneal reflexes, and he may have an irregular pupillary reaction to light or complete loss of pupillary reflexes. The thermal, respiratory, or other vital regulatory mechanisms in the brain may be disturbed. In the presence of such disturbance the prognosis is usually poor.

Unconsciousness may be caused by systemic disease or toxemia affecting the brain. In vascular diseases such as cerebral hemorrhage or cerebral emboli there may be enough damage to brain tissue from anoxia to cause unconsciousness. The pressure of expanding space-occupying cerebral lesions such as subdural hematomas and intracranial tumors also may cause unconsciousness. Other causes are head injuries with primary damage to the cerebrum or pressure from edema; overdoses of sedatives and narcotics, alcohol, and anesthetizing agents; severe fluid and electrolyte imbalance; and altered metabolic states. Unconsciousness is also seen in some functional diseases of the nervous system and in diseases such as epilepsy, in which there is a disturbance of brain physiology.

Although special care for the unconscious patient is directly related to the cause of the condition, gen-

■ STUDY QUESTIONS

1 As a result of your experience in the hospital, list the equipment that you would need in preparing a room for the admittance of an unconscious patient.

2 Review your basic physical needs in a 24-hour period. Do they differ from the needs of one who is unconscious? If so, how?

3 Review the following basic nursing procedures: mouth care, gavage, throat suctioning, enemas, positioning, and skin care.

eral care does not vary with the cause. In this chapter only the general nursing care will be discussed. Nursing problems related to unconsciousness in specific diseases are discussed in appropriate chapters.

In caring for the unconscious patient the nurse must make provision for meeting his physical and spiritual needs and his family's emotional and spiritual needs. The objectives of patient care are to continually observe and assess the patient's degree of awareness and responsiveness, to maintain normal body function, and to prevent complications that will impede full recovery when consciousness is restored. The nurse must remember that the patient cannot do anything for himself or even ask for help. He cannot, for example, change his position if he is uncomfortable, strained, or cramped. Nurses caring for unconscious patients should keep in mind the bodily needs they meet for themselves each day and should also recall the requests that conscious patients make for little extra comforts.

The patient who is unconscious because of anesthesia usually receives care in the recovery room. The critically ill, unconscious patient usually is cared for in the intensive care unit. When his condition stabilizes, he returns to a general care unit.

■ OBSERVATION AND ASSESSMENT
Observations

The nurse is an invaluable member of the health team in the area of ongoing observation and assessment of the patient with a change in level of awareness. Detailed observations of any change should be reported and recorded, since the cause of the patient's change in consciousness may be obscure. Such things as a slight change in the patient's orientation to his environment, stiffness of the neck, or flaccid limbs may provide the physician with information that will aid him in making a diagnosis.

In describing and recording the level of awareness of the patient it is not enough for the nurse to use such terms as "lethargic," "confused," "stuporous," and "semicomatose." These and other similar terms are not precise enough for valid assessment of the level of unconsciousness. Therefore it is essential that the nurse describe objectively and specifically those behaviors and responses that clearly indicate the level of awareness of the patient. Nursing assessment should be guided by the patient's response to auditory, visual, painful, or tactile stimuli.[12]

Guides to patient assessment

1. Is the patient oriented as to time, place, and person? Does he know where he is, who he is, the day or time, or how long he has been in the hospital?

2. Does he respond to stimuli in his environment such as noise, light, or spoken words?

3. Does he lie quietly, or is he restless? Is his restlessness continuous or only in response to specific stimuli?

4. Does the patient respond verbally? Describe his verbal responses: are they clear, one-word responses, complete sentences, groans, or mumbles? Are the responses appropriate or unusual?

5. Are his actions in accord with his verbal response?

6. How does the patient respond to simple commands such as, "Raise your left hand"? Does he follow people with his eyes? Does he respond to complex questions or commands?

7. Can he move all four of his extremities? Is he able to grip or squeeze your hand on command? Is muscle response equal on both sides of the body?

8. Are his movements purposeful? Does he change position automatically? How does he respond to nursing measures such as bathing or the taking of vital signs? Are his movements accompanied by any other response such as groans, words, or facial grimace?

9. How does the patient respond to painful stimuli? What is his response to such things as pinching of skin or muscle of the arm, stroking of the sole of the foot, or administration of injections?

Additional observations

Observations over and above those made while giving patient care may be ordered. The physician may wish the vital signs, the pupillary response, and the level of consciousness determined at periodic intervals. A rising blood pressure correlated with a slowing of the pulse rate is indicative of increasing intracranial pressure and should be reported at once. Any marked change in the character of the pulse or respirations or any decrease or increase in the level of consciousness should be reported.

The pupillary response is checked by opening the upper eyelid and flashing a light into the eye from the outer aspect inward toward the nose. Each eye should be tested separately. Irregular reaction of either eye or "fixed" pupils should be reported, since these responses suggest increased intracranial pressure.

The corneal response is tested by the physician. He will need a wisp of sterile absorbent cotton for this procedure. The patient who has lost the corneal reflex will not blink when the cornea is touched.

■ THE ENVIRONMENT AND THE FAMILY

The appearance of the unconscious patient and his surroundings is very important to members of his family. Not being able to communicate with a loved one is very difficult for them. Seeing that the patient looks comfortable, however, and that he is in a neat and pleasant room may give assurance to the family.

The room should be well ventilated, and the temperature should be kept at about 21° C. (70° F.). The very young and the very old patient may be more comfortable in a warmer temperature, 26° C. (80° F.). Since patients with depressed states of consciousness are often more disturbed in darkness, it is best to keep rooms well lighted at all times.[3] If a member of the family is remaining with the patient, a comfortable chair should be provided. He should be told where the rest room is, where he may eat, and where the public telephone is located. If the patient remains unconscious for a long time, other family members should be urged to share the time spent with him. Sometimes they can be encouraged to come only for short periods of time each day. They should be assured that they will be notified at once if there is any change in the patient's condition. The nurse should help them conserve their physical resources, for the patient who recovers after a period of unconsciousness needs much care and attention during convalescence.

Members of the patient's family frequently have many questions. If the nurse cannot answer them, the family should be referred to others who can. Explanations of treatments such as would be given to the patient if he were conscious should be given to members of the family. Explaining helps to allay some of their fears and helps them to understand and to feel they have a part in the patient's care. If the family wishes, the spiritual adviser should be called. He may help the patient and give the family comfort and emotional help. If religious medals are significant to the patient and his family, they may be attached to the head of the bed or secured in such a way that they are not lost. Often the patient wears a medal on a chain around his neck, and many hospitals do not require that it be removed unless necessary for a treatment or an examination such as a radiograph.

Hearing is probably the last of the critical faculties to be lost in unconsciousness. On regaining consciousness, many patients have reported conversations they heard when other faculties were obliterated by anesthesia. Conversation of persons close to the patient should be no different than if the patient were conscious. Members of the family and other visitors may need to be reminded of this fact. Because the patient may be able to hear, he should be told what is going to be done to him; for example, he should be told when he is going to be turned or given mouth care.

■ MANAGEMENT OF THE UNCONSCIOUS PATIENT
Maintenance of an adequate airway

In order to provide good pulmonary ventilation, the unconscious person should be placed on his side or in the prone position. It is unsafe to leave an unconscious patient unattended if he is lying on his back because his tongue may fall back and occlude the air passages. He may also have more difficulty swallowing or otherwise handling his secretions if on his back. When the patient is placed on his side or abdomen, a small, firm pillow rather than a soft one should be used under the head so that there is no danger of his becoming accidentally smothered as a result of his face being buried in the pillow. Since the patient is unable to blow or otherwise clear his nose, the nasal passages may become occluded with mucus. Cleansing or suctioning of the nasal passages of patients who have had brain surgery or who have suffered a head injury should not be done without a physician's order, but in other instances the nose should be swabbed gently first with a moistened applicator and then with one lightly lubricated with mineral oil. If the mucous membranes of the nose and mouth become unusually dry, humidification of the room air is useful.

Excess mucus may need to be suctioned from the mouth or the nasopharynx. A No. 14 or 16 Fr. catheter is commonly used for this procedure. The mouth should be held open with a padded tongue blade. Ideally, a fenestrated catheter or Y tube attachment should be used so that no suction is applied as the catheter is inserted. (See Fig. 11-8.) If the tube is to be inserted through the nose, it should be lubricated with water-soluble lubricating jelly. The mucus is aspirated by covering the opening in the catheter or by covering the Y valve with the fingertip, rotating the catheter, and withdrawing it gently.

If there is any question about the patient's ability to maintain an adequate airway, a cuffed endotracheal tube is inserted. This may be followed by an elective tracheostomy if the patient is expected to be unconscious for a prolonged period of time. Most physicians consider it safer to insert an endotracheal tube first, since this assures them of a patent airway before a tracheostomy is attempted. A cuffed endotracheal tube will not only provide an adequate airway and make removal of tracheobronchial secretions easier, but it will also permit positive pressure ventilation as necessary and will seal off the digestive tract from the trachea and thereby prevent aspiration.[21] When a cuffed tube is used, the cuff will have to be deflated *at least* 5 minutes every hour. (See p. 592 for care of patient with an endotracheal tube and p. 612 for care of patient with a tracheostomy.)

Maintenance of circulation

Circulation of blood is enhanced by muscle movement. The patient must not be left in a position that restricts circulation to any part of the body; for example, lying for any length of time with an acute angle bend at the knee joint will produce enough pressure on the popliteal artery and accompanying veins to impede circulation to the lower leg. A definite routine for frequent turning and for exercise not only improves circulation and helps maintain muscle tone but also helps to prevent hypostatic pneumonia or atelectasis. In addition, it maintains a normal range of joint motion and helps prevent formation of vascular thrombi. Scheduled turning of the unconscious patient at specific intervals by an assigned team of nurses and/or auxiliary personnel assures maintenance of these physiologic functions. A checklist with the patient's name and the position changes needed at specific intervals is also useful. Bony prominences should be protected from direct pressure by soft padding, and bedclothes should be kept dry, clean, and wrinkle-free. Sheepskin pads, Gelfoam pads, flotation pads, or flotation mattresses may be helpful in preventing pressure sores. Reddened areas (except on lower extremities) should be gently massaged and should be noted in the nursing care plan and in the nursing notes on the patient's chart so that they will receive special care.[20] Wrapping the lower extremities from toe to thigh with Ace bandages or applying antiembolism stockings may help prevent venous stasis in the lower extremities. Stockings or Ace bandages should be changed at least once every 8 hours to allow for inspection of the skin.

Moving and positioning

A turning sheet should be used in moving an unconscious patient. It not only helps to maintain the patient's body alignment by allowing the entire trunk to be moved at the same time but also lessens the strain on the nurse's or attendant's back. A turning sheet is a large sheet folded lengthwise and then in half. It should be placed under the patient so that it reaches from above the shoulders to below the buttocks. The technique for placing a turning sheet under the patient is the same as for placing a drawsheet there. In preparing to turn the patient, remove the top bedclothes so that they will not be in the way and so that the alignment of the patient's body can be easily seen. Two nurses are needed to execute the turn—one on each side of the bed. Roll the sheet edges up close to the patient's body and grasp them firmly. (See Fig. 33-11.) Gently roll the patient onto his back, and then lift or pull him on the sheet toward the side of the bed opposite that to which he is to be turned. Bend the knee that will be uppermost after the patient is turned. The nurse who will be facing the patient after he is turned should then grasp the far side of the turning sheet and roll the patient toward her onto his side, pulling the hip and shoulder well under him. Check to see that the spine is straight, the neck is not bent, and the lower leg is straight. Place firm, plastic-covered pillows under the uppermost arm and leg. They should support the

entire extremity and be of such a height as to prevent abduction or adduction of the arm or leg. The uppermost leg should be flexed with the knee at right angles to the hip. To prevent foot drop, the foot of the straightened leg should be firmly dorsiflexed against a foot block at scheduled intervals. The lowermost arm should be flexed at the elbow and placed palm up flat on the bed. The fingers of the hand that rests on the pillows should be allowed to curve gently over the edge of the pillow. The wrist, however, must be supported on the pillow to prevent wrist drop. The fingers should never be continuously hyperextended or tightly clenched, and sometimes it is advisable to maintain the hand in its position of function by placing a roll of 3-inch bandage in the palm and curling the fingers around it. If the thumb tends to fall forward, it may be supported in a position of common use by attaching a tab of cloth to the hand roll and using it as a supportive bandage (Fig. 10-1). If the unconscious patient is placed correctly in a side-lying position, a pillow to support his back is unnecessary.

If the patient does not move, all the extremities should be put through the complete range of joint motion at least twice each day. When he is turned each hour, the extremities on one side may be passively exercised. Such a routine assures passive exercise to all extremities. In turning the patient, extreme care should be taken to prevent strain on joints.

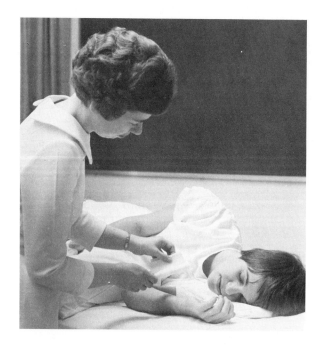

FIG. 10-1. The nurse is preparing to wipe the mouth of an unconscious patient. Note that the patient is lying on her side supported by pillows and that her right hand is curled about a hand roll with the thumb held in pronation.

The patient may be turned directly onto his abdomen for short periods. When he is in this position, his feet should extend over the edge of the mattress to prevent pressure on the toes, and his head should be turned well to the side. Usually no pillow is necessary under the head, but a small one may be slipped under the abdomen to prevent excessive pressure on the chest. This is sometimes needed to relieve pressure on the breasts of women. Turning the unconscious patient is facilitated by the use of the Stryker frame or the CircOlectric bed.

Skin care

The unconscious patient should be thoroughly bathed with warm water each day. In order to prevent dryness of the skin, superfatted soaps or bath oils such as Alpha Keri are helpful. The skin should be briskly washed and dried to stimulate circulation. In some hospitals, patients who have been unconscious for some time are lifted into a bathtub several times a week since this measure seems to control the development of decubiti remarkably well. Three people trained in doing a three-man lift are needed for the procedure. Care must be taken not to injure the patient in moving him to the tub or to place undue strain on the nurses. Shallow tubs at bed height with access on three sides are preferable but not essential.

If the skin is dry despite the special care just described, it should be lubricated daily with lanolin, cold cream, or moisturizing lotions. The feet should be lubricated each day since poor circulation from lack of activity causes the skin to become dry and the nails to harden and become horny. Alcohol is drying to the skin and should not be used. The fingernails and toenails should be short and clean. As the depth of unconsciousness becomes more shallow, many patients scratch themselves.

The hair should be neatly combed. If a woman's hair is long, it is usually more manageable and attractive in braids. If unconsciousness persists, the physician may permit a shampoo, provided that the movement involved is not harmful to the patient. Shampoos should be given at least every 2 weeks to patients who are unconscious for long periods of time.

Mouth care

Since the unconscious patient tends to be a "mouth breather," the mouth often becomes dry. Therefore mouth care should be given every 2 to 4 hours. Dentures should be removed and safely stored until the patient is fully conscious. The patient's own teeth should be brushed at least twice a day. A child's toothbrush is more easily used than an adult's. The inside of the mouth, the gum line, and the tongue should be inspected daily, using a flashlight and a tongue depressor, and the mouth should be cleaned thoroughly every 2 to 4 hours with normal saline or an aromatic alkaline mouthwash solution. One study has questioned the use of glycerin and lemon juice because of its drying effect on the oral mucosa.[26] The mouth must be held open with a padded tongue blade and is then cleansed with a piece of gauze wrapped around a toothbrush, a tongue depressor, or a cotton swab. Covering exposed mouth tissues with petroleum jelly may help prevent dehydration in patients who are mouth breathers.[16] The nurse's fingers should never be put in the patient's mouth. The hold on the jaw may loosen and allow the jaws to close down on the fingers, and a human bite may cause severe infection. The lips should be coated with a lubricant such as cold cream or petroleum jelly to prevent cracking.

Eye care

The patient's eyes should be carefully inspected several times a day. If they appear irritated, if the corneal reflex is absent, or if the lids are incompletely closed, they should be covered with an eye shield. If an eye shield is not available, a circle of transparent x-ray film, 9 cm. in diameter, may be used by slitting it to the middle and overlapping the edges of the slit to make a cone-shaped shield. All the edges of the x-ray film shield should be bound with cellophane tape to prevent irritation of the skin, and the shields may be held in place with cellophane tape. An equally effective eye shield can be made from a small piece of plastic food wrap.

"Butterfly" adhesive strips may be used to close the eye. The physician may order an eye irrigation. Physiologic solution of sodium chloride is commonly used. The eye should always be irrigated away from the inner canthus so that the return flow is away from the other eye. If the patient tends to open his eyes at intervals, there also may be an order for instillation of a drop or two of mineral oil or methyl cellulose, 0.5% to 2% solution, in each eye daily to protect the cornea from lint and dirt and to provide moisture and lubrication. Sometimes the physician may order the administration of a broad-spectrum antibiotic such as neomycin eye ointment prophylactically. Neglect of eye care can lead to drying of the cornea and eventual blindness.

Food and fluids

The comatose patient cannot be given fluids or food orally since he does not swallow normally and would aspirate fluid into the lungs. He may be fed by intravenous infusion; however, it is difficult to meet all his nutritional needs in this manner. Therefore many physicians feel that it is preferable to use a nasogastric tube and to give small amounts of liquid containing all essential foods. (See p. 127 for preparation of these feedings.) Only about 100 to 200 ml. should be given, and this amount should be given every 2 to 3 hours. If the stomach is overfilled, the patient may vomit and aspirate with serious consequences. The amount of residual stomach contents should be checked before each feeding. If the residual is greater than 75 to 100 ml., it may indicate that the patient is receiving too much fluid at each feeding or that the digestive process is not progressing as rapidly as it should. The feeding should be delayed or omitted in the event of significant residual stomach contents. All feedings should be followed with about 50 ml. of water to clear the tube. Additional water may be ordered and given periodically in order to meet the desired fluid intake for the patient. Tube feedings should be cool when given.

If a cuffed endotracheal tube or tracheostomy tube is used, the cuff should be inflated before the feeding is administered to prevent possible aspiration and remain inflated for 30 to 45 minutes after the feeding. The nasogastric tube should be removed at least every 5 days and inspected. The distal end of rubber and plastic tubes becomes rigid and may traumatize the stomach mucosa.[9] Usually the physician inserts the tube. However, if the nurse is expected to insert the tube, specific instructions in the correct method should be given. After the tube is inserted, it is customary to test its placement in the following ways: place it under water and check for the presence of air bubbles, which would indicate that it is in the lungs instead of in the stomach; aspirate a little fluid to prove that it is in the stomach or inject up to 5 ml. of air through the tube while listening with a stethoscope over the stomach. If the tube is in the stomach, the sudden rush of air will cause a swooshing or popping sound. For details on care of equipment and technique for this procedure, see fundamentals of nursing textbooks. The patient who has a nasogastric tube inserted needs special care of the nose to prevent crusting and ulceration. The nose should be cleaned and inspected daily, and the tape holding the tube kept clean and replaced as necessary. Tincture of benzoin applied to the nose before the tape is applied will help hold the tape more firmly and will protect the skin. For patients requiring a slow, constant rate of delivery of food through the nasogastric tube, a mechanical pump is available. The pump may be adjusted so that it delivers from 40 to 200 ml. of food/hour into the stomach.

If it appears that the patient may be unconscious for a prolonged period, a gastrostomy may be performed. A feeding catheter with an inflated balloon tip is inserted into the stomach through an abdominal incision. The tube is sutured in place, and the balloon is kept inflated to anchor it in the stomach. A small dressing is placed around the tube insertion site and is changed daily or more often if needed. When feeding the patient, the same precautions should be observed as for feeding via a nasogastric tube. This includes proper positioning of the patient, checking for tube placement and for residual stom-

ach contents, and inflating the cuff on an endotracheal or tracheostomy tube.

If the patient responds to verbal stimuli and has a gag reflex, fluids may be put into the back of the mouth through an Asepto syringe to which is attached about 2 inches of rubber tubing to obviate the danger of the patient's biting down on the tip of the syringe. He may have to be reminded to swallow each mouthful. Suction should be readily available in case he shows signs of choking.

Hyperthermia

When the heat-regulatory center in the hypothalamus is disturbed, the patient's temperature will rise suddenly. This is known as hyperthermia. It may occur after trauma to vital centers, and it often occurs in the last stages of chronic medical illness (such as uremia) when the body relinquishes vital controls prior to death. The temperature of any unconscious patient should be taken rectally every 4 hours, and if it is elevated, it should be taken at least every 2 hours. Elevation of temperature may also be a sign of complications such as pneumonia, wound infection, dehydration, or urinary tract infection. The nurse should carefully observe the patient for any signs that might indicate the onset of complications.

When elevation of temperature is caused by the improper functioning of the heat-regulatory center, the nurse can help compensate for the loss of this natural control. If the temperature is over 38.4° C. (101° F.), some bedclothes should be removed, and sometimes the patient should be covered only by a sheet. Occasionally the patient's gown and sheet are removed and only a loincloth and breast covering are used. Aspirin or acetaminophen (Tylenol) may be dissolved and inserted through a nasogastric or gastrostomy tube, or it may be introduced into the rectum as a suppository. Fluids may not be forced if the physician feels that increasing fluid intake may increase intracranial pressure. If the temperature continues to rise despite conservative treatment, ice bags may be applied to the groin and axillae. Alcohol sponge baths often are ordered, and fans placed slightly to the side of the patient may increase evaporation. If fever still persists following this treatment, the patient may be placed on an electrically controlled cooling mattress in an attempt to reduce his temperature. (See discussion on hypothermia, p. 209.) If an air-conditioned room is not available, the patient may be placed in an oxygen tent for its cooling effect. The room should be kept cool so that body heat will be lost from the skin surfaces. As shivering increases the metabolic demands on the body, it should be prevented either by warming the patient or giving a drug such as chlorpromazine (Thorazine) at regular intervals. If the patient's temperature goes over 40° C. (104° F.), it should be taken every hour until it returns to and remains at a lower level. Some-

190

times, if the elevation is due to increased intracranial pressure, a lumbar puncture is performed in order to remove cerebrospinal fluid and decrease pressure. Unabated high temperature eventually will cause death.

Hypothermia

The unconscious patient may have a temperature that is too low. This condition may occur when vital centers are depressed but control has not yet been lost. The unconscious patient who does not move produces less normal body heat and is likely to have a low temperature and to need extra covering. The nurse should feel the patient's feet to determine circulation in the extremities and to judge whether or not adequate external warmth is being supplied.

Problems of elimination

The unconscious patient often has both urinary and fecal incontinence. A Foley catheter or external drainage apparatus may be used to control urinary incontinence (Chapter 9). Because of frequent urinary tract infections in patients with indwelling catheters, tidal drainage may be instituted, or the catheter may be irrigated at specified intervals with a solution such as Neosporin G. U. Irrigant (1: 1,000). If the use of these devices is contraindicated, the nurse should try to determine the patient's normal voiding schedule and place him on a bedpan or put a urinal in place according to this schedule. The skin should be kept dry and clean to prevent decubiti and add to comfort (Fig. 9-4). The urinary output should be measured. If measurement is impossible because of incontinence, output should be estimated by recording each time the patient is incontinent and whether or not a large amount of urine was voided (p. 176).

The unconscious patient usually is given an enema every 2 or 3 days to help prevent fecal incontinence and formation of impactions. The patient who is fed through a nasogastric tube may be given juices that have a laxative effect, such as prune juice. Sometimes a mild cathartic such as milk of magnesia, citrate of magnesia, psyllium hydrophilic mucilloid (Metamucil), a concentrate of senna (Senokot), or dioctyl sodium sulfosuccinate (Colace) is ordered and can be given through the nasogastric tube. In giving the enema the nurse may need to hold the patient's buttocks together to prevent premature expulsion of fluid. When it is desirable for the enema to be expelled, the patient should be turned onto a bedpan, with special care taken to support the back and to prevent pressure damage to the skin from weight against the pan. A firm pillow protected with water-resistant material is best for this purpose. The lower abdomen should then be massaged gently from right to left. Sometimes it is necessary to siphon fluid from the lower bowel, in which case the enema may have to be repeated. The physician may order bisacodyl suppositories (Dulcolax). A bowel movement usually occurs within half an hour after their insertion. Glycerin suppositories also may be used.

If the patient has a vaginal discharge, it should be reported to the physician. Sometimes cleansing douches are ordered. The patient who is menstruating will need perineal care every few hours.

Prevention of accidents

Precautions should be taken to prevent accidents to unconscious patients. No external heat such as hot-water bottles or heating pads should be used. Padded side rails should be kept on the bed, since the patient might have a convulsion or suddenly move when not expected to do so. If a convulsion is anticipated, a padded tongue blade should be kept at the bedside. If a convulsion occurs, the padded tongue blade should be inserted at the side of the mouth between the molar teeth. Manual pressure at the angle of the jaw sometimes makes it easier to open the mouth. Forceful attempts at inserting the padded tongue blade can result in broken teeth or lacerations of the mouth. The unconscious patient should be observed at least every half hour. If his condition is critical, he may need to be observed every 15 minutes or to be attended constantly. Diazepam (Valium), 5 to 10 mg., paraldehyde, 5 ml., or sodium phenobarbital, 30 to 60 mg. ($^1/_2$ to 1 grain), may be ordered for overactivity, excitability, or when seizures occur. Any patient who is unconscious and receives sedation must be observed closely for signs of depression of vital functions. A certain amount of restlessness is desirable, as it encourages deeper respirations and the patient is more likely to move about in bed.[17]

If the patient is semiconscious, he may be placed in a chair twice a day. This improves circulation and prevents pulmonary and circulatory complications. To prevent him from falling, the nurse should apply a chest harness type of Posey belt or tie a twisted drawsheet about his waist and to the back of the chair. The nurse must make certain that the patient is placed in as near a proper sitting position as possible. The spine should be straight, he should be sitting on his buttocks, and his feet should be flat on the floor. The head and arms will need to be supported. The reason for getting the patient out of bed should be carefully explained to the family.

■ CONVALESCENCE

A patient may recover completely after being unconscious for several weeks. He will gradually return through the stages of unconsciousness, and he often first responds verbally to a familiar face or voice. Efforts should not be made to arouse him until the level of unconsciousness has lightened. He may be unable to speak, may be partially paralyzed, or may have other losses, and the rehabilitation program will be planned accordingly. If he has been well cared for while he was unconscious, so that pressure sores, contractures, or corneal ulcer was prevented from developing, he should have a shorter hospitalization.

During convalescence, definite rest periods should be planned each day. If the patient becomes overtired, he will tend to regress. He will need the encouragement and security of knowing that family and friends are concerned and interested in his recovery. He also will need to be reoriented because his memory may be blank for the time immediately before and during unconsciousness. The nurse can assist in the reorientation of the patient by explaining where he is and what has happened to him. As soon as possible, the patient should be involved in making decisions about his daily activities. Each small accomplishment of the patient, such as assisting with his bath, turning himself, etc., should be allowed and encouraged, even though it may add to nursing time needed to complete the daily care of the patient.

■ DEATH OF THE PATIENT

Many patients die without regaining consciousness. Kubler-Ross[15] has written extensively on the stages

of dying as experienced by the patient and family, and these same reactions are evidenced by the family of the unconscious patient who has died. In addition to showing grief at the loss of a loved one, the family may also express anger at the deceased for "giving up" or anger at the physician for not saving the patient. If the onset of unconsciousness is sudden, without warning, and the patient dies, the family may feel guilty that the deceased was not comforted and that final concerns and thoughts were not shared. If the care of the unconscious patient has been long, the family may view the financial investment as a waste and may express anger about this.

Just as the family is comforted when any patient dies, so should the family of the unconscious patient be supported. The nurse should provide privacy, time, and emotional support to a family who might be showing sorrow, grief, and anger. The family members may express their feelings by crying, talking, or even indicating relief that the ordeal is over.

After the body has been bathed, family members may want to see the body and an opportunity should be provided for them. A clergyman can be summoned if the family indicates that this would be helpful. The nurse may also help arrange for other family members to be called and for transportation home for the family.

REFERENCES AND SELECTED READINGS*

1 *Bardsley, C., and others: Pressure sores, a regime for preventing and treating them, Am. J. Nurs. **64:**82-84, May 1964.
2 Barron, J., Prendergast, J. J., and Jocz, M. W.: Food pump—new approach to tube feeding, J.A.M.A. **161:**621-622, June 1956.
3 Beeson, P. B., and McDermott, W., editors: Cecil-Loeb textbook of medicine, ed. 13, Philadelphia, 1971, W. B. Saunders Co.
4 Best, C. H., and Brobeck, J. R.: The physiological basis of medical practice, ed. 9, Baltimore, 1973, The Williams & Wilkins Co.
5 Brooks, H. L.: The golden rule for the unconscious patient, Nurs. Forum 4(3):12-18, 1965.
6 Butts, C. A., and Canney, V. E.: The unresponsive patient, Am. J. Nurs. **67:**1886-1888, Sept. 1967.
7 Byrne, J. J., editor: The management of shock and unconsciousness, Surg. Clin. North Am. **48:**247-459, April 1968.
8 Carini, E., and Owens, G.: Neurological and neurosurgical nursing, ed. 6, St. Louis, 1974, The C. V. Mosby Co.
9 *Davenport, R. R.: Tube feeding for long-term patients, Am. J. Nurs. **64:**121-123, Jan. 1964.
10 Eckenhoff, J. E.: The care of the unconscious patient, J.A.M.A. **186:**541-543, Nov. 1963.
11 *Fuerst, E. V., and Wolff, L. V.: Fundamentals of nursing, ed. 5, Philadelphia, 1974, J. B. Lippincott Co.
12 *Gardner, M. A. M.: Responsiveness as a measure of consciousness, Am. J. Nurs. **68:**1034-1038, May 1968.
13 *Gibbs, G. E.: Perineal care of the incapacitated patient, Am. J. Nurs. **69:**124-125, Jan. 1969.

14 Gray, V. R.: Grief, Nursing '74 **4:**25-27, Jan. 1974.
15 Kubler-Ross, E.: On death and dying, London, 1969, Macmillan Publishing Co., Inc.
16 Lite, T., DiMalo, D. J., and Bruman, L. R.: Gingival pathoses in mouth breathers, Oral Surg. **8:**382-391, April 1955.
17 Luessenhop, A.: Care of the unconscious patient, Nurs. Forum 4(3):6-11, 1965.
18 MacBryde, C. M., and Beacklow, R. S.: Signs and symptoms, ed. 5, Philadelphia, 1970, J. B. Lippincott Co.
19 *Olson, E. V., and others: The hazards of immobility, Am. J. Nurs. **67:**779-797, April 1967.
20 *Pfaudler, M.: Flotation therapy: flotation, displacement, and decubitus ulcers, Am. J. Nurs. **68:**2351-2355, Nov. 1968.
21 Phipps, W. J., and Barker, W. L.: Respiratory insufficiency and failure. In Meltzer, L. E., Abdellah, F. G., and Kitchell, J. R., editors: Concepts and practices of intensive care for nurse specialists, Philadelphia, 1969, The Charles Press, Publishers.
22 *Redman, B. K., and Redman, R. S.: Oral care of the critically ill patient. In Bergersen, B. S., and others, editors: Current concepts in clinical nursing, vol. 1, St. Louis, 1967, The C. V. Mosby Co.
23 Reitz, M., and Pope, W.: Mouth care, Am. J. Nurs. **73:**1728-1730, Oct. 1973.
24 *Rodgers, H. M.: Flotation therapy: a water pillow, too, Am. J. Nurs. **68:**2359-2360, Nov. 1968.
25 *Thornhill, H. L., and Williams, M. L.: Flotation therapy: experience with the water mattress in a large city hospital, Am. J. Nurs. **68:**2356-2358, Nov. 1968.
26 *Van Drimmelen, J., and Rollins, H. F.: Evaluation of a commonly used oral hygiene agent, Nurs. Res. **18:**327-332, July-Aug. 1969.
27 Williams, S. R.: Nutrition and diet therapy, ed. 2, St. Louis, 1973, The C. V. Mosby Co.

*References preceded by an asterisk are particularly well suited for student reading.

11 Surgical intervention

■ When an individual is confronted with the need for surgical intervention and all its related experiences, the result may be a period of anxiety and stress for the patient and his family. A high level of stress occurs when a sudden illness or accident precipitates an ambulance ride to the hospital and results in emergency surgery. Likewise, it may be equally stressful for the patient who must endure a period of observation and undergo numerous tests prior to surgery. The patient who must have repeated surgery also faces frustrations and fears that may intensify his reactions.

Although some operations are considered to be minor procedures by hospital personnel, surgery is always a major experience in the life of the patient and his family. Surgery is usually performed in a hospital. Although the patient knows that many wonderful things are done in hospitals, a hospital is still a place where one goes to have serious operations and where one may lose freedom of action and identity. In our society many people also die in the hospital. An operation is associated in the patient's mind with pain, and often with an anesthetic and its unpleasant side effects. Surgery also represents a physical encounter for the patient in which he is at a distinct disadvantage in that he cannot strike back or avoid the encounter in the usual manner. The patient may fear exposure of his body, sharing of his emotions with strangers, and simply losing control. A surgical procedure may imply maiming or loss of a part of the body, which is a damaging blow to self-esteem and to the concept of self. Above all, surgery often raises fears of what will be found during the operation and how this may alter the patient's life or even curtail it.

The nurse is an essential member of the health care team, which attempts to make surgery a more tolerable experience for the patient. Nurses contribute to the functioning of the team in many ways. Ob-

■ STUDY QUESTIONS

1 What general reactions do you believe you would have if told that you must have immediate surgery? To whom would you wish to talk? Have you observed these reactions in any close member of your family? If so, describe them.

2 What general physical deficiencies can you identify that might necessitate a delay in surgery?

3 What are safe and effective ways to cleanse the skin? Can the skin be made sterile?

4 Review the charts of several patients on your clinical unit who have received anesthetic agents. What kinds of anesthetic agents were used? How were they administered?

5 Talk to two patients on your clinical unit who have recently received anesthetic agents. Did they express fear? What vivid recollections do they have?

6 What is the significance to the circulatory system of a sudden drop in blood pressure?

7 Review the circulation of the blood and the physiology of respiration.

8 Review the dangers of prolonged bed rest. What techniques have you learned for helping patients to get into and out of bed? What safety measures should be taken?

9 What disturbances of physiology can occur when the patient cannot take solids or liquids orally?

10 List the nursing measures you have learned that may assist a patient to void.

taining, assessing, and sharing appropriate data about the patient preoperatively is an integral part of the nurses' contribution. Sometimes the surgeon knows the patient and his family well; many times he does not. The public health nurse who sees the patient in various community settings, the nurse in the hospital clinic, the nurse on the scene at the time of an emergency, and the nurse caring for the patient in the hospital environment can contribute by accurate recording and reporting of pertinent information. The nurse may also assist in providing the patient with educational materials and explanations that make the entire experience of hospitalization and surgery a more positive one for him and his family. For example, nursing personnel on the clinical units should prepare patients for such things as x-ray procedures and routines that they will encounter postoperatively, while operating room nurses should visit patients preoperatively to acquaint them with the routines that will be carried out when they arrive in the operating room environment. The nurse also contributes in giving physical and emotional care during the operative period and by being sensitive to the needs of the surgical patient at all times. Some of the skills and abilities essential to effective contributions by the nurse are discussed in this chapter.

The purpose of care during the preoperative period is to prepare the patient, both physically and psychologically, to withstand the effects of anesthesia and surgery. The time allowed for this preparation depends on the condition of the patient and the type of surgery to be performed. It may be very short, or it may extend into weeks. The physician may initiate this preparation by discussing the patient's need for surgery with him; however, he relies on nurses for much assistance and delegates certain responsibilities to them. The nursing staff can contribute substantially to the patient's physical and emotional welfare and can greatly influence his preoperative progress. The surgeon's orders for preparation for surgery should be carefully reviewed and carried out in such a way as to provide the greatest possible comfort and safety for the patient.

The nurse will need to draw on basic knowledge of human behavior, normal physiology, and the development of disease processes in order to assist the patient to understand the need for the anticipated surgery. This knowledge also enables the nurse to make pertinent observations and to share them with appropriate members of the health team.

■ PSYCHOLOGIC PREPARATION FOR SURGERY

Preparation for hospital admission

Preparation for surgery should begin as soon as the physician makes a diagnosis and decides that an operation is necessary. From that moment on the patient and his family are faced with the decision of accepting this treatment and its consequences. The physician should tell the patient and his family that the operation is necessary, explain why it must be performed, what will be done, and what the probable outcome will be. He discusses duration of hospitalization, cost, length of absence from work, and disabilities or residual effects that may be expected. An appointment for admission to the hospital is then made. The date for admission is influenced by the acuteness of the patient's illness, the hospital treatment needed preoperatively, and the amount of time the patient requires to make necessary arrangements regarding his family, financial matters, and work.

The patient needs to know when to arrive at the hospital, where to go, and what information to have available. The admitting clerk will ask about his employment, insurance, and hospital plans. He should know that the business office can help him make arrangements for paying his bill and that he can consult a social caseworker about family, financial, and convalescent problems. He should be told what toilet articles and clothing to bring with him. He will be interested in knowing the visiting hours and how his family may contact him. He should be encouraged to think through any problems that may arise and to plan for them. It is current practice to permit a parent to accompany a child to his hospital bed, to remain with him during his first day and evening in the hospital, and on the morning of the operative day to be with him until he goes to the operating room. Some hospitals allow parents to visit the child while he is in the recovery room. This, of course, may not be appropriate for complex procedures such as open heart surgery.

Fear of surgery

Although patients may or may not express it, almost all of them have some fear of surgery. It can be a fear of the unknown, or it can be a fear based on something they have heard friends or relatives say about their operative experiences. They may have had personal contact with someone who died as a result of an operation. They may be afraid of the diagnosis. They may have fears about anesthesia, pain, disfigurement, disability, or death. The older patient often worries about becoming a burden to his family.

The nurse may be able to help the patient talk about his fears and should give him every opportunity to ask questions. If feasible, the same nurse or member of the nursing team should be assigned to care for the patient each day preoperatively so that he feels he is known as an individual by at least one person on the nursing staff. Such sustained personal contact often makes it easier for the patient to share his real feelings about his impending surgery. Preoperative patients who are helped to understand and cope emotionally with their need for surgery are undoubtedly spared much anxiety. The nurse should keep the patient and his family well informed and explain each procedure and examination (Fig. 11-1).

Information should be shared with the patient in a competent and unhurried manner. If it is appropriate, the nurse can make arrangements for the patient to talk with other patients who have successfully recovered from similar surgery. The patient's family may need to be reminded of the importance of their visits to the patient. Frequent visits will assure him that he is wanted and loved. On the other hand, if the patient is seriously ill or unduly apprehensive, too frequent visits may prevent him from getting adequate rest. Often the patient has great confidence in his spiritual adviser and gains much comfort from speaking with him. If the patient wishes, the nurse can make arrangements for a visit from the hospital chaplain.

Patients will obviously differ in their emotional reactions to surgery and some may demonstrate behavior reflecting extreme apprehension or depression. If the patient cries frequently, withdraws from others, refuses to eat, or is not sleeping, the nurse should attempt to obtain clues from him as to what meaning this behavior has for him. Symptoms of unusual emotional reactions should be carefully documented and then reported to the surgeon. Patients who are extremely frightened often respond poorly to surgery and frequently develop postoperative complications. Unless the operation is an emergency, the surgeon may delay the surgery.

The child should be told in simple language appropriate to his age and his development level what to expect before and after the operation and what the operative procedure will be (Fig. 11-2). The child, like the adult, should have individualized instruction. Sometimes the preparation should be gradual, and storybooks about hospitalization and anesthesia are available and are useful for parents to use. Unless the child is old enough to have developed a perspective as to time, a small amount of factual information given shortly before the operation is best. Knowing too far ahead may only confuse the child, since his concept of time is immediate and he does not grasp the significance of a waiting period. Parental participation in preoperative care should be encouraged. The child should never be told untruths. Honesty and simplicity concerning tests, preparations, surgery, stitches, and pain encourage the child to trust those who will be caring for him. He should know that the experience may not be entirely pleasant, but the positive aspects of the situation should be stressed. Placing a child in a room with other children usually helps him adjust to hospitalization more easily, and telling him (if it is true) that his mother will be at his bedside when he awakens helps a great deal to comfort him and allay fear. When possible the child should be allowed to bring his favorite toy, blanket, or other comfort symbol with him to the hospital. He should also be allowed to take this object to the operating and recovery rooms. One mother reassured her child that she would be returning by leaving her purse with him. Since he knew that his mother valued her purse, he knew that she would be coming back to get it.

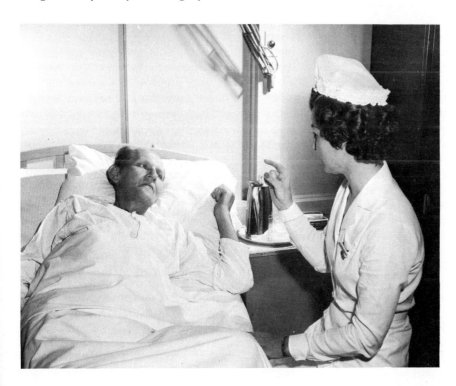

FIG. 11-1. The nurse supplements the physician's explanation of the operation and postoperative care.

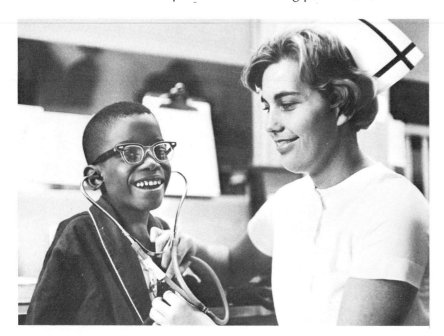

FIG. 11-2. Depending on the child's age and development, he may be shown what it is hoped will be accomplished by surgery. (Courtesy Muhlenberg Hospital, Plainfield, N. J.; photo by Warren R. Vroom.)

Preoperative information

The nurse should know what information has been given to the patient so that she can answer his questions intelligently. Many patients hesitate to ask the physician to repeat information and are often too upset to understand all they have been told or to ask questions. Thus they frequently turn to the nurse for clarification and reinforcement of such information. The nurse may also be questioned about the surgeon's competence, the number of people who have recovered from a similar operation, and about the hospital. Answers should be given factually and in a manner that will inspire confidence in the surgeon, the nursing staff, and other hospital personnel.

Some patients and their families are more frightened by what they do not know or by the unexpected than by what is explained to them and planned with them. Others function better not knowing and will say so if they are given the opportunity. Almost all persons, however, are apprehensive about the preparation for an operation and benefit from some explanation. The responsibility for giving preoperative instructions to the patient belongs primarily to the nurses who care for him in the hospital. However, the nurses in the outpatient department, physician's office, and public health agency also share this responsibility and should tell the patient as much as they can about the preoperative period. The patient and his family should be told how extensive the preoperative preparation will be and approximately how long it will take. The purpose of the physical examination, radiography, and other tests should be explained to them. The patient should be told about preoperative treatments such as shaving and preparation of the operative area, medications, the enema (if one is ordered), and why fluids and food will be withheld. He should know if he will awaken

in a recovery room, if an oxygen tent, suction unit, drainage tubes, IPPB, or other equipment may be used, and if intravenous fluids will be given. If it will be necessary for him to spend time in surgical intensive care, the patient and his family should be informed about the many kinds of monitoring equipment that may be used. The patient's family should also be told when they will be allowed to visit him. He should be instructed in any special exercises that he must do postoperatively such as breathing deeply, coughing, contracting and relaxing the leg muscles, and turning. In order to be sure that the patient completely understands these exercises he should do a return demonstration of them for the nurse.

The patient and his family should be told that frequent blood pressure recordings and other special observations and treatments are the rule, lest they be considered a sign of poor progress. He should also be told that the physician may think it best for him to be out of bed soon after surgery but that assistance in moving and walking will be given.

Preoperative visits. Preoperative visits by the operating room nurse are an important adjunct in preparing the patient for surgery as well as providing the operating room nurse with data that can be used to increase and enhance the effectiveness of nursing care given in the operating room. The operating room nurse should work with the unit nurses in order to know what the patient has already been told. The patient and his family should be told the approximate length of the surgery and the length of the postanestheia recovery period so that they do not become overly anxious. This knowledge also helps the family to plan their time so that they will be available when the patient can have visitors. The operating room nurse should answer questions about the operating room; what the patient will see, hear, and smell before he goes to sleep; and briefly what to expect in the recovery room. The nurse should answer questions regarding the surgical procedure in general terms, while encouraging the patient to clarify specifics with the surgeon. The patient should be offered reassurance when possible, especially regarding the competency of the operating room staff and the measures that will be taken to assist in his recovery. The critical data that the operating room nurse has collected such as hearing impairments, language barriers, obesity, heart disease, etc. will be used to plan for the needs of the patient during surgery and should be passed on to the recovery room nurses in order to provide continuity of care.

When the patient is scheduled to remain in the hospital for only a few hours postoperatively, he and his family will need to be given instructions for postoperative care prior to admission to the hospital. At this time the patient has not received medication to lessen his alertness, and a family member usually is present. These instructions should be reviewed with the patient and his family postoperatively.

■ THE OPERATIVE PERMIT

Informed consent

The patient will be asked to sign a statement indicating that he consents to have the operative procedure performed. This consent implies that the patient has been provided with the knowledge necessary to understand the nature of the procedure to be carried out as well as the known and possible consequences of the procedure. The patient should be informed of the options available to him and the risks associated with each. The patient has thus given his "informed consent" for the procedure to be carried out when he signs the permit. The signed consent protects the hospital and the surgeon against claims that unauthorized surgery has been performed and that the patient was unaware of the potential risks of complication involved. The permit also protects the patient from undergoing unauthorized surgery.

Sometimes the patient wishes to talk to a close family member before signing an operative permit. If so, the nurse should assist him in contacting the relative. If serious, extensive, or disfiguring surgery must be anticipated, the patient may wish to leave the hospital for a short time to confer with relatives or attend to business affairs before he signs the permit. The nurse should realize that signing the operative permit is a very serious step for the patient and one that is taken much more easily when the nurse conveys warmth, friendliness, and sympathy for him at this time of decision.

Permission should be obtained for each operation performed and is usually obtained for major diagnostic procedures that involve entering a body cavity such as thoracentesis, cystoscopy, and bronchoscopy. For the consent to be valid, the person giving it

must be mentally competent. If a patient is determined to be incapable of understanding or is intoxicated, a relative or guardian must sign for him. When mental incompetence has been determined on the basis of a judicial or court determination, permission must be obtained from the legal guardian appointed by the court. The legal guardian may be an individual, an institution, or an agency. If the legal guardian is not available, a court of competent jurisdiction may authorize the operative procedure. The written permission must be witnessed by an authorized person, and who this person can be may vary from one institution to another. If a patient is unable to sign his legal signature, he may write an "X" after which is noted "his mark." In this event, two witnesses are required. In an emergency situation the surgeon may operate without written permission of the patient or his family, although, time permitting, every effort should be made to contact a family member. Consent in the form of a telegram or telephone call is permissible in this situation. It is customary to require the signature of a parent or legal guardian for a minor child. An "emancipated minor," that is, one who is married and/or earning his own livelihood and retaining the earnings, can sign his own permit. The signature of the husband or wife of a married minor is also acceptable. Parenthood alone does not emancipate a minor. Consent for a procedure on the child of an unwed minor parent must be obtained from the adult who is next of kin to the unwed parent. A special informed consent form for a therapeutic abortive procedure and/or an operative procedure that has the express purpose of terminating reproductive capacity may be required. This form usually requires the signature of the patient and his or her spouse.

The nurse is usually responsible for seeing that the operative permit is signed and attached to the patient's chart when he goes to the operating room. The signature should be obtained without pressure and before the patient receives sedation. The patient may refuse to undergo an operation, and it is his privilege to do so.

The nurse should note whether or not a permit has been signed at least a day before an elective operation is scheduled. If it has not been signed or if the patient is reluctant to sign it, the nurse should notify the surgeon at once. The ultimate responsibility for obtaining the necessary permission for an operation rests with the surgeon.

■ PHYSICAL ASSESSMENT AND PREPARATION FOR SURGERY

Both surgery and anesthesia produce changes in the body, and the patient must be in the best possible physical condition to withstand these changes. The cardiovascular, respiratory, and renal systems may be depressed by general anesthetics and therefore are carefully evaluated before surgery. A history of the patient's past and present illnesses is obtained, and a complete physical examination, including laboratory tests, is made to ascertain the patient's physical status and to discover coexisting diseases that might alter the patient's response to surgery or his recovery. Routine radiographs of the chest are taken to be sure that the patient does not have any lung disease that would complicate the operative course or be aggravated by anesthesia. Difficulties associated with inadequate oxygen supply through the lungs and of cardiac function are the ones most often encountered during anesthesia. If the patient is elderly, a measure of his vital capacity may be taken. This precaution is taken because it is sometimes difficult for the elderly patient to obtain enough oxygen, his rib cage having become firmer and alterations having occurred in all the tissues of the respiratory tract, particularly of the lung parenchyma (alveoli). Patients with chronic obstructive pulmonary disease will usually have pulmonary function tests and blood gas studies prior to surgical intervention. Signs of any upper respiratory infection must be noted by the nurse and reported. Usually the surgeon prefers not to operate on any patient of any age within 1 week of his having had symptoms of a cold or other upper respiratory infection.

The patient's urine is always examined preoperatively to detect the presence of urinary tract infection or of any other disease condition that may become a serious problem during and after the operation. For example, the presence of sugar may indicate diabetes mellitus; albumin or a low specific gravity may indicate chronic renal disease; and acetone, particularly in a small child, may indicate starvation and dehydration. Any of these conditions will greatly alter the treatment that is needed before, during, and after surgery. Blood tests such as a complete blood count, hemoglobin determination, and bleeding and clotting time determinations will help ascertain whether or not the patient has a chronic infection or has signs of anemia or other blood dyscrasia. Any one of these conditions may produce difficulties during the operation or interfere with wound healing and thus prolong convalescence. If major surgery is anticipated, blood typing and crossmatching, including determination of the Rh factor, is always done so that a transfusion of blood may be given at once if needed. If the patient is beyond middle age, a blood sugar test may be done to rule out the presence of mild or incipient diabetes, which, if present and untreated, may lead to such postoperative complications as delayed wound healing and infections. Determinations of blood volume are often made preoperatively so that blood and other fluids lost during the operation may be replaced more exactly and the dangers of shock and other complications minimized. An ECG is usually ordered for adult surgical patients and particularly for those patients with a history of cardiac disease. The ECG is especially helpful in determining any cardiac damage or in interpreting arrhythmias.

When the preliminary examinations establish that there is a coexisting disease, a more intensive study is done. Although it may not always be possible to cure coexisting diseases before surgery, knowledge of their presence will influence the care given to the patient in the preoperative period, during the operation, and postoperatively. For instance, efforts are made to bring cardiac disorders and diabetes mellitus under control prior to surgery or general anesthesia. Patients with bronchiectasis or emphysema are frequently treated with aerosol inhalations, IPPB treatments, and postural drainage. They will also have to stop smoking. Many days may be required before the patient with chronic obstructive respiratory disease becomes sufficiently improved to reduce chances of a fatal outcome or undesirable postoperative sequelae. The nurse plays an important role in preparing the patient for preoperative tests, in seeing that the tests are completed, and that the results are filed in the chart before the patient goes to surgery.

During the time that tests are being performed and the patient is being prepared as fully as possible for the anticipated surgery, the nurse should observe him, try to get to know him, and report any significant findings to the physician. Sensitivity to a medicine or an allergic response to adhesive tape, iodine, or merthiolate may not be reported by the patient when he talks to the physician, yet may be mentioned to the nurse. The potent phenothiazines (Thorazine, Vesprin, Stelazine) can cause hypotension and tachycardia during anesthesia, while diazepam (Valium) is not recommended prior to bronchoscopy or laryngoscopy as it may increase the cough reflex and cause laryngospasm. If the patient is receiving any tranquilizer in the hospital or has taken them at home, this should be noted on the chart and reported to the anesthesiologist or the surgeon before the patient goes to surgery.

Nutrition

The patient should be in the best possible nutritional state before undergoing surgery. Dehydration and poor nutrition at the time of surgery have been found to adversely influence the operative prognosis, particularly in infants and in elderly persons. When there is a protein deficiency, wounds heal slowly and there is decreased resistance to infection. A lack of vitamin C also retards wound healing. Excessive vomiting or diarrhea preoperatively will dehydrate the patient and cause electrolyte imbalance. Chronic illness and a poor appetite make a patient a poor candidate for any surgery. When emergency surgery must be done on patients whose nutritional status is poor, an intravenous infusion of fluid containing glucose is started before the patient receives an anesthetic agent.

Every effort is made to correct nutritional deficiency before surgery. A well-balanced diet will be ordered for the patient, and he may receive supplementary protein and vitamins. The nurse should always know how well the patient is eating and should consult with the physician about any problems that may arise. The nurse should explain the importance of restoring and maintaining good nutrition and should encourage the patient to eat the proper foods. When he expresses likes and dislikes or does not eat well, the nurse should ask the dietitian to talk with him so that satisfactory adjustments in his diet can be made. The patient's family may be permitted to bring him special foods that he particularly enjoys. When the patient cannot tolerate food orally, he is given fluids containing glucose, vitamins, and electrolytes parenterally. If marked protein deficiency exists, he may be given transfusions of whole blood or of blood plasma.

■ PREOPERATIVE MANAGEMENT

Preoperative orders

When the patient is ready for surgery, the physician writes orders for the immediate preoperative preparation. In many hospitals these orders cancel all previous ones. The nurse should consult with the physician at this time to see that the orders meet all the patient's needs. Care must be taken that orders for important treatments such as postural drainage or for medications such as digitalis preparations, insulin, steroids, or other hormones are not inadvertently canceled. After the physician tells the patient and his family that the operation is scheduled, the nurse may begin preparing the patient by explaining the procedures and treatments that will be done and supplementing the information given to the patient by the physician.

Diet

Adult. Unless the patient is on a special diet he may have a regular meal the evening before surgery. If the surgery is scheduled late the next day or is going to be performed under local or spinal anesthesia, the doctor usually permits a light breakfast and fluids up to 6 hours before the operation. If the surgery is to be under general anesthesia, fluids usually are permitted until midnight, and the adult patient is told that he must not take anything orally after this time since there is danger that he may vomit while under anesthesia. If he vomits, he may aspirate stomach contents into his lungs. If the patient's mouth becomes very dry while waiting for surgery, a piece of moist gauze may be used to wet his lips. If the nurse discovers that the patient has taken food or fluids immediately before the opera-

tion, she should inform the surgeon, as this will necessitate rescheduling of the surgical procedure.

Child. Differences in the metabolic rate of the infant and the child from that of the adult require that preoperative feeding regimens differ substantially. The metabolic rate is so rapid in children that withholding feedings makes them not only restless and hungry but dehydrated. Their glycogen reserve is proportionately less than that of the adult, so that starvation is tolerated less well and signs of acidosis such as acetone in the urine may occur if some carbohydrate is not given regularly. Therefore infants usually receive formula up to 4 hours prior to anesthesia. Children over the age of 2 can have clear fluids up to 4 hours prior to anesthesia. No child under 8 years of age should be without supplemental glucose for more than 6 hours preoperatively. In the child a smaller proportion of the body fluid is in the intravascular compartment so that changes in body fluids are less well tolerated. More fluid is lost, too, through skin evaporation in the infant and child than in the adult. This greater fluid loss results from the fact that although the infant's body weight is only approximately 5% of an adult's weight, his skin surface, from which evaporation is occurring constantly, is 15% of an adult's skin surface. Before major surgery is started on an infant, a phlebotomy or cutdown and insertion of a fine polyethylene tube usually is done on a vein so that fluids containing glucose and electrolytes can be given without interruption during and following surgery.

Preparation of the skin

Thorough cleansing of the skin surrounding the operative area is carried out preoperatively in order to decrease the entrance of bacteria into the wound from the skin surface at the time of surgery. The bacterial count of the skin can be substantially and progressively reduced by daily cleansings with hexachlorophene preparations. Some surgeons may advise their patients scheduled for elective surgery to use such a product at home several days prior to admission. Cleansing of the skin with the same product should be continued after admission and until surgery. Such a routine is particularly desirable in preparation for orthopedic surgery, since infections of the bones and joints are serious and may lead to permanent dysfunction. It should be noted that hexachlorophene is a chlorinated phenol compound that is insoluble in water but soluble in organic solvents such as alcohol and aqueous zephiran, which will thus remove the effect of the hexachlorophene. Other aspects of surgical asepsis are discussed on p. 79.

Shaving the skin lessens the likelihood of wound infections because it removes the hair to which bacteria may cling. Extreme care must be taken that the skin is not cut during shaving, because cuts are open wounds that can become infected. Most hospitals now use disposable skin preparation sets that are discarded after use. If such sets are not available, an autoclaved razor and new blade should be used for each patient. These measures are necessary to prevent the transmission of serum hepatitis (SH virus) by an inadequately sterilized razor.

The skin should be lubricated with hexachlorophene (pHisoHex), and the hair should be shaved in the direction in which it grows. This part of the skin preparation may be carried out in the operating room or on the patient care unit. The decision of where, when, and by whom the skin preparation is performed is determined by the philosophy and policies established by each hospital. Regardless of where the shave is done, the nurse should explain to the patient the purpose and routine of the procedure. Also, the nurse should be responsible for teaching all personnel who shave patients the correct technique and the importance of not cutting the skin. During the procedure the nurse should make sure that the patient is provided with comfort, safety, and privacy. The patient's body should be maintained in good alignment, utilizing special supports for positioning if needed. During the procedure the nurse should observe the general condition of the patient's skin. If there is any contraindication to the procedure such as lesions, irritations, or evidence of infection, the surgeon should be notified and his instructions followed.

It should be remembered that regardless of the method or products used, the purpose of the preoperative skin prep is to free the operative site of as many bacteria as possible. Thus personnel who carry out this preparation should be made fully aware of the importance of what would seem to be a routine task. Every effort should be made to minimize discomfort and embarrassment of the patient by carrying out the skin preparation in a considerate, orderly, and professional manner.

Usually the surgeon leaves instructions as to how large a skin area he wishes to have prepared. In other instances, the nurse prepares an area specified by hospital procedure for a particular operation. The area to be prepared will be more extensive than actually required for the incision. This allows for a margin of safety and prevents the skin adjacent to the wound from being a source of contamination during draping. If it should become necessary to extend the incision, this can be safely done. Shaving of the skin usually is omitted in the infant and young child. When orders for preparation of the skin are written, the following areas are usually prepared for surgery.

Abdominal procedures. If the patient is a woman, the skin from below the breasts to and including the pubic area is shaved. If the patient is a man, the skin from the nipple line to and including the pubic area is shaved. The umbilicus is cleansed thoroughly with hexachlorophene and water.

Chest procedures. The skin on the affected side from the spine to beyond the midline of the anterior chest and from the clavicle to the crest of ilium is shaved.

Radical mastectomy. The skin from the spine on the affected side to beyond the midline anteriorly and from the clavicle to the umbilicus is shaved. The axilla and the arm on the affected side down to the elbow should also be shaved.

Rectal procedures. The skin within a 6- to 8-inch radius around the rectum is shaved.

Gynecologic procedures. The skin from the umbilicus to and including the pubic area and the perinium is shaved.

Kidney procedures. The skin on the affected side from the spine to beyond the midline anteriorly and from the nipple line to the pubic area is shaved.

Neck surgery. The skin from the chin to the nipple line and to the hairline of the face on both sides is shaved.

Head surgery. The head usually is shaved in the operating room by the surgeon. Long hair should be saved and given to the patient or his family.

Orthopedic procedures. When surgery on the limbs is to be carried out, the entire extremity on the affected side is prepared to facilitate draping and manipulation. Preparation usually includes one joint above and one joint below the operative site.

Other operations. Areas to be prepared for other operations will be specifically ordered by the surgeon. Operations for amputations and spinal surgery require preparation dependent on the extent of the patient's disease and the preference of the surgeon.

Preparation of the bowel

Whether or not an enema is given preoperatively depends on the circumstances as well as on the personal preferences of the surgeon. If the patient has had a normal bowel movement the day before the operative day, and if the anticipated surgery does not involve the gastrointestinal tract and early mobilization is expected, it is now common practice to omit an enema preoperatively. Enemas are seldom ordered for children preoperatively. They are ordered when the surgery involves the gastrointestinal system or the pelvic, perineal, or perianal areas. Any enema given should be effectual. If it is not, the physician must be so informed. If the enema is to be given until the returns are clear, the nurse should ask the physician how many enemas he wishes the patient to have. Repeated enemas tire the patient, upset electrolyte balance, and irritate the rectal and bowel mucosa. Rest periods between enemas are beneficial to the patient, and enemas given slowly often produce better results and thus reduce the number necessary.

Sedation

It is important that the patient rest the night before surgery. Barbiturates such as Seconal, Nembutal, Amytal, and phenobarbital may be ordered for this purpose. Chloral hydrate and Dalmane are nonbarbiturates that are also commonly used. Other drugs such as tranquilizers may be given 1 or 2 days before surgery to decrease anxiety. Small doses of sodium phenobarbital may be ordered for children. Barbiturates are given after all preoperative treatments have been completed. They sometimes cause the patient to become confused, and it is advisable to put side rails on the bed, especially if the patient is elderly. The nurse should instruct the patient to call during the night instead of getting out of bed if he wishes something. The patient should be observed frequently during the night, and if he cannot sleep, it may be helpful if the nurse remains with him for a while and tries to make him as comfortable as possible. If a second barbiturate or any medication for pain is needed, it must be given at least 4 hours before the preoperative medication is due. This precaution will minimize any respiratory depression caused by the cumulative effect of these medications. If it is too late to give the patient medication safely and if he is apprehensive or has pain, the surgeon should be consulted.

Care of the patient on the day of surgery

Care on the morning of surgery depends on the time of surgery and the practices of each institution. Many surgeons feel that patients should be allowed to sleep as long as possible and to rest undisturbed until shortly before the administration of preoperative medication. Consequently, a bath or shower may be taken the evening before surgery instead of the next morning.

The nurse is chiefly concerned with observing the patient's emotional state, checking his physical condition, safeguarding his belongings, and physically preparing him to receive anesthesia. Unless he is sleeping, the nurse should visit with him early and explain all procedures. This will help to allay fear. If the operation is to be delayed even for as short a time as $1/2$ hour, both the patient and his family should be informed.

It is advisable that the patient is not unduly stimulated by visitors before surgery. The patient's choice of whom he wants to see should be taken into consideration whether it be family members or a close friend. The nurse should arrange a short time of privacy for the patient and his visitors. (A parent is usually encouraged to remain with a child.) The patient may desire a visit from a chaplain on the morning of surgery. If the patient is very anxious about the operation and expresses fear about its outcome, the nurse should notify the surgeon or anesthesiologist. Patients who are extremely apprehen-

sive tolerate surgery poorly, and the operation may have to be delayed or canceled.

When the patient awakes or is awakened on the morning of surgery, his vital signs (temperature, pulse, respirations, blood pressure) are taken and recorded. The nurse observes the patient and questions him about how he feels. Signs and symptoms of upper respiratory infections and expressions of new or different pain should be referred to the surgeon. Anesthesia and surgery aggravate such conditions and may cause postoperative complications.

The patient should be given sufficient time to bathe, brush his teeth, and change to a hospital gown before he is called to the operating room. The woman patient is advised to braid her hair if it is long. Most hospitals provide surgical patients with cloth or disposable paper caps when they are transferred to the surgical suite. This practice not only maintains surgical asepsis but protects the patient's hair if he vomits while recovering from anesthesia. Hairpins are removed because they may become dislodged and injure the patient's scalp and because they may cause sparks during administration of anesthetic agents. Patients are also asked to remove nail polish, as it may be necessary to observe nail beds for signs of hypoxia. This is particularly important if an extremity is to be operated on such as an arm or leg, as postoperative checks for adequate circulation to toes or fingers are very important. Religious medals or rosary beads taken to the operating room should be pinned to the patient's gown or secured to the bedpost. All jewelry and money should be taken from the bedside and locked up. The patient is permitted to wear a wedding ring, but it should be taped or tied securely to the hand.

Most anesthesiologists prefer that dentures and removable bridges be removed before the patient goes to the operating room since, as the muscles relax under anesthesia, these prostheses may fall away from the gums and drop back into the pharynx, causing respiratory obstruction. The removal of dentures also prevents their being broken accidentally. Dentures taken from the patient should be labeled immediately with the patient's name and room number and placed in a container in a safe place. Other prostheses such as false limbs or eyes should also be removed, labeled, and placed in safekeeping. If the patient wears a hearing aid, the operating room nurse who will be caring for the patient should be informed. The device may be left with the patient so that the operating room staff can communicate with him in the crucial minutes before surgery. The operating room nurse should remove the device after the patient is asleep and make sure that it goes with him to the recovery room. If the patient does not speak English, an attempt should be made to locate a translator who can accompany him to the operating room and remain with him until anesthesia is induced. Many larger hospitals have foreign language registries of employees who can be called on for such assistance.

The patient should void shortly before going to the operating room to prevent urinary incontinence due to muscle relaxation during the operation. An empty bladder is particularly important in abdominal or pelvic surgery, since it permits a better view of the abdominal cavity and decreases the chances of inadvertent injury to the bladder. Since restriction of fluids causes dehydration, the patient may not be able to void immediately before surgery. Voiding during the preoperative night is sometimes recorded, for this may help determine whether or not catheterization is necessary. If the bladder must be kept in a collapsed state throughout the operation or if the patient has a condition which will interfere with urination postoperatively, an indwelling catheter is inserted and attached by tubing to a closed drainage system.

The surgeon may order the application of elastic bandages (Ace bandages) to both legs and thighs before the patient goes to surgery. These should be wrapped beginning at the toes and working upward. Antiembolic stockings of various lengths are frequently ordered as an alternative to regular elastic bandages. These are very important for patients who have pronounced varicosities, are elderly, are to have surgery that may be time-consuming or that involves removal of any of the pelvic organs, are having a procedure performed that will not allow them to ambulate for a period of time postoperatively, or have a history of embolic formation. This measure helps to prevent the stasis of blood in the veins of the lower extremities by exerting pressure on them and thus lessens the chances of the development of thrombophlebitis. It also assists in preventing shock by keeping blood that might pool in the extremities in the circulating blood system.

Preanesthetic medications

Preanesthetic medication refers to the administration of drugs to decrease anxiety, provide a smoother induction of anesthesia, provide smoother maintenance of anesthesia, and diminish undesirable reflexes during emergence from anesthesia. The medications most commonly used for this purpose include barbiturates, narcotics, and anticholinergic drugs such as atropine. Phenothiazines and tranquilizers may also be prescribed. These drugs are usually given in combination and have several purposes.

Pentobarbital and secobarbital are the barbiturates prescribed most frequently. They minimally depress respiration and circulation and decrease the patient's apprehension. Barbiturates may be ordered alone, given in combination with other drugs, or given before other preanesthetic medications.

The most commonly used preanesthetic narcotics

are morphine and meperidine (Demerol). Morphine assists in reducing anxiety and tension and is one of the drugs of choice if pain is present before surgery. The usual dosage is 8 to 10 mg. intramuscularly. Meperidine in 50 to 100 mg. doses intramuscularly is also commonly used for preanesthetic medication. Both drugs produce depression of respirations. Anticholinergic drugs such as atropine and scopolamine are frequently given in combination with these narcotics. These drugs act to reduce secretions and prevent reflex parasympathetic action on the heart. When the patient receives these drugs, he should be told that his mouth will feel dry.

Phenothiazine derivatives, promethazine and triflupromazine being the most popular, are sometimes used for preanesthetic medication. They are usually combined with a barbiturate or narcotic and are used because of their sedative, antiarrhythmic, antihistaminic, and antiemetic properties.

These medications are generally administered $1\frac{1}{2}$ to 1 hour before the induction of anesthesia. Because the anesthesiologist has timed the preanesthetic medication so that its maximal effects take place before the administration of the anesthesia, any delay in its administration should be reported immediately to him or to the surgeon. Atropine alone is the drug usually ordered for the infant. Occasionally antibiotics are given for their prophylactic effect. They must be given at the exact time specified so that drug levels in the blood will be at their peak during the height of the operation.

After the medication is given, the patient should be carefully observed for signs of respiratory or circulatory depression caused by a sensitivity to the drug or by an overdosage. Because opiates make the patient feel drowsy, lightheaded, and unsteady on his feet, he should stay in bed after they are administered. Some hospitals require that side rails be in place at this time. The patient should be told to call the nurse if he needs anything and reminded not to smoke, as he may fall asleep and drop the cigarette in his bed. The nurse should have completed all preoperative procedures before the medication is given. Noise and confusion should be avoided, and the patient's environment should be kept quiet until he is taken to the operating room. Finally, it should be emphasized that drugs should never be used as a substitute for reassurance and adequate explanations. Studies have shown that the administration of preanesthetic medication without any attempt at psychologic preparation may render the patient drowsy but does not reduce his anxiety.

Recording

The preoperative recording should be accurate and complete. It should contain information on the nurse's notes and the nursing care plan to provide a baseline for observations and nursing care postoperatively. For example, if the patient has any irregular coloring of the nail beds or a slight cyanosis, the condition should be recorded because it would be significant postoperatively. If the patient has any physical limitations or sensory deficits, these should be noted. It is helpful to the recovery room nursing staff if vital signs, especially blood pressure, are recorded more than once preoperatively, as this provides them with more baseline data to compare with postoperative findings. If the patient is exceedingly restless and active preoperatively, his behavior should be recorded so that after surgery it may be understood better. The chart must also contain all the information that the surgeon and the anesthesiologist need at the time of surgery. It is essential that the nurse chart the time the medication was given, the patient's temperature, pulse, and respiratory rate, the time he last voided, whether dentures were removed, and any treatments that were given. The operative permit should be attached to the patient's chart. The nurse should check to be sure that all laboratory, x-ray, and ECG reports are in the chart. If the patient was admitted the evening prior to surgery, it is extremely important to see that the laboratory reports are back and that they are within normal limits. Any abnormality in laboratory findings should be reported to the surgeon before the patient is taken to the operating room. Charts from previous admissions should also be sent with the patient.

Transportation to the operating room

The surgical patient is usually transported to the operating room on a stretcher or in some instances in his bed. The stretcher should be well maintained and in good working condition at all times. It is washed and made up with fresh linen between each patient use. To protect the patient from falling, each stretcher should have restraint straps for over the body and side rails. Stretchers used for transporting children have head and foot rails in addition to side rails. Foot extensions must be available for use with the patient who is over 6 feet tall and extends beyond the end of the stretcher. Personnel transporting the surgical patient must identify themselves to the clinical unit nursing staff and request assistance. The unit nurse assigned to prepare the patient for surgery checks the patient record, accompanies the transportation attendant to the patient's bedside, and signs the patient identification form. Before the patient is transported from his room the patient identification form is attached to the stretcher or bed. The patient is made comfortable with a pillow under his head and a cotton blanket as a cover. Woolen or synthetic blankets must never be sent to the operating room because they are a source of static electricity.

Patients should be protected from drafts, and if the patient holding area in the operating room is kept cool, additional blankets may be needed.

Children may be transported on a stretcher, or in the case of the tiny infant the isolette incubator may be used. The temperature of the operating room must be adjusted for infants and children. The pediatric patient under 12 years of age should be placed on a heating-cooling unit to monitor and maintain the body temperature (see Fig. 11-4).

After the patient arrives in the operating room suite, there should be a minimum of delay, noise, and physical disturbance. The professional nurse responsible for the patient during the operative period should greet the patient by name and identify herself/himself; review the patient record; and check patient identity through identification bracelet, patient record, and asking the patient his name. In the preoperative period the professional nurse in the operating room must assess the patient and his needs in order to develop a plan of care for the operative period.

The patient's family

The patient's family or close friends who plan to be with him the day of surgery should be made aware of the schedule and plans for the day. The nurse should share with the patient and his family the time the patient is scheduled for surgery, the time the patient will leave his room, where the family should wait while the patient is in the operating and postanesthesia recovery room, how they will receive information about the patient after surgery is completed, the length of time the patient is expected to be in the recovery room, policies related to recovery room visitation, and plans for the patient if transfer to an intensive care unit is anticipated postoperatively. If the family does not plan to stay in the hospital during the operative period, they should be made aware of the importance of leaving a phone number where they can be reached.

The patient and his family should be prepared for the use of any special equipment or devices that may be used in the care of the patient postoperatively, that is, oxygen, drainage tubes from catheters, intravenous fluids, monitors, etc. If they are prepared for these nursing care activities, it will lessen the anxiety level of both the patient and his family in the immediate postoperative period.

■ ANESTHESIA
USE

Anesthesia must be given by an experienced person who has been trained in the administration of anesthetic agents. Although surgical nurses do not administer anesthetic agents, they may be called on to assist the physician on the clinical unit or in a specialized area of the hospital such as the emergency room. Therefore nurses should understand anesthetic agents and their purposes and effects. The nurse should also be able to answer questions the patient may have regarding the anesthetic to be administered during surgery. It is essential for the nurse to have an understanding of the preanesthetic preparation of the patient and the effects of anesthetic agents given during the operative phase in order to provide effective nursing care in the postoperative period.

Anesthesia implies amnesia (loss of memory), analgesia (insensibility to pain), hypnosis (artificially produced sleep), and relaxation (rendering a part of the body less firm or rigid). Anesthetic agents that produce unconsciousness and are given by inhalation or intravenous injection are referred to as general anesthetics. Regional anesthesia produces a loss of sensation in a discrete area of the body while the patient remains conscious. Regional anesthetic agents applied to the body surface (topical) and those injected around nerves interfere with the initiation and transmission of nerve impulses; thus the patient experiences no pain.

CHOICE

The choice of anesthesia is based on many factors: the physical condition and age of the patient; the presence of coexisting diseases; the type, site, and duration of the operation; and the personal preference of the anesthetist. The anesthesiologist (a physician with specialized training in anesthesia) evaluates each patient carefully and selects the anesthetic agents best suited for that individual. Within limits of feasibility, an important factor to consider when selecting the anesthetic to be administered is the preference of the patient; that is, many patients may have a preference for spinal, local, or general anesthesia.

An apprehensive patient may not respond well to a regional anesthetic. In some instances patients having intravenous anesthetics may respond with depression of respirations. Spinal and regional anesthetics are not practical for children as they have difficulty in holding still.

ANESTHESIA AND THE PATIENT

Patients have many anxieties and fears related to anesthesia. They may fear going to sleep and not waking up or they may simply have a fear of the unknown. They frequently express a dislike of ether because of a previous experience and the pungent odor of the agent. They may be apprehensive regarding the effectiveness of the anesthesia and fearful of experiencing pain during the surgical procedure. Patients frequently have concern about nausea and vomiting that may occur postoperatively as a result of the anesthesia. Other fears associated with anesthesia may relate to talking and revealing personal information, anticipation of a mask being placed over the face, or having an anesthetic that would not

induce unconsciousness, that is, spinal anesthesia.

Most fears can be dispelled if the patient and his family are well informed about the anesthesia selected for use and the care taken by the physician in assessing the patient's physical condition. The patient should be encouraged to discuss any questions or concerns about the anesthesia with either the anesthesiologist or surgeon.

The nurse can assure the patient and his family that recovery from anesthesia is usually uneventful. They should be made aware that the patient is under close surveillance while under anesthesia and in the immediate postoperative period. The nurse can reassure the patient that he will not be left alone until he has fully recovered from the effects of anesthesia. Very few patients talk while under anesthesia, and what is said is usually unintelligible, so that talking need not be of great concern to the patient. Persistent anxiety on the part of the patient regarding his anesthetic should be discussed with the surgeon and anesthesiologist.

GENERAL ANESTHESIA

General anesthesia is produced by inhalation of gases or vapors of highly volatile liquids or by injection into the bloodstream of anesthetic drugs in solution. Certain drugs that produce general anesthesia such as thiopental sodium (Pentothal sodium) are used to put the patient to sleep and are almost always supplemented with other agents to produce surgical anesthesia. Other general anesthetic agents such as ether do produce surgical anesthesia but are very irritating to the respiratory tract.

Such irritation prolongs the introductory stages of anesthesia. Frequently a combination of inhalation anesthetic agents such as nitrous oxide and oxygen may be used with curare and a narcotic. The choice of agents will depend on the anesthesiologist's judgment and the individual patient's needs.

General anesthesia affects all the physiologic systems of the body to some degree. It affects chiefly the central nervous, respiratory, and circulatory systems. The anesthesiologist judges the depth of anesthesia by the changes produced in these systems. These changes are best observed by monitoring heart rate with the precordial stethoscope, by ECG, blood pressure, and respiratory rate, and by blood gas determinations. Stages of anesthesia are best seen with diethyl ether. Stage I extends from the beginning of the administration of an anesthetic to the beginning of the loss of consciousness. Stage II, often called the stage of excitement or delirium, extends from the loss of consciousness to the loss of eyelid reflexes. If the patient is very apprehensive or was not given premedication correctly or on time, this stage, usually of short duration, may last longer. The patient may become excited and struggle, shout, talk, laugh, or cry. Stage III, the stage of surgical anesthesia, extends from the loss of the lid reflex to cessation of respiratory effort. The patient is unconscious, his muscles are relaxed, and most of his reflexes have been abolished. Stage IV is the stage of overdosage or the stage of danger. It is complicated by respiratory and circulatory failure. Death will follow unless the anesthetic is immediately discontinued and artificial respiration performed. The nurse may find that some patients recovering from the effects of general inhalation anesthesia pass through stage II before becoming fully conscious and are very noisy and restless.

Inhalation anesthesia

Inhalation anesthesia is produced by having the patient inhale the vapors of certain liquids or gases. Oxygen is always given with these anesthetic agents. The gas mixture may be administered by mask, or it may be delivered into the lungs through an endotracheal tube inserted into the trachea. The use of the endotracheal tube is called endotracheal intubation. Intubation assures an airway that can be used to aerate the lungs when the chest wall is open. The endotracheal tube has a balloon that is inflated after insertion. The balloon fills the tracheal space, lessening the chance of aspiration of gastric contents. Regardless of the skill of the anesthesiologist, an endotracheal tube cannot help causing some irritation to the trachea and subsequent edema. Because the child's trachea is smaller, edema may more easily obstruct the lumen. Therefore signs of sudden respiratory difficulty are more likely to occur postoperatively in the child than in the adult. The child's respiratory pattern must be observed carefully when an endotracheal tube has been used. Signs of respiratory embarrassment such as cyanosis or difficulty in inspiring must be reported to the surgeon at once.

Ether. Ether is a volatile, flammable liquid. It has a very pungent odor that is disagreeable to many patients. It is irritating to the mucous membranes of the pulmonary tract and the first and second stages of anesthesia are prolonged. For this reason a rapid-acting, nonirritating drug such as thiopental sodium may be used to produce sleep before ether is administered. Ether is a relatively inexpensive drug. It is used for many operations because it provides excellent muscle relaxation and has a greater margin of safety than some of the other anesthetic agents.

Recovery from anesthesia with ether may be prolonged, especially if a large amount of the drug was used. The patient will require constant supervision until completely awake. Because of ether's irritating qualities, large amounts of mucus may be present, in which case the patient must be suctioned frequently. Since vomiting often occurs after the administration of ether, the patient should be placed on his side to prevent aspiration of any vomitus. If the

foot of the bed is elevated, gravity will aid the flow of mucus and vomitus from the throat and mouth. Before anesthesia is started, an isotonic eye ointment in a petroleum base is frequently instilled into the eyes to prevent irritation. If an irritation does occur, it should be immediately checked and, if serious, an ophthalmologist consulted. Redness or blistering of the skin, which sometimes occurs around the site of the mask, is caused by the combination of ether, moisture, and pressure. This condition can be unsightly and uncomfortable for the patient. Petroleum jelly or other ointments may be applied as ordered to relieve discomfort. When the patient has recovered from anesthesia, he should be encouraged to breathe deeply and to cough productively to clear secretions from the bronchi. Since the odor of ether may be disturbing to others, patients recovering from anesthesia should not be close to other patients.

Nitrous oxide. Nitrous oxide is a nonirritating, odorless, colorless, nonflammable gas. Nitrous oxide should be given with no less than 30% oxygen. The patient becomes anesthetized quickly and recovers rapidly. This gas may be used for dental surgery and as a supplemental agent when ether is to be administered.

Nitrous oxide is also used extensively with halothane and methoxyflurane to supplement their actions. In low concentrations, nitrous oxide may provide adequate anesthesia even for intra-abdominal procedures in patients who are in profound shock, debilitated, or who are critically ill and cannot tolerate other anesthetic agents. If an excessive amount of this gas is administered, there is the possibility of hypoxia. Patients having open chest surgery should have arterial oxygen determinations when inhaling high percentages of nitrous oxide. It is a relatively inexpensive anesthetic agent.

Cyclopropane. Cyclopropane is a highly flammable and pleasant-smelling gas that quickly produces unconsciousness and produces adequate relaxation for most abdominal surgery. Because it is associated with cardiac irritability and causes arrhythmias, it should be used with caution in patients with cardiac diseases. Postoperatively, the patient's pulse rate and cardiac rhythm should be checked frequently for any irregularities that might occur as a result of receiving cyclopropane gas. Emergence excitement is common. Nausea, vomiting, and headache may also occur in the postoperative period. During the administration of this gas, extreme care must be taken to prevent the production of any electric charge that might cause it to be ignited. Operating room procedures should be consistent with those for other hazardous environments.

Halothane. Halothane (Fluothane) is a highly potent, nonflammable, colorless liquid with a sweet smell somewhat resembling chloroform. It is easily inhaled and usually administered through special vaporizers with nitrous oxide and oxygen. Halothane is nonirritating; thus irritation to the larynx is reduced and laryngospasm is infrequent. Induction of anesthesia is usually much faster than with ether and the rate of emergence is more rapid.[37] An important clinical feature of halothane is the low incidence of postoperative nausea and vomiting. Emergence from anesthesia may be accompanied by shivering, probably of neurologic origin rather than the lowered body temperature commonly found.[24] Halothane can depress the circulation when high concentrations are given. It is also a respiratory depressant. A minimum of 30% oxygen should be present in the inspired mixture.[94] Disadvantages are that it is expensive, tends to depress respiration and circulation, and may cause hepatic failure.[37] There is some evidence that in certain very rare individuals, exposure to halothane may lead to sensitization so that subsequent halothane anesthesia may be followed by severe, and indeed fatal, jaundice. Some authorities recommend omitting halothane from the anesthesia sequence if multiple administrations for the same patient are anticipated.[94]

Methoxyflurane. Methoxyflurane (Penthrane) is a clear, colorless liquid with a characteristic fruity odor. It is a nonexplosive and nonflammable agent under normal conditions of clinical anesthesia. It is a halogenated ether and induction is prolonged. This may be overcome by injecting a quick-acting drug such as thiopental sodium before administration of methoxyflurane. Emergence from anesthesia is slow, and the need for analgesic drugs in the immediate postanesthesia period may be lessened. Methoxyflurane is associated with renal toxicity in a dose-related manner. Nausea and vomiting may occur postoperatively but to a lesser degree than after cyclopropane or ether.

Enflurane. Enflurane (Ethrane) is a clear, colorless, nonflammable liquid that has a mild, sweet odor. It is fluorinated ether used for inhalation anesthesia. Induction and recovery from anesthesia with enflurane are rapid. It does not appear to stimulate excess salivation or tracheal-bronchial secretions, and pharyngeal and laryngeal reflexes are readily deadened. Enflurane reduces ventilation and decreases blood pressure as the depth of anesthesia increases. It provokes a sigh response reminiscent of that seen with diethyl ether. Heart rate remains relatively constant.

Muscle relaxation is adequate for intra-abdominal operations at normal levels of anesthesia, and if greater relaxation is necessary, minimal doses of muscle relaxants may be used. All commonly used muscle relaxants are compatible with enflurane. Enflurane may be used for induction and maintenance of general anesthesia. It is contraindicated when the patient is subject to seizure disorders or has a known sensitivity to enflurane or other halogenated anesthetics.

Intravenous anesthesia

Thiopental sodium. Thiopental sodium (Pentothal sodium) is the drug used most frequently for induction of anesthesia. It produces unconsciousness quickly. Recovery is rapid if the total dose is small. Thiopental may also be given to relieve severe, prolonged convulsive states. Laryngeal reflexes are not depressed at light levels of narcosis, and laryngospasm may occur with stimulation of the larynx. Signs of laryngospasm are apprehension, stridor (a harsh whistling sound), retraction of the soft tissue about the neck, and cyanosis. If these signs appear in the postanesthesia period, the nurse should notify the physician immediately. If large doses of thiopental have been used, the patient may sleep for a long period of time and should be observed for signs of respiratory depression. Some individuals appear to awaken quickly only to return to the anesthetized state when undisturbed.[24] The blood pressure may drop suddenly and should be checked frequently. Thiopental is detoxified in the liver and excreted by the kidneys. Therefore in patients with liver or kidney disease this drug should be used with caution.

Thiopental is used primarily to produce sleep before an inhalation anesthetic is administered. The major advantage of this agent is the smooth induction afforded the patient. This anesthetic agent may be used for brief surgical procedures such as closed reduction of a fracture or a dislocation or incision and drainage of an abscess.

Droperidol and fentanyl. Droperidol and fentanyl (Innovar) are the combination of a potent tranquilizer (droperidol) and a powerful narcotic analgesic (fentanyl). Surgical anesthesia is produced quickly and recovery is smooth and rapid. In most patients, orientation returns quickly without restlessness or emergence delirium. Incorporating droperidol and fentanyl into the anesthetic regimen will usually result in a lower incidence of postoperative nausea and vomiting. Because of its apparent lack of toxicity to the liver, kidneys, and heart, it can be given intermittently throughout a surgical procedure. Due to the tranquilizing component, droperidol, the patient requires less analgesia in the postanesthesia recovery room. Patients should be observed for hypoventilation during the immediate recovery period and may need to be urged to breathe. Postoperative narcotic orders should be reduced to one-third or one-fourth the usual amount. Droperidol and fentanyl may be used as premedication, as an adjunct to general anesthesia, alone, or with regional anesthesia.

Ketamine. Ketamine is a nonbarbiturate, parenteral anesthetic agent. The anesthetic state characterized by ketamine is termed *dissociative anesthesia*. It is a substance permitting surgical operations on patients who may appear to be awake since movement may occur and the eyes remain open. However, the individuals are anesthetized so far as recollection or awareness is concerned. Ketamine is chemically related to the hallucinogens, and unpleasant dreams during awakening and extending into the postoperative period may constitute a drawback.[24] To overcome these effects a small dose of a barbiturate is given—or more important the patient is left undisturbed during the emergence phase.[94]

Ketamine produces profound analgesia but does little to block visceral pain, which eliminates its usefulness for intra-abdominal or intrathoracic procedures unless supplemented by an inhalation agent.[24] It is useful in diagnostic procedures such as neuroradiology and for superficial procedures of short duration. Ketamine has been most valuable in the anesthetic management of children and young adults.[24] Contraindications for the use of ketamine include patients with upper respiratory infections, prior cerebrovascular accident, hypertension, and psychiatric disorders.

MUSCLE RELAXANTS

Certain drugs such as *d*-tubocurarine chloride (curare), succinylcholine chloride (Anectine), pancuronium bromide (Pavulon), and gallamine triethiodide (Flaxedil) are neuromuscular blocking agents used to provide muscle relaxation. They are employed for facilitating endotracheal intubation and may also be given as adjuncts to provide sufficient relaxation of abdominal muscles.[37]

These agents cause respiratory depression or paralysis; thus the patient must be observed closely for signs of respiratory distress during and after administration of the drug. Patients developing respiratory problems will require intubation and mechanical ventilatory assistance. All patients who are paralyzed with muscle relaxants require skilled airway management with the capability of endotracheal intubation until the patient is able to maintain his own respirations.

The drug *d*-tubocurarine is injected intravenously in the form of solutions. About one third of the amount administered is excreted unchanged in the urine, whereas the rest is metabolically altered. It is probably still the most important competitive neuromuscular blocking agent.[37]

Succinylcholine chloride is a valuable agent for producing short periods of muscular relaxation. The short duration of action of succinylcholine may be attributed to its rapid metabolic degradation. Facilities for artificial respiration are essential since this appears to be the only effective antidotal measure to apnea.[37]

Pancuronium bromide is approximately five times as potent as *d*-tubocurarine chloride. It has little effect on the circulatory system. The most frequently reported observation is a slight rise in pulse rate. A major portion of administered pancuronium bromide is excreted unchanged in the urine.

Gallamine triethiodide is a synthetic drug that has an atropine-like effect on the cardiac branch of the vagus nerve and can produce considerable tachycardia.[37] It is excreted unchanged in the urine and is not the agent of choice in the presence of poor renal function.

REGIONAL ANESTHESIA

Regional anesthesia is produced by the injection or application of a local anesthetic agent along the course of a nerve, thus abolishing the conduction of all impulses to and from the area supplied by that nerve. The patient experiences no pain in the operative area and remains awake during the entire procedure because the anesthetic affects a particular region only; it does not affect cortical functions.

Regional anesthesia is used for treatments, diagnostic measures, examinations, and surgery. The nurse usually assembles the equipment necessary for the administration of the drugs used to produce anesthesia, assists the physician during the procedure, and observes the patient for reactions to the anesthetic or to the procedure.

The drugs used to produce regional anesthesia are usually called local anesthetics. Examples are procaine (Novocain), cocaine, tetracaine (Pontocaine), dibucaine (Nupercaine), and lidocaine (Xylocaine). When these drugs are absorbed into the bloodstream, they cause stimulation of the central nervous system and depression of the heart. Therefore care is taken that they are given in a localized area and in the smallest dose necessary to produce anesthesia. A barbiturate is usually given before the drugs are administered to reduce patient anxiety. Epinephrine may be added to the solution of local anesthetic drugs to produce vasoconstriction in the area of the injection. Vasoconstriction tends to reduce the rate of absorption, to extend the length of anesthesia, and to reduce hemorrhage. Epinephrine should not be added to solutions when nerve block of the digits is contemplated.

The nurse must observe the patient carefully for signs of excitability (laughing, crying, excessive talking), twitching, pulse or blood pressure changes, pallor of the skin, and respiratory difficulties. At the first sign of these toxic reactions an intravenous injection of a short-acting barbiturate such as thiopental sodium should be ready for the physician to administer. Oxygen may also be necessary, and it is important that a patent airway be maintained. If the reaction is due to an idiosyncrasy to the drug, circulatory failure may occur, and emergency measures such as artificial respiration must be started. Patients should be questioned regarding any previous sensitivity to these drugs, and skin tests are usually advocated before their administration.

Regional anesthesia of the limbs can be achieved by injecting an anesthetizing agent such as lidocaine into a vein in the limb to be anesthetized. A tourniquet is applied to the limb to prevent the distribution of the anesthetizing agent throughout the body.[23,43]

Topical anesthesia. Topical anesthesia is accomplished by applying or spraying a local anesthetic drug such as cocaine or lidocaine directly on the part to be anesthetized. It is used for surgical procedures on the nose and throat and to eliminate pharyngeal and tracheal reflexes during bronchoscopy and similar procedures. Topical anesthesia may be used in genitourinary procedures (urethral meatotomy, cystoscopy) and to provide anesthesia of the lower urethra.

Infiltration anesthesia. Infiltration anesthesia is accomplished by the injection of the anesthetic drug directly into the area to be incised or manipulated. This method is used for minor procedures (incision and drainage, thoracentesis). Nerve block is regional anesthesia in which the drug is injected into or around the nerve a short distance from the site of the operation. This method may be employed for patients having tonsillectomies, dental procedures, or plastic surgery.

In an epidural block the drug is injected into the epidural space and affects a band around the body, depending on the area of the vertebral columns and the dose of the drug. When a caudal block is performed, the drug is injected into the caudal canal lying below the cord and affects the nerve trunks that supply the perineal area.

In a pudendal block a long 20- or 22-gauge spinal needle attached to a Luer syringe is passed just below and beyond the ischial spine. Solution is then injected to anesthetize the internal pudendal nerve. The needle is partially withdrawn and then inserted laterally toward the ischial tuberosity, where more solution is injected, followed by infiltration of the labia in the same manner, which is repeated on the opposite side. Perineal muscles relax in a few minutes and the skin of the perineum is anesthetized.

Spinal anesthesia. Spinal anesthesia is accomplished by the injection of a local anesthetic drug in solution into the subarachnoid space, which contains spinal fluid (Fig. 11-3). The anesthetic drug acts on the nerves as they emerge from the spinal cord. Depending on the type of anesthesia desired, the injection is made through the second, third, or fourth interspace of the lumbar vertebrae. Anesthesia is quickly produced and provides good relaxation of muscles.

Spinal anesthesia is used for surgery of the lower limbs, perineum, and lower abdomen and sometimes for surgery in the upper abdomen such as removal of the gallbladder. It is not used for operations on the upper part of the body because it causes paralysis of the diaphragm and the intercostal muscles used in respiration. A "saddle block" is a low spinal block commonly used in vaginal deliveries. With this block, analgesia rarely extends above the tenth dermatome. The patient may be unable to move her legs for 2 to 8 hours following induction of the anesthetic. With spinal anesthesia the patient may be conscious of pulling sensations throughout the operation, but he experiences no pain. Occasionally a feeling of faintness and nausea occurs because of these sensations. One of the limitations of spinal anesthesia is that the patient may be awake during the operation, although the preoperative medication may make him quite unaware of his surroundings. A screen restricts his vision in the operating room, and a towel may be placed over his eyes. The conversation and activities of the members of the operating room staff should be carried on with his consciousness in mind.

It is a nursing responsibility to remind other members of the surgical team that the patient is awake and that some topics of conversation may be upsetting to him. In some hospitals a sign "Patient

Fig. 11-3. Patient in lateral position for spinal anesthesia.

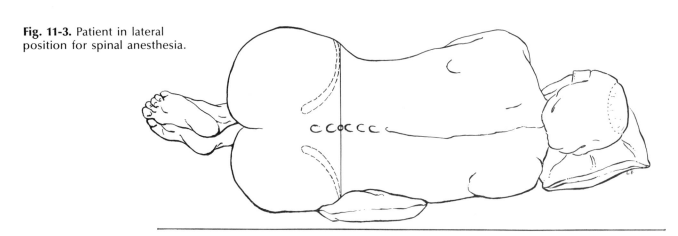

is Awake" is posted both in the operating room and outside the door.

Because of the sympathetic blockade, hypotension may occur with these anesthetic techniques. Vasopressor drugs such as epinephrine hydrochloride may be given if a drop in blood pressure occurs.

Following spinal anesthesia, the patient should be quiet in bed in a supine position. Since sensation may not return to the anesthetized area for an hour or two, the nurse must see that the patient sustains no injuries such as burns from hot-water bottles during this time. The nurse must always be alert for signs of respiratory or circulatory depression. Although the patient is conscious, his blood pressure, pulse, and respirations should be checked frequently. Hypotension may occur as a result of relaxation of the vascular bed.

Headache following spinal anesthesia will be reduced if the patient does not sit up or assume the erect position for 8 hours. Spinal headache is thought to be due to leakage of spinal fluid from the puncture in the dura or to sterile chemical meningitis. It usually occurs 24 hours after the puncture and is more common in women than in men. It may last several days, and occasionally it persists for weeks or months. The nurse should not suggest the possibility of this complication to the patient. If it does occur, the patient complains of a throbbing, pulsating headache that is aggravated by a change to the upright position or by merely coughing or sneezing; an ice bag may bring relief. To lessen discomfort, analgesics and sedatives should be given as ordered. Hydration of the patient is of great importance since it will aid in the replacement of spinal fluid. Increased oral intake should be encouraged. If the patient is receiving nothing orally, intravenous fluids will be ordered.

When the effects of the anesthetic wear off, the patient occasionally complains of a backache. His pain may be the result of the position in which he was placed on the operating table or of the insertion of the needle at the time of the puncture. The complaint is treated symptomatically, and heat applied locally often brings relief.

FIRE, EXPLOSION, AND ELECTRICAL SAFETY

Certain anesthetizing agents such as ether and cyclopropane are flammable and explosive. Therefore extreme caution must be taken at all times to eliminate electric charges that could ignite or explode these agents. Fire and explosion hazards have decreased in recent years as new nonflammable anesthetic agents have been developed, and flammable agents are used with much less frequency. The nurse should be aware of these dangers before entering the operating room suite. All personnel entering the operating room must strictly adhere to the dress code regulations. Conductive shoes or boots are worn in this area.

Today the greatest hazard to the life of the surgical patient is the electrical one. The present concerns revolve around the grounding systems in operating and recovery rooms and the increasing use of electrical monitoring equipment. All electrical equipment used in the operating room area must be grounded, and the nurse should consult with the anesthesiologist before activating the equipment.

INDUCED HYPOTHERMIA
Local hypothermia

Induced local hypothermia refers to the lowering of the temperature of only a part of the body such as a limb. It is used largely to produce surgical anesthesia prior to amputation of a limb affected by arteriosclerotic gangrene. Elderly, debilitated patients and patients who have diabetes are most likely to be treated with this anesthesia. Advantages of this method are that physical shock to the patient is minimal, no inhalation anesthesia is required, and the lowered temperature reduces cell metabolism.

The extremity is packed in ice and anesthesia is usually obtained in $1\frac{1}{2}$ to 3 hours. The duration of anesthesia produced by this method is approximately 60 minutes. The patient may be experiencing pain from the diseased limb and the weight of the ice makes him more uncomfortable; thus there is a need to administer a barbiturate or narcotic before initiating the procedure.

Another method for producing hypothermia in an extremity is through the use of a blanketlike device consisting of coils that contain circulating water. Thus the temperature of the water can be lowered to produce hypothermia and raised when the limb is to be rewarmed.

General hypothermia

General hypothermia for the patient in surgery is rarely used today. It refers to the reduction of body temperature below normal to reduce oxygen and metabolic requirements. Hypothermia is now being used widely for a variety of illnesses when extremely high temperatures occur. For example, patients with neurologic disease causing a high temperature may be kept in a state of relatively mild hypothermia (30.6° to 35° C. or 87° to 95° F.) for as long as 5 days.

If hypothermia is to be used as an adjunct to anesthesia during surgery, the patient usually is given meperidine hydrochloride and atropine sulfate 45 minutes to 1 hour before the procedure is to begin. Provision is made for monitoring temperature readings from different parts of the body, preferably the esophagus and rectum, by placing electric thermometers in these areas. In addition, the heart is monitored with an electrocardiograph to detect cardiac arrhythmias produced by lowered temperature, and the brain is monitored with an electroencephalograph to detect cerebral anoxia. The care of the patient at this time is under the supervision of the operating room team. The temperature is lowered by one of the following methods.

External hypothermia may be produced by applying crushed ice around the patient, by totally immersing the patient in ice water, or by exposing him to the cooling effects of special blankets. The most widely accepted method of hypothermia today is the use of cooling blankets. The patient is placed on and may be covered by body-sized vinyl pads containing many coils. The pads are connected to a reservoir filled with alcohol and water. A pump fills the coils and circulates the solution through the coils in the pad. A recording thermometer monitors the patient's temperature, and an electric unit heats or cools the solution to a preset temperature (Fig. 11-4).

Extracorporeal cooling, a method of bloodstream cooling, consists of removing the blood from a major vessel, circulating it through coils immersed in a refrigerant, and returning it to the body through another vessel. Bloodstream cooling is the fastest method for producing hypothermia and is used primarily for patients who are undergoing surgery. The patient is given heparin to prevent the blood from clotting during the procedure.

Nursing intervention during prolonged hypothermia. If he is conscious, the patient who is to undergo hypothermia for an elevated temperature needs reassurance that the procedure will not be too uncomfortable. Because the treatment is relatively new and is often erroneously conceived by the laity, the patient may have fears and apprehension that should be reported to the physician so that he can answer specific questions that may be causing worry. When hypothermia is to be continued for several days, any of the external methods for producing hypothermia may be used. Before the procedure is started, the patient is given a complete bath and a thin coating of oil or cream may be applied to the skin; a cleansing enema may also be ordered. While the temperature is being lowered to the desired level and for as long as the procedure is continued the patient is observed closely. Any irregularities of pulse, temperature, or blood pressure must be reported at once. It is expected that all of these vital signs will lower gradually. If they rise, drop too suddenly, or fluctuate, the physician should be notified. The temperature is monitored by a rectal thermometer to determine whether or not a desired temperature (usually between 30° and 32° C. or 86° and 89.6° F.) is maintained throughout the treatment.

Shivering is a complication of hypothermia that should be avoided because peripheral vasocontriction is accompanied by an increase in body temperature, circulation rate, and oxygen consumption. Usually shivering occurs when the temperature is

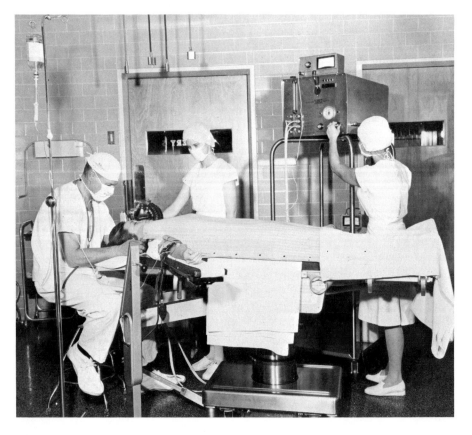

FIG. 11-4. Hypothermia can be produced by means of a cooling blanket. Cold alcohol and water are circulated through the coils by a pressure pump. (Courtesy Gorman-Rupp Industries, Inc., Bellville, Ohio.)

lowered to 30° C. (86° F.). To prevent shivering, chlorpromazine hydrochloride (Thorazine) usually is administered before the treatment is started and is repeated as often as every 2 hours if shivering continues. Since urinary output is decreased when the body temperature is reduced to 32° C. (89° F.), a retention catheter (Foley type) is inserted before hypothermia is started so that output can be measured carefully and recorded. Because the gag and other reflexes may be depressed, food and fluids are not given orally. Fluids containing glucose and electrolytes are given intravenously and usually through a polyethylene catheter that has been sutured into a vein. Depending on the method being used to produce hypothermia, the patient may be fed by means of a nasogastric tube. The patient's skin must be observed for signs of pressure, edema, and discoloration. He should be turned at least every 2 hours, and footboards and pillows should be used to prevent strain on joints and to maintain proper body alignment. Often the patient is placed on a CircOlectric bed to make possible a complete change in position.

Good oral hygiene is necessary, and dried secretions should be removed from the nares. If corneal reflexes are diminished and eye secretions reduced, the eyes may need to be cleansed and covered to protect them as described on p. 189.

The cooling agent or blankets are removed at the termination of hypothermia and regular blankets are applied. The patient is usually allowed to warm at his own rate. The temperature must be observed carefully as it approaches normal, and blankets must then be removed. The thermometer is removed when the temperature becomes stable.

■ POSITIONING THE PATIENT FOR SURGERY

The responsibility for positioning the patient on the operating room table is one shared by the nurse, surgeon, and anesthesiologist. The nurse must be aware of the position required for each surgical procedure and understand the many physiologic changes that occur as the anesthetized patient is placed in a particular operative position.

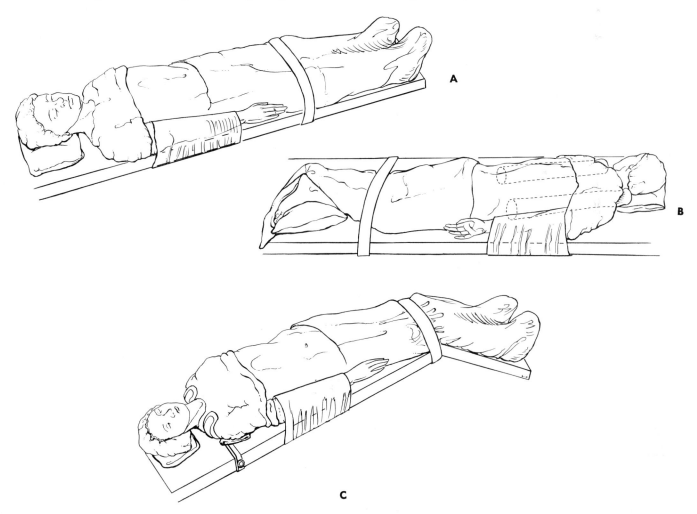

FIG. 11-5. Three commonly used operative positions. **A,** Supine. **B,** Prone. **C,** Trendelenburg.

No matter what position is to be assumed, good positioning is important to (1) adequately expose the operative area; (2) make the patient accessible for induction of anesthesia and administration of intravenous solutions or drugs; (3) minimize interference with circulation due to pressure on a body part; (4) provide protection from injury to nerves due to improper positioning of arms, hands, legs, or feet; (5) provide for the maintenance of respiratory function by avoiding pressure on the chest to allow for adequate ventilation of the lungs and by holding the jaw forward to keep it from dropping on the chest; and (6) provide for the patient's individuality and his privacy by proper draping. A brief discussion of the commonly used operative positions and some of the precautions that are necessary follow.

Supine. In the supine position the patient lies flat on his back with arms at his side, palms down with fingers extended and free to rest on the table, and legs straight with feet slightly separated (Fig. 11-5, A). This is the most commonly used position in the operating room and is used for hernia repair, exploratory laparotomy, cholecystectomy, gastric and bowel resection, and mastectomy. Attention must be given to proper support of the patient's neck and jaw to assure the maintenance of a patent airway.

Prone. In the prone position the patient lies on his abdomen with his face turned to one side and his arms at his side with palms pronated and fingers extended (Fig. 11-5, B). The arms should be well protected and carefully positioned to prevent ulnar or radial nerve damage. Elbows may be slightly flexed to prevent overextension of the shoulders. The patient's feet should be elevated off the table with a small pillow or blanket roll to prevent plantar flexion and pressure on the toes. Body rolls should be placed under each side of the patient to raise the chest and permit the diaphragm to move freely and the lungs to expand. When the patient is in the prone position, the restraint strap is placed below the knee. It is important that the patient's head and neck be positioned properly to assure a patent airway. This position is used for surgery on the back, spine, and rectal area. The patient is anesthetized in the supine position and then placed in the prone position. This position should be assumed gradually and usually four persons are required to turn the patient safely. Details of the turning process can be found in specialized texts and articles.[3,57]

When the surgery is completed, the patient will be returned to the supine position. This should be done gradually and slowly to allow the patient's cardiovascular system to adjust to the change in position. Rapid turning of the patient can cause a precipitous drop in the blood pressure.[57]

Trendelenburg. In the Trendelenburg position the patient's head and body are lowered into a head-down position. The knees are flexed by "breaking" the table, and the patient is held in position by padded shoulder braces (Fig. 11-5, C). This position is used for operations on the lower abdomen and the pelvis to obtain good exposure by a displacement of the intestines into the upper abdomen. The upward position of the viscera decreases the movement of the diaphragm and interferes with respiratory excursion. For this reason this position is not maintained any longer than necessary. The operating room table should be returned to a normal position very slowly so that the patient's cardiovascular system has time to adjust to the shift in position. When the patient is in the Trendelenburg position, blood pools in his upper torso and the blood pressure rises. As the patient is lowered to a normal position, the venous supply is shunted to the legs and a sudden drop in blood pressure may occur.

Reverse Trendelenburg. As the name implies, in this position the head is elevated and the feet are lowered. This position may be used to obtain better visualization of the biliary tract in surgery. The patient must be properly supported by a footboard, body restraints, and a lift sheet around the arms. Since blood will tend to pool in the lower extremities, caution should be used in slowly returning the patient to a normal position. A sudden influx of the pooled blood from the feet can cause an overloading of the cardiovascular system. Obviously this would be of most concern in elderly patients or in those with preexisting cardiovascular problems.

Lithotomy. In the lithotomy position the patient lies on his back with his buttocks to the break in the operating table. After the patient is anesthetized the thighs and legs are flexed at right angles and then simultaneously placed in stirrups (Fig. 11-6, A). This prevents injury, which can occur to the muscle if each leg is flexed and placed in the stirrup separately. The hands and arms may be placed over the patient's chest and secured by his gown or positioned on armboards at his side. They should not extend beyond the break in the table as they may be injured when the table is manipulated. The lower section of the table is then lowered. This position is used in perineal, rectal, and vaginal surgery.

In this position the patient has blood from his legs shunted into his torso and upper extremities. If the patient must remain in the lithotomy position any period of time, Ace bandages are often wrapped around each leg prior to surgery to lessen pooling and thrombus formation. Because of increased pressure on the sacral area, these patients may also develop pressure areas with redness and maceration of the skin.[57]

When the surgery is completed, the patient's legs must be gradually returned to a normal position. As in the Trendelenburg position, rapid lowering of the legs may cause a sudden drop in blood pressure as part of the total blood volume is shunted back into the legs.

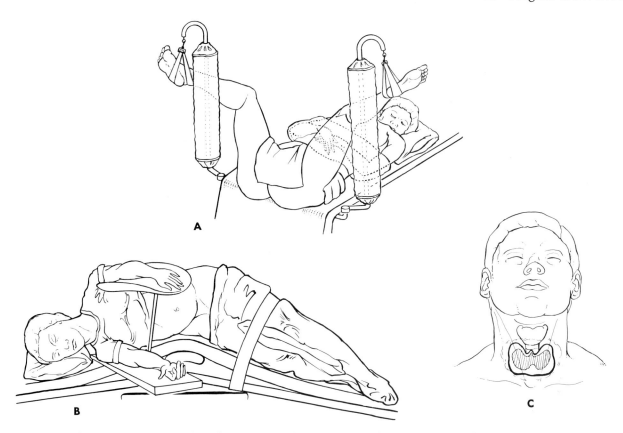

FIG. 11-6. Three operative positions for specialized surgery. **A,** Lithotomy. **B,** Lateral. **C,** Thyroid exposure.

Lateral positions. Various versions of the lateral position are used for surgery on the kidney and the chest. The kidney position (Fig. 11-6, *B*) is used for nephrectomy and pyelolithotomy. As can be seen in Fig. 11-6, *B*, this position puts pressure on the lower arm and leg and blood pools in these areas. The position of the chest allows the upper lung to move more freely than the lower lung. This can interfere with pulmonary ventilation as the two lungs function differently. (See the current literature for further discussion of these problems.[57])

Other positions. Special positions may be necessary to place the operative site in the best possible position. One example of this would be the thyroid exposure (Fig. 11-6, *C*). In this position the patient lies on his back with his head hyperextended and a small sandbag, pillow, or thyroid rest under his neck and shoulders to provide exposure of the thyroid gland.

Special operating tables and attachments are frequently used for genitourinary, rectal, bone, endoscopy, and brain surgery. The operating room nurse, anesthesiologist, and surgeon must be well informed in the use of such tables and attachments and be aware of the desired position for each surgical procedure.

In the past few years more attention than ever has been paid to the proper positioning of the patient to minimize the physiologic changes that occur in the sedated and anesthetized patient. The nurse who is aware that these changes can occur will be more alert to situations in the operating room that can adversely affect the recovery of the patient.

■ NURSING INTERVENTION IN THE IMMEDIATE POSTANESTHETIC PERIOD

The immediate postanesthetic period is a critical one for the patient. He must be observed diligently and must receive intensive physical and psychologic support until the major effects of his anesthetic have worn off and his overall condition stabilizes. The nurse is largely responsible for the care of the patient at this time and must be prepared to meet his specific needs as they arise.

It is the practice in most hospitals that any patient who has received general, dissociative, or regional anesthesia is taken to a postanesthesia recovery room after surgery where he can be given continuous attention for a period of time. In some instances the patient who has had local anesthesia but who requires close observation in the immediate postoperative period may also be cared for in the recovery room. In such an area, specially prepared nursing personnel and all the equipment that may be necessary for the care of the postanesthetic patient are readily available. Ideally, the recovery room is located on the same floor as the operating rooms or in the immediate vicinity. If there is no recovery room, the nurse must prepare the patient's clinical unit with as much equipment as may be needed, considering the individual patient who will be returning to the unit.

Baseline assessment of the patient

The patient should be accompanied to the recovery room or to his clinical unit by the anesthesiologist and another member of the operating room professional staff. While the anesthesiologist remains at the bedside, the nurse begins assessment of the patient by obtaining his vital signs (blood pressure, pulse rate, respiratory rate). Measuring the vital signs also includes evaluation of the pulse volume and regularity, airway patency, symmetry of chest expansion, depth of respirations, and color of the skin. The patient's level of consciousness and ability to follow commands should also be ascertained at this time.

Once it has been determined that the patient's circulatory and ventilatory functions have remained adequate after the transfer from the operating room, the nurse receives reports on the patient's condition from members of the operating room team before assuming responsibility for his care. This report should include: the surgical procedure performed and why; anesthetic agents, narcotics, muscle relaxants, and drugs used for reversal of muscle relaxants; complications encountered during surgery and treatment instituted; blood loss and blood and fluid administration; and pertinent preoperative physical and/or psychologic problems. Information pertaining to the patient's preoperative status may already have been obtained if a preoperative patient visit was made by recovery room nursing personnel.

Following the report, the nurse completes the overall assessment of the patient. The temperature is taken. The surgical site is inspected for dressings and for the presence of drainage or frank bleeding. Tubes and catheters, including intravenous infusion lines, are evaluated for patency. Drainage tubes are connected to proper collection containers and the character of all drainage is noted. The patient who has received regional anesthesia is evaluated as to his ability to move the extremity(ies) and recognize touch in the areas anesthetized. Finally, assessments specific to the surgical procedure performed are carried out, and the physician's order sheet is checked for other instructions and orders for treatments and medications that need to be initiated.

It is essential that there is complete and accurate recording of the immediate postanesthetic course so that those who continue management of the patient have a thorough picture to refer to as necessary. The recording should start with a summary of the patient's status when he is admitted from the operating room, that is, the baseline assessment. Thereafter, changes in the patient's status as determined by frequent reassessments need to be noted. All medications, fluids, and treatments the patient receives during this time must be recorded so that there will be no duplication that might prove harmful to the patient.

Ongoing nursing intervention

Much of the ongoing nursing care provided in the immediate postanesthetic period is dependent on the particular surgical procedure performed and is discussed elsewhere in this text (see specific disease entities and surgical procedures). There are, however, nursing care goals that are the same for all postanesthetic patients: maintenance of pulmonary ventilation, maintenance of circulation, and protection from injury and promotion of comfort.

Maintenance of pulmonary ventilation. The goal of respiratory care for the postoperative patient is to maintain pulmonary ventilation that is adequate to prevent hypoxemia (a deficiency of oxygen in the blood) and hypercapnia (an excess of carbon dioxide in the blood). In the immediate postanesthetic period, two of the most common causes of inadequate pulmonary exchange are airway obstruction and hypoventilation.

Airway obstruction most frequently occurs as a result of the tongue, which is relaxed from anesthesia, falling back against the pharynx or as a result of secretions or other fluids collecting in the pharynx, trachea, or bronchial tree. While caring for the postanesthetic patient, it is essential for the nurse to recognize that all noisy breathing (for example, snoring, gurgling, wheezing, crowing) is indicative of some type of airway obstruction. It is equally important, however, for the nurse to realize that obstruction can occur without being accompanied by noise.

The most desirable position to ensure maintenance of a patent airway depends on the size and condition of the patient, the anesthesia used, the surgery performed, and the amount of experienced nursing care that is available. Ideally, the patient should be in a position so that he can breathe normally with full use of all portions of his lungs and so that vomitus, blood, and mucus can drain out and will not be aspirated. Until protective reflexes have returned, the best position for the majority of patients is a side-lying or semiprone position with the head tilted back and the jaw supported forward. It is important to remember that aspiration can occur unless the *whole body* is turned. Turning the patient's head when his chest and shoulders remain in the back-lying position is useless. Although the side-lying position somewhat diminishes chest expansion, it has the advantages of helping to keep the tongue forward and promoting the drainage of secretions and other fluids outside the mouth. The disadvantage related to chest expansion can be minimized by turning the patient frequently and by raising the flexed upper arm and placing it on a pillow. The supine position with head hyperextended permits fullest expansion of the lungs, but as noted, it is dangerous because of its potential for aspiration or obstruction from secretions. Unless absolutely necessary, this position should not be used before the patient's pharyngeal reflexes have returned and he is able to manage his own secretions. When the supine position must be used, all supplies for suctioning as well as personnel to perform the procedure must be available at the bedside at all times.

An oro- or nasopharyngeal airway is often left in place following the administration of a general anesthetic to keep the passage open and the tongue forward until pharyngeal reflexes have returned. These artificial airways are made of rubber, plastic, or metal. They should be removed as soon as the patient begins to awaken since their presence can be irritating and can stimulate vomiting or laryngospasm. If an artificial airway is ineffective or if one is not in place, the majority of obstructions due to the tongue falling back can be alleviated by holding the patient's jaw up and forward or by positioning him on his side as described previously. When absolutely necessary to clear the airway, the nurse can open the patient's mouth by pushing at the angle of the jaw with the thumbs and have someone insert a padded tongue depressor between the back teeth. The tongue can then be brought forward by grasping it with a piece of gauze. An endotracheal tube may need to be inserted by the physician if there is considerable difficulty maintaining a patent airway.

Excessive secretions from the nasopharynx or tracheobronchial mucosa can also lead to partial or complete airway obstruction. Unless the patient can manage these secretions by coughing them up and expectorating them, they must be removed by suctioning. Pharyngeal suctioning is often all that must be done (Fig. 11-7). If intratracheal suctioning is necessary, sterile technique should be used and the patient should be hyperventilated with 100% oxygen before and after each introduction of the catheter into the trachea. Rarely, but occasionally, a bronchoscopy may be needed to remove secretions, especially if they are very inspissated. When thick secretions are a problem or potential problem, the humidity of the air breathed should be increased to keep secretions as thin as possible and to prevent dry air from further irritating the already irritated respiratory passages.

Postoperative hypoventilation results from numerous causes. Respirations can be directly de-

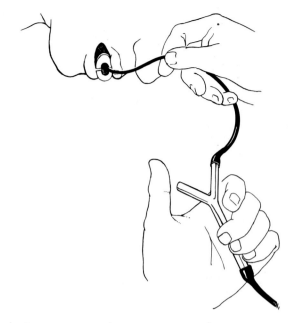

FIG. 11-7. Inserting catheter into airway of unconscious patient. The Y tube valve is left open until the catheter is inserted and in place. The Y opening is then occluded with the thumb and the secretions are aspirated.

pressed by drugs, which may have been administered preoperatively, intraoperatively, or postoperatively. These drugs include inhalation and intravenous anesthetic agents, narcotics, tranquilizers, and sedatives. The residual effects of muscle relaxants and of high spinal or epidural anesthesia in which paralysis of the lower rib cage muscles results can limit the patient's power to breathe. Incisional pain, obesity, gastric dilatation, and constrictive surgical dressings also can interfere with lung expansion and thus with respiratory exchange.

Oxygen is usually given postoperatively because after anesthesia almost all patients have decreased pulmonary expansion and areas of atelectasis, both of which result in hypoxemia. Oxygen is administered by nasal cannula or catheter, disposable face mask or shield, or endotracheal or tracheotomy tube if one is in place. How long postoperative oxygen therapy should be continued depends on the individual patient. As a general rule, all patients should receive oxygen at least until they are conscious and able to take deep breaths on command. Prolonged oxygen therapy should be guided by arterial blood gas determinations. Patients with thoracic or upper abdominal incisions or with preexisting pulmonary disease may be given oxygen for several hours, perhaps until the next day. Special care must be taken when administering oxygen to patients with chronic obstructive pulmonary disease so that hypoxemia, which is their stimulus to breathe, is not entirely removed. Any patient experiencing shivering, which increases oxygen consumption, should receive oxygen therapy until the shivering has ceased.

To help maintain normal levels of arterial blood gases and to counteract hypoventilation, all patients need to be encouraged to breathe deeply at frequent intervals. Ideally the patient will take three or four deep inhalations every 10 to 15 minutes. If the patient is unconscious or if he will not breathe deeply when stimulated, the nurse can hyperventilate his lungs passively using a breathing bag and mask.

When hypoventilation exists to the extent that hypercapnia is present, the patient must have respiratory assistance. Drug therapies that might be indicated include narcotic antagonists such as nalorphine or naloxone to counteract the respiratory depressant effects of the opiate, reversal agents such as neostigmine or edrophonium to counteract the effects of nondepolarizing muscle relaxants, and narcotics themselves if pain is causing the patient to splint his respirations. With obesity, elevation of the head of the bed is often helpful in relieving pressure on the diaphragm. Nasogastric tubes may be inserted to relieve gastric distention. Constrictive dressings must be loosened. When these measures are ineffective in improving ventilation and in instances of excessive respiratory depression from depolarizing muscle relaxant drugs or from high spinal anesthesia, the patient may need to be intubated and receive mechanical ventilator assistance.

Maintenance of circulation. Hypotension and cardiac arrhythmias are the most commonly encountered cardiovascular complications of the immediate postanesthetic period. Early recognition and management of these complications before they become serious enough to diminish cardiac output is dependent on frequent assessment of the patient's vital signs. The blood pressure, pulse, and respirations are usually taken every 15 minutes until stable, then every half-hour for 2 hours, and then every 4 hours until ordered otherwise. In many hospitals the monitoring of vital signs every 15 minutes extends for as long as the patient is in the recovery room and for at least 1 hour after he leaves the recovery room. The rate, volume, and rhythm of the pulse should be carefully observed and the character and rate of respiration noted.

Moving the patient from the operating room table to his bed, jarring during transport, reactions to drugs and anesthesia, loss of blood and other body fluids, cardiac arrhythmias, cardiac failure, inadequate ventilation, pain, and residual sympathectomy from conductive anesthesia are among the many factors that will cause circulatory changes that may result in lowering the blood pressure. A mild decrease in the patient's blood pressure from his normal preoperative range is not uncommon during the early postoperative period. It is usually well tolerated in healthy patients and does not require treatment.

Shock, however, must be prevented because the brain, heart, kidneys, and other vital organs do not tolerate long periods of hypoxemia. A weak, thready pulse with a significant drop in blood pressure may indicate hemorrhage or circulatory failure. The surgeon and/or anesthesiologist should be notified at once if any of these signs occur, especially if the patient's skin becomes cold, moist, pale, or cyanotic or he suddenly becomes restless or apprehensive. Oxygen therapy should be started to increase the oxygen saturation of the circulating blood. Unless contraindicated, the patient's legs should be elevated to facilitate venous return. Blood, plasma, or other intravenous fluids usually are ordered to increase the blood volume when the hypotension is due to hypovolemia. Vasopressor agents may be used when vasodilation is apparent. Digitalis preparations or other inotropic agents may be administered if the decrease in blood pressure is due to cardiac failure.

When a cardiac arrhythmia is detected, it is important for the nurse to ascertain if the patient has a history of such a disturbance. Arrhythmias unchanged from those that existed preoperatively usually do not require treatment. When there is no history of a cardiac irregularity but one has developed postoperatively, the nurse should immediately assess the patient to determine if he is ventilating adequately. Oxygen should be started while the physician is being notified. A patient who is exchanging gases poorly should receive ventilatory assistance with a bag and mask. Hypoxemia and hypercapnia are common causes of postoperative cardiac arrhythmias, especially premature beats and sinus tachycardia. These arrhythmias often can be suppressed by adequate ventilation. Frequent premature beats of ventricular origin, which are not decreased by oxygen therapy, are usually treated with drugs such as intravenous lidocaine (Xylocaine) or procainamide (Pronestyl). The sinus bradycardia that may follow the administration of neostigmine (Prostigmine) or edrophonium (Tensilon) is counteracted by the administration of atropine. Other common causes of postoperative cardiac arrhythmias include pain, hypovolemia, gastric distention, and acidosis. In the event that a life-threatening arrhythmia such as ventricular fibrillation or cardiac asystole occurs, resuscitation efforts must be started immediately.

Protection from injury and promotion of comfort. Following anesthesia, side rails on the stretcher or bed are generally placed in the up position and are left so until the patient is fully awake. Although the patient is constantly watched, it is possible for him to turn suddenly and throw himself from the bed. Hot-water bottles, heating pads, heat lamps, or cast driers must be used with great care while the patient is unconscious or semiconscious so that burns do not occur. When infusions are being given, the patient's arm should be secured on an armboard if the needle is in an area where it could be easily dislodged. Physical restraints are seldom used if the patient is restless. Instead, the nurse should remain with the patient and guide his movements so he does not hurt himself. Restraints can be frightening to the semiconscious individual and may stimulate him to struggle violently to get away from them. The patient should be turned frequently and placed in good body alignment to prevent nerve damage from pressure and muscle and joint strain due to lying in one position for a long period of time. The nurse must be constantly aware that unconscious patients and those recovering from spinal or epidural anesthesia have loss of sensation and are unable to indicate discomfort.

The immediate postanesthetic period is often a frightening time for the patient. Psychologic support is imperative for his physical as well as his emotional well-being. While awakening from anesthesia, the patient needs frequent orientation as to where he is and reassurance that he is not alone. He also needs to know that his operation is over and that he is recovering from anesthesia satisfactorily. Procedures carried out should be carefully explained to him even when it appears that he is not alert. Patients who receive this type of support frequently recover from anesthesia faster, with fewer complications, and with less incisional pain. The patient who has had regional anesthesia needs the same information and needs to be reassured that the sensation and movement in his extremities will return.

Incisional pain is a common complaint after surgery, and from the patient's point of view it is probably the most significant postoperative complication. It is discussed in detail elsewhere (Chapter 8). In the immediate postanesthetic period, narcotic analgesics should be given for pain when warranted, but should be done so with the realization that pronounced depression of the respiratory, circulatory, and/or central nervous systems may follow. Because the patient generally has not completely recovered from the effects of anesthetic agents, the first postoperative dose of a narcotic is usually reduced to about one-half the dose he will be receiving after he has fully recovered from anesthesia. Pain medication for restlessness should be given only after it has been determined that the restlessness is not a result of hypoxia.

Discharge from the recovery room

Multiple criteria can be used to determine when a patient has sufficiently recovered from anesthesia to be transferred from the recovery room. At discharge the patient's vital signs should be stable and indicative of adequate respiratory and circulatory function. He should be awake or easily aroused and able to call for assistance if needed. Any complications encountered, including excessive wound drainage, vomiting, fever, pain, or inadequate urinary output as well as complications specific to the type of surgery performed, must have been thoroughly evaluated and must be under control. The patient who has had regional anesthesia should have motor as well as partial sensory return to all areas that were anesthetized. Acutely ill patients who cannot adequately fulfill these criteria are usually transferred to an intensive care unit.

Before discharging a patient, the recovery room nurse needs to determine that there is adequate nursing staff available on the clinical unit to receive and care for him. All pertinent information concerning the patient's status must be communicated to the nurse who will be continuing to provide his postoperative nursing care.

■ GENERAL POSTOPERATIVE CARE

Preparation for return of the patient to the clinical unit

Before the patient returns to the clinical unit from the postanesthesia recovery room, the nurse should prepare the room to facilitate meeting the patient's needs in the immediate postoperative period. The bed should be made so that the patient can be moved easily from stretcher to bed. The bed should have added protection in areas where drainage may be expected to occur and sufficient covers to ensure patient warmth.

The patient's room should be cleared of any unnecessary equipment and a clear passageway provided for approach to the bed by the stretcher. Equipment that will be needed should be placed in readiness. This equipment will depend on the type of surgery and might include such items as an intravenous pole, emesis basin, tissues, sphygmomanometer, and stethoscope. The recovery room nurse should alert the unit staff of any specialized equipment such as suction or oxygen that may be needed.

The nurse on the clinical unit should show the greatest consideration to the patient's family during the time that he is in the operating and recovery rooms. The family should be informed of the patient's progress, particularly when the patient's return to the unit has been delayed. Information that can be shared with the patient's family helps to lessen their anxiety.

Most surgeons discuss the results of the operation with the family immediately after the surgery and also visit the patient, telling him briefly what was found and reassuring him about his condition. The family is frequently highly anxious concerning the patient's condition and may not perceive or understand all that the surgeon tells them. The patient frequently experiences periods of amnesia during the hours when he first regains consciousness and may not remember what he has been told. The nurse needs to know what information was given to the patient and family so as to be able to answer their questions. The family also needs to know what to expect when the patient returns to his bed on the unit.

Return of the patient to the clinical unit

The recovery room nurse generally calls the unit when the patient is ready to be transferred and reports on the patient's condition. When the patient arrives, the unit nurse should accompany him to his room and assist with a smooth transfer from stretcher to bed.

Assessment of the patient's status. The nurse should make an immediate assessment of the patient to collect data concerning his general condition. The following data should be obtained:

Respiratory status	Patency of airway, depth, rate, and character of respirations
Circulatory status	Vital signs, color and temperature of skin, pedal pulses if indicated
Neurologic status	Level of alertness
Wound	Presence of drainage on dressings, presence of tubes from dressing that need to be connected to drainage systems
Tubes	Intravenous—rate, amount in bottle, tubing not entangled from transfer; presence of other tubing (e.g., nasogastric tube, indwelling catheter), type, patency of tubing, connection of appropriate containers, character and amount of infusion or drainage
Comfort	Patient position—facilitation of good ventilation; position of comfort, head slightly elevated unless contraindicated; presence of pain, nausea, or vomiting
Safety	Necessity for side rails

Additional data collection. Once the initial patient assessment is completed, the nurse should collect the following data from the patient's record:

Surgical notes	Postoperative diagnosis, type of surgery performed, anesthesia, problems incurred during surgery, estimated blood loss, amount of fluid replacement, presence of drains, condition of patient when leaving surgical suite
Recovery room summary	Level at which vital signs stabilized (for comparison of present vital signs), course of patient while in recovery room, type and time of medications given, time and amount of urine if patient voided

Planning patient care. The nurse utilizes the collected data to identify the specific needs of the patient in the postoperative period. The preoperative condition of the patient, type of surgery performed, and strengths and resources of the patient are determining factors influencing the occurrence of postoperative discomforts or complications. In planning the patient's care, therefore, the nurse needs to utilize previously collected data plus knowledge of factors related to specific types of surgery (as illustrated in succeeding chapters of this text) and of predisposing causes of postoperative complications. Specific plans for care should be written on the nursing care plan and observations made during the patient assessment should be charted.

■ COMPLICATIONS AND THEIR PREVENTION

Much of the nursing care given postoperatively is directed toward the prevention of complications, and this care should be started as soon as the patient returns from the operating room. The nurse should know what complications can develop, how to help prevent them, and their early signs and symptoms.

Respiratory complications

The most common respiratory complications are bronchitis, atelectasis, and pneumonia. *Bronchitis* is an inflammation of the bronchi. *Atelectasis* is the blockage of air to a portion of the lung, causing this portion to collapse. *Pneumonia*, a bacterial infection, often follows atelectasis. Signs and symptoms of these complications usually develop within 24 to 48 hours after surgery. There is usually a rise in the patient's temperature and in his pulse and respiratory rates. He may or may not complain of chest pain, cough, or difficulty in breathing. Cyanosis may occur, and the patient may be restless and apprehensive. These complaints should be brought to the physician's attention immediately.

Although most patients experience some respiratory irritation following intubation and inhalation anesthesia, respiratory complications most frequently occur in patients who smoke heavily; in those who suffer from chronic respiratory diseases such as bronchitis, emphysema, or bronchiectasis; or in those who are very young, elderly, debilitated, or obese. They are most likely to occur after high abdominal operations when prolonged inhalation anesthesia has been necessary and vomiting has occurred during the operation or while the patient is recovering from anesthesia. Gastric contents are known to be extremely irritating to the lungs, and most patients who aspirate vomitus postoperatively develop respiratory complications.

If the postoperative patient is kept on his side or in a semiprone position until he is fully awake, has the respiratory passages suctioned when necessary, is turned frequently, and is encouraged to breathe deeply and to cough productively, respiratory complications usually can be prevented. Even after awakening from anesthesia, the back-lying position is not advisable for the elderly patient sleeping soundly under sedation or for any patient with a history of sinusitis or chronic postnasal drip, since there is danger of aspiration of infected material from the nasopharynx.

Following inhalation anesthesia, bronchial secretions usually are increased. Unless the mucus is removed, the bronchioles will become obstructed and atelectasis will occur. The lungs may be inadequately aerated because of incomplete excursion of the chest. Preanesthetic and postoperative medications, anesthesia, and shock tend to depress respirations. Tight abdominal dressings or binders tend to inhibit normal action of the abdominal muscles and the diaphragm, causing the lung bases to remain uninflated. In the elderly patient, firming of the rib cage and loss of elasticity of chest structures increase this problem. Surgical trauma, especially after high abdominal operations, may lead to injury of fibers of the phrenic nerve, causing the diaphragm to become flaccid and relaxed. Pain in the incision or fear of pain may prevent the patient from fully expanding his chest cavity on inspiration. The patient then tends to have shallow respirations and to compensate for the restricted intake of air by breathing rapidly. Any factors that limit the full expansion of the lungs encourage the development of atelectasis because the ability to expel bronchial exudates and to aerate the lung is decreased. As the air is absorbed behind the occluded bronchioles, more exudates are produced and consolidation of this portion of the lung usually occurs. This condition is known as pneumonitis or inflammation of the lung.

Turning. If the patient lies in one position with continuous pressure from his weight against the chest wall, proper ventilation and drainage of secretions on that side of the chest are not possible, and atelectasis can develop. Atelectasis can be prevented by changing the patient's position frequently while he is on bed rest. Turning and changing of position provide for better ventilation of the lungs by encouraging deep respiration and drainage of secretions. The patient should be turned at least every 2 or 3 hours. His position may usually be rotated in the following manner: side, back, side, abdomen. When turning is restricted by the nature of the operation, he should be moved within the specified limitations. Although turning may increase pain in the incision, the nurse can use techniques that will cause as little discomfort as possible such as turning the patient in one smooth movement. When the patient is able to cooperate in turning, the nurse can help him to first move his head and trunk to the side of the bed and then move his buttocks and lower extremities. The patient then is in a good position to roll onto his side or abdomen. Good body mechanics should be used to protect both the patient and the nurse from injury, and the nurse should not attempt to move a helpless or very heavy patient without assistance. When the desired position is attained, the patient should be placed in good body alignment with all dependent parts supported to prevent pull on the incision and unnatural strain on muscles and joints. Pillows placed against the back and abdomen and between the legs may make the patient more comfortable in a side-lying position. Unless contraindicated, the head of the bed should be elevated slightly. The schedule for turning the patient should be interrupted only when he is out of bed for several hours at a time and should be discontinued only when medical examination indicates that his lungs are clear and expanding fully. Radiographs may be taken to verify the return of the lungs to normal function.

Deep breathing and coughing. When the patient coughs productively, he expels any mucous secretions blocking the bronchi. Deep breathing often causes the patient to cough, and it assures complete ventilation of the lungs. The frequency for deep breathing and coughing exercises to be carried out by the patient depends on the presence of any of the predisposing factors to respiratory complications. The greater the possibility that these complications may occur, the more frequently the exercises should be carried out. Thus an elderly patient with a history of lung disease who smokes and has just had high abdominal surgery may need to carry out coughing and deep breathing exercises as often as every 15 to 30 minutes during the first few hours postoperatively. All patients who have had inhalation anesthesia should be asked to deep breathe and cough at least every 2 hours during the early postoperative period. Coughing may be contraindicated in a few instances such as following brain, spinal, or eye surgery. The nurse should assess each patient considering the predisposing factors present in the situation as well as assessing the present respiratory status. As the patient becomes more active and the risk of complications decreases, ventilation exercises can be spaced farther apart.

The patient can be taught abdominal breathing, in which he relaxes his abdominal muscles as he breathes in and thus causes his diaphragm to go down, and contracts his abdominal muscles as he breathes out and thus draws the diaphragm up. The nurse can determine whether or not he is breathing correctly by placing her hand lightly on his abdomen as be breathes. The abdomen should rise with inspiration and fall with expiration. This type of breathing permits the diaphragm to descend fully and the entire lung to expand. If there are secretions in the bronchi, deep breathing will stimulate coughing and expectoration of the mucus. The patient should be asked to do the breathing exercises at frequent intervals himself.

Since most patients find coughing painful after surgery, they need encouragement and assistance. Some surgeons advocate the administration of narcotics before coughing is begun. Narcotics decrease the cough reflex, however, and heavily sedated patients should be encouraged to cough more frequently. The nurse can promote patient comfort during coughing by "splinting" the operative area with a drawsheet or towel (see Fig. 22-16), small pillow, or placement of the nurse's hands firmly on either side of the incision and exerting slight pressure. Such splinting prevents excessive muscular strain around the incision. If the patient must remain flat in bed while he coughs, restraining bedclothes and pillows should be removed from around the chest. If he is permitted to sit up in bed, a pull rope attached to the foot of the bed will help him assume and maintain a sitting position while coughing. The patient should be encouraged to cough deeply and productively. If the first attempt is not successful, he should rest and then try again.

Other measures may be indicated to increase pulmonary ventilation with high-risk patients. A rebreathing tube such as the Adler or Dale-Schwartz tube uses the principle of the patient rebreathing expired air, which is higher in carbon dioxide content. The increased carbon dioxide stimulates the respiratory center to increase the depth of breathing, thus increasing the amount of inspired air. Blow bottles are another method often favored by a patient because he can view his own progress. The patient blows through a tube, forcing fluid to flow from one bottle to another. The goal is to try to move approximately 800 ml. of fluid with one breath. The patient is forced to take a deep breath in order to accomplish this and the pressure of the fluid produces forced expiration against resistance. An IPPB machine may be ordered by the physician to assist the patient who cannot cough effectively (p. 567). An adequate fluid intake will help liquefy secretions, and humidity may need to be added to the patient's inspired air.

It is often exceedingly difficult to induce children to breathe deeply and to cough. A variety of games such as blowing balloons, soap bubbles, feathers across a table, or colored water from one bottle to another (Fig. 11-8) may be used to encourage children to breathe deeply and cough.

Coughing at regular intervals should be continued until the lungs are clear of all secretions. The condition of the lungs is determined by auscultation, percussion, and radiographic examination. If excessive amounts of secretions are present and the patient is unable to cough productively, nasopharyngeal suctioning may be indicated. Tracheobronchial suctioning should only be carried out by a physician or nurse who is specially trained to do so (p. 591). If these means are ineffective, the physician may have to pass a bronchoscope to remove pulmonary secretions.

Circulatory complications

The formation of clots in the veins of the pelvis and the lower extremities is a fairly common and potentially serious postoperative complication. It is thought to be due to impairment of the venous flow of blood and to trauma or irritation of walls of the veins. Additional factors related to anesthesia and surgery may play a part in the development of this complication following an operation. Most surgeons believe that early ambulation helps prevent the development of venous complications. This conviction, along with the knowledge that moving freely and getting out of bed soon after an operation are beneficial to all body systems, accounts for the emphasis on early ambulation for almost all operative patients. Venous stasis occurs in the lower trunk and extremities as a result of muscular inactivity, of postoperative respiratory and circulatory depression, and of

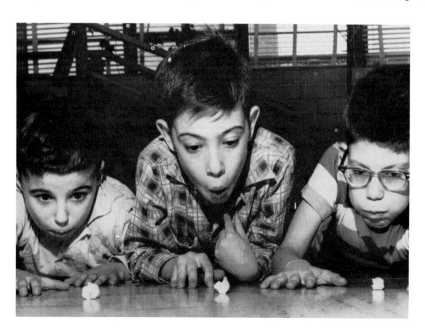

FIG. 11-8. A variety of games such as blowing wads of paper across the room may be used to get children to breathe deeply and to cough. (Courtesy Today's Health, American Medical Association, Chicago, Ill.; UPI photo.)

increased pressure on blood vessels from tight dressings, intestinal distention, and prolonged maintenance of a sitting position. Other contributing factors are obesity, cardiovascular diseases, debility, malnutrition, foci of infection, and old age. Vascular complications occur much more frequently in adults than in children, although they can and do occur in adolescents. Varicose veins predispose the patient to the development of vascular complications. In an effort to prevent this development it is now routine practice in many hospitals to have all elderly patients and those with evidence of varicosities wear elastic bandages (Ace bandages) or elastic stockings when in bed and when walking for the first time. Elastic bandages should be applied smoothly with even pressure from the foot to the knee, midthigh, or groin and should be rewrapped whenever they become loose, usually two to three times daily. Elastic stockings should be removed at least once daily to permit washing of the legs.

Phlebothrombosis and *thrombophlebitis* are the most common circulatory complications. The two terms are sometimes used interchangeably and they may be difficult to distinguish since inflammation almost always follows the formation of a thrombus as well as the obstruction of a blood vessel. The term "phlebothrombosis" usually designates a clot formed in one of the larger veins without inflammation of the vein and sometimes giving no symptoms of inflammation. Postoperatively it often forms in a vein of the foot or the calf, where it may cause pain on dorsiflexion of the foot (Homan's sign). However, pain does not always occur. The thrombus is soft, loosely attached distally, and its free end floats in the blood. As it enlarges, the thrombus, or a portion of it, may break loose from its attachment and may be carried by the bloodstream to the lungs, heart, or brain and cause a sudden fatal embolism. A common site for an embolism to lodge is the lungs (pulmonary embolism), where it causes sudden sharp, upper abdominal or thoracic pain, dyspnea, shock, and frequently death (p. 581). Phlebothrombosis is the most common cause of pulmonary embolism.[46] Because of the danger of dislodging a clot, even if the patient has no symptoms, the nurse should never massage the muscle portion of a postoperative patient's limbs without a written order. If a patient is noted to be massaging his leg, the nurse should question him about his discomfort and report it to the physician. If the patient complains of pain in the foot, the calf of the leg, or the thigh on walking, he should be put to bed at once and advised to keep the limb quiet, and the physician should be notified.

In thrombophlebitis the clot develops and becomes firmly attached to a vein wall and increases until it occludes the lumen of the vein. Because of the firm attachment of the clot, thrombi are not likely to break loose and enter the bloodstream. It is be-

lieved to occur most often in vessels irritated or inflamed by pressure or other factors. It occurs in either deep or superficial veins, where it is accompanied by pain and local tenderness. If a superficial vein is involved, thrombophlebitis can be noted as a reddened line along the vessel route, which feels firm on gentle palpation. If it forms in the femoral or iliac veins, the entire limb becomes swollen, pale, and cold. There is usually exquisite tenderness along the course of the vein. The swelling and coldness are caused by lymphatic obstruction and arterial spasm. The patient's temperature often rises. If the thrombophlebitis is confined to the saphenous vein, the accompanying edema is not so marked, but pain and tenderness are just as severe, and heat and redness can be noted along the inflamed vein. The development of the thrombi prolongs the patient's convalescence. He is confined to bed, and intensive treatment is begun (p. 392).

Postoperative exercises and early ambulation. Nursing measures to help prevent thrombus formation should be initiated at once after the operation. Bed exercises and early ambulation are known to minimize the effects of venous stasis caused by bed rest, and they usually are contraindicated only in the presence of thromboembolic diseases or after vascular surgery such as anastomosis of a blood vessel. Specific exercises for the upper extremities are not usually necessary since the patient uses his arms in eating, bathing, combing his hair, and reaching for articles on his bedside stand or overbed table. (For specific exercises when needed, see p. 811.)

Exercises of the lower extremities are particularly important in the prevention of venous stasis and should be performed until the patient is up and walking about several hours a day (Fig. 11-9). He should be taught to bend his knees, to lower them, and to push the backs of the knees hard against the bed. The nurse's hand can be slipped under the popliteal area while the patient pushes hard against it. The same thing can be accomplished by having the patient alternately contract and relax his calf and thigh muscles. This should be done at least 10 times, and a brief period of rest should follow each contraction and relaxation. The cycle is contract, relax, and rest. Leg exercises should also include flexion, extension, adduction, and abduction of the leg and extension, flexion, and rotation of the foot. A footboard placed at the bottom of the bed, against which the foot can rest in the normal walking position and against which the patient can push firmly, will help prevent foot drop and provide additional exercise. Whenever possible, the patient should lie on his abdomen for $\frac{1}{2}$ hour two or three times a day to prevent blood from pooling in the pelvic cavity. This position also prevents contracture at the hip joint. Until he is permitted out of bed, he should have supervised exercise at least every 4 hours, but he should be en-

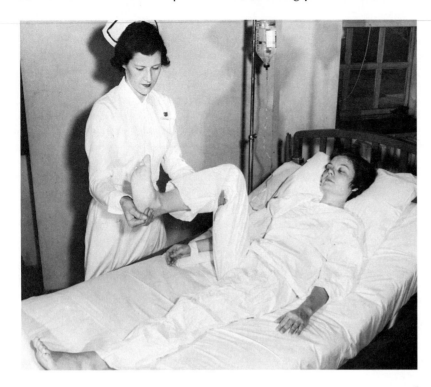

FIG. 11-9. Supervising the postoperative patient in bed exercises. Here the nurse assists the patient as she bends the knee and dorsiflexes the foot.

couraged to do the exercises more frequently than scheduled and to move his legs about in bed as much as possible. The bed should be made so that the bed linen does not restrict the patient's movements. If the patient is unable to do these exercises actively, they should be done passively by the nurse.

If the patient has responded well to surgery and does not show excessive fatigue, ambulation usually is started within 24 hours after surgery. Before ambulating, the nurse should assist the patient to sit on the side of the bed and dangle his legs. Once he has become accustomed to being in an upright position, he may be helped out of bed. At first he should walk only a short distance and should not be pushed beyond his physical ability. The distance walked should be increased each time, and usually the patient is encouraged to walk two or three times a day. When the patient becomes tired he should return to bed.

The nurse should assist and supervise the patient in getting out of bed and walking until he is able to do this without difficulty or danger of injury to himself. Early ambulation should not consist of sitting in a chair at the bedside, since this posture may cause increased stasis of blood in the lower extremities. If the patient is permitted to sit in a chair, he should be advised to stand up frequently and walk about. When he is sitting, he should elevate his legs on another chair to prevent pooling of venous blood in the lower extremities. The legs should be supported from the knees to the ankles, but there should be no pressure against the popliteal area. Some surgeons have advised the use of rocking chairs postop-

eratively since the movement necessary to rock the chair provides excellent exercise for the legs.

Most patients are more confident if there are two people to help when they get up for the first time. However, by using good body mechanics, one nurse can help most postoperative patients out of bed for the first time without personal injury or injury to the patient. The nurse should walk beside the patient, linking arms so that his palm is up and the nurse's palm is down. If the patient becomes weak, the nurse can then slide her arm up into the patient's axilla and, by moving her outer leg to the side, provide a wide enough base of support to balance the patient against her hip until help arrives.

When the nurse helps the patient up for the first time, his condition should be appraised carefully to see what problems are involved. The aged patient usually has difficulty getting up because of stiff joints and muscle weakness. Patients who have arthritis or arteriosclerosis or who have been on prolonged bed rest may need extra time to become ambulatory. They should sit on the edge of the bed and dangle their feet for short periods before walking is attempted. Their progress may be slow, and they should be observed with special care for signs of fatigue. They may need assistance longer than most patients. The fact that any patient is to be out of bed at intervals should never be taken by the nurse as a sign that he is able to care for himself.

Young children usually recover quickly from the effects of surgery and often sit up and walk around in their cribs without urging. Older children occasionally are fearful of injuring the operative site and must be encouraged to leave the bed and move about freely.

Treatments need not interfere with helping the patient out of bed. If the patient is receiving an infusion, the bottle of infusion fluid can be hung on a movable pole that can be wheeled by the nurse as the patient walks. Permission is usually given by the physician to clamp off nasogastric tubes for a short period of time. Urethral catheters should remain attached to the closed drainage system. Plastic drainage bags make ambulation for these patients possible.

Pain. Pain in the incision is a common postoperative complaint. The patient often becomes aware of this pain as soon as he awakens from anesthesia. It usually lasts 24 to 48 hours after surgery, but it may continue longer, depending on the surgery performed, the pain threshold of the patient, and his psychologic response to pain. Most of this pain arises from trauma to the somatic nerve fibers in the skin. It is sharp and localized. Muscles and fascia are also supplied with somatic nerve fibers, and extensive dissection or prolonged retraction of these tissues will produce deep, long-lasting pain. Pain in the operative area may be aggravated by skin sutures, tight dressings, swelling of the incision during healing, and the presence of infection or hematomas in the wound. Continuous and severe pain can produce anxiety, restlessness, sleeplessness, anorexia, and irritability. Its presence can also prolong convalescence since it may interfere with return to activity.

It is not always possible to prevent the occurrence of pain, but it can be alleviated so that the patient is relatively comfortable. Patients who have had adequate preoperative instructions and who have confidence in the surgeon, in the nurses, and in the outcome of the surgery usually have less postoperative pain than the apprehensive patient because they have less tension. Infants and young children usually recover from symptoms of pain more quickly than older people. Pain can be relieved by nursing measures and/or by the administration of narcotics. The patient's position often aggravates wound pain by causing pressure or pull on the incision. A change of position, elevation of the head of the bed, loosening of restraining sheets, and support of dependent parts of the body may give relief. Dressings that are binding or casts that are too tight should be reported to the physician so that they can be loosened or removed.

In addition to making the patient as comfortable as possible, it is usually necessary to give a narcotic. Considerable nursing judgment is required in administering postoperative orders for narcotics. However, the nurse should keep in mind the need to have the patient free enough from pain so that he can breathe deeply, cough, and turn without too much difficulty. The patient who is in pain often splints his chest, breathes shallowly, and fails to move about in bed adequately. Although narcotics such as morphine can depress the patient's respirations, they can be given quite safely to most postsurgical patients whose respiratory rate is over 16/minute. Meperidine hydrochloride may cause a drop in blood pressure. Therefore the patient's blood pressure should be monitored closely after the drug is administered. This is especially important if the patient's blood pressure has been low or unstable. If the nurse is in doubt about giving a narcotic for pain, the surgeon should be consulted. Most surgeons prefer that their patients be kept fairly comfortable for the first few hours postoperatively since they feel this facilitates postoperative nursing care and recovery of the patient.

Narcotics can be given every 3 to 4 hours during the first 12 to 36 hours postoperatively without danger of addiction, but they may cause urticaria, restlessness, nausea, and vomiting. Therefore the patient should be observed for any untoward reaction. A patient who has received a narcotic shortly before getting out of bed to walk should be supervised closely since the action of the drug may cause him to become dizzy or faint. The need for narcotics should decrease after 48 hours, and continuous, severe pain after this time should be reported to the physician.

■ CARE OF THE WOUND

Most surgical wounds are clean, closed wounds that heal rapidly with a minimum of scarring. After the incision has been sutured, the incised skin surfaces are quickly glued together by strands of fibrin and a thin layer of clotted blood. Plasma seeps onto the surface, forming a dry protective crust. There should be a very small amount of serous drainage from such a wound, and after a few hours all seepage onto the dressing should cease.

Occasionally surgeons leave an operative wound uncovered, believing that healing progresses best when the wound is exposed to air. Usually, however, for psychologic reasons and to prevent trauma, the wound is covered in the operating room with a dry sterile dressing. Medicated sprays form a protective, transparent film on the skin and are being used as dressings over clean incisions. The film lasts 3 to 4 days; it may be removed with acetone or will form flakes and peel off eventually. This type of dressing is particularly useful in covering wounds in children. Some surgeons and pediatricians believe that sedatives and analgesic drugs in small carefully measured doses should be given to children postoperatively to prevent pronounced pain and restlessness. The nurse should assess the need for restraints with a small child who may be tampering with the wound or dressing. The age of the child, ability to reason, presence and anxiety level of family members, type of surgery, actions of medications given, and safety of the child are factors utilized by the nurse in assessing the need for any type of restraint that might be necessary.

Drains may be inserted at the time of surgery to allow fluids such as bile, pus, and serum to drain from the operative site and prevent the development of deep wound infections (Fig. 11-10). They may exit directly from the incision or through a separate small incision known as a stab wound. The nurse should check with the surgeon or look on the operative sheet to determine the exact location of drains in order to know the type and amount of drainage to expect. Drainage from stab wounds may be profuse, and a catheter that can be attached to low suction may be used as the drain.

If there is no drainage, the dressing does not need to be changed until the sutures are removed. The suture line is weakest during the third to sixth day after surgery. After this time there is union of deep tissues as a result of fibroplasia and collagen deposition. Increase in wound strength progresses rapidly from the sixth to the fourteenth day and then continues slowly for some months. Although wound union is only relatively firm until after the sixth postoperative day, the sutures permit the patient to cough, turn, and get out of bed without danger of wound separation. It is important for the patient to know this fact. Otherwise he may be reluctant to participate in such activities for fear of harming the incision. Skin sutures (black silk thread, fine wire, or metal skin clips) are removed from abdominal wounds on about the seventh postoperative day, from neck and face wounds on about the third to the fifth postoperative day, and from wounds of the ex-

tremities on the eighth to tenth postoperative day. Retention sutures made of heavy wire and placed deep into muscle tissue usually are not removed until the fourteenth to the twenty-first postoperative day. Most patients become apprehensive when they know the sutures are to be removed. They may be told that they will have little, if any, pain during the procedure. Unless there is some seepage of fluid after the sutures are removed, a dressing is not necessary, and the area may be washed.

The most exact attention to good aseptic technique is essential in caring for all wounds, since organisms can be introduced from the environment into wounds, including those already infected. (For the correct technique in changing dressings see texts on fundamentals of nursing.) Care must be taken that a drain is not inadvertently removed when the dressings are changed. Neither must the drain be permitted to slip into a deep wound, where probing, with possible trauma to the wound, might be needed to remove it. Thin drains such as Penrose drains are usually anchored with a large safety pin that cannot enter the wound opening. A piece of gauze dressing is placed under the pin to keep it from direct contact with the skin about the wound. Using Montgomery straps simplifies changing the dressings and eliminates the repeated removal of adhesive tape from the skin. If the drainage is irritating to the skin, the skin should be washed frequently with soap and water and a protective ointment may be applied. The character and amount of drainage should be recorded, and any change in the amount, color, or consistency should be reported to the surgeon. The patient should be told the reason for the drainage so that he does not become alarmed when he sees it on the dressing or on his gown. Drains are shortened gradu-

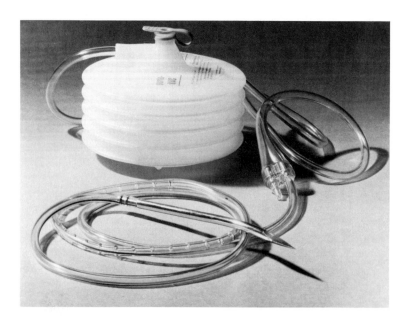

FIG. 11-10. Porto-Vac portable wound suction unit consists of bellows with top port, drain plug, and side port; x-ray opaque wound tube with needle attached; and connector tube. The needle, with wound tube attached, is placed in the wound and brought out through healthy tissue near the wound. After the wound tube is cut from the needle, it is assembled to the connector tube. To establish vacuum, the connecting tube is attached to the side port of the bellows, the drain plug on top of bellows is opened, the bellows are depressed against a solid surface, and the drain plug reinserted. Drainage is removed by opening drain plug, inverting bellows, and pouring fluid out. (Courtesy Howmedica, Inc., Medical Division, Rutherford, N. J.)

ally and are removed when the drainage has diminished sufficiently. The opening caused by the drain heals in a few days.

Hemorrhage from the wound

Although hemorrhage from the wound is most likely to occur within the first 48 hours postoperatively, it may occur as late as the sixth or seventh postoperative day in apparently normal wounds, and after a much longer time if the wound is infected. Hemorrhage occurring soon after operation may be due to the slipping of a ligature or the mechanical dislodging of a clot, caused, for example, by vomiting after a tonsillectomy. Hemorrhage may also be caused by the reestablished blood flow through vessels that, if the patient's blood pressure was low or if a tourniquet was used during the operation, were not noticed and properly obliterated. Hemorrhage after a few days may be due to sloughing of a clot or of tissue, to infection, or to erosion of a blood vessel by a drainage tube.

The nurse should inspect every postoperative dressing frequently. If bright red blood is present, the area should be outlined with a pencil so that the rate of increase can easily be determined. The surgeon should be notified at once. The dressings then should be checked at 15-minute intervals or more often to determine the rate of bleeding, and the patient should be observed for other signs of hemorrhage such as fall in blood pressure, rise in pulse and respiratory rates, restlessness, pallor, weakness, and cold, moist skin. If the bleeding is profuse, the nurse should apply a pressure dressing and remain with the patient until the surgeon arrives. The nurse should remain calm so that the patient is not unduly alarmed. The patient's blood pressure should be taken in order to help determine the extent of the hemorrhage. The nursing staff should gather equipment that the physician may need such as infusion fluid, material for drawing blood for typing and crossmatching, shock blocks, and dressing equipment. The physician usually treats a wound hemorrhage by applying pressure on the wound to occlude the bleeding vessels and, if necessary, administering an infusion to replace fluid loss. A hemostatic gelatin sponge such as Gelfoam soaked in saline solution is sometimes used to control wound bleeding. The sponge is applied to the bleeding site, and pressure is exerted for 2 to 4 minutes. It is left in place and, over a period of several weeks, is absorbed. As absorption occurs, drainage from the wound may appear dark, and pieces of black material may be on the dressing occasionally.

When severe wound hemorrhage occurs, the patient is taken immediately to the operating room, where the wound is opened and the bleeding vessel ligated. If a preanesthetic medication is ordered, the nurse should check to see when the last narcotic was given. Under pressure of the emergency there is danger that the patient may receive an overdose of narcotic, thus causing respiratory and circulatory depression and prohibiting the administration of an anesthetic. Since the patient often becomes frightened by the hemorrhage and the subsequent emergency procedures, the nurse should make every effort to reassure him and to keep noise, confusion, and technical discussions at the bedside to a minimum.

Infection

Wound infections are fairly common postoperative complications. The causative organisms often are staphylococci and streptococci that have been introduced into the wound. Wound infections are more prevalent in debilitated and obese patients possibly because the blood supply to the site of operation may be impaired. From 3 to 6 days after surgery the patient begins to have a low-grade fever, and the wound becomes painful and swollen. The nurse should be alert for purulent drainage on the dressing. Complaints of persistent pain in the incision should be reported to the physician, who may change the dressing to inspect the wound. If spontaneous drainage of the wound does not occur, and if there is definite evidence of infection, the surgeon may choose to open a portion of the healed incision to facilitate drainage. Wound discomfort usually disappears when this procedure is done. The nurse usually is asked to change the dressings as necessary.

A culture and sensitivity study may be made of the fluid obtained from an infected wound, and the administration of appropriate antibiotics is started either immediately or when the report of culture growth is obtained. For superficial wound infections, sterile, warm, wet dressings may be ordered. (See fundamentals of nursing texts for the procedure.) Sometimes infected wounds have to be irrigated or have packing that must be changed at intervals (p. 61).

Dehiscence and evisceration

Wound disruption (dehiscence) is a partial to complete separation of the wound edges. Wound evisceration is protrusion of abdominal viscera through the incision and onto the abdominal wall. These complications often are brought to the nurse's attention by the patient's complaint of a "giving" sensation in the incision or of a sudden, profuse leakage of fluid from the incision. On inspection, the dressing will be found to be saturated with clear, pink drainage. The wound edges may be partially or entirely separated, and loops of intestine may be lying on the abdominal wall (Fig. 11-11). These complications may occur at any time through the fourteenth postoperative day, but they usually occur between the sixth and the eighth day. They are thought to be due to cachexia, anemia, advanced age, hypoproteinemia, dehydra-

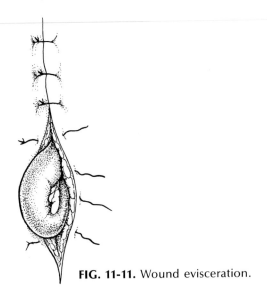

FIG. 11-11. Wound evisceration.

tion, infection, or excessive vomiting, retching, and coughing.

If the patient experiences either a wound dehiscence or wound evisceration, he should be put to bed in a low Fowler's position and told to remain quiet, not to cough, and not to eat or drink anything until the surgeon arrives. Protruding viscera should be covered, preferably with a warm, sterile saline dressing. The nurse should observe the patient for signs of shock (increased pulse and respirations, decreasing blood pressure, cold, moist skin, restlessness). The surgeon will redress the wound after inspection and start an infusion if shock is present or incipient.

The treatment for wound dehiscence and wound evisceration is immediate closure of the wound under local or intravenous anesthesia. Since the patient is likely to be in shock, he is taken to the operating room in his bed, and preanesthetic medication usually is not given. These serious complications are potential threats to the patient's life, involve a second operation, and prolong convalescence, although usually the wound heals surprisingly well following the secondary closure.

■ RETURN OF URINARY FUNCTION

If the patient is well hydrated, urinary function usually returns within 6 to 8 hours after surgery. Although 2,000 to 3,000 ml. of intravenous solution usually is given on the operative day, the first voiding may not be more than 200 ml., and the total urinary output for the operative day may be less than 1,500 ml. The small amount of urinary output, in relation to fluid intake, is due to the loss of body fluid during surgery and to perspiration, hyperventilation, vomiting, and increased secretion of antidiuretic hormone (ADH) due to the stress response to sur-

gery. As body functions stabilize and fluid and electrolyte balance returns to normal, however, the ratio of intake to output should also return to normal. This process may take about 48 hours, and during this time a record is kept of the intake and the time and amount of each voiding. If the urinary output is less than 500 ml. in 24 hours, this fact must be reported to the surgeon, since the decreased urinary output may be due to a decrease in the glomerular filtration rate secondary to shock or a reaction to the anesthetic or other drugs.

Occasionally, after extensive surgery in elderly patients or other patients who have shown signs of shock immediately following surgery, a retention catheter (Foley catheter) is inserted before the patient awakens from anesthesia. Urine is then collected in a sterile calibrated container and the surgeon may wish to be notified if the output is less than 30 ml./hour. This decrease in output may indicate impending renal failure, which should be prevented by immediate measures to raise the patient's blood pressure. Measures might include giving whole blood, blood volume expanders, and other fluids and vasopressors such as metaraminol bitartrate (Aramine).

Some patients are unable to void after surgery and may thus experience severe discomfort. The difficulty may be due to the recumbent position, nervous tension, the effects of anesthetics that interfere with bladder sensation and the ability to void, the use of narcotics that reduce the sensation of bladder distention, the pain caused by movement onto the bedpan, or pain at the site of operation if it is near the bladder or urethra. Inability to void is a common occurrence following surgery on the rectum or colon and following gynecologic procedures since the innervation of the bladder musculature may be temporarily disturbed, and local edema may increase the difficulty. Voiding may be facilitated by nursing measures such as forcing fluids, placing the patient on the bedpan at regular intervals, running the water in the sink while the patient is on the bedpan, pouring warm water over the perineum, having the patient use a straw to blow bubbles into a glass of water, and assuring the patient of privacy. Many men can void if they are allowed to stand at the side of the bed. Women can often void if allowed bathroom privileges. If these measures are not effective, the physician may order catheterization. Because of the emotional trauma to the young child, the possibility of reproductive tract infections in men, and the danger of urinary infection to all patients, the physician may delay catheterization longer than the usual 8 hours postoperatively in the hope that the patient will void normally. If the bladder is palpable over the pubic bone and suprapubic pressure causes discomfort, however, catheterization is usually ordered to prevent stretching of the vesical wall. Marked and prolonged distention of the bladder may cause infection of the urinary system and atony of the bladder muscles, resulting in inability to void later. If the patient must be catheterized repeatedly after an operation, a Foley catheter usually is inserted into the bladder and fluids are forced. Good perineal care of a patient with an indwelling catheter will help to prevent ascending infection. Bacteria can move up the outside of the catheter by means of capillary action.

Occasionally a patient voids frequently but in small amounts. This condition is known as "retention with overflow." The overdistended bladder expels just enough urine to relieve the pressure within it temporarily. The condition should be reported to the physician, who will probably order the patient catheterized for residual urine. Since a large volume of residual urine is a good medium for bacterial growth, a Foley catheter may be left in place for several days. Otherwise catheterization usually is performed every 6 to 8 hours until the residual urine left in the bladder after voiding is less than 50 ml.

Postoperative urinary tract infection can usually be avoided by emptying the bladder completely at each voiding, preventing bladder distention, and using sterile, nontraumatic technique when catheterizations are necessary. Staphylococcal infection of the urinary tract, a common complication of catheterization, is thought to be most often caused by poor technique in performing the procedure. Patients who must be on prolonged bed rest, who have had urinary tract infections in the past, who are elderly, or who have had operations on the pelvic organs are especially prone to bladder and kidney infections. Special attention should be given to the amount and quality of their urinary output, and they should drink at least 3,000 ml. of fluid a day unless this measure is contraindicated by age or by cardiac or renal dysfunction. Symptoms such as a burning sensation in the bladder and urethra during or after urination, frequency, chills, fever, malaise, and anorexia may be indicative of urinary tract infection and should be reported to the physician.

■ RETURN OF GASTROINTESTINAL FUNCTION

Following surgery, gastrointestinal function returns to normal more quickly if the patient's usual diet can be resumed at once. Fluids (not chilled) and food are often given as tolerated after the patient has reacted fully from the anesthesia and all sensations of nausea and vomiting have passed. There is some evidence that iced fluids tend to cause gaseous distention and distress. Most children can take clear fluids the evening of the operative day and a soft diet the day after surgery. With careful attention to giving suitable fluids and foods orally in frequent small amounts, the need for parenteral fluids may be obviated. There is general agreement that the best way

to supply essential foods to all patients is orally, and some surgeons believe that the patient should eat solid food because mastication promotes flow of saliva, which aids digestion and stimulates the stomach to empty. This process, in turn, stimulates peristalsis in the lower tract. Discomfort from accumulation of flatus and the need for enemas and other treatment for distention and constipation can probably be reduced further by the patient's moving about freely in bed and by early ambulation. Ingestion of solid food also helps to prevent the occurrence of nonepidemic parotitis, a painful inflammation of the salivary glands that occurs occasionally in debilitated patients who have poor oral hygiene and who also may be dehydrated. If the patient has had operative treatment of a fracture of a bone, surgery of the chest, or a simple herniorraphy, for example, food usually is given as tolerated. No patient, however, should be urged to eat solid food for a day or two following anesthesia and surgery. Urging solid food when the patient has no appetite may induce vomiting, which will cause pain and distress and may lessen the desire to eat.

Since a quick return to good nutritional status speeds wound healing, the patient should be encouraged to eat a well-balanced diet as soon as he can tolerate one. It is estimated that a caloric intake of 50% more than the basic caloric requirement for the individual is needed to provide for energy expended in early ambulation and for reparative processes.[44] An attractive, well-balanced general diet should be served, and the patient should be allowed to select what appeals to him. After even a few days of enforced starvation, the patient may be somewhat indifferent to food. It may take 2 or 3 days on a well-balanced general diet to overcome this condition, brought on, in part at least, by lack of food. Special surgical diets usually are ordered only after gastric or bowel surgery. Special diets for medical conditions such as diabetes mellitus or cardiac insufficiency should be resumed as soon as possible after surgery.

When surgery has been performed on the gastrointestinal tract or on the closely related organs within the abdomen, fluids and foods are not given until peristalsis returns. A nasogastric tube may be inserted preoperatively and left in place for approximately 24 hours if surgery has been performed on the gallbladder and for approximately 2 to 4 days if an operation has been performed on the stomach. A nasogastric or a Miller-Abbott tube may be inserted and left in place approximately 2 to 5 days if surgery has been done on the small or the large bowel. These decompression tubes, attached to suction, remove flatus that may cause tension on the operative site or fluids and secretions that may accumulate. Because these tubes remove secretions containing electrolytes and because they cause general discomfort, they are removed as soon as possible. While they are in use the patient is given nothing orally, and he is given fluids intravenously that contain nutrients and electrolytes to meet, as nearly as possible, his daily needs and to restore losses caused by use of the decompression tube. However, it is impossible to meet metabolic needs fully by giving fluids parenterally except by hyperalimentation (Chapter 5). By using modified gastric tubes (Abbott-Rawson or Olander-Puestow) it is possible to decompress the stomach as necessary following gastric surgery and yet supply liquid feedings into the jejunum. The use of these tubes thus provides better nutrition. The greatest care should be taken that tubes used for decompression do not cause further nausea, since it increases the danger of serious postoperative respiratory complications. (For care of the patient having gastric or intestinal decompression, see p. 656.)

The patient who is taking no fluids or foods orally should have frequent oral care. If he is receiving sufficient fluids intravenously, thirst should not be a problem. Chewing gum or sucking on small pieces of hard candy or ice often helps to allay thirst and keeps the patient's mouth moist.

The return of normal peristalsis is verified when the bowel sounds are heard on auscultation. The passage of flatus by rectum or a spontaneous bowel movement also indicates the return of peristalsis and should be recorded and reported. When peristalsis returns, the patient usually is given clear fluids first. If he tolerates them well, he can usually progress rapidly to other foods.

Vomiting

Postoperative vomiting is one of the most distressing problems that the patient encounters. In addition to the discomfort it causes, severe vomiting or retching can be harmful to the operative wound. Usually it is due to the effects of certain anesthetics on the stomach or to eating food or drinking water before peristalsis returns. Psychologic factors also contribute to vomiting. It is not unusual for the patient who expects to vomit postoperatively to do so.

To prevent danger of aspiration, the patient who is vomiting should lie on his side. He should be advised not to take food or fluid for several hours and to lie quietly in bed. The emesis basin and soiled bed linen should be removed, and oral care should be given. When vomiting has subsided, sucking on chips of ice, taking sips of ginger ale or hot tea, or eating small amounts of dry, solid food may relieve nausea. Sometimes, trimethobenzamide hydrochloride (Tigan), an antiemetic, or prochlorperazine dimaleate (Compazine) or promethazine hydrochloride (Phenergan) may be administered.

Persistent postoperative vomiting is usually a symptom of pyloric obstruction, intestinal obstruc-

tion, or peritonitis. This type of vomiting tires the patient, puts a strain on the incision, and causes excessive loss of fluids and electrolytes. Projectile vomiting of gastric contents occurs in the presence of pyloric obstruction. In intestinal obstruction the vomitus is fecal in nature, and it usually flows continuously and effortlessly from the patient's mouth. If persistent vomiting occurs, a nasogastric tube is passed, and the stomach is lavaged. The tube may be left in place and attached to suction to keep the stomach empty. The patient is not given anything orally, and intravenous fluids containing electrolytes are administered to replace the fluid and electrolyte loss.

Hiccoughs

Hiccoughs interfere with eating and sleeping and are among the most exhausting postoperative complications. The exact cause of postoperative hiccoughs is not known, but it is known that dilation of the stomach, irritation of the diaphragm, peritonitis, and uremia cause either reflex or central nervous system stimulation of the phrenic nerve. Fortunately the hiccoughs are not a common postoperative complaint. They usually disappear within a few hours. They may be relieved by such a simple measure as having the patient breathe his own carbon dioxide at 5-minute intervals by inhaling and exhaling into a paper bag held tightly over his nose and mouth. Carbon dioxide inhalations, using 5% carbon dioxide and 95% oxygen, may also be ordered for 5 minutes every hour. If dizziness occurs, they should be discontinued, since an overdose of carbon dioxide may cause convulsions and coma. Aspiration of the stomach will stop hiccoughs caused by gastric dilation. Chlorpromazine hydrochloride is used to treat mild cases of hiccoughs. If the hiccoughs are persistent and do not respond to these treatments, local infiltration of the phrenic nerve with 1% procaine may be necessary, or in extreme cases surgical crushing of the phrenic nerve may be done.

Abdominal distention

Postoperative distention is a result of an accumulation of nonabsorbable gas in the intestines caused by a reaction to the handling of the bowel during surgery, by swallowing of air during recovery from anesthesia and as the patient attempts to overcome nausea, and by passing of gases from the bloodstream to the atonic portion of the bowel. Distention will persist until the tone of the bowel returns to normal and peristalsis resumes. It is experienced to some degree by most patients after abdominal and renal surgery.

"Gas pains" are caused by contractions of the unaffected portions of the bowel in an attempt to move the accumulated gas through the intestinal tract. The patient complains of discomfort, and if the distention is high in the abdomen, he may have difficulty in breathing. High distention may be due to stomach dilatation and can be relieved by aspiration of fluid and gas from the stomach with a nasogastric tube. Ambulation often stimulates the return of peristalsis and the expulsion of flatus. Gas in the lower bowel may be removed by a lubricated rectal tube inserted into the rectum. This tube should be inserted just past the rectal sphincter and should be removed after approximately 20 minutes. If necessary, it may be used every 4 hours. Heat applied to the abdomen in the form of a hot-water bottle or heating pad may be ordered in conjunction with the use of a rectal tube. A Fleet's enema is often effective in relieving gas pains postoperatively. If this fails, small carminative enemas of milk and molasses or of glycerin, magnesium sulfate, and water sometimes are ordered to stimulate the expulsion of flatus. If the distention progresses and the flatus is not expelled after 48 hours, a *paralytic ileus* is suspected. This condition is the complete absence of bowel tone and is caused by the anesthetic, by a generalized infection such as peritonitis, or by other factors. The patient is given nothing orally, and nasogastric suctioning is started and continued until peristalsis returns.

Defecation

After abdominal surgery, the nurse should record the time when the patient first passes flatus and when a bowel movement occurs so that the surgeon is kept informed of the patient's progress. The first spontaneous bowel movement usually occurs 4 to 5 days after surgery and indicates that normal gastrointestinal function has returned. Unless there are symptoms of fecal impaction or intestinal distention, no attempt is made to hasten bowel evacuation. The patient who is eating normally, drinking adequate fluids, walking about, and going to the bathroom routinely will usually have a bowel movement without an enema. When an enema seems necessary, a Fleet enema or a small soapsuds enema usually will stimulate defecation. If the patient is constipated, an oil retention enema followed by a soapsuds enema may be necessary.

While caring for the postoperative patient, the nurse should question him about the expulsion of flatus or the occurrence of a bowel movement, since a delay in bowel evacuation beyond 4 or 5 days postoperatively may be a symptom of paralytic ileus or intestinal obstruction.

Postoperative diarrhea may occur. Since it may be caused by a fecal impaction, it should be reported to the physician. If the patient has severe burns of the buttocks or has undergone extensive rectal or pelvic surgery, bowel movements may be intentionally delayed for several days by the administration of paregoric or opium orally.

■ PREPARATION FOR DISCHARGE FROM THE HOSPITAL

Discharge planning is an important part of nursing care postoperatively. Plans for the patient's discharge may have been discussed and begun preoperatively, but most of the teaching, arrangements, and preparations are done after surgery. The patient, his family, and the members of the health team responsible for the care of the patient during his hospitalization should participate in the long-range planning.

As a result of the early resumption of ambulation and a nutritious diet, most patients regain their strength rapidly, and the average hospital stay following surgery is less than 2 weeks. During this time the patient and his family should be prepared for any care that must be given at home, and any necessary arrangements for convalescent care should be completed several days prior to discharge. The patient should be helped to become as self-sufficient as possible before being discharged so that he does not have to depend any more than necessary on the assistance of relatives and friends.

Soon after surgery the nurse should consult with the physician regarding the anticipated discharge plans for the patient. The nurse should assess the patient's ability to participate in the care to be given at home, the interest and the desire of the family to help, and the home situation and its facilities. Whenever possible, both the patient and a member of his family should be taught all treatments and exercises that must be done at home. Sometimes arrangements should be made for a member of the family to come to the hospital to observe and perhaps practice procedures, to talk to the dietitian, to consult with the physician, to discuss problems with the social case worker, and to plan with the nurse about home care. The patient and his family should have ample opportunity to ask questions.

The nurse should try to anticipate any problems that might arise and help the patient and his family plan for them. For example, if a colostomy irrigation must be given and there are no bathroom facilities, extra equipment will be necessary so that it can be done in the room available. If the patient is reluctant or unable to give himself an injection, some member of the family must be taught how to give injections, or arrangements must be made for a public health nurse to give them. If the patient does not understand English, an interpreter may be needed to explain diets, medications, or treatments. If dressings are needed, the patient should be given a 48-hour supply to take home unless a family member has already obtained them from the hospital. The patient and his family must know where in the community they can get dressings and other needed materials. If treatment of almost any kind is to be done at home, it is advisable for the nurse to discuss with the surgeon and with the patient the advisability of having a public health nurse visit the patient in his home soon after he leaves the hospital. A written referral should be made, and the report returned by the public health nurse helps the nurse in the hospital to learn how effective her teaching of the patient has been.

If the patient lives alone or has no relatives or friends to care for him, he may need to go to another hospital for further treatment or for terminal care, or he may need nursing home care. Since these institutions usually have long waiting lists and since it takes time to arrange for such transfers, referrals should be made as early as possible. Thus, as soon as the need for a specific type of care is established, the physician should discuss it with the patient and family. If the health team includes a social worker, he will explore community resources, present alternate plans (if there are any) for consideration, and help with the referral. Both the patient and the family may need a great deal of support to help them accept the plan that seems best.

On discharge the patient is given an appointment for a follow-up examination in the surgeon's office or in the outpatient department of the hospital. This appointment is usually for 1 or 2 weeks after discharge. The nurse should make sure that the patient understands the importance of returning for the medical examination and that he can make arrangements to come in at this time.

With modern surgical techniques the wound is well healed by the time of discharge from the hospital. Therefore the convalescent period usually is relatively short, and most patients may return to their usual activities and occupation within 2 to 4 weeks postoperatively. During this time the patient should rest when he becomes tired and should increase his activity gradually. When the patient visits the physician after discharge, the healing of the wound and the patient's general physical condition are checked. Depending on the outcome of this examination and the type of work the patient does, the surgeon will decide when it will be desirable for him to resume his usual activities.

REFERENCES AND SELECTED READINGS*

1 American College of Surgeons: Manual of pre-operative and post-operative care, ed. 2, Philadelphia, 1971, W. B. Saunders, Co.
2 Anderson, H. C.: Newton's geriatric nursing, ed. 5, St. Louis, 1971, The C. V. Mosby Co.
3 *Ballinger, W. F., and others: Alexander's care of the patient in surgery, ed. 5, St. Louis, 1972, The C. V. Mosby Co.
4 *Barnett, L. A.: Preparing your patient for the operating room, A.O.R.N.J. **18:**534-539, Sept. 1973.
5 Beal, J. M., and others: Intensive and recovery room care, New York, 1969, Macmillan Publishing Co., Inc.
6 Bergersen, B. S.: Pharmacology in nursing, ed. 12, St. Louis, 1973, The C. V. Mosby Co.
7 *Berry, E. C., and Kohn, M. F.: Introduction to operating room technique, ed. 4, New York, 1972, McGraw-Hill Book Co.
8 *Betschman, L. I.: Handbook of recovery room nursing, Philadelphia, 1967, F. A. Davis Co.
9 *Bird, B.: Psychological aspects of preoperative and postoperative care, Am. J. Nurs. **55:**685-687, June 1955.
10 *Breckenridge, F. J., and Bruno, P.: Nursing care of the anesthetized patient, Am. J. Nurs. **62:**74-78, July 1962.
11 *Brinling, T.: Tearing down a wall, Am. J. Nurs. **71:**1406-1409, July 1971.
12 *Brownsberger, C.: Emotional stress connected with surgery, Nurs. Forum **4:**46-55, 1965.
13 Bushnell, S. S.: Respiratory intensive care nursing, Boston, 1973, Little, Brown & Co.
14 *Carnes, M. A.: Postanesthetic complications, Nurs. Forum **4**(3):46-55, 1965.
15 *Carnevali, D. L.: Pre-operative anxiety, Am. J. Nurs. **66:**1536-1538, July 1966.
16 *Case, T. C., and Giery, R. A.: Surgery in patients between

80 and 100 years of age, J. Am. Geriatr. Soc. **12:**345-349, April 1964.
17 *Castillo, P.: Care of the patient under local anesthesia, A.O.R.N.J. **18:**283-285, Aug. 1973.
18 Clark, R. B.: The case for spinal anesthesia, Am. J. Nurs. **67:**294-297, Feb. 1967.
19 Cole, W., and Mason, J. H.: Surgical aspects. In Cowdry, E. V., editor: The care of the geriatric patient, ed. 3, St. Louis, 1968, The C. V. Mosby Co.
20 *Collart, M. E., and Brenneman, J. K.: Preventing postoperative atelectasis, Am. J. Nurs. **71:**1982-1987, Oct. 1971.
21 Creighton, H.: Law every nurse should know, ed. 2, Philadelphia, 1970, W. B. Saunders Co.
22 Davis, L., editor: Christopher's textbook of surgery, ed. 10, Philadelphia, 1972, W. B. Saunders Co.
23 Dickler, D. J., Friedman, P. L., and Susman, I. C.: Intravenous regional anesthesia with chloroprocaine, Anesthesiology **26:**244-245, March-April 1965.
24 Dripps, R. D., Eckenhoff, J. E., and Vandam, L. D.: Introduction to anesthesia, ed. 4, Philadelphia, 1972, W. B. Saunders Co.
25 Dumas, R. G., and Leonard, R. C.: The effect of nursing on the incidence of postoperative vomiting, Nurs. Res. **12:**12-15, Winter 1963.
26 Dumas, R. G., and others: The importance of the expressive function in preoperative preparation. In Skipper, J. K., and Leonard, R. C., editors: Social interaction and patient care, Philadelphia, 1965, J. B. Lippincott Co.
27 Egbert, L. D., Laver, M. B., and Bendixen, H. H.: The effect of site of operation and type of anesthesia upon the ability to cough in the postoperative period, Surg. Gynecol. Obstet. **115:**295-298, Sept. 1962.
28 Egbert, L. D., and others: Reducing postoperative pain by encouragement and instruction of patients, N. Engl. J. Med. **270:**825-827, 1964.
29 Eisele, J. H.: Recognizing and treating respiratory problems in the surgical patient, A.O.R.N.J. **17:**80-87, May 1973.

*References preceded by an asterisk are particularly well suited for student reading.

30 *Field, L. W.: Identifying the psychological aspects of the surgical patient, A.O.R.N.J. **17:**86-90, Jan. 1973.

31 Fitzmaurice, J. B., and Sashara, A. A.: Current concepts of pulmonary embolism: implications for nursing practice, Heart & Lung **3:**209-218, March-April, 1974.

32 Flatter, P. A.: Hazards of oxygen therapy, Am. J. Nurs. **68:**80-84, Jan. 1968.

33 Fuerst, E., and Wolff, L.: Fundamentals of nursing, ed. 5, Philadelphia, 1974, J. B. Lippincott Co.

34 Ginsberg, F., and others: A manual of operating room technology, Philadelphia, 1966, J. B. Lippincott Co.

35 *Glenn, F.: Surgical care of the aged, J. Am. Geriatr. Soc. **10:**927-931, Nov. 1962.

36 Goodman, L. S., and Gillman, A.: The pharmacological basis of therapeutics, ed. 4, New York, 1970, Macmillan Publishing Co., Inc.

37 Goth, A.: Medical pharmacology, ed. 7, St. Louis, 1974, The C. V. Mosby Co.

38 *Goulding, E. I., and Koop, C. E.: The newborn, his response to surgery, Am. J. Nurs. **65:**84-87, Oct. 1965.

39 *Gruendemann, B., and others: The surgical patient: behavioral concepts for the operating room nurse, St. Louis, 1973, The C. V. Mosby Co.

40 *Halsell, M.: Moist heat for relief of postoperative pain, Am. J. Nurs. **67:**767-770, April 1967.

41 Hanamey, R.: Teaching patients breathing and coughing techniques, Nurs. Outlook **13:**58-59, Aug. 1965.

42 *Hardiman, M. A.: Interviewing? Or social chit-chat? Am. J. Nurs. **71:**1379-1381, July 1971.

43 *Harris, W. H., Slater, E. M., and Bell, H. M.: Regional anesthesia by the intravenous route, J.A.M.A. **194:**1273-1276, Dec. 1965.

44 Hayes, M. A.: Postoperative diet therapy, J. Am. Diet. Assoc. **35:**17-18, Jan. 1959.

45 *Healy, K. M.: Does preoperative instruction make a difference, Am. J. Nurs. **68:**62-67, Jan. 1968.

46 Hopps, H. C.: Principles of pathology, ed. 2, New York, 1964, Appleton-Century-Crofts.

47 Johnson, J., and others: Psychosocial factors in the welfare of surgical patients, Nurs. Res. **19:**18-29, Jan.-Feb. 1970.

48 Leithauser, D. J., Gregory, L., and Miller, S. M.: Immediate ambulation after extensive surgery, Am. J. Nurs. **66:**2207-2208, Oct. 1966.

49 Le Maitre, G., and Finnigan, J. A.: The patient in surgery, Philadelphia, 1970, W. B. Saunders Co.

50 Lindeman, C. A., and Van Aerman, B. H.: Nursing intervention with the presurgical patient—the effects of structured and unstructured preoperative teaching, Nurs. Res. **20:**319-332, July-Aug. 1971.

51 Linehan, D.: What does the patient want to know? Am. J. Nurs. **66:**1066-1070, May 1966.

52 Linton, R. R.: Venous thrombosis, pulmonary embolism, and varicose veins, J.A.M.A. **183:**198-201, Jan. 1963.

53 *Lipman, M.: Informed consent and the nurse's role, R. N. **35:**50, Sept. 1972.

54 Lisboa, J. M.: Role of the special care unit nurse in a preoperative teaching program, Nurs. Clin. North Am. **7:**389-395, June 1972.

55 Litsky, B.: Infection control and hospital design, Supervisor Nurse **3:**23, Feb. 1972.

56 Mezzanotte, E. J.: Group instruction in preparation for surgery, Am. J. Nurs. **70:**89-91, Jan. 1970.

57 *Minckley, B. B.: Physiologic hazards of position changes in the anesthetized patient, Am. J. Nurs. **69:**2606-2611, Dec. 1969.

58 *Mitchell, J. A., and Cragin, C. L.: Informed consent—a doctor's dilemma, A.O.R.N.J. **18:**810-826, Oct. 1973.

59 Modell, W., editor: Drugs in current use, New York, 1969, Springer Publishing Co., Inc.

60 *Moore, C., and Marion, R.: Working with children and their families to help them through a long-anticipated surgical experience. In Bergersen, B., and others, editors: Current concepts in clinical nursing, St. Louis, 1967, The C. V. Mosby Co.

61 Murphy, J. W., Riu, R., and Ponka, J. L.: Local anesthesia for gastric surgery in aged patients, J. Am. Geriatr. Soc. **16:**673-679, June 1968.

62 Mustard, W. T., and others: Pediatric surgery, 2 vols., ed. 2, Chicago, 1969, Year Book Medical Publishers, Inc.

63 Nett, L. M., and others: Acute respiratory failure, Am. J. Nurs. **67:**1847-1856, Sept. 1967.

64 *Nielsen, M. A.: Intra-arterial monitoring of blood pressure, Am. J. Nurs. **74:**48-53, Jan. 1974.

65 *Norris, C. M.: The work of getting well, Am. J. Nurs. **69:**2118-2121, Oct. 1969.

66 Norris, W., and Campbell, D.: A nurses' guide to anesthetics, resuscitation and intensive care, ed. 5, London, 1972, E & S Livingstone, Ltd.

67 *Nursing care of the patient in the O.R., Somerville, N. J., 1972, Ethicon, Inc.

68 Olson, E. V., and others: The hazards of immobility, Am. J. Nurs. **67:**779-797, April 1967.

69 *Patrick, H.: Electrical hazards in the operating room, A.O.R.N.J. **18:**1127-1130, Dec. 1973.

70 Powell, M.: An environment for wound healing, Amer. J. Nurs. **72:**1862-1865, Oct. 1972.

71 *Powers, M. E., and Storlie, F.: The apprehensive patient, Amer. J. Nurs. **67:**58-63, Jan. 1967.

72 Rhoads, J. E., and others: Surgery: principles and practices, ed. 4, Philadelphia, 1970, J. B. Lippincott Co.

73 Sasahara, A. A., and Foster, V. L.: Pulmonary embolism, Amer. J. Nurs. **67:**1634-1641, Aug. 1967.

74 Schmitt, F. E., and Woolridge, P. J.: Psychological preparation of surgical patients, Nurs. Res. **22:**108-116, March-April, 1973.

75 Schwartz, S. and others: Principles of surgery, New York, 1969, McGraw Hill Co.

76 Scully, H. F., and Martin, S. J.: Anesthetic management for geriatric patients, Amer. J. Nurs. **65:**110-112, Feb. 1965.

77 Shaw, W. M.: Positional control of immediate postanesthetic vomiting, Anesthesiology **26:**359, May-June 1965.

78 Simeone, F. A.: Shock, Amer. J. Nurs. **66:**1286-1294, June 1966.

79 *Smith, R. B., Petruscak, J., and Solosko, D.: In a recovery room, Am. J. Nurs. **73:**70-73, Jan. 1973.

80 Smith, R. M.: Anesthesia for infants and children, ed. 3, St. Louis, 1968, The C. V. Mosby Co.

81 *Stahl, W. M.: Major abdominal surgery in the aged patient, J. Am. Geriatr. Soc. **11:**770-780, Aug. 1963.

82 *Tinker, J. H., and Wehner, R. J.: Postoperative recovery and the neuromuscular junction, Am. J. Nurs. **74:**74-75, Jan. 1974.

83 *Traver, G. A.: Assessment of thorax and lungs, Am. J. Nurs. **73:**466-471, March 1973.

84 Walter, C. W.: Safe electric environment in the hospital, Bull. Am. Coll. Surg. **54:**4, July-Aug. 1969.

85 *Wang, K. C., and Howland, W. S.: Cardiac and pulmonary evaluations in elderly patients before elective surgery, J.A.M.A. **166:**993-997, March 1959.

86 Warren, R.: Surgery, Philadelphia, 1963, W. B. Saunders Co.

87 *Webb, W. R.: Management of pulmonary complications, Hosp. Med. **1:**16-22, Oct. 1965.

88 Weiler, Sister C. M.: Postoperative patients evaluate preoperative instruction, Am. J. Nurs. **68:**1464-1467, July 1968.

89 Williams, S. R.: Nutrition and diet therapy, ed. 2, St. Louis, 1973, The C. V. Mosby Co.

90 Willig, S. H.: The nurse's guide to the law, New York, 1970, McGraw-Hill Book Co.

91 Winter, P. M., and Lowenstein, E.: Acute respiratory failure, Sci. Am. **221:**23-29, Nov. 1969.

92 *Wolfer, J. A., and Davis, C. E.: Assessment of surgical patients preoperative emotional condition and postoperative welfare, Nurs. Res. **19:**402-414, Sept.-Oct. 1970.

93 Wright, I. S.: The treatment of thrombophlebitis, J.A.M.A. **183:**194-198, Jan. 1963.

94 Wylie, W. D., and Churchill-Davidson, H. C.: A practice of anesthesia, ed. 3, Chicago, 1972, Year Book Medical Publishers, Inc.

95 *Zepernick, R. G.: New trends in anesthesia, Nurs. Forum **4**(3):41-45, 1965.

12 Plastic surgery

■ Plastic surgery has been attempted for centuries. Surgery of this kind was performed prior to the era of the Roman Empire. Hindu records describe some good results from efforts to alter deformities caused by disease or other misfortune. In the sixteenth century, Italian surgeons did remarkable work in plastic surgery, and there was interest in the emotional aspects of facial deformities. The discovery of anesthetics and of the cause of infection enabled surgeons to make strides in this field. Disfigurements resulting from World Wars I and II challenged the imagination of surgeons so that new techniques were developed.

There is every reason to believe that plastic surgery will become a more important part of medical care as time goes on. The main purposes of such surgery are to restore function, prevent further loss of function, and cosmetically improve the defects caused by deformities present at birth, from disease, or from trauma. Plastic surgery such as skin grafting may be performed as an emergency measure in severe burns. It is also performed for cosmetic improvement.

Although medical science has made progress in learning the causes of some developmental anomalies (for example, it has been learned that German measles contracted during the first trimester of pregnancy may cause anomalies in the infant), it is not possible at the present time to prevent the occurrence of many defects at birth. Many birth defects such as cleft lip and cleft palate require plastic surgery. The cause of cancer is still unknown, and extensive surgery will continue to be used until a better method of treatment is discovered. Following surgical treatment for this disease, plastic surgery often is necessary. Trauma such as that sustained in automobile accidents often necessitates plastic surgery, and it seems likely that the number of people requiring such treatment will increase. Plastic surgery is often needed following loss of skin and scarring from burns. *Keloid tissue,* the thick weltlike masses of overgrowth of scar tissue, which most commonly occur in dark-skinned persons, will often require plastic surgery. Posttraumatic scars in which subcutaneous tissues are separated from, or are adherent to, underlying structures such as bone may be corrected by plastic surgery.

The two aspects of plastic surgery, reconstruction and correction, are evident in most plastic surgical treatment. Often several medical specialists care for patients needing reconstructive and corrective surgery. The dental surgeon, the ear, nose, and throat specialist, and the plastic surgeon may all work together, for example, in treatment of the child who has a cleft lip and a cleft palate.

■ IMPLANTS AND TRANSPLANTS

In plastic surgery the surgeon may use, in addition to the patient's own tissues, inert materials and tissues from other human beings. Inert substances must

■ STUDY QUESTIONS

1 What reaction does the average person have when he encounters someone with a facial abnormality? What types of work would probably not be available to the person with such a deformity? List as many recreational activities as you can that would be difficult or impossible for a person who has a marked deformity of the right hand.

2 Review the anatomy of the skin. How does skin differ from granulation tissue? Describe how new skin forms at the edges of a wound. On what does the elastic quality of skin depend?

3 What is meant by an autoimmune reaction?

4 Review the procedure for using sterile, moist compresses.

meet several criteria. They must not be irritating or contribute to the development of cancer, they should be an appropriate consistency for their intended use, and they should not deteriorate or change their shape and form with time. A large variety of substances has been used in the past, including wax, metal, ivory, and bone that has been rendered inert by boiling. In recent years materials such as Teflon and silicone have been used extensively, since they appear to be nonirritating and they retain their form indefinitely.

For many years reconstructive procedures have been attempted in which the tissues of other human beings are used. To be successful, these procedures require adequate surgical treatment. Furthermore, the grafted tissue must grow and carry on normal function. In recent years great strides have been made in the technical aspects of tissue transplants. Success in the transplantation of major organs such as the heart, lung, kidney, and liver has been reported. However, less success has been achieved in inducing the body to accept and make part of itself the tissue it receives. Long ago it was observed that skin grafts taken from another human being appeared to do well for a short time. Eventually, however, and usually within 4 to 15 days, they underwent changes and died. It is believed that the graft from another person (homograft transplant) acts as an antigen, causing the host to produce antibodies and to develop a sensitivity to it. When a second homograft is used, it is rejected more quickly than the first, thus substantiating the belief that sensitivity to the foreign protein (antigen) is present. Many questions regarding the autoimmune reaction are not yet answered, and results of studies on experimental animals have not always been entirely consistent. Until medical science solves the riddle of the autoimmune reaction and learns how to deal with it, the transplantation of body organs and any tissue from one person to another will be fraught with problems. The least difficulty is encountered with tissues such as the cornea of the eye that have a very limited blood supply. Attempts are made to combat the body's sensitivity by giving immunosuppressive drugs. When these are given, grafted tissues have survived for years in some instances. Azathioprine (Imuran) and 6-mercaptopurine are given at the time of surgery, and if rejection threatens, actinomycin C and prednisone are given in large doses. (See pp. 369, 480, and 726 for further discussion of specific organ transplants.)

■ GENERAL PRINCIPLES OF MANAGEMENT

The nurse has two important functions relating to patients needing plastic surgery. These functions are to direct persons who may benefit from plastic procedures to appropriate medical care and to serve as an important member of the team caring for the patient undergoing reconstructive and corrective procedures.

Directing the patient in seeking appropriate care

Many people do not know that it is possible to correct a congenital defect. Some parents may delay seeking medical care for a child with a defect due to a congenital anomaly because of their own guilt feelings. They may hope that somehow, miraculously, the child will "outgrow" the condition. Often they do not realize that the normal development of the child depends on the early treatment of some conditions. A defect may interfere with the use of a part of the body so that normal growth does not take place. This result follows the principle that form follows function; for instance, a child's deformed and therefore unused hand does not grow at the same rate as the hand that is used normally. Contractures of joints and atrophy of muscles occur with disuse, thus increasing the defect and handicap; for example, facial asymmetry can result from contractures in the neck that prevent uniform action of the muscles of both sides of the face even though the muscles themselves are not affected.

Parents need to know that healthy emotional development in the child is dependent on normal physical appearance. When a defect is allowed to persist, there may be emotional maladjustment that will affect the child's entire life. For example, conspicuous patches of brightly discolored skin present at birth and known as birthmarks or port-wine stains are quite common. These stains, particularly if they are on the face or neck, cause the child great emotional distress and sometimes lead to serious personality maladjustment. Yet many people do not know that they may sometimes be effectively treated by tatooing.

A patient's emotional reaction to a deformity or defect must not be underestimated. One's pride in himself, his ability to think well of himself, and to regard himself favorably in comparison with others are essential to the development and maintenance of a well-integrated personality. Every person who has a defect or a handicap, particularly if it is conspicuous to others, suffers from some threat to his emotional security. The extent of the emotional reaction and the amount of maladjustment that follows depend on the individual's makeup and his ability to cope with emotional insults. Disfigurements almost invariably lead to disturbing experiences. The child who has webbed fingers may be ridiculed at school; the adolescent girl who has acne scars may be self-conscious and avoid social situations; and the young man with a posttraumatic scar on his face may be refused a salesman's job. Under any of these circumstances it is not unusual for the individual to withdraw from a society that is unkind. The defect may be used to justify failure to assume responsibility or to justify striking out against an unkind society by such reactions as becoming a "problem child" or, in some extreme cases, a criminal.

Plastic surgery may require repeated and long hospitalizations that may place serious financial strain on the patient and his family if they must assume responsibility for the major part of the expense. Clinic nurses, public health nurses in the community, social workers, and welfare agency personnel can help in preparing the patient for this problem and in helping him to meet it. If the patient is an adult, leaves from employment, financial support while undergoing treatment, and plans for convalescent care and rehabilitation are examples of problems that must be faced in many instances. The patient should be encouraged to discuss his problems freely, since their solution does affect his medical treatment.

Many parents do not know that financial resources are available to cover costs of plastic surgery for children. Every state in the country has a plan for medical care of crippled children. This program is partially supported by matching funds from the federal government, administered by the Office of Child Development (formerly the Children's Bureau) of the Department of Health, Education and Welfare, which was created soon after the first White House Conference on Child Care, held in Washington, D. C., in 1909. Children and adolescents up to 21 years of age with defects requiring plastic surgery are eligible for care under his plan. If the nurse encounters a child who might benefit from medical treatment the family can be encouraged to discuss this with their physician. If the family has no personal physician, the local hospital may conduct a clinic or may recommend a physician designated to care for eligible children in the area or the state. Small community hospitals may not have clinics of their own but may refer patients to larger hospitals or special clinics in nearby cities. In larger communities the school nurse is usually well informed about available resources.

Preparation for surgery

It is believed that any plastic surgery for an obvious defect is justified if it helps the patient to feel he has a better chance for recognition among his fellowmen. The plastic surgeon may reshape a nose or repair a deformed hand so that an emotionally stable person will have more assurance among others. However, it is foolish to assume that reconstructive surgery alone will correct a basic personality problem. It has been learned that some people blame an apparently trivial physical defect for a long series of failures in their lives when the major defect lies within their personalities. Because of this possibility, the patient is usually carefully studied before surgery is planned. It is necessary to know what the patient expects the surgery to accomplish before the physician can decide whether or not such expectations are realistic and if surgery should be performed.

It is also necessary to learn about the social standards and cultural mores of the community in which the patient lives and his adjustment to them. His economic contribution as a citizen and as a member of a family, his characteristic pattern in interpersonal relationships, and whether or not he has previously sought medical treatment for the particular problem should be assessed. The nurse and the social worker are often called on to assist the surgeon in his efforts to learn as much as possible about the patient. By observing and recording the patient's behavior at home, in school, in the clinic, on arrival at the hospital, and during preparation for surgery, the nurse can assist the surgeon in his study of the patient. Sometimes the help of specialists in psychology and psychiatry is sought. Before surgery, the surgeon will tell the patient what probably can be done and what changes are possible. It is important that the nurse know what the patient has been told so that misunderstandings and misinterpretations can be avoided. The nurse can increase the patient's confidence in his surgical treatment by answering his questions and repeating explanations as often as necessary.

The patient who is admitted to the hospital for plastic surgery may have extensive scarring and deformity and may be exceedingly sensitive to scrutiny by the people he encounters. On the other hand, the patient may have little apparent deformity, and it may be difficult to understand why the patient wishes to have surgery. The nurse cannot possibly know what the disfigurement means to the individual patient and should avoid judging whether or not surgery is necessary. Nurses may be inclined to concentrate their efforts on the more physically ill patients. Yet it is important for nurses to learn about each patient who is to have plastic surgery and to assure him of their interest.

The patient should be in the best possible physical condition before plastic surgery. A diet high in protein and vitamins prior to elective surgery is thought to help in the "take" or healing of the graft. Hemoglobin and clotting times are usually determined, and the blood protein level is assayed because a normal blood protein level has been found necessary for satisfactory growth of grafted tissue.

The wound that is to receive the graft must be free from infections that would delay healing, lead to more scar tissue formation, or cause death of the graft. Infection is treated by the administration of antibiotics and by the use of warm soaks and compresses. A sterile physiologic solution of sodium chloride is the solution most often used. Before skin grafting is attempted, any dead tissue that is adherent to the wound is removed by debridement; otherwise this tissue will interfere with the graft's healing.

The *donor site* (the area from which skin is to be taken) is washed with a germicidal soap the evening before surgery, and this cleansing may be repeated the morning of operation. Frequently the site is shaved in the operating room after the patient is anesthetized so that the damage of cutting the skin is minimized. Strong antiseptics are avoided because they may irritate the skin. If the *recipient site* (the area that is to receive the graft) is not an open wound, it is cleansed in the same way.

It is important to explain to the patient the measures used to prepare him for surgery, and he should be prepared for the postoperative experience. It must be repeatedly explained to him that the immediate results may not meet his expectations. The patient may become alarmed and discouraged if he has not been prepared for the normal appearance of skin grafts and reconstructed tissue immediately after surgery. Postoperative tissue reaction may distort normal contours, suture lines may be reddened, and the color of the newly transplanted skin may differ somewhat from that of surrounding skin. The appearance of the surgical area changes as the edema decreases and the suture line becomes less reddened and indurated. Six months after surgery the scar will be less noticeable than at 6 days or 6 weeks postoperatively.

The patient frequently needs support when he sees the operative site for the first time. The nurse is present when dressings are removed and assesses the reaction of the patient so immediate and future nursing intervention can be planned and implemented. If it is not possible to remove all mirrors to prevent the patient from inspecting the results of facial surgery, dressings may be left on longer than necessary to cover wounds. Members of the patient's family should also know what to expect so that they will not be unduly worried and so that they can give support to the patient if apprehension occurs.

■ SPECIAL PROCEDURES FOR CONTRACTURES

Plastic surgeons make excellent use of the natural elastic quality of normal skin. Operations known as *Z-plasty* and *Y-plasty* are often performed. Scar tissue can often be removed, and the Z-shaped or Y-shaped incision enables the surgeon to undermine adjacent skin, draw the edges together, and cover the defect without using skin from another part of the body (Fig. 12-1). These procedures are naturally limited by the size of the scar and its location, since elasticity of skin varies in different parts of the body. Z-plasty and Y-plasty procedures are suitable for such locations as the axilla, the inner aspects of the elbow, and the neck and throat. They are not so useful in treating defects on the back or on the palmar surfaces of the hand because the skin in these areas cannot be undermined and stretched.

■ TYPES OF GRAFTS AND RELATED CARE

Nearly all plastic surgery requires moving tissue from one part of the body to another. The moved tissue, or graft, is known as an *autograft,* and skin, bone, cartilage, fat, fascia, muscle, or nerves may be taken. Tissue transplanted from another person is called a *homograft (allograft).* It can be obtained from living persons, or it can be taken from persons shortly after death. Tissue taken under the latter circumstances can be used only if cancer or an infectious disease was not present. The use of homografts may be necessary when the patient's condition is poor and autografting is impossible. For example, the patient may be in shock but require the covering of large burned areas by grafted skin. The survival time of homografts varies from a few days to a number of weeks. Depending on the tissue used and the recipient site, the transplanted tissue will then die and slough or be absorbed and replaced by the host's own developing tissues. They are used only as temporary grafts.

Heterografts (xenografts) consist of tissue from another species. They are rejected by the recipient

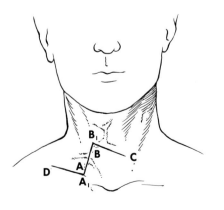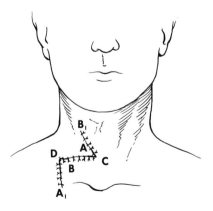

FIG. 12-1. By means of Z-plasty operations, scar tissue can be removed and defects can be covered without the need to transplant skin.

and are used only in special cases. For example, if tissue in banks is not readily available, it may be more feasible to use heterografts to cover the open wounds of patients with massive burns. The transplant acts as an antigen, and the body forms antibodies against it that prevent growth and function of the graft. When bone, cartilage, or blood vessels are obtained from sources other than the patient, they do not become part of the patient's body but act as a framework around which the body usually lays down cells of its own. The graft is then gradually absorbed over a period of time.

Plastic surgery may be performed by means of free grafting—cutting tissue from one part of the body and moving it directly to another part. It may also be done by leaving one end of the graft attached to the body to provide a blood supply for the graft until blood vessels form at the new place of attachment. The surgeon selects skin for grafting that is similar in texture and thickness to that which has been lost. He studies the normal lines of the skin and its elasticity to avoid noticeable scars. Scar tissue contracts with time, and in normal circumstances this process is good because it produces a complete closure of the line of injury. However, in some cases scar tissue may contract in such a way that surrounding tissues are pulled out of normal contour, and distortion may result. The plastic surgeon is an artist as well as a surgeon, and he studies cosmetic and many other aspects of the patient's problem before he decides on the type of graft or plastic procedure that will be most effective.

Free grafts

Free grafts are those that are lifted completely from one site and placed at another site. There are several types of free grafts, each with its advantages and limitations. Split-thickness grafts consist of the epidermis and varying thicknesses of the dermis. Full-thickness grafts include the entire dermis and epidermis (Fig. 12-2).

Thin split-thickness grafts (Ollier-Thiersch grafts), which have only a very thin layer of the dermis, are of limited use since they contract easily, often become shiny and discolored, and have poor wearing qualities. They are often used to replace mucous membrane in reconstructive surgery of such areas as the mouth and vagina. Appropriate means to prevent excessive contraction of the graft as it heals must be taken. Thin split-thickness homografts may be used to cover large burned areas to reduce the loss of body fluids. Within a few weeks the grafts can be removed and replaced with intermediate or thick split-thickness autografts.

Intermediate and *thick split-thickness grafts* are widely used. These grafts have a thicker layer of dermis attached to the epidermis and do not wrinkle, contract, or become discolored as easily as the thin split-thickness graft. The donor site is able to reepithelialize completely, since the deeper layers of the dermis have been left intact. These split-thickness grafts can be used to cover almost any part of the body. They can be cut into large pieces with a dermatome set to ensure a uniform thickness of the graft, and these can then be cut into smaller

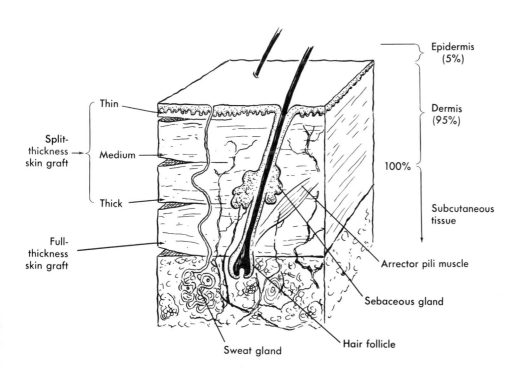

FIG. 12-2. Diagram of the layers of the skin involved in various types of skin grafts. The thickness of epidermis and dermis pictured here are typical of that found on the lateral thigh of an adult. (Redrawn from Graab, W. S., and Smith, J. W.: Plastic surgery, Boston, 1968, Little, Brown & Co.)

pieces to correspond to the size of the area to be grafted.

Full-thickness grafts (Wolfe's grafts) are used primarily to cover small areas where matching skin color and texture are important, such as on the face. One disadvantage of the full-thickness graft is that only a moderate-sized piece of full-thickness skin can survive as a free graft under the best circumstances because the blood supply cannot become established quickly enough to provide essential nutrition. For nourishment these grafts depend entirely on existing lymph until their own blood supply can be established. It takes at least 2 weeks for blood supply to become established, although it is usually possible to tell within a week whether the graft is going to survive. If the graft dies, the skin is irretrievably lost to the body, since regeneration of skin at the donor site is not possible. If possible, the surrounding skin at the donor site is usually undermined so that the skin edges can be brought together, and grafting of the donor site is not necessary. This means that full advantage may have been taken of the elastic quality of the skin, and another graft probably cannot be taken from the same place for some time.

Skin flaps

When a large and deep defect is to be covered, a skin flap or pedicle flap may be used. "Sliding," "rotating," or "tubed" are some of the terms used to identify various types of grafts that are never completely removed from the body at any one time, thereby maintaining a direct vascular supply for nourishment of the tissue. Skin flap grafts may include skin and subcutaneous tissue and sometimes fat and cartilage or bone. Depending on the relative locations of the donor and the recipient sites, the skin graft may be released from the donor site on three sides. For example, it may be slid sideways directly over the recipient site and sutured in place, or it may be lifted and sutured to another area of the body such as a skin flap from the abdomen being sutured to the hand or arm. This type of grafting is called *primary grafting*. If the skin graft is to be moved a considerable distance, and primary grafting is not feasible, the edges of the graft are often sutured together to form a tube. This graft is known as a *tubed pedicle* or *suitcase handle graft* (Fig. 12-3). This modification lessens the danger of the flap becoming infected and permits tissues such as fat or cartilage to be easily transferred. This type of graft may be used to cover a defect on the back of the neck with skin from the abdomen. For example, the piece of skin taken from the abdomen may be grafted to the wrist. Then, when circulation is safely established there, the attachment on the abdomen may be released and attached to its final location on the neck. The attachment on the wrist is maintained until cir-

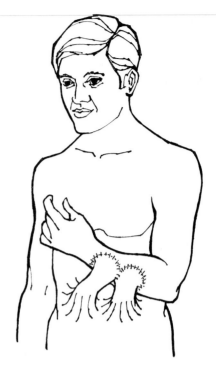

FIG. 12-3. Bilateral tubed pedicle flaps from the abdomen to the forearm. At a later operation they will be detached from the forearm and spread to cover burned areas on the trunk.

culation is established in the neck, at which time the graft is freed from the wrist and the tube opened and sutured into place to cover the defect. Circulation from the new attachment is often tested by putting a rubber-covered clamp or tourniquet about the pedicle close to its oldest attachment and noting the color and warmth of the pedicle at intervals of 10 to 15 minutes. Usually it takes 3 to 6 weeks for new blood vessels to become established. These grafts are less likely to die than are free grafts, but strangulation can occur from pressure, and tissue can be lost from infection. Tubed pedicle grafts are often taken from the abdomen, where fat and subcutaneous tissue are available, to support skin areas of the body that are subject to pressure such as the heel, the sole of the foot, and the palm of the hand. The piece of skin taken is fairly narrow, and adjacent skin is undermined so that edges can be sutured together. When this wound has healed, a small gauze dressing is usually placed between the tubed pedicle and the suture line to keep the area dry and free from the accumulation of dead skin.[8]

■ POSTOPERATIVE MANAGEMENT

The patient undergoing plastic surgery may not have a life-threatening disease; but time, discomfort, and economic and emotional factors are involved. Sometimes a procedure that is not successful cannot be repeated because necessary skin is lost and too much scar tissue may have formed. Moreover, the patient undergoing extensive reconstructive surgery has usually suffered a great deal both physically and emotionally. His ability to cope with the disappointment of unsatisfactory results may be limited.

In addition to general supportive care of any patient who has had surgery, the nurse has special responsibilities necessary to assure the success of the plastic surgery procedure. Maintaining pressure dressings as requested, preventing infection of grafted areas, and applying compresses to stimulate circulation to the graft all require meticulous nursing attention.

The operative areas

A graft must be in constant contact with the underlying tissue in order to attach itself and to grow. Anything that comes between the undersurface of the graft and the recipient area such as a discharge caused by infection, excess serous fluid, or blood will float the graft away from close contact and may cause it to die. To prevent floating, some surgeons insert tiny drains at strategic spots along the edges of the graft, or a small catheter is inserted on the edge of the graft under the recipient skin and attached to suction to remove the fluid.

If the recipient site is a clean wound with no infection, the graft usually is sutured with many fine sutures to hold it in place and in contact with the normal skin adjacent to it. If the recipient site is known to be infected, only a few scattered sutures, if any, may be used, and the grafted site may not be dressed. The area is inspected frequently to see if the skin is adhering to the underlying tissue. If fluid collects under the skin graft, it is removed by aspiration with a sterile needle and syringe or the fluid is rolled to the wound edge with a sterile applicator.

A wide variety of materials are used as dressings.

The choice depends on the kind of graft and the surgeon's preference. Petrolatum, Furacin, Adaptic gauze, or Telfa dressings are often selected. Silver foil may also be used. Often the graft is covered with a piece of coarse-mesh gauze that is anchored to the adjacent skin edges with an elastic bandage (Elastoplast) to give firm, gentle pressure and to immobilize the area. The first dressing may be covered with a compress of sterile normal saline solution. Because the compress is moist, it fits the contour of the wound better. Continuous pressure is necessary to keep the graft adherent to the recipient bed, but pressure should not be so firm as to cause death of the graft. Marine sponges, rubber sponges, cotton pads, and mechanic's waste may be applied as outer dressings by the surgeon to provide the desired amount of pressure. Occasionally the sutures anchoring the graft at the skin edges are left uncut and brought over a pressure dressing to hold it firmly against the graft (Fig. 12-4). The graft site is elevated when possible and protected from pressure and motion. The nurse should be certain that dressings do not become loosened so that pressure is reduced and that the patient does not lie on these dressings or in any other way increase the pressure on them. When flap grafts are used, slings and casts may assure immobilization and help to keep parts of the body in the correct relationship for healing (Fig. 12-5).

Some surgeons believe that grafts are stimulated in their effort to establish blood supply by the use of warm, moist compresses, and sterile normal saline solution is usually ordered for this purpose. The greatest care must be taken that infection is not introduced when compresses are being changed and moistened. Hands must be washed before dressings are handled or compresses changed. Meticulous technique is followed so that infection does not occur. Care is taken so that the newly grafted skin is not traumatized. The temperature of the compress solution should not be over 40.5° C. (105° F.), and

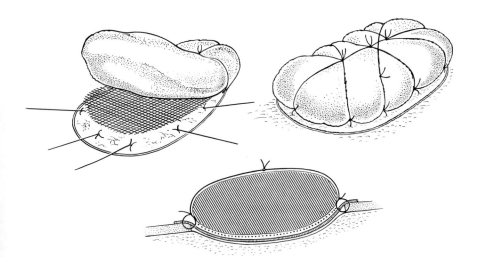

FIG. 12-4. Tieover dressing used as a pressure dressing on skin graft. (Modified from McGregor, I. A.: Fundamental techniques of plastic surgery and their surgical applications, ed. 4, Baltimore, 1969, The Williams & Wilkins Co.)

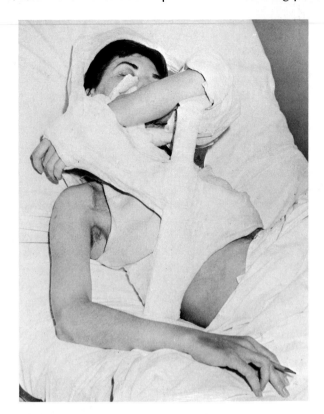

FIG. 12-5. Plastic operations sometimes require the patient to be in extremely awkward positions. Eating, mouth hygiene, and communicating with others are problems in caring for this patient. Note the pencil used for communicating.

compresses should be applied with sterile forceps. Compresses may sometimes be covered with a sterile petroleum jelly dressing and moistened by gently directing fluid from a sterile Asepto syringe under the edge of the dressings. Sterile tubes with tiny openings (Dakin's tubes) may also be placed through the outer compresses to provide a means of moistening the inner dressings without disturbing them and without introducing infection.

The patient may be placed on an oscillating bed in order to improve circulation to the graft as well as to help prevent circulatory complications such as thrombophlebitis. Some physicians prescribe vasodilating drugs such as tolazoline hydrochloride (Priscoline), nicotinic acid, papaverine hydrochloride, and alcohol in a further attempt to produce vasodilation at the recipient site.

When split-thickness grafts have been used, the donor site (often the anterior surface of the thigh) may be a greater source of discomfort to the patient than the recipient site. A Telfa dressing or Furacin petrolatum gauze may be applied to the area and then protected by a firm outer dressing, which is anchored with an Elastoplast bandage that does not encircle the thigh lest it hamper circulation. Or the

dressing is secured by wrapping the leg with Kerlix or an elastic bandage. Some plastic surgeons remove the outer dressing in 2 days and others wait 2 weeks. The patient has intense pain for a short period when the outer dressing is removed from the donor site. A more recent method of treatment is to cover the area with one firm layer of gauze anchored firmly at the edges and leave it exposed to the air. It is believed by some surgeons that healing occurs faster with this method and that there is less danger of death of the deeper skin layer, which must develop the new outer skin layer.[17] If this open method is used, the patient must be supervised carefully so that he does not injure the donor site, since this will cause severe pain. A heat lamp may be used to hasten drying of the donor site. A bed cradle is used to prevent pressure from bedclothes and to allow the donor site to be exposed to the air. Analgesic drugs such as dextropropoxyphene hydrochloride (Darvon), acetylsalicylic acid (aspirin), meperidine hydrochloride (Demerol), and pentazocine (Talwin) may be needed for pain and should not be withheld during the first few days postoperatively.

The nurse should observe the dressings at both the recipient and the donor sites for drainage and bleeding. Dressings are also checked to make sure that they are secure and that they have not become too tight because of local edema, thus interfering with circulation. Inner dressings on the recipient site are changed by the surgeon 1 to 2 days after surgery, and it is usually possible to know then whether or not the result of the operation is satisfactory. Sutures may be removed at this time. When a dressing is no longer necessary, lanolin or cold cream may be applied to the donor site to relieve dryness and discomfort.

The patient requiring a cast

The patient who must be in a cast for one or more stages of plastic surgery requires special care. Sometimes it is helpful preoperatively for the patient to assume the position that will be necessary for the next stage of the procedure so that he may become accustomed to a posture that may cause tedious strain on joints and muscles. Immediately after application and frequently thereafter, the cast must be examined for cracks or breaks that will interfere with support for the graft, and it must be carefully checked to make certain that no excessive pressure is being exerted. Pillows can be used to give support and to lessen strain on body parts. Sometimes overbed bars and side rails help the patient to shift his position if he has one free arm and is otherwise able to do so. The patient who is in an extensive cast for several weeks must be reminded to do muscle-setting exercises for limbs in the cast and to actively exercise the limbs that are not confined.

Arrangements should be made for the patient to

see what goes on around him. Sometimes this is made possible by changing his position in bed or the position of the bed in the room. In some instances putting the patient "head to foot" in the bed is helpful. A mirror may be attached to the bed and arranged at such an angle that the patient can see at least a part of the room if his head, neck, and shoulder movements are restricted by a cast.

The patient requiring lengthy hospitalization

Activities must be planned to keep the patient busy and to keep his mind from his discomfort. The patient should be referred to the occupational therapy department if the hospital has one. If such therapy is not available, or if the patient is unable to engage in hand work, then passive activities such as listening to the radio, reading, and watching television should be arranged. Even the patient who appears to be in a very complicated cast and in an awkward position can be placed on a stretcher or wheeled in his bed to a solarium or to other locations where he may have a change of scene and engage in some activity with others. Members of the patient's family should be encouraged to visit him as much as possible and to try in every way to help maintain his community relationships that have been temporarily interrupted by his hospitalization. Arrangements should be made for patients of school age to continue their schoolwork so that they will not be behind their peers following the rehabilitation period.

The nurse may also help the patient to think along constructive lines in regard to what he will do when surgery is completed. Since a long period of rehabilitation is sometimes necessary, it is important to keep the patient in the best possible physical condition so that he will be ready to undertake specific rehabilitation activities and not require corrective therapy for disabilities acquired during hospitalization. For example, the patient who is having extensive skin grafting for a large traumatic wound on one leg should not be found to have foot drop on the unaffected limb when reconstructive procedures are completed.

The patient may tire of the hospital menu and may need to be encouraged to eat a well-balanced diet to promote healing of the graft, to reduce the chance of infection, and to maintain muscle strength during hospitalization. If he is on bed rest for a long time, it is important that bulk food be eaten in sufficient quantities to help elimination and plenty of fluids be taken so that complications of the renal system do not develop.

■ TATTOOING

Tattooing has been found useful in plastic surgery for changing the color of grafted skin so that it more closely resembles the surrounding skin. This treatment is usually given on an ambulatory basis. Pigment is carefully selected and blended with the normal skin coloring by a skilled technician who then impregnates the grafted skin, using a tattooing needle. The procedure is painful, since no anesthetic is used. Sometimes the patient is given a sedative such as phenobarbital or is instructed to take such medication approximately 1 hour before coming to the clinic or the physician's office. Prior to the tattooing, the skin is cleansed with a gauze sponge moistened with alcohol or normal saline solution. There may be a slight serous oozing from the skin after the treatment and it should be left to dry and crust. Sometimes a piece of sterile gauze can be placed over the tattooed area, and an ice bag may be applied if severe discomfort follows the treatment.

Tattooing is usually done in several stages. The amount done at one time depends on individual circumstances such as the location of the part treated and the emotional reactions of the patient. For example, treatment of the skin close to the eye is often quite painful and is extremely trying for the patient. Therefore usually only a small amount of tattooing is done at one time. Children may be given a general anesthetic for treatment around the eyes. Grafted skin may change in color with time, so tattooing done for the purpose of changing the color of grafted skin may have to be repeated.

Port-wine stains that are too large to treat by excision and grafting have also responded to this method of treatment with excellent results. The whole area may be treated at one time and the treatments repeated so that the color changes slowly. This is a tedious procedure if the stain is large and dark but, finally, in some cases the stain is barely apparent to the casual observer.

■ DERMABRASION AND CHEMICAL PEELING

Dermabrasion

Pockmarks, scars from acne, and certain other disfiguring marks may be removed from the skin by abrasive action. The variable results depend on the type and extent of the condition, but there is usually noticeable improvement in the patient's appearance (Fig. 12-6). Preoperatively the patient is prepared by the surgeon for the degree of improvement to be expected so that his expectations are realistic. He is also informed about the face bandage he may wear, postoperative swelling, discomfort, crusting, and the erythema, which may persist for several weeks. The procedure is performed under local or general anesthesia, depending on the size of the area to be treated, the individual patient, and the preference of the surgeon. It may be done in the clinic, the surgeon's office, or the hospital, again depending on the extent of the procedure and the preference of the physician.

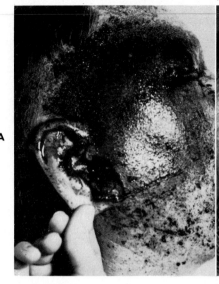 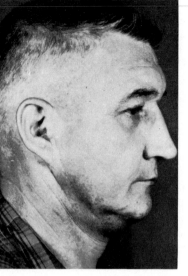

FIG. 12-6. A, Meticulous cleansing and dermabrasion were required to remove impregnated bits of galvanized metal. **B,** Postoperative view of patient 17 years after dermabrasion. (From Havener, W. H., Saunders, W. H., and Keith, C. F.: Nursing care in eye, ear, nose, and throat disorders, St. Louis, 1974, The C. V. Mosby Co.)

Hospitalization is necessary if a general anesthetic is used.

The skin is washed with germicidal soap for several days prior to surgery, and then a nonirritating aqeous antiseptic such as benzalkonium chloride is used to prepare the skin in the operating room.[28] Ethyl chloride or other less flammable spray anesthetics such as Frigiderm are used most often for local anesthesia. After the skin preparation has been completed, the skin is stretched and its superficial layers are removed either by sandpapering or by using an abrasive machine (Dermabrader). If the procedure has not been extensive and oozing is slight, the area may be left uncovered. Usually it is covered either with an ointment or by compresses moistened with an antiseptic solution such as benzalkonium chloride and then by a pressure dressing that covers the entire face except for the eyes, nose, and mouth. Prepared dressings that adhere less readily to the skin surface, such as Telfa dressings, are also used.

If the patient has had a general anesthetic, he must be turned to his side to prevent the dressing from becoming wet or contaminated in the event of vomiting or excessive salivation. The dressing should be checked for signs of bleeding, and the patient must be observed for signs of respiratory embarrassment, which may be caused by pressure from the dressing. A pressure dressing usually is removed after 48 hours, and the patient is discharged to return to the physician's office or the clinic. Washing the face and shaving are seldom permitted until all the crusts have fallen away, but some physicians permit the patient to wash his face gently with a mild soap as soon as the dressing has been removed. If the patient's face feels dry after healing has occurred, gentle lubrication with substances such as cold cream usually is advised. Dermabrasion may be done in stages. At least 2 weeks and often longer may intervene between treatments.

Chemical peeling

Chemical peeling is a newer approach to changing the condition of the skin. There are specific indications for dermabrasion and for chemical peeling and some indications overlap. Chemical peeling is particularly suited for removing fine wrinkles of the face. A special chemical solution is applied to the skin, and then a waterproof tape mask is applied to the area. As the solution is applied, the patient experiences a brief burning sensation. Later, after the mask is applied, the burning pain returns and medication for relief of the pain is frequently necessary. When the mask is removed, the skin is edematous and weeping. A crust develops that separates spontaneously as the skin underneath leaks. Following the procedure, the skin of the person is sensitive to direct and indirect sunlight for a period of 3 to 6 months.[2]

■ MAXILLOFACIAL SURGERY

Maxillofacial surgery is a specialty requiring a surgeon with unusual preparation and nurses with special knowledge and experience. Maxillofacial surgery received impetus as a result of the injuries sustained in World War II and the increase in radical surgery now being done for malignancies of the head and neck. The surgeon works closely with the dental surgeon and with the specialist in problems of the nose and throat. Preventing infection, ensuring an adequate airway, and providing nourishment for the patient are some of the greatest nursing problems. (For details of nursing care, see p. 617.)

The emotional reactions of patients who undergo extensive maxillofacial surgery are severe, and one of the biggest nursing problems is attempting to keep

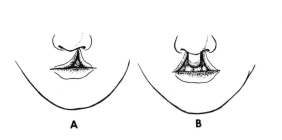

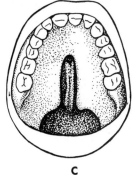

FIG. 12-7. Cleft lip and palate. **A,** Single cleft of lip. **B,** Double cleft of lip. **C,** Cleft of posterior palate.

up the patient's morale. The patient may be helped by seeing someone else who has undergone a similar operation with a good result and who has made good adjustment. When damage has been so great that reconstruction with living tissue is impossible, it is sometimes possible to construct prosthetic parts of the face that are so true to natural color and contour that they are not easily detectable. For example, a side of the nose may be replaced by a prosthetic part that is colored to match the patient's skin and disguised with marking to resemble skin.

■ BIRTH DEFECTS

Birth defects can occur in any part of the body. Providing they are treated at the proper time in the child's life, most of them can be improved a great deal by reconstructive procedures and some can be corrected entirely. The most important nursing responsibilities lie in helping to place children with birth defects under specialized medical care. These responsibilities are discussed in the first part of this chapter. Anomalies of the urogenital system are fairly common and are discussed in Chapter 20 and more fully in pediatric nursing texts and specialized medical texts on these subjects. Musculoskeletal anomalies and deformities are among the more common anomalies and are discussed fully in specialized nursing texts on orthopedic nursing.

Cleft lip and *cleft palate* are among the most common birth defects (Figs. 12-7 and 12-8). Cleft lip usually is repaired surgically soon after birth. Some surgeons repair the defect in the first few days of life before the baby leaves the hospital. In some cases the repair is done when the infant is 6 to 8 weeks old and there is more tissue available for the repair. A second operation often is necessary but does not imply that the first one was not successful. A cleft palate is a much more difficult defect to treat than a cleft lip. It is repaired as early as possible, depending on the extent of the defect and the condition of the child. Most specialists believe that it should always be repaired by the time speech is attempted. The many nursing problems that are encountered in teaching mothers to feed and care for an infant with

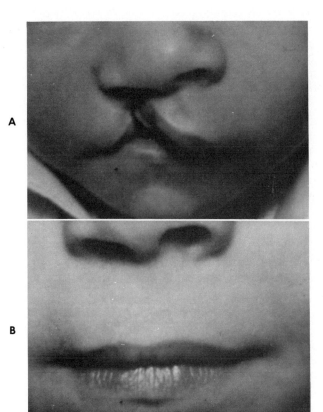

FIG. 12-8. A, Patient with almost complete cleft lip. **B,** Three years after surgery. (From Brauer, R. O.: In Georgiade, N. G., editor: Symposium on management of cleft lip and palate and associated deformities, vol. 8, St. Louis, 1974, The C. V. Mosby Co.)

this defect and that the nurse needs to know to care for a child who has had a cleft lip or cleft palate repaired are included in pediatric nursing texts and current periodicals and will not be included here.

■ COSMETIC SURGERY

Reconstructive surgery of the nose, *rhinoplasty,* is the most common cosmetic surgical procedure. Bone and cartilage may be removed from the nose if it is irregular, or they may be inserted if a defect such as a saddle nose is being corrected (Fig. 12-9). A local anesthetic is often used for these procedures unless it will interfere with a study of contours during the operation. In this case an intravenous or a rectal anesthetic may be used. The incision is usually made at the end of the nose inside the nostril so that it is not conspicuous. A nasal splint made of plaster, tongue blades, or crinoline may be used for protection. Immediately after surgery there will be ecchymosis and swelling around the eyes and nose. Ice compresses and an ice bag may be used to help prevent these reactions. The patient must anticipate

waiting several weeks before evaluating the final result of the surgery.

Another common operation for purely cosmetic effect is removal of some of the cartilage from the ears in order to flatten them against the head. This procedure is relatively simple for the plastic surgeon and requires only a short hospitalization.

Rhytidoplasty is commonly called "facelifting." An incision is made at the hairline, and excess skin

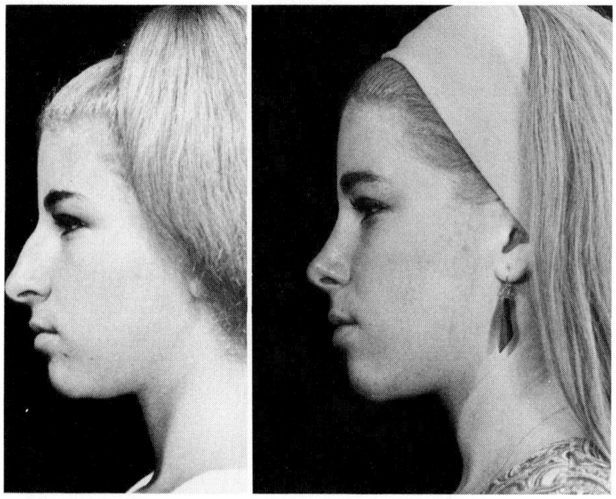

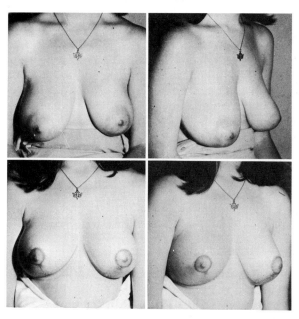

FIG. 12-10. Surgical correction of a moderate degree of hypertrophy and ptosis in a 20-year-old patient via nipple transposition procedure. Top: Preoperative views. Bottom: Postoperative views. (From Wise, R. J.: In Masters, F. W., and Lewis, J. R., Jr., editors: Symposium on aesthetic surgery of the face, eyelid, and breast, vol. 4, St. Louis, 1972, The C. V. Mosby Co.)

FIG. 12-9. A, Preoperative appearance of 16-year-old girl. **B,** Postoperative appearance 1 year after rhinoplasty. (From Peck, G. C.: In Masters, F. W., and Lewis, J. R., Jr., editors: Symposium on aesthetic surgery of the nose, ears, and chin, vol. 6, St. Louis, 1973, The C. V. Mosby Co.)

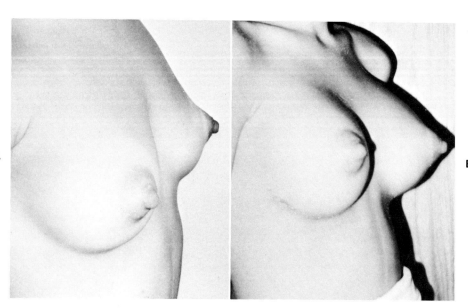

FIG. 12-11. A, Preoperative appearance of the patient. **B,** Early postoperative appearance following augmentation with the Silastic mammary prosthesis, new seamless design, medium size. (From Gerow, F. J.: In Masters, F. W., and Lewis, J. R., Jr., editors: Symposium on aesthetic surgery of the face, eyelid, and breast, vol. 4, St. Louis, 1972, The C. V. Mosby Co.)

is separated from its underlying tissue and removed. The remaining skin is pulled up and sutured at the hairline, thus removing wrinkles and giving firmness and smoothness to the face. A gentle pressure dressing is then applied and left in place for 24 to 48 hours. The patient is often discharged at this time and sutures are removed later in the surgeon's office. The patient frequently needs medication for pain in the postoperative period because of the extent to which the tissue has been undermined.

Mammoplasty can be done to improve the appearance of a woman's breasts. Some women develop conspicuously large and pendulous breasts that they wish to have reduced in size. Large breasts are embarrassing to some women and make it difficult for them to participate in sports, maintain good posture, and buy clothes that fit. Such women often respond to reconstructive surgery remarkably well (Fig. 12-10). Cosmetic surgery of the breast may also be done to make unusually small breasts larger (Fig.

12-11). A variety of plastic materials may be used for this procedure.

Reconstructive surgery of the breast is usually a major procedure and requires the use of general anesthesia. A variety of dressings are used postoperatively and some of them restrict arm motion. The patient must be instructed not to use her arms to lift herself since this strain on the pectoral girdle must be avoided. The nipples should be checked frequently for signs of vascular insufficiency and either pallor or venous congestion of the nipples should be reported at once. The patient is advised to wear a firm, supporting brassiere both night and day for several months after surgery. It is important that the fit be such that firm, constant support is provided when the patient is in the prone position. If the patient cannot make necessary adjustment in brassieres she already owns or cannot buy satisfactory ready-made brassieres, she may need to have some specially made. Large department stores usually provide this service.

REFERENCES AND SELECTED READINGS*

1 Atkinson, H. C.: Care of the child with cleft lip and palate, Am. J. Nurs. **67**:1889-1892, Sept. 1967.
2 Baker, T. J., and Garden, H. L.: Chemical face peeling and dermabrasion, Surg. Clin. North Am. **51**:387-402, April 1971.
3 Castillo, P.: The younger look: rhytidectomy, A.O.R.N.J. **8**:41-45, Nov. 1968.
4 Converse, J. M., editor: Reconstructive plastic surgery, Surg. Clin. North Am. **47**:261-556, April 1967.
5 Conway, H.: Skin grafts—the techniques, Am. J. Nurs. **64**:94-97, Nov. 1964.
6 Cronin, T. D., and Brauer, R. O.: Augmentation mammoplasty, Surg. Clin. North Am. **51**:441-452, April 1971.
7 Edwards, B. F.: Endoprostheses in plastic surgery, Am. J. Nurs. **64**:123-125, May 1964.
8 Grabb, W. C., and Smith, J. W.: Plastic surgery, Boston, 1968, Little, Brown & Co.
9 Hurwitz, A.: About faces, Am. J. Nurs. **71**:2168-2171, Nov. 1971.
10 Iverson, P. C., and Staneruck, I. D.: Dermal abrasion and nursing care after dermal abrasion, Am. J. Nurs. **57**:860-864, July 1957.
11 Jones, G. P., editor: Care of the plastic surgery patient, Nurs. Clin. North Am. **2**:475-510, Sept. 1967.
12 *Knorr, N. J., Hoopes, J. E., and Edgerton, M. T.: Psychiatric-surgical approach to adolescent disturbance in self image, Plast. Reconstr. Surg. **41**:248-253, March 1968.
13 *Macgregor, F. C.: Selection of cosmetic surgery patients, Surg. Clin. North Am. **51**:289-298, April 1971.

14 Macgregor, F. C., and others: Facial deformities and plastic surgery, Springfield, Ill., 1953, Charles C Thomas, Publisher.
15 McGregor, I. A., and Reid, W. H.: Plastic surgery for nurses, Baltimore, 1966, The Williams & Wilkins Co.
16 McGregor, I. A.: Fundamental techniques of plastic surgery, ed. 5, Baltimore, 1972, The Williams & Wilkins Co.
17 Moyer, C. A., and others: Surgery—principles and practice, ed. 4, Philadelphia, 1970, J. B. Lippincott Co.
18 *Nayer, D. D.: Skin grafts—the patient, Am. J. Nurs. **64**:98-101, Nov. 1964.
19 Rees, T. D., editor: Cosmetic surgery, Surg. Clin. North Am. **51**:265-531, April 1971.
20 Rees, T. D., and Wood-Smith, D.: Cosmetic facial surgery, Philadelphia, 1973, W. B. Saunders Co.
21 Rhoads, J. E., and others: Surgery—principles and practice, ed. 4, Philadelphia, 1970, J. B. Lippincott Co.
22 *Rosillo, R. H., and others: The patient with maxillofacial cancer: psychologic aspects, Nurs. Clin. North Am. **8**:153-158, March 1973.
23 Sabiston, D. E., editor: Davis-Christopher's textbook of surgery, ed. 10, Philadelphia, 1972, W. B. Saunders Co.
24 *Shapiro, C. S., and others: Nursing care of the cleft-lip/cleft-palate child, R.N. **36**:46-60, Aug. 1973.
25 Strombeck, J. O.: Reduction mammoplasty, Surg. Clin. North Am. **51**:453-470, April 1971.
26 Welty, M. J., and others: The patient with maxillofacial cancer: surgical treatment and nursing care, Nurs. Clin. North Am. **8**:137-151, March 1973.
27 Williams, S. R.: Nutrition and diet therapy, ed. 2, St. Louis, 1973, The C. V. Mosby Co.
28 Wood-Smith, D., and Porowski, P. C., editors: Nursing care of the plastic surgery patient, St. Louis, 1967, The C. V. Mosby Co.

*References preceded by an asterisk are particularly well suited for student reading.

13 Special needs of the chronically ill

Extent and effect of chronic illness
Differences between acute and chronic illness
Management of the chronically ill person
The chronically ill person and his family
Rehabilitation
Patterns and facilities for continuing care

■ Prevention and control of chronic diseases is one of the major health problems in the United States today. The incidence of chronic diseases and mortality from chronic diseases have increased since the beginning of the nineteenth century, with the most rapid increase occurring in recent years. This increase has been brought about by a number of developments, one of the first of which was general improvement in sanitation, which led to reduction of many infections that, prior to this time, had cut short the lives of many persons at a relatively early age. A pronounced reduction in deaths caused by the acute communicable diseases and infections came about as organisms became better known, immunizations against many of them were developed, and drugs to combat many organisms were found. In 1900 the leading causes of death were pneumonia and influenza, tuberculosis, and those diseases classified as gastritis. *Today the leading causes of death are diseases of the heart, malignant neoplasms, and vascular lesions of the central nervous system.*

There has been a tendency among health workers to equate chronic disease with old age. While it is true that most elderly people have one or more chronic diseases such as arteriosclerosis, osteoarthritis, and diabetes mellitus, chronic disease is also common in the younger age group. Because of the strides made in pediatric medicine, children who 30 years ago would have died for lack of knowledge and treatment of certain diseases such as cystic fibrosis are now living longer with chronic diseases. The life span at all age levels has increased, and the number of people in each age group has increased as the population as a whole has grown. Predictions of the number of persons who may be afflicted with chronic illness in the future must be based on predictions of population growth based on fertility rates. Fertility rates, however, have been found to be quite unpredictable and do not change as might be expected. For this reason the Bureau of the Census makes two sets of predictions based on fertility rates—one that supposes a high level of fertility and the other a lower level. On either basis the predictions are that by 1980 the largest proportion of the population will consist of persons 5 to 19 years of age.[19] *Based on these predictions and present figures, it is estimated that by 1980 there will be 39.5 million more people than at present who will have one or more chronic conditions, and that 24.4 million of these will be under 35 years of age.*[19]

■ **STUDY QUESTIONS**

1 Review the case histories of patients on a medical or surgical ward in your hospital. What proportion has a chronic illness as either the primary or secondary diagnosis? What proportion has more than one chronic condition? What age group is affected most by multiple diseases?

2 Consult your notes on social and community health aspects of nursing, and review what you learned about the facilities for care of the chronically ill patient in your immediate community. What is the total patient capacity of these facilities, and what percentage of the total population of the city or town could hope to receive care from them if necessary? How are these facilities supported financially?

3 What kinds of patients do you think are most in need of rehabilitation? Select a patient from one of the hospital wards to illustrate rehabilitation needs.

4 From what you have learned of anatomy, outline in detail the physical movements necessary in order to rise from a sitting position in a chair to a standing position. Describe how you would assist a patient to a standing position while allowing him the opportunity to help himself.

■ EXTENT AND EFFECT OF CHRONIC ILLNESS

According to the National Health Survey, 73.8 million people have one or more chronic conditions. The National Health Survey list of chronic diseases included asthma, allergy, tuberculosis, bronchitis, emphysema, sinusitis, rheumatic fever, arteriosclerosis, hypertension, heart disease, cerebral vascular accident and other vascular conditions, hemorrhoids, gallbladder or liver disease, gastric ulcers, kidney stones, arthritis, prostate disease, diabetes mellitus, thyroid disease, epilepsy or convulsions, spinal disease, cancer, chronic dermatosis, and hernia.

During 1969 and 1970 an estimated average of 23,237,000 persons, about 11.7% of the civilian, non-institutionalized population of the United States, were reported to be limited to some extent in performing normal activities as a result of chronic disease or impairment. Of these, approximately 33.3% are under the age of 17 years, 35.8% are 17 to 44 years of age, 21.7% are 45 to 64 years of age, and the remaining 9.2% are 65 years and over. Heart conditions, arthritis, rheumatism, and visual impairment were reported to be among the chief causes of limitation of activity. Of the total number limited in activity, 2.9% are unable to carry on their major activity (work, keep house, or go to school); 6.2% have limitation of some kind but can still carry out their major activity; and 2.6% have limitations but not in their major activity. The remaining 88.3% have no limitations. Within these percentages, however, there is an age variation. Only 0.2% of those under 17 years of age are unable to carry on their major activity, while 16.4% of those 65 years and over are unable to carry on their major activity.[49]

Further, persons with chronic illness who are limited in mobility as well as in ability to carry on their major activity are likely to have a greater number of "bed-disability days" (time actually confined to bed). During the period from July 1957 through June 1961 approximately 18 million people had their activity limited due to chronic illness; and of these, about 4.7 million had mobility limited to some degree. Those who had only activity limitations had bed-disability days ranging from 12.7 to 62.5 days/year. Those who had the additional limitation of mobility had bed-disability days ranging from 31.9 days/year if they had difficulty getting about alone to 131.3 days/year if they were confined to the house. The average number of bed-disability days for those who could not move about alone was 41.8 days/year.[48]

The inability to work or to move about influences greatly the kind of medical treatment and health supervision needed by persons who have chronic illness. Some need only periodic medical examination and perhaps continuing treatment with drugs. Others may require complete physical care. Some have a disease that progresses very slowly without remissions, while others may have episodes of acute illness and then seem comparatively well for a time. Each person requires thorough consideration to determine the stage of his illness and the course his disease is likely to take. To help the patient appropriately, the nurse should be able to distinguish between these phases of illness.

■ DIFFERENCES BETWEEN ACUTE AND CHRONIC ILLNESS

An acute illness is one caused by a disease that produces symptoms and signs soon after exposure to the cause, that runs a short course, and from which there is usually a full recovery or an abrupt termination in death. Acute illnesses may become chronic. For example, a common cold may develop into chronic sinusitis. A chronic illness is one caused by disease that produces symptoms and signs within a variable period of time, that runs a long course, and from which there is only partial recovery. The symptoms and general reactions caused by chronic disease may subside with proper treatment and care. This period during which the disease is controlled and symptoms are not obvious is known as a *remission*. However, at a future time the disease becomes more active again with recurrence of pronounced symptoms. This is known as an *exacerbation* of the disease. A chronic disease is characterized by remissions and exacerbations and slowly progressive physical changes. Many emotional, social, and economic implications of chronic illness will be mentioned later in this chapter.

Acute exacerbations of chronic disease often cause the patient to seek medical attention and may lead to hospitalization. Distinction must be made between acute illness and an acute phase of a chronic illness. The needs of a patient who has an acute illness may be very different from those of the patient with an acute exacerbation of a chronic disease. For example, a young person may enter the hospital with complaints of fever, chest pain, shortness of breath, fatigue, and a productive cough. If the diagnosis is pneumonia, the patient usually can be assured of recovery after a period of rest and a course of antibiotic treatment. However, if the diagnosis is rheumatic heart disease, and if the patient is being admitted to the hospital for the third, fourth, or fifth time, the reassurance needed will not be so definite, clear-cut, or easy to give. In this instance it will be necessary for the nurse to begin planning care that will extend beyond the period of hospitalization, taking into consideration many aspects of the patient's total life situation. The concerns of the patient who has had repeated attacks of illness will be very different from the concerns of the one who has a short-term illness.

Further, the nurse must be aware of the needs of

patients who are admitted to the hospital with an acute illness but who also have an underlying chronic condition. For example, the elderly patient who enters the general hospital with pneumonia may receive treatment for the pneumonia and recover from his illness. However, he may still be hampered by the arteriosclerotic heart disease and arthritis that he has had for years. These two chronic conditions may have been aggravated by the acute infection, or the patient's return to his former activity may be hindered by joint stiffness resulting from enforced bed rest and inactivity. The nurse who considers the patient's several diagnoses can help in preventing new problems associated with his chronic illness.

Early detection of chronic illness

Relatively little is known about how to prevent chronic illness. Predisposing characteristics or habits that help to identify the person likely to develop a particular chronic disease have been studied extensively. By altering habits of eating, rest, activity, or smoking, the course of certain chronic diseases such as emphysema or cardiac disease may be changed. Unfortunately many chronic conditions begin without the individual's awareness of significant physiologic changes. An important step in prevention is early detection of these changes.

Screening programs and periodic health examinations are two methods that have helped to identify persons who are "high risks" and considered more likely to develop certain chronic diseases. Simple tests are offered to all citizens of the community or to selected groups such as workers in industry, children at school, women, or men. Some of the more familiar screening tests are chest x-ray examinations to detect heart disease, cancer or tuberculosis; urine or blood sugar tests to detect possible early signs of diabetes; and blood pressure determinations to detect hypertension.

Screening tests may be offered to apparently well persons who have no particular symptoms. Often in the course of interviews with persons coming to these screening programs, signs and symptoms of chronic illness are obvious to the interviewer although the person has either attached no meaning to them, ignored them, or attributed them to some other cause. Careful questioning about daily activities frequently uncovers discomforts such as joint pain, backache, swelling of the ankles, shortness of breath, and other signs that may indicate early and chronic disease.

The *interview* accompanying a screening test can be as important in detection as the test itself. The nurse responsible for planning screening programs should try to ensure the inclusion of an interview as part of the program. Conferences scheduled with parents in order to discuss their children offer ideal circumstances and opportunity for the nurse in the hospital clinic or community agency to offer counseling, health guidance, health appraisal, and appropriate referral for diagnosis.

Screening tests differ from diagnostic tests in that the latter are used either to establish the presence of disease or to rule it out. Nurses should know the diagnostic facilities available in their community and encourage the public to use them. Earlier medical treatment is now sought by families who carry medical, hospitalization, or group health insurance, but most persons need help in understanding the importance of early detection.

■ MANAGEMENT OF THE CHRONICALLY ILL PERSON

The management of the chronically ill person today is focused on *prevention and reduction of disability and on enabling the person to remain a socially functioning individual in every respect.* Some of the disability seen among the chronically ill might have been prevented if prompt, aggressive, suitable medical and nursing care had been available at the onset of illness. Many of the difficulties that limit the chronically ill may not have been caused by the disease but may have developed because of immobility during the acute phase of the illness.

Keeping the patient's body in good alignment, maintaining muscle tone, and preventing contractures are physical measures that every nurse must bear in mind constantly while working with any patient. A careful plan of rest and activity helps to preserve physical resources and to make the day purposeful. If assistance is needed, the nurse or a trained assistant can help the patient with the activity.

Much was said in Chapter 1 about the nurse's need for self-knowledge and self-understanding as well as the need for understanding the patient. This concept is particularly important in caring for the chronically ill. Before nurses can help patients to help themselves, they need to distinguish between their own values, standards, and goals and those of the patient. In day-to-day contact with a patient who is making little or no progress the nurse may be tempted to make plans for his future because of a sincere interest in helping him. This is particularly true when the patient is about the same age as the nurse. The nurse may feel that something must be done to speed progress. Helping the patient to help himself (for example, in getting out of bed independently) is progress. The nurse may become frustrated by the feeling of wanting to do something or wanting to see some marked change. However, there must be recognition on the part of the nurse that management of the chronically ill patient requires a slow-moving, persistent pace with possibly little or no change for a long time. The patient's physical and mental condition must be maintained at its present level or improved, and effort must be made to further his progress and to encourage his and his family's acceptance of his condition. His eagerness and readiness to progress will be determining factors of his future. The "doing" in the care of the chronically ill patient is not always an active, physical "doing" with the hands. Many times the maintenance of a positive approach and attitude and a demonstration of real interest are the greatest help to the patient.

Nursing assessment

Since medical diagnoses do not accurately reflect the physical capacity of the chronically ill person, the use of a *physical profile system* may be instituted as a guide for those working with the patient.[29] The patient is graded considering six categories: (1) physical condition such as cardiovascular, pulmonary, gastrointestinal, genitourinary, endocrine, or cerebrovascular disorders; (2) upper extremities, including the shoulder girdle, and cervical and upper dorsal spine; (3) lower extremities, including the pelvis, and lower dorsal and lumbar sacral spine; (4) sensory components relating to speech, vision, and hearing; (5) excretory function, including the bowels and bladder; and (6) mental and emotional status. The grades for each of these categories range from 1 to 4. Grade 1 indicates no expected difficulty. Grade 2 indicates a minor difficulty that does not preclude normal activity but that may require occasional medical supervision. Grade 3 indicates a difficulty that requires medical and/or nursing supervision but that does not prevent limited activity. Grade 4 indicates severe impairment requiring constant and complete care.

The nurse should assist in making the evaluation of each patient and in interpreting it to others who may care for him or who may be making plans with him. The "Patient Information Guide for the Nurse," included in Chapter 1, can be useful to the nurse in carrying out this responsibility. The nurse can use the guide in planning for nursing care, both immediate and long term, and will find it useful in assisting the family to make realistic plans for the patient's care. Since a chronic condition is not static, reassessment should be made at regular intervals to indicate improvement or regression.

Nursing intervention

Recognizing what is meaningful to the patient is one of the first steps toward helping him to help himself. Personal needs become of paramount importance to the chronically ill patient. Meeting these physical needs provides a way for the nurse to convey to the patient her interest in his progress and welfare. By helping the patient to take his own bath, to attend to toilet needs, and to groom himself, the nurse can give him some sense of accomplishment

and help him to maintain his self-esteem. Helping him to be dressed appropriately is important. Patients who are in their homes or in substitute homes should be encouraged to dress in regular, comfortable street clothing rather than in pajamas or gowns. Visitors coming into the home and members of the family who constantly see them dressed in bedclothes think of them as sick and are reminded of the illness. Seeing them dressed as they ordinarily would be helps to maintain normal attitudes, relationships, and expectations. An appropriately dressed housewife seated in a wheelchair paring vegetables is much more conducive to ordinary, cheerful conversation with neighbors than one who is dressed in a gown, robe, and slippers sitting with her hands idle.

Nursing care of chronically ill patients requires alertness of feeling, seeing, and hearing. Continued warmth and interest are necessary to the well-being of a chronically ill person. Very often it is the nurse who helps the patient change and become highly motivated. It may be taxing to listen to the same person and to say the same things day after day, but the nature of chronic illness may require this attention, and the way in which the nurse responds will convey warmth and interest. The world of a chronically ill person, whether he is in the hospital or elsewhere, becomes narrowed and circumscribed. He treasures and is interested in those things and those people who are close about him. His conversations may be largely about himself, his immediate environment, a few close objects, and the persons who are close to him. Although he is confined to bed and to his room, others can keep him up-to-date on outside news. Many patients welcome hearing about outside

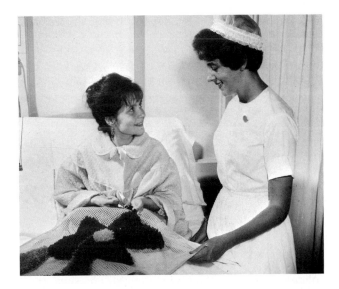

FIG. 13-1. Occupational therapy provides the patient with purposeful activity. Interest shown by the nurse encourages the patient to complete the project.

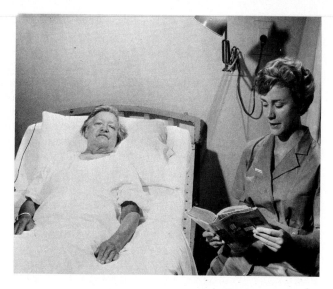

FIG. 13-2. Volunteers can often be recruited to read to disabled patients.

events, but others may not be able to think beyond themselves. Newspapers, magazines, radio, and television help patients to keep up their interest in others and in outside world events. Creating something with their own hands also helps some patients (Fig. 13-1).

Public libraries in many communities provide facilities for disabled persons. Ceiling projectors for books, books of current interest printed in large type, and recordings of books and music are often available on loan. Volunteer workers may act as readers both in hospitals and in homes (Fig. 13-2). Many libraries have elevators and ramps that make library facilities available to the person who is unable to climb stairs and may make taking a person to the library in a wheelchair possible. The publication *Books for Tired Eyes** should be of interest to nurses.

Some communities have organized "friendly visiting programs" in which volunteer workers go to the hospital or the home to provide companionship and to do errands for patients. The nurse should evaluate the advisability of such a plan, and sometimes the physician should be consulted. "Visitors" are not advisable for all patients and should be selected carefully. Often the nurse can help the visitor to give appropriate help to the patient.

Activity with a purpose, no matter how small the activity may be, is desirable for the chronically ill person. One may hear the patient say to friends that he does not have time to visit because he has to take care of the plants, do personal laundry, or perform some other task that may seem unimportant to the casual observer. Actually, to the patient these jobs may appear to be the most important in the world.

*Published by the American Public Library Association.

■ THE CHRONICALLY ILL PERSON AND HIS FAMILY

Most persons with a chronic or long-term illness can be cared for at home and actually prefer to be at home, where family and friends are close by and where they can still contribute something to family life. They all require medical supervision. The arrangements that can be made vary greatly and depend on the needs of the individual and the facilities available. Many persons are ambulatory and during remissions are able to visit their local clinic. Others manage with visits from their personal physicians and with a periodic diagnostic workup done in the office or with the assistance of a technician who goes into the home. Public health nurses from voluntary and official agencies help the chronically ill in their homes. Many chronically ill persons with disabilities also visit special rehabilitation units of hospitals or outpatient centers for daily or periodic instruction and practice in physical skills and job training.

The nurse who visits the home to assist the individual and/or family member to accomplish daily care will need to give special attention to helping the family understand the patient. The chronically ill person is very often misjudged by even the closest members of his family because of lack of understanding. The nurse needs to help the person's family to understand his limitations and his necessary restrictions. Both the individual and his family may benefit from association with others who have had similar experiences. The chronically ill and their families often meet together in organized groups to share experiences. For example, there are organizations for persons who have an ostomy and for persons who have multiple sclerosis. There has been a recent growth of such groups because of the increase in chronic illness and because people are reluctant to accept the isolation that chronic illness may impose.

Marked changes often take place in family living as a result of chronic illness. Families often find themselves drawn closer together, and new relationships develop. For example, when it is suddenly learned that the mother has a heart condition, the husband and teenage children may rally to assist in household chores. All seem to work together with a special purpose in mind. On the other hand, family members may drift apart and be incapable of helping one another. Chronic illness may threaten an individual's basic emotional stability, and the whole situation may be unbearable to others. Sometimes the individual's emotional needs may not have been apparent to the family early in the illness, but when such needs grow obvious, relatives feel inadequate in the situation. The length of illness, periodic hospitalization, increased financial burdens, and emotional and social burdens are sometimes more than families can withstand. Public assistance is accepted by many families, whereas others find it degrading.

Many persons struggle on their own to assume the full financial burden and consequently expose other members of the family to lower standards of nutrition, housing, and care. Many times relatives move in with one another, arguments develop, and family ties are strained or broken. Some accept public and other assistance without reservation and make little attempt to help themselves.

The effects on individuals and their families are numerous and varied. Usually the individual and the family as a whole will respond in a manner similar to that in which they have reacted to problems in the past. However, the first impact of the disability may nearly immobilize both the individual and his family. For example, a person who is almost totally helpless as a result of an accidental spinal cord injury may seem to have no interest in learning ways to help himself. His family may react in the same way and be of little help to him. At this time both the individual and his family need interest and support from professional persons. With this reassurance the individual may learn that he can do some activities such as bathing part of his body and combing his hair. This small success may be stimulating enough to strengthen his motivation so that he and his family may make amazing strides in thinking through and working out future problems themselves. In order for their planning to be realistic and ultimately functional, medical and paramedical personnel must teach them the total physiologic ramifications of the disability as well as methods of coping with the ramifications.

The chronically ill person is most often an individual who determines to live his life although his problems may seem insurmountable to the professional people who care for him. Each nurse working with chronically ill persons has seen that many times life has meaning for the individual even though it may not be apparent to the nurse. Nurses with this understanding can help make the person's life more satisfying and can positively influence the attitudes of the family, professional co-workers, and the public.

The cost of disability

Every effort should be made to prevent disability in any person who has a chronic illness. Disability can be devastating to the individual, his family, and the community, and it takes its toll in the nation's productivity. Most individuals who are unable to work must be supported by others, either from private or from public funds.

There are 2 million adults between the ages of 18 and 64 years who are unable to work because of chronic disabilities.[19] *There are an additional 3.5 million who are partially limited in ability to work. About 800,000 of the totally disabled persons are now receiving benefits under the Social Security Administration's Old-Age, Survivors, and Disability Insurance Program. An additional 400,000 disabled persons receive public assistance from the Aid to the Permanently and Totally Disabled Program.*

The cost of hospitalization rises yearly. Frequent or extended hospital stays and medical expenses can be devastating for patients and their families if they are inadequately insured or if they can no longer qualify for insurance programs. Many are reduced to seeking public assistance merely to survive. Placement in quality nursing homes is frequently financially impossible for patients or their families to manage. The cost of medications to control or maintain a patient's health status may require major portions of the family budget. The goal, then, of maintaining the patient in the best possible condition relative to his illness must be the primary concern of each nurse who works with such a patient. A good program of maintenance is the best way to help the patient avoid excessive financial drain caused by unnecessary or preventable complications. Further, if the availability of means by which the patient's goals may be achieved is limited by inadequate financial resources, the ingenuity of the nurse may be greatly taxed to find substitute means for achieving the goals.

The ability of the individual family to pay its own way is determined in part by which member of the family becomes disabled. Studies show that if the wife is disabled, the family suffers less economic deprivation. However, money is only one consideration. Each disabled person and his family are subjected to great personal and emotional losses that must also be dealt with. Loss of self-esteem, loss of status within the family, feelings of rejection, and feelings of helplessness are only a few. These can be more devastating than economic deprivation.

The death rate of the disabled population is high. For persons under 50 years of age, the death rate is 10 times that of the total population between the ages of 25 and 49 years. The death rate for disabled persons between the ages of 50 and 54 years is higher than for all persons in the general population who are 75 to 84 years of age. Two thirds of the disabled persons are men.

■ REHABILITATION

Rehabilitation has been defined by many persons, and each definition seems to express the particular viewpoint of the person or organization offering it. "Rehabilitation is an adjustment to living"[31] is one simple definition. An expanded definition is as follows: "Rehabilitation is the process of assisting the individual with a handicap to realize his particular goals, physically, mentally, socially, and economically."[31] The purpose or extent of rehabilitation ranges from employment or reemployment for the handicapped person to the more limited achievement of developing the ability to give his own daily care. This latter accomplishment can be just as important to the individual as earning money and may represent his greatest life achievement. This might be true, for example, for a person who was born with a severe physical handicap such as cerebral palsy.

Success in learning to adjust to living with a disability will depend on the person's premorbid personality and total life experience and premorbid family relationship as well as the current behavior and motivation the person presents. Certainly some rehabilitation can occur in any health agency; nevertheless, the greater the number of rehabilitation disciplines working cooperatively with the individual, the greater is his chance of achieving his highest potential. The rehabilitative process, as any form of education, is involved as deeply in the motives and purposes of the teacher as those of the learner.[45]

The person with a disability, whether it is obvious to others or unrecognizable to them, should not be viewed from the standpoint of his disability alone. Usually his greatest need is for comprehensive health services and continuing care. *Comprehensive care* has been defined as "care that is provided to the patient according to his needs in an appropriate, continuous, and dynamic pattern.[36] Accommodating the plan of care to the needs and goals of the individual is the essence of comprehensive care.

The nurse in rehabilitation

The concepts of comprehensive nursing management and rehabilitation can be considered synonymous. Helping the patient and his family to help themselves is an integral part of nursing care. The nurse who is working with patients who have disabilities has two major responsibilities: first, to see that disability from disease is limited as much as possible and, second, to see that a rehabilitation program is planned and implemented. Limitation of disability requires attention to the prevention of complications, to early recognition of symptoms of exacerbations or complications, and to the prevention of deformity. For patients with chronic illnesses, the onset of exacerbations or complications is frequently subtle, marked by minute changes in functional ability or general performance or attitude. Nurses who work closely with such patients and who understand the pathophysiology of the patients' diseases are frequently the first to recognize initial signs of difficulty and make provision for appropriate intervention.

The second responsibility, planning and implementing a program of rehabilitation in accordance with the patient's goals, is a process in which the nurse is intimately involved. Nursing personnel are likely to be in contact with a patient and his family for a greater period of time each day than are members of any other single discipline on the rehabilitation team. Both in the hospital and the home the nurse is in an excellent position to plan a reasonable care program with the patient as well as teach the patient, his family, and if necessary his employer about his limitations and rehabilitative expectations.

Much of the nursing activity in the rehabilitation process is no different from the nursing care given to all patients. The assistance that the nurse will be able to give the patient and his family will depend on an ability to understand self, personal feelings, and personal behavior as well as the behavior of the patient, his family, and other professional team members. Chapter 1 includes a discussion of these basic understandings. Additionally, the patient in a rehabilitation program must often learn and practice special physical techniques to strengthen muscles and to improve mobility. Such measures as physical exercise to improve walking, activities to improve self-care abilities, and the use of prostheses require of the physical and occupational therapists special knowledge and technical skills. To be effective in the rehabilitation process, the nurse must have an understanding of the techniques used by the various therapists in order to be able to plan and work cooperatively with the therapist in caring for the patient and to be in a position to help the patient use these physical techniques in carrying out the activities of daily living.

The nurse must assume responsibility for teaching the patient and family as well as helping them utilize what is taught them by members of other disciplines. Such things as appropriate bowel and bladder programs, providing proper diet and fluid requirements, and implementing new methods of bathing and maintaining skin integrity fall within the domain of nursing concern and knowledge. Initially, nursing personnel may assume almost total responsibility for performing these activities for the patient. After assessing patient needs in these areas, the nurse formulates, implements, and evaluates a teaching plan in much the same way as do therapists from other disciplines.

One of the most important aspects of giving continuing care to a patient with a disability is the nurse's own attitude, perseverance, and expectations. Improvement may be slow and the patient may reach a "plateau" in his progress. Such a time can be critical for the patient because he may become discouraged and not wish to continue with his program of care. The nurse's encouragement can often sustain the patient so that he will not regress in any respect until some improvement is noted.

Teamwork in rehabilitation

The number of professional people required to assist the patient and his family with rehabilitation will vary. Most often the patient, his family, the phy-

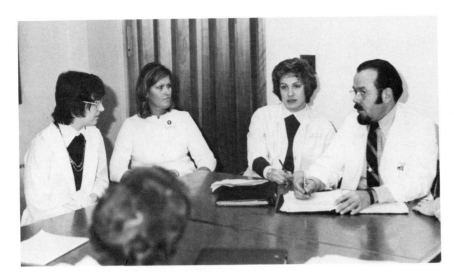

FIG. 13-3. The team approach to rehabilitation is essential. Here, the physician, nurse, physical therapist, social worker, and occupational therapist review a patient's program and progress.

sician and the nurse can work out a practical plan. If a patient's problems are complex, a social worker and perhaps a psychiatrist may be necessary. Specific physical limitations of the patient may require the services of a psychiatrist, physical therapist, occupational therapist, or speech pathologist. If learning a new type of job is a part of the patient's adjustment, a vocational counselor may be needed. Teamwork requires that each member of the group be able to use his special knowledge and skill and understand the value of his contribution to the patient's care. In addition, each team member needs some understanding of each of the other professional person's functions and contributions.

One of the cooperative efforts of the team is to meet regularly to thoroughly evaluate the patient and the abilities he has to use. Based on this assessment, the patient and the team devise a plan to help him readjust, compensate, and learn new ways of managing self-care and living. A typical rehabilitation team consists of a physician, nurse, medical social worker, vocational counselor, psychologist, speech pathologist, occupational and physical therapists, and case worker from the patient's social agency. In Fig. 13-3 some of the members of this team review a patient's rehabilitation program.

Patient motivation

The most important contributions to his rehabilitation are made by the patient himself. The patient, the physician, the nurse, the social worker, the occupational therapist (Fig. 13-4), and sometimes others planning together can arrive at the best goal for his future, but the patient's attitudes, acceptance, and direction of motivation are the most important considerations. If he cannot accept his disability, whatever it may be and however extensive it may be, attempts at rehabilitation usually are hindered. The patient is the person who really makes the decisions, and he changes within himself at his

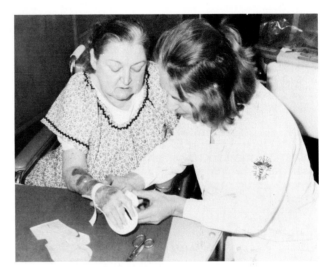

FIG. 13-4. The occupational therapist makes a resting splint for a patient whose hands are severely deformed by rheumatoid arthritis. The splint will be worn by the patient in an effort to prevent further deformity.

own pace. If he is agreeable to suggestions but makes little or no effort to try them, one should question if he really has accepted the suggestions.

The patient's behavior from day to day in small ways can be the first indication of the direction of positive motivation. For example, if he makes every effort to resume normal daily activities such as feeding himself, bathing, and dressing, one can be quite certain that he is a person with a sincere desire to be independent. As he becomes ready for more advanced activities such as ambulation and work in the occupational therapy shop, he needs continuing genuine interest and support from the nurse and others (Fig. 13-5 to 13-6). As obstacles present themselves, he may be able to accept them and eventually overcome them. The patients who are truly motivated toward helping themselves never seem to give up

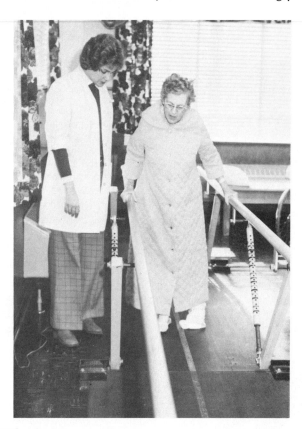

FIG. 13-5. The physical therapist begins the patient's ambulation training by teaching her to walk with the support of the parallel bars. The patient's left foot is wrapped in a towel to remind her not to bear weight on it.

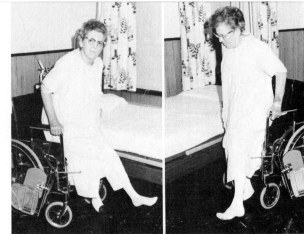

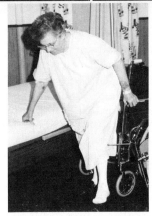

FIG. 13-6. **A,** The patient executes a transfer from bed to chair. She is nonweight bearing on her left leg; thus she moves toward her right, or strong side. **B,** Here the patient moves back into bed from the wheelchair, again leading with her right, or strong side. She pushes up from the chair using the arms of the chair for support. **C,** Having attained her balance, she places her right hand on the bed for support, pivots on her right foot, and sits down. Elderly patients in particular need time and encouragement to learn proper, safe transfer techniques. Leaving the shoe off the affected foot can be a reminder to the patient not to place the foot on the floor.

and find ways of accomplishing activities that professional personnel might believe impossible. However, there are some patients who, when faced with an added burden, cannot accept it and give up trying. Guidance and support for the families of such patients becomes tremendously important.

Special services for rehabilitation

Patients with very complex problems of rehabilitation may need to receive care at specialized centers for rehabilitation, or care at home may be combined with visits to a day rehabilitation center. Rehabilitation centers and services have developed quite rapidly since World War II. There are various types of centers: teaching and research centers (centers located in and operated by hospitals and medical schools), community centers with facilities for inpatients, community outpatient centers, insurance centers, and vocational rehabilitation centers. In addition to centers that provide multiple services for the physically disabled, there are specialized centers for rehabilitation of the blind, deaf, mentally ill, and mentally retarded. Most centers offer a wide range of services that usually fall into three areas:

Medical Area
Physical and medical evaluation
Physical therapy
Occupational therapy
Speech therapy
Medical supervision of appropriate activities

Psychosocial Area
Evaluation
Personal counseling
Social service
Psychometrics
Psychiatric service
Recreational therapy

Vocational Area
  Work evaluation
  Vocational counseling
  Prevocational experience
  Industrial fitness of programs
  Trial employment in sheltered workshops
  Vocational training
  Terminal employment in sheltered workshops
  Placement

Advantages of organized programs. Patients participating in organized programs of therapy have an opportunity to see and be with others who have similar or more extensive disabilities. Often they progress more rapidly when they realize that others have similar difficulties and are overcoming them. Group therapy often arouses a competitive spirit, and a formerly reluctant person may become willing and diligent. On the other hand, the nurse, physician, and therapist need to be alert to those patients who have the opposite reaction. A patient who sees others advance in activity while he either does not improve or progresses very slowly may become so discouraged that he gives up trying.

Activities are scaled so that the individual can see his own progress in comparison with his beginning abilities. Patients may take an active interest in keeping their own scores. After a program of therapy has been planned and is scheduled as to time of day, the patient can help to keep himself on the schedule by having a copy of it at the bedside. The nurse can help him gradually assume more and more responsibility for getting himself ready for scheduled activities.

A master plan of activities for all patients on the unit can be a useful device for nurses, physicians, and therapists. The plan can be kept in a central place on the unit and should list name, activity, and time of activity for each patient. This type of plan is helpful, too, when a patient's progress is to be re-evaluated.

In the community a public program for vocational rehabilitation has been serving the nation since 1920 in a partnership between the state and the federal governments. Services for disabled persons are provided by state divisions of vocational rehabilitation. The federal government, through the Social and Rehabilitation Service (SRS), administers grants-in-aid and provides technical assistance and national leadership for the program. Opportunities and services are available in each of the 50 states, the District of Columbia, and Puerto Rico. All persons of working age with a substantial job handicap resulting from either physical or mental impairment are eligible for help or assistance. The purpose of this service is to preserve, develop, or restore the ability of disabled persons to earn their own living. The individual services offered are medical care, counseling and guidance, training, and job finding. Thirty-six states have separate rehabilitation programs for the blind.

Application for such services can be made to the Social and Rehabilitation Service or to the agency in the state for serving the blind.

■ PATTERNS AND FACILITIES FOR CONTINUING CARE

It is impossible to include here all of the many facilities that provide continuing care. Only those programs that have been developed or emphasized recently will be considered.

Outpatient care. The term "ambulatory care" is used interchangeably with the term "outpatient care." Persons who are able to come to a patient care facility outside their own homes very often attend outpatient clinics. The number of persons receiving care solely in the outpatient service has increased tremendously and is still growing. A good outpatient service constitutes one of the most important elements of the hospital's contribution to community health. Many persons receive all their medical care under these auspices, whereas others come only for diagnosis or follow-up care. Increased use of outpatient emergency services is one of the most rapidly developing practices at the present time.

Home care. Until fairly recently the home was the place where medical treatment was given. Well-to-do persons rarely thought of going into a hospital, and they received the services of a private physician in their own home. The family was responsible for the day-to-day care. Poor families were among the first persons to use hospitals. The philosophy of home care can be traced as far back as 1796, when the Boston Dispensary provided medical care to the sick poor. One of the first institutions to study and demonstrate the advantages of continuous medical care for patients at home was the University Hospital in Syracuse, New York, in 1940. The Montefiore Hospital Home-Care Program in New York City started their services in 1947, and within a year the New York City Department of Hospitals initiated similar programs in five city hospitals. By 1950 eleven additional New York City hospitals offered this service. In 1960 some 30 cities had 45 coordinated home care programs, caring for approximately 5,000 patients.[21] By 1965 there were some 60 coordinated home care programs in the United States.

One of the most obvious reasons for the development of home care programs was to provide care to patients with long-term illnesses who did not need the around-the-clock services of an institution and yet might be too ill to go to an outpatient service. Caring for patients at home is what the individual and his family often want, and it also releases hospital beds for use by acutely ill patients.

The coordinated home care program provides comprehensive patient care for persons who otherwise might not receive it. The specification that the program is coordinated means that it is centrally administered and, through coordinated planning, evaluation, and follow-up procedures, provides physician-directed medical, nursing, social and related services to selected persons at home. This program can be offered either by a hospital or by a community agency such as a local health department.

Most patients have been in the hospital before referral to home care and often have had short hospital stays for acute exacerbations or complicated treatments interspersed with periods at home. This service provides care that could not be equaled easily in institutional care. Not only does the patient have the security of knowing that he is counted as a part of the hospital census and will receive continuing care, but he also has the satisfaction of being cared for in his own environment by a group of professional people who know him, his family, and his total situation.

Home care is not the solution for all patients. The present trend is toward smaller dwellings, and adequate space for the patient and other members of the family may be at a premium. The choice of home care or institutional care will depend largely on the desires of the patient and his family. Despite many inconveniences, some families wish to have the patient with them. The family's understanding of the patient and his situation and their ability to assist one another will make a great difference. Not only may space be inadequate, but many times it is impossible to have a member of the family in attendance with the patient during the day. Members of the family who work cannot afford to sacrifice jobs to stay with the patient. However, many families find it easier financially to have the patient at home and are able to make satisfactory arrangements even though the facilities are limited.

Some communities now provide portable meals (Meals-on-Wheels) for homebound persons. Most programs provide one hot meal daily and unheated food for at least one other meal. The cost differs widely and depends on the services offered, such as special diets, and on the sponsorship of the plan. Volunteer groups frequently act as delivery messengers. The local public health nursing service usually participates actively in the plan by selecting suitable patients and by being a resource for the workers who encounter health problems on their "rounds." This service alone often makes it possible for a chronically ill person to remain at home.

Home Health Aid services. Home Health Aid services have developed with the increased use of home care plans and particularly since Medicare plans have come into existence. The greater number of persons eligible for Home Health Aid services under Medicare has spurred the growth of such services, not because the services were not needed before but because the cost of such services would have been

prohibitive for most of the persons who needed them. Medicare makes payment for such services available to a large number of persons. When there is a demand for service and a means of paying for the service, there are usually agencies that will begin providing the service. Home health aides are being trained in many states and are assigned to home care through a central office that coordinates plans of care often in collaboration with public health nursing agencies. The public health nurse assists by evaluating the home situation and the patient's need for physical personal care. Consequently, the public health nurse supervises the home health aide in continuing care.

Homemaker services. Homemaker services also have developed with the increased use of home care plans. These services are increasingly in demand in many communities and may be sponsored by a public or voluntary health or welfare agency that employs personnel to furnish homemaker service to families with children and to the person who is convalescing, aged, or acutely or chronically ill. Women homemakers are trained to assist in homes where the mother or other responsible family manager is temporarily unable to perform her usual responsibilities because of illness or absence.

Institutional resources. Many patients and families have to resort to institutional care for the patient because their own facilities are not suitable, no member of the family can be in attendance during the day, or the kind of care needed by the patient requires close professional supervision. A large or a limited selection of outside facilities may be available, depending on the community. These include chronic disease hospitals, skilled care facilities, convalescent homes, rest homes, homes for the aged, and nursing homes.

Foster homes. Care in foster homes is a relatively new service that is now being widely used in many communities. Carefully selected families volunteer to take chronically ill persons into their own homes and provide the nonprofessional care that is needed. The family is paid either by the patient or his family, from public funds, or by some social agency. The plan is primarily for those patients who have no family and who cannot live alone, but who neither desire nor need institutional care.

Nurse's role in continuing health care. The nurse may be involved in continuing health care in a number of ways: as a supervisor of home health aides; as a public health nurse or visiting nurse involved in a primary rehabilitative program in the home; or as a hospital nurse concerned about the care a patient will be receiving after he leaves the hospital, particularly in situations where the patient's rehabilitation program is not completed or where rehabilitation is not possible. The nurse must know the community resources available to the patient in order to interpret to him and his family what resources he may be able to obtain, the types of services from which he may benefit, and what kinds of referrals he needs for obtaining those services. When care is to be continued beyond the hospital setting, the hospital nurse should clearly communicate (with the patient's permission) to the continuing care agency those data pertinent to the care of the patient that will provide continuity in the transfer of services. Teamwork and continuity are the keys to successful rehabilitation services for patients, and they must be practiced at all stages of the patient's care if the patient is to realize his fullest potential.

REFERENCES AND SELECTED READINGS*

1 Anderson, H. C.: Newton's geriatric nursing, ed. 5, St. Louis, 1971, The C. V. Mosby Co.
2 Areawide planning of facilities for rehabilitation services, Report of the Joint Committee of the Public Health Service, Publication no. 930-B-2, Washington, D. C., 1963, U. S. Department of Health, Education and Welfare.
3 Barker, R. G., and others: Adjustment to physical handicaps and illness: a survey of the social psychology of physique and disability, New York, 1953, Social Science Research Council.
4 Christopherson, V. A.: Role modifications of the disabled male, Am. J. Nurs. **68:**290-293, Feb. 1968.
5 Cockerill, E., and Margolis, H. M.: The concept of disability, J. Chronic Dis. **3:**167-169, Feb. 1956.
6 Council on Medical Service, Committee on Aging: Report on conferences on aging and long-term care, Chicago, 1965, American Medical Association.
7 *Crate, M.: Nursing functions in adaptation to chronic illness, Am. J. Nurs. **65:**72-76, Oct. 1965.
8 Ford, A. B., and others: Results of long term home nursing: the influence of disability, J. Chronic Dis. **24:**591-596, Sept. 1971.
9 Garrett, J. F., and Levine, E. S.: Psychological practices with the physically disabled, New York, 1962, Columbia University Press.
10 *Goffman, E.: Stigma, Englewood Cliffs, N. J., 1963, Prentice-Hall, Inc.
11 Gordon, G., editor: Proceedings: Conference on medical sociology and disease control, New York, 1966, National Tuberculosis Association.
12 Guidelines for the practice of nursing on the rehabilitation team, New York, 1965, American Nurses' Association.
13 Hirschberg, G. G., and others: Rehabilitation: a manual for the care of the physically disabled and elderly, 1964, J. B. Lippincott Co.
14 *Hurd, G. G.: Teaching the hemiplegic self-care, Am. J. Nurs. **62:**64-68, Sept. 1962.
15 Katz, S., and others: Studies of illness in the aged: the index of A.D.L.: a standardized measure of biological and psychosocial function, J.A.M.A. **185:**914-919, Dec. 1963.
16 Kolb, L. C.: Disturbances of body image. In Arieti, S., editor: American handbook of psychiatry, vol. 1, New York, 1959-1966, Basic Books, Inc., Publishers.
17 *Kottke, F. J., and Anderson, E. M.: Deterioration of the bedfast patient, causes and effects and nursing care, Public Health Rep. **80:**437-451, May 1965.
18 Ladieu, G., and others: Studies in adjustment to visible injuries, evaluation of help by injured, J. Abnorm. Psychol. **42:**169-192, 1947.
19 Lilienfield, A. M., and Gifford, A. J., editors: Chronic diseases and public health, Baltimore, 1966, The Johns Hopkins University Press.
20 Litman, T. J.: An analysis of the sociologic factors affecting the rehabilitation of physically handicapped patients, Arch. Phys. Med. Rehabil. **45:**9-16, Jan. 1964.
21 Littauer, D., Flance, I. J., and Wessen, A. F.: Home care, Hospital monograph series no. 9, Chicago, 1961, American Hospital Association.
22 *Madden, B. W., and Affeldt, J. E.: To prevent helplessness and deformities, Am. J. Nurs. **62:**59-61, Dec. 1962.
23 Martin, N.: Nursing in rehabilitation of physically disabled. In Beland, I. L., editor: Clinical nursing: pathophysiological and psychosocial approaches, ed. 2, New York, 1970, Macmillan Publishing Co., Inc.
24 Martin, N., King, R., and Suchinski, J.: The nurse therapist in the rehabilitation setting, Am. J. Nurs. **70:**1694-1697, Aug. 1970.
25 Mead, S.: Rehabilitation. In Cowdry, E. V., editor: The care of the geriatric patient, ed. 3, St. Louis, 1968, The C. V. Mosby Co.
26 *Morris, E. M.: Choosing a nursing home, Am. J. Nurs. **61:**58-61, Jan. 1961.
27 Morrisey, A. B.: Rehabilitation nursing, New York, 1951, G. P. Putnam's Sons.
28 *Morrissey, A. B., and Zimmerman, M. E.: Helps for the handicapped, Am. J. Nurs. **53:**316-318, March 1953; **53:**454-456, April 1953.
29 *Moskowitz, E., and McCann, C. B.: Classification of disability in the chronically ill and aging, J. Chronic Dis. **5:**342-346, March 1957.
30 Myers, J. S.: An orientation to chronic disease and disability, New York, 1965, Macmillan Publishing Co., Inc.
31 National Health Forum: Changing factors in staffing America's health services, New York, 1954, National Health Council.
32 *Olson, E. V., editor: The hazards of immobility, Am. J. Nurs. **67:**780-797, April 1967.
33 Palmer, I. S., guest editor: Nursing in long term illness, Nurs. Clin. North Am. **5:**1-84, March 1970.
34 Questions and answers on health insurance for the aged, medical and related aspects of the new program and how it will operate, Social Security Administration, Washington, D. C., 1965, U. S. Department of Health, Education and Welfare.
35 *Riffle, K. L., guest editor: The patient with long term illness, Nurs. Clin. North Am. **8:**571-681, Dec. 1973.
36 Ryder, C. F.: The chronic disease era, J. Miss. State Med. Assoc. **4:**96-101, March 1963.
37 Schreiber, F. C.: Dental care for long-term patients, Am. J. Nurs. **64:**84-86, Feb. 1964.
38 Shapiro, L.: Rehabilitation stalemate, Arch. Gen. Psychiatry **15:**173-177, Aug. 1966.
39 *Sister M. Willa: Nursing in rehabilitation, J. Nurs. Educ. **4:**15-23, April 1965.
40 *Skinner, G.: The nurse—key figure in preventive and restorative care, Hospitals **35:**52-56, Jan. 1961.
41 Skipper, J. K., and others: Physical disability among married women: problems in the husband-wife relationship, J. Rehabil. **22:**16-19, Sept.-Oct. 1968.

*References preceded by an asterisk are particularly well suited for student reading.

42 *Sorensen, K., and Amis, D. B.: Understanding the world of the chronically ill, Am. J. Nurs. **67**:811-817, April 1967.

43 *Stoeckle, J. D., and others: Medical nursing clinic for the chronically ill, Am. J. Nurs. **63**:87-89, July 1963.

44 Stryker, R.: Rehabilitative aspect of acute and chronic nursing care, Philadelphia, 1972, W. B. Saunders Co.

45 Talbot, H. S.: A concept of rehabilitation, Rehabil. Lit. **22**:358-359, Dec. 1961.

46 Terry, L. L.: Health needs of the nation, Public Health Rep. **76**:845-851, Oct. 1961.

47 The expanding role of ambulatory services in hospitals and health departments, Bull. N. Y. Acad. Med. **41**:1-158, Jan. 1965.

48 U. S. Department of Health, Education and Welfare, Public Health Service: Vital and health statistics—bed disability among the chronically limited, National Health Survey, July 1957-June 1961, Series 10, no. 12, Washington, D. C., Sept. 1964.

49 U. S. Department of Health, Education and Welfare, Public Health Service: Vital and health statistics—limitation of activity due to chronic conditions, National Health Survey, 1969 and 1970, Series 10, no. 80, Washington, D. C., April 1973.

50 Weeks, L. E., and Griffith, J. R., editors: Progressive patient care, an anthology, Ann Arbor, Mich., 1964, The University of Michigan Press.

51 Whitehouse, F. A.: The utilization of human resources: a philosophic approach, Chest **30**:606, Dec. 1956.

52 Williams, S. R.: Nutrition and diet therapy, ed. 2, St. Louis, 1973, The C. V. Mosby Co.

53 Wright, B. A.: Spread in adjustment to disability, Menninger Clin. **28**:198-208, July 1964.

14 Accidents, emergencies, and disasters

Accidents

Accidents in the United States claimed 114,000 lives in 1970. Accident costs amounted to around $27 billion. This figure includes medical expense, insurance and claim settlement, damage to motor vehicles, property loss in fires, certain indirect costs of work accidents, and wage loss. Motor vehicles accounted for the greatest number of accidental deaths in all age groups under 75 years in 1970, and accidents of all kinds were the leading cause of death for individuals 1 to 37 years of age in the same year. There was a 27% increase in the number of accidental deaths between 1958 and 1968; accidents were the fourth most important cause of death (exceeded only by heart disease, cancer, and strokes) in all age groups during 1970.[1] It is important to note here that the recent imposition of the 55 mile/hour speed limit in a move to conserve energy has reduced considerably both the number of automobile accidents and the number of deaths from such accidents. Since it appears that this restricted speed limit will continue, it is expected that the accident rate may decrease instead of increase as in the past.

Many injured persons spend months and years seeking some degree of rehabilitation. The Cleveland Press, April 29, 1970, reported on a study by the Department of Transportation, which concluded that the American automobile insurance system has largely failed. The report stated that "in the case of 22% of the seriously injured accident victims, another family member was forced to find a job, 14% had to move to cheaper housing, 30% had to draw on savings and 28% had to borrow money. . . ." According to the deputy assistant transportation secretary, 45% of the victims were forced to change their standard of living. He said that this report gives some insight "into the human sufferings associated with the losses."

The chief of the Division of Accident Prevention, Public Health Service, has described the accident as "a phenomenon of diverse, often multiple etiology, often the result of an occurrence or series of occurrences, chronologically remote from the accident itself."[37] Accidents are, for the most part, preventable and require attention not only to their causes and the environment in which they occur but also to the victim's physical, social, and psychologic state as well as to his readiness to avoid accidents through attainment and application of public education.

■ STUDY QUESTIONS

1 Based on reports in the daily papers, list what you believe to be the most common causes of accidents.
2 What provisions are there in your hospital for the reporting of accidents within the hospital? What action is taken when an accident occurs? By whom is the action taken?
3 What are some precautions taken in your unit to prevent accidents to patients?
4 List potential accident hazards that are found in the average home.
5 What is the civil defense program in your hospital, in your community, and in your state?
6 What are the common causes of accidents to older patients?
7 What poisonous snakes are found in the area where you live?

■ PREVENTION OF ACCIDENTS

Prevention is the keynote to success in dealing with the problem of accidents. Accident control has been acknowledged as a major public health goal, and both the American Public Health Association and, in the United States, the Public Health Service are active in promoting accident prevention. In addition, some communities have organized citizen committees that have been helpful in conducting surveys of accident hazards in homes.

Teaching accident prevention and participating in programs for accident prevention are responsibilities of all members of the health team, including physicians, nurses, and health educators. Nurses are essential members of this team. Their influence can be felt in many areas because they are represented in schools, in industry, in the home, in the hospital, and elsewhere in the community. Space does not permit a detailed description of the many ways in which a nurse can contribute in this important health field, but a few examples will be given for some areas. Many references are available. The nurse can turn to the National Safety Council, which has a monthly publication, *Home Safety Review,* and a yearly bulletin, *Accident Facts.* An excellent way for the nurse to keep informed in this field is to read regularly the *Statistical Bulletin* of the Metropolitan Life Insurance Company. Nurses can contact their local health department for health education materials and for information on other sources, such as the many excellent publications on accident prevention prepared by life insurance companies and industrial organizations. Engineers are often invaluable resource people for consultation on structural hazards at home and in the community. The safety committee in the nurse's own hospital or public health agency may be of help. Finally, nurses must use their own resourcefulness and imagination in preventing accidents.

Home and community

Nurses can help in accident prevention whether they are actively practicing nursing in a hospital or community nursing agency or whether they are not currently practicing professionally. Lay individuals and lay groups often turn to nurses for assistance and guidance in learning of community needs and of how they may best contribute in accident prevention. They should be able to point out good sources of general information on the national level, such as the reports of the National Safety Council. The local or county health department, the local police department, the visiting nurse association, the welfare and health council, or similar agencies are all good sources of help. The nurse should assure the layman that his voice will be heard provided it is directed to the right authorities and may point out that groups have a stronger voice than individuals. Parent-teacher associations, various religious and social organizations, and many other groups are interested in the

problem of accident control. Efforts should be made to use existing agencies and groups and to work with them in order that the sincere efforts of small groups of enthusiastic citizens will not be dissipated. Phases of accident prevention that should be of community interest include (1) teaching of accident prevention in the public schools, (2) better control and inspection of homes for the aged, (3) rigid enforcement of driving regulations, (4) improvement of street lighting and traffic signals at busy intersections, (5) periodic inspection of all automobiles, and (6) promotion of laws pertaining to fire-proofing of buildings and laws protecting the public from flammable clothing, potentially harmful toys, and similar items.

Accidents in and about the home cause almost one third of all accidental deaths each year. Falls account for about half the number, and fires, burns, and poisonings account for most of the remainder. Many aged persons who fall do so when walking from room to room. Some fall because of heavily waxed floors, loose rugs, poor lighting, scattered toys, and other conditions that could have been corrected. A fair number of fatal home accidents occur as a result of the popular "do it yourself" movement. People are falling from roofs, windows, high ladders, and steps and are being fatally burned or otherwise injured while using solvents and cleansing agents without proper knowledge of their hazards. The number of electric appliances used in the home has increased the danger of electric shock and fire from overloaded circuits. Many persons die in fires caused by burning cigarette ashes left on furniture or rugs and by cigarettes that are dropped as the smoker falls asleep. Attention needs to be given to teaching homeowners with older heating systems to have the equipment checked periodically for gas leaks and other unsafe features.

The public health nurse may be called on to evaluate the patient's home for accident hazards prior to his leaving the hospital. Very often such patients are those with physical disabilities. This kind of request provides the nurse with an ideal opportunity to teach not only the patient but also members of his family about general accident prevention as well as specific measures for the safety of the patient.

Child abuse

The nurse working in the emergency department must consider the possibility of child abuse when children, especially those under the age of 3 years, are seen with injuries such as bruises, fractures, or burns. When child abuse is suspected, the professional staff members have a responsibility to protect the child from further injury by reporting their suspicions. At the same time it is important that help be sought for the parent or parents involved. In several communities, groups have been organized for parents who are child abusers. Since it has been found that most parents who abuse their children were abused children themselves, this form of group therapy is often helpful in assisting parents to ventilate deep-seated feelings. Information about local groups can be obtained from child welfare agencies. One group working in this area is CALM (Child Abuse and Listening Mediation, Inc.), located in California.*

Hospital

In the hospital the nurse should take an active part in accident prevention. The danger of accidents to hospital patients has increased in recent years. The turnover of patients is much more rapid, and the patient has less time to adjust to his new environment. Early ambulation of patients has added to accident hazards. Most important is the great increase in the proportion of elderly patients. Many are in their eighties and even their nineties. An infinite number of improvements could be made in general hospitals that might reduce accidents, and they vary with each situation. For example, handrails should be installed in the corridors of medical and surgical units, where patients now walk about each day. Stools should be placed in showers, beside tubs, and in washrooms. Chairs with arms should replace the straight, armless ones sometimes used. A nurse's call system should be installed in all bathrooms so that the patient may call for assistance if needed.

Careful study of nursing practice and of the quality of nursing care may reveal good suggestions for accident prevention. For instance, one large hospital[†] analyzed a group of accidents in which patients fell out of bed. The two main causes of the falls were attempts to climb over the side rails and attempts to reach for a bedpan or other piece of equipment on the bedside table when the table or the bed had free-rolling casters. Obvious solutions seemed to be the use of Hi-Lo beds and the removal of casters on beds and bedside tables. The change to Hi-Lo beds must be made gradually, since few hospitals can afford to replace all beds at once.

Study of the patients who attempted to climb over side rails showed that most of them were aged and that many had received barbiturate sedation. Again, measures for prevention of accidents seemed obvious. Aged patients should be placed in Hi-Lo beds and in a location where they will have frequent observation. After having slept for 60 years in a low bed, they cannot remember that they are in a high hospital bed; like Rip Van Winkle, they awake to find many changes. Since sedation may make a patient confused and disoriented, elderly patients should be given fewer sedatives than young persons. It is better to rely on nursing measures such as a warm drink, a backrub, a cheerful word, attention to ventilation, and control of noise to ensure a good night of sleep. Environmental cues such as a night light help to compensate for sensory deprivation in a person whose senses are waning.

The danger of accidental injury or death from fire must be constantly borne in mind by all hospital personnel. If smoking is permitted in patient units, the nurse should caution patients who smoke to be careful and should be on the alert for signs of lack of caution. Many hospitals no longer permit smoking except in a sitting room, porch, or solarium. If the patient has physical and/or emotional limitations that make his conduct unpredictable, and if the physician feels that he should be permitted to smoke, the nurse or an auxiliary nursing staff member should remain with him while he smokes. Conscientious participation by all nurses in regular fire drills is necessary in case a fire should occur.

Emergencies

Every nurse should be conversant with the general principles of first aid and, if a physician is not present, should be prepared to assume leadership when accidents occur. First aid is defined as immediate and temporary care given the victim of an accident. Some general principles have application to most accident situations. The nurse can teach these principles to patients and to their relatives. Booklets such as *The American Medical Association First Aid Manual*[‡] should be useful in helping the public learn the practical steps in first aid. In order to improve emergency care, nurses working in some hospital emergency departments are involved in teaching basic emergency measures to ambulance attendants and members of police and fire department rescue squads.

In the following discussion a distinction will be made between the first aid given by the nurse at the scene of an accident and the nursing care given in the hospital. Usually standing orders guide nursing actions in schools, industries, and public health agencies. Emergency treatment of medical emergencies, including postoperative shock, pulmonary embolism and edema, heart attack, convulsions, cerebrovascular accident, and severe burns, will be considered in chapters relating to the body systems involved.

---

*P.O. Box 718, Santa Barbara, Calif. 93102.

†Unpublished study, The New York Hospital–Cornell Medical Center.

‡Prepared jointly by the American Medical Association's Council on Occupational Health and the Department of Community Health and Health Education of the Division of Environmental Medicine and Medical Services (30¢ each).

■ GENERAL PRINCIPLES OF MANAGEMENT

The first thing to do when an accident occurs is to remain calm and to think before acting, then to step forward and identify oneself as a nurse to the patient and onlookers. Take the patient's pulse; this act will establish the nurse as a person of experience and it will *reassure* the patient if he is conscious. Untrained yet overzealous individuals can be helpful when diplomatically asked to report the location and nature of the accident by telephone to the local police department and physician and to stop traffic or direct people away from where the patient lies. Usually it is best for the police to call the ambulance.

If the patient is conscious, talk to him and assure him that help is on the way. Because physical shock accompanies all traumatic injuries, the injured person should be kept lying down. He may be covered with a light blanket or another covering. *If circumstances permit* and the possibility of spinal injury is remote, a second blanket may be pushed under him with a long flat object. This will conserve body heat and may make him more comfortable. He should be reassured that someone is concerned about him.

Should the nurse be in doubt about the extent of the injuries, the patient should not be moved. However, if the nurse believes it is safe to move the patient, assistance should be obtained from those at the scene. It is the responsibility of the nurse to be sure that the patient is moved gently and that good body alignment is maintained with special attention to the injured part. Clear and firm directions should be given to those willing to help.

Breathing

The best way to tell whether or not the patient is breathing is to watch the movement of the chest and the nostrils and to feel for flow of air from the mouth or nose. If the patient is not breathing, stretch him out on his back and loosen any tight clothing around his neck or chest. Any obstruction to breathing must be removed at once, and if the patient vomits, his head must be turned to one side. His head should be tilted backward to attempt to enlarge the airway to the trachea, but the tongue must be kept forward to prevent its obstructing the air passage. Artificial respiration should be started at once.

The accepted method of artificial respiration at the present time is mouth-to-mouth or mouth-to-nose breathing.[5] First, any foreign matter in the victim's nose and mouth must be removed with a finger or a finger covered with cotton material. The procedure is then as follows:

1. Tilt the victim's head back and pull or push the jaw into a jutting-out position (Fig. 14-1)
2. If the victim is a small child, place your mouth over his mouth and nose and blow gently (Fig. 14-1). If the victim is an adult, open your mouth wide and place it over the victim's mouth while pinching his

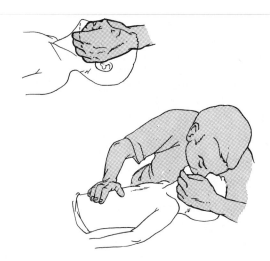

FIG. 14-1. Correct method of mouth-to-mouth breathing in a child. Note that the victim's chin is held forward. Air entering the stomach is removed by gentle compression.

nostrils, or close his mouth and place your mouth over the victim's nose; blow vigorously. Watch to see the chest rise as air enters.

3. Remove your mouth, turn your head to the side and listen for return rush of air.
4. If the chest does not expand or if there is no air return, check position, turn the victim quickly on his side, and slap him between the shoulder blades to loosen foreign matter. Return him to the back-lying position and remove any material from his mouth or nose.

For a child the rate of blowing should be approximately 20 times/minute, blowing puffs of air from the cheeks. For an adult it should be 12 times/minute, blowing air taken in after a deep inspiration. A piece of gauze or other material such as a handkerchief can be placed between your mouth and the victim's. With vigorous blowing, this does not diminish the air blown into the victim's lungs.

Artificial respiration should be continued until the patient has started to breathe or has been pronounced dead. It may be continued for 4 hours or more. Although a few gasping breaths on the part of the patient are most heartening to the person giving artificial respiration, they should not be taken as an indication that artificial respiration can be stopped. Patients may take one or two breaths and then stop breathing again. The patient must be watched carefully for at least an hour, and assistance must be given as needed. A cyanotic and then deep red flush will suffuse the entire face when breathing is resumed. If prolonged artificial respiration is required, the person doing the breathing should be relieved periodically to prevent him from becoming hyperventilated and fainting.

Cardiopulmonary resuscitation (external cardiac massage accompanied by artificial respiration) is

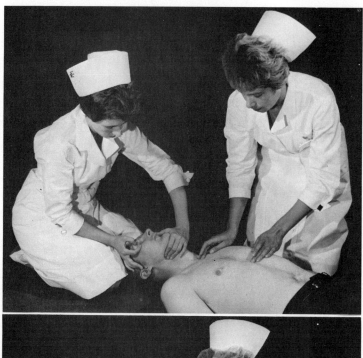

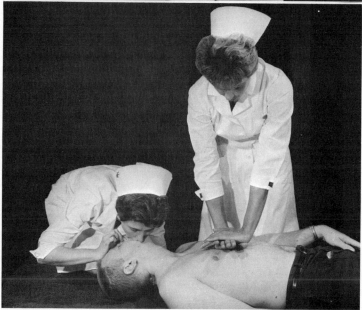

FIG. 14-2. Cardiopulmonary resuscitation. **A,** One nurse is checking for carotid pulse and dilation of the pupils while the other nurse locates the xiphoid process and supraclavicular notch. **B,** As one nurse does mouth-to-mouth breathing, the other applies external rhythmic pressure to the sternum. Note the first nurse's hand under the patient's neck to maintain hyperextension. The second nurse completely releases the pressure after each sternal compression to give the heart a chance to refill.

now considered an emergency procedure and has been found to be as satisfactory as internal cardiac massage in restoring heart action. Nurses and other hospital personnel should be specially trained if they are expected to carry out this procedure as part of their job. There is no doubt that persons who have had special preparation in this procedure have saved many lives by taking immediate action in the interval before medical assistance arrived.

Because cardiopulmonary resuscitation has become a widely accepted emergency procedure, even those nurses who would not ordinarily be called on to do the procedure during their working hours may wish to learn it in order to be prepared for emergency situations in their own homes or community. Ob-

viously no nurse should ever attempt the procedure without special training in the technique involved.

Cardiopulmonary resuscitation is best done by two persons, one who will breathe for the patient and the other who will massage the heart (Fig. 14-2). The usual steps are as follows: (1) Place the victim face up on a hard surface such as the floor. (2) Check the carotid or femoral artery for pulse, the pupils for dilation, and the airway for signs of breathing. (3) By palpating the sternum, locate the xiphoid process and the supraclavicular notch. (4) Tilt the head back to ensure an open airway and give five to six deep breaths either mouth-to-mouth or mouth-to-nose and then recheck the pulse. (5) If there is no pulse, start cardiac massage by placing the heel of one hand just above the xiphoid process, with fingers spread and raised, and the other hand on the first one; press down firmly, depressing 1½ to 2 inches. Repeat this procedure once per second, maintaining the ratio of one mouth-to-mouth respiratory excursion to five depressions. Check the pupils for dilation frequently. If no pupillary contraction occurs within 5 minutes, it is usually considered useless to continue cardiopulmonary resuscitation.

When there is only one person to do both the artificial resuscitation and the cardiac massage, the most important thing to remember is that unless there is oxygenated air in the lungs the massage is useless. While it is extremely difficult for one person to perform cardiopulmonary resuscitation, it has been done successfully. Prepare the patient as above and start the resuscitation with two deep breaths. Then switch positions and compress the chest 15 times. Return to the mouth and give two deep breaths.[63] Continue this routine until help arrives. Obviously, however, one person cannot do this over an extended period of time.

Cardiac massage will maintain the victim's blood pressure until the cause of the cardiac or pulmonary arrest can be determined and treated by the physician. Previously diseased hearts are less likely than normal ones to resume spontaneous sinus rhythm.

Hemorrhage

Bleeding may be external or internal. Severe external bleeding must be treated at once. Quickly run your hands over the entire body surface, being sure to check under the patient. Any pronounced bleeding will have saturated the clothing and can be noted in this way. Cut or tear away the clothing and expose the wound. Cover the wound with several layers of sterile dressing or the cleanest material available. Apply pressure over the dressing with the extended hand. Elevate an extremity that is bleeding. Most bleeding can be controlled in this way, but bleeding from a cut artery may require the use of pressure on a major blood vessel over a bony prominence, proximal to the point of hemorrhage (Fig. 14-3). Digital pressure is most effective when three fingers are used rather than the thumb or only one finger.

A tourniquet may be used if bleeding will not stop by using the other methods. The tourniquet should be at least 1 inch wide, and it should never be made of a material that might cut the flesh (such as a rope or a wire). Tighten the tourniquet just above the wound, tight enough to stop the bleeding but no tighter. Once the tourniquet is applied it should be released only by a physician, no matter how long it has been in place. A notation should be made and attached to the patient, giving the location of the tourniquet and time of application. A large T on the forehead, made with lipstick, identifies the patient as having a tourniquet on. The person who applied

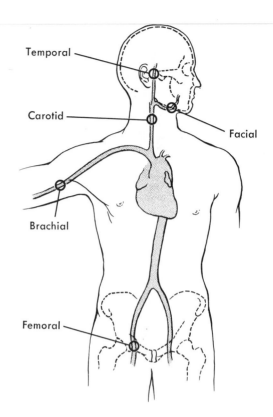

FIG. 14-3. The pressure points—locations at which large blood vessels may be compressed against bones to help control hemorrhage.

the tourniquet should see that the patient receives immediate medical assistance and should accompany him if he has to be moved to receive medical help.

Internal bleeding may be identified by a weak rapid pulse, thirst, sighing respirations, cold clammy skin, and dizziness. If internal bleeding is suspected, keep the patient flat and quiet and apply ice packs if materials are available.

Fracture

It is best not to move the patient or the affected part when a fracture is suspected. Nerves, blood vessels, and other tissues may be damaged, and pain and shock will increase. Fractures of the skull usually are accompanied by loss of consciousness, unequal pupil dilation, heightening color of the face, and, in the case of a fracture at the base of the skull, bleeding or draining serous fluid from the nose and/or ears. Only loose, fluffy dressings may be used on bleeding head wounds as pressure on the damaged area may increase pressure on the damaged brain.

Fractures of the extremities very often will be pinpointed by the conscious patient. Fractures should be suspected if the limb is out of alignment, edematous, or very painful. A compound fracture should be covered loosely with a sterile dressing and a tourniquet placed, but not tightened, above the wound.

Moving the patient. When a fracture is suspected, it is preferable that the patient, especially the injured part, not be moved. If it is necessary to move the patient before medical help arrives, the fractured extremity should be immobilized. Immobilization may be accomplished by the use of splints. Splints may be improvised from a variety of materials such as pillows, pieces of board, and rolled-up newspapers. Even rifle barrels, golf clubs, and tennis rackets have been used by resourceful persons. A heavy magazine makes an excellent splint for the wrist. Lacking even this, many pages of the daily newspaper serve almost as well.

Before the patient is moved, the splints should be prepared and all persons who are to help must know what to do and how to work together. If the fracture is within a joint, the entire limb may be very carefully supported, placed on a splint such as a pillow, and bandaged securely. If the fracture is in the shaft of the bone, gentle traction and countertraction will usually be needed. One person may support the part above the fracture and one may exert a steady, firm pull until the splint has been applied and secured with improvised bandages above and below the site of fracture. Enough bandages should be used to secure the splint and immobilize the whole limb. In some instances (for example, when strong muscle pull is involved, as in fracture of the femur), a steady pull away from the body must be maintained.

No matter how expertly the emergency care has been given, improper handling and careless transportation often add to the severity of the original injuries, increase shock, and frequently endanger life. Various carriers can be used in emergencies, but the stretcher is the preferred device. Stretchers may be improvised from blankets, coats, poles and cloth, or planks of wood. At least three but preferably four people should work together as gently and steadily as possible to lift an injured person onto a stretcher. The fourth person works opposite the other three and places his hands under the thighs and shoulder of the injured person and assists in raising him. While the patient rests on the knees of the three members of the team, the fourth person places the stretcher under the patient.

Fracture of the spine. All questionable injuries to the neck and back, even in the absence of signs of paralysis, should be treated as a fracture of the spine. Paralysis in the unconscious person may be determined by pinching or pricking the toes or fingers with a pin or other sharp object. The patient with injury to the spine requires the most exact care in handling if he must be moved. Forward or backward bending of the spine must not be allowed to occur because it may cause pressure on the spinal cord and immediate death. A door makes the best temporary splint. It takes at least six persons working in perfect harmony to move the patient safely.

The patient with a fracture of the neck or of the lower spine should not be rolled if he is lying on his back. He should be slid carefully sideways onto the board or splint. One person (preferably a physician) kneels at the patient's head and, holding the head securely with his hands under the jaws, exerts a firm, steady pull. A second person supports the patient's feet, again exerting a firm, steady pull. The other members of the team draw the patient's body onto the stretcher or splint. At no time must his head be allowed to bend forward, backward, or to the side. His head and body must move as one piece, and there must be very firm support under his shoulders so that sagging, which will cause forward bending of the neck, cannot occur. If the patient is found lying on his face, he is usually rolled very carefully onto his back and onto the splint. Again, traction is applied to his head so that his spine is kept straight; forward, backward, or sideways bending is avoided. A folded blanket is laid on the splint at the level of the thoracic spine before the patient is placed on it so that the normal position of the spine is maintained when the patient is in a backlying position. (For hospital care of patients with fractures, see p. 916.)

Other injuries

Puncture wounds of the chest must be covered immediately, and manual pressure applied to seal off the wound. Penetrating objects must be left in place, supported and padded until medical attention can be obtained. Covering the wound and leaving penetrating objects in place prevents atmospheric pressure from forcing air into the opening and collapsing the lung.

The unconscious person

If a person is found unconscious either in his home or on the street, he should be examined for signs of having bitten his tongue, as so often happens in convulsions, and for a fruity odor to the breath (presence of acetone), which may indicate diabetic ketoacidosis. Patients subject to convulsions and those with diabetes mellitus are usually advised to carry identifying information on their persons. The odor of poisons such as phenol and iodine and of alcohol can be detected on the breath. When an odor of alcohol is detected, it should not be assumed that the cause of unconsciousness has been determined. The environment should be carefully inspected and relatives and friends interviewed for evidence of the cause of the patient's condition. The patient should be examined for signs of injury, particularly of the head. The skin should be checked for signs of drug injection. No attempt should be made to give anything by mouth to an unconscious person. A physician should be called and immediate arrangements should be made to get the patient to a hospital. Unconsciousness with marked decrease in respirations is common in patients with diazepam (Valium), morphine, heroin, and barbiturate poisoning and in carbon monoxide poisoning. Artificial respiration may be given while awaiting arrival of an ambulance.

■ BITES

Animal bites

The most common animal bites are those of dogs, cats, and rats. Dog bites are particularly dangerous, since dogs are the most common carriers of the deadly disease hydrophobia, or rabies. Cat bites are likely to cause infection because the cat's mouth contains many pathogenic bacteria and because the long, sharp teeth make a deep wound that may become sealed off. Human bites easily become infected because of the very high bacterial count in the human mouth.

The first-aid treatment for all animal bites is extremely thorough washing with soap and hot water for 5 to 10 minutes. Running water should be used. Tetanus toxoid and/or antitoxin may be given. If the bite is deep and if the animal is suspected of having rabies, the wound must be made to bleed and may even be probed, depending on circumstances and how soon medical aid will be available. Strong caustic medications should not be applied. Detergent solutions, however, have been found to be very effective in cleaning wounds from animal bites. The wound should be covered with a piece of sterile or clean gauze, and the advice of a physician sought at once. The physician will decide whether or not treatment for rabies is necessary. The offending animal should always be kept alive until the advice of a physician has been obtained. If it is a household pet and the circumstances indicate that the bite was accidental, the animal will usually be confined and observed for a week to 10 days. If the animal must be killed immediately for the protection of others, the brain should not be damaged and must be sent to a laboratory for examination. If an animal suspected of having rabies is at large, the police department and the health department must be notified at once.

Rabies. Rabies is a fatal acute infectious disease caused by a virus that travels along nerve pathways to the brain. The disease has been known for centuries. In the twentieth century B.C. the Eshnunna code of ancient Mesopotamia set forth strict regulations about the obligations of dog owners who let mad dogs bite persons, thereby causing death.[34] Rabies is most commonly acquired from dogs, but it can be carried by any animal that nurses its young. In the United States it is fairly common in dogs, skunks, bats, foxes, coyotes, racoons, and cats. There has never been a case of human rabies reported in the United States following exposure to infected mice or rats.[2] The economic loss from rabies among cows is significant, even though the cow is not a common source of the disease in man.

Infection always occurs through an open break in the skin caused by the bite of an infected animal. Clothing gives some protection because the animal's teeth are wiped by the garments. Because the saliva is infectious for several days before the onset of symptoms in the affected animal, it is exceedingly important that all suspected animals be caught and kept under inspection for 10 days. If the animal shows symptoms that are strongly suggestive of rabies and is destroyed or dies, its brain is sent to a laboratory for examination. The presence of Negri bodies in the brain of an animal is conclusive evidence of rabies.

Acute rabies can be prevented in man by adequate treatment. Some persons who are exposed will not contract the disease. However, since the disease is always fatal if it develops, the treatment is always given if the offending animal is known or suspected to have rabies. In the United States more than 30,000 people receive the vaccine every year.* If bites have been sustained about the head, the injections will very likely be started at once, since the incubation period seems to be shorter than when the bite is on other parts of the body. Antirabies treatment is usually given if the animal has escaped and is suspected of having rabies.

Treatment consists of copious flushing the wound with water alone, soap and water, or detergent and water. Quaternary compounds such as benzalkonium chloride (Zephiran) may be used.[2] Some experts feel that the immediate and thorough local treatment of all bite wounds is the most effective means of preventing rabies.[2] Both rabies vaccine and antirabies serum are available for prophylaxis against rabies in those who have been bitten. In severe bites both the vaccine, which produces active immunity, and the hyperimmune serum, which produces passive immunity, are used. There are two vaccines approved for active immunization—Duck Embryo Vaccine (DEV) and Nervous Tissue Vaccine (NTV), and either type may be given. However, the lower frequency of central nervous system reactions with DEV make it preferable to NTV.[2] The injections are given subcutaneously in rotating sites in the abdomen, lower back, and lateral aspects of the thighs for 14 to 21 days, depending on the severity of the bite.

The antirabies serum is in horse serum and since horse serum causes allergic reactions in at least 20% of those receiving it, hypersensitivity testing must be performed before it is administered. It should be given as soon as possible after exposure. The dose is 1,000 units (one vial intramuscularly per 40 pounds of body weight. At least one half of this dose

---

*The Plain Dealer, Cleveland, June 1, 1970.

is used to infiltrate around the wound and the remainder is given intramuscularly.[2]

The control of rabies is a public health responsibility. The police and health departments must be notified at once if a rabid animal is thought to be at large. In England and the Scandinavian countries the disease has been almost entirely eliminated by rigid enforcement of laws that prohibit allowing dogs to run about unleashed. Rabies could be controlled by compulsory vaccination of all dogs and cats kept as household pets, capture and confinement of stray animals, and destruction of wild animal reservoirs of infection under the supervision of wildlife experts. Annual vaccination of all dogs is required in some states and counties. How long the immunity lasts following vaccination is not known for certain. Immunization in man is thought to last about a year and in animals up to 39 months.

The public should know that not all rabies-infected animals are "mad." There are two types of rabies. In one type the animal may be restless, barking, and biting. In the other, so-called "dumb" rabies, the animal may be quiet and stay close to its master. In the latter type, paralysis, which begins in the throat and lower jaw, may lead the animal's owner to suspect that something harmful has been swallowed. If he tries to investigate the trouble, some of the highly infectious saliva may enter an abrasion on his hand.

Another name for rabies is *hydrophobia*. The incubation period of the disease in man is from 10 days to more than a year.[11] The involvement, as in animals, is in the central nervous system. The disease is ushered in with a few days of melancholia, depression, pain at the site of the animal bite, and a feeling of impending danger. Acute symptoms (difficulty in swallowing, excessive salivation, muscle spasm, often maniacal fear, difficulty in breathing, and convulsions) then appear. A terrific, painful spasm of the muscle of deglutition occurs when there is an attempt to swallow water—hence the name hydrophobia. Even the mention of water is often enough to bring on an attack. Aerophobia is also present, and convulsions can be produced by a draft of air on the skin. Death from rabies has been reduced in the United States to several cases per year.

The nursing care of the patient with acute rabies is difficult but of short duration. Most patients die from heart failure or respiratory difficulty within 3 or 4 days of the acute onset of symptoms. The patient is restless, irritable, and fearful, with episodes of uncontrolled fear and mania alternating with periods of calm. Every effort is made to keep the patient quiet. The room is darkened, and noises in the halls outside the room should be eliminated. Side rails are placed on the bed and are sometimes padded to help prevent injury during episodes of uncontrolled thrashing about. Sedatives, including chloral hydrate, morphine, and the barbiturates, are given.

Anesthetics may be given intravenously. Fluids often are given intravenously, and it is important to bandage the arm securely on a board to prevent injury in the event of a convulsion or an attack of mania while a needle is in the vein. The head of the bed is sometimes lowered in an attempt to facilitate drainage of saliva, and often suctioning must be used. All persons caring for the patient should be aware of contamination with saliva, and a gown and rubber gloves should be worn.[2] Relatives of the patient must be prepared for the fact that the patient cannot talk. Sometimes the visits of relatives bring on severe painful muscle spasm in the throat of the patient, who is usually conscious up to the time of death even though he is unable to speak.

Insect bites

Insect bites are more serious in children than in adults. Multiple bites have caused serious systemic reaction and even death of children. If the reaction is severe or prolonged, medical aid should be sought at once. The bites of wasps and bees are among the most common of insect bites and occasionally cause serious and even fatal reactions. A dressing of sodium bicarbonate and water often gives relief, since formic acid is present in the material injected by these insects. A weak solution of household ammonia also decreases pain and is safe to use.

A tick is best removed by holding the hot end of a previously lighted match to it, thereby causing it to withdraw its mouthpiece. Sudden removal of a tick will result in its mouthpiece being left in the skin. A drop of turpentine placed on the insect is also effective and without fire hazard. Ticks are the vectors of Rocky Mountain spotted fever and Colorado tick fever. If the person bitten lives in an area where these diseases are endemic, medical advice should be sought.

Mosquito bites are important because one species of mosquito (*Anopheles*) is active in the transmission of malaria and encephalitis and because the bites of mosquitoes and similar insects sometimes cause troublesome infections. The greatest danger of infection is in elderly persons with poor circulation in whom bites on the legs may lead to infected ulcers that heal with extreme difficulty. The best treatment for the nuisance and discomfort of mosquito bites is prevention, largely by avoiding highly infested areas and wearing protective clothing when one must be exposed. A mosquito net worn over a broad-brimmed hat when outdoors and the use of a large net canopy when sleeping provide good protection. Draining of swamps where mosquito larvae live helps in some areas. Oil of citronella and many trade preparations are useful as repellents, but none are completely effective. Lotions containing calamine and phenol help to allay the itching and discomfort accompanying the bites.

The bites of poisonous spiders and other poisonous insects such as scorpions are treated in a manner similar to treatment of snakebite.

Snakebites

There are four kinds of poisonous snakes in the United States. Three of them, the copperhead, the cottonmouth moccasin, and the rattlesnake, belong to the group known as pit vipers and are distinguished by a pit resembling a second nostril between the eyes and the nostril and by a broad, flat, triangular head. Everyone should know the kinds of poisonous snakes found in the part of the country in which he lives and how to recognize them. The copperhead, named for its color, is about 3 feet long, and is found in the eastern and southern states. The cottonmouth moccasin is grayish in color and blends with its surroundings. It is found in marshy country in the southeastern states. Rattlesnakes are probably found in every state in the United States and are responsible for the largest number of bites and the largest number of deaths. One antivenin is effective for all pit vipers.

The fourth poisonous snake, the coral snake, is small with coral, yellow, and black rings encircling its body. It is found in North Carolina and other southern states, particularly around the Gulf of Mexico. The snake is shy and seldom bites, but its venom is deadly and affects the nervous system. No specific antivenin is prepared for the bite of the coral snake, but cobra antivenin, kept in most zoos, is effective.

Poisonous snakes in North America will almost always move away when disturbed and will not bite unless suddenly molested without warning. Snakebites can often be prevented by wearing high leather boots and thick trousers when walking through snake-infested areas. Heavy gloves should be worn and the greatest care taken when climbing because hands may be placed on ledges that cannot be seen, and reptiles often sun themselves on rocky ledges.

The bite of a poisonous snake is distinguished by two fang marks above the horseshoe-shaped array of tooth marks. Immediate severe pain and swelling distinguish the bite of a poisonous snake from that of a nonpoisonous one, even when swelling and discoloration are so sudden as to make the fang marks impossible to see. The wider the space between the fang marks, the larger the snake (sometimes unseen) and the more intensive the treatment should be.

The first-aid treatment for snakebite is the immediate application of a tourniquet just above the bite. This tourniquet should not be tight enough to prevent venous return in deep vessels or arterial supply to the part but should be tight enough to prevent superficial venous circulation of blood and lymph, thus stopping absorption of the poison. In severe cases, if swelling appears above the tourniquet, the tourni-

quet is reapplied above the level of edema, or a second tourniquet may be used. Incision into the bite must be made immediately, and the cut should be made in the direction of nerves and blood vessels to prevent injury to them. A pocketknife or any sharp instrument, sterilized if possible by flaming with a match, can be used. If emergency snakebite equipment* is not available, suction must be applied by mouth. This procedure is safe, since the venom is not poisonous if swallowed. Suction should be continued constantly for at least 30 minutes and then for 15 minutes out of each hour until medical aid is found. The patient should lie quietly to lessen circulatory flow and absorption of the poison. Since shock may develop from the poison, he should be kept warm. Medical aid should be sought at once. About 15% of the persons bitten by poisonous snakes die without treatment.[5] If a snakebite kit is available, antivenin should be given at once. If a physician is not available or is delayed, whoever is at the scene should inject at least half of the ampule into the tissue around and above the bite and the rest intramuscularly in any nonedematous muscle. Warm fluids can be given. Alcohol is contraindicated since it may speed up the absorption of venom. Signs of poisoning are palpitation, weakness, shortness of breath, nausea and vomiting, and dimness of vision. Occasionally the venom from the snake is injected directly into a blood vessel and fatal reaction may occur within 15 minutes.

When the patient who has been bitten by a snake arrives at the hospital, the nurse should anticipate that stimulants such as caffeine may be ordered. Intravenous infusions of glucose and normal saline solution may be ordered for those patients who are dehydrated, who have low blood pressure, and in whom liver damage is suspected. Tetanus toxoid is usually administered, and antibiotics are given to combat infection. Since there is horse serum in antivenin, a reaction may be anticipated in some patients who have been treated at the scene of the accident. Usually skin testing for sensitivity to horse serum is done before additional antivenin is used in the hospital. Occasionally massive sloughing of tissue occurs following snakebite. This type of wound heals very slowly and in severe cases may necessitate amputation.

■ POISONING

Drugs and chemicals

Three fourths of all fatal accidents from poisoning occur in the home. Poisoning is the third-ranking cause of home accidents among people of all ages.

---

*Snakebite kits contain a suction cup, tourniquet, razor blade, iodine, ampule of antivenin powder, vial-syringe of sterile distilled water, and instructions.

Poisoning by solids and liquids was the cause of 3,000 deaths in 1970, an increase of 11% from 1969.[1] In small children, poisoning usually results from accidental ingestion of poisonous substances. The Food and Drug Administration established regulations in 1970 that required that hazardous medicines be enclosed in containers with child-proof safety closure caps. The cap must be squeezed in or pushed down before it can be released. Originally the Safety Packaging Law applied to aspirin and drugs containing aspirin. Later it was extended to include narcotics and barbiturates; as of April 16, 1974, all prescription drugs are included with the exception of nitroglycerin and isosorbide dinitrate (Isordil). In adults, poisoning commonly occurs from not checking medications and from suicide attempts. Most large cities now have poison control centers in the emergency departments of hospitals where emergency information and supplies are kept. This program is sponsored by local health departments and is under the supervision of specialized pediatricians. These centers act as resources for physicians and provide immediate telephone directions to citizens.

Barbiturates are often recorded as the cause of accidental death by poisoning. In a 17-month period ending in December 1972, there were 1,711 barbiturate suicides and 3,475 overdoses and injury cases reported in 32 states. Because of the high potential of the abuse of certain barbiturates, the U. S. Justice Department's Drug Enforcement Agency (DEA) (formerly the Bureau of Narcotics and Dangerous Drugs) established stricter control methods for five of the barbiturates. As of December 17, 1973, prescriptions for amobarbital (Amytal), pentobarbital (Nembutal), secobarbital (Seconal), sodium amobarbital (Amytal sodium), and Tuinal may not be refilled. In addition, these drugs must be stored in a locked narcotic cabinet.

Another activity of the Drug Enforcement Administration was project DAWN (Drug Abuse Warning Network), which was set up to gather data on drug abuse. This project surveyed approximately 750 emergency rooms from July to October of 1973 in an attempt to learn the most common substances cited as the reasons for drug abuse visits to emergency departments. The survey showed that the six most commonly abused substances were diazepam (Valium), alcohol (in combination), aspirin, heroin, chlordiazepoxide (Librium), and secobarbital. These reports reinforce the need for nurses to take an active role in discouraging the public from the injudicious use of drugs. It is also important that the public be reminded to store all drugs and other dangerous substances out of reach of children.

Drug cabinets, kitchen cupboards, and laundry closets are the places from which poisons most often are taken. Strychnine poisoning from eating rodent poisons or laxatives containing strychnine occurs quite often. Disinfectants such as phenol, iodine, bichloride of mercury, and creosol are easily taken by children if these substances are not locked away. Sleeping and tranquilizer tablets left on bedside tables and in handbags are a potential source of trouble. The "do it yourself" movement has brought more paints, solvents, dyes, stains, turpentine, bleaches, and paint removers into the home, and suburban living has increased the danger of poisoning from insecticides. The public constantly needs to be reminded to keep poisons of all kinds conspicuously labeled, stored in cupboards, separate from foods, and placed out of the reach of children. Most manufacturers list the constituents of their products on the outside of the container. Some do not. The public should be encouraged to buy only those products whose contents are noted on the container, since medical treatment in the event of accidental poisoning may be delayed while the physician attempts to learn what poison must be dealt with.

First-aid treatment in poisoning consists of trying to find out what poison was taken, diluting the poison, removing it from the stomach if possible, and getting in touch with a physician or a poison control center. Lives have been saved by quick common-sense treatment while awaiting medical help. For example, if bichloride of mercury, a deadly poison, can be removed from the stomach within 15 minutes, the patient will usually live. On the other hand, when a strong acid such as phenol or a strong alkali such as lye has been taken, further damage and even rupture of the esophagus may be caused by vomiting. If strychnine has been taken, convulsions may be brought on by vomiting. If in doubt, give something bland by mouth and seek medical assistance.

When poisoning is suspected, first examine the mouth of the patient for signs of burns and for any poison that can be removed and saved for study. Note the breath for an odor such as that of kerosene or phenol. The poison can be diluted by giving large amounts of fluid by mouth, provided the patient is conscious and able to swallow. Do not try to remember the specific antidote for each poison, but if the container is nearby, naturally one would read the label for the antidote recommended. Give milk, egg, soap and water, plain water, soda and water, mustard and water, or other fluid that is on hand. The important thing to do is to give plenty—usually 6 or 7 glasses—and then produce vomiting by tickling the back of the throat. After a few minutes, repeat the process. *If it is known that an alkaline substance has been taken, give an acid such as vinegar or lemon juice. If an acid has been taken, give an alkaline substance such as baking soda or starch and water.* After the stomach has been washed out thoroughly, give a bland liquid such as milk. Then get in touch with the physician, who will give directions as to what to do next and may suggest that a saline laxative be given.

In the hospital the nurse need not know the specific antidote for each poison. The emergency departments of most general hospitals have a list and keep the common antidotes as well as equipment for washing out the stomach on hand. Common poisons and their antidotes are given in pharmacology and toxicology texts.

Good nursing care of the acutely poisoned patient may make the difference between a favorable and a fatal outcome. The patient should be kept warm and watched extremely carefully for changes in physical signs such as rapid, thready pulse, respiratory changes, cyanosis, diaphoresis and other signs of collapse, vasogenic shock, or impending death. Changes must be reported to the physician at once. Vital signs should be checked every 15 minutes for several hours. Nausea, vomiting, and abdominal pain should be noted, and all vomitus should be observed for signs of blood and should be saved for study. Stools and urine must be checked for abnormal constituents such as blood. Intravenous infusions that have been ordered must be administered at the prescribed rate.

When poisoning has resulted from an overdose of opiates, barbiturates, tranquilizers, or other sedatives, efforts must be made to keep the patient awake. A cup of strong coffee may be given every hour if it can be swallowed and retained. Strong coffee may also be ordered to be given as a retention enema. It is not good treatment to walk the patient about because this simply tires him and may cause complete exhaustion. Renal dialysis may be used in an effort to speed up excretion of the drug (p. 473).

If the patient has marked depression of respiration, oxygen may be given, and sometimes a mechanical ventilator is necessary. A suction machine should be on hand at all times, for sometimes deep suctioning of the bronchial tree is necessary in an effort to prevent atelectasis. If the patient is unconscious, his position must be changed every hour, and he should be turned completely on alternate sides to provide drainage from each bronchus. Occasionally the head of the bed is lowered to encourage drainage of bronchial secretions. Death from barbiturate poisoning is likely to be delayed. Many patients live 2 or 3 days before death occurs. Death from poisoning by gas, however, is much more sudden. The patient who is in the hospital recovering from carbon monoxide poisoning must be observed very carefully for the first 24 hours. Some patients who appear to have responded favorably to artificial respiration and oxygen die of heart failure several hours after some level of consciousness has been restored.

The person who has been known to take poison in a suicide attempt presents additional nursing problems. Such a patient must not be left alone under any circumstances. He should be in a room where windows are equipped with bars or stops if one is available. On awakening, the patient has not only his original problem to face but also the discomfort and the emotional impact of learning that he has failed in his suicide attempt. Patients in these circumstances have been known to jump out of a window when it was not thought possible that they had the strength to get out of bed. Others have attempted to electrocute themselves or to carry out their original aim of self-destruction by other means. Precautions used for mentally ill patients should be observed (p. 152).

Environmental pollutants

In recent years the total environment has become a source of poisoning to all living things. The air we breathe may contain irritating and noxious fumes such as sulfuric acid, and the water we use may contain untreated sewage. Deadly chemicals such as pesticides, radioactive substances, and injurious drugs may be ingested by the animals we use for food. Increased world population, subsequent crowding, increased industrial activity with production of detergents, pesticides, and quantities of industrial wastes and limited world control of radioactive wastes all have contributed to this problem. The treatment for this poisoning is to treat its cause by education, legislation, and all other feasible means. The nurse should take leadership in informing the public of the seriousness of the present situation. For further discussion, see Chapter 3.

Food poisoning

Acute food poisoning. Each year a large number of people, many of whom eat away from home, suffer acute gastrointestinal upsets due to food poisoning. Acute food poisoning is usually caused by a toxin produced by certain strains of *Staphylococcus aureus*. This toxin causes immediate irritation to the gastrointestinal tract, hence the name "enterotoxin." Illness is not caused by eating foods that are simply "old" and that have been subject to bacterial action. In many parts of the world (for example, in England, where "seasoned" game is popular), "spoiled" foods are ingested without harm. Pathogenic organisms must be present and active to produce disease. Cooking will destroy the organisms and stop the production of enterotoxin but will not destroy the poison that has already been formed.

Acute food poisoning can be prevented by rigorous enforcement of sanitary practices in eating establishments and by teaching the public to take sensible precautions, particularly when eating in restaurants and attending picnics during hot weather. Staphylococci are carried on the hands of workers and inadvertently deposited on food. Food handlers should not be allowed to work if they have even minor infections on their hands or if they do not meet requirements for washing the hands. Foods that are handled and allowed to remain without refrigeration before being cooked or eaten are the most dangerous. For example, chicken that has been removed from the bone and left for some time before creamed chicken is prepared, potatoes that have been peeled and left standing before potato salad is prepared, and seafood that has been removed from the shell by hand some time before being eaten all provide excellent opportunities for the pathogenic organisms to produce enterotoxin.

Signs of acute food poisoning include salivation, cramping, nausea, vomiting, and diarrhea. Signs and symptoms usually appear from 1 to 6 hours after eating the offending food, the length of time depending on the amount of food eaten and the amount of enterotoxin present. In severe cases there may be lassitude, headache, dehydration, rapid pulse, and prostration. Treatment is supportive and may include intravenous fluids and measures to combat shock if present.[2] Usually fluids such as tea, boiled milk, and broth are tolerated within a short time. If diarrhea is severe, drugs such as bismuth and camphorated tincture of opium are ordered, and fluids may be given intravenously.

Mushroom poisoning. Poisonous mushrooms are the most common cause of death from poisoning by food. It is best to teach the public that there is no sure way to tell whether or not a wild mushroom is safe to eat. All mushrooms found in the free state should be looked on with suspicion, and only those grown under cultivation should be eaten. Deaths occur each year from the consumption of mushrooms by persons who either thought they were experts in determining a safe variety or listened to other so-called experts.

Signs and symptoms of mushroom poisoning are severe abdominal pain, nausea, vomiting, diarrhea, and prostration occurring usually within $1/2$ to 24 hours after eating the mushroom. The first-aid treatment should be the same as for drug poisoning: give fluids and induce vomiting, keep the patient warm, and notify a physician at once. One ounce of magnesium sulfate may be given in water by mouth, and enemas can also be given to remove any poison still in the intestinal tract.

In the hospital the care is symptomatic. Fluids are given intravenously. The position for shock and suctioning may be ordered, and side rails are used if convulsions occur. Moist compresses may be ordered if lacrimation is excessive. The patient should be attended constantly, since he is fearful of death.

Botulism. Botulism is a very serious form of food poisoning caused by neurotoxins A, B, E, and F produced by an anaerobic, spore-forming organism, *Clostridium botulinum.* Improper home canning is often the cause of poisoning with A and B toxins,

since the spores can resist several hours of ordinary cooking. Even intermittent cooking is not considered safe. People should not can any foods at home unless pressure-cooking methods are used. Agricultural colleges and home economics departments in most states distribute booklets on home canning, and the nurse should encourage their use. The neurotoxin, unlike the enterotoxin produced by a strain of *Staphylococcus,* is destroyed by cooking. It is not destroyed by mere heating. Foods should be cooked for 10 to 15 minutes, depending on the density of the solid food, before they are safe to eat.

There is no emergency first-aid treatment suitable for botulism poisoning except to notify the physician at once and to make preparations to move the patient to a hospital. If the symptoms are severe, the patient may not tolerate being moved. All persons who are suspected of having eaten the contaminated food should be reached, for it is in early treatment of persons least affected that the best results are obtained. Symptoms usually appear within 24 to 48 hours after ingestion of the food, and their severity depends on the amount of infected food eaten. There may be constipation, lassitude, headache, and double vision. Nausea and vomiting are often absent. As further damage to the nervous system occurs, there are difficulty in swallowing, lowered voice, and finally inability to talk or to swallow and muscular incoordination. Treatment consists of supportive care and the administration of large doses of antitoxin. Antitoxin cannot undo damage that has been done, but it helps to prevent further damage. The mortality rate from botulism in the United States is approximately 65%, with patients usually dying within 3 to 16 days of the onset of symptoms. Fortunately this type of poisoning is now quite rare.

Nursing the victim of botulism poisoning includes keeping the patient quiet, usually in a darkened room. Other aspects of nursing care are similar to those described for patients with mushroom poisoning.

■ REACTIONS TO THE SUN'S HEAT

Sunburn. Sunburn can occur even when the sun cannot be seen, since rays are able to filter through clouds. Reflection of rays from water increases the danger of burning. The best prevention for sunburn is careful, gradual exposure to the sun's rays and avoiding the midday hours, when the rays are hottest. Some trade preparations, such as those containing para-aminobenzoic acid, are helpful in keeping out harmful rays, and olive oil, cocoa butter, and many creams and ointments are useful. Cool compresses may be used to ease discomfort from sunburn. If chills, fever, edema, or blistering occur, the advice of a physician should be sought.

Heat cramps. Heat cramps are sudden muscle

pains caused by excessive loss of sodium chloride in perspiration during strenuous exercise in hot weather. The best treatment is prevention by taking extra salt when severe exertion is anticipated. The immediate treatment consists of salty fluids and foods by mouth, extra water, and rest for a few hours.

Heat exhaustion. Heat exhaustion is vasomotor collapse due to inability of the body to adequately supply the peripheral vessels with sufficient fluids to produce the perspiration needed for cooling and yet meet vital tissue requirements. The condition usually follows an extended period of vigorous exercise in hot weather, particularly when the person concerned has not had a period of acclimatization. The symptoms are faintness, weakness, headache, and sometimes nausea and vomiting. The skin is pale and moist. Temperature is normal or subnormal. Heat exhaustion can often be prevented by taking extra salt and extra fluid during hot weather and by tempering physical activity during very hot weather. Emergency treatment consists of lowering the patient's head, preferably by placing him with the head lower than the body. He should be in the coolest spot available. Fluids should be given, and preferably they should contain salt. If the attack has been severe, the patient should rest for several hours before resuming activity.

Heatstroke (sunstroke). Heatstroke is a serious condition in which excessive body heat is retained, and it requires immediate emergency treatment. It is due to a failure of the perspiration-regulating mechanism in the hypothalamus. The person undergoing vigorous exercise in intense heat may perspire profusely for some time and then become dehydrated and fail to produce sufficient perspiration to maintain normal body temperature. The skin is dry, hot, and flushed in contrast to the pale, moist skin of the person suffering from heat exhaustion. The patient becomes confused, dizzy, and faint and may quickly lose consciousness.

There is probably no greater medical emergency than heatstroke. Without treatment almost 100% of heatstroke victims will die, but with prompt and vigorous treatment almost as many will recover. The patient must be moved to the shade, preferably to a cool room, and a physician must be notified at once. The patient's temperature should be taken as soon as possible. Treatment to reduce the temperature must be started immediately. The best method of doing this is to place the patient in a tub of cold water and to massage the skin vigorously to bring more blood to the surface for cooling. Spraying the body with cold water from a garden hose is often effective. Ice should be placed on the head and cold drinks given by mouth if the patient is conscious and can swallow. Pouring cold water on the patient and fanning him helps in the absence of tubs and sprays.

If the elevated temperature is allowed to persist, serious permanent damage is done to the brain and the entire nervous system. A temperature of 40.5° C. (105° F.) or more means that treatment is essential. Treatment should be continued until the temperature has been lowered to 39.9° C. (102° F.), and it must then be checked carefully for several hours for sudden rise. The patient should respond when the temperature lowers. Failure to do so may indicate that brain damage has occurred. Patients do not recover from heatstroke as quickly as from heat exhaustion. Often there is faulty heat regulation for days and a lowered tolerance to heat for years and sometimes for the rest of the patient's life. The person who has had heatstroke should be advised to plan his living so that repeated long exposures to heat are avoided.

■ FROSTBITE

Frostbite occurs most often on the nose, cheeks, ears, toes, and fingers. Sometimes an individual will not know that he has been frostbitten since he cannot see the part, although it will feel numb and will appear white on inspection. The frozen parts should not be rubbed with snow or cold water as was formerly thought desirable, because if this is done, the frozen crystals of body fluid will traumatize cell walls and may cause serious damage to them. Good first-aid treatment consists of taking the patient to a warm room, keeping him warm, and giving him warm drinks. Alcohol is sometimes recommended. The frozen part should be thawed as quickly as possible by immersing it gently in warm, but not hot, water or by wrapping it in warm blankets. Massage must be avoided because it damages tissues. The use of direct heat in any form, such as placing the part near a warm stove, is harmful because it increases metabolism, thereby taxing blood supply demands that are already seriously reduced. When the part thaws, the patient should be advised to exercise it gently. Blisters that form should not be disturbed. As thawing occurs, pain may be severe. Aspirin may be given for the pain. The patient should be taken to a physician or a hospital as soon as possible. The care for frostbite is then similar to that needed in vascular disease of the extremities. Efforts are made to decrease the oxygen needs of the tissues while the healing takes place, to improve blood supply by the use of drugs, and to prevent infection if there are open lesions. Some tissues may eventually die and have to be debrided as healing occurs.

Frostbite can usually be prevented by better attention to the clothing worn out-of-doors in intemperate weather. It is more likely to occur in the aged and debilitated person or the one with poor circulation. In the colder states of the United States it also occurs fairly often among teenagers who conform to local styles in regard to clothing, such as no hats or covering for the ears.

■ ASPHYXIATION

The common causes of asphyxiation are inhalation of carbon monoxide gas, inhalation of fumes from burning buildings, drowning, and electric shock. If carbon monoxide or toxic fumes are encountered, it is useless to hold a cloth over the nose, as is so often done by persons who enter burning buildings. While this procedure may screen out some smoke and smoke particles, it does not screen out carbon monoxide or other toxic fumes. The victim of carbon monoxide or other toxic gas poisoning should be moved at once into fresh air, and artificial respiration should be started. Emergency aid, including a pulmotor, should be sent for.

The victim of drowning should be placed on his back with his chin forward. It is not necessary to elevate his feet in an attempt to drain water out of the respiratory passages. The important thing to do is to begin artificial breathing while other aid is being sought. Nothing takes the place of artificial respiration.

Electric shock accidents become more numerous as man uses more electricity to operate equipment in his home and at work. Immediate first aid consists of removing the person from contact with the live wire, with the rescuer being careful to avoid contact with the electric charge. The rescuer must never have direct contact with the body of the victim because the charge may be transmitted. He should use a long, dry stick and stand on a dry board. Also, asbestos or some other material or heavy, dry gloves should be used when moving the victim away from the wire. Artificial respiration should be started at once and a physician summoned. Artificial respiration should be continued even when there is no evidence of response. Some patients have responded after as long as several hours. Ventricular fibrillation is not uncommon following electric shock. The nurse should observe the victim for cardiac arrest secondary to fatal cardiac arrhythmia and provide external cardiac massage while the patient is immediately taken to a hospital where his heart will be defibrillated.

■ FOREIGN BODIES
In the eye

The eye should not be rubbed when a foreign body has entered it. Hands should be thoroughly washed before attempting first-aid measures. The inner surface of the lower lid should be examined first. If the foreign object is not there, then gently bring the upper lid down over the lower lid (many foreign bodies lodge on the undersurface of the upper lid).

If this is not effective, lavage the eye, using an eyecup, a medicine dropper, or a drinking glass. This measure often suffices to wash away the offending material. The patient can usually feel and tell approximately where the irritation is. If it appears to be under the upper lid, the lid should then be inverted. The procedure is as follows. Prepare an applicator by anchoring a shred of clean cotton on a toothpick and moistening it with tap water. Then, preferably standing behind the patient, grasp the upper lashes firmly and invert the lid over a match, pencil, or other convenient object. Standing behind the patient is favored by some because it allows for better control if the patient should jerk and permits one to use a sidewise approach to the lid with the applicator, again avoiding danger if the patient should move quickly. The exact method used depends on individual manual dexterity and right- or left-handedness.

If the foreign body is on the cornea and is not removed by irrigation, or if marked irritation remains but no foreign object is seen and removed, it is best to close the eye, cover it with a piece of cotton, and anchor the cotton with cellophane tape. The patient should then seek a physician at once. Foreign bodies embedded in the cornea can lead to serious consequences because of the danger of infection and ulceration. They should never be removed by the uninitiated. Metallic objects are of particular danger because rusting, which is extremely irritating to the eye tissues, may occur.

Chemicals accidentally introduced into the eyes should be washed away with copious amounts of plain water. Many persons whose vision could have been saved by this simple remedy are now blind. Use a cup or glass and pour the water from the inner to the outer part of the eye. The eye must be held open since the patient will not be able to do this himself. Sometimes it is best to put the victim's head under a faucet if one is available and to use large amounts of running water. A drinking fountain is ideal for this purpose. An eyecup does not ensure diluting the chemical sufficiently and should not be used. Lavage should be continued for several minutes, and after 15 minutes the procedure should be repeated. The patient should then be taken at once to a physician.

In the ear

When a foreign object has entered the ear canal, the first thing to do is to attempt to identify it. The outer ear is held up and back in an adult and down and out in a child. This straightens the ear canal and makes it possible, with good lighting, to see as far as the eardrum. The patient must be cautioned not to try to dislodge the object since such an attempt may push it farther into the ear. Children must be constantly observed and may need to be restrained. Occasionally the foreign object (for example, a wad of material or cotton) may be removed with tweezers if it can be readily seen and has free ends. Some authorities believe that it is permissible in first-aid treatment to attempt to get behind the object with a bent hairpin, but this practice may be dangerous in the hands of the uninitiated. Irrigation of the ear is often a fruitless practice because it seldom dislodges a foreign body that is firmly anchored. If the object turns out to be a bean, a pea, or any other substance that swells, irrigation may cause further damage. The best procedure is to take the patient to a physician.

The best treatment for insects in the ear is to drop a little oil or strong alcohol into the ear canal. Water should not be used because it makes the insect more active, which will increase pain. Insects can sometimes be enticed out of the ear canal by a flashlight held to the ear. The light from matches should not be used because of the danger of burns.

In the nose, throat, and esophagus

Foreign bodies in the nose are usually placed there by children during play. If they are visible, one may attempt to remove them with a fine forceps or a pair of tweezers. If a foreign body has passed into the posterior nose or pharynx, it is best to take the patient to a physician.

Food and other material may become lodged in the throat and interfere with breathing, necessitating emergency treatment. The best procedure is to place the patient on his face, with the head lower than the feet, and to slap him briskly between the shoulders. Children may be treated by picking them up by their heels, which usually suffices to cause them to cough and dislodge the foreign object.

Recently a "choke saver," an instrument shaped somewhat like a crochet hook, has been used to remove lodged food such as pieces of steak. In one state there is legislation pending that will make it mandatory for all food establishments to have a "choke saver" on the premises for emergency use.

Another technique for removing lodged food is being tried experimentally. In this manuever the rescuer stands behind the victim and grasps him firmly with both arms just above the belt line. The rescuer then grasps his own right wrist with his left hand and strongly presses into the victim's abdomen. This forces the diaphragm upward, compressing the lungs, and hopefully expelling the lodged food. The same procedure of compression can be used with the victim lying prone or supine.[33a]

Surprisingly large objects can pass the larynx and go into the trachea and bronchi. Sometimes they cause immediate respiratory difficulties, whereas at other times the aspirated object (a peanut, for example) may remain in the lungs for some time and lead to a mistaken diagnosis of asthma or cause an abscess before it is discovered. Removal of these objects is discussed on p. 551.

Foreign objects that lodge in the esophagus are usually fish or chicken bones. The choking and discomfort are very distressing. First aid consists of keeping the patient as quiet as possible and encouraging him not to swallow or struggle to dislodge the object. A physician should be notified at once. Foreign objects in the esophagus are removed relatively easily by means of esophagoscopy. There is danger of fatal mediastinitis following perforation of the esophagus by a foreign object, and antibiotic drugs are given to prevent this.

Disasters

Disaster nursing has become increasingly important because of the occurrence of a relatively greater number of natural disasters such as hurricanes, tornados, fires, and floods in recent years and because each year finds nations of the world with larger and more powerful means of mass destruction. The main differences between damage caused by atomic attack and that caused by other major disasters such as severe explosions are extent of damage and the spread of radioactive substances. In the following discussion, consideration will be given particularly to nursing preparation for, and conduct during, disaster resulting from atom bombing. Emphasis will be placed on the principles of disaster nursing that remain relatively constant from year to year and that apply, in varying degrees, to all major disasters. It is a foregone conclusion that information confined

within the covers of a book cannot possibly be completely up-to-date. However, pamphlets are released at frequent intervals by national, state, and local agencies responsible for keeping professional workers and the public informed about new dangers that may have to be faced, and they include changes in methods of treatment and management in the event of disaster. At the request of the Armed Forces Medical Services the National Academy of Sciences' Research Council appointed a committee on disaster studies, which does research, encourages communication and planning among students of disaster, and offers consultation services on civil defense. The Department of Sociology, Disaster Research Center, Ohio State University, is doing disaster field studies to determine the responses of community-wide organizations to disaster.

Nurses cannot begin too early in their professional preparation to think seriously of their particular responsibility in national disaster. In general this responsibility consists of knowing what overall plans are being made on national, state, and local levels and how nurses may best define their roles within these plans. Nurses should be prepared to help the public understand what to do if there is a natural disaster or bombing attack. The professional nurse will be looked to by others for leadership and guidance in time of disaster. Because nurses are members of the largest single professional group in the health field, they will be in contact with many people. The sphere of activity of the nurse covers a wider range than that of members of most professional groups who will be in positions of leadership. In time of disaster, professional nursing duties will include direct care of the sick and injured, the teaching of lay persons to care for themselves and others, supervision of practical nurses, medical aides, and other workers, and assistance in the field of sanitation and disease prevention. Decentralization of cities and relocation of perhaps thousands of people will present challenges to all health workers because there will be interruption of sanitary controls for milk and water and for the disposal of wastes.

■ OVERALL PLANS

Overall disaster planning for a country as large as the United States is a major undertaking and is dependent on public and private organizations working in close cooperation with each other. The Division of Emergency Health Services, under the Department of Health, Education and Welfare, is the official national agency concerned with health aspects of national defense, natural disasters, and day-to-day emergency medical care. Some functions of this division are to encourage states to establish civil defense commissions, to furnish part of the funds needed for supplies, and to arrange for civil defense forces from one state to aid those of another state in the event of bombing within its boundaries. This division works closely with other groups, including other governmental departments such as the Department of Agriculture, the military services, other divisions of the Public Health Service, the American Medical Association, the American National Red Cross, the American Hospital Association, and the national nursing organizations. It serves regional, state, and local civil defense organizations in a guidance capacity. Specific activities include helping to prepare literature and helping to develop courses for professional groups such as physicians, dentists, and nurses. It also sponsors the assembling of improvised hospitals, each of which will be able to care for over 200 patients. These hospitals will be located close to probable target areas. It is assigned

the responsibility for assembling such essential equipment as transfusion sets, dressings, plasma and blood volume expanders, and drugs and equipment to determine radiation contamination (survey meters, dosimeters, and dosimeter readers). The state civil defense commissions carry out similar functions on a state level, providing supplies and developing plans for training professional workers as well as for educating the public. Responsibility for health aspects of civil defense within states is usually delegated to the state health department. Local communities may have their own organization, the Emergency Medical Service.

Certain highly populated cities and industrial areas throughout the country have been designated as target areas because they are most likely to be attacked. Communities near these target areas have been designated as support areas, and in the event of an attack their medical forces will go immediately to the assistance of the attacked area without direction from the state. Additional help will be sent as needed by the state and is termed state-directed aid. If further help is needed, the Division of Emergency Health Services will direct aid from other nearby states.

All nurses should learn about the Emergency Medical Service in their hospital and community. This information can usually be obtained by enrolling in courses in medical and nursing aspects of medical defense offered by the local civil defense organization. Here knowledge can be tested to some extent in practical experience. Membership in local units of the National League for Nursing and the American Nurses' Association is important as a means of learning of new developments in disaster nursing. Local organizations of the two associations, sometimes assisted by the state, may sponsor and conduct institutes and refresher courses for their members. The professional nurse may contribute to lay education by teaching courses sponsored by the Division of Emergency Health Services and the American National Red Cross (for example, home nursing and first-aid courses and courses for nurse's aides) or by teaching medical self-help training courses to community groups (a program designed by the United States Office of Civil Defense with the objective of reaching one member of every American family).

Nurses' attendance at local civil defense meetings is valuable for them and for others. They should not, however, offer their services as a plane spotter or a Geiger count checker, for instance. The reason is simply that their special training in care of the injured will be so badly needed if disaster occurs that they will not be available for duties that can be handled by nonnurses. Nurses should know specifically where and how to report in the event of disaster and should be prepared to go quickly. Most nurses who work in general hospitals should be quite well oriented by their institutions. The Joint Committee on Accreditation of Hospitals now requires that all hospitals wishing to qualify for accreditation have a written plan for their institutions in the event of disaster and that they practice the plan three times each year. It is probable that in the future there will be more detailed planning within general hospitals and better orientation of the professional members of the staff for their particular assignments.

Nurses who are not attached to a hospital or an emergency medical unit should listen for radio instructions and proceed immediately to the nearest assignment depot in the area in which they happen to be. Nurses who live a considerable distance from their place of regular work should know the location of the assignment depot and of secondary-aid stations in their living area. Nurses with children should make some provision for care of their children so that they may make themselves available in the shortest possible time.

Nurses should carry their personal identification as a nurse and wear a Civil Defense armband if they have one. In addition, it is advised that they have with them a flashlight with batteries, bandage scissors, a dozen safety pins, a hypodermic syringe and needle, indelible pencil, matches, a small package of tissues, a small notebook, and lipstick for skin marking.

▨ EDUCATING THE PUBLIC FOR PROTECTION

Everyone should know the basic rules for self-protection in the event of sudden enemy attack, how to prepare for disaster, and how to protect oneself immediately following a bombing. The nurse should include this information in teaching health education to all patients and in contacts with laymen.

The American public does not give first priority to learning to cope with the hazards that will be present in atomic disaster. Despite the thousands of booklets and pamphlets distributed on the subject, the average citizen does not know the most fundamental steps that may be necessary for his survival. Just as the patient often delays going to the physician when he fears cancer lest his suspicions be confirmed, so he fails to heed the constant public reminders of what he should know to help assure his survival.

Many pamphlets give simple but complete explanations and rules to go by in preparation for disaster and during disaster. *Survival Under Atomic Attack,* a pamphlet released by the United States government, is excellent for the average layman.

Families living in or near target areas should set aside materials for an emergency. These materials should include two flashlights, a battery radio, a first-aid kit, canned food to last 2 weeks, bottled and canned fluids, a can opener, a bottle opener, spoons, newspapers, and paper dishes. A large bottle of drinking water should be stored (ideally several gallons) and changed weekly. In addition, a container of water should be available for washing in case anyone is exposed to radiation dust, because water may suddenly be cut off or contaminated. A garbage can with a tight cover and a pail for human wastes are necessary. Disposable plastic bags will also be helpful.

Every citizen should have a transistor (battery) radio that can be used in a national emergency. The radio should be turned on and instructions awaited if a bombing is threatened. Windows and doors should be closed and blinds drawn, all electric equipment should be turned off, and pets should be brought indoors. The family should then proceed to the basement. Many people fear that they may be trapped in the cellar, but it has been shown that this danger is much less than that which will be encountered by staying above ground in the event of an atomic bombing. When a bomb is known to have been exploded, the family should remain in the basement until advised by radio that it is safe to go outdoors.

It is important to know what to do when at work or out-of-doors at the time of a bombing. Despite the tremendous fear of radiation in this country, by far the greatest number of deaths and severe injuries in an atomic bombing will come from blast and heat. The following three rules, if followed, will save many lives.

1. Try to put a wall between yourself and the bomb, judging that the bomb will be dropped in the most industrialized area. Even a ditch or a gutter is better than no protection.

2. Fall flat on your face, bury your face in your arm, and if possible pull something over your head and hair.

3. Stay there until things are quiet. Do not rush out to look around. Explosive radiation lasts about a minute after a bomb has exploded and may easily affect persons within a mile of the center of the attack unless they have been quite well protected.

Lingering radiation is due to the presence of many fine particles of "ashes" or leftover fission products that may remain in the vicinity of the bombing for an indefinite time. These particles usually rise high in the air and spread over a wide area and may not be concentrated enough to do harm to persons a few miles from the site of the bombing. Lingering radiation dust is extremely difficult to remove from houses, and it is advised that windows broken by the blast be covered with a blanket or cardboard to prevent as much dust as possible from entering the house. If a large amount of radiation dust is present, some will undoubtedly filter into the house. If the explosion occurred underwater or if water reservoirs were exposed to large amounts of radiation dust, the water will be seriously contaminated. So far there is no known simple or effective method for decontaminating such water, and if a major bombing occurs, the water supply may present an extremely serious problem, although the use of shale, coagulant, and settling gives promise of effectiveness. Persons who are at home should draw water immediately and put it into covered, clean containers because the water in the immediate mains will not be contaminated by radioactive substances and may suffice for emergency needs. Thereafter it is not advisable to use water from taps until advised by radio of its safety. Even if water is not contaminated by radioactive substances, it may be contaminated by bacteria following damage to sewer systems. Bacterial contamination can be overcome by boiling the water, but boiling will not remove radioactive contamination.

Although radiation is a real danger following a bombing, it should not prevent one from assisting others. Anyone who is out in the open shortly after a bombing should keep his head and other parts of the body covered. On coming into the house, he should shed his outer clothing, including his shoes, at the doorway and should scrub thoroughly with soap and water. If possible, he should then be checked for the amount of radioactive contamination still present, particularly on exposed parts of the body, and the scrubbing process should be repeated if necessary.

The public is urged not to telephone during a disaster. The radio will give instruction for the precautions and cleanup measures that are necessary for each vicinity. A safe rule to follow if in doubt, however, is to err on the side of caution. Food that has been uncovered during a bombing should be discarded. Food in wrappers and fruits and vegetables with skins are safe, though the outer wrappings or peelings should be carefully removed and discarded. The outsides of cans as well as utensils, furniture, and any equipment that has not been in tightly closed cupboards or drawers should be washed thoroughly.

The public should know that mass evacuation of cities may seriously affect water and other sanitary facilities. Foods and fluids of all kinds should be cooked if there is any doubt about contamination. Disaster conditions often threaten mass epidemics of diseases such as typhoid.

■ IMMEDIATE SERVICES IN EVENT OF BOMBING

Patients whom the nurse will encounter in disaster will not differ very much from those seen in everyday practice. It will be the numbers of injured and the severity of the injuries that will be different as well as the working conditions. It is estimated that one atomic bomb could kill 80,000 persons and wound 80,000 more. Of the injured it is estimated that approximately 12,000 will be in shock, 12,000 will suffer radiation illness, 27,000 will be severely burned, and 13,000 will have fractures, open wounds, and crushing injuries. It is almost impossible to think in these numbers and to plan how work can be carried out with the confusion and tensions that will be present. Major obstacles will be dislocation of transportation, communication, light, and water supply.

It must be understood by all nurses that tremendous adjustments in basic thinking will have to be made if an atomic bombing should occur. It will not be possible even to begin to do all that might be desirable for everyone. Whatever is best for the largest number must be done. The dying should be made as comfortable as possible, but the available facilities must be used for those whose possibility of survival is best. Some careful techniques will have to be discarded, and the nurses will have to rely heavily on their knowledge of basic principles rather than specific procedures. They will have to improvise and use whatever is available. For example, one syringe may have to be used for several patients, with only the needle being changed. Nurses must remember that prompt action will save many lives. Those who are available to help will be less likely to suffer emotional reactions if they are kept busy with definite tasks. In the first few hours of disaster, treatment will have to be routine and simple. Much of it will have to be performed by unskilled workers, whereas nurses will have to do many things usually done by physicians. The ability to keenly appraise the physical condition of people will be a valuable asset in time of disaster. Nurses are the only people with this skill with the exception of physicians. Decisions that must be made will include who must be constantly attended, who can be moved, and who is not responding to therapy and will need further assistance.

It is expected that nurses will serve where professional response is most needed during a disaster. There will not be time for consideration of choices and probably not even time to use all skills to the best advantage. It is hoped that physicians will be in charge of all aid stations. It is possible, however, that a nurse may have to take charge until a physician arrives. Nurses will be assigned from their designated assignment depots to secondary-aid stations, permanent hospitals, improvised emergency hospitals, and holding stations. Secondary-aid stations are established at designated places outside target cities as part of preparation for disaster. First-aid stations will be determined by groups sent out from the secondary-aid station after the bombing. Permanent hospitals will be hospitals in the target city that are suitable for use. Improvised emergency hospitals will be temporary facilities set up in school buildings, garages, or any other place with suitable space at a considerable distance from the bombed area. In field studies of natural disasters, persons transporting injured victims often bypass temporary first-aid stations in their urgency to go to the nearest familiar hospital.

Stretcher teams will go from the first-aid station, give first aid, and bring the wounded to the secondary-aid station, where the important function of sorting and identifying casualties is done. This function is called *triage.* Classification for treatment has been listed in four priorities as follows:

Priority I   Persons requiring outpatient care only

Priority II   The moderately injured and ill, whose chances of recovery are good following immediate definitive treatment

Priority III The injured and ill whose chances of recovery are not jeopardized by delayed definitive treatment

Priority IV   The critically injured or ill, who require extensive, complicated, time-consuming or material-consuming procedures, and the persons who are beyond help

The physician should be responsible for triage and should decide which patients should receive immediate treatment, which should be sent to secondary-aid stations, and which should be sent to remote stations. He should also determine which should be transported by litter and which may be treated as "walking wounded." If no physician is available, a nurse will substitute. The general rules taught in all first aid should be followed: treat suffocation, severe hemorrhage, shock, severe wounds, burns, fractures, and dislocations in that order. Judgment in estimating the severity of the injury must be used along with this rule. Treatment will not usually be given at the triage station, but each patient will be tagged and the injuries noted on the tag. Priorities in triage may change, depending on the help and facilities available and on individual patients' responses.

Injuries may be any of the following: injury caused by blast of the nuclear weapon, traumatic injuries resulting from flying parts of physical structures, burns from the initial bombing or flash burns from the heat from explosions, radiation injuries from explosive radiation, or poisoning from nerve gas or other poisons. Emotional reactions will also occur.*

In first-aid stations and secondary-aid stations nurses may be called on to do things usually done by physicians, such as prescribing medications, starting intravenous infusions, giving anesthetics (if they have had some preparation), suturing lacerations, debriding wounds, applying pressure dress-

*Committee on Disaster and Civil Defense: First aid for psychological reactions in disasters, Washington, D. C., 1964, American Psychiatric Association.

ings, dressing burns, applying and readjusting splints, and directing the disposition of patients. It is to be hoped that the nurse will not be so occupied with medical procedures that observing patients for changes in vital signs is neglected. The nurse may also be needed to search for and help persons who are injured and in need of care yet who are too frightened to leave their homes or places of hiding.*

Morphine has been stockpiled in disposable Syrettes, each containing 30 mg. ($\frac{1}{2}$ grain). Penicillin has also been stockpiled, and chlortetracycline hydrochloride (Aureomycin), 250 mg.; oxytetracycline (Terramycin), 250 mg.; and phenobarbital are available. Dried plasma has been stocked in containers ready for the addition of sterile distilled water and normal saline solution. Sodium citrate has been stocked in powdered form, ready for use by addition of unsterile water. This solution is given by mouth to persons who can take fluids orally.

Shock. Hypovolemic shock will be a major problem, particularly in the first few hours following the explosion, and should sometimes have first priority in treatment, sometimes even taking precedence over hemorrhage. Shock will probably be due to trauma that may or may not have caused external laceration. Blood loss may be external or internal and may be due to crushing injury or fluid loss from burns. Shock may be partially prevented and controlled by stopping hemorrhage, giving medication for pain if the patient is not already in shock, splinting fractures before moving patients, covering burns, dressing open wounds, preventing loss of body heat, and giving fluids by veins, by hypodermoclysis, or by mouth. The lower limbs should be elevated above the level of the trunk.

Hemorrhage. The care of the patient with hemorrhage will not differ from that given in any emergency situation. Once applied, a tourniquet is not removed until a nurse or physician checks the patient for cessation of bleeding. Removal of the tourniquet must be done where facilities are available to control the bleeding. Whenever a tourniquet is applied in the field or in a first-aid station, a large T is marked on the forehead of the patient with a lipstick. He then will receive priority in transportation to a secondary-aid station.

Burns. Patients burned in disaster have been classified into three groups: the hopelessly burned, the severely burned, and the moderately burned. Attention in disaster will be given first to the severely burned, since the hopelessly burned will not be expected to survive. Treatment includes prevention of infection by giving antibiotics, alleviation of pain, and replacement of body fluids. A special burn dressing has been stockpiled in large quantities as part of

*See reference 6, which defines the American Nurses' Association expectations of the nurse's role in disaster.

civil defense emergency medical supplies. It consists of a cellulose pad covered with a layer of cotton and faced with extremely fine gauze. The gauze is placed next to the burn, and the dressing is then held in place with a tensile yarn roller bandage, included in the burn package. Burn dressings are provided in two sizes. When applying dressings, it is important to bandage the neck loosely, never to leave two skin surfaces in contact, to cover the burned area completely, and to avoid overlapping of the cellulose dressing, since an overlap may cause uneven pressure. The pressure of the outer yarn bandage should be firm, gentle, and even. (For further details on care of patients with severe burns, see p. 791.)

Wounds, lacerations, and fractures. Many patients will have open chest wounds, wounds of the face and neck, and penetrating abdominal wounds as well as fractures of the skull and other bones of the body. Abdominal viscera must be kept moist. If sterile water or normal saline solution is not available, plasma or even unsterile water may be used to moisten dressings applied over the protruding viscera. No penetrating objects or debris should be removed, the patient should not be given fluids by mouth, and he should be sent at once to a secondary-aid station.

Open chest wounds can sometimes be closed by applying wide adhesive tape (3-inch) in a crisscross fashion. A small, dry dressing should be placed over the opening, and the adhesive tape should extend approximately 4 to 6 inches on each side of the wound so that good traction can be obtained and so that the wound can be kept airtight. If the patient is having difficulty in breathing, he should be placed on his injured side, with the head and shoulders elevated. If he does not have difficulty in breathing or injury to contraindicate this, he should be placed in shock position, with the body flat and lower limbs elevated about 45 degrees.

Severe wounds of the mouth and jaw often cause obstruction of breathing after an hour or more when swelling occurs. Under no circumstances should tight bandages or slings be applied to severe wounds of the jaws, mouth, or throat, since they may cut off passage of air as edema occurs. Patients should be transported in a face-down position. In some instances it is safest to insert an airway before the patient is moved. Airways are stocked in the supplies for emergency medical units.

Blood clots and obstruction must be removed before an airway is used. The airway is inserted concave side down, by directing it along the tongue, which is held forward, and by moving it carefully back and slightly from side to side until the guard comes in contact with the teeth. It is then tied in place or anchored with adhesive to prevent its slippage out in transit.

Some debridement of large open wounds is necessary to prevent infection. Even with large doses of

antibiotics, infection cannot be prevented if much dead tissue is left. The nurse who is not familiar with suturing or who does not have suture equipment may make excellent use of strips of adhesive tape to hold wound edges together. Pieces of adhesive tape are notched and folded over in the center portion and are applied so that the center part passes over the wound. This center portion is flamed before the adhesive tape is applied. Adhesive tape of any width can be used, depending on the location and size of the wound. The skin must be dry, and usually several strips, or "butterflies," are used (Fig. 14-4). Wounds on the lips and other parts of the face are often very satisfactorily cared for in this way. Skin clips can be used easily by nurses who are not familiar with the technique of suturing.

The care of fractures is similar to that necessary in any accident situation, with the exception that many patients with fractures will also have severe burns and may be suffering from radiation effects or other injuries. The enormous number of persons with fractures will make the need for improvised equipment very great. Pieces of wood from destroyed buildings, doors, canes, umbrellas, ironing boards, and magazines are a few of the materials that may be used.

Obstetric emergencies. A bombing disaster will cause many pregnant women to abort and many to deliver their babies prematurely. They will be sent

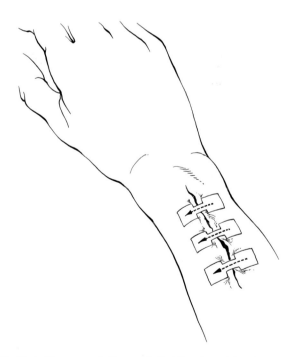

FIG. 14-4. The use of "butterfly" adhesive strips to approximate the skin edges in a laceration of the forearm. Note the irregular wound edges and the placement of the adhesive. Arrows indicate the direction of pull used to partially close the wound.

to the secondary-aid stations to be delivered, and nurses may be the only professional persons available. No materials have been stockpiled for this situation, and nurses or persons in attendance will have to improvise to the best of their ability. A shoelace, a piece of string, or a piece of bandage may have to be used to tie the cord. A lay person may be called upon to check the fundus for an hour or more, and the mother may then be treated as a "walking wounded" and returned to her home or sent to a permanent hospital. It is very important that the mother and baby be identified. Identification bands for both mother and baby can be made of cloth, and information on each should include the name of the father, the address, the sex of the baby, and the time and place of birth. If at all possible the baby should be kept with the mother. If the delivery has been such that there is danger of infection, an antibiotic may be given.

Radiation. Radiation injury may come from gamma rays and neutrons released as the explosion occurs (*initial* radiation). This type of injury is most likely to affect persons who had insufficient protection between themselves and the blast and who have suffered severe burns and flash injuries. Or it may result from irradiated strontium, known as strontium 90 or radiostrontium, which is part of the mushroomlike cloud that rises and is dispersed widely (fallout). Strontium 90 is acquired through inhalation, by ingesting food that either contains or is externally contaminated with radioactive substance, or by drinking contaminated water.

Radiation illness probably will not become apparent until several hours or even days after exposure. Persons affected may have nausea, vomiting, and malaise within a few hours of exposure. Since it may be difficult to distinguish the person with early and severe radiation illness from the one with severe emotional reaction, all persons suspected should have immediate bed rest and should be sent as quickly as possible to a hospital where treatment can be given as necessary. More detailed descriptions are available in specialized publications.[44]

If the exposure has been lethal, severe vomiting and diarrhea will occur within a few hours. Since the entire body may be exposed in an atomic bombing, the reactions that occur first probably will be systemic and may cause death while no skin reaction or other external reaction is evident. Other symptoms of severe radiation illness are severe inflammation and sometimes sloughing and hemorrhage of the mucous membrane of the mouth and throat, hemorrhage spots under the skin, and loss of hair. A severe leukopenia quickly follows exposure to large amounts of radiation.

There is no specific treatment for radiation illness. The patient needs the same care as one who receives radiation treatment for a specific illness (p. 296). This care may include rest, antibiotics, protection from superimposed infection, blood transfusions, fluids and electrolytes, and a bland diet that is high in calories.

Nerve gas damage. Nerve gases are the substances that are most likely to be used in chemical warfare. They are colorless to light brown and can be released in either liquid or vapor form. They have a slightly fruity odor or else are odorless. If inhaled in large amounts, they may cause death within a few minutes by producing overstimulation of the centers of respiration and circulation. Symptoms include excessive salivation, constriction of the pupils, dimness of vision, pain in the eyeballs, coryza, cyanosis, coughing, circulatory disturbances, and convulsions. Atropine sulfate should be given at once in large doses (2 mg. or $\frac{1}{30}$ grain). It has been stockpiled in tablets of this strength. Clothing should be removed and the skin washed with sodium bicarbonate in water. If sodium bicarbonate is not available, plain water should be used. Because clothing is highly contaminated by liquid gas, care should be taken to avoid contamination of others with such clothing. The victim of nerve gas poisoning should be hospitalized as soon as possible.

Emotional reactions. The stresses placed on all who survive a major disaster are almost beyond our comprehension, so that it is difficult to think through the problems and to plan for care. The emotional reactions will affect physicians, nurses and all others giving aid as well as all survivors. Members of the medical and related staffs will be less likely to show signs of emotional effects than others because they will have more knowledge of what is happening and will be busy. These persons are most likely to experience fatigue responses. The American Psychiatric Association has outlined the major types of reactions that are likely to occur and has suggested methods of management.

1. Normal reaction. There may be a normal reaction of tremor, profuse diaphoresis, pallor, and nausea associated with an automatic fight-flight response that soon disappears.

2. Acute panic. This reaction is one of the most serious of the reactions and must be dealt with immediately, since in time of crisis it is acutely "contagious." It has been demonstrated repeatedly that in times of disaster one person in panic can set off a chain reaction and cause untold damage. The person in panic is devoid of judgment and is inordinately but not purposefully active. He cannot be reasoned with and makes wild attempts to flee. Horses in panic have been known to rush back into a burning barn and be killed, and such behavior is not too different from that of human beings in panic. Panic must not be confused with rapid exit from a point of danger. This is sensible, provided it is orderly and purposeful. The person in true panic must be re-

strained, usually by force, and should be firmly held by medical aides until he can be removed to a place where his influence on others will not be dangerous. Persons who have experienced disaster should be segregated from those who have not because they may easily become panicky at threat of further disaster. Although it is serious and contagious, sociologists doing field studies of natural disaster find panic to occur only when an individual perceives his exit of escape is blocked and is given no information to the contrary. Panic does not often occur when communication is adequate.

3. Depressed reactions. Persons who have depressed reactions will be slowed down or numbed. They will sit and stare into space and will be completely oblivious to what is going on around them. These patients must be protected, since they will not move to help themselves.

4. Overly active response. These persons will be very active, possibly joking inappropriately or laughing hysterically, be unable to concentrate on one job, and be a disturbing influence upon the person in command of the location.

5. Severe bodily reactions. These persons may not be able to use a limb and may have nausea and vomiting as a result of fear of radiation exposure.

In management of patients and others who are suffering from emotional effects, the nurse should apply the basic principles of psychiatric nursing. It is well to remember that there will be serious limits to what any one person can do. The nurse should observe each patient and decide what can be done in the particular situation and what is best for the patient and the group. It is useless to argue with the patient, to expect him to stand up better under strain than he has done, or to imply that any of his beliefs of physical limitations are not real. Kindness and gentleness are important. Most patients with emotional reactions are afraid, and they respond to a genuine kindly interest in them and an honest attempt to understand how they feel. Patients should be kept busy if at all possible. The patients in panic must be restrained, the dazed ones given routine things to do in as quiet an environment as possible, and the overly active ones assigned to tasks that require moving about. Patients with an imagined major physical defect can often help with a task with which their imagined problem does not interfere, such as writing identification tags if they believe that their lower limbs are affected.

Chlorpromazine (Thorazine) has been stockpiled for use by medical workers and may be used to treat those who have severe or prolonged emotional reactions. This drug relieves nausea and vomiting, releases tension, and lessens anxiety.

The most important point in nursing management and in prevention of emotional reactions is the poise and conduct of the nurse. Just as one person in panic can upset a crowd, so one calm, collected person can quiet a group.

REFERENCES AND SELECTED READINGS*

1 *Accident facts, Chicago, 1971, National Safety Council.
2 American Academy of Pediatrics: Report of the Committee on Infectious Diseases, ed. 17, Evanston, Ill., 1974, The Academy.
3 American Hospital Association: Principles of disaster preparedness for hospitals, rev. ed., Chicago, 1971, The Association.
4 American National Red Cross: Disaster handbook for physicians and nurses, Washington, D. C., 1966, American National Red Cross.
5 *American National Red Cross: First aid textbook, ed. 5, Washington, D. C., 1962, American National Red Cross.
6 *American Nurses' Association: Nursing in disasters, Am. J. Nurs. 60:1130-1133, Aug. 1960.
7 Anderson, G. W., Arnstein, M. G., and Lester, M. R.: Communicable disease control, ed. 4, New York, 1962, Macmillan Publishing Co., Inc.
8 Baer, E.: Civil disorder: mass emergency of the 70's, Am. J. Nurs. 72:1072-1076, June 1972.
9 Baker, G. W., and Chapman, D. W., editors: Man and society in disaster, New York, 1962, Basic Books, Inc.
10 Beall, Fr., A. C., Noon, G. P., and Harris, H. H.: Surgical management of tracheal trauma, J. Trauma 7:248-256, March 1967.
11 Beeson, P. B., and McDermott, W., editors: Cecil-Loeb textbook of medicine, ed. 13, Philadelphia, 1971, W. B. Saunders Co.
12 *Bergersen, B. S., and Krug, E. E.: Pharmacology in nursing, ed. 12, St. Louis, 1973, The C. V. Mosby Co.
13 Brooks, E.: Preparation of nurses for action in disaster, Int. Nurs. Rev. 9:23-25, July-Aug. 1962.
14 Butrico, F. A.: Early warning systems concerned with environmental contaminants, Am. J. Public Health 59:442-447, March 1969.
15 Cosgriff, J. H., Jr.: Emergency nursing, Supervisor Nurse 5:30-37, March 1974.
16 Council on Environmental and Public Health: Immunization, J.A.M.A. 204:156-158, April 1968.
17 Crawford, O. E.: Eye injuries in a chemical plant, Nurs. Outlook 3:447-449, Aug. 1955.
18 *Department of Defense, Office of Civil Defense: In time of emergency: a citizen's handbook on nuclear attack, natural disasters, H-14, Washington, D. C., March 1968, U. S. Government Printing Office.
19 *Division of Health Mobilization, Public Health Service: The role of the nurse in national disaster, Publication no. 1071-1-5, Washington, D. C., 1965, U. S. Department of Health, Education and Welfare.
20 *Dolman, C. E.: Botulism, Am. J. Nurs. 64:119-124, Sept. 1964.
21 Dreisbach, R. H.: Handbook of poisoning, diagnosis and treatment, ed. 7, Los Altos, Calif., 1971, Lange Medical Publications.

---

*References preceded by an asterisk are particularly well suited for student reading.

22 Eckert, C., editor: Emergency room care, Boston, 1967, Little, Brown & Co.

23 Eiseman, B.: Combat casualty management in Viet Nam, J. Trauma 7:53-63, Jan. 1967.

24 Elliman, V. B., editor: Disaster nursing, Nurs. Clin. North Am. 2:285-358, June 1967.

25 *Emergency medicine (special fifth anniversary edition): Common emergencies in daily practice, Feb. 1974.

26 Erdman, K.: Keeping the consumer informed, FDA, Ohio's Health, vol. 19-22, July-Aug. 1973.

27 Fletcher, B. D., and Brogdon, B. G.: Seat-belt fractures of the spine and sternum, J.A.M.A. 200:167-68, April 1967.

28 Flint, T. J.: Emergency treatment and management, ed. 4, Philadelphia, 1970, W. B. Saunders Co.

29 Frazier, C. A.: Diagnosis and treatment of insect bites, Ciba Clin. Sym. 20:75-101, July-Aug.-Sept. 1968.

30 Garb, S., and Eng, E.: Disaster handbook, ed. 2, New York, 1969, Springer Publishing Co., Inc.

31 Gordon, J. E., editor: Control of communicable disease in man, ed. 11, New York, 1970, American Public Health Association.

32 Green, M.: Immediate management of accidental poisoning in children, Hosp. Med. 3(4):114-118, April 1967.

33 Hanlon, J. J.: An ecologic view of public health, Am. J. Public Health 59:4-11, Jan. 1969.

33a Heimlich, H. J.: Pop goes the café coronary, Emergency Med. 6:154-155, June 1974.

34 Hill, G. J. II, editor: Out-patient surgery, Philadelphia, 1973, W. B. Saunders Co.,

35 *Igel, B. H.: First aid, programmed instruction, 1964, Palo Alto, Calif., Behavioral Research Laboratories.

36 Imburg, J., and Hartney, T. C.: Drowning and the treatment of nonfatal submersion, Pediatrics 37:684-698, April 1966.

37 Iskrant, A. P.: The epidemiologic approach to accident causation, Am. J. Public Health 52:1708-1711, Oct. 1962.

38 Karas, J. S., and Stanbury, J. B.: Fatal radiation syndrome from an accidental nuclear excursion, N. Engl. J. Med. 272:755-761, April 1965.

39 Kerr, A.: Orthopedic nursing procedures, ed. 2, New York, 1972, Springer Publishing Co., Inc.

40 *Kilpatrick, H. M.: The frightened patient in the emergency room, Am. J. Nurs. 66:1031-1032, May 1966.

41 Kossuth, L. C.: Vehicle accidents: immediate care to back injuries, J. Trauma 6:582-591, Sept. 1966.

42 *Kummer, S. B., and Kummer, J. M.: Pointers to preventing accidents, Am. J. Nurs. 63:118-119, Feb. 1963.

43 *Magnussen, A.: Who does what—in defense, in natural disaster, Am. J. Nurs. 65:118-121, March 1965.

44 *Mahoney, R. F.: Emergency and disaster nursing, ed. 2, New York, 1969, Macmillan Publishing Co., Inc.

45 Mandelbaum, I., Nahrwold, D., and Boyer, D. W.: Management of tornado casualties, J. Trauma 6:353-361, May 1966.

46 *Manheimer, D. I., and others: Fifty thousand child-years of accidental injuries, Public Health Rep. 81:519-533, June 1966.

47 Marcus, H.: The accident repeater: a comparative psychiatric study, Int. J. Indust. Med. Surg. 37:768-773, Oct. 1968.

48 McGonagle, L. C.: Psychological aspects of disaster, Am. J. Public Health 54:638-643, April 1964.

49 Miller, R. R., and Johnson, S. R.: Poison control now and in the future, Am. J. Nurs. 66:1984-1987, Sept. 1966.

50 Moore, W. S.: A new classification system for disaster casualties, Hospitals 41:66-72, Feb. 1967.

51 Nabbe, F. C.: Disaster nursing, Paterson, N. J., 1961, Littlefield, Adams & Co.

52 *Parrish, H. M.: Incidence of treated snakebites in the United States, Public Health Rep. 81:269-276, March 1966.

53 *Peszczynski, M.: Why old people fall, Am. J. Nurs. 65:86-88, May 1965.

54 Pratt, M. K., and Thompson, L. B.: Five cared for five hundred, Am. J. Nurs. 67:1684-1687, Aug. 1967.

55 Reider, F.: Medical self-help training program, Public Health Rep. 80:283-286, April 1965.

56 Reynolds, W. A., and Lowe, F. H.: Mushrooms and a toxic reaction to alcohol: report of four cases, N. Engl. J. Med. 272:630-631, March 1965.

57 *Robischon, P.: The challenge of crisis theory for nursing, Nurs. Outlook 15:28-32, July 1967.

58 *Russell, F. E.: Injuries by venomous animals, Am. J. Nurs. 66:1322-1326, June 1966.

59 Sandlick, H.: Emergency care of the injured, Am. J. Nurs. 62:93-96, Dec. 1962.

60 *Scheffler, G. L.: The nurse's role in hospital safety, Nurs. Outlook 10:680-682, Oct. 1962.

61 *Skellenger, W. S.: Treatment of poisoning in children, Am. J. Nurs. 65:108-112, Nov. 1965.

62 Slater, R. R.: Triage nurse in the emergency department, Hospitals 44:50-52, Dec. 1970.

63 Standards for cardiopulmonary resuscitation and emergency cardiac care, J.A.M.A. 227:796-797, Feb. 1974. (Supplements available from local chapters of the American Heart Association; 10¢ each if 100 or more copies ordered.)

64 *Stewart, R. D.: Poisoning from chlorinated hydrocarbon solvents, Am. J. Nurs. 67:85-87, Jan. 1967.

65 *Sullivan, C. M., and Eicherly, E. E.: Civil defense in a nuclear age, Am. J. Nurs. 65:121-125, Nov. 1965.

66 *Sullivan, C. M., Elliman, V. B., and National League for Nursing: What price survival? The bridge between disaster and mass casualty nursing, Nurs. Outlook 8:128-135, March 1960.

67 U. S. Public Health Service: Directory of poison control centers, Washington, D. C., 1965, National Clearinghouse for Poison-Control Centers, U. S. Public Health Service.

68 Verhulst, H. L., and Cratty, J. J.: Childhood poisoning accidents, J.A.M.A. 203:1049-1050, March 1968.

69 *Wagner, M., guest editor: Emergency nursing, Nurs. Clin. North Am. 1:377-466, Sept. 1973.

70 Wilson, W. J.: Heat injury, Am. J. Nurs. 60:1124-1125, Aug. 1960.

71 Wintrobe, M. M., and others, editors: Harrison's principles of internal medicine, ed. 7, New York, 1974, McGraw-Hill Book Co.

72 Wright, W. H.: How one poison control center works, Am. J. Nurs. 66:1988, Sept. 1966.

15 Malignant diseases

■ Cancer is a disease that is much publicized and greatly feared in our society. However, the nature of the nurse-patient interaction often fosters a close feeling on the part of the patient, and as a result, the nurse may be entrusted with patient confidences concerning feelings about cancer that are not shared as readily with other members of the health team. For this reason it is extremely important that all nurses examine their own feelings about cancer and work them through by discussing them openly with members of the health team. Nurses who have worked through their own feelings about cancer are in a much better position to be of assistance to patients than those who have not done so.

The nurse must be aware of current knowledge in prevention, control, and treatment of cancer and be able to apply this information in a variety of settings. Teaching about prevention is not limited to the hospital or clinic setting but takes place in industry, at P.T.A. meetings, and in other public forums. In addition to teaching about prevention, the nurse has an active role in treatment and control programs in all the settings in which patients are found. Patients and their families look to the nurse for assistance and guidance in all phases of illness from detection to terminal care. To be effective in helping patients and their families, the nurse needs to understand the emotional impact that the diagnosis of cancer has on the patient and his family.

■ FACTS ABOUT CANCER

It is estimated that in 1975, 665,000 persons in the United States will be diagnosed for the first time as having cancer.[3] During this year more than 1 million Americans will be under medical treatment for the disease, while 365,000 persons will die from it. The latter figure represents an average of 975 persons a day, or more than one person every 2 minutes, who will succumb. Cancer ranks second only to heart disease as the cause of death in the United States.

Figures from the National Center for Health Statistics reflect an increase in the cancer death rate from 161.4/1,000 deaths in 1971 to 166.8/1,000 deaths in 1972. The accelerated rate was blamed on greater exposure to cancer-causing chemicals in the environment.[4] The *1974 Cancer Facts and Figures* reports that whether this upward trend will continue remains uncertain and can only be determined as yearly figures become available (Table 15-1).

Although in general cancer shows no respect for economic or social status, there are some variations with regard to race and sex as well as age. The rea-

■ STUDY QUESTIONS

1 Review the differences between benign and malignant tumors. What are the important characteristics of malignant growths? How are tumors classified, and how are they usually named? What features of a growth help to determine the degree of malignancy? What is meant by metastasis, and how does it occur?

2 Review the principles and techniques used in medical aseptic technique (isolation).

3 What facilities such as home care programs and hospitals for chronically ill patients are available in your community for care of the patient with cancer in the terminal stages?

4 What is the physical law of inverse-square?

5 Review the gonadal and pituitary hormones. What preparations of male and female hormones are often given? How are they administered?

6 What close family member has had cancer? Did he know the diagnosis? Consider his total reaction to his illness. What was the reaction of his family to his illness?

sons for some of these variations are obvious while others remain obscure. The *1975 Cancer Facts and Figures* states, "For almost 40 years—since 1936—the age-adjusted death rate has been declining slowly but steadily among American women, a drop of 13 percent. During the same period, the male death rate has increased about 40 percent. The decline among women is traceable to a sharp reduction in mortality from cancer of the uterine cervix, a readily detectable disease. The rise among men is due mainly to a 1,400 percent increase for lung cancer—which is a largely preventable disease."[3] It is revealing to note that there has been an increase in the incidence of lung cancer in women from 6 to 12 cases/100,000 between the years 1947 to 1969. This appears to be related to increased smoking by American women.

Although more than half of all the deaths due to cancer occur in persons over 65 years of age, cancer is the leading cause of death in women ages 30 to 54, and more school-age children die of it than any other disease. It is estimated in 1975 more than 3,500 children under the age of 15 will die of cancer; about half that number will die of acute leukemia.

The death rate from cancer involving the female genital tract has dropped from between one third to

Table 15-1   Reference chart: leading cancer sites, 1974*

Site	Estimated† new cases 1974	Estimated deaths 1974	Warning signal: if you have one, see your doctor	Safeguards	Comment
Breast	90,000	33,000	Lump or thickening in breast	Annual checkup, monthly breast self-examination	Leading cause of cancer death in women
Colon, rectum	99,000	48,000	Change in bowel habits, bleeding	Checkup, including proctoscopy, especially for those over 40 years of age	Highly curable disease when digital and proctoscopic examinations are included in checkups
Lung	83,000	75,000	Persistent cough, lingering respiratory ailment	Heed facts about smoking, annual checkup, chest x-ray film	Leading cause of cancer death among men, largely preventable
Oral (including pharynx)	24,000	8,000	Sore that does not heal, difficulty in swallowing	Annual checkup	Many more lives should be saved because mouth is easily accessible to visual examination
Skin	8,000‡	5,000	Sore that does not heal, change in wart or mole	Checkup, avoidance of overexposure to sun	Readily detected by observation and diagnosed by simple biopsy.
Uterus	46,000§	11,000	Unusual bleeding or discharge	Checkup, including pelvic exam with Pap test	With wider application of Pap test, many more lives can be saved from cervical cancer
Kidney and bladder	43,000	16,000	Urinary difficulty or bleeding: consult doctor at once	Annual checkup with urinalysis	Protective measures for workers in high-risk industries help eliminate causes of these cancers
Larynx	10,000	3,000	Hoarseness, difficulty in swallowing	Checkup, including mirror laryngoscopy	Readily curable if caught early
Prostate	54,000	18,000	Urinary difficulty	Annual checkup, including palpation	Occurs mainly in men over 60, can be detected by palpation and urinalysis at checkup
Stomach	23,000	14,000	Indigestion	Annual checkup	A 40% decline in mortality in 20 years, reasons yet unknown
Leukemia	21,000	15,000	A cancer of blood-forming tissues characterized by abnormal production of immature white cells. Acute leukemia strikes mainly children and is treated by drugs that have extended life to as much as 10 years. Chronic leukemia strikes usually after age 25 and progresses less rapidly. Drugs or vaccines that might cure or prevent cancers probably would be successful first for leukemia and lymphomas.		
Lymphomas	28,000	20,000	These diseases arise in the lymph system and include Hodgkin's disease and lymphosarcoma. Some patients with lymphatic cancers can lead normal lives for many years.		

*From Cancer News **27**:12, Fall-Winter 1973-1974.

†Based on the National Cancer Institute's Third National Cancer Survey.

‡Estimates vary widely, from 300,000 to 600,000 or more for superficial skin cancer.

§If carcinoma in situ of the uterine cervix is included, cases total over 86,000.

one half of the rate of 25 years ago, and there is ample evidence that the use of the Papanicolaou test to detect lesions of the cervix before symptoms develop has made early treatment of cancer of the cervix yield a high rate of cure.

A report on 3-year survival rates given at the 1972 National Cancer Conference indicated improvement in rates among white Americans since 1940 for cancers of the bladder, brain, breast, cervix, body of the uterus, larynx, thyroid, and prostate; chronic and childhood leukemia; Hodgkin's disease; melanoma; and multiple myeloma. The report noted "little or no improvement in life expectancy" for patients with cancer of the lung and pancreas.

Although the incidence of cure of cancer has not improved materially over recent years, there is reason to believe that the rate of cure could be improved substantially if there were earlier recognition and more complete reporting of early signs. Success in treatment of many cancerous lesions such as those of the esophagus, stomach, and lung awaits better and more sensitive diagnostic aids to detect the lesions in their early stages. In some parts of the body such as the skin and cervix, early recognition and prompt treatment of suspicious lesions are possible and often result in permanent cure. Multimedia programs in public information are conducted nationally by the American Cancer Society in an attempt to reach people where they live, where they work, and where they meet to persuade them to consult their physicians at the early recognition of a warning signal and to have annual checkups that could lead to earlier diagnosis, treatment, and therefore more cures.

■ CHARACTERISTICS OF TUMORS

Normal tissue contains large numbers of mature cells of uniform size and shape, each containing a nucleus of uniform size. Within each nucleus are the chromosomes, a specific number for the species, and within each chromosome is *deoxyribonucleic acid* (DNA). DNA is a giant molecule whose chemical composition controls the characteristics of *ribonucleic acid* (RNA), which is found both in the nucleoli of cells and in the cytoplasm of the cell itself and which regulates cell growth and function. When ovum and sperm unite, the DNA and RNA within the chromosomes of each will govern the differentiation and future course of the trillions of cells that finally develop to form the adult organism. In the development of various organs and parts of the body, cells undergo differentiation in size, appearance, and arrangement, so that the histologist or the pathologist can look at a piece of prepared tissue through a microscope and know the portion of the body from which it came.

A *malignant* cell is one in which the basic structure and activity have become deranged in a manner that is unknown and from a cause or causes that are still poorly understood. It is believed, however, that the basic process involves a disturbance in the regulatory functions of DNA. It is known that the DNA molecule is affected by radiation in certain instances, and it is speculated that it may be affected by other things also.

A characteristic of malignant cells that can be observed through a microscope is a loss of differentiation, or a *likeness* to the original cell (parent tissue) from which the tumor growth originated. This loss of differentiation is called *anaplasia,* and its extent is a determining factor in the degree of malignancy of the tumor. Other characteristics of malignant cells that can be seen through a microscope are the presence of nuclei of various sizes, many of which contain unusually large amounts of chromatin (hyperchromatic cells), and the presence of mitotic figures (cells in the process of division), which denotes rapid and disorderly division of cells. These are some of the criteria used to grade malignant tumors. A grade I tumor is the *most* differentiated (most like the parent tissue) and therefore the *least* malignant, whereas grade IV is the least differentiated (unlike parent tissues) and has a high degree of malignancy. These classifications are useful to the physician in knowing whether or not the tumor may be expected to respond to radiation treatment as well as in planning all other aspects of the patient's treatment. Usually malignant tissue is slightly more sensitive to irradiation than normal tissue. In radiation therapy a dose that is tolerable to normal tissue while destroying tumor tissue is sought. However, normal cells recover more rapidly and more completely than malignant cells and this difference is fully exploited by the radiotherapist in order to obtain a successful therapeutic result.

Malignant tumors have no enclosing capsule, and thus they invade any adjacent or surrounding tissue, including lymph and blood vessels, through which they may spread to distant parts of the body to set up new tumors *(metastases).* Unless completely removed or destroyed, they tend to recur after treatment, and their continued presence causes death by replacing normal cells and by other means not fully understood.

There is a great deal of difference in the rate of growth of malignant tumors. Occasionally one grows so slowly that it can be removed completely after a long period of time. This characteristic accounts probably for the good results obtained in a few circumstances even when treatment had been delayed. No physician, however, ever relies on this possibility to justify delay in treatment. Occasionally a malignant tumor grows slowly for a long time and then undergoes change, and the rate of growth increases enormously.

Cancer was recognized in ancient times by skilled

observers who gave it the name "cancer" (crab) because it stretched out in many directions as the legs of the crab. The term is somewhat general and is used interchangeably with malignant tumor or malignant neoplasm. It denotes a tumor caused by abnormal cell growth. Forms of cancer are found in plants and in other animals as well as in man.

Malignant tumors may arise from any or all of the three embryonal tissues from which all other tissues are formed. These embryonal tissues are as follows: (1) the *ectoderm,* from which arise the skin and the glands within it, and the entire nervous system including the eyes; (2) the *mesoderm,* from which develop the muscles, bones, fat, cartilage, and other connective tissue; and (3) the *entoderm,* from which develop the mucous membrane lining and the cellular elements of the respiratory tract, the gastrointestinal tract, and the genitourinary tract as well as the cellular elements of other internal organs such as the liver and the spleen.

The term *"carcinoma"* denotes a malignant tumor of epithelial cells, and the term *"sarcoma"* denotes a malignant tumor of connective tissue cells. When a malignant tumor contains all three types of embryonal tissue, it is called a *teratoma.*

Benign or *nonmalignant* tumors are composed of adult or mature cells growing slowly and in an orderly manner within a capsule, not invading surrounding tissues, causing harm only by pressure, remaining localized and not entering the bloodstream. Benign tumors do not recur on removal and cause

death only by their pressure on vital structures within an enclosed cavity such as the cranium.

Tumors derive their names from the types of tissue involved (Table 15-2), but classification of malignant tumors is difficult, since many contain several types of cells and may have benign tissue incorporated within them as well. They are named also for general characteristics of the tumor. The scirrhous carcinoma, for example, is a common malignant tumor developing in the breast and is so named because of the large amount of fibrous connective tissue surrounding the active cells, giving a firmness to the tumor that is detectable when it is palpated.

■ CANCER RESEARCH

Although a tremendous amount of money and research effort goes into attempts to learn the cause and true nature of cancer, as yet the cause of the disease is unknown. However, each year more is learned about cell behavior and cell growth, and it is expected that eventually the actual cause of abnormal cell growth probably will be found.

Cancer research workers are active in a variety of fields, and it finally may be shown that several factors act together in the development of abnormal cell growth. It is believed that certain chemical compounds may have cytoxic (toxic to cells) effects that contribute to the development of cancer. It is known that certain toxic damage to cells, such as is caused by repeated exposure to substances containing radi-

Table 15-2 Types of tumors

Type of cell or tissue	Benign tumor	Malignant tumor
Epithelium		
Skin, outer layers	Papilloma	Squamous cell carcinoma
Skin, pigmented layer (melanoblasts)	Nevus	Malignant melanoma
Glandular epithelium	Adenoma	Adenocarcinoma
Muscle	Myoma	Myosarcoma
Connective tissue		
Fibroblast	Fibroma	Fibrosarcoma
Cartilage	Chondroma	Chondrosarcoma
Bone	Osteoma	Osteosarcoma
Fatty tissue	Lipoma	Liposarcoma
Endothelial tissue		
Blood vessels	Hemangioma	Hemangiosarcoma
Lymph vessels	Lymphangioma	Lymphangiosarcoma
Nerve tissue		
Neuroglia	Astrocytoma	Glioblastoma
Medullary epithelium		Medulloblastoma
Lymphoid and hematopoietic tissue		
Lymphocytes		Lymphosarcoma
		Lymphatic leukemia
Myelocytes		Multiple myeloma
		Myeloid leukemia

um, can cause cancer. It is also known that cancer may follow chronic irritation of any part of the body. Examples are cancer of the lip in pipe smokers and cancer of the skin over the bridge of the nose or behind the ears in people who wear glasses. Many years ago it was observed that skin cancers developed more often in men who were employed as chimney sweeps in English homes in which coal was burned in fireplaces. It was then learned that when the suspected substance (methylcholanthrene) contained in the sweepings was repeatedly painted on the ears of experimental animals, cancer developed. Then it was noted that this carcinogen was somewhat similar in chemical structure to some of the hormones. This observation led physicians to experiment with removal of the ovaries in women who had cancer of the breast and later to give male hormones to men who had developed cancer of the prostate. Hormone treatment is used at the present time for many forms of cancer in both sexes, and although it does not cure the disease, it sometimes retards the activity of abnormal cell growth to a remarkable degree.

There appears to be a genetic factor involved in the predisposition to develop cancer and in the determination of the part of the body attacked. This factor has been conclusively demonstrated in experimental animals by repeated breeding of mice from cancerous and noncancerous strains. A strain of mice has been developed in which almost all the mice develop breast cancer, an indication that heredity may affect the tendency to develop cancer, although many other factors may be involved. Evidence obtained through animal experimentation does not necessarily prove that human beings react in the same way, but it raises the possibility that they may do so.

The possibility that viruses may contribute to the development of cancer has been raised repeatedly and is undergoing intensive study at the present time. In the animal laboratory it has been demonstrated that some substance in the milk of the mouse from a carcinogenic strain can be transmitted to the young who ingest this milk. In a high proportion of cases, baby mice from noncarcinogenic strain, put to nurse immediately at the breast of a mouse from a carcinogenic strain, will later develop cancer.

Throughout the last 10 years in cancer research immunologists have been increasingly aware of the role of the immune system in the natural history and therapy of malignant disease. They suggest that it may be possible to strengthen the cancer patient's own natural response so that the body itself would be able to destroy malignant cells. Researchers in this field have established that human neoplasms contain tumor-specific antigens not found in normal adult cells, that the immune response to tumor-specific antigens is important in controlling the development and progression of human neoplasia, and that

the immune response can induce regression of human neoplasms. Early results of clinical trials using nonspecific immunotherapy with BCG (the bacillus of Calmette and Guérin) in the treatment of selected neoplasms such as skin carcinomas and malignant melanomas appear encouraging. The progress made to date indicates that immunotherapy has potential as a new form of cancer treatment used as an adjunct to definitive cancer surgery, radiation therapy, or chemotherapy.

■ PREVENTION AND CONTROL

Prevention and control of cancer depend largely on use of present knowledge to avoid these conditions that are known to predispose to the development of the disease and to educate the public to have thorough periodic physical examinations and to seek attention promptly if any signs of cancer appear. The nurse is important in any program for prevention and control of cancer. Charles S. Cameron, the medical and scientific director of the American Society for the Prevention of Cancer, once said: "If cancer control is to make the progress so urgently called for, the nurse will have to assume more and more responsibility, as a community-minded citizen, for the development of broad cancer education programs among the general public. The success of control measures depends in large measure on developing a public with higher awareness, better understanding, and a more constructive attitude toward the disease."*

Prevention

Sources of chronic irritation that may lead to cancer should be avoided. Effort is being made in industry to protect workers from coal-tar products known to contain carcinogens. Masks and gloves are recommended in some instances, and workers are urged to wash their hands and arms thoroughly to remove all irritating substances at the end of the day's work. Industrial nurses participate in intensive educational programs to help workers understand the need for carrying out company rules that may help to prevent cancer.

There are many ways to prevent irritation that may lead to cancer. It is possible that cleanliness of the skin is helpful, particularly for persons who live and work in highly industrial environments where the soot content in the air is high. Prolonged exposure to wind, dirt, and sunshine may lead to skin cancer. Skin cancer on the face and hands is particularly frequent among farmers and cattle ranchers who have fair complexions and who do not protect themselves from exposure.

Any kind of chronic irritation to the skin should

---

*From A cancer source book for nurses, New York, 1963, American Cancer Society, Inc.; reprinted by permission of the American Cancer Society, Inc.

be avoided, and moles that are in locations where they may be irritated by clothing should be removed. Shoelaces, shoe tops, girdles, brassieres, and shirt collars are examples of clothing that may be a source of chronic irritation. Glasses, earrings, dental plates, and pipes that are in repeated contact with skin and mucous membrane may contribute to cancer. Chewing food thoroughly is recommended to lessen irritation in the throat and stomach. Cancer in the mouth is sometimes associated with rough jagged teeth and the constant irritation of tobacco smoke. The habit of drinking scalding hot or freezing cold liquids is thought to be irritating to the mouth and to the esophagus. Indiscriminate use of laxatives is thought to have possible carcinogenic effects on the large bowel.

Encouraging women to breast-feed their babies, if there are no contraindications, may contribute to the prevention of cancer of the breast. Cancer of the breast is reported to be unknown among Eskimo women and to be relatively rare among Japanese women. Both groups practice breast-feeding, and it is believed that this factor may be responsible for the favorable record, although the relationship is still unproved.

There is now no question that excessive smoking is linked with the increased incidence of lung cancer. More and more reports are appearing that incriminate moderate and heavy cigarette smoking as a predisposing factor in the development of lung cancer, which now causes 14 times as many deaths each year as it did 30 years ago. In 1975 lung cancer will kill approximately 81,000 persons in the United States (63,500 men and 17,600 women).[3] These figures represent an increase of 3% in males and an increase of 10% in females over the 1973 figure. Although the rate of increase of lung cancer in men has been alarming, separate and independent studies have noted a rise in the rate of lung cancer (and heart disease) in women. The rise appears to parallel an increase in women smokers, particularly teenage girls, over the last 5 years. In 1968 the number of girl smokers between the ages of 12 and 18 was about half the number of teenage boys who smoked. By 1972 there was only a 2.4% difference. The rise in number of women smokers has captured the attention of cigarette manufacturers, who have increased their advertising efforts in this direction to the point of designing cigarettes expressly for women. An enormous amount of effort is being made by both private and public agencies concerned with the health of the public to alert everyone, smokers as well as nonsmokers, to the dangers of cigarette smoking.

After the release of the Surgeon General's Report on Smoking and Health in 1964, The National Interagency Council on Smoking and Health was formed. This group, composed of 27 public and private health, educational, and youth organizations,

has as its major objective combating smoking as a health hazard. Several of these participating organizations have produced films and other educational materials that are available to schools, organizations, and individuals. Assistance in securing films and other materials can be obtained from the Library, National Clearinghouse for Smoking and Health, Public Health Service.* One of the main concerns of the Interagency Council is how to convince young people not to start smoking. A new film, "Breathing Easy," was produced by the American Lung Association† especially for the preteen group. The American Cancer Society is designing smoking cessation clinics for places of employment and for schools. Antismoking education drives in schools are conducted through school courses, assemblies, and exhibits.

As of January 2, 1971, no cigarette advertising is permitted on either television or radio. On the same date the warning on cigarette packages was changed from "Caution: cigarette smoking may be hazardous to your health" to "Warning: The Surgeon General has determined that cigarette smoking is dangerous to your health." While the campaign to convince people to stop smoking has been slow and arduous, there has been change noted in smoking patterns. There is a trend toward increased use of filter cigarettes and pipes among smokers. The two thirds of the population who are nonsmokers have been active, and in some instances successful, in getting smokers to refrain from smoking in public places such as specified sections of airline services and public buildings. In 1972 the Surgeon General of the United States declared that smoking in the presence of a nonsmoker might be considered an act of aggression. Experiments have shown that cigarette smokers in a crowded, ill-ventilated room or automobile can raise the level of carbon dioxide to the point that all within the area can experience trouble discriminating time intervals and visual and sound cues as well as difficulty with eye-hand coordination. Action in the form of bills, ordinances, and restriction on smoking and the sale of tobacco in places of public assembly are being instituted at all levels on a nationwide basis.

Nurses have a responsibility, both as well-informed citizens and as professional persons, to be aware of the most recent antismoking programs and to interpret them to the public. One of the best ways for nurses to do this would be to stop smoking themselves. Although there are no figures available on the number of nurses who have stopped smoking, the American Cancer Society estimates that 50,000 physicians have done so.

Air pollution caused by smoke, industrial fumes, and exhaust from automobiles, jet airliners, etc., has received considerable attention as a public health

---

*5401 Westbord Ave., Bethesda, Md. 20016.
†1740 Broadway, New York, N. Y. 10019.

hazard, and many groups are now actively involved in working to control pollution of the air. It is widely accepted that air pollution contributes to the incidence of many respiratory diseases and that the conditions of individuals with these diseases are made worse when air pollution is high.

The search for carcinogenic agents is a continuous one. In late 1969 cyclamates, which were widely used as a sugar substitute, were banned when experimental studies revealed that in high doses they could produce cancer of the bladder in mice.

Control

More widespread knowledge of cancer and a more positive attitude toward the disease are essential for the control of the disease. Despite all the public announcements that have been made in the last few decades, there are still people who think of cancer as a disgraceful disease that must be hidden from others. Cancer is talked about in whispers by some people who look on it as a punishment for past sins, a shameful disease, or a disgrace to the family. This attitude stems partly from the fact that cancer in its terminal stages often is a painful and demoralizing disease that is sometimes accompanied by body odor and other signs of physical decay that are deeply etched on the consciousness of friends and relatives. Actually there is no characteristic odor of cancer, although diseased tissue that breaks down and becomes infected with odor-producing organisms will be as unpleasant as any other infected wound. The essential point—so often missed by the public—is that this tragic situation is by and large an unusual one.

Some people fear cancer and shun persons who have the disease because they believe it is contagious. Scientific speculation on the possibility that a virus may be the cause has added to this fear. At this time there is no conclusive evidence that a virus or any other communicable agent contributes in any way to the development of cancer.

The positive aspects of cancer should be emphasized. It is estimated that approximately one third of the persons for whom a diagnosis is made are cured by medical treatment. Another third could perhaps be cured by medical treatment if diagnosed early enough. Only a third, therefore, have cancer occurring in locations in which the disease advances beyond permanent medical aid before sufficient signs appear to warn the patient of trouble. In spite of these facts, however, some persons think it is useless to report symptoms early, since they believe that if they do have cancer they cannot be cured. It can only be hoped that the recent publicity given to well-known persons who have been treated for cancer will help overcome some of these beliefs. If nothing else, the open discussion of the diagnosis and treatment in all types of media should result in a better informed public than ever before.

Warning signals of cancer

Everyone should know the seven danger signs of cancer and should report them immediately to his physician: (1) any sore or lesion in the mouth or anywhere else in the body that does not heal within 2 weeks, (2) a lump or mass in the breast or anywhere else in the body, (3) any unusual bleeding or discharge from any body orifice, (4) any change in size, color, or appearance of a wart or a mole, (5) persistent indigestion or difficulty in swallowing, (6) persistent hoarseness or cough that does not clear up within 2 weeks, (7) any change in normal bowel habits. It should be emphasized in all health teaching that any of these signs should be investigated medically but also that their occurrence does not necessarily mean that the patient has cancer.

A very common misconception that leads the patient to ignore symptoms is a belief that a disease as serious as cancer must be accompanied by weight loss. Weight loss is usually a late symptom of cancer, yet the patient often remarks, "I wasn't losing weight so I thought nothing serious could be wrong." Another reason for neglect of cancer is that it may not cause pain, and, again, the patient takes the absence of pain as a sign that his indisposition is minor. It must be repeatedly emphasized to the public that pain is not an early sign of cancer and that cancer may be far advanced before pain occurs.

All people should know the most common sites of cancer. In women they are the breast, uterus (cervix), skin, and gastrointestinal tract (Table 15-1). All women should be taught to examine their breasts each month immediately after the menstrual period. Women past the menopause should designate a day on their calendars regularly for this examination. Such self-examination (Fig. 30-3) is a much better method of detecting early cancer than is an annual physical examination. (See p. 804 for details of self-examination of the breast.) Mammography, a soft tissue radiograph of the breast, is used as an aid in detecting cancer of the breast before clinical signs and symptoms are evident[17] (Fig. 30-1). See Chapter 30 for further discussion of carcinoma of the breast.

Women of all ages should know the importance of reporting any abnormal vaginal bleeding or other discharge occurring between menstrual periods or after the menopause. (See p. 510 for details of early symptoms of cancer of the female reproductive system.)

All women should have a pelvic examination annually, and a cervical smear should be taken for testing by the Papanicolaou method. Some physicians advise that the Papanicolaou test be done every 6 months for women over the age of 30. The nurse should encourage all women to visit their doctor regularly for this test and to request that the test be done if it has inadvertently been overlooked by the physician. The Papanicolaou test represents an enormous step forward in the early diagnosis of cancer of the cervix. It is also useful in diagnosing cancer in other parts of the body such as the lungs. The value of the test lies in the fact that abnormal malignant cells that are sloughed off in the early stages of a cancer of the endothelium may be identified from secretions about the lesion. The sloughing of these particular cells usually occurs before the lesion has invaded the deeper structures, and if the test is done early, the cancer may be diagnosed and removed before metastasis occurs.

The most common sites of cancer in men are the skin, lungs, gastrointestinal tract, and prostate gland. All men 40 years of age and over should have an annual physical examination that includes search for diseases in these locations. In many cancer detection clinics, proctoscopic examinations are done on all men 35 years of age or over because of the high incidence of cancer of the lower bowel in men of this age group.

Further information about cancer of specific organs can be found in appropriate chapters in Section II of this book.

Facilities for education and care

Cancer detection is not inexpensive. Education of the public often includes convincing them that this is a sound investment in their total health care program. Some cities have cancer detection centers where a complete physical, chest radiograph, Papanicolaou smear, breast examination, proctoscopy, urinalysis, and blood count are performed for a moderate fee. Nurses should also be aware of clinics in their area where patients needing such resources may be referred. The nurse needs to teach that there is no quick or certain cure for cancer. Despite all the public education and all efforts of the medical profession to control the extravagant claims of a few unethical practitioners, there are still some people who rely on quick "cure" remedies prescribed by quacks. The best hope for cure of cancer lies in immediate medical attention if danger signs appear. If a person who suspects he has cancer has no private physician or feels that he cannot afford one, he should report to his local health department and seek referral to a suitable hospital or to a local cancer detection clinic. The state or local branch of the American Cancer Society will have complete directives on facilities as to location, services available, and financial arrangements.

In dealing with a patient who has delayed seeking early medical treatment, the nurse must give hope and encouragement to him and his family. Sometimes guilt, a feeling of hopelessness, or a fatalistic attitude will cause further delay in pursuing a suggested course of medical diagnosis or treatment.

The nurse should know of sources of information and help for persons who have cancer. There is one large national voluntary organization, the American Cancer Society, Inc.,* which has branches in all states and in 11 major cities. It was organized in 1913 as the National Society for the Control of Cancer with the major objective of combating the fear, shame, and ignorance that were outstanding obstacles in the early treatment of the disease. The huge organization, which receives large annual bequests and gifts, has expanded its functions and now has several objectives. It finances research to seek the cause of cancer and to develop better methods of treatment. It publishes booklets and pamphlets for the use of physicians and nurses, and it stimulates better preparation of professional people in the care of patients with cancer by sponsoring institutes and programs for special groups. Information about booklets and pamphlets may be obtained by writing directly to the main office of the society or to the state or local offices.

In addition, the American Cancer Society strives constantly to educate the public. It works intensively through magazines, women's clubs, insurance companies, state departments of health, and medical and nursing organizations in an effort to reach all the population with the educational message of how cancer may be prevented and controlled. A large amount of literature for the laity is prepared and distributed annually. Also, many excellent films for use in public education are made available.

The American Cancer Society also performs services for patients and their families. Branches in most communities provide assistance for cancer patients who cannot afford to pay for adequate care and for those who, although they can presently afford to pay, will eventually leave their families with too great a financial burden. Depending on how much local support is given to the society, the services may include dressings, transportation to and from clinics and physicians' offices, special drugs such as expensive hormones, blood, prostheses, and the loan of expensive equipment such as hospital beds. In some communities, homemaking, visiting nurse, and rehabilitation services are also provided. Of the money collected, 60% remains with the local chapter for the community's use. Patients and their families should know about these services before their own resources are depleted, and local citizens should be urged to support the society generously. Many of these agencies do not use the term "cancer" in their title so that patients who do not know their diagnosis may be safely referred to them.

In addition to the American Cancer Society, some large cities have other voluntary organizations that serve only cancer patients; for example, Cancer Care, a large voluntary organization in New York City, confines its activities solely to the tremendous needs

---

*Headquarters: 291 E. 42nd St., New York, N. Y. 10017.

of patients with advanced cancer and to the needs of their families. The nurse who works in a small community or a rural area may learn of the resources available to cancer patients through local or state health departments.

Lists of available films for both professional and lay use can be obtained from the American Cancer Society and from state and local health departments. Some insurance companies such as the Metropolitan Life Insurance Company and the John Hancock Insurance Company prepare very useful pamphlets on control of cancer and the care of persons who have the disease. These pamphlets are useful to nurses in conducting health education programs and in teaching relatives of a patient with cancer how to care for him.

Federal recognition of the need to give intensive assistance to educational programs in cancer was evident in 1926, when Congress proclaimed April of each year as National Cancer Control Month. In 1937 the National Cancer Institute was created within the National Institutes of Health. This institute, with generous support from the federal government, conducts an extensive program of research in the field of cancer.

■ NURSING INTERVENTION

A sound personal philosophy and an objective, positive attitude toward the disease based on real knowledge will help the nurse who is caring for the patient with cancer. The nurse should be able to give support and hope to the patient and to his significant others. Although compassion is necessary, inspiring false hope should be avoided. The nurse must try to understand the fears experienced by the patient as he awaits diagnostic procedures or other treatment— fear of hospitals, fear of pain, fear of radical surgery with mutilation, fear of expense that cannot be met, and fear of death, with all that it means to him. In working with the patient the young and inexperienced nurse should not hesitate to turn to an instructor, head nurse, or supervisor with problems that appear too great to handle alone.

A nurse's kindly interest in the patient as an individual often helps him. Many patients must undergo extensive diagnostic examination and surgery in large medical centers a long distance from their homes. Some patients have reported that, although they were confident that they were in "good medical hands," such confidence did not make up for the feeling that they were not always known as individuals. They needed desperately to feel that at least one person knew and understood them as individuals. Some patients experience near panic at the thought of their loved ones' coming to visit and being unable to locate them. The nurse who works with the patient in the community, in the small hospital, or in the

physician's office can help the patient by preparing him for what he may experience in the large center. In most instances it is best for the patient to be accompanied by a relative or a close friend. It should also be recognized that even a patient in familiar surroundings may feel very much alone when awaiting diagnostic tests or surgical treatment for known or suspected cancer.

The nursing staff needs to know whether or not the patient has been told that he has cancer. This information should be recorded on the nursing care plan and discussed with other health team members. This will ensure that the patient does not receive different answers to the same questions from physicians, nurses, social workers, and other health team members. Some hospitals have partially overcome this problem by having regular meetings of all the members of the professional staff at which the information given to each patient is reviewed. If meetings of this type are not being held, the nurses or nursing staff should take the initiative in planning such a meeting. Often other health team members are concerned about the approach to be taken with the patient with cancer and are appreciative of an opportunity to discuss their feelings.

The emotional climate produced during the period of diagnostic examination and initial treatment is very important in determining whether or not the patient will continue diagnostic examination, treatment, or repeated follow-up care after discharge. The care he receives in the hospital may shape his attitudes toward his disease and may determine whether or not he can return home and either care for himself or be cared for by his family. An important nursing function in care of the patient with cancer is building up his faith in the physician and in the clinic or the medical center where he receives care. The patient needs to feel certain that everything possible is being done for him and that new measures will be tried if there is any promise whatsoever of their being helpful.

Members of the medical profession differ in their opinions as to whether or not the patient with cancer should be told the diagnosis. Decision usually depends on the patient, his family, and the physician. The present trend is toward telling the patient he has cancer, although studies show that fewer than 50% of physicians tell their patients.[43] Many spiritual advisers recommend telling the truth. However, some patients may not want to know the diagnosis. They may ask and then answer their own question negatively. Some do not ask for the diagnosis because they do not wish to have confirmed what they already suspect. Some insist on knowing the diagnosis and are preoccupied with every detail of their progress and treatment in a detached but completely abnormal fashion. Finally, there are some who wish to know the facts and who can accept them in a realistic way when given an opportunity to discuss their feelings with others. Some physicians prepare the patient over a period of time and tell him the complete truth when they feel it is best to do so. Psychologic reactions depend on the emotional makeup of the individual and are as varied as man's ability to face stress and threats throughout life. Since disclosure of the diagnosis lies entirely with the discretion of the physician, the nurse cannot tell the patient or his family. The nurse can, however, refer to the physician any questions, misinformation, or apprehensions that the patient or his family have expressed. This will often help the physician to decide what course of action seems best. Any sudden severe depression or expressed thoughts of suicide should be reported at once. Often a patient's fears are communicated to a nurse long before he summons the courage to question the physician.

The patient needs something to keep him occupied while he is awaiting completion of diagnostic tests and treatment and between steps of treatment such as surgery or x-ray therapy. Usually he fares best in a room with other patients, where there is more going on and less time for introspective thought. Most patients are able to concentrate only on conversation, music, newspapers, and light games at this time. Some patients may like to do work with their hands, such as crocheting or working with leather. If there is no occupational therapy department from which supplies may be obtained, the nurse may arrange for members of the patient's family to provide them.

The family also needs to keep busy while awaiting the results of diagnostic tests and the outcome of surgery or of other treatment. One woman, on learning that her husband had far-advanced carcinoma, went home immediately and made his favorite cake, even though he was in the hospital and unable to enjoy it. Psychologic relief may sometimes come from keeping occupied with usual daily activities. Anxious relatives also receive satisfaction from doing things that the patient would do if he could, thus preserving parts of cherished routines. Taking the dog for his daily walk is an example. Members of the family often need direction in their activity when they have just learned that a loved one has cancer. They may need to talk over immediate and long-term plans with someone not close to the family situation. The nurse can sometimes be this listening person. At other times the family can best be served by a social caseworker, who will help them talk through and think through a course of action.

■ SURGICAL TREATMENT

The best treatment for cancer at the present time is complete surgical removal of all malignant tissues before metastasis occurs. Surgery must often be extensive and may require adjustment for the patient beyond that needed in many other conditions. The patient with cancer does not have the privilege of electing surgery, as he may in some diseases. This fact alone makes him feel trapped and seriously threatened. He does not have time to accustom himself gradually to the idea of how the surgery may change him and how it may affect his way of life. The patient must often face the prospect of mutilating surgery with only the hope and not the certainty that it will cure the cancer and save his life. He may be more concerned about his family than he is about himself. Obviously he needs sympathy and understanding when he and his family are attempting to accept the news and the immediate surgical treatment that the surgeon recommends. The operative procedures and nursing care for cancer involving the particular systems are discussed in the appropriate chapters and will not be included here.

■ RADIATION

Ionizing radiation consists of electromagnetic waves or material particles that have sufficient energy to ionize atoms or molecules (that is, remove electrons from them) and thereby alter their chemical behavior.[58] In adequate amounts it destroys the cells. Radiation is used medically for diagnosis, treatment, and research.

General facts

Every living thing from the beginning of time has been exposed to small amounts of radiation from the sun and from certain natural elements in the earth, such as uranium, that emit gamma rays in the process of their decay. This is called *natural background radiation.*[58] No problem regarding radiation existed until after 1895, when the roentgen-ray (x-ray) machine was developed and became widely used in diagnosis of disease. The development of this machine was followed by the discovery of radium and the use of both radium and x-rays for treatment of diseases such as cancer. With developments in the field of nuclear energy, it has been possible to produce radioactive isotopes of a number of the elements, although only a few of them, such as gold, cobalt, and phosphorus, have medical application at the present time. The problem of overexposure and possible harm to patients and to the personnel caring for them has increased greatly with the increased use of x-rays in diagnosis and treatment and the more recent use of radioisotopes in diagnosis and treatment. Also, radiation in the environment resulting from atomic testing has become a widely feared and much debated subject in many parts of the world.

No one really knows how much exposure to radiation is safe for persons working with patients and for patients having repeated x-ray films taken for various purposes. Relatively small amounts of exposure have produced serious damage in experimental animals, but man has not lived through enough generations of relatively high exposure for conclusive evidence of safe levels to be obtained. It is reasonable to assume that the less exposure one has the better. This does not mean that a patient receiving radiation treatment should not receive adequate nursing care. There are ways to protect persons from exposure, and hospitals are required to have protective procedures and guides for persons who care for patients receiving radioactive materials. All nurses should be familiar with the procedures used in the institution in which they are employed.

The ionizing effect of radiation on the body cells remains, so that exposure is cumulative throughout life. Exposure of the entire body enormously increases the amount of radiation received. For this reason, all of the body except the part being treated is protected from exposure when relatively high doses are given for therapeutic purposes.

The National Committee on Radiation Protection has accepted 5 R (roentgens, or units of measurement) per year as the maximum permissible dose considered safe for well people over 18 years of age.[36] The United States National Academy of Sciences and the United Nations have estimated that the average person receives a total of 3 to 5 R from background radiation between birth and 30 years of life. They also estimate that additional exposure for medical and dental work probably doubles this amount in the Western world. The amount of exposure the patient receives from a series of x-ray films taken for diagnostic purposes depends on the machine used and the technical skill involved. Usually the fluoroscopic examination entails more exposure than the radiograph. To prevent excessive exposure with fluoroscopy, the physician allows time for his own eyes to accommodate to the darkened room so that he can then observe the patient with a lower intensity of the machine. The exposure of the average nurse working in a hospital and occasionally assisting a patient while a radiograph is taken is almost negligible.

Systemic reactions to excessive radiation exposure are leukopenia, leukemia, and sterility or damage to the reproductive cells. Leukemia is an occupational disease among radiologists, with one study showing that its incidence was nine times higher among radiologists than among other physicians.[36] Because of the increased risk, badges are worn by persons whose daily work exposes them to radiation. The badge, which contains photographic film capable of absorbing radiation, is developed each month. A darkening or blackening of the film indicates excessive exposure. Personnel who are becoming overexposed are removed, at least temporarily, from direct contact with radiation.

Because of the possible danger to the fetus, particularly between the second and sixth weeks of life,

radiographs are seldom taken on pregnant women. If they must be taken, the lower abdomen is protected carefully. Also, pregnant women usually are not employed in x-ray departments or in caring for patients receiving radioactive materials internally.

Nurses who work where they are exposed to x-rays repeatedly or who care for patients receiving radioactive substances must take responsibility for learning how to protect themselves from too much exposure.

The radiation used medically consists of alpha, beta, and gamma rays (Fig. 15-1). Alpha and beta rays cannot pass through the skin. Therefore exposure to them must come from taking them into the body through the mouth by careless handling of drainage or body wastes and by not washing hands thoroughly after touching any materials that may be contaminated. Gamma rays, however, have been found to penetrate several inches of lead, although lead shielding offers a considerable degree of protection. X-rays, which are similar to gamma rays, require lead protection.

Radiation can be delivered to the patient by exposure to rays externally *(external radiation),* either from an x-ray machine or from cobalt 60, which has been made radioactive artificially, or by placing material from which radiation emanates, such as radium, radon seeds, radioactive cobalt (^{60}Co), or radioactive gold (^{198}Au), within a body cavity or within the tissues *(sealed internal radiation).* Another way to give internal radiation is to administer radioactive materials intravenously or orally, so that they are distributed throughout the body *(unsealed internal radiation).*

Radiation delivered externally (including x-rays) can do harm to persons working with the patient *only during* the time that the patient is being treated. This is true also of the radiation from some radioactive substances used for other methods of treatment, as will be described later. Patients with internal radiation who emit gamma rays, however, may expose other persons to radiation for varying periods of time, and the time one can be exposed safely to the patient is important in planning care. The time interval required for the radioactive substance to be half dissipated is called its *half-life* (Table 15-3). This period varies extremely widely, but as the end of the half-life is reached, danger from exposure decreases.

There are three ways by which exposure to radiation can be controlled. These are *time, distance,* and *shielding.* All emanations are subject to the physical law of *inverse-square.* For example, if a person stands 2 feet away from the source of radiation, he receives only one fourth as much exposure as when standing only 1 foot away. At 4 feet he receives only one sixteenth of the exposure. Therefore increasing the distance from the emanations decreases the exposure (Fig. 15-2). When a patient such as an infant must

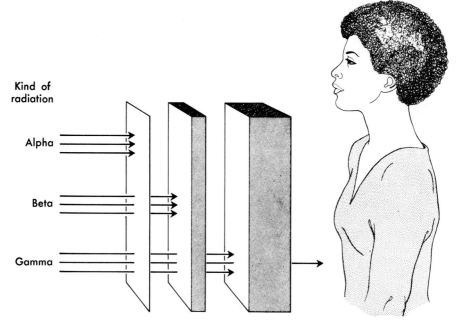

FIG. 15-1. Relative penetrating power of the three types of radiation. (From Bouchard, R., and Owens, N. F.: Nursing care of the cancer patient, ed. 2, St. Louis, 1972, The C. V. Mosby Co.)

Table 15-3 Characteristics and uses of some commonly used radioactive agents

Radiation source	Half-life (where applicable)	Rays emitted	Appearance or form	Method of administration
X-ray	—	Gamma	Invisible rays	X-ray machine
Radium	1,600 years	Alpha Beta Gamma	In needles, plaques, molds	Interstitial (needles) Intracavitary (plaques, molds)
Radon	4 days	Alpha Beta Gamma (low intensity)	In seeds, needles	Interstitial (seeds, needles)
Cesium 137	33 years	Beta Gamma	In needles, capsules	Interstitial (needles) Intracavitary (capsules)
Cobalt (^{60}Co)	5 years	Beta Gamma	External (cobalt unit) Internal (needles, seeds, molds)	Machine (teletherapy) Interstitial (needles, seeds)
Iodine (^{131}I)	8 days	Beta Gamma (low intensity)	Clear liquid	By mouth
Phosphorus (^{32}P)	14 days	Beta	Clear liquid	By mouth, intracavitary, intravenous
Gold (^{198}Au)	3 days	Beta Gamma	Purple liquid	Intracavitary
Iridium (^{192}Ir)	74 days	Beta Gamma (low intensity)	In needles, wires, seeds	Interstitial
Yttrium (^{90}Y)	3 days	Beta	Beads, needles	Interstitial

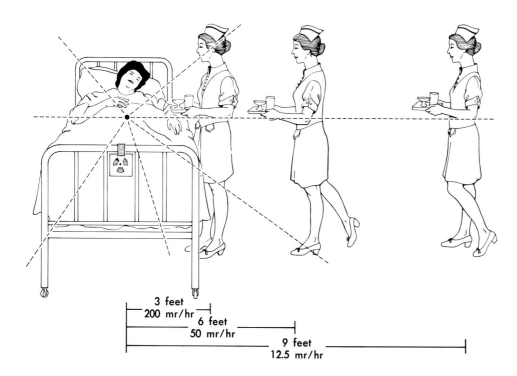

FIG. 15-2. Nurse nearest source of radioactivity (the patient) is exposed to more radioactivity. (From Bouchard, R., and Owens, N. F.: Nursing care of the cancer patient, ed. 2, St. Louis, 1972, The C. V. Mosby Co.)

3 feet
200 mr/hr
6 feet
50 mr/hr
9 feet
12.5 mr/hr

be held for x-ray treatment, the nurse or person who holds him must be careful to keep at arm's length or as far away as possible and to avoid having any body part in the direct path of the rays. *Lead-lined gloves and a lead apron, which act as a shield to reduce exposure, should be used by anyone who attends patients during x-ray treatment or during examination by fluoroscopy.*

When the nurse knows the kind of substance used, the kind and amount of rays it emits, its half-life, and its exact location in the patient and considers these facts in relation to control of exposure, safe and adequate care for the patient can be planned.

Radiotherapy and cancer

Radiotherapy is the term used when forms of radiation are employed in the treatment of disease. Radiotherapy has been used in the treatment of cancer for about 70 years, whereas surgery has been used for hundreds of years. The principal radiation agents used are x-ray, which consists of electromagnetic radiation produced by waves of electrical energy traveling at a very high speed; radium, which is a radioactive isotope occurring freely in nature; and the artificially induced radioactive isotopes produced by bombarding the isotopes of elements with highly energized particles in a cyclotron. One of the most useful of these radiation agents is radioactive cobalt (cobalt 60, irradiated cobalt), which is now used in external radiation therapy. Because of its lower cost, it is largely replacing radium for sealed internal use.

Radiotherapy is effective in curing cancer in some instances. In other instances it controls the cancer cells for a time. Because it may deter the growth of cancer cells, it may relieve pain even when extension of the disease is such that cure is impossible. Radiotherapy is based on the known fact that malignant cells are more sensitive to radiation than normal cells. Therapeutic doses of radiotherapy are calculated to destroy or delay the growth of malignant cells without destroying normal tissue. Rotation of either the target site in the patient or the radiation beam makes it possible to deliver a high total dose to the tumor, while at the same time only part of the dose reaches the noncancerous tissue surrounding it.

To many people, radiotherapy and cancer are synonymous. It is natural, then, that the patient may react with panic to news that this treatment is necessary. Sometimes the patient is told that the treatment is necessary "to cure a growth that may become cancerous if not so treated." Often he does not really believe this statement. The nurse should give the patient who is about to receive radiation therapy an opportunity to talk about the therapy and to ask questions.

Because radiation therapy causes depression of the hematopoietic system and in turn a low white blood cell count, the patient should be protected from infection. If the patient is at home and receiving treatment on an ambulatory basis, he and his family should be cautioned to avoid persons with upper respiratory or other infections. In the hospital he should never be in the same room with patients who have these conditions. Antibiotic drugs may be ordered to be given prophylactically both during and following a course of treatment.

External radiotherapy. The patient who is to have

x-ray or radioactive cobalt therapy needs an adequate explanation so that he will know what to expect before, during, and after the treatment. He may have heard that the treatment causes nausea or skin burns or irritation. If he asks about these problems, the nurse should explain that with the carefully controlled dosages now given they seldom occur. Usually patients are not told of these possible complications unless they occur. It is helpful if nurses can observe a patient receiving therapy since this will enable them to answer the patient's questions about the therapy more intelligently. The patient should know that he will be placed on a table in a room by himself and that the equipment, although somewhat similar to what he has probably seen during a routine x-ray examination, will be larger and more complicated. He should also know that the radiologist or the radiotherapist will be stationed outside the room, will observe him throughout the treatment, and can communicate with him via an intercommunication system. After the radiologist has positioned the patient, the patient must remain absolutely still. This is a very trying experience for many patients and the sympathetic understanding of the nurse will be appreciated. The patient should also be told that there is no pain associated with radiation therapy.

In medical centers where hyperbaric oxygen chambers are available, patients may receive radiation therapy while receiving hyperbaric oxygen. The rationale for this combined therapy is that malignant cells, in which the oxygen tension is increased, are more susceptible to the effects of radiation. At the same time the sensitivity of normal cells to the radiation effects is not increased.[4,39,40] Several excellent references on the use of hyperbaric oxygen can be found in the bibliography at the end of this chapter.

In giving treatment, rays can be directed at the tumor from several different angles so that normal tissue has a minimum of exposure. The areas through which rays pass are known as *ports*. Different ports may be used on different days, or the position may be changed at intervals during a daily treatment so that only a certain amount is given through each of several ports. The patient may be placed on a rotating device such as a rotating chair so that, although the tumor mass receives the full dose of radiation, skin areas receive less exposure.

The patient may be curious as to how many treatments he will receive. It is best not to give a definite answer. Radiation dosages may be difficult to estimate accurately if the growth is deep within the body. Sometimes treatment must be discontinued because of local skin reaction or other reasons. Thus the patient who has been told the number of treatments planned to assure successful recovery may become depressed when treatment is discontinued. The patient also becomes concerned if he learns he is to receive more treatments than were originally planned.

Skin preparation for external radiation therapy includes removal of any ointment and dressing and thorough cleansing of the skin. This procedure usually is followed by an alcohol rub. After this preparation, nothing should be used on the skin. The area to be treated is usually outlined by the radiologist at the time of the first treatment. Occasionally a small tattoo mark is used instead of the conspicuous skin markings when treatment is given to exposed parts of the body. Marks must not be washed off until the treatment is completed because they are important guides to the radiologist (Fig. 15-3). If the patient is ambulatory, he is instructed not to wash the skin in the area being treated or remove the marks. Sponge bathing of other parts of the body must replace showers and tub baths. A vegetable fat or oil may be ordered to protect the affected skin.

Medicated solutions or ointments and even powders that may contain heavy metals such as zinc are not permitted on the skin until the series of treatments is completed because they may increase the radiation dosage. Cornstarch may be used instead of powder.

When treatment is directed toward abdominal organs or any deep tissues, there is almost always some skin reaction. There may be itching, tingling, burning, oozing, or sloughing of the skin. The term "burn" should never be used in referring to this reaction since it implies incorrect dosage. Reddening may occur on or about the tenth day, and the skin may turn a dark plum color after about 3 weeks. The skin may also become dry and inelastic and may crack easily. Usually the radiologist should be con-

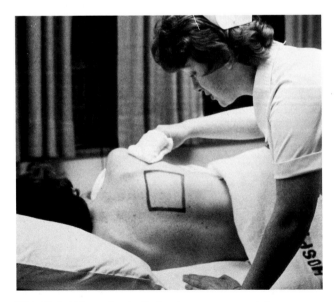

FIG. 15-3. When the bath is given, care must be taken not to remove skin markings used to guide the radiologist in giving x-ray treatment.

sulted about the appropriate care. The area may be cleansed gently with sterile mineral oil, but crusts should not be removed. Lanolin or petroleum jelly may be used to protect the area, and healing ointments containing vitamins A and D and healing oils such as cod liver oil may be used if breakdown of superficial tissues occurs. Healing usually starts approximately in the fifth week of treatment and should be complete about a month later.

Ointments are best applied by spreading them on a piece of sterile gauze and fastening the gauze to the patient's clothing. If this procedure is not possible, dressings may be bandaged loosely or anchored to healthy skin outside and beyond the treatment ports. If tape must be used instead of bandage, cellophane tape should be used instead of adhesive tape because it is less irritating to skin. In removing dressings the greatest care must be taken to pull toward the middle of the area and thus avoid any pull on affected skin. Dressings should be loose to permit circulation of air and to avoid pressure on the skin.

Because the skin exposed to radiation treatment may become irritated and break down easily, it should be protected from constricting clothing or friction of any kind. For example, the patient receiving treatment to the trunk should not wear a girdle, a garter belt, or a constricting trouser or skirt belt during the period of treatment and for several weeks thereafter. During the period of treatment, the patient should avoid excesses of heat and cold to affected skin surfaces. Hot-water bottles and ice caps should not be used, and exposure to the sun should be avoided. Some physicians advise that no water be used on the skin for at least 2 weeks after the completion of treatment.

If the radiation dosage has been high and blanching or discoloration of the skin has resulted, the physician may advise the patient to avoid exposure to temperature changes for several years. The patient may have to take much cooler baths or showers than formerly, and he may have to avoid sunbathing or any other extreme of temperature. If x-ray treatment has been given to a woman's face, she must be cautioned regarding the use of cosmetics to cover discolored skin. They may contain heavy, irritating oils and should not be used until the physician believes they are safe.

When treatment must be given to any part of the head, women patients may ask about the danger of loss of scalp hair and men about loss of beard. Whether or not hair will return after falling out depends on the amount of radiation received. Specific questions should be referred to the physician. Attractive scarves and wigs are useful for women patients who must receive large doses for palliative purposes, with permanent baldness resulting, or until such time as the normal hair returns.

Gastrointestinal reactions to radiation therapy are more common when treatment includes some part of the gastrointestinal tract or when the ports lie over this system. The patient may have nausea, vomiting, anorexia, malaise, and diarrhea. This difficulty is not discussed with the patient before treatment is started because it is thought that the power of suggestion may contribute to symptoms. However, almost all patients who receive moderate or large doses of radiation have these symptoms in varying degrees. Intravenous solutions of glucose in physiologic solution of sodium chloride are used for nausea, anorexia, and dehydration. Pyridoxine (vitamin B_6), dimenhydrinate (Dramamine), chlorpromazine (Thorazine), and trimethobenzamide hydrochloride (Tigan) relieve symptoms in some patients. Camphorated tincture of opium (paregoric) may be used to control the diarrhea, but drugs such as bismuth subcarbonate are not given because they contain a heavy metal that will increase radiation dosage.

Many patients find that resting just before meals and lying down immediately after eating help to control nausea and vomiting. Frequent small meals instead of the usual three a day should also be tried. Some patients find that it helps to avoid food for 2 or 3 hours before and about 2 hours after each treatment. Sour tasting beverages and effervescent liquids may also relieve nausea. Usually breakfast is the meal best tolerated. Therefore it should be substantial, and the patient should be encouraged to eat as much as possible. Problems related to radiation therapy in specific locations are discussed in the appropriate sections of this book.

Internal radiotherapy. Whether or not the patient receiving internal radiation will be on radiation precautions and the nursing time with him restricted depends on the amount of radioactive material used, its location, and the kinds of rays being emitted (Table 15-3). Special precautions may be taken if more than a tracer diagnostic dose has been given. Hospitals in which therapeutic doses of radioactive isotopes are administered are required to have someone on the staff who functions as a radiation safety officer. Quite often this person is a physicist. The radiation safety officer determines the precautions to be observed in each situation. Most hospitals have printed instruction sheets stating the precautions to be followed for each substance used. Personnel should be fully acquainted with all precautions and should be supervised in carrying them out. Generally the patient will be placed in a single room or in a double room with another patient who is also receiving radioactive therapy. A radiation precaution sign should be placed on the door to the patient's room and visitors should be restricted.

The nurse and all others who come in direct contact with the patient for any length of time may wear an isolation gown and rubber gloves and a film badge under the gown to determine the amount of exposure received. Occasionally no direct contact with the patient is permitted. If so, the patient's room must be equipped with an intercommunication system and all supplies he may need during his isolation. The room should have a window through which the patient can be observed and through which he can see other people. It should have a telephone so that he can talk to family members if he is able and wishes to do so. Food and other items the patient desires or needs usually are passed into the room through a special porthole.

It is important to explain the routine to the patient and the reason for the precautions that are to be taken. He is being kept in his own room for the period of isolation so that danger of contamination to others is minimized and so that his reaction to the radioactive substance can be studied and controlled. He should know that isolation is temporary, and he should be told specifically when restrictions will be removed. The patient should be told that members of the nursing staff will be available for anything that he needs, but that they will work quickly and will only remain in the room long enough to carry out essential activities. The patient should be assisted in notifying his significant others about the restriction on visitors and how long it will last.

The patient should know how the radioactive substance he takes is eliminated lest he fear that he will be dangerous to other people indefinitely and become concerned about social isolation or about the possibility of harming his loved ones when he returns home. He should have a radio or television in order to keep in contact with outside happenings, and a communication system between the patient's room and the nurses' station helps. The patient needs to see the nursing staff, however, and if treatment permits, they should speak to him from the open doorway. If isolation is complete, they should come to the observation window frequently and speak to him via the intercommunication system.

There are many things the nurse can do to add to the patient's physical and emotional comfort during the period of restricted nursing contact. Before treatment is given, his immediate environment should be checked. Are the bed and bedside table in the most convenient location for self-help? Can any arrangement be made so that the patient may draw his own blinds or curtains? Are extra covers readily available? Does the patient have reading material and is the lighting adequate and conveniently located? Are plants and flowers receiving care, and is it possible to arrange their location so that the patient may care for them himself if he feels able?

Before treatment requiring a period of precaution or isolation is started, the patient should have a complete bath so that bathing may be omitted for a few days. The bed should be made with clean linen and all personal linen should be fresh. If the patient is very ill and requires help in turning and moving, a turning sheet may be placed under him so that the nursing staff can turn him and raise him in bed in a short time and with little close contact. Sometimes a laxative or an enema is ordered to obviate the need for an enema or attention to bowel elimination for a few days. If treatment requires lying still in a specified position, measures for comfort should be anticipated. For example, if the patient is receiving treatment to the cervix and must lie on her back, a small pillow should be provided to use against the curve of the back *before* fatigue and discomfort become a major problem. This measure helps to lessen the nursing time needed to massage the patient's back and to assist her with any very slight change of position that may be permitted.

Trips made in haste into the patient's room are disturbing to him psychologically because they imply that he is not acceptable to others. The nurse who plans thoughtfully might deliver a letter, a telephone message, an ice cap, fresh water, and the newspaper and make pertinent observations in much less time than the one who plans less well and must make several trips into the patient's room. Social isolation for the patient by too infrequent visits to him must be avoided whenever possible. Brief communication with him from an open doorway is permissible to assure him that he has not been forgotten.

Many patients anticipate cure from radioactive isotopes. The nurse can learn what the patient understands about the treatment and should report any misunderstandings on his part to the physician.

Nurses wishing to know about radioactive substances can obtain information from the Division of Radiological Health of the Public Health Service or from their state health department. Several drug companies also publish pamphlets which contain helpful information.

Sealed internal radiotherapy. Radium, a naturally occurring radioactive isotope, and cobalt and iridium that have been made radioactive artificially are used to deliver sealed internal radiotherapy to certain malignant lesions that can be expected to respond to this kind of treatment. These radioactive substances may be used in the form of molds, plaques, needles, wires, special applicators, or ribbons that are carefully placed and left in position for a specified length of time (Fig. 15-4). Emanations from the radioactive substances may also be sealed in tiny gold tubes (seeds) and left indefinitely within the tissues into which they are inserted (Fig. 15-5). The half-life of the seeds is much less than that of the substances from which their emanations came. Radium is extremely costly, and its use is being replaced with the use of radioactive cobalt and other radioactive materials.

A fairly common site for the implantation of seeds

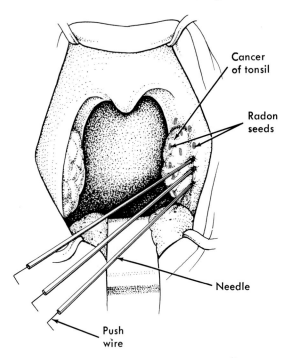

FIG. 15-5. Radium emanations may be sealed in tiny gold tubes (radon seeds) and left indefinitely within the tissues into which they are inserted. This schematic drawing shows insertion into the tonsil.

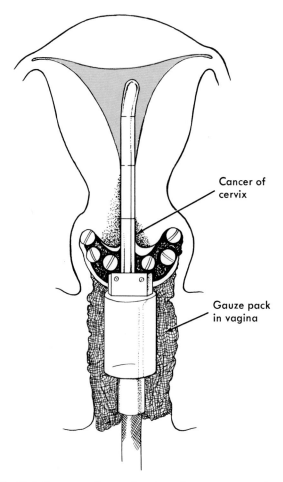

FIG. 15-4. Ernst applicator in place for treatment of cancer of the cervix. Note the gauze packing in the vagina to help maintain the applicator in position.

is the mouth. Plaques and molds also are used for lesions in the mouth. (For the nursing care of patients having treatment in this location, see p. 637.) Sealed internal radiation also is used widely in treatment of cancer of the cervix (p. 526).

Safe practice for the nurse caring for a patient receiving sealed internal radiotherapy depends on the principles of time, distance, and shielding discussed on p. 293. Radioactive materials for sealed internal therapy usually are kept in a lead-lined container in the radiology department and are inserted into the patient in the operating room. They should never be touched with bare hands. When the nurse handles these products, a pair of forceps at least 14 inches long is used and the radioactive materials are held at arm's length and above waist level. A pair of forceps should be kept in the patient's room for use in case the radioactive implant should become dislodged.

Sealed radioactive material is often reused. On removal from a patient the radioactive material should be cleansed using the precautions just described and returned to the radiology department in a lead-lined

container at once so that it may be safe from accidental handling or loss. Even if it is not to be reused, it is returned in a lead-lined container. To prevent accidental loss in cleansing, radioactive material is cleansed in a basin of water instead of in an open sink. If a brush must be used, it must be grasped with forceps so that close contact with the material is avoided.

Exposure is sometimes termed *external* in that it can occur only by direct exposure to the encased radioactive substance. It cannot result from contact with linen, vomitus, or urine or from touching the patient. Knowing where the radioactive material is implanted helps the nurse to plan activities of care. If, for example, the substance is in the patient's mouth, there is less exposure if one stands toward the foot of the bed. If it is in the uterus or bladder, standing at the head of the bed is safer.

Sloughing of tissue and subsequent hemorrhages are complications that must be considered when radiation is used in any form. Hemorrhage is not mentioned to the patient, but if he is ambulatory, he is told that he should call the physician at once should any sloughing of tissue occur.

Unsealed internal radiation. Unsealed internal radiation is delivered to the patient by mouth as an "atomic cocktail" or as a liquid instilled into a body cavity. Exposure for persons caring for the patient can result from direct contact with emanations from the substance in the patient *(external exposure)* or from contact with the patient's discharges that contain the radioactive substances *(internal exposure)*. It may be inhaled, ingested, or absorbed through the skin. The exposure varies with each of the substances used, and safety for the nurse and for other persons caring for the patient depends on a thorough knowledge of the substance used and its action within the body. Many times, if only tracer doses (very small amounts) of radioactive substances are used, as is often done for diagnostic purposes, no precautions are necessary.

The substances used most often at the present time are radioactive iodine (^{131}I), radioactive phosphorus (^{32}P), and radioactive gold (^{198}Au). None of them cures cancer, but they sometimes control the disease to some extent and lessen pain. They are used in selected cases of cancer along with other forms of treatment such as surgery and x-ray therapy.

Radioactive iodine (^{131}I) is a clear liquid with a half-life of 8.1 days. Originally it was hoped that it might destroy malignant cells in the thyroid gland, but results of its use have been disappointing because malignant thyroid cells do not concentrate iodine as well as normal thyroid cells. Therefore the treatment of the original tumor in the thyroid gland or its areas of metastasis with radioactive iodine is not effective. However, it is often used in conjunction with surgical removal of the thyroid gland. Radioactive iodine is also used extensively in the study and diagnosis of disease of the thyroid and to treat hyperthyroidism. Also, researchers are experimenting with it in other diagnostic tests. Radioactive iodine-tagged albumin has proved useful in locating tumors in the brain, and it is frequently used to determine blood volume.

In diagnostic procedures a tracer dose of the radioactive iodine either is taken by mouth or is injected intravenously as radioactive iodine-tagged albumin. The scanner, an instrument that is very sensitive to radioactivity, is then passed over the body to locate areas that have retained the radioactive substance. The tests may be dependent on the percentage of the dose picked up (blood volume) or on the rate of excretion (hyperthyroid studies). This is only one example of the advances that have occurred in the diagnostic use of radioactive isotopes. The scanning technique, which permits the mapping of organs by the detection and measurement of radioactive substances, plays an important part in the evaluation of the patient with cancer. (See Figs. 26-1 and 32-9.)

When used for treatment, radioactive iodine is given in larger amounts. Most of the radioactive iodine is eliminated through the kidneys, but small amounts will be present in sputum, vomitus, perspiration, and feces. Special precautions are needed only for the urine, which usually is collected in a lead-lined container. It is transported daily on a special cart to the radioisotope laboratory, where it is stored until it can be disposed of safely. An indwelling catheter may be inserted before the radioactive iodine is given, and it may be released at intervals to drain directly into the container. If the insertion of a catheter is not considered advisable, patients may be instructed to empty their urinal or bedpan directly into the container. It is important that all urine be collected carefully, because it is the quantitative determination of the amount of radioactive substance excreted that determines when the patient may be removed from isolation. The nurse should find out the approved hospital procedure to safely care for any urine that may be spilled on the floor accidentally.

No linen or equipment should be removed from the room until it is monitored with a Geiger-Müller counter for contamination. If the isolation gown and linen show contamination, they are placed in a special container labeled "radioactive" and stored in lead containers in the isotope laboratory, or they are burned. Dishes are washed thoroughly and then monitored, or else paper dishes are used and then burned. In some institutions the dishes are sent to the kitchen if the monitor reading is less than 6 milliroentgens (mR) per hour. If the nurse's skin should become contaminated, it should be washed thoroughly with soap and water and then monitored. If contamination remains, washing should be continued until monitoring shows that additional cleansing is not necessary. Because washing is essential to prevent or to lessen contamination, the patient must be in a room that has running water.

When the patient is removed from isolation, all equipment is monitored and carefully scrubbed by attendants who have been instructed in safe methods by persons who are in charge of the administration of the radioactive substance. It is then remonitored. The room is aired until monitoring shows that radioactivity is negligible and that the room is safe for any other patient. Airing takes at least 24 hours.

Radioactive phosphorus (^{32}P) is a clear liquid with a half-life of 14 days. It is used in the treatment of polycythemia vera and leukemia. It may be given intravenously, orally, or directly into a body cavity. Sources of contamination are vomitus and seepage from wounds. There is no danger from external exposure because the beta rays emitted by this substance are absorbed by the patient's body. Vomitus and dressings are placed in a lead-lined container and taken to the radioisotope laboratory for disposal. Care of contaminated equipment and the procedures used when staff members are exposed by contamination on the skin are similar to those described for radioactive iodine contamination.

Radioactive gold (^{198}Au) is a purple liquid with a half-life of 2.7 days. It is used largely for treatment of cancer of the lung that has caused effusion into the pleural cavity and for peritoneal ascites due to generalized carcinoma. It is injected into the body cavity, and the patient is turned every 15 minutes for 2 hours so that the radioactive gold will be spread evenly within the cavity. In addition to beta rays, the substance emits gamma rays, so that special isolation precautions may be necessary to prevent external exposure.

If a purple stain appears, it indicates that some of the radioactive gold is escaping from the wound or the site of injection. Wearing rubber gloves, the nurse should apply dressings over the site of injection or the seeping wound. Linen that has been in contact with the wound or the site of injection should be placed in a special container clearly marked for care in the isotope laboratory or other facilities provided by the hospital. Dressings and cleansing tissue should be burned immediately or sent for disposal in special containers to the isotope laboratory.

The patient who receives radioactive gold is usually terminally ill. If he dies soon after receiving [198]Au, a notation that the patient was receiving radioactive gold immediately before death should be made on a tag, and the tag should be conspicuously placed on the body for the protection of the coroner and the mortician. If the nurse has any questions about precautions that should be taken, the person in charge of radioisotopes in the institution should be consulted.

■ CHEMOTHERAPY

Surgery and radiation, when used with early diagnosis, are still the most important treatments for cancer. However, some cancers, either by their nature or by their extent at the time of diagnosis, are too widespread to be treated successfully with surgery or radiation or both. For these patients, the chemical control of the cancer is the primary therapeutic method. The effectiveness of drug therapy in cancer has been best demonstrated in the treatment of the lymphomas and leukemias. At present the potential for controlling metastatic cancer with chemotherapeutic agents is undergoing intensive study and research.

Among the major conceptual advances in the treatment of cancer in the past decade have been those of combination chemotherapy, the realization that the stage of mitotic activity of the cancer target cell may determine the metabolic effects of chemotherapeutic agents, and the realization that dose scheduling of drugs is as important as the drug itself in achieving therapeutic benefit and lessening the toxic response by normal tissue.[38]

The goal in using combination chemotherapy is to produce an effect that is greater than that from the sum of each agent alone (synergism). An example of synergism in cancer chemotherapy is the combination of vincristine and prednisone in acute lymphocytic leukemia. By using the drugs singly, the observed remission rate is approximately 80%, whereas combination therapy effects a 90% remission rate. Combination chemotherapy decreases the potential for the development of resistant cells. There is less likelihood of the evolution of mutations resistant to several drugs than of mutations resistant to single drugs. Only a combination of drugs may be capable of destroying all the malignant cells.

Combination chemotherapy is of greatest advantage when it is used to exploit different toxicities of the chemotherapeutic agents used. Suppression of bone marrow activity is an important limiting factor in the use of these agents. By using combinations of drugs that have different toxicities to bone marrow, the dose of each drug can be given in combination at full dose.[60]

Zubrod states that "chemotherapy has arrived at a stage where it is clearly responsible for producing normal life expectancy in 10 of the 100 or more types of cancer. These are generally cancers of the young and are uncommon, yet high on the list of causes of childhood deaths. In a number of more common tumors of older age groups, chemotherapy is producing an increasing percentage of complete remissions of significant duration—milestones on the road to normal life expectancy."[63] The effectiveness of chemotherapy in cancer has been best demonstrated in the treatment of the lymphomas and leukemias. The trend today is to the use of a dose schedule of antitumor drugs in combination and as an adjunct to other treatment modalities. Cancer chemotherapy is gradually being confined to special centers where experience and facilities are concentrated. Many such centers around the world are actively devising and testing multiple drug schedules for all forms of advanced cancer and are applying more sophisticated techniques of biochemistry and cell kinetics directly to the problems of human cancer. There are five large classes of chemotherapeutic agents in use today; these are the alkylating agents, antimetabolites, hormones, antibiotics, and plant alkaloids. A discussion of each follows.

Alkylating agents (mustards). These agents act on already formed nucleic acids. Interference with the function of the nucleic acids, particularly DNA, accounts for the inhibition of proliferative activity of certain normal and neoplastic cells. The various types of nitrogen mustards in use have essentially similar action on normal and malignant cells. They differ mainly in local tissue irritation, degree of stimulation of the vomiting center, absorption from the gastrointestinal tract, and, consequently, routes of administration. At effective dosage levels all produce some degree of bone marrow depression.

The administration of these drugs involves proper psychologic preparation of the patient as well as a frank discussion of their possible effects. Nursing intervention at this point must be supportive. There are times when the nurse may strongly disagree with such radical drug therapy, and such an attitude can be easily transmitted to the patient. Preparation of the patient for the administration of Mustargen, for example, can greatly aid in its effectiveness or at least diminish some of its side effects. Mustargen is usually given in the evening. Supper is either omitted or is limited to fluids. Administration of an antiemetic drug and a sedative prior to the treatment may prevent nausea and vomiting. Meticulous intravenous technique must be observed to prevent infiltration and consequent necrosis. The dose is adjusted according to the patient's weight and also his previous experience, if any, with agents that depress bone marrow. Adequate fluid intake is felt by some to prevent hyperuricemia, thought to be a consequence of sudden cytolysis.[55] If hyperuricemia is considered to be a serious threat, allopurinal, a drug inhibiting uric acid formation, is given several days before chemotherapy is begun.

Antimetabolites. The antimetabolites act by interfering with the synthesis of chromosomal nucleic acid necessary for new tumor cell production. This group includes 6-mercaptopurine, 5-fluorouracil, cytosine arabinoside, and the folic acid antagonists such as methotrexate. Their toxic reactions include anorexia, oral ulceration, gastrointestinal disturbances such as diarrhea, and bone marrow depression.

Hormones. It is believed that steroid hormones may determine the time of development or "trigger" the growth of certain malignant tumors, providing other factors within the cell are present. They may also be necessary for the continued growth of certain tumors of the secondary sexual gland tissues. Attempts to alter the hormonal influences on the tumor consist of either removing the glands producing the hormones (ovaries, testicles, adrenal glands) or the endocrine gland controlling their secretion (pituitary gland) or negating the action of these respective hormones by giving their antagonists. Thus men having carcinoma of the prostate may be given a female hormone such as stilbestrol, and women who have carcinoma of the breast with metastasis may be given a male hormone such as testosterone. These persons may also be given large doses of hormones of their own sex to prevent stimulation of the pituitary gland and to prevent their own sex glands from producing the hormone.

Adrenocorticosteroids such as hydrocortisone or prednisone are used as a specific therapy for certain leukemias, lymphomas, multiple myeloma, other blood dyscrasias, and metastatic cancer of the breast. They are also often employed terminally in many diverse cancers for their nonspecific ability to temporarily improve appetite and sense of well-being. Toxic manifestations include gastrointestinal bleeding, congestive heart failure due to sodium and water retention, iatrogenic Cushing's syndrome, diabetes mellitus, osteoporosis, psychosis, and increased susceptibility to infections (p. 82).

Antibiotics. Actinomycin D is produced by a species of *Streptomyces*. It has been used to control metastasis of Wilms' tumor (nephroblastoma), testicular tumors, and choriocarcinoma. Side effects include bone marrow depression and gastrointestinal irritation. Infiltration during intravenous administration produces a severe local irritation.

Plant alkaloids. Vincristine and vinblastine are plant alkaloids that act as mitotic inhibitors. In addition to transient bone marrow depression, these drugs may cause nausea and vomiting, alopecia, severe constipation, paralytic ileus, and peripheral neuritis.

If it seems that the toxic effects of these agents have been stressed rather than the therapeutic effects, it is only because they lend themselves to summarization and also because the nurse must be concerned with creating an environment in which these agents can be safely used. The bone marrow depression and the subsequent leukopenia and thrombopenia require that the patient be protected from infection and trauma. Oral ulcerations may occur as a result of the effects on the mucous membrane, and effective methods of coping with the problems of oral hygiene need to be instituted. The general effect of nausea and vomiting challenge the nurse and dietitian in the maintenance of adequate nutrition. Cancer chemotherapy nursing is difficult and many times discouraging; however, it is expected that chemotherapy for cancer will grow in importance and effectiveness as the result of continued research in this area.

Infusion. Most of the chemotherapeutic drugs may be given as an intravenous infusion for their general suppressive effect on an advanced malignancy. More recently they have been given in this way at the time of surgery for their suppressive effect on any malignant cells that might be released into the circulation or remain at that time. They may also be given by infusion along with radiation therapy in order to hasten or increase its effect.

Perfusion. By means of several variations of a procedure known as perfusion, it is now possible to deliver an extremely large dose of one of the alkylating agents directly to a tumor. *Intra-arterial perfusion* differs from the usual intravenous method only in that the drug is introduced under pressure and inserted into an artery flowing directly into the area to be treated. Thus the full strength of the drug reaches the tumor before it enters the general circulation and is distributed throughout the body.

302

Intra-arterial perfusion is used for cancers of the head and neck, for liver metastasis, and as adjuvant chemotherapy with radiotherapy for advanced cancer of the cervix. This method provides for prolonged administration and exposure of neoplastic cells to the drug at a time when rapid mitosis is occurring (Fig. 15-6). Complications to be watched for

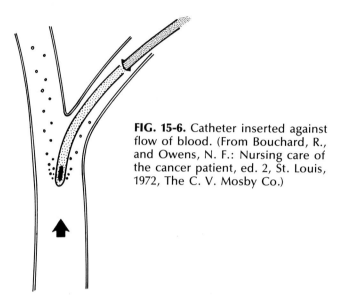

FIG. 15-6. Catheter inserted against flow of blood. (From Bouchard, R., and Owens, N. F.: Nursing care of the cancer patient, ed. 2, St. Louis, 1972, The C. V. Mosby Co.)

are hemorrhage from the artery at the site of injection, either during or after the treatment, and renal failure. If a lesion in the head is being treated, temporary baldness may occur on the affected side several weeks after treatment and may be most distressing to the patient. Ulceration of the mouth also occurs and makes frequent mouth care necessary. It may become a real challenge to find enough suitable foods to maintain the patient's nutritional status. Intra-arterial infusion can be accomplished on an ambulatory basis by means of portable infusion pump slipped over the patient's head and anchored at the waist (Fig. 15-7).

In the special technique known as *extracorporeal perfusion*, or *isolation perfusion*, a portion of the body to be treated may be isolated in its blood supply from the rest of the body during the time of treatment. This measure makes it possible to give much larger doses more directly to the tumor than would be tolerated if they were introduced into the general circulation. For example, a tumor of the lower limb can be treated by applying a tourniquet to the upper portion of the thigh. The drug is injected directly into an artery leading to the tumor, and venous blood is removed from the area being treated through a catheter, circulated through an oxygenator to provide oxygen, and then returned under pressure to the artery.

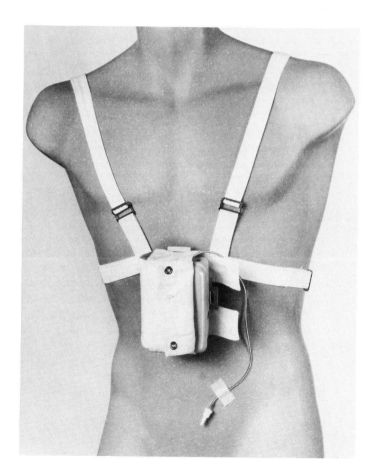

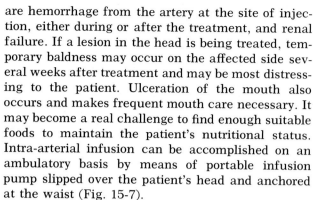

FIG. 15-7. Torso showing lightweight battery-operated infusion pump. Flow rate is variable and may be set exactly by means of a plug-in meter. The power pack supplies current to operate the pump for 7 days without recharging or replacement. (Courtesy Sigmamotor, Inc., Middleport, N. Y.)

After the drug has been circulated for the prescribed length of time, the blood in which the drug was circulated may or may not be replaced by a fresh transfusion, depending on the condition of the patient, the amount of drug used, and its toxicity.

If the tumor to be treated is in the abdomen or lower pelvis, an abdominal operation may be required, and the entire procedure becomes much more difficult. The blood supply to the cancerous area is isolated and blocked from systemic circulation by means of pneumatic tourniquets and clamps to prevent distribution of the drug throughout the body. Catheters are inserted into the artery and vein supplying the area to be treated, and the agent is introduced through the arterial catheter as near to the tumor as possible. The venous catheter is attached to a pump oxygenator that provides for oxygenation of the blood and pumps it back into the arterial system through the arterial catheter. This procedure is essential for tissue viability (Fig. 15-8). When the treatment is complete and fresh blood has been supplied by transfusion if necessary, the vessels are unclamped, catheters and tourniquets are removed, and the surgical wound is closed.

Postoperative concerns are related to the local tissue tolerance and the amount of leakage of the agent used. Local tissues can be permanently damaged, and thrombosis and phlebitis may occur at or near the sites of treatment. Reactions of significance appear as tanning, erythema, or blistering of skin over tissues that have been perfused. These reactions resemble toxic reactions to radiation. The toxic effects of leakage may cause bone marrow depression, and infection such as septicemia can occur. The general signs of circulatory disturbance that sometimes occur after cardiac surgery should be watched for and reported promptly if they occur (p. 366). Renal function must be checked carefully. Following extracorporeal perfusion of an extremity, color and warmth of the extremity must be observed. Pain in the extremity is a danger sign and often indicates that there has been severe tissue damage.

The patient who undergoes perfusion procedures needs thoughtful care and encouragement. Usually his disease is advanced and the procedure is only palliative, although it is done only when there is reasonable assurance that metastasis has not spread throughout the body. Sometimes the patient develops lesions elsewhere after the growth seemed to be controlled satisfactorily by perfusion.

■ NURSING SUPPORT OF THE PATIENT WITH UNCONTROLLABLE CANCER

When all possible surgery and maximum radiation therapy have failed to control cancer, the patient and his family have many special problems. They need encouragement and help in living as normally as possible, in planning for the late stages of the patient's illness, and in adjusting to death and its implications for the family.

Before nurses can help the patient and his family, they must have developed a mature philosophy that allows acceptance of death as an eventual reality for

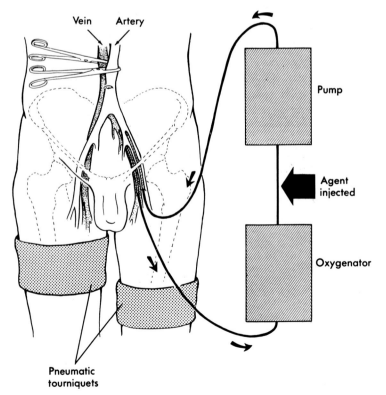

FIG. 15-8. Schematic drawing showing regional perfusion for a pelvic tumor. (From Bouchard, R., and Owens, N. F.: Nursing care of the cancer patient, ed. 2, St. Louis, 1972, The C. V. Mosby Co.)

everyone. This philosophy is usually not acquired overnight. For most persons it requires experience with death and dying and the opportunity to discuss feelings openly with supportive colleagues. The nurse needs to develop a working philosophy about death in order to be of the greatest assistance to the dying patient and his significant others. The many excellent references available on death and dying indicate clearly that it is a subject of major interest to all persons involved in care of the terminally ill. Many of these references are listed at the end of this chapter and should be helpful to the nurse who is not experienced in working with the dying. Kubler-Ross[33] has described the dying process as occurring in five stages: (1) denial and isolation, (2) anger, (3) bargaining, (4) depression, and (5) acceptance. The knowledge that these same stages usually occur in the staff caring for the patient as well as in the patient and his significant others should help the nurse understand better the actions of various members of the health team. Problems are particularly likely to occur when the patient and his significant others are at different stages in the grief process. Often the patient reaches the stage of acceptance before family members, as in the following situation:

A 60-year-old woman, whose daughter was a nurse, went to surgery for a breast biopsy. On the first postoperative day, she asked her daughter whether the breast had been removed and was told that it had. From that point on there was no question in the patient's mind and in the minds of her three adult children that she had cancer. The patient, who was quite religious, accepted the diagnosis with equanimity and faith that the surgery would prove successful. Two years later she developed metastasis to her spine and had to be rehospitalized. At this time she asked her daughter whether she thought she would ever go home. Since mother and daughter had always been close, the daughter answered truthfully, "I don't think so." The mother replied, "I am very tired and am looking forward to a good rest."

During the later phases of the patient's illness, it became apparent that the woman's husband had not accepted the seriousness of his wife's illness, for he kept asking when she would be going home. His children had talked with him about the fact that she probably would not be returning home. Still he persisted in asking when she would be discharged. The surgeon was informed of the husband's failure to accept the terminal nature of his wife's illness and an appointment was made for him to talk with the surgeon. When the husband returned from the physician's office, he angrily demanded of his children, "Why didn't you tell me she was going to die?"

This case is an example of selective hearing by which some persons protect themselves from unpleasant information. Even though the patient knew she was dying and her children and other relatives realized that her illness was terminal, the husband had blocked this knowledge from his conscious awareness. Thus it is important for the nurse to understand how the patient and his family are accepting his illness so that nursing intervention will be appropriate to the situation.

At the present time there is a great deal of discussion concerning whether or not the patient who has uncontrolled cancer should be told. The feeling is increasing among religious workers, students of social psychology, and psychiatrists that the patient should be told. The statement often made by physicians, "Can the patient stand to know?" may eventually be changed to "Can the patient stand not to know?" There is evidence that to many persons the uncertainty of not knowing their situation is much more upsetting than knowing the truth. There appears to be no relationship between telling the patient and increase in suicide. In one study the reverse was true.[43]

Despite general feelings on the subject, the final decision to tell or not to tell the patient that he has uncontrollable cancer and is going to die rests with the physician. The majority of physicians still do not tell their patients. One detailed study indicates that their reasons are related much more to their own attitudes and emotional reactions than to their concern about the patient's reactions.[43] The nurse may help by discussing with the physician the reactions of the patient and the feelings he expresses, but must acknowledge the physician's final responsibility. It is the nurse's responsibility and sometimes a real challenge to accept this situation and work effectively for the ultimate benefit of the patient within the seeming limitations it may impose.

Kubler-Ross worked extensively with dying patients and the medical and nursing staffs caring for these patients in a large medical center. Patients were invited to participate in a conference attended by the medical and nursing personnel. The patients were encouraged to express their feelings about having a fatal illness. In this setting, many patients were helped to accept their own death. At the same time the medical and nursing personnel gained more insight into their own feelings about dying and about working with the dying patient. This increased their sensitivity to the individual patient and made it possible for them to be more supportive to many of these patients.[26,33,34]

Since most nurses will not have an opportunity to participate in experiences like the one just described, alternate methods of working through feelings should be provided. Recently the introduction of audio visual materials such as "Perspectives on Dying"* have become available. These tapes can be used to stimulate discussion among health team members and are often helpful in assisting physicians as well as nurses to express their feelings about death.

The patient who knows he has cancer with uncontrollable metastasis often asks about the length of time he may expect to live. Since life is precious to every normal person, it is safe to assume that this

---

*Concept Media, 1500 Adams Ave., Costa Mesa, Calif. 92626.

question is on every patient's mind even though he may not ask it directly. Although no absolute answer can be given, the physician can give the best estimate of life expectancy, and such questions should be referred to him. The nursing staff must know what the patient has been told so that they can reinforce the information.

Very occasionally there is a mistake in diagnosis, or the disease is in some way arrested for a long time. If the patient assumes that one of these occurrences may take place in his case, the nurse should not try to help him face probable reality. The nurse must, however, avoid encouraging false hopes. Many patients accept their prognosis philosophically, with the hope that a cure for cancer will be found before their disease is far advanced. Some patients are better able to accept the situation if their religious faith can be strengthened. The nurse must encourage the patient and his family to live each day as fully as possible without looking too far ahead. Sometimes patients with cancer have few symptoms and are able to carry on quite well until shortly before death.

Patients with uncontrollable cancer should resume their regular work if they can possibly do so, for work makes them feel as though they are still an active part of their group and worthy of the approval of others. It was said many centuries ago that employment is man's best physician, and this concept applies particularly to persons whose existence is seriously threatened by cancer. Social activities and all experiences associated with normal family life should be continued whenever possible. There is probably no better service the nurse can give to the patient with uncontrollable cancer than to help him to continue in any way possible. Family members often need guidance in seeing the patient's need to live as normally as possible. Sometimes the patient appears almost unduly concerned with the details of some aspect of his immediate treatment and almost oblivious to his entire problem. Such a patient senses that success with the immediate treatment is his only way to remain up and about or carrying on as well as he is at that time.

The patient with uncontrollable cancer often worries about whether or not he will have severe pain and whether or not such pain can be alleviated. He should know that medical science now has several ways of controlling pain. Hormones, radiation therapy, and a number of analgesic drugs are available and helpful in most instances. Synthetic substitutes

for the opiate drugs make it possible to alternate drugs so that their benefit is not lessened by tolerance and so that toxic reactions can be avoided. Members of the patient's family are sometimes told of operations that can be performed if pain becomes too severe to control by other means (p. 881).

The patient may be haunted by fear of brain involvement, loss of mental faculties, and the possibility that he may become completely helpless and dependent on others. By these fears he expresses one of man's basic wishes—the wish to leave the world with as much dignity as possible. The nurse should urge the patient and his family to discuss such fears with the physician. The patient may feel that the physician is too busy and that his questions are too trivial to justify the use of the physician's time. Such questions, however, are not trivial at all, and a satisfactory answer to them adds tremendously to the patient's peace of mind. Metastasis to the brain in persons who have other metastases is somewhat rare, and some patients suffer more from fear of damage to the brain than is justified. The patient should know that good general hygiene, good nutrition, being up and about for part of each day, and doing deep-breathing exercises with attention to posture all help to prevent helplessness. A positive approach to all problems certainly shortens the time of helplessness and makes the patient more content.

At least half of all deaths from cancer occur in the patient's home. Planning for home care of the patient without completely disrupting the rest of the family takes the concerted efforts of many people. The patient must always be consulted, and his wishes should be respected in the early stages of the disease. In the final stages, he is too ill to be bothered or concerned with making decisions. In the hospital the physician, the social worker, and the nurse must work together with the local community nursing agencies, such as the American Cancer Society, to ensure continuity of care from the hospital to the home. The principles governing suitability for home care are similar to those for any patient receiving home care, although the patient with cancer may not live as long as many others with chronic long-term illnesses. The patient must be under medical supervision; it must be possible to give the care he needs in his home, he must want to be home, his family must want him home and be able to assist with care, and the home facilities must be suitable. (For further details on home care, see p. 255.)

REFERENCES AND SELECTED READINGS*

1 *American Cancer Society, Inc.: A cancer source book for nurses, New York, 1963, The Society.

*References preceded by an asterisk are particularly well suited for student reading.

2 *American Cancer Society, Inc.: Essentials of cancer nursing, New York, 1963, The Society.
3 American Cancer Society, Inc.: 1975 cancer facts and figures, New York, 1974, The Society.
3a *American Cancer Society, Inc.: Proceedings of the national conference on cancer nursing, New York, 1974, The Society.

4 Augenstein, D.: Hyperbaric oxygen radiation therapy, Nurs. Forum 12(3):324-335, 1968.

5 Barber, J. C., King, H., and Mason, M. J.: Cancer rates and risks, Washington, D. C., 1964, U. S. Department of Health, Education and Welfare.

6 *Barckley, V.: The crisis in cancer, Am. J. Nurs. 67:278-280, Feb. 1967.

7 Beattie, E. J., Jr.: Philosophy of cancer care, Surg. Clin. North Am. 49:213-216, April 1969.

8 Behnke, H. D., editor: Guidelines for comprehensive nursing care in cancer, New York, 1973, Springer Publishing Co., Inc.

9 *Boeker, E. H.: Radiation safety, Am. J. Nurs. 65:111-116, April 1965.

10 *Boeker, E. H., editor: Symposium on radiation uses and hazards, Nurs. Clin. North Am. 2:1-113, March 1967.

11 Bouchard, R. E., and Owens, N. F.: Nursing care of the cancer patient, ed. 2, St. Louis, 1972, The C. V. Mosby Co.

12 Browning, M. H., and Lewis, E. P., compilers: The dying patient: a nursing perspective, New York, 1972, The American Journal of Nursing Co.

13 Browning, M. H., and Lewis, E. P.: Nursing and the cancer patient, New York, 1973, The American Journal of Nursing Co.

14 Croll, M. N., and Brady, L. W., editors: Recent advances in nuclear medicine, New York, 1966, Appleton-Century-Crofts.

15 *Donaldson, S. H., Fletcher, W. S., and Nowak, P. A.: The treatment of cancer by isolation perfusion and nursing care in isolation perfusion, Am. J. Nurs. 64:81-88, Aug. 1964.

16 *Downs, H. S.: The control of vomiting, Am. J. Nurs. 66:76-82, Jan. 1966.

17 Egan, R. L.: Mammography, Am. J. Nurs. 66:108-111, Jan. 1966.

18 Fitzpatrick, G. M., and Shotkin, J. M.: Pelvic perfusion, Am. J. Nurs. 61:79-81, June 1961.

19 Gahart, B. L.: Intravenous medications: a handbook for nurses and other allied health personnel, St. Louis, 1973, The C. V. Mosby Co.

20 *Geis, D. P.: Mothers' perceptions of care given their dying children, Am. J. Nurs. 65:105-107, Feb. 1965.

21 George, M. M.: Long-term care of the patient with cancer, Nurs. Clin. North Am. 8:623-631, Dec. 1973.

22 Greenwald, E. S.: Cancer chemotherapy, N. Y. State J. Med. 72:2541-2556, Oct. 1972.

23 Greenwald, E. S.: Cancer chemotherapy, ed. 2, Flushing, N. Y., 1973, Medical Examination Publishing Co., Inc.

24 Harrop, M., editor: Nursing in cancer, Nurs. Clin. North Am. 2:585-690, Dec. 1967.

25 Hilkemeyer, R.: Intra-arterial cancer chemotherapy, Nurs. Clin. North Am. 1:295-307, June 1966.

26 Hoffman, E.: "Don't give up on me!" Am. J. Nurs. 71:60-62, Jan. 1971.

27 Isler, C.: The cancer nurses: how the specialists are doing it, R.N. 35:28-34, Feb. 1972.

28 *Karnofsky, D. A.: Cancer quackery: its causes, recognition and prevention, Am. J. Nurs. 59:496-500, April 1959.

29 *Kautz, H. D., Storey, R. H., and Zimmerman, A. J.: Radioactive drugs, Am. J. Nurs. 64:124-128, Jan. 1964.

30 *Kegeles, S. S., and others: Survey of beliefs about cancer detection and taking Papanicolaou tests, Public Health Rep. 80:815-823, Sept. 1965.

31 Klagsbrun, N. C.: Communications in the treatment of cancer, Am. J. Nurs. 71:944-948, May 1971.

32 *Kneisl, C. R.: Thoughtful care for the dying, Am. J. Nurs. 68:550-553, March 1968.

33 Kubler-Ross, E. K.: On death and dying, New York, 1969, Macmillan Publishing Co., Inc.

34 Kubler-Ross, E. K.: What is it like to be dying? Am. J. Nurs. 71:54-61, Jan. 1971.

35 *Kyle, Sister M. Willa: The nurse's approach to the patient attempting to adjust to inoperable cancer—effective thera-peutic communication in nursing, Clinical Session 8, 1964, American Nurses' Association.

36 *Lieben, J.: The effects of radiation, Nurs. Outlook 10:336-338, May 1962.

37 *Livingston, B. M.: How clinical progress is made in cancer chemotherapy research, Am. J. Nurs. 67:2547-2554, Dec. 1967.

38 Modell, W., editor: Drugs of choice 1972-1973, St. Louis, 1972, The C. V. Mosby Co.

39 Molbo, D. M.: The nurse's role in hyperbaric therapy. In Bergersen, B. S., and others, editors: Current concepts in clinical nursing, vol. 1, St. Louis, 1967, The C. V. Mosby Co.

40 Molbo, D., and vonElk, J.: Hyperbaric oxygenation. In Meltzer, L. E., Abdellah, F. G., and Kitchell, J. R., editors: Concepts and practices of intensive care, Philadelphia, 1969, The Charles Press, Publishers.

41 *Moore, G. E.: Cancer: 100 different diseases, Am. J. Nurs. 66:749-756, April 1966.

42 Niles, A. G., and Paulen, A. E.: A humanistic approach to nursing care, Supervisor Nurse 4:42-44, July 1973.

43 *Oken, D.: What to tell cancer patients: a study of medical attitudes, J.A.M.A. 175:1120-1128, April 1961.

44 Pearson, O. H., and Lubic, R. W.: Adrenalectomy and hypophysectomy and nursing care after adrenalectomy and hypophysectomy, Am. J. Nurs. 62:80-86, April 1962.

45 Prosnitz, L. R.: Radiation therapy-treatment for malignant disease, R.N. 34:42-47, March 1971.

46 *Quimby, E. H.: Safe handling of radioactive isotopes in medical practice, New York, 1960, Macmillan Publishing Co., Inc.

47 *Regan, P. F.: The dying patient and his family, J.A.M.A. 192:666-674, May 24, 1965.

48 *Rhoads, P. S.: Management of the patient with terminal illness, J.A.M.A. 192:661-665, May 24, 1965.

49 Robbins, S. L.: Basic pathology, Philadelphia, 1971, W. B. Saunders Co.

49a Rodman, M. J., and Smith, D. W.: Clinical pharmacology in nursing, Philadelphia, 1974, J. B. Lippincott Co.

50 *Rumerfield, P. S., and Rumerfield, M. J.: What you should know about radiation hazards, Am. J. Nurs. 70:780-786, April 1970.

51 Shepardson, J.: Team approach to the patient with cancer, Am. J. Nurs. 72:488-491, March 1972.

52 Silverstein, M. J., and Morton, D. L.: Cancer immunotherapy, Am. J. Nurs. 73:1178-1181, July 1973.

53 Teitelbaum, A. C.: Intra-arterial drug therapy, Am. J. Nurs. 72:1634-1637, Sept. 1972.

54 Turnbull, F.: Pain and suffering in cancer, Can. Nurse 67:28-30, Aug. 1971.

55 Ultmann, J.: Chemotherapy of lymphoma, Semin. Hematol. 3:131-153, April 1966.

56 Vanden Bergh, R. L., and Davidson, R. P.: Let's talk about death, Am. J. Nurs. 66:71-75, Jan. 1966.

57 *Vernick, J., and Lunceford, J. L.: Milieu design for adolescents with leukemia, Am. J. Nurs. 67:559-561, March 1967.

58 Warren, S.: Ionizing radiation and medicine, Sci. Am. 201:154-176, Sept. 1959. (Entire issue devoted to radiation, including articles on what it is, its circulation in the body, and how it affects the cell, evolution, and the whole animal.)

59 *Welsh, M. S.: Comfort measures during radiation therapy, Am. J. Nurs. 67:1880-1882, Sept. 1967.

60 Wintrobe, M. M., and others: Harrison's textbook of medicine, ed. 7, New York, 1974, McGraw-Hill Book Co.

61 *Wygant, W. E., Jr.: Dying, but not alone, Am. J. Nurs. 67:574-577, March 1967.

62 *Zaino, C.: Eliminating the hazards from radiation, Am. J. Nurs. 62:60-61, April 1962.

63 Zubrod, C. G.: The basis for progress in chemotherapy, Cancer 30:1474-1479, Dec. 1972.

16 Communicable diseases

■ A communicable disease is an illness that is caused by an infectious agent *(pathogen)* or its toxic products. The pathogen may be transmitted directly to a susceptible person *(the host)* by an infected person or animal, or it may be transmitted through an intermediate animal host *(a vector)* or something in the inanimate environment contaminated by it, such as the milk or water supply. The origin of the infectious agent is known as the source. In order for disease to occur, the pathogen must be present in the environment and it must be able to be transmitted to a person susceptible to it. It also must be virulent enough to overcome the body's defenses against it. The prevention and control of communicable disease either in an individual or in a community depend on application of knowledge of the interdependence of the host, the infectious agent, and the environment. Alteration in any one of these factors may cause disease or allow it to occur.

Since the turn of the century, significant changes have occurred in the prevention and control of communicable diseases. Increased knowledge about causative organisms, development of immunizing agents, and more successful treatment with the introduction of antibiotics have changed the nature and extent of the problem in many countries, including the United States.

However, additional factors such as urbanization, increased mobility, decreased levels of acquired immunity, and resistance to antibiotics and insecticides

■ STUDY QUESTIONS

1 Plan a teaching program to encourage new parents to have their babies receive the recommended immunizations.

2 Plan a teaching program to encourage susceptible members of the public to participate in influenza immunization.

3 If you were working in an immunization clinic, what conditions would contraindicate a person's receiving immunization for influenza? Poliomyelitis? Measles?

4 What is the danger of giving immunizing agents that are prepared from chicken or duck embryos? What question should the patient be asked in order to avoid the possibility of an untoward reaction?

5 What is the danger of giving antibodies in horse serum? What is the procedure that should be followed prior to injecting this type of solution?

6 Active immunization might be described as "giving one a small local infection." Review the signs and symptoms of local infection in various age groups (Chapter 4).

7 What are the most common means by which diseases are transferred from one person to another? How are they transferred from animals to man?

8 What are some of the provisions of the sanitary code in your community and of the laws in your state that protect against communicable disease?

9 Look up the characteristics of the agent causing (a) scarlet fever, (b) mumps, (c) hepatitis, (d) malaria, (e) trichinosis, (f) Rocky Mountain spotted fever, and (g) ringworm. On the basis of the information, plan the isolation measures, if any, needed to control spread of the disease. Where would you look for the source of the disease and how could it be controlled?

10 Assume that there has been an outbreak of food poisoning in a school. What is the most probable source? What measures would help to reduce the possibility of a recurrence?

11 If there were an outbreak of diarrhea in a nursery, what precautions would you take? Why?

are creating new epidemiologic concerns. Despite the significant increase in our knowledge of communicable diseases, there remain many countries throughout the world in which communicable disease constitutes a major health problem.

The Center for Disease Control (formerly the Communicable Disease Center) of the Public Health Service has classified communicable diseases in the United States into three categories. Category A includes diseases that require only constant surveillance. Much of the natural history of these diseases is known; if preventive measures are applied regularly, the diseases occur infrequently, and when they do occur, there are control measures for immediate use. This group includes such diseases as cholera and malaria. Category B includes diseases occurring more frequently and requiring more intensive application of preventive measures. This group includes such diseases as brucellosis and tuberculosis. Category C is the largest and most important. For this group of diseases, effective preventive measures still need to be developed. Diseases such as infectious mononucleosis and salmonellosis are included. Of 50 communicable diseases occurring in the United States, 7 are in category A, 11 in category B, and 32 in category C.[22]

Although regional variations in occurrence of communicable disease may be caused by differences in causative factors, perhaps the greatest variation is related to the application of measures for prevention and control. One of the primary objectives of the World Health Organization (WHO) is to improve and standardize measures of disease prevention and control throughout the world. Its Epidemiological Intelligence Service in Geneva, Switzerland, receives immediate notification of outbreaks of communicable disease throughout the world and therefore is able to warn countries of impending *epidemics* (massive outbreaks of disease). It also gives them advice as to control measures. *The Weekly Epidemiological Record* has been published by this group (originally part of the League of Nations) since 1925.

With the increase in speed and amount of travel to all parts of the world, the possibility of the spread of communicable diseases to new areas or to areas presumed safe has become great, and relaxation of surveillance or of application of controls can cause drastic changes in the occurrence of communicable diseases. Thus the use of measures for the general promotion of health as well as specific methods of prevention and control should be emphasized continually.

Progress in prevention, control, and treatment of communicable diseases has produced changes in nursing responsibilities. Today education of the public about control of communicable disease is a primary responsibility. The nurse must help to ensure that the gains of the past 50 years are maintained by teaching sanitary practices in the homes, interpreting community efforts in sanitation, and encouraging immunization against diseases for which this protection is available. Nursing responsibility includes interpreting to the public new and needed controls and thereby gaining support for programs for communicable disease control. This teaching may be done at the bedside of the hospitalized patient, in the clinic, in the school, in the patient's home, or in other community settings. The nurse also may direct the investigation of persons suspected of having contracted communicable disease and of their relatives, friends, or other contacts, and the nurse may care for or teach others to care for persons who are ill with communicable disease.

■ PRINCIPLES OF COMMUNICABLE DISEASE CONTROL

Agents that cause communicable diseases

The agents that cause communicable diseases in man depend, at least partially, on man for the proteins essential for their life cycle and, in the process of obtaining them, produce disease in him (p. 72). These disease-producing agents may be classified as bacteria, rickettsiae, protozoa, fungi, helminths (worms), and viruses. The following is a list of some of the diseases produced by specific organisms in each category.

Bacteria

Brucellosis
Chancroid
Cholera
Diarrhea of newborn
Diphtheria
Gas gangrene
Gonorrhea
Meningococcal meningitis
Pertussis
Plague
Pneumococcal pneumonia
Staphylococcal infections
Streptococcal infections
  (scarlet fever)
Syphilis
Tetanus
Tuberculosis
Typhoid and paratyphoid
  fever
Yaws

Rickettsiae

Q fever
Rickettsial pox
Rocky Mountain spotted
  fever
Typhus

Protozoa

Amebic dysentery
Kala-azar
Malaria
Trichomonas vaginitis

Fungi

Blastomycosis
Candidiasis
Histoplasmosis
Monilial vaginitis
Ringworm
Thrush

Helminths

Filariasis
Hookworm
Pinworm
Schistosomiasis
Tapeworm
Trichinosis

Viruses

Chickenpox
Common cold
Diarrhea of newborn
Encephalitis
German measles
Hepatitis
  (infectious and serum)
Herpes zoster
Influenza
Lymphogranuloma venereum
Measles
Mumps
Poliomyelitis
Psittacosis
Rabies
Smallpox
Trachoma
Yellow fever

Nurses should know the communicable diseases that are prevalent in the region in which they work and become thoroughly acquainted with the characteristics of the agents that cause them. This knowledge will guide them in helping with control measures.

Planning control measures

The principles basic to invasion of human beings by pathogens are outlined on p. 79. They should be reviewed in conjunction with this section.

In planning control measures it is important to know about the *physical characteristics* of the agent, that is, whether it can live outside the human body, whether it can remain inactive for periods of time and still exist *(sporeformers),* whether its activity is seasonal or climatic in nature, whether it requires passage through an intermediary host *(in which it lives)* such as a mosquito in order to complete its life cycle, and whether it needs an intermediary agent *(on which it lives)* such as a tick, louse, or flea in order to spread. This information gives clues that will aid in looking for the source of the infectious agent and in determining the appropriate control measures. For example, if the source is environmental, such as water or flies, controls need to be exerted over these factors. However, if the disease is spread by human beings via "droplets" of mucus or via hands, the infected persons must be isolated. Sometimes, in order to control the disease, the original environmental source may need to be eliminated and the infected persons isolated. For example, an outbreak of typhoid fever originating from the milk supply must be controlled in this way.

Knowledge of where the organism obtains its nourishment and reproduces—*its biologic characteristics*—provides a guide in determining who may be susceptible to attack. Viruses, for instance, feed on deoxyribonucleic acid (DNA), a giant molecule found in the nucleus of living cells, and consequently can live only on healthy cells. Viruses, therefore, rarely complicate diseases that cause tissue breakdown. On the other hand, bacteria can live on cells that are broken down, and bacterial diseases frequently attack tissue that has already been damaged by disease, infection, or trauma. Many infectious organisms can live only on specific tissues or produce disease only after reaching these tissues. Others require specific conditions for reproduction, such as the absence of oxygen or the passage through an intermediary agent. Some organisms, although they reproduce in man, can be transferred from one person to another only by a vector. Medical treatment often is based on decreasing the organism's ability to use food. Antibiotic drugs, hyperbaric oxygen, and hypothermia all operate on this principle. If an intermediary host or a vector is essential, elimination of it will bring the disease under control.

If one knows the source of the pathogen and how it gets into the body *(portal of entry),* on what tissue it reproduces, and how it leaves the body *(portal of exit),* necessary isolation procedures or reverse precautions can be used. The purpose of isolation is to prevent the passage of the pathogen causing the communicable disease from infected persons to others. Because individuals can carry infectious organisms in and on their bodies without having disease themselves, it is essential that susceptible people be protected against passage of these organisms to them. This is the purpose of protective (reverse) isolation procedures, which are described in detail on p. 80, and it constitutes the basis for health teaching of such measures as handwashing and sanitary procedures related to food, water, sewage, vermin, and insects such as flies and mosquitoes. Sanitary codes have been established by law to control potential environmental sources of infection such as food, water, and sewage. The pasteurization of milk and the determination of the bacterial count of public water supplies and swimming facilities are examples of measures required by the codes.

Prevention of the spread of highly virulent organisms is exceedingly important. Knowledge of the *chemical characteristics* of the pathogen gives clues as to its virulence. Organisms that produce toxins usually cause serious disease that is difficult to control because the toxin is spread throughout the body by the bloodstream. Methods of artificial immunization against these organisms are being sought constantly, and as they become available, the public should be urged to use them. Chemical characteristics also influence the viability of the pathogen (its resistance to destruction). Knowledge of this viability is essential for determining adequate decontamination processes.

It would be impractical in a book of this type to try to discuss each communicable disease in relation to its control. The American Public Health Association publishes a manual* containing the facts about the common communicable diseases occurring in the world. It is a valuable addition to every nurse's bookshelf. Because of the rapid reproduction of pathogens, genetic mutations that change the characteristics of the organisms appear rather frequently, and therefore it is important to use current information in the control of communicable disease. Another excellent source of information is the manual published every 3 to 4 years by the American Academy of Pediatrics and commonly referred to as *The Red Book.*† Information on any communicable disease

---

*Control of communicable diseases in man, American Public Health Association, 1015 Eighteenth St. N.E., Washington, D. C. 20036.
†Report of the Committee on Infectious Diseases, American Academy of Pediatrics, P.O. Box 1034, Evanston, Ill. 60204.

found in the world can be obtained from the *Epidemiological and Vital Statistics Reports* of the World Health Organization.

Immunization

It is sometimes possible and desirable to enhance the body's defenses against disease-producing organisms artificially. This is known as immunization, and immunization programs have played and continue to play a primary role in the control of infectious disease throughout the world. The body can be stimulated to produce antibodies against some specific diseases without actually having the disease *(active artificial immunity).* Temporary protection sometimes can be provided by injecting antibodies produced by other persons or other animals into the bloodstream of a human being *(passive artificial immunity).*

Active immunity. Active immunity can be acquired by artificially injecting small numbers of attenuated (weakened) or dead organisms of specific types or modified toxins from the organisms into the body. This procedure is known as *inoculation.* A long-term antigen-antibody response similar to that described on p. 77 is produced without the person's having the infectious disease. This method is highly effective and desirable in preventing infectious disease. If 90% of the population is protected against organisms that require continued passage through human beings in order to reproduce and live, the disease caused by the organism can be virtually eliminated because there are too few susceptible hosts for the organism to thrive. Smallpox has been eliminated from the United States in this way. This type of protection of a group is called *herd immunity.* It is ineffectual, however, against organisms such as tetanus bacilli that can exist independently of man, and in this instance each person must be immunized to be protected. If the disease is one not prevalent in the environment, such as smallpox in the United States, or is not spread from person to person by direct contact, such as tetanus, the inoculation must be repeated at regular intervals to maintain protection (p. 312). This inoculation is called a *booster dose,* and usually one tenth of the original inoculating dose is sufficient.

An inoculation causes a histamine response. Local symptoms of inflammation (redness, tenderness, swelling, sometimes ulcerations) appear at the site of the injection, and symptoms of widespread tissue involvement (slight febrile reactions, general malaise, muscle aching) for a day or two are common. The initial inoculation produces delayed symptoms because tissues must become sensitized to the antigen. There is an accelerated and less severe systemic reaction to subsequent inoculations because antibody production is stimulated at once. The local reaction also is less severe than that following the initial inoculation because the organisms have less opportunity to produce inflammation.

An inoculating substance containing a disease-producing organism is called a *vaccine.* It is produced in the laboratory by exposing the pathogens to heat, cold, chemicals, or repeated cycles of growth to decrease their ability to produce disease while still retaining their ability to stimulate antibody production. Organisms that are not killed but only made less virulent are called *attenuated organisms.* Vaccines for poliomyelitis (Sabin vaccine), rabies (Pasteur treatment), yellow fever, and measles are prepared from organisms that have been attenuated by repeated cycles of growth in laboratory animals. The bacilli that cause typhoid, paratyphoid, cholera, plague, whooping cough, and influenza are injected after being killed by heat, as is the Salk vaccine for poliomyelitis. In some cases the body also will manufacture antibodies against a virulent pathogen if it is exposed to a less virulent pathogen with similar characteristics. For instance, an injection of cowpox virus will produce an active immunity against the smallpox virus. The vaccine for tuberculosis (BCG) is made from an attenuated bovine strain of the tubercle bacillus. The procedure of introducing vaccine into the body is called *vaccination.*

An inoculating substance containing a modified toxin of a specific pathogen is called a *toxoid.* It is produced in the laboratory by treating the toxin chemically so that its toxicity is decreased but its antibody-producing properties are maintained. Diphtheria toxoid and tetanus toxoid are widely used, and streptococcus and staphylococcus toxoids are available.

Immunization programs. Active artificial immunization against many bacilli and viruses is now available. Every person should be encouraged to avail himself of the protection advised by health officials in his local area. He also should be advised to keep a permanent record of the date of each immunization.

In the United States the Public Health Service recommends that all children be immunized against diphtheria, pertussis (whooping cough), tetanus, mumps, rubella, poliomyelitis, and measles. The injections are started when the baby is 2 months old, and 0.5 ml. of DPT, a combination of diphtheria, pertussis, and tetanus vaccines, is given monthly for 3 months and followed by a reinforcing dose a year later. To be certain of immunity to tetanus, a booster dose of toxoid is recommended at the time of entrance into school and every 10 years thereafter. Since the immunity conferred by the toxoid has proved to be long lasting, annual booster injections are unwarranted. Puncture wounds, animal bites, and wounds likely to be contaminated with soil or manure are indications for giving tetanus toxoid. However, if the person is known to have received the toxoid within the past years, the inoculation could be omitted. Passive prophylaxis is needed for unimmunized individuals who have sustained crushing injuries, burns, or penetrating wounds. Individuals who have had no tetanus toxoid for many years and who are seen more than 24 hours after sustaining injuries that could cause tetanus should be provided with passive immunization. Tetanus immune globulin (TIG), 250 to 500 units intramuscularly, is recommended. Equine antitoxin (TAT), 3,000 to 5,000 units, may be given if TIG is not available. The antitoxin injection should be preceded by appropriate history taking and sensitivity testing.[2]

Routine vaccination against smallpox is no longer recommended by the Public Health Service. Because of the low incidence of smallpox, the side effects and complications of the vaccine have become of greater concern than the danger of acquiring the disease. However, vaccination is recommended for individuals living or traveling in countries where smallpox is endemic. The World Health Organization report of 1972 indicated an increase in the number of cases of smallpox from 1971 to 1972, causing some concern among epidemiologists.

Immunization against poliomyelitis may be started when the infant is 6 weeks of age or older. Salk vaccine is now rarely used, but the nurse should be familiar with the schedule by which it is given to help parents determine whether their children had a complete course. This is essential for protection. Two injections of Salk vaccine are given 1 month apart, a third injection 7 months later, and a booster dose in a year. Immunization with oral Sabin vaccine is now recommended. To provide maximum protection it should be started 2 or 3 months before the "polio season." Trivalent Oral Poliovirus Vaccine (TOPV), which contains Sabin strains types I, II, and III, is usually given. Two drops of the vaccine are taken orally either on a cube of sugar, in a small amount of distilled water, or with a spoonful of corn syrup. The first dose of trivalent vaccine is given at approximately 2 months of age; the second and third at 6- to 8-week intervals. A fourth dose should be given at approximately 18 months of age. For infants, three doses of trivalent vaccine are recommended. For the primary immunization of older children and adults, trivalent vaccine is given with an interval of 8 weeks between the first two doses, followed by a third dose 6 months to 1 year later. In the event that monovalent vaccine is used, it is given to the infant 1 to 2 months apart in the following order: type I, type III, and type II. Approximately 1 year later a single booster dose of a trivalent preparation is administered.[1,2]

Measles (rubeola) vaccine is not given until the child is 12 months old because antibodies from the mother make it unnecessary. One injection is given. Children who have not been immunized as infants can be given measles vaccine at any age.[2]

Immunization to protect against other disease is given on a selective basis; that is, groups at a high risk are immunized. Because of the prevalence of influenza and its potential for causing death, the Public Health Service recommends immunization against influenza for the aged and persons with chronic cardiac, respiratory, metabolic, and renal disease. Initial protection is obtained by giving two injections of the vaccine 2 weeks apart beginning in October or November. Infants and children up to 6 years of age are given three small doses, the first and second doses 2 weeks apart and a third dose 2 months later. Yearly booster doses are needed to maintain immunity.

In 1966 the Public Health Service announced that a new vaccine against German measles (rubella) had been developed. Studies since then indicate that 95% of the susceptible individuals vaccinated develop antibodies; however, the titers are lower than those following natural infection. The duration of immunity has not been established, but it is likely to be long term. Live rubella virus vaccine is recommended for children between 1 year of age and puberty, regardless of whether there is a history of German measles. School-age children (between 5 and 9) should have priority since they are the major source of virus dissemination in the community.

As a preventive measure, women in the childbearing years should be tested for rubella antibodies. If no antibodies are present and it is certain that the woman is not pregnant, rubella vaccine is given. The woman should agree not to become pregnant for at least 2 months after vaccination.[2]

At the present time, immunization against typhoid fever is only recommended when there is exposure to a typhoid carrier in the household, when there is an outbreak of typhoid in a community, or when traveling to countries where typhoid is endemic.[2]

Passive immunization. Antibodies produced by other persons or by other animals such as the horse, cow, and rabbit can be introduced into the bloodstream of a person to protect him against attack by a pathogen. This protection is *temporary,* usually lasting only a few weeks, and stimulates no production of antibodies by the recipient. It is called *artificial passive acquired immunity.* Artificial passive immunization is given to a person who has been exposed to a disease and has no natural or artificial active immunity. It usually is given before the disease develops, but it may be given to modify the symptoms of a disease. However, for effectiveness after the disease has developed, it must be administered early, before extensive damage to body tissues has occurred.

Passive immunization usually is reserved for situations in which the disease would be detrimental to the person. For example it is rarely given to prevent a disease such as chickenpox or mumps in children because they are at an optimum age for the body to produce antibodies with minimal histamine response. On the other hand, an adult exposed to the same disease often would be given antibodies because adults may have a severe histamine response. Immunization is given to all age groups exposed to pathogens that cause serious diseases such as hepatitis, poliomyelitis, diphtheria, tetanus, or rabies. Antivenins, which are given to people bitten by poisonous snakes or black widow spiders, also are passive immunologic products.

Products used for passive immunization may be specific to the disease. Antitoxins and immune animal and human sera are examples. The whole blood of a patient who has recently recovered from a disease against which antibodies are produced also may be used. Antitoxins are available for diphtheria, tetanus, botulism, gas gangrene, and the venom of snakes. Immune animal serum is available against the *Haemophilus influenzae* virus and rabies; human immune serum is available for mumps, measles, pertussis, poliomyelitis, and tetanus.

Immune serum globulin (ISG), or gamma globulin, is an antibody-rich fraction of pooled plasma from normal donors. The rationale for pooling plasma is that someone among the donors will have had the diseases and will have developed antibodies against them. The globulin fraction of the plasma is believed to carry the antibodies, and because it is known not to transmit the virus of hepatitis, it is considered safe to use. Because of occasional side effects, it is now recommended that the use of immune serum globulin be limited to those disorders in which its efficacy has been definitely established. These are measles prophylaxis or modification, viral hepatitis type A (infectious hepatitis) prophylaxis or modification, and antibody deficiency diseases. Immune serum globulin is considered to be of questionable value in the following situations: (1) prevention of rubella in the first trimester of pregnancy, (2) prevention or modification of varicella in certain high-risk patients, (3) prevention or modification of viral hepatitis type B (serum hepatitis) after accidental inoculation, and (4) life-threatening bacterial infections.[2]

Special human immune serum globulins are derived from the sera of persons previously immunized or convalescing from specific diseases. Tetanus Immune Globulin (Human) is of value in prophylaxis and treatment of tetanus. Vaccinia Immune Globulin (Human) is used in the prophylaxis and treatment of vaccinia complication and for smallpox. Pertussis Immune Globulin (Human) and Mumps Immune Globulin (Human) are of uncertain or unproved value in the prevention and treatment of pertussis and mumps, respectively.

Nursing responsibilities in immunization. Probably the greatest responsibility of the nurse in immunization programs is to teach the public the advantages of immunization and encourage widespread participation in programs recommended by the local public health officer. Every September an immunization survey is conducted by the Center for Disease Control of the Public Health Service and the Bureau of the Census. The 1972 survey revealed that 24.4% of children from 1 to 4 years of age had not completed diphtheria-pertussis immunization and 37.1% had not received adequate immunization against poliomyelitis. Of this latter group, 10.7% had not received polio vaccine of any kind. Of these children, 34% had not been vaccinated against measles.[38] From these figures it is obvious that there is still much work to be done if immunization protection is to reach all children. This is particularly true since there is considerable discrepancy between the immunization levels in poverty and nonpoverty areas. Since immunization is almost always available free of charge, it would appear that factors other than cost may be involved.

In teaching it is advisable to provide the public with the following information: against what disease protection is being given, why immunization is desirable, and when booster doses should be obtained.[16] The relative safety of the immunization and the advantages of immunization early in life should be stressed.

The nurse is responsible for assessing patients prior to immunization because there are some contraindications to receiving certain immunizing substances. Those that are prepared in chicken or duck embryos may cause an allergic reaction in persons who are allergic to eggs. Many people are allergic to horse serum, and substances containing horse serum, such as tetanus antitoxin, should never be given unless a small amount of the substance has been injected intradermally (a sensitivity test) and after 20 minutes produces no "hive" reaction about the injection site (p. 94). Active immunologic products should not be given while a person has a cold or other infection because the histaminic reaction from the immunization will be greater than usual.

Children with histories of allergy often are *not* given routine immunization against diseases for which there is herd immunity, because the danger of severe allergic response to the immunization is greater than the danger of contracting the disease. These children should be immunized against diseases such as tetanus, however, and immunization is achieved by giving the vaccine or toxoid in small doses over a period of several weeks or months. The package inserts accompanying the immunologic product should always be read carefully to determine the indications, precautions, and side effects.

Before the person leaves the clinic, he or his family should be instructed as to the expected effects and told to contact his physician or to report to a hospital emergency room if any other symptoms develop. He should be cautioned not to scratch any lesion produced by an inoculation. If a severe local reaction with redness, swelling, and tenderness occurs, the physician may order the application of hot, wet dressings. If the lesion is open, these dressings should be sterile.

When antitoxins, antisera, or antivenins are given, the patient should be kept under observation for 20 to 30 minutes. Symptoms of severe allergic response (p. 94) usually will appear within that period of time.

■ CONTROLLING CONTACT WITH SOURCES OF INFECTION

Communicable disease sometimes can be controlled by limiting the contacts of infected persons with others and by identifying potential susceptible hosts so that they can be protected prophylactically. The nurse often is called on to help with these measures.

All patients with known infection should be isolated as necessary to decrease the possibility of their infecting others. When there is a known epidemic of airborne disease such as influenza, scarlet fever, or measles, health officials may close public meeting places such as schools and theaters in an attempt to minimize the spread of the disease by persons who are in the incubation stage. The nurse often must interpret this restriction to the public and try to gain their cooperation. Without it, groups may continue to gather, and spread of the disease will not be halted. During this period the public also should be urged to practice good general hygiene in relation to rest, food, exercise, and fresh air so that optimum resistance to infection is maintained. Keeping rooms well ventilated and with air moderately humid and avoiding chilling also may deter invasion by airborne pathogens.

Sometimes an infected person has a communicable disease such as tuberculosis or syphilis that he may have transmitted to persons with whom he has been in close contact. To ensure that these persons (the *contacts*) receive early and adequate treatment and to prevent their infecting others, the nurse may be asked to help trace them and encourage them to seek medical attention. This procedure, requiring the utmost tact, is described on p. 538.

Mass screening often is done to identify groups that have a high risk of contracting diseases such as scarlet fever, diphtheria, and tuberculosis because they have no resistance to the disease-producing organism. The *Schick test* is done to detect susceptibility to diphtheria, and the *Dick test* is done to detect susceptibility to scarlet fever. A prescribed amount of toxoid is given intradermally on the forearm. A positive reaction (a red, indurated area at the site of injection appearing in 24 to 48 hours and lasting 4 or 5 days) to either of these tests indicates susceptibility to the disease. Artificial active immunization should be given to persons with a positive

Schick test, and persons with a positive Dick test should try to avoid contact with anyone who has scarlet fever. If they become exposed, they should seek medical attention at once. Usually antibiotics are given. The *tuberculin test* can be done by various techniques. A positive reaction to this test indicates that the person at some time has had contact with the tubercle bacillus, but it does not indicate that he has had active tuberculosis. However, positive reactions in children under the age of 2 years usually indicate active disease. (See p. 560 for a complete discussion of this test, the prophylactic measures used for persons whose reaction is negative, and the further screening of those who have positive reactions.) The nurse working in the community often is asked to teach the public about the need for this type of screening, and the public health nurse frequently is responsible for scheduling screening clinics in the community at regular intervals. The nurse may read and record the test results and is responsible for directing persons who need further treatment or follow-up to the proper facilities and for explaining the need for this continued care to them.

■ PLANNING NURSING INTERVENTION FOR THE PATIENT WITH A COMMUNICABLE DISEASE

General care. In general the nursing care of a patient with a communicable disease is the same as that needed by anyone with a generalized infection (p. 84). Rashes and skin lesions frequently accompany such childhood diseases as measles, chickenpox, and scarlet fever. Care of wounds, which may be involved, is described on p. 86.

Isolation. The patient with a communicable disease may require medical aseptic techniques *(isolation)*. In planning care, therefore, the nurse first needs to determine the characteristics of the pathogen involved to determine whether or not the patient needs to be isolated and, if so, what type of isolation is needed. The determining factor is the method by which the pathogen is transmitted from person to person. The types of isolation are strict isolation, respiratory isolation, enteric precautions, and wound precautions.

Strict isolation is recommended only for highly communicable diseases that are spread by direct contact and airborne routes of transmission. A few examples of diseases requiring strict isolation are diphtheria, plague, and smallpox. Strict isolation requires that the patient is in a private room with the door kept closed; gowns, masks, and gloves are worn by all persons entering the room; hands are washed on entering and leaving the room; and all articles in the room must be placed in impervious plastic bags and double-bagged for disinfection or sterilization.

Respiratory isolation is recommended to prevent transmission of organisms by droplets or droplet nuclei that are coughed, sneezed, or breathed into the environment. Some of the diseases for which respiratory isolation is recommended are chickenpox, herpes zoster, measles, mumps, and whooping cough. Tuberculosis no longer requires respiratory isolation; the reasons are explained in Chapter 22. The precautions to be practiced in respiratory isolation include placing the patient in a private room with the door closed. Masks are worn only by persons susceptible to the disease, and gowns and gloves are not necessary. Tissues and dressings are placed in a paper or plastic bag, sealed, and then placed in an impervious plastic bag before removal from the room.

Enteric precautions are recommended for patients with cholera, viral hepatitis (infectious and serum), salmonellosis (including typhoid fever), and shigellosis. The purpose of enteric precautions is to prevent transmission of disease through direct or indirect contact with infected feces or heavily contaminated articles. Pathogens are spread from infected hands to the mouth, where they are ingested. In this type of isolation the emphasis is placed on proper handwashing, gown technique, and excreta precautions. Gloves are recommended by some experts because of the fear that proper handwashing will not be practiced consistently.

Wound and *skin precautions* are used to prevent cross-infection from infection transmissible from wounds and heavily contaminated articles. It is recommended for infected burn wounds, gas gangrene, impetigo, and other wounds with purulent drainage. The emphasis is on proper handwashing before and after patient contact, and gloves are recommended for persons having direct contact with the infected area. A private room is desirable but not required. Dressings should be closed securely in an impervious plastic bag, double-bagged, and incinerated. Contaminated linen should also be double-bagged, and mattresses and pillows should be covered with impervious plastic.

If the pathogen is found in excreta or drainage and can be passed to others by food or through open wounds, flies that might transmit the infection to others must be prevented from entering or leaving the patient's room. If the pathogen must pass through a vector in order to complete its life cycle and be transmitted to human beings, as, for example, the pathogen that causes malaria passing through the *Anopheles* mosquito, then protecting the patient with mosquito netting is the only precaution needed—and this only if he is in an area where *Anopheles* mosquitoes are present.

In caring for any patient with a communicable disease requiring isolation, careful and thorough handwashing after any contact with the patient or the equipment in his room is mandatory. The Public Health Service has published a manual establishing guidelines for isolation techniques in hospitals.* This manual is a valuable source of information for all nurses.

Prevention of complications. Many of the communicable diseases commonly prevalent today are caused by viruses. Special care should be taken to protect patients with viral diseases from exposure to bacteria, because cells damaged by viral infection have increased susceptibility to bacterial invasion. Because bacterial complications frequently accompany viral diseases, and because bacteria are prevalent in hospitals, physicians may prefer to treat patients with viral diseases at home. Ear infections, meningitis, and encephalitis of bacterial origin are common complications of measles, and staphylococcal pneumonia is a common sequela of viral influenza.

Toxin-producing bacterial diseases such as streptococcal sore throat, scarlet fever, rheumatic fever, and diphtheria frequently cause serious secondary disease of the heart or kidneys. Patients with these diseases usually are given antibiotics and are kept relatively quiet until the blood sedimentation rate returns to normal.

Home care. Unless the pathogen is highly contagious, patients with communicable diseases frequently are cared for at home. The public health nurse often is asked to teach the mother or some other family member how to care for the patient and how to protect herself and other family members; other nurses may be consulted by friends and neighbors about protection. The same principles apply in the home as in the hospital. A smock or coverall may be used to protect the clothes, and a mask can be improvised from any closely woven, absorbable white material, or disposable ones can be bought at a pharmacy. All liquid wastes can be flushed down the toilet. Garbage and other wastes from the room should be burned. If local laws prohibit burning of rubbish, the wastes should be wrapped in several layers of newspaper and tied securely with string before discarding in a rubbish container. Dishes should be boiled for 10 minutes before washing. If the laundry must be isolated, it can be boiled for 10 minutes and then washed. When the patient has recovered, the room should be thoroughly aired. Depending on the type of illness, the walls, floor, and furniture may need to be washed well with a detergent or disinfectant and warm water. If materials that cannot be washed, such as books and toys, have been contaminated, leaving them in the sun and air for 24 to 48 hours usually provides sufficient protection.

---

*Isolation techniques for use in hospitals, Publication no. 2054, Washington, D. C., 1970, Public Health Service.

REFERENCES AND SELECTED READINGS*

1 *Ager, E. A.: Current concepts in immunization, Am. J. Nurs. **66:**2004-2011, Sept. 1966.

2 American Academy of Pediatrics: Report of the Committee on the Control of Infectious Diseases, ed. 17, Evanston, Ill., 1974, The Academy.

3 Anderson, G. W., Arnstein, M. G., and Lester, M. R.: Communicable disease control, ed. 4, New York, 1962, Macmillan Publishing Co., Inc.

4 Benson, M. E.: Handwashing—an important part of medical asepsis, Am. J. Nurs. **57:**1136-1139, Sept. 1957.

5 *Carroll, L. D.: Problems in acute communicable disease control, Nurs. Outlook **2:**593-595, Nov. 1954.

6 Communicable diseases and vector control in 1972, WHO Chronicle **27:**301-313, 1973.

7 Control of communicable disease in man, ed. 11, New York, 1970, American Public Health Association.

8 Diplovax—a new oral polio vaccine, Med. Lett. Drugs Ther. **14:**57-58, 1972.

9 Dubos, R. J., and Hirsch, J. G., editors: Bacterial and mycotic infections of man, ed. 4, Philadelphia, 1965, J. B. Lippincott Co.

10 *Frances, B. J.: Current concepts in immunization, Am. J. Nurs. **73:**646-649, April 1973.

11 *Frye, C.: Viral hepatitis—a risk to nurses, Can. Nurs. **69:**33-36, July 1973.

12 Gell, P. G. H., and Coombs, R. R. A., editors: Clinical aspects of immunology, ed. 2, Philadelphia, 1968, F. A. Davis Co.

13 *Getting, V. A.: Food-borne diseases, Nurs. Outlook **2:**364-367, July 1954.

14 Hoeprich, P. D.: Infectious diseases, New York, 1972, Harper & Row Publishers, Inc.

15 Horsfall, F. L., and Tamm, I.: Viral and rickettsial infections of man, ed. 4, Philadelphia, 1965, J. B. Lippincott Co.

16 Immunization, J.A.M.A. **204:**156-160, April 1968.

17 Influenza, Med. J. Aust. **1:**1073-1074, June 1973.

18 Influenza vaccine: U. S. Public Health Service, Ann. Intern. Med. **77:**425-426, Sept. 1972.

19 *International quarantine, World Health, Feb. 1964, p. 24.

20 Kempe, C. H., and Benenson, A. S.: Smallpox immunization in the United States, J.A.M.A. **194:**161-166, Oct. 1965.

21 Lane, J. M., and others: Deaths attributed to smallpox vaccination, 1959 to 1966, and 1968, J.A.M.A. **212:**441-444, April 1970.

22 Leavell, H. R., and Clark, E. G.: Preventive medicine for the doctor in his community, ed. 3, New York, 1965, McGraw-Hill Book Co.

23 Lilienfeld, A. M.: Epidemiology of infectious and non-infectious disease: some comparisons, Am. J. Epidemiol. **97:**135-147, March 1973.

24 Marks, M. I., and others: Immunization today—a review, Can. Med. Assoc. J. **108:**1413-1417, June 1973.

25 Measles vaccines, recommendations of Public Health Service Advisory Committee on Immunization Practices, Ann. Intern. Med. **76:**101-104, Jan. 1972.

26 *Morrison, S. T., and Arnold, C. R.: Patients with common communicable diseases, Nurs. Clin. North Am. **5:**143-155, March 1970.

27 Piszozek, E. A., and others: Smallpox vaccination, J.A.M.A. **22:**1185, Nov. 1972.

28 Rawland, H. A. K.: Going abroad, Br. Med. J. **2:**639-642, June 1972.

29 *Redeker, A. G.: Viral hepatitis: current concepts, Postgrad. Med. **53:**77-81, Jan. 1973.

30 Riley, R. L., and O'Grady, F.: Airborne infection, New York, 1961, Macmillan Publishing Co., Inc.

31 *Rogers, F. B., editor: Studies in epidemiology, New York, 1965, G. P. Putnam's Sons.

32 *Roueche, B.: Eleven blue men, New York, 1953, Berkley Publishing Corp.

33 *Shaw, W. E.: Nursing and nurse training in venereology, Nurs. Times **69:**635-637, May 1973.

34 Smith, D. H., and Peter, G.: Current and future vaccines for the prevention of bacterial diseases, Pediatr. Clin. North Am. **19:**387-412, May 1972.

35 *Steele, J. H., and Carroll, L. D.: Animal diseases transmissible to man, Nurs. Outlook **4:**156-161, March 1956.

36 *Steele, J. H., and Lester, M. R.: Rabies and rabies control, Am. J. Nurs. **58:**531-536, April 1958.

37 U. S. Department of Health, Education and Welfare, National Communicable Disease Center in cooperation with the Bureau of the Census: United States immunization survey—1967, 1968, Washington, D. C., Dec. 1968, U. S. Department of Health, Education and Welfare, Public Health Service.

38 U. S. Department of Health, Education and Welfare, Public Health Service: U. S. immunization survey—1972, Publication no. (HSM) 73-8221, Atlanta, 1973, Center for Disease Control.

39 Webster, B.: Changing patterns in the organization of venereal diseases service in the U. S. A., Br. J. Vener. Dis. **49:**141-143, April 1973.

40 Weibel, R. E., and others: Rubella vaccination in adult females, N. Engl. J. Med. **280:**682-685, March 1969.

41 Williams, S. R.: Nutrition and diet therapy, ed. 2, St. Louis, 1973, The C. V. Mosby Co.

42 World Health Organization: International sanitary regulations, ed. 3, Geneva, Switzerland, 1966.

*References preceded by an asterisk are particularly well suited for student reading.

Nursing care related to patients with specific medical and surgical problems

17 Cardiovascular diseases

■ Survival, growth, reproduction, and productivity of the human organism depend on a balance between movement of nutrients to the cells and of wastes away from the cells. In health, this end is accomplished by the efficient functioning of three factors: a pump (the heart), a circulatory circuit, and a fluid medium (the blood). Disease or structural alterations of any one of these three factors may hinder the transport system and ultimately affect the survival of the organism. This chapter deals with the heart, the diseases that affect its functioning, and the management of patients with cardiac disease.

More people in the United States are affected, directly or indirectly, by cardiovascular disease than by any other illness. It is difficult to determine the exact prevalence of cardiac disease (and the associated vascular conditions such as cerebrovascular disease and peripheral vascular disease) in a community or in the entire country. Diagnostic techniques have not yet been developed that can be used in mass screening for all types of cardiovascular disease. Many persons do not know that they have heart disease until severe symptoms develop.

Cardiovascular diseases cause more deaths than all other diseases combined. In 1971, out of a total of 1,921,000 deaths in the United States, almost 60%, or 1,013,000, were caused by cardiovascular diseases and 740,170 by diseases of the heart.[124] Thus at the present time it can be safely predicted that unless some remarkable events occur to change the present trend, at least one out of every two persons alive in the country today will die of cardiovascular disease.

Deaths caused by cardiac disease vary with age. Congenital malformations of the heart and closely related vascular system are the cause of over 90% of the deaths from these causes in children under 5 years of age and of more than one third of persons 5 to 24 years of age. By far the most common cause of death from heart disease after the age of 25 years is ischemic heart disease (coronary artery disease), which accounted for 677,260 deaths in 1968.[124]

Despite some advances in prevention and treatment, the incidence of heart disease continues to be high. Approximately 10 million persons in the United

■ STUDY QUESTIONS

1 Diagram the main chambers of the heart and the adjacent blood vessels. Trace the flow of blood through these structures, and review the normal physiology of the cardiovascular system.

2 What medications improve, regulate, or stimulate heart action? How are these administered?

3 What is the normal daily intake of sodium chloride? What common foods are high in sodium content?

4 Review the nursing care needed by a patient receiving oxygen.

5 What can the nurse do to help prevent valvular heart disease? Congenital heart disease?

6 Review the coagulation process. What is the difference between clotting or coagulation time and prothrombin time? Which test is used with heparin? With warfarin sodium (Coumadin)? Why?

7 Review the electrophysiology of the heart.

8 Why is the measurement of urinary output important in a patient with a myocardial infarction? Why are rectal procedures discouraged in these patients?

9 What is the rationale for the use of diuretics in cardiac disease? What are some of the hazardous side effects of this therapy?

10 Review and practice cardiopulmonary resuscitation.

States, including 500,000 children, have heart disease.[104] Most of the advances in treatment deal with amelioration of heart disease and not with removal of its causes.[120] Research efforts continue in attempts to find effective medications, but results from use of the medications now available have not always been beneficial over long periods of time. For example, widespread use of antibiotics has produced drug-resistant strains of bacteria and drug-resistant persons. Medications used to lower the cholesterol levels in the blood and perhaps reduce the incidence of coronary artery thrombosis are not wholly satisfactory, and some new drugs that produce vasodilation in animal studies have not proved helpful to man. Heart surgery is publicized widely and is a valuable treatment at times, but at present it is practicable for less than 1% of all patients with heart disease.[104]

■ PREVENTION

Although at this time a "cure" is not usually possible for patients with heart disease, development of the disease can be prevented in many persons, and many of those who have heart disease can be helped to live happy, useful, and long lives. Immunization against acute infectious diseases such as diphtheria, scarlet fever, and measles and control of infections through selectively used antibiotics have contributed much to the decreased incidence of infectious complications such as pericarditis, endocarditis, and myocarditis. The incidence of syphilitic aortitis has decreased because of early case findings and prompt treatment. State health departments now provide physicians with immune serum globulin (ISG) for women in the first trimester of pregnancy who have been exposed to German measles and who will not consider therapeutic abortion should they develop the disease. The routine use of ISG is no longer recommended, since the development of rubella viremia is not prevented and the symptoms of the disease, if it does occur, may be masked by ISG administration.[1a] Newer laboratory tests for determining whether a pregnant woman has been infected with rubella are discussed on p. 312. Because school-age children are the major source of rubella infection in the community, the best method for preventing rubella in pregnant women is to vaccinate children. It is hoped that the widespread campaign to have all children between the age of 1 and puberty immunized against rubella will decrease the incidence of German measles among pregnant women and thus reduce the number of congenital anomalies or therapeutic abortions.

Since streptococcal infections are frequently complicated by rheumatic fever with heart involvement, educational programs stressing the importance of early and adequate treatment of these infections have been directed at the medical professions and the general public. The incidence of rheumatic heart disease is being decreased by vigorous educational and prophylactic programs. Through the joint efforts of local heart associations and local health departments, penicillin for prophylactic use has been made available at a reasonable cost to families who have children with rheumatic heart disease. Since dental extractions and surgery may activate a bacterial infection in the heart, efforts have been made by dentists and surgeons to prevent bacterial endocarditis in persons with known diseases of the heart. Antibiotics are usually given prophylactically before and following surgery.

Unfortunately at the present time there are no certain measures that can be taken to prevent ischemic heart disease (coronary artery disease), which is by far the most prevalent disease of the heart in the United States today. Some measures that may possibly prove to be preventive in the future are discussed later in this chapter.

Research in prevention

Although the causes of many types of heart disease are not yet known, extensive epidemiologic studies and research are being carried on currently in an attempt to determine preventive measures. Organizations such as the American Heart Association are financing research to uncover further information on the causes of heart disease and to develop new methods for its treatment. As part of the National Institutes of Health, supported by the federal government and under the United States Public Health Service, the National Heart Institute is conducting an intensive study on the cause, control, and treatment of heart disease. Vital statistics are being studied carefully in an attempt to discover whether such factors as sex, occupation, constitutional make-up, ethnologic background, or dietary patterns are associated with certain types of heart disease. Grants have been made to study the effects of new drugs on the heart, to perfect techniques that will make cardiac surgery possible for more patients, and to study the mechanisms by which heart diseases affect the tissues. Future studies of many people in their own home and community setting, to learn how diet, living practices, regular exercise, and many other aspects of living affect heart disease, will require the help of nurses who are particularly skilled in working with people.

In recent years there has been increasing concern about the gap between medical research and new knowledge and its application to patient care. President Johnson appointed a Commission on Heart Disease, Cancer, and Stroke to study this problem. As a result of its report, Congress passed and the President signed, in October 1965, a bill establishing Regional Medical Programs for Heart Disease, Cancer, Stroke and Related Diseases. The Regional Medical

Programs had many objectives, all of which were designed to improve the knowledge of physicians and nurses and thereby improve patient care. Most of these programs have been phased out, but many health professionals attended programs sponsored by them.

Role of the nurse in prevention. The informed nurse can play an important role in the prevention of heart disease and its disabilities. First is the role in primary prevention. In this role the nurse participates in immunization programs and in public education programs emphasizing immunization, good hygiene, and proper nutrition. As a public health nurse, office nurse, hospital nurse, or parent, the nurse can impress on parents the importance of seeking medical care for children with diseased tonsils and carious teeth. The nurse can encourage people with infectious disease to stay in bed and to have medical care and can support the use of an ECG as part of a routine physical examination.

The second role is in case finding. The nurse is often in a position to assess patients and to observe symptoms that may be significant in the detection of heart disease or may pick up clues of significant symptoms from details of family history. Frequently it is the alert nurse who can help persons with undiagnosed heart disease to obtain medical attention.

A fatalistic attitude about heart disease and a conviction that nothing can be done about heart attacks, which "just happen," prevent many persons from reporting early signs of heart disease to their physicians. Since early medical treatment could often prevent or delay progress of the condition, this is doubly unfortunate. Persons who are unfamiliar with the symptoms often ignore them or attribute them to some other cause. Nurses can help to prevent the development of serious heart disease by teaching the public the early signs of possible heart disease and by urging prompt referral to physicians when they occur. For example, attacks of shortness of breath or unexpected dyspnea on exertion, feelings of pressure in the chest, awakening in the night with consciousness of heart action or distress, and discomfort resembling indigestion that is relieved by sitting up are reasons to see a physician even though the cause may be found to be trivial. Most persons have read magazine articles about anginal attacks with pain. They should be taught that pain is *not* a common sign of coronary artery disease. Dyspnea and signs of cardiac decompensation occur much more often. Many elderly persons hesitate to report symptoms because they believe that nothing can be done for them because of their age. Again, this idea is very seldom accurate. A friendly interest on the part of the nurse and assurance that medical care can be helpful will often lead them to seek medical treatment. By working closely with the parents of children with rheumatic disease, nurses can help

them to care for the children and encourage them to cooperate with medical follow-up and with long-term programs for prevention of recurrences.

The nurse needs to understand the many fears to which patients and families might be subject, so that they can be helped to have a clearer understanding of the positive aspects of the situation. One of the biggest problems to be met in educating the public on heart disease is overcoming fear. Awareness of the fact that the heart is necessary to life makes most people view heart disease differently from diseases of other organs. Much of the publicizing of heart disease in magazine articles, television programs, and films depicts the fatality more than the control of the disease. Although public education measures are intended to motivate people to have physical examinations and to use discretion in eating, exercising, resting, not smoking, and checking symptoms with their physician, they create threats for some people. Some persons who are told that their symptoms are suggestive of heart disease often continue to worry when diagnostic tests prove nothing, and they cannot accept the fact that nothing is wrong. The person who has had one heart attack may live in fear of another and be prevented from resuming his place as a useful member of society. Others cannot find work because employers are afraid to hire them. Heart associations, health departments, and insurance companies spend large sums of money each year for educational publications on heart disease in an attempt to overcome these problems.

The nurse needs to face realistically any personal fear about heart disease before good care can be given to patients and families. Helping others see the positive side of the picture, such as the fact that many who have heart attacks recover almost completely and are able to live relatively normal lives, also helps the nurse. The nurse should try to gain patients' cooperation in following medical advice, helping them to see how they themselves can participate in keeping well. Much of this ability stems from the nurse's own confidence in and a realistic approach to treatment of heart disease.

Some families in which a member has heart disease live in fear of a repeated heart attack, particularly because they realize that they do not know what to do in such an emergency. The nurse should know the signs and symptoms of heart diseases and also the kind of emergency care the patient's family can give. Family members usually can be taught to act wisely in an emergency if the physician and the nurse are explicit and certain of what should be done. Some families find little consolation in being told to call an ambulance or to call the police or fire department, but if they also know the position in which to place the patient and perhaps how to administer medication, they will react better in an actual emergency. Although emergencies may be expected, the nurse should help the patient who has cardiac disease and his family to develop a wholesome attitude toward his condition so that they can lead relatively normal lives and not live in constant expectation of disaster.

■ CARDIOVASCULAR ASSESSMENT

Nursing assessment of a patient's cardiovascular system is an integral part of the overall assessment obtained prior to planning nursing care. While depth of assessment varies with preparation and experience of individual nurses, certain data should be obtained by all nurses. These include blood pressure, heart rate (elicited from the first and second heart sounds) and heart rhythm, presence or absence of peripheral arterial pulses, capillary filling, color of skin, lips, and nail beds, and presence or absence of edema in the lower extremities. The means used to obtain this data are inspection, palpation, and auscultation.

Cardiac auscultation always should be carried out systematically (Fig. 17-1). The first heart sound (S_1), caused by closure of the mitral and tricuspid valves, is heard best when the diaphragm of a stethoscope is placed over the apex of the heart (fourth or fifth intercostal space to the left of the sternum). This sound correlates with ventricular contraction and coincides with the arterial pulse. The second heart sound (S_2), caused by closure of the aortic and pulmonic valves, is heard best when the diaphragm of a stethoscope is placed either over the second right

intercostal space (aortic component) or the second or third left intercostal space (pulmonic component). The first and second heart sounds are heard as the familiar "lub-dub." Heart rhythm is determined simply by listening to the regularity of the "lub-dubs."

Vascular auscultation usually means measurement of arterial blood pressure. This is done with a sphygmomanometer and stethoscope. Initial blood pressure measurements should be taken on both arms, and all measurements should be recorded according to the sounds of Korotkoff; that is, the first, fourth, and fifth phases of sound are included in the reading (for example, 120/80/74). The first phase of the Korotkoff sounds is a tapping sound and is the initial one heard as the cuff is deflated. The fourth phase occurs when the tapping of the third phase becomes muffled and the fifth phase occurs as sound disappears entirely. It is felt that the true diastolic pressure is between the fourth and fifth phases. Deviation from the normal sounds of Korotkoff can indicate cardiac or vascular abnormalities.

Peripheral arterial pulses, which indicate circulation to body parts, are palpated systematically, usually from head to foot in the following sequence: carotid, brachial, radial, femoral, popliteal, posterior tibial, and dorsalis pedis. Palpation should be gentle, especially in patients who have diminished circulation to an area and in the elderly, so that circulation is not further compromised. Pulses on both sides of the body should be compared as to presence and equality.

Capillary filling, commonly called blanching, is another indicator of peripheral circulation and

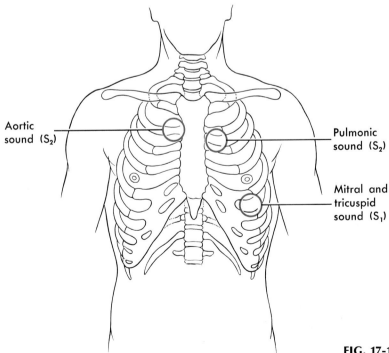

FIG. 17-1. Auscultation of heart sounds.

Aortic sound (S_2)

Pulmonic sound (S_2)

Mitral and tricuspid sound (S_1)

should be tested in all nail beds. This is done by pressing the thumbnail against the edge of a patient's fingernail or toenail and then quickly releasing it. The normal response is whitening (blanching) of the area when pressure is applied and return of color when pressure is released.

A further indication of cardiovascular status is the color of skin, lips, and nail beds. This information is obtained through inspection of the patient's skin, particularly around his lips and on his extremities, and by inspection of lips, oral mucosa, and nail beds.

Finally, a very important indicator of cardiovascular function is the presence or absence of peripheral edema, especially in the feet, ankles, and legs. This is determined by inspection of the body parts and palpation. These steps should be carried out systematically, comparing one side of the body with the other.

Along with the physical assessment, the nurse should obtain a brief cardiovascular history from the patient or his family. This should include (1) family history of heart disease or hypertension, (2) chest discomfort of any kind, (3) the relationship of discomfort to activities of daily living such as eating or exercise, (4) leg cramps related to exercise such as walking, and (5) previous health problems.

■ DIAGNOSTIC PROCEDURES
Signs and symptoms

Heart diseases are diagnosed by the clinical signs and symptoms. Laboratory tests and an x-ray examination are helpful mainly in confirming the diagnosis, determining the course of the disease, indicating complications, showing residual effects, and predicting the results of treatment. The nurse may be directly or indirectly involved in these tests and examinations. The nurse should know why a particular test or observation is being made and what it will contribute to the diagnosis. This information will help the nurse be better able to explain the test to the patient. The nurse can help in the diagnosis by carefully observing and recording signs and symptoms while working with the patient. The character as well as the rate of the *pulse* is important. The pulse may be markedly irregular, or there may be an irregularity that recurs in the same pattern. The pulse may be abnormally rapid or unusually slow. The apical and the radial pulse may not be the same, since sometimes the heart contracts ineffectually, and little blood is pushed out into the arteries. The *respirations* may be labored, and this difficulty may be increased by certain positions or activities. The patient may have *pain* in his arms, chest, neck, upper back, shoulders, or epigastrium. It is important for the physician to know the location and type of pain as well as the activity that caused it. The pa-

tient's *color* and its relationship to activity, position, shortness of breath and pain should be observed. The presence of *edema* of the tissues and increase or decrease of edema related to activity, position, or fluid and salt intake should be recorded. Many of these signs and symptoms are subtle and will be missed if one is not especially looking for them.

Blood analysis

Blood count. A complete blood count is made on all patients with heart disease. In bacterial endocarditis an anemia persists as long as inflammation is active. The blood count, therefore, guides the physician in determining when the patient's physical activity can be increased. The red blood cell count and the hemoglobin level are observed carefully in patients with heart disease that involves intracardiac shunts, for such observations enable the physician to determine how well the blood is being oxygenated. Adequate oxygenation of the blood is a major problem in cardiac disease since the diseased heart may not be able to adequately circulate the blood through the lungs. If there has been a myocardial infarction, which causes death of a portion of the heart muscle, the white blood cell count is usually elevated, because the presence of necrotic tissue anywhere in the body causes leukocytosis.

Blood sedimentation rate. The blood sedimentation rate is determined by a nonspecific test that measures the rate at which red blood cells settle in a glass test tube. It is used to follow the course of inflammation and infection. It is often used to monitor the progress of patients who have rheumatic heart disease or some other inflammatory condition of the heart. A decrease in the sedimentation rate usually indicates that the condition of a patient with an infection is improving.

Prothrombin time. A prothrombin time determination is a blood test that indicates the rapidity of blood clotting. This test is done routinely on patients receiving anticoagulant therapy with drugs such as bishydroxycoumarin (Dicumarol), warfarin sodium (Coumadin, Prothromadin) or a combination of heparin and one of these drugs. A daily prothrombin time is usually done to determine the dosage of the anticoagulant. The coumarin derivatives affect the formation of prothrombin as well as other coagulation factors. With decreased prothrombin activity, the prothrombin time will be prolonged. The nurse should be sure that the blood for the prothrombin time is drawn and that the results are on the patient's chart. Often the physician will attempt to increase the prothrombin time to 2 to 2½ times the normal range of 11 to 18 seconds.

Coagulation time. This test measures the time required for venous blood coagulation. The normal range is 9 to 12 minutes. This test is used particularly with patients on heparin therapy, since this drug affects the formation of thrombin from prothrombin as well as prevents the agglutination and disintegration of platelets and release of thromboplastin.[7]

Blood urea nitrogen. A blood urea nitrogen (BUN) test, used to determine kidney function, is usually made to learn whether kidney function is disturbed as a result of impaired cardiac output or as a result of other causes. The normal range is 9 to 17 mg./100 ml. of blood.

Serum cholesterol. Serum cholesterol tests usually are made in order to determine the cholesterol level in the blood. People with a high cholesterol level are known to have a high incidence of coronary artery disease. Considerable research is being done on the relationship between elevated cholesterol levels and coronary artery disease. The normal levels are considered to be between 150 and 280 mg./100 ml. of blood.[6]

Urinalysis

A routine urinalysis is done on all patients with heart disease. This test includes a description of the color, pH, specific gravity, protein content, glucose content, and sediment of the urine specimen. It is used to determine the effects of the cardiac disease on kidney function and to determine the existence of concurrent renal or systemic diseases such as glomerulonephritis, hypertension, or diabetes mellitus.

Enzyme tests

Enzyme level measurements are helpful in determining the existence of damage to the cardiac muscle as in myocardial infarction. When the muscle cells are damaged or destroyed by the disease process, these enzymes are released into the blood. The transaminases are present in many tissues throughout the body (as are all the other enzymes mentioned), but serum glutamic oxaloacetic transaminase (SGOT) is somewhat more predominate in the heart, and serum glutamic pyruvic transaminase (SGPT) occurs in greater quantities in the liver. The normal SGOT range is 10 to 40 units, but in an acute myocardial infarction the level may increase to 50 to 500 units within 24 hours. Another enzyme present in cardiac muscle is lactic dehydrogenase (LDH). This enzyme has five isozymes of which LDH-5 occurs in greater quantities in the heart. The other isozymes of LDH (1, 2, 3, 4) occur more predominately in the liver, spleen, lung and pancreas, and kidney, respectively.[40] LDH levels peak about 12 hours after an infarction. The normal level ranges from 165 to 300 units, but in an infarction the level may rise from 2 to 10 times normal. Creatinine phosphokinase (CPK) levels are now frequently used in diagnosing a myocardial infarction, since they show an increase within 2 to 5 hours of the infarction.

Electrocardiogram

An electrocardiogram (ECG, EKG) is a record of the electrical activity of the heart muscle. Certain drugs such as digitalis and quinidine as well as exercise and anxiety produce changes in the ECG similar to those seen in disease. Therefore, if the patient is receiving such a drug or if the patient is anxious, the cardiologist should be so informed.

Electrodes, or leads, are placed against the patient's skin on the extremities and the thorax and then connected by wires to a recording galvanometer. They are usually placed on both forearms, on one or both lower legs, and over the precordial area, but many variations may be ordered.[42] A special electrode jelly is rubbed onto the portion of the skin on which the electrode, a small strip of metal, is strapped. The patient lies down or sits while the ECG is made, and he should be relaxed. If it is his first ECG, an explanation of the procedure should be given. If the patient is hospitalized, a technician may come to the bedside to do this procedure. The recording machine may be brought to the bedside, and in some institutions the wires are plugged into special wall outlets that transmit recordings to a central location, or "heart station."

The nurse should understand the ECG in order to be able to explain the procedure to the patient and to understand the significance of the tracings (Fig. 17-2). The electric currents spreading in a wavelike pattern over the heart proceed in an orderly cycle if the heartbeat is normal. The cycle normally begins with impulses from the sinoatrial (SA) node. The SA node controls the heart rate and is the pacemaker. However, any part of the myocardial tissue has the ability to initiate impulses and may take over under abnormal circumstances.

The initial impulse spreads from the SA node through the muscles of the atria by way of internodal tracts, causing them to contract, and is directed obliquely to the atrioventricular (AV) node, then down the bundle of His, spreading along the left and right branches to reach the terminal fibers, the Purkinje system. The Purkinje fibers spread throughout the muscles of the ventricles, and the ventricles contract as the electrical impulse reaches this last point. There is a period of muscular rest while the ventricles fill with blood, and then the cycle is repeated.

For purposes of assessment, recording, and reporting, the deflections appearing on an ECG, which represent electrical activity generated during the cardiac cycle, have been designated P, Q, R, S, and T waves. They are recorded by using electrodes placed on the surface of the body. Because the flow of electrical forces (vector) spreads in several directions, the ECG must be recorded in different planes. When a cardiac monitor is used, recording is done from only one plane or lead, usually equivalent to lead II or V_1.

The graph paper used for recording is divided by horizontal lines, which measure voltage in millivolts, and vertical lines, which measure time in seconds. Thus the P wave represents the electrical impulses initiated in the SA node and the spread through the atria. If these waves are normal in size and shape (Fig. 17-2), one can assume that the impulse began at the SA node. If the waves are absent or unusual in shape, the impulse began outside the SA node.

The *P-R interval* is designated as the period between the start of the P wave and the beginning of the QRS complex. It indicates the time it takes for the original impulse to reach the ventricles and initiate contraction. The latter may be referred to as *depolarization.* During this time (usually not exceeding 0.2 second), the impulse has passed through the atria and the AV junction. If the time exceeds 0.2 second, a conduction delay is considered to have occurred in the AV junction. If the P-R interval is shorter (less than 0.1 second), then it may be that the current reached the ventricle through a shorter-than-normal path.

The *QRS complex* generally consists of three waves, an initial downward deflection (Q wave), an upward deflection (R wave), and a second downward deflection (S wave). This complex reflects the time necessary for the impulse to spread through the bundle of His and its branches. This impulse usually takes less than 0.12 second. An increased amount of time indicates that the ventricles have been stimulated in a delayed, abnormal manner, such as in a bundle-branch block.

The *S-T segment* is the time interval between completion of depolarization and repolarization (recovery) of the ventricular muscles. If there is injury to the muscle, as in myocardial infarction, the S-T segment may be elevated or depressed, while the T wave may be inverted and shortened or prolonged.

The T wave is the recovery phase after contraction (repolarization).

The ECG shows the electrical forces of the heart, which may or may not be disturbed by a pathologic process. It does not show the actual physical state of the heart or its function. Its most important diagnostic use is the identification of abnormal rhythms and coronary heart disease. Since the rhythm may be normal even in the presence of serious heart disease, a single ECG often is not significant, and repeated tracings may be necessary before evidence of disease can be detected. ECG's may also be done at intervals to follow the course of disease. These repeated examinations may be upsetting to the patient unless he understands why so many must be made.

Radiograph of the chest

A radiograph of the chest may be taken to determine the size and shape of the heart and the aorta. Calcifications in the pericardium, heart muscle, valves, or large blood vessels also can be visualized in such an x-ray film, which is sometimes called a *cardiovascular film.* Chest radiographs will also reveal any lung congestion associated with cardiac disease.

Special tests

Special procedures and tests may be ordered to gain additional information concerning certain heart diseases. If known infection is present or if the patient has a transient fever of unknown origin, blood is drawn for culture and sensitivity studies in an effort to learn the causative organism and the antibiotic that will be most effective in treating it. Multiple blood cultures are ordered for patients who have suspected endocarditis. The most scrupulous attention to aseptic technique must be observed in any procedure in which a blood vessel is entered. Nurses have a major responsibility because they often prepare equipment and assist during the procedure.

Venous pressure. Venous pressure is the pressure exerted by the circulating blood against the venous walls. It is elevated in congestive heart failure, in acute or chronic constrictive pericarditis, and in venous obstruction caused by a clot in a vein or external pressure against a vein, as when the jugular vein is manually compressed. The measurement of venous pressure is particularly helpful after open heart surgery in detecting hypervolemia, hypovolemia, congestive failure, and cardiac tamponade.

Venous pressure may be determined in several ways.[2] The easiest of these is examination of the neck veins. Normally these veins are collapsed above the level of the suprasternal notch when the person is sitting with his head elevated 30 to 45 degrees. With increased venous pressure, the veins are distended in this position. The veins on the dorsum of the hand

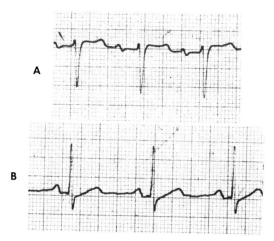

FIG. 17-2. A, Normal ECG in lead V₁. **B,** Normal ECG in lead II.

also provide a ready source of information about venous pressure. While the person is sitting, the hand is held below the level of the heart, and the veins become distended. Normally, as the hand is raised to the sternal notch, the veins collapse. With increased venous pressure, the veins will remain distended even if the hand is raised above the notch.

Central venous pressure. To obtain an accurate central venous pressure (CVP) reading, particularly useful in the patient with heart disease, a catheter is inserted into a major vein and threaded through the superior vena cava into the right atrium. The catheter is attached by a three-way stopcock to an intravenous infusion and a water manometer (Fig. 17-3). The intravenous solution (usually 5% glucose in water) is allowed to drip slowly into the vein to keep the vein open. When a reading is to be taken, the stopcock is opened to the manometer and the manometer is filled with the intravenous solution. Then the stopcock is turned to the venous opening. The fluid level in the manometer should fluctuate with each respiration. The fluid is allowed to stabilize before a reading is taken, and the highest level of the fluid column is then used for the reading. As soon as the reading is taken, the stopcock is turned to the

solution position, and the infusion is continued. For the CVP reading to be accurate the patient must be relaxed, and the zero point of the manometer must always be at the level of the right atrium, which in most people is level with the midaxillary line. If the patient cannot be flat in bed, the zero point on the manometer is adjusted to the level of the right atrium in a sitting position. Any change in the patient's position requires that the zero point be reset. The initial CVP reading and the position that the patient was in when it was taken should be recorded, as these will serve as a baseline for comparison with subsequent readings. For each reading the patient should be placed in the same position, since even a slight change in position alters the CVP. The physician should be informed promptly if there is a significant change in the reading. A high or rising reading usually indicates that the contractility of the heart is impaired; congestive failure and pulmonary edema may occur. A low or falling reading indicates inadequate blood volume (hypovolemia); fluid replacement may be necessary. The normal range for CVP is from 4 to 10 cm. of water. The catheter insertion site should be kept scrupulously clean to minimize the possibility of phlebitis. Changing the dressing daily

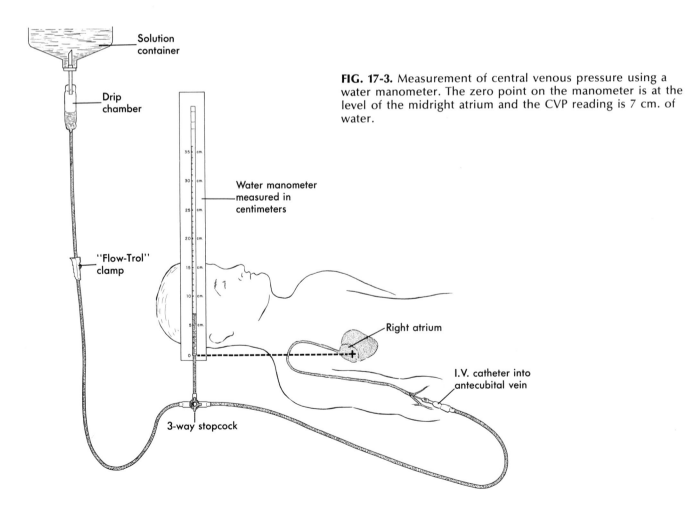

FIG. 17-3. Measurement of central venous pressure using a water manometer. The zero point on the manometer is at the level of the midright atrium and the CVP reading is 7 cm. of water.

after cleansing and application of a bactericidal ointment are helpful. Patient movement is not restricted as long as the catheter and tubing are secured adequately and intravenous flow maintained.

Peripheral venous pressure can also be measured, and the normal peripheral pressure ranges from 60 to 120 mm. of water. This procedure is used much less than formerly and the reader is referred to hospital procedure manuals for details.

Circulation time. Circulation time is determined by the amount of time it takes a patient to taste a substance such as sodium dehydrocholate (Decholin sodium) injected intravenously. The normal arm-to-tongue time is 15 seconds or less. Circulation time is prolonged in congestive heart failure. To do this test, the following equipment is necessary: a stopwatch, a sterile 5 ml. syringe, a no. 19 needle, a tourniquet, an ampule of sodium dehydrocholate, sucrose, or calcium chloride, a solution such as benzalkonium chloride or 70% alcohol, and sponges to cleanse the skin. The nurse should explain carefully to the patient his part in this test and may be asked to record the time interval between the injection of the drug and the time that the patient tastes it. Special variations on this test may be used.

Angiocardiogram. An angiocardiogram is a radiograph of the heart and its vessels made after the intravenous injection of a radiopaque substance. It outlines the chambers of the heart and the large blood vessels and enables the physician to see how these chambers function. The meal preceding the x-ray procedure is omitted, and the patient is given a sedative such as phenobarbital sodium about ¹/₂ hour before going to the x-ray department. The sedative helps to alleviate apprehension. After injecting a local anesthetic, the physician makes a skin incision over the antecubital vein and then inserts a no. 19 needle, attached to a syringe, into the vein. The dye is forced rapidly into the vein, and a series of radiographs is taken as the solution flows through the heart, pulmonary vessels, and aorta (Fig. 17-4).

Some patients are sensitive to substances containing iodine, such as sodium acetrizoate (Urokon sodium) and iodopyracet (Diodrast), which may be used as the radiopaque substance. Nausea is a frequent untoward reaction, and urticaria, shortness of breath, or severe anaphylactic reaction may occur. If the patient has a history of asthma or other allergic reactions, this test is seldom done. Any systemic reaction to the dye usually occurs immediately, and an antihistaminic drug such as tripelennamine hydrochloride (Pyribenzamine) or epinephrine (Adrenalin) and oxygen should be readily available.

Leakage of the dye outside the vein may cause irritation and sloughing of tissue. Thrombosis of the

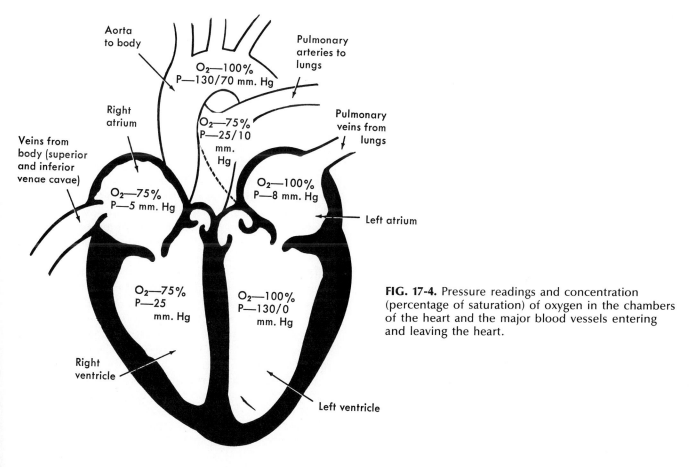

FIG. 17-4. Pressure readings and concentration (percentage of saturation) of oxygen in the chambers of the heart and the major blood vessels entering and leaving the heart.

vein at the site of the injection may occasionally occur.

When the patient returns from the x-ray department, nursing action includes inspection of incision for bleeding and irritation and recording of findings. The nurse also should include in succeeding assessments inspection and palpation of the arm to detect phlebitis or thrombosis of the vein. If this occurs, warm, moist compresses usually are ordered. The vein normally is tender, and the patient may have difficulty bending his arm. He should be reassured that this condition is temporary and that it probably will disappear within 24 hours.

Selective arteriography. Selective visualization of the aorta and its major arterial systems enables the physician to study a particular vessel closely. For example, in a patient with renal hypertension, the renal arteries including very fine intrarenal branches can be studied. The physician can study the pathologic anatomy of the coronary arteries and their branches and by this means plan a course of treatment that is best for the particular patient.

Initial preparation of the patient usually is done by the physician, who gives an explanation of the procedure. The nurse reinforces this explanation and assists the patient to express his feelings and concerns. Simple diagrams of the heart and coronary arteries (right coronary artery [RCA], left coronary artery [LCA] and its branches, left anterior descending artery [LAD], circumflex coronary artery [CCA]) usually are helpful in teaching the patient. On the day the procedure is to be performed the patient receives nothing by mouth. A sedative is given to help relieve anxiety. Local anesthesia is used and the patient is placed on a special fluoroscopic table that tilts from side to side.

Usually the femoral artery or the brachial artery is used. The site of puncture is infiltrated with procaine hydrochloride. The technique of entry to the artery is known as the *percutaneous catheter placement technique.* A special needle is inserted, and a long, flexible spring guide is passed through the needle for about 15 cm. At this point the needle is removed, and an arterial catheter is threaded over the spring guide into the artery. The guide and the catheter are advanced until the desired position is reached, and then the guide is withdrawn. A few milliliters of a radiopaque substance are injected through the catheter so that the tip of the catheter can be seen under the fluoroscope, and at the same time the patient is observed for signs of sensitivity to the radiopaque substance, such as chills, tremor, or shortness of breath. Since the radiopaque substance is eliminated very quickly by the kidneys, rapid films are taken by means of a special camera that makes it possible to take four to six pictures per second. This type of film is known as a *cinefluorogram.*

On completion of the examination by means of films, the catheter is withdrawn, and manual pressure is applied over the puncture site for about 5 minutes. A pressure bandage is applied, and the patient is returned to his room. Usually the pressure bandage is removed in approximately $1/2$ hour, and an Ace bandage is applied firmly. After 48 hours this bandage may be removed and a small strip of adhesive tape used. Providing that the patient has no local or systemic reactions to the examination, he may be up and about within several hours of returning to his room.

After the patient has returned to his room, the nurse takes his blood pressure (on the opposite arm if the brachial artery has been used) every 15 minutes for 2 hours and inspects the puncture site for bleeding. Findings are recorded and reported. Chance of hemorrhage from the puncture site is much greater than would be the case if a vein had been opened. If bleeding does occur, the nurse should apply pressure firmly an inch above the site of bleeding and notify the physician immediately.

Cardiac catheterization. Cardiac catheterization is the procedure of passing a catheter into the heart to study heart function. Cardiac catheterization, once limited to study of the right side of the heart, has been improved and is now used to study the left side of the heart also. *Right cardiac catheterization* is done when congenital heart disease is suspected, but it may also be used to evaluate certain acquired heart conditions such as tricuspid stenosis and valvular incompetence. Blood samples and blood pressure readings are taken, ECG studies are done, and radiographs of the right heart chambers and the pulmonary arterial circulation are made. The physician who obtains the patient's written permission should explain the procedure to him. The nurse should reinforce this explanation and must know what the physician tells the patient, since often the latter is not told exactly what will be done lest he become unduly anxious. Even with careful explanation most patients are apprehensive. The meal prior to the procedure is withheld. A sedative is given the evening before and the morning of the procedure, and an antibiotic drug such as penicillin may be given the day before, the day of, and the day following the procedure. Young children may be given a general anesthetic. For adults a local anesthetic is injected over the vein to be used. A cutdown similar to that for an angiocardiogram is done, usually using the antecubital vein.

A sterile radiopaque catheter similar to a ureteral catheter, but 100 to 125 cm. in length, is passed into the incision in the vein and through the vein into the superior vena cava, through the right atrium and the right ventricle, and into the pulmonary artery. The course of the catheter is followed by fluoroscopy, and radiographs may be taken at any point. An ECG is monitored on an oscillograph, and pressures can be checked regularly. As the catheter is passed through the various vessels and cardiac chambers, samples of blood are taken to study the oxygen content, and blood pressures are recorded (Fig. 17-4). When there is an interatrial septal defect, the oxygen content is higher in the blood of the right atrium than in the superior or inferior vena cava. In certain heart conditions such as pulmonary or mitral stenosis, the pressure readings within the heart may be elevated three to four times above normal.

The patient has no pain during a right cardiac catheterization, but he usually is extremely alert and anxious. He may feel the passage of the catheter, and he may complain of a feeling of warmth and of a fluttering sensation around the heart. He also may have a tendency to cough as the catheter is passed up the pulmonary artery. When he returns from the examination, he is usually quite exhausted and needs rest since the procedure takes from 1 to 3 hours. He may resume his regular activity as soon as he desires, but his pulse and blood pressure are usually taken every 15 minutes for 1 hour and then every half hour for 3 hours. Tachycardia or arrhythmia should be reported to the physician. The temperature may be slightly elevated for 4 to 6 hours after the procedure, and the patient may complain of some discomfort at the site of the cutdown. It should be inspected at hourly intervals for several hours to note any bleeding or inflammation. If a local thrombophlebitis occurs, it is treated with warm, moist sterile compresses.

In *left cardiac catheterization* a catheter is passed through the aorta from either the brachial or femoral artery using fluoroscopic visualization. After the catheter reaches the aorta, it then is passed around the aortic arch, down the ascending aorta, and through the aortic valve into the left ventricle. Care of the patient is the same as that for a patient having selective arteriography.

In addition to study of the left side of the heart, study of the coronary arteries also is done by fluoroscopy with passage of a peripheral arterial catheter. After the catheter is passed into the aorta, it then is guided into the left and right coronary arteries. Once the catheter has been placed in the artery, dye is injected to outline coronary circulation. Care of the patient having this procedure also is the same as that for a patient having selective arteriography.

Risks during cardiac catheterization are slight, although complications can occur. Cardiac arrhythmias, thrombophlebitis, and local infection are the most common complications. Right cardiac catheterization may be done in the radiology department, but left cardiac catheterization and coronary arteriography usually are performed in a specially equipped laboratory.

Memory of the experience often is vivid, and the patient can describe in detail what was done. This ability to recall so vividly may be due to the amount and size of the equipment that is used, the number of personnel needed to do the procedure, fear of the catheter and its placement in the blood vessels and heart, the anticipation of something going wrong, and thoughtless discussion by persons performing the procedure. The time required for the catheterization may also have affected the patient. The patient's tension is increased by lying rather still for several hours while procedures are done, by instructions given back and forth among physicians and technicians, by changes in voice tones of personnel, and by equipment noises. If the patient is allowed to talk about his reactions, his preoccupation with them may be at least partially relieved.

Echocardiogram. In echocardiography the heart is bombarded with high-frequency ultrasonic energy. This technique of ultrasound makes it possible to determine the presence or absence of certain kinds of heart pathology in a noninvasive manner. In this regard it is safer than cardiac catheterization; thus, whenever possible, echocardiography is carried out first and then followed with cardiac catheterization as necessary. There is no special preparation for the test, but the patient must be cooperative and able to lie quietly. The patient is positioned on a table so that he is slightly turned to his left side with his head elevated about 15 degrees. The echocardiogram takes about 30 minutes to complete as it must be carried out very precisely. The data obtained appear as lines and spaces on an oscilloscope. These lines and spaces represent bone, cardiac chambers and valves, the septum, and muscle. The oscilloscope findings are photographed and become a permanent graphic record of the findings.

Echocardiography is most valuable in determining (1) the presence of pericardial effusion, (2) the function of cardiac valves, especially the mitral valve, (3) the presence of cardiac tumors, (4) left ventricular function, and (5) the presence of congenital heart disease.

Ballistocardiogram. A ballistocardiogram is a record of the headward-footward movement of the body of a person during systolic ejection of the blood from the heart into the aorta and pulmonary arteries. When a ballistocardiogram is ordered, the patient is placed on a special table that is so delicately balanced that any vibration of the body can be recorded by a machine attached to the table. There is no special preparation for this test other than explaining the procedure to the patient. The patient simply lies quietly on the table. He may be aware of the vibrations and may be startled by them. The ballistocardiograph is thought to be more sensitive in some instances than an electrocardiograph. It may be used to measure cardiac output as well as to study the force of contraction of the heart.

Graphic procedures. Many other tests have been

and are being developed. Two of them are phonocardiography, which produces an electrical record of the heart sounds, and electrokymography, which produces a record of the border movements of the heart.

■ CLASSIFICATION OF HEART DISEASES

Heart diseases may be divided into two general groups: those that are congenital and those that are acquired after birth. Congenital heart disease follows an abnormality of structure caused by error in fetal development. Acquired disease may affect the heart either suddenly or gradually. There may be damage to the heart from bacteria, chemical agents, or diminished blood supply. For example, inflammation may cause scarring of heart valves, muscle, or outer coverings that may impair the heart's function. Any changes in the coronary vessels supplying the heart muscle may decrease its efficiency.

Heart disease may also be classified according to a specific cause such as rheumatic fever, bacterial endocarditis, or hypertension. It may be classified according to anatomic change such as valvular scarring or according to a physiologic abnormality such as arrhythmia.

Despite the varied methods of classification, progression of any of these diseases may lead to cardiac arrhythmias and/or cardiac failure. Varying degrees of cardiac arrhythmia and cardiac failure are the cause of many of the symptoms commonly associated with the various cardiac diseases, but with early diagnosis and treatment these complications need not develop.

Congenital heart disease

Congenital heart disease is discussed in detail in pediatric nursing books and will only be reviewed briefly here. Congenital heart disease occurs in about 3 of every 100 live births and accounts for about 50% of deaths caused by congenital defects in the first year of life.[91] Heart defects may be caused by heredity (defects inherent in the genes), vitamin deficiency, or the occurrence of a viral infection such as German measles in the first trimester of pregnancy. However, in the majority of cases the cause is unknown.

The nurse should be familiar with the signs and symptoms of congenital heart disease. One of the nurse's most important contributions can be case finding. Signs and symptoms of congenital heart disease may include abnormal heart murmurs, varying degrees of cyanosis, shortness of breath, generalized poor development, and clubbing of fingers and toes. The child may have no visible symptoms, such as may occur in an interatrial septal defect, and a heart murmur may be discovered during physical examination. Infants with defects such as those that occur in tetralogy of Fallot will become cyanotic soon after birth.

Congenital heart diseases usually are classified as (1) those that cause cyanosis such as tetralogy of Fallot, transposition of the great vessels, and tricuspid atresia and (2) those that do not cause cyanosis such as coarctation of the aorta, aortic stenosis, patent ductus arteriosus, interatrial septal defects, interventricular septal defects, and pulmonary stenosis (Fig. 17-5). *Tetralogy of Fallot* consists of four defects: a ventricular septal defect, pulmonary stenosis, right ventricular hypertrophy, and overriding aorta. This combination produces cyanosis, and the infant is often referred to as a "blue baby." In *transposition of the great vessels,* the aorta arises from the right ventricle instead of the left, and blood is pumped back into the circulation without having received any oxygen from the lungs. If complete congenital *atresia* (occlusion) of the *tricuspid valve* is present, there is no direct communication between the right atrium and the right ventricle. The right atrial blood is shunted through a foramen ovale, or an atrial defect, into the left atrium, where it is

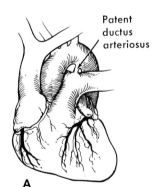 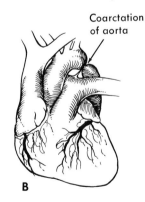 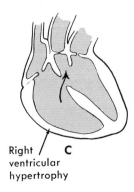 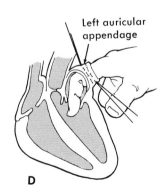

FIG. 17-5. Some common anomalies of the heart. **A,** Communication between the aorta and the pulmonary artery found in patients with patent ductus arteriosus. **B,** Abnormality found in coarctation of the aorta. Note the engorgement above the constriction. **C,** Abnormal opening between the right and left ventricles that exists when a ventricular septal defect is present. **D,** Technique used in a mitral commissurotomy for adhesions of the mitral valve.

mixed with pulmonary venous blood. A *coarctation of the aorta* is a localized stricture just below the origin of the left subclavian artery, causing the blood pressure in the blood vessels above the constriction to become elevated and in those below the constriction to become lower than the pressure above the constriction. *Aortic stenosis* is a fusing of the commissures of the aortic valve, which obstructs the flow of blood from the left ventricle. A *patent ductus arteriosus* permits the shunting of oxygenated blood from the aorta back to the pulmonary artery. In *interatrial septal defects* the foramen ovale, or normal opening in the atrial septum, fails to close shortly after birth as it should, and blood returning from the lungs to the left atrium shunts over to the right atrium. An *interventricular septal defect* is an abnormal opening between the right and left ventricle through which blood from the left ventricle is shunted into the right ventricle and is recirculated through the pulmonary artery and lungs. *Pulmonary stenosis* is a narrowing of the pulmonary valve, which decreases the amount of blood flowing into the lungs.

Congenital heart disease no longer necessarily has an unfavorable prognosis. More accurate diagnosis and evaluation of cardiac defects is now possible by means of angiocardiograms and cardiac catheterization. In the last two decades, advances in anesthesiology and surgical techniques have made correction of many congenital anomalies possible, and subacute bacterial endocarditis, one of the most frequent complications, can now be arrested with penicillin or other antibiotics. The prognosis in congenital heart disease, however, varies. Patients who are treated before development of serious complications such as retarded growth, heart muscle hypertrophy, or heart failure have better prognosis than if treatment is delayed. The nurse should urge parents of children with suspected anomalies of the heart to seek early medical care.

Medical treatment is preventive and supportive. The child should be protected from exposure to infections, and when they occur, he should be treated by a physician. Antibiotics usually are prescribed for infections and before and after dental therapy and surgery. Most operations attempt to repair the defect, either by closing an abnormal opening or removing or opening an abnormal obstruction. Unless the infant will not survive without surgery, as may happen when a tetralogy of Fallot is present, most surgery is postponed until early childhood. The operative mortality is low and the results good after most of these procedures.

Pericarditis

Pericarditis is an inflammatory process of the pericardium. It may be an isolated event or it may be a manifestation of a disease elsewhere in the body. Acute pericarditis may be caused by viral or bacterial infections, chemical changes, connective tissue diseases, neoplastic processes, myocardial infarction, or trauma. A predominate clinical manifestation is pain with fever, chills, and fatigue. Shortness of breath may also occur. This acute process may be accompanied by an outpouring of fluid into the pericardial sac (pericardial effusion). Whether this happens rapidly or gradually, the patient will experience pericardial tamponade with resulting cardiac failure and cardiogenic shock (p. 352). The general treatment for acute pericarditis is treatment of the infection with appropriate antibiotics. Surgical drainage of the pericardial sac may be necessary.

In chronic constrictive pericarditis, dense scar tissue, often impregnated with calcium deposits, forms within the pericardial space and interferes with heart action during diastole. The cause of this disease is unknown, although it is suspected that the disease is infectious in origin and that perhaps a virus may be the cause.[6] The disease is primarily one of adults; children are much less frequently affected.[6] Signs and symptoms may include all those of congestive heart failure, making it difficult for the physician to make an accurate diagnosis.[6] Chronic constrictive pericarditis may be cured or markedly improved by surgery.

Pericardectomy (pericardial resection, decortication of the heart). A pericardectomy is the removal of the scar tissue and pericardium that are adherent to the heart. The pericardium is separated carefully from the myocardium and removed. Almost at once, many of the patient's symptoms are relieved. A chest catheter is usually inserted for drainage postoperatively. The nursing care of patients undergoing a pericardectomy is similar to that of those having other cardiac surgery. It is discussed in detail later in this chapter.

Myocarditis

Myocarditis is an inflammatory disease of the myocardium, which may occur with a wide variety of systemic diseases including viral and bacterial infections and allergic and hypersensitivity reactions. It is clinically manifested by precordial or substernal discomfort and possibly shortness of breath. Frequently there is an accompanying arrhythmia such as tachycardia or premature beats (Fig. 17-6), and occasionally there is an increase in the SGOT level. The medical treatment involves treatment of the underlying disease with appropriate drugs such as antibiotics and corticosteroids and management of the arrhythmia to prevent heart failure and cardiogenic shock.

Subacute bacterial endocarditis

Subacute bacterial endocarditis is a serious complication of heart diseases. Organisms in the blood-

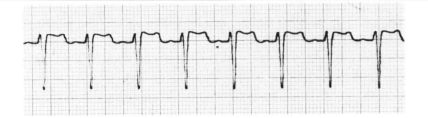

FIG. 17-6. Sinus tachycardia (lead V₁). Rate is 115, rhythm regular, QRS complex normal, P-R interval normal, T wave upright.

stream invade the heart. The valves are most often involved, being covered with vegetations or products of bacterial degeneration. During healing after active infection, the cardiac valves may become scarred, resulting in functional difficulty and eventual heart failure, although the infection itself is cured. The most common organism affecting the heart is the *Streptococcus,* and its invasion is usually preceded by rheumatic involvement of the cardiac valves or by a congenital heart anomaly. Diseased teeth and gums also seem to predispose to infection and subacute bacterial endocarditis.

The patient usually has recurring bouts of fever and malaise, often dating from an attack of "flu." He may have petechiae (small capillary hemorrhages) in the conjunctiva, in the mouth, and on the legs, and his fingers may be clubbed if the infection occurs in the presence of congenital heart anomaly. If the disease is untreated, it progresses rapidly to heart failure from valvular inefficiency or injury to the myocardium. Death may follow within 1 or 2 months of onset as a result of emboli to the lungs, kidneys, brain, or spleen or as a result of heart failure. Ninety percent of patients with subacute bacterial endocarditis can now be cured by the administration of massive doses of penicillin and/or other antibiotics. It is important to identify the organism by blood culture prior to treatment in order to aid in selection of proper antibiotics. Treatment is usually continued for 2 to 6 weeks, and the patient is kept on bed rest during this time and for some time afterward. Prevention of bacterial endocarditis by early and adequate treatment of infections, especially streptococcal infections, and by the administration of prophylactic doses of antibiotics to patients with known heart disease before and after tooth extractions and operations is extremely important. After recovery, patients are usually maintained on daily prophylactic doses or oral penicillin for life.

Rheumatic fever and rheumatic heart disease

Acute rheumatic fever with clinical symptoms follows from 0.3% to 3% of hemolytic streptococcal infections.[103] The streptococcal infection that leads to rheumatic fever is usually caused by *group A streptococci,* and almost always it is the respiratory system that is first affected. The severity of the infection and complications are usually greater in persons who are undernourished and who live in crowded urban households. Approximately one half of all streptoccocal infections do not give rise to symptoms, and the only accurate way to detect presence of infection is to take a throat culture.

Rheumatic fever is still one of the most important infections of childhood. Although mortality and morbidity rates for the disease have decreased, it is difficult to estimate the true incidence. The rates for rheumatic fever are highest among persons who have recently moved from rural to urban living.[103] Susceptibility to rheumatic fever has a definite familial tendency, but patterns vary. It is probable that both environment and heredity contribute to susceptibility. The peak incidence occurs during the late winter and early spring.

About 90% of first attacks of rheumatic fever occur among persons 5 to 15 years of age. The age of greatest risk is 8 to 10 years. It is relatively rare for an attack of rheumatic fever to occur before the age of 2 years or after 25 years of age. Since immunity is not developed by an attack of rheumatic fever, attacks of the disease can recur. Streptococcal infections precipitate recurrences in 25% to 50% of children with a past history of the disease. Approximately 20% of patients have a recurrence within the first 5 years after the initial attack, but the likelihood of recurrence decreases with age. Recurrence is relatively rare after 20 years of age.

The clinical manifestations of rheumatic fever are varied, but the most common type of onset is the sudden occurrence of fever and joint pain. Other manifestations include involvement of the heart and pericardium, abdominal pain, and skin changes as well as anorexia, weight loss, weakness, and fatigability. For details of the development and the treatment and nursing care of rheumatic fever with joint involvement, see p. 935.

Acute rheumatic heart disease is an acute inflammatory reaction. It may involve (1) the lining of the heart, or endocardium, including the valves, resulting in scarring, distortion, and stenosis of the valves, (2) the muscle of the heart, or myocardium, where small areas of necrosis develop and heal, leaving scars (Aschoff bodies), or (3) the outer covering of the heart, or pericardium, where it may cause adhesions to surrounding tissues. The development of symptoms of chronic rheumatic heart disease in later life depends on the location and severity of the damage and other factors. Probably somewhat less than 10% of patients with rheumatic fever develop rheumatic heart disease, and about one half of those with rheumatic heart disease have mitral stenosis.[26] It is possible for rheumatic fever and rheumatic heart disease with mild symptoms to go undiagnosed, or the disease may be subclinical, with no noticeable symptoms occurring. Thus the discovery of rheumatic heart disease is made years later. Careful recall of illness in childhood may include a recollection of "growing pains," confirming the likelihood that the patient had rheumatic fever during childhood.

About 20% to 40% of persons who have acute rheumatic heart disease are disabled or have life shortened from this cause. The nurse should understand rheumatic fever—its origin and its consequences in order to help either to prevent the rheumatic infection or to prevent the development of the complications of heart disease.

Prevention. Rheumatic heart disease cannot be prevented unless its precursor, rheumatic fever, and in turn its precursor, a hemolytic streptococcal infection, are prevented. Learning that group A hemolytic streptococcal infections precede rheumatic fever has led to treatment that has greatly reduced the incidence of rheumatic fever, but *primary prevention*—the prevention of streptococcal infections—still needs particular emphasis. When children, teenagers, or young adults have sore throats, the nurse should encourage prompt medical attention so that a throat culture can be taken and the cause found. By means of special health education programs, high school and college students may be taught the importance of reporting *any* sore throat because some streptococcal infections do not cause serious discomfort. Parents of younger children often are unaware that illnesses apparently caused by a simple cold or a mild sore throat can be serious and may lead to rheumatic fever. The nurse should emphasize the importance of identifying the organism in any infection of the throat. A child who has a persistent sore throat that appears red and inflamed should not attend school or mingle with other children until a throat culture has been taken and the causative organism identified.

Sore throats and other upper respiratory infections caused by the group A hemolytic streptococcus usually respond to prompt and adequate treatment with penicillin or the sulfonamides. The nurse working with the child's family in the community or in the clinic should know the condition of the child and the treatment he is receiving. The nurse should encourage parents to complete the course of treatment, which is likely to be neglected if an oral form of the drug is prescribed. When symptoms subside and the child seems better, parents may become careless and may omit the later doses of medication. Treatment should continue for at least 10 days even though clinical signs have abated.[1a]

Secondary prevention of rheumatic fever is achieved largely through antistreptococcal prophylaxis. Oral penicillin, one tablet of 200,000 or 250,000 units, taken twice daily is the treatment of choice. An alternate treatment is a long-acting, injectable penicillin, 1,200,000 units of benzathine penicillin G, intramuscularly every 4 weeks. If the child is sensitive to penicillin, sulfonamides are given. Whether or not a child has evidence of carditis, some physicians prescribe prophylactic treatment to be taken continuously for several years or longer, depending on the child's physical condition. Careful examination of the child at periodic intervals is made to determine continuing treatment.

Although the nurse and physician can stress to the patient that he should avoid people with colds and sore throats, this goal is often difficult to achieve within families with young children and among school-age children. Adherence to a regimen of the daily prophylactic dose of penicillin, obtaining adequate sleep and rest, eating well-balanced meals, and protection from exposure to dampness and cold will usually be the most effective method for prevention of further attacks of fever.

Taking prophylactic medication daily after an acute attack of rheumatic fever can be very difficult for the patient. The nurse can help families to work out ways of remembering to take the medication. It is easier for everyone in the family if the patient considers taking his medication to be part of his daily personal care, as, for example, brushing his teeth. If the medication is forgotten for 1 or 2 days, the nurse should try to learn from the family the real reason why it was omitted so that it will be taken more readily in the future. The nurse should avoid being judgmental and should realize that taking such a drug regularly can be a disturbing experience for some people. Adolescents often do not take their medication, particularly if parents remind them repeatedly and, as is sometimes the case, the adolescents feel that parental wishes are not important. Often, encouragement from a nurse such as the school nurse or a nurse in the hospital or the home who cared for an adolescent when he was ill with the fever and with whom he feels comfortable can be much more effective than parental admonitions.

Prophylactic rheumatic fever programs have been made increasingly available with the help of the Office of Child Development of the Department of Health, Education and Welfare. Extensive studies have been carried out by the Division for Study and Control of Heart Disease of the Public Health Service and by the American Heart Association.

Care of the patient. The typical picture of the acutely ill child who has had rheumatic fever and rheumatic heart disease has changed in the past decade. The very ill child with high temperature, severe joint pain, greatly dilated heart, and slow response to available treatment is now seldom seen. It is believed that improved social and economic conditions generally as well as the advent of antibiotics are responsible for this epidemiologic trend.

The treatment and care of a child with an attack of rheumatic fever is largely symptomatic. It includes good general care and understanding of the child (see pediatric texts) and care of the patient with acute joint pain (p. 935). Salicylates and bed rest are usually required. However, the length of time that the patient must remain in bed has been somewhat reduced in recent years. Occasionally corticosteriods are given to control joint inflammation, and the child is allowed up and permitted to attend school. Usually, however, ambulation is gradual; the length of time for convalescence varies according to the individual child and the results of laboratory tests.

Children with rheumatic fever and rheumatic heart disease are often cared for at home, and medical care is given at the physician's office, in a hospital clinic, or in a preventive clinic of a local health department. Unless the child is seriously ill, hospitalization is not advised, providing suitable home care is available. The public health nurse is often called on to visit the child in his home in order to help his family to plan adequate and safe care for him and to prepare him for the measures that will probably be advised to prevent future attacks. If the child is confined to bed, family members may need help in providing bedside care, including attention to good body alignment in bed and moving painful joints (Fig. 33-1). The most taxing time for parents and child usually comes when symptoms have decreased or disappeared but modified activity is still recommended by the doctor. Quiet yet stimulating and satisfying activities, games, and toys, help to pass the time enjoyably while avoiding exertion. When the child is allowed out of bed, supervision may be needed but has to be given with the utmost care to avoid frustration and resentment on the part of the child.

Children who have rheumatic heart disease are usually advised by the physician to lead a relatively normal, unrestricted existence in which only vigorous, competitive athletics are prohibited. The recommendations are specific for the individual patient and his particular situation, and they vary a great deal. If heart damage has been severe and permanent damage is likely, the nurse should help the child's parents to direct the child's interest toward activities that can become satisfying and rewarding and yet are not strenuous. For example, artistic interests developed from childhood might lead to skills that earn recognition and a livelihood or to a variety of other satisfying occupations that are within the person's physical capacity.

Overprotection by parents is sometimes a serious problem. The nurse needs to be understanding and accepting of the parents' fears and concerns and provide sufficient time to allow discussion of them. The reason for overprotection may be very complex at times, and the nurse may need to seek consultation in order to understand and work through the problem with the parents. The nurse may refer the parents to a medical social worker, if one is available, or work with the physician in seeking psychiatric consultation.

Valvular heart disease

Valvular heart disease, particularly mitral stenosis and mitral regurgitation, may develop from rheumatic endocarditis. Other causes of valvular incompetence include bacterial endocarditis, syphilis, congenital malformation of the valves, and rupture of the chordae tendineae. With valvular dysfunction, there are pressure changes within the heart as well as pulmonary and peripheral circulatory changes. The dysfunction may eventually lead to cardiac failure, cardiac arrhythmias, and cardiogenic shock.

Mitral stenosis. About one half of the patients with rheumatic heart disease have mitral stenosis.[26] After repeated attacks of rheumatic fever, rheumatic nodules grow on the mitral valve at the line where the valves meet. The valves thicken and fuse together, the chordae tendineae shorten and thicken, and the valve opening narrows from 4 to 6 cm.[2] to 1 cm.[2] or less.[26] There is increased pressure in the left atrium, which is reflected to the pulmonary vessels and the right ventricle, and the load on the right heart may lead to right-sided heart failure. Signs and symptoms include shortness of breath on exertion progressing to orthopnea, pulmonary edema, and hemoptysis. The patient usually becomes incapacitated, and without treatment death usually occurs between 30 and 50 years of age.

Treatment varies with the degree of severity of the disease. Conservative treatment includes limitation of activity to decrease the work load on the heart, sodium restriction, use of diuretics, and digitalis. Surgical treatment is used as the symptoms limit the patient's activity. Mitral commissurotomy is often the first step. Mitral commissurotomy is the fracturing (breaking apart) of the stenosed leaves (commissures) of the mitral valve, which is located between the left atrium and the left ventricle. At the present time most surgeons operate on the patient who has simple mitral stenosis by the closed technique. In this operation the thorax usually is entered through a left anterolateral incision. The fourth rib is partially resected to give adequate exposure, and then the heart is entered through the left auricular appendage. The surgeon inserts his finger through the incision into the atrium and through the mitral valve (Fig. 17-5). He then makes several attempts to release the leaves of the mitral valve either with his finger, with a special knife, or with a transventricular dilator.[26] At this point he will know whether or not the operation can be expected to relieve the patient's symptoms. Sometimes it is impossible to release the stenosed valve because of excessive calcium deposits around it or because of other pathologic conditions. If any clots are found, they are removed to prevent their escape into the general circulation.

If the operation has been successful, there will be a decline in the pulmonary pressure, reduction of the heart size, and a gradual diminishing of the symptoms previously experienced. Many patients who have been semi-invalids are able to return to a relatively normal life. In some patients, however, the stenosis may recur after varying periods of time, and the symptoms may become worse than preoperatively. The surgeon then may attempt to relieve the stenosis by doing open heart surgery. If the valve is calcified or severely deformed, it may be replaced with an artificial ball valve. One type consists of a silicone rubber ball, a cage of stainless steel, and an outer ring of Teflon fabric.

The nursing care of the patient undergoing mitral commissurotomy is similar to that of other patients having other cardiac surgery. It is discussed in detail later in this chapter.

Aortic stenosis. Aortic stenosis usually is caused by rheumatic fever. The disease attacks the valve cusps, which become stiff and calcified and obstruct blood flow. There is an elevation of left ventricular pressure and low cardiac output. Even though the obstruction may be substantial, the patient may have few clinical symptoms for some time. Some patients complain of fatigue, faintness, and angina, and radiographs may show a heart either of normal size or with slight enlargement of the left ventricle. Untreated aortic stenosis will contribute to, and often finally cause, congestive heart failure. ECG changes may be the only evidence of the severity of the stenosis.

Surgery for aortic stenosis is done with the use of extracorporeal circulation, which permits full visualization of the operative area. The aortic valve may be repaired by three methods: the calcium may be removed and the fused commissures opened; the aortic valve sometimes is reconstructed by removing one cusp and rebuilding a valve consisting of only two cusps; or part or all of the valve may be removed. When part or all of the valve is removed, artificial cusps may be stitched into normal position of the valve, or ball valves similar to those designed for the mitral valve may be used.[26] The nursing care before and after operation is the same as for patients having heart surgery for other causes.

Cardiovascular syphilis

Cardiovascular syphilis usually occurs from 15 to 20 years after the primary syphilitic infection. Since the highest incidence of primary syphilis is among persons in their early twenties, patients with symptoms of cardiovascular syphilis are usually over 35 years of age. If the primary infection is not treated, approximately 10% of persons affected will develop syphilitic aortitis or aneurysm.[6]

It is the aim of health organizations and medical personnel to treat all persons with syphilis before they develop cardiovascular disease or any of the other complications of late syphilis. Primary syphilis can be arrested. However, once syphilis has affected the aorta and the valves of the heart, little can be done except to treat the patient symptomatically. The treatment of primary syphilis is discussed on p. 538.

In cardiovascular syphilis the spirochetes attack the aorta, the aortic valve, and the heart muscle. The portion of the aorta nearest the heart is usually affected, and the elastic wall of the aorta becomes weakened and bulges. This bulge is known as an aneurysm. As the aneurysm grows, it may press on neighboring structures, such as the intercostal nerves, and cause pain. Aneurysms may also be present without symptoms. Evidence may be discovered on x-ray examination. There is a possibility that the aneurysm may rupture as it increases in size, and the patient is encouraged to avoid strenuous activities that might cause a sudden increase in the pressure exerted against the bulging vessel. Surgical resection of the aneurysm can sometimes be done (p. 388).

Syphilis may also attack the aorta more diffusely, causing aortitis. The aorta becomes dilated, and small plaques containing calcium are laid down. Patients may complain of substernal pain associated with exertion due to constriction at the orifices of the coronary arteries. Thrombi may develop along the aorta, and emboli may occur, resulting in severe complications such as myocardial infarction or cerebral emboli.

Spirochetes may also attack the aortic valve, causing it to become scarred. This causes aortic insufficiency, and the patient may have a bounding pulse and a high systolic blood pressure because of the extra effort demanded of the ventricles to pump blood into the systemic circulation. Heart failure eventually occurs.

The use of penicillin in the treatment of the patient with cardiovascular disease is thought to possibly prolong life, since penicillin destroys any active organisms and permits healing to occur. Treatment at this stage, however, will not restore damaged aortic tissue or damaged aortic valves, and extensive scarring may occur. The patient with cardiovascular syphilis should be given guidance in planning his activities of daily living and in selecting work that places the least possible burden on the damaged heart and aorta. In certain cases of aortic insufficiency, surgery is possible.

Hypertension and hypertensive heart disease

An estimated 17 million adults in the United States were found to have definite hypertension and 10.5 million adults to have hypertensive heart disease during a health examination survey.[52] Hypertension is one of the most common causes of heart diseases, and it affects all age groups. However, incidence of both hypertension and hypertensive heart disease rises with age. The patient is said to have hypertension when the resting systolic blood pressure reading is consistently over 160 mm. Hg and the diastolic pressure is over 90 mm. Hg.[6] The elevation of the diastolic pressure is of greater significance than that of the systolic pressure. The diastolic pressure more closely indicates the pressure exerted on the arterial walls by the circulating blood exclusive of the additional pressure caused by the contraction of the left ventricle, the pulse pressure.

The incidence of hypertension varies considerably around the world. In the United States the incidence is higher among blacks than among whites; it is also found at an earlier age in blacks, especially black women. Although the reasons for this are not well understood, some experts believe it may be caused by environmental factors that force the black to repress feelings of hostility and rage. Some clinicians are concerned that the incidence of hypertension in blacks is reaching epidemic proportions.

The cause of most cases of hypertension is unknown. Hypertension of unknown etiology is commonly classified as *essential hypertension.* In a small percentage of cases, causes have been found, including increased stroke volume of the heart (from anemia or thyrotoxicosis), disorders of the central nervous system (poliomyelitis, neoplasms, inflammatory lesions), disorders of the adrenal gland (pheochromocytoma, Cushing's syndrome), disorders of the kidney, toxemia of pregnancy, and coarctation of the aorta.

Malignant hypertension (accelerated hypertension) refers to hypertension that is severe and rapidly progressive, resulting in fibrinoid necrosis, especially of the heart, kidney, brain, and eye. The patient often has papilledema and retinal exudates and hemorrhages. The eye changes are rated according to severity from 1+ to 4+. Unless medical treatment is successful, the course is rapidly fatal and most persons do not survive longer than 2 years. Causes of death in malignant hypertension are secondary to fibrinoid necrosis of the kidney, heart, brain, and eyes. Thus the patient may succumb to uremia, myocardial infarction, congestive failure, or a cerebral vascular accident. Malignant hypertension is seen most often in blacks, especially men under age 40 years.

There are two main factors that control arterial blood pressure: cardiac output (strength, rate, rhythm of heartbeat and blood volume) and peripheral vascular resistance (diameter of blood vessels and viscosity of blood). These factors are directly affected by the sympathetic nervous system, the endocrine system (particularly the adrenal medulla), and the kidney. The sympathetic nervous system regulates the smooth muscle of the blood vessels, causing a change in peripheral resistance (either vasoconstriction or vasodilatation), and may be stimulated by an environmental stressor, adrenal hormones, or the central nervous system (such as impulses from the carotid sinus). Epinephrine increases the force of cardiac contraction and thereby affects cardiac output; norepinephrine causes vasoconstriction, which increases peripheral resistance.

With increased blood pressure, the vessels tend to constrict, causing increased peripheral resistance. The constricted systemic arterioles offer greater resistance to the flow of blood from the arteries into the capillaries and veins. The arterial pressure rises to compensate for this increased resistance. The cardiac output remains normal in volume, but blood must be pumped by the heart at an increased pressure to counteract resistance and thus maintain flow. Two pathologic changes occur in time. The walls of the arterioles thicken, and the left ventricle, which has to work increasingly harder to push against the resistance, becomes hypertrophied. Eventually the left ventricle may no longer be able to pump the blood out of the heart adequately, and congestive heart failure develops. Inadequate blood supply through the coronary arteries may cause symptoms of angina pectoris, or acute myocardial infarction may occur.

Hypertension may be present for years before the patient has any symptoms. Since no prevention or specific treatment is known, physicians feel that it is best only to tell patients that they have a tendency toward high blood pressure and to reassure them that it may not cause any difficulties for many years. Until symptoms appear, follow-up examinations may be suggested for every 6 months to a year. No restrictions are placed on activity, except that young people are encouraged to participate in individual sports instead of group sports lest they feel impelled to overexert themselves so as not to let down their teammates. Moderation in all activities should be the rule, as it should be for all people. Excess in food, alcohol, tobacco, tea, and coffee should be avoided, and adequate rest should be obtained. If the patient has a tendency to become overly tense, he should be encouraged to talk to someone who will listen to his problems—a physician, a member of his family, a friend, a minister, a nurse, a social worker, or a psychiatrist. The physician may discuss the problem with members of the family to obtain their cooperation in freeing the home environment of tension-creating situations, since emotional upsets increase the constriction of the already narrowed arterioles.

Symptoms appear when tissues beyond the constricted arterioles receive too little blood or when a constricted arteriolar wall ruptures. The heart, the brain, the kidneys, and the eyes most often give rise to symptoms. One of the first symptoms of hypertension may be headache. The headache is usually occipital and is commonly present in the early morning. Sometimes the headache is severe enough to awaken the patient from sleep. There may also be fatigue or shortness of breath on exertion. The patient may experience loss of vision, have a cerebral vascular accident or a peripheral arterial embolism, or develop kidney or heart failure. *Angina pectoris* is also common.

A variety of laboratory tests may be made on patients with hypertension in an attempt to determine the cause. Complete kidney and endocrine studies often are done. If the cause cannot be found, the status of the heart, eyes, kidneys, and nervous system are determined and recorded on the patient's record as a guide in evaluating the course of the disease.

If the cause of the hypertension can be determined, and if it is amenable to treatment, curative treatment is started. The treatment of essential hypertension and of hypertension caused by irreversible changes is usually palliative, and it may be divided into medical therapy and surgical therapy. The purpose of both types of treatment is to decrease the blood pressure, thus delaying the onset of serious complications. Sometimes the patient may be hospitalized, but often he is treated on an ambulatory basis.

Medical management. Treatment for hypertension includes bed rest, sedatives, antihypertensive medications, diuretics, and low-sodium and weight-reducing diets. Bed rest may lower the blood pressure slightly, and it is usually part of the initial treatment of a patient with severe symptoms of hypertension. Sedatives such as phenobarbital or diazepam (Valium) are often given to relieve tension and to foster rest. Some long-term sustaining measures for adequate rest and relaxation may be needed. Often patients with hypertensive disease are hardworking, driving, and ambitious in their everyday life. They constantly push themselves in activities. Modifications in their daily habits of work, exercise, and rest are advisable along with prescribed medications.

The physician makes a very careful selection of medications to treat hypertension. Caution is necessary not only because of the particular stage of the person's illness but also because of the possible side effects of some of the medications. An ideal antihypertensive preparation should decrease the resistance of the arterioles and lower the blood pressure. It should not decrease the output of the heart. However, no medication with these ideal effects is available.

Medications commonly used in the treatment of hypertension fall into several categories, including sympathetic nervous system depressants, such as the alkaloids of rauwolfia; selective sympathetic nervous system inhibitors such as guanethidine sulfate, methyldopa, or hydralazine hydrochloride, which block postganglionic nerves to arterial smooth muscle; veratrum preparations such as Alkavervir and protoveratrine, which inhibit vasoconstriction; ganglionic blocking agents such as hexamethonium chloride and pentolinium tartrate; amine oxidase inhibitors, which suppress the release of norepinephrine from peripheral sympathetic neurons; and the thiazides, which reduce the amount of water, sodium, and chloride in the body and may augment the effect of other antihypertensive preparations.[7]

Even with the mildest of these preparations, side effects occur. The nurse should give patients the opportunity to discuss symptoms in general and should recognize those that may be due to the particular hypertensive medication the patient is taking. Often such symptoms occur, but the patient or members of his family attribute them to his general ill health, his age, or possibly his personality. One of the more serious side effects is mental depression. Other patients may become increasingly tense. The significant symptoms to look for are described with the following specific treatments.

Rauwolfia serpentina (Raudixin) or partially purified fractions from it, such as alseroxylon, may be used in treating mild or moderate forms of hypertension. *Alseroxylon,* 4 mg. orally, is usually given at bedtime each day. It takes several weeks to obtain a maximum effect from this medication, and severe hypotension is not likely to occur. Both the systolic and the diastolic blood pressures are lowered. Dizziness and headache are relieved, but the patient often complains of nasal stuffiness in the morning. This congestion is relieved by antihistaminic preparations. Since alseroxylon may make the patient drowsy, he should be cautious while driving or working around machinery. The appetite is stimulated, and the patient may gain weight. Since the stimulation of the parasympathetic nerves causes increased bowel motility, nausea, vomiting, and diarrhea may occur. The side effects of the medication subside readily on reduction of dosage or withdrawal, but the hypotensive action continues for several weeks. *Reserpine* is a purified alkaloid of *Rauwolfia serpentina.* Some of the trade names for this preparation are Serpasil, Rau-Sed, and Reserpoid.

Hydralazine hydrochloride (Apresoline) is used for patients with moderate or early malignant hypertension. It reduces the blood pressure by acting directly on the arterioles, where it relaxes the smooth muscle of the vessel wall. It causes an increase in cardiac output and increases the blood flow through the kidney, but the latter action is often transient.

The medication is given orally in gradually increasing doses. The patient is usually started on 40 to 50 mg. of the medication a day, given in divided doses. The dosage may be increased to as much as 800 mg./day. While the patient is receiving this preparation, his blood pressure should be checked frequently. Nausea, vomiting, headache, tachycardia, tingling of the extremities, malaise, nervous tension, depression, and hypotension on standing may be toxic reactions. Any of these symptoms should be reported to the physician. Although the depression is often very distressing for the patient, the physician may decide not to discontinue the medication, since with continued treatment the depression seems to decrease.

Guanethidine sulfate (Ismelin) is a potent antihypertensive agent, which has fewer side effects than the ganglionic blocking agents. It causes a release and subsequent depletion of norepinephrine from the postganglionic nerve endings. Because of its sustained effect, only one dose of the medication is required daily. The initial dose is usually 10 to 25 mg. daily, which is increased weekly until the desired therapeutic effect is reached. Maintenance doses vary from 10 to 75 mg. daily.[7] The most common side effect is postural hypotension. Therefore the patient's blood pressure is taken in lying, sitting, and standing positions. The patient should also be instructed to sit up slowly when arising and to sit down and lower his head if he feels faint. Diarrhea is also a common side effect and may be distressing enough to the patient to cause the physician to discontinue the medication. Guanethidine has prolonged action and its effects may persist for as long as 7 to 10 days after it is discontinued. It is commonly given in conjunction with the thiazide diuretics and/or one of the other antihypertensive agents such as methyldopa.

Methyldopa (Aldomet), like guanethidine and reserpine, causes a pronounced decrease in tissue norepinephrine.[15] The mechanism for this action is not well understood, however. Methyldopa lowers blood pressure primarily by reducing peripheral vascular resistance.[15] It is used to treat persons with moderate to severe hypertension. The initial dose is usually 500 mg. daily with increments of 250 mg. weekly or biweekly until the desired effect is obtained. It is given three times a day, and the daily maintenance dose is from 500 to 3,000 mg. Although postural hypotension is not a common side effect, it can occur; therefore the blood pressure should be taken in the lying, sitting, and standing positions, especially while the optimum dose is being determined. Other side effects include sedation (usually transient), dry mouth, nasal congestion, fluid retention, and edema. Acquired hemolytic anemia has been a rare side effect. Side effects are usually relieved when the dosage is reduced. When fluid retention and edema occur, a thiazide diuretic is commonly given with methyldopa.

Pentolinium tartrate (Ansolysen), mecamyla-mine hydrochloride (Inversine), and chlorisonda-mine chloride (Ecolid chloride) are potent hypotensive agents that produce ganglionic blockage. These medications inhibit the transmission of nerve impulses through both the sympathetic and the parasympathetic ganglia, preventing vasoconstriction and thereby causing an increase in blood flow and a drop in blood pressure. Pentolinium tartrate is given orally, intramuscularly, or subcutaneously. The initial oral dose is usually 20 mg., and the total daily dose may vary from 60 to 600 mg. The initial parenteral dose is 2.5 to 3.5 mg. Toxic signs include dry mouth, blurring of vision, faintness and transient nausea, constipation, and retention of urine. The blood pressure should be taken in the lying, sitting, and standing positions before a dose of a ganglionic blocking agent is administered. The difference between the lying and standing blood pressure often determines the dose of the medication to be given.

The chlorothiazide derivatives so widely used as diuretics are also effective in the treatment of hypertension. They may be given alone in the treatment of mild hypertension or in combination with antihypertensive agents in moderate and severe hypertension. Although toxic reactions are not common, electrolyte disturbances, especially hypokalemia, can occur. Therefore supplementary potassium is often given. Foods high in potassium and low in sodium, such as orange juice and bananas, are often prescribed, or potassium chloride may be ordered. When the thiazide diuretics are discontinued, the patient may have an abrupt rise in blood pressure; thus many patients are maintained on thiazides indefinitely. The medication can be given daily or several times a week.

Diet. The physician may request that the patient with hypertension restrict sodium intake. At one time severe reductions in sodium intake to levels of 500 or 200 mg. daily were prescribed frequently. Development of new antihypertensive medications and diuretics has changed this approach to therapy. It is now usual for the physician to prescribe a moderate limitation in sodium intake together with a medication regimen. This combination works synergistically and is an easier regimen for patients to follow. Diets severely restricted in sodium are difficult for patients to manage because of loss of palatability, cost of special food items, and the common presence of sodium as a flavoring and preserving agent in American food and cooking customs. In addition, patients consuming very low levels of sodium should be watched for evidence of sodium depletion. Persons limiting sodium intake to moderate or low levels and taking diuretics should be watched for evidence of electrolyte imbalance or potassium depletion. Most salt substitutes contain potassium and some contain a small amount of sodium. Salt substitutes should be recommended only with the physician's knowledge and consent.

A mild sodium restriction, 2 to 3 Gm., is frequently prescribed and entails control of salt, baking soda, brine, and monosodium glutamate intake. Some salt may be used in cooking, but none at the table and foods very high in salt such as potato chips or pretzels are avoided. A moderate restriction, 1 Gm., requires limiting the intake of foods naturally rich in sodium such as carrots and celery as well as the restrictions outlined above.

Control of weight is a component of treatment for hypertension. The obese patient needs to reduce calories, and a weight reduction diet is frequently ordered. The physician may also limit the patient's use of alcohol, tobacco, tea, and coffee.

Surgical management. Bilateral resection of some of the sympathetic fibers (sympathectomy) may be done to block stimuli to the blood vessels they innervate. The vessels, in turn, dilate, increasing the flow of blood through the body and lowering the blood pressure. However, a sympathectomy does not always give the desired result in the patient with hypertension. Now that medications to lower blood pressure are available, surgery is seldom done for hypertension.

If coarctation of the aorta is suspected as the cause of hypertension, an aortogram may be made to determine the location and nature of the obstruction. This type of lesion can be corrected surgically, providing relief of hypertension in the upper part of the body. Another cause of hypertension amenable to correction by surgical treatment is an abnormality of the arterial circulation of one kidney. This vascular abnormality may be congenital or acquired. Renal arteriograms make definite diagnosis possible, and removal of the affected kidney or correction of the vascular abnormality may cure the hypertension. Endocrine neoplasms such as tumors of the adrenal gland produce large amounts of epinephrine or norepinephrine and may cause intermittent or constant arterial hypertension. Removal of the tumor may bring about a cure of the hypertension.

Ischemic heart disease (coronary artery disease)

Ischemic heart disease is the number one health problem of our times. Of the 745,360 deaths from heart disease in 1968, 677,260 were due to ischemia. Of these deaths, 368,340 were attributed to acute myocardial infarction, 303,810 to chronic ischemic heart disease, and 150 to angina pectoris and asymptomatic ischemic heart disease.[124]

There are indications that the death rate from myocardial infarction may be leveling off in white males. From 1968 to 1972 the death rate dropped 8.7%, from 441 deaths/100,000 persons to 427 deaths/100,000 persons. The rates also appear to be declining for black males. Despite this improvement, there were 700,000 deaths from myocardial infarction in 1974. Although the reason for this decrease is not proved, some clinicians believe that it is related to a decrease in smoking by American men since the mid-1950's.* Deaths from ischemic heart disease appear to be higher in the United States than in some other countries. It is also believed that lesions leading to ischemic heart disease are developing at an earlier age. For example, it was found that 77.3% of young men of the average age of 22 years who were killed in the Korean War had gross pathologic changes in the coronary arteries, and 10% had evidence of advanced disease.[39] Ninety percent of the persons who develop symptoms of ischemic heart disease are between the ages of 40 and 70 years. The incidence is much higher in men than in women until the menopause is reached, and then women appear to quickly lose their poorly understood immunity.

Coronary artery disease is caused by a narrowing or obstruction of the coronary arteries, resulting in a reduction of blood supply to the myocardium. In most instances, atherosclerosis and general arteriosclerosis cause the narrowing and/or obstruction in the coronary arteries. As atherosclerosis develops, yellowish, fatty material composed largely of cholesterol is gradually deposited as plaques along the walls of the arteries, causing them to become fibrotic, thick, calcified, and narrowed in their lumen. This condition may cause a temporary anoxia of the myocardium, such as occurs in angina pectoris, or it may cause a complete obstruction of the blood supply to a portion of the myocardium, such as occurs in myocardial infarction. The resultant damage to the heart muscle may cause severe cardiac complications such as congestive heart failure and arrhythmias, or it may cause cardiac standstill and immediate death. If the obstruction is only slight, the blood supply may not be reduced significantly and the disease may be asymptomic. Autopsies on patients who died from other causes frequently show some obstruction in their coronary arteries.

Symptoms of congestive heart failure may develop in persons who have had mild symptoms of ischemic heart disease or in those who have had an acute coronary attack with myocardial infarction if the heart muscle has been seriously damaged.

Although an enormous amount of research (both epidemiologic and in the laboratory) is being conducted in order to learn the cause of ischemic heart disease, at the present time the cause is unknown. Certain characteristics, however, have been singled out as being common in persons who have or who will develop coronary atherosclerosis. They include (1) family history of coronary artery disease, (2)

*From The Cleveland Press, Jan. 24, 1975, reporting a statement by Dr. Jeremiah Stamler at the American Heart Association meeting.

hypertension, (3) a high level of blood serum cholesterol, (4) gout, (5) diabetes, (6) overnutrition, or obesity, (7) excessive smoking, (8) muscular build with heavy bones, and (9) sedentary existence.[81]

Individuals who have most of these conditions are considered to be "high risk" for coronary heart disease. These characteristics of the high-risk group have been studied intensively, and summaries of some investigations are included in current texts.[39] One of the most comprehensive studies conducted (in Framingham, Massachusetts, under the sponsorship of the National Heart Institute) attempted to outline the observations and determinations by which risk of heart attacks can be expected. These findings consider age, the level of serum cholesterol, blood pressure, ECG abnormalities, vital capacity, and cigarette smoking. The study showed the following: A man in his fifties has four times the risk of attack as a man in his thirties. A man with a serum cholesterol level above 240 mg/ml. of blood has more than three times the risk of a man with a serum cholesterol level below 200 mg. An individual with systolic blood pressure greater than 160 has four times the risk of one with systolic pressure of less than 120. An individual with an ECG abnormality has two and one-half times the risk of one with a normal ECG. An individual with a low vital capacity has approximately twice the risk of one with a high vital capacity, and one who smokes has almost twice the risk of the nonsmoker.

Prevention. The nurse has a very real responsibility to contribute to the prevention of coronary artery disease by general health education of people. It appears likely that good health practices established in childhood in regard to diet, exercise, and not smoking can contribute to better health in later years and perhaps to the prevention of coronary artery disease. Formation of habits or the established patterns of behavior in regard to food and exercise are developed in the younger years and can persist during a lifetime. Poor habits well established are difficult to change, and coronary artery disease may be advanced when adulthood is reached. If teenagers and young adults can be convinced that they should stop smoking, their risk would be lessened, and they would help materially in setting a good example to younger children. There seems to be increasing evidence that exercise is important in the prevention of coronary artery disease, and there is general agreement that regular moderate exercise contributes to good general health and better functioning of many body systems. Yet many people in the United States do not exercise at all. Teenagers should plan to obtain in young adulthood a somewhat modified form of the exercise they receive in the usual school activities. Our present way of life, in which we ride to work in automobiles, spend working hours sitting down in many cases, and then spend evenings sitting in front of a television set,

may need modification to allow for more exercise.

Persons who have had physical examinations and who may have some evidence of coronary artery disease can often benefit from changing health practices, and it is a nursing function to help them make changes. Even if damage already done cannot be reversed, further damage may be prevented or delayed.

Because there is much interest in the association of coronary artery disease with a high-fat diet, the nurse may be asked for information about this relationship by the general public and patients. At the present time there is a great deal about this subject that is uncertain, controversial, or unknown. An enormous amount of research is presently under way. In addition to the laboratory work, studies are being made of the eating patterns of large units of the population, so that some definite evidence of the relationship of diet to coronary artery disease may be forthcoming in the near future. While research continues to seek answers, the nurse must meet responsibilities in counseling; emphasis should be given to the development of sound food practices, as discussed in Chapter 6. Dietary fads should be avoided. Not only are fads often expensive, but they are sometimes injurious to health.

To date it has not been definitely proved that *any* food has *any* effect on the development of arteriosclerosis, atherosclerosis, and coronary artery disease. There are some facts or circumstances, however, that appear to indicate that there may be some relationship between diet and coronary artery disease: (1) The national dietary average for fat consumption is at an all-time high in the United States, with approximately 50% of our dietary calories being derived from fats, (2) studies show that populations that consume low-fat diets generally have been found to have lower blood serum cholesterol levels than those consuming high-fat diets, and there seems to be a strong correlation between high-fat consumption and the death rate from coronary heart disease, and (3) it is known that the atheromatous lesions of atherosclerosis contain free cholesterol, that certain dietary constituents have been found to increase the concentration of blood cholesterol, that blood cholesterol level is lowered when fats containing a high proportion of polyunsaturated fatty acids (especially linoleic acid) are substituted for the more saturated fats, and that a high-fat meal induces hypercoagulability of the blood for several hours.

Cholesterol in the body comes from two sources: it can be taken into the body directly via food or it can be manufactured by the liver and intestine.[30] Approximately 0.8 Gm. of cholesterol is manufactured by the liver each day. Cholesterol is involved in lipid transport and excreted with bile salts into the intestine to participate in the digestion and absorption of fats. The complex process by which cholesterol is manufactured, distributed, and eliminated is not very well understood, although it is widely believed that the inherited endocrine system plays a definite part because of its effect on the metabolic processes. Studies have shown that when a large amount of saturated fat is eaten, the cholesterol level in the blood tends to rise. When the saturated fats are replaced by polyunsaturated fats, the blood cholesterol level tends to fall.

Since the American population appears to have a high risk of coronary artery disease, many physicians and health groups believe that the general public should modify its patterns of smoking, physical exercise, and eating. The American Heart Association has endorsed a policy recommending some modification in diet for everyone—reducing the fat content of the diet from 40% to 50% of calories to about 35%; substituting polyunsaturated fat for saturated fat; and maintaining body weight at normal levels. Rigorous changes in diet are not recommended and not all clinicians agree on the need for change on the basis of current evidence.

On the other hand, many physicians do recommend that persons from families with a history of coronary artery disease and persons with a history of coronary artery disease, myocardial infarction, elevated serum cholesterol levels modify their habits to reduce risk. They reason that a change for these groups is justified even though more evidence is needed, since the risk is high and the measures might be beneficial. Turpeinen[122] in a review of studies on secondary prevention, concluded that "adherence to a serum cholesterol-lowering diet is followed by a decreased incidence of new coronary events." Weight control, particularly reduction of excessive body fat, is also recommended.

Dietary counseling has been directed in particular to calorie control and fat control. Total caloric intake is adjusted to meet needs and to permit weight loss when necessary. The fat content of the diet is maintained at moderate levels (one third of dietary calories), and polyunsaturated fats are used. Some sources of polyunsaturated fat are corn, cottonseed, soy, and safflower oils and margarines incorporating these oils in liquid form. Oils that have been hydrogenated contain more saturated fat, as do coconut oil, butterfat, and animal fats. Recently, attention has been focused on the carbohydrate content of the diet as well, particularly on the intake of simple sugars. During the past 70 years, there has been a general decrease in the amount of carbohydrate eaten by the American public, but a dramatic increase in the proportion of sugar to starch.[39] It has been suggested that this dietary practice as well as the increased consumption of animal fats may be related to the high risk of coronary artery disease in the general population.[76,137] The amount of sucrose (table sugar) consumed as candy, ice cream, and sweet desserts contributes to dental caries and to excessive calorie intakes as well, without providing any benefit other than flavor. Limitation of sugar intake has been a recommendation in general health education counselling for years. The increase in sugar intake as well as the level of obesity and coronary artery disease in the population has some health education implications for nurses.

In the last decade, attention has been directed to the identification and treatment of *hyperlipidemia.* Increased concentrations of certain plasma lipids have been associated with increased risk of atherosclerosis as well as with certain undesirable aspects of hyperlipidemia per se. Coronary risk is related to the plasma concentration of β-lipoproteins, which carry about two thirds of the total plasma cholesterol, and possibly to the concentration of pre-β-lipoproteins. The hyperlipoproteinemias have been classified on the basis of clinical and laboratory data into five types with recommendations for therapy.[38,71] The conditions may be primary (familial) or secondary to some other condition or process. The goal of therapy for the majority of patients is reduction of the rate of development of atherosclerosis. Some clinicians are urging that blood lipid testing be done and that preventive therapy begin early in childhood.

Therapy varies for the classification of hyperlipoproteinemia, as does drug and supportive treatment, although weight control is advocated. Obesity appears to contribute to the clinical expression of hyperlipidemia, and many clinicians consider reduction to normal weight the first goal of therapy. For the patient with type I hyperlipoproteinemia, dietary fat is limited to 15% or less of total calories. The type of fat makes no difference, although medium-chain triglycerides may be used if necessary to increase fat levels above 15% of calories. For persons with type II or III hyperlipoproteinemia, the amount of fat in the diet is kept at moderate to normal levels, but the kind of fat is controlled. The level of polyunsaturated fat is increased, that of saturated fat decreased, and dietary cholesterol may be limited. Persons with type IV hyperlipoproteinemia are often obese. Weight reduction alone may reduce serum lipids. The fat content of the diet is kept at normal levels and the carbohydrate reduced. This type is referred to as *carbohydrate-induced hyperlipoproteinemia.* Persons with type V hyperlipoproteinemia are also obese; weight reduction is the most effective form of therapy and appears to improve response to drug therapy.

More work on the identification and classification of hyperlipidemia and extended trials of diet and drug therapy are needed. The nurse should be aware of this rapidly developing area and alert to new information and interpretation as the body of knowledge concerning the hyperlipidemias increases.

Coronary endarterectomy. In some instances it is possible to surgically remove fatty deposits from the walls of the coronary arteries. This procedure is known as coronary endarterectomy. It is possible to enter the right coronary artery without placing the patient on cardiopulmonary bypass, but extracorporeal circulation must be used for left coronary artery surgery.[26] A more recent development is the "gas endarterectomy." In this procedure a jet of high-pressure carbon dioxide is forced through the coronary artery after the patient is placed on cardiopulmonary bypass. The jet of carbon dioxide loosens the fatty deposits from the arterial wall and makes it easier for the surgeon to remove the fatty plaques after opening the coronary artery. The care of these patients is the same as that of any other patient having cardiac surgery (see p. 363 for details of nursing care). Coronary endarterectomy is used to treat selected patients with severe atherosclerosis in an attempt to prevent coronary thrombosis and myocardial infarction.

Angina pectoris. Angina pectoris is a serious cardiac disorder. Although it is usually caused by atherosclerosis of the coronary vessels, the incidence of agina pectoris is high in patients with hypertension, diabetes mellitus, thromboangiitis obliterans, polycythemia vera, periarteritis nodosa, and aortic regurgitation due to syphilis or rheumatic heart disease. It is characterized by paroxysmal retrosternal or substernal pain, often radiating down the inner aspect of the left arm. The pain is often associated with exertion and is relieved through vasodilation of the coronary arteries by means of medication or by rest. It is believed to be caused by a temporary inadequacy of the blood supply in meeting the needs of the heart muscle. The location and severity of the pain vary greatly, but the same pattern recurs repeatedly in a given individual. The frequency and severity of the attacks usually increase over a period of years, and less and less exertion may cause pain. No matter how mild the attacks, they may be complicated at any time by acute myocardial infarction, cardiac standstill, or death. The diagnosis of angina pectoris may be confirmed by ECG's taken at rest, after exercise, or preferably during an attack.

Management. Management of the patient with angina pectoris is based on the symptoms and is individualized for each patient. The success of the treatment in achieving a comfortable and worthwhile existence for the patient depends on educating him to live within his limitations, being guided by the pain. The nurse as well as the physican should participate in the teaching program. Since the patient often is not hospitalized, the nurse in the physician's office or in the clinic carries the major nursing responsibility for helping the patient with angina pectoris. He is taught to cease effort immediately on experiencing pain and to rest for several minutes after the pain has subsided. *Nitroglycerin tablets* placed under the tongue and allowed to dissolve in the saliva often relieve the pain by causing vasodilation of the coronary arteries. Usually tablets containing 0.4 mg. (1/

150 grain) of the drug are prescribed. Effects should be noticed in 2 or 3 minutes, but if pain persists, the dose may be repeated two or three times at 5-minute intervals. Other nitrite preparations are available, but most patients prefer nitroglycerin since it is less expensive and causes fewer side effects. Perles of *amyl nitrite* come in 3 ml. doses and are preferred by some patients because the action is immediate. The perle is crushed into a handkerchief, and it should be inhaled no more than three times. Pentaerythritol tetranitrate (Peritrate) is a long-acting preparation that is taken twice daily. One tablet is taken on arising and another 12 hours later. Isosorbide dinitrate (Isordil) is another nitrite prescribed and is available in sustained-release tablets, which last 12 hours. Nitrite preparations cause flushing of the skin because of capillary dilation. The pulse and respirations increase, and the blood pressure may fall slightly. Many patients develop severe headaches from the use of nitrites. This difficulty can usually be overcome by decreasing the dosage. Some patients use nitroglycerin prophylactically when they have no choice but to undertake some activity that usually causes pain. The action lasts for about $\frac{1}{2}$ hour. The patient with angina pectoris should always carry a nitrite preparation with him. He may use it freely since the effects do not decrease with usage, and it is not habit-forming. Many patients are reluctant to use the medication for various reasons and must be encouraged to do so by careful discussion of their objections.

A xanthine preparation such as theophylline ethylenediamine *(aminophylline)* or theobromine may be given three or four times a day to produce a prolonged vasodilation. Since these preparations frequently cause nausea and vomiting, they should be given after meals or with food.

Diet. If the attacks of anginal pain are precipitated by eating, six small meals taken at evenly spaced intervals, rather than three average meals, may give relief. If the patient is overweight, a low-caloric diet may be prescribed. The physician may suggest that the patient drink 15 to 30 ml. (½ to 1 ounce) of brandy or whiskey several times a day to dilate the blood vessels. Physicians usually advise the patient not to smoke since nicotine has a vasoconstrictive effect.

Activity. Most patients with angina pectoris can tolerate mild exercise such as walking and playing golf, but exertion such as running, climbing hills or stairs rapidly, and lifting heavy objects causes pain. The pain is likely to be evoked more easily in cold weather since the vessels normally constrict to conserve body heat. When the patient with angina pectoris must be exposed to the cold, he should err on the side of being too warmly clad. It is unwise for him to sleep in a cold room, and walking against the wind and uphill should be avoided because these activities increase the work load of the heart and cause pain.

Since excessive emotional strain also causes vasoconstriction by releasing epinephrine into the circulation, emotional outbursts, worry, and tension should be minimized. The patient may need continuing help in accepting situations as he finds them. The family, the spiritual adviser, business associates, and friends can sometimes help. An optimistic outlook helps to relieve the work of the heart. Many patients who learn to live within their limitations live out their expected life span in spite of the disease. Helping a patient to adjust to living with this disease can be most rewarding for the family, the patient, the physician, and the nurse. Fear of impending catastrophe is almost a characteristic of anginal pain, and many patients believe each episode of pain is a "heart attack." Therefore reassurance and education are extremely important.

Acute myocardial infarction. Acute myocardial infarction is caused by sudden blockage of one of the branches of a coronary artery. It may be extensive enough to interfere with cardiac function and cause immediate death, or it may cause necrosis of a portion of the myocardium, with subsequent healing by scar formation or fibrosis. A *coronary thrombosis,* in which the blood supply is interrupted by the formation of a thrombus in the coronary artery, may occur. *Coronary occlusion* is a more general term because it includes other causes of blockage of a coronary artery. Blockage may be caused by sudden progression of atherosclerotic changes or by prolonged constriction of the arteries. Myocardial infarction usually follows an acute occlusion of a coronary artery.

Acute myocardial infarction is the most common cardiac emergency. The mortality rate for a first attack is about 20%[23] although this percentage is decreased to 15% or less when patients are cared for in well-run coronary care units that are equipped to handle the slightest change in the patient's condition.[2] The patient typically complains of a sudden, severe, crushing or viselike pain in the substernal region. This pain may radiate into the left, and sometimes the right, arm and up the sides of the neck. At other times it may simulate indigestion or a gallbladder attack, with abdominal pain. The patient often becomes restless, gets up and paces about the room, throws open the windows, or has a sudden urge to have a bowel movement. He often feels that he is dying, and his skin becomes ashen and clammy. He may become short of breath and cyanotic and show signs of severe shock. The pulse is usually rapid, and it may be barely perceptible. The blood pressure usually falls, and the patient may collapse.

To confirm the diagnosis, the blood sedimentation rate and the enzyme levels (SGOT, SGPT, LDH, CPK) of the blood serum are determined, and an ECG is made. The ECG may show no changes for several days but then usually shows changes indicative of a myocardial infarction. These changes include the appearance of large Q waves, elevated S-T segments, and inverted T waves. The blood sedimentation rate and enzyme levels are elevated, and the blood cholesterol level often is elevated (p. 323).

The major objective in caring for the patient who has had an acute myocardial infarction is to provide him with physical and mental rest and to prevent complications such as arrhythmias, cardiac rupture, or congestive heart failure and shock. The damaged heart may be able to maintain basal activity, but additional strain may cause it to fail. The length of time the patient will be kept on bed rest varies. Some physicians order strict bed rest for a week or more, while others allow their patients up for commode privileges within a few days. If the patient has no complications, he may gradually resume normal activities. During this period, collateral circulation has had a chance to develop, and the necrotic tissue in the myocardium has healed, forming a fibrotic scar. The convalescent period for most patients following a coronary occlusion is 2 or 3 months.

Nursing assessment. In the acute period, nursing assessment includes verification of data (such as vital signs, presence of edema, and respiratory symptoms) obtained in the emergency department as well as continued collection of data through inspection (identification of cyanosis), palpation (determination of peripheral pulses and edema), and auscultation (identification of clearly audible breath sounds, apical pulse, and blood pressure). Nursing assessment also includes identification of normal and abnormal cardiac rhythms on the cardiac monitor (p. 345). All of the data obtained are then recorded and reported for use by all members of the health team. Within the first 24 hours the temperature may become slightly elevated, and leukocytosis occurs. It is unusual for the temperature to be over 38.5° C. (101° F.), and any further elevation should be reported to the physician because it may be caused by a complication such as a pulmonary infarction. The fever and leukocytosis are normal reactions to tissue necrosis.

Most patients with myocardial infarction will have an intravenous infusion started as an emergency access route to a vein. The nurse is then responsible for seeing that this system is maintained and that the infusion rate does not overload the patient's cardiovascular system.

Management. The nurse has a major responsibility for providing the patient with rest. The plan of care can be instrumental in the accomplishment of this crucial objective. Initially the patient is bathed, shaved, and assisted in most activities. Many patients react to this routine with tension, anxiety, and resentment. Explanations as to the reasons for this care as well as explanations of procedures are helpful in gaining the patient's cooperation, relieving his anxiety, and providing rest. Relief of pain is also important in providing rest.

The physician usually orders morphine sulfate or meperidine hydrochloride (Demerol) to be given at frequent intervals until the pain is relieved. If the patient complains of dyspnea, is cyanotic, or has severe pain, oxygen usually is given. If pain continues, the physician may order theophylline ethylenediamine (aminophylline) or papaverine hydrochloride. Since both of these drugs relax smooth muscle, they help to dilate the coronary vessels. Positioning the patient to relieve pain and facilitate breathing (semi-Fowler's position) may also be helpful.

Providing a quiet, unrushed atmosphere is a challenge for the nurse, but essential in providing rest for a patient. Visitors may have to be limited and the nurse is often responsible for observing and regulating situations in which the patient becomes tense or upset. Explaining visiting restrictions to the family and friends as well as to the patient is necessary. Although bed rest is the usual method of obtaining rest for a patient with myocardial infarction, *"armchair care"* may be ordered. The rationale behind this treatment is that the work load on the heart is lessened by the person's being in an upright or semi-upright position.[112] It has been shown that a larger blood volume tends to "pool" in the pulmonary vessels when the patient is in a prone position, and it is believed that this condition may increase strain on the heart that may be relieved by permitting more blood to flow into the lower extremities, as when the patient sits up.

The provision of armchair care does not imply that rest for the patient is less important or that activity is permitted. The patient must be lifted very carefully into a comfortable armchair or special cardiac chair for the length of time designated by the physician. Since getting out of bed has been found to be an activity that requires a large amount of energy under normal circumstances,[67] the nurse and the persons helping must not allow the patient to exert himself. He must be cautioned repeatedly to relax and to let the nursing staff do the lifting and moving, and he must be helped to relax by the calm and confident way in which they go about moving him. When in a chair, the patient must be protected from chilling, and he must be observed closely for change in his vital signs that would indicate increased cardiac work load. Sometimes a low footstool is used to elevate the feet slightly, and some patients are more secure and comfortable with a light restraint, such as a loose drawsheet, across the front of the chair to give them security when they relax and sleep.

To decrease the possibility either of further extension of the thrombus or of embolic complications, the patient who has had a myocardial infarction may be given an anticoagulant such as bishydroxycoumarin (Dicumarol) for 3 or 4 weeks. While he is receiving anticoagulants, the physician will order a periodic prothrombin time determination. The dosage of the anticoagulant is based on this determination. The prothrombin time is maintained at approximately 30 seconds, or 10% of normal.[6] If the prothrombin time should drop below 10%, there is danger that the patient will bleed profusely from minor cuts such as shaving nicks or from gum injuries sustained while brushing his teeth. Hematuria may also occur. The nurse should be alert for any signs of excessive or unusual bleeding and report them to the physician. If bleeding should occur, the patient may be given vitamin K preparations or a small blood transfusion.

The prognosis of a patient who has had an acute myocardial infarction is always guarded until about 4 weeks after the attack. There is danger of such complications as pulmonary or systemic embolism, cardiac rupture, cardiac standstill, ventricular fibrillation, irreversible shock, and acute pulmonary edema. The first 2 weeks are considered the most dangerous, and patients who survive the third week usually recover from the attack.[6] The degree of residual disability cannot be predicted, however, and some patients are permanently incapacitated with severe angina pectoris or congestive heart failure. Many patients may return to normal or near normal activity, and perhaps 60% to 80% of patients who have recovered can return to some employment.

Since the patient who has a myocardial infarction is quite likely to be in the prime of life and to have become suddenly ill, the nurse should anticipate that he may have many worries and concerns related to his business and to his family. It is often better for the patient if he is allowed to make some arrangements or at least is told what arrangements are being made. The family, a business partner, or the social service worker may be able to give the help needed so that the patient can be more relaxed. The decision in this regard, however, is the physician's. He often orders rather heavy sedation for the patient who seems exceedingly upset over business or personal matters.

The myocardial necrosis usually heals within 6 weeks. Therefore the patient may be told to remain on limited activity for the duration of this period. The program varies with each patient. Hill and stair climbing are ususally some of the last activities in which the physician permits the patient to engage, because they add to the work load of the heart substantially. Walking is considered a desirable exercise, and increased distances can be walked daily. This activity also helps to combat the weakness and fatigue that result from muscle disuse. However, a patient may be allowed to do too much for himself and to return to activity too quickly because he appears to be quite well. His appearance may also make it more difficult for the family to comprehend fully the seriousness of the situation and the very real possibility of repeated attacks or death for the patient who does not respect his condition and live in moderation both physically and emotionally. A patient may also be made an invalid for the rest of his life needlessly. Since there is evidence that exercise is beneficial in myocardial disease, return to work may be much better for the patient than a long period of enforced inactivity and leisure. It has been found that more myocardial infarctions occur during leisure hours than at work.[23]

Before the patient is discharged, he and his family should be instructed concerning appropriate activities, how to follow a pattern of living in moderation, and how to recognize when activity or emotional strain is too great. The patient should know that if he has any further symptoms, rest is of prime importance and that the physician should be contacted at once. He should remain under close medical supervision.

■ CARDIAC ARRHYTHMIAS

Cardiac rhythm, the sequence of heartbeats, is normally controlled by the sinoatrial node, sometimes called the "pacemaker." The stimulus initiating the beat arises in the sinus node, which is located in the right atrium; spreads over the atria, inducing their contraction; and then spreads through the atrioventricular junction and over the bundle branches to stimulate simultaneous contraction of both ventricles.[6] Both the rate and the rhythm of the heartbeat are usually regular but may vary under certain circumstances. These variations may be a normal physiologic response, may have no clinical importance, or may be a symptom or a complication of organic heart disease. Although some arrhythmias do not cause any symptoms, they are noticeable to the patient and cause apprehension. He may describe the sensations as a "flutter," a "turning over" of the heart, "pounding" or "palpitation" of the heart, or "skipping" of the heart. He often feels weak or faint. If he feels his pulse, he may be aware that it is very rapid and irregular or perhaps very slow. Patients with extremely slow pulse rates, however, are less likely to have symptoms.

Patients with cardiac irregularities should be urged to seek medical attention. If, after a thorough examination, the physician finds nothing organically wrong, the patient should be urged to live normally.

Cardiac irregularities in patients hospitalized with organic heart disease should be reported to the physician immediately, since they may become incompatible with life. The pulse rate of a hospitalized patient with cardiac disease should be taken by a professional nurse for a full minute several times a day to note any marked increase or decrease in the rate, the presence of alternating strong and weak beats (pulsus alternans), coupling of beats (two together followed by a pause), or other irregularities in the rhythm. Abnormal rates and rhythm in a patient with heart disease often mean that the left ventricle is not pumping adequate blood into the systemic circulation to take care of body needs. Congestive heart failure may then occur.

Cardiac monitors

It is becoming more common for nurses in general hospitals to encounter cardiac monitors. As intensive cardiac care units are established, this equipment becomes concentrated in one area staffed by specialized personnel. However, a staff nurse on a general ward may be expected to care for a patient on a cardiac monitor. It is therefore necessary for the nurse to know the purpose of the monitor and how to interpret the various cardiac rhythms displayed on the screen. This section will deal briefly with the common arrhythmias. For further study the reader is referred to more specialized texts.[2,42]

As described in the previous section on ECG's, an ECG tracing usually consists of five major wave deflections: P, Q, R, S, and T. These deflections are recorded on graph paper, with the horizontal lines measuring voltage and the verticle lines measuring time (Fig. 17-2). On the time axis, each small square represents 0.04 second; the time between the heavy lines is 0.20 second. On the voltage axis, each small square represents 0.1 mV.

In interpreting an ECG tracing, it is helpful to approach each tracing systematically. One suggested approach is to determine (in the following order) the (1) rate (2) rhythm (3) occurrence of a P wave (4) P-R interval (5) QRS interval (6) Q-T interval, and (7) the basic cardiac rhythm and presence of any abnormalities. A normal sinus rhythm, as in Fig. 17-2, has a rate of 60 to 100, a regular rhythm (regular R-R intervals), with P waves before each QRS, a P-R interval of 0.12 to 0.2 second, a QRS interval of 0.06 to 0.1 second, and a Q-T interval of 0.32 to 0.4 second. There are several methods of determining the rate. Count the number of beats in a 6-inch strip of ECG (a 6-second time interval) and multiply by 10; count the number of small squares between two heartbeats (the R-R interval) and divide 1,500 by this number; or count the number of large squares between two heartbeats (the R-R interval) and divide 300 by this number. When there are differences in the R-R interval, the rhythm is irregular. Analysis of the other parameters may indicate the mechanism of this irregularity.

When the patient is being monitored, the nurse is responsible for regular patient care, attention to the patterns on the monitor, and special care of the electrode areas on the patient's chest to provide clear

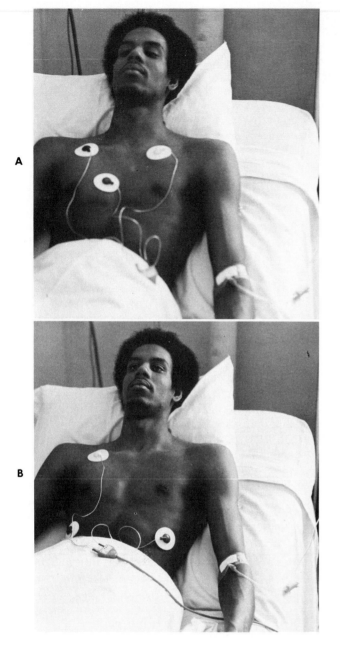

FIG. 17-7. A, Placement of ECG electrodes on anterior chest wall for lead V₁. The grounding electrode is on the upper right chest, negative electrode on the upper left chest (midclavicular lines), and positive electrode on the right fourth intercostal space (sternal border). **B,** Placement of ECG electrodes on anterior chest wall for lead II. The grounding electrode is on the lower right chest, positive electrode on the lower left chest (anterior axillary lines), and negative electrode on the upper right chest (midclavicular line).

monitor patterns and to prevent skin irritation. The electrodes should be removed and the area washed and dried at least once every 24 hours or as recommended by the manufacturer. The electrode paste and electrodes can then be reapplied (Fig. 17-7) and

the patient reattached to the monitor. The electrode site usually is changed daily to avoid skin irritation.

Common arrhythmias

Sinus tachycardia. The most common rhythm disturbance of the heart is sinus tachycardia (Fig. 17-6). It is characterized by a heartbeat of more than 100 contractions/minute and is a normal physiologic reaction to exercise, fever, fear, excitement, or any other condition in which the basal metabolism is increased, thus necessitating a greater supply of blood. For example, tachycardia is common in patients with anemia, pulmonary tuberculosis, rheumatic fever, hyperthyroidism, myocardial infarctions, congestive heart failure, and hemorrhage. The patient may be unaware of the accelerated heart rate, or he may complain of palpitations. The physician may order sedatives to relieve annoying symptoms. When the underlying cause is corrected, the heart rate returns to normal. If this condition is allowed to persist, heart failure may occur.

Sinus bradycardia. In sinus bradycardia (Fig. 17-8) the heart rate falls to 60 beats/minute or slower. A heart rate as slow as this is common in young adult men and in trained athletes. Bradycardia also normally occurs during sleep. It may also occur in patients with brain lesions and in patients receiving digitalis because of the drug's action in slowing the heartbeat. On withdrawal of digitalis, the heart rate will return to normal. Bradycardia may not require treatment. However, a patient may be treated by removal of the underlying cause, by medication such as atropine, or by cardiac pacing.

Heart block. In atrioventricular (A-V) heart block, normal stimuli arise in the sinoatrial node, but they are blocked or delayed on their way through the A-V junction. This may occur occasionally without evidence of organic heart disease or in digitalis toxicity, infectious diseases, coronary artery disease, and myocardial infarction (from occlusion of the right coronary artery).

The passage of a stimulus from its point of initiation in the right atrium to the ventricles normally takes less than 0.2 second.[6] If there is any interference in its passage, the ventricles do not contract when expected, and thus a heart block has occurred. It may be only partial or it may be complete. The patient with complete A-V heart block may have no symptoms once the block is established because, although no impulses from the atria reach the ventricles, the ventricles have adjusted by setting up their own rate. This rate is usually very slow (20 to 40 beats/minute). During the period before complete block occurs, however, the patient may have symptoms known as the *Adams-Stokes syndrome*. He may faint and have convulsive seizures, and on exertion he may feel dizzy and weak. This syndrome may be treated by giving epinephrine, 1:1,000 (0.5 to 1

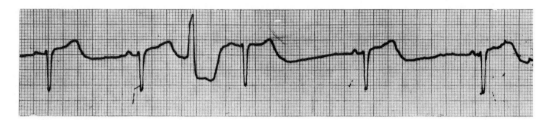

FIG. 17-8. Sinus bradycardia with sinus arrhythmia and premature ventricular beat (lead V₁). Rate varies from 38 to 50, rhythm irregular, QRS complex normal, P wave preceeding beats 1, 2, 4, 5, and 6. Note that beat 3 is a premature ventricular beat, no P wave, wide QRS complex, T wave deflection opposite that of the QRS.

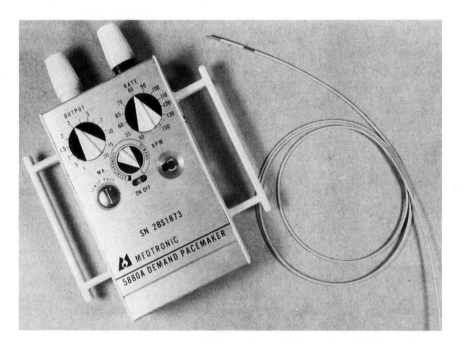

FIG. 17-9. Temporary (external) pacemaker. The pulse generator is battery powered. The electrode is passed into the heart before being attached to the pulse generator.

ml.), during acute seizures and then ephedrine sulfate, 20 to 30 mg. three times a day. A preparation more frequently used is isoproterenol hydrochloride (Isuprel), 10 to 15 mg. (¹/₆ to ¹/₄ grain) tablets, administered sublingually. Isoproterenol has a stimulating effect on the heart, resulting in better conduction of electrical impulses, an increased ventricular rate, and improvement of blood circulation. When the block is due to an acute inflammatory disorder, as in acute rheumatic fever, steroids may be given. There is some evidence that steroids given intravenously may promote normal conduction in patients with acute myocardial infarction who develop heart block.[6] Physicians usually advise patients with heart block to avoid strenuous exercise but otherwise to lead normal lives. Heart block in a patient with arteriosclerosis or a myocardial infarction is indicative of progressive heart damage.[6]

Pacemaker. The artificial pacemaker is an electrically operated mechanical device that electronically stimulates atrial or ventricular heart action, but is used most often in the ventricles.[51] It can be adjusted to stimulate the ventricular contractions either constantly and at a normal rate or only when normal impulses are not forthcoming or fall below a rate set by the physician. There are both temporary and permanent pacemakers. In temporary pacing the pulse generator is usually located externally in a self-contained battery (Fig. 17-9). In permanent pacing the pulse generator is implanted subcutaneously (Fig. 17-10). The pacemaker may be used as an emergency measure in event of sudden heart block, as a safety measure following cardiac surgery, or in medical illness when it is suspected that heart block may occur.

In temporary pacing there are several methods of placing an electrode in the heart. Usually an electrode catheter is inserted through an antecubital, external jugular, or subclavian vein and passed into the superior vena cava, the right atrium, the tricuspid valve, and then the right ventricle. Pacing electrodes also may be placed by insertion of needles through the chest wall into the heart muscle. The electrodes or pacing catheter then are connected to the external pulse generator.

Another method of regulating the heart rate is the

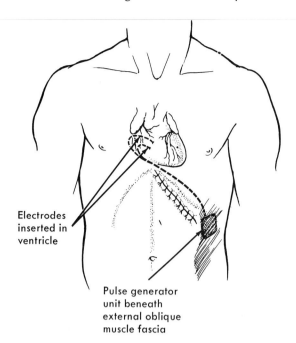

Electrodes
inserted in
ventricle

Pulse generator
unit beneath
external oblique
muscle fascia

FIG. 17-10. The pacemaker may be implanted subcutaneously in the upper abdominal area and the electrodes directed through the diaphragm into the myocardium of the heart.

use of needles inserted into the heart through the chest wall and connected by wires to an external pacemaker. Needles also may be placed in the myocardium at the time of surgery and connected by wires brought out through the skin to the external pacemaker. The ECG of a patient with a pacemaker will show the pacing stimulus (Fig. 17-11).

The maintenance and operation of the external pacemaker is the responsibility of the physician, but the nurse must understand its use and be able to care for the patient when it is used. In addition to providing general nursing care, the nurse must continually assess functioning of the pacemaker and safety of the patient and prevent avoidable complications. Assessment includes inspecting the catheter insertion site for irritation or infection, inspecting the pulse generator and electrode terminals to be certain that insulation is intact, identifying that the pulse generator is attached to the patient so as to prevent disconnection of the electrodes, and identifying the pacing stimulus on the cardiac monitor and ECG. Prevention of avoidable complications includes support of the extremity (if the pulse generator is attached there) to prevent external rotation that can displace the electrode, prevention of infection, and identification and immediate reporting of any pacemaker malfunction. The nurse also should reinforce information given by the physician as well as provide emotional support to the patient.

External pacemakers are unsatisfactory for long-term use because infection will travel along the elec-

trode wires. Several types of implantable (internal) pacemakers are available. One type uses mercury cells as its source of power and is estimated to last 5 years.[26] The unit, which is encased in Teflon, is implanted in the subcutaneous tissues of the chest or other adjacent areas of the body. Its electrode wires extend through the chest wall and the electrodes are implanted in the myocardium, usually the left ventricular wall[48] (Fig. 17-10). Another type of implantable pacemaker is a tiny, self-contained, transistorized unit measuring 6 cm. in diameter and 1.5 cm. in thickness (Fig. 17-12). The internal pacemaker delivers from 8 to 15 volts to the heart muscle at regular intervals and may last for as long as 5 years. Batteries or cells in the set can be replaced without disturbing the electrodes by making a small surgical opening in the tissue directly over the pacemaker.

Any patient who uses an internal pacemaker should have careful medical and nursing supervision. If the patient returns home, a referral to the public health nursing agency in his community is often needed. Many patients do suprisingly well with this seemingly complicated form of treatment. However, any part of the equipment may act as a foreign body and cause local or systemic reaction. The patient who develops any pain or tenderness at the point of insertion or of attachment of any piece of the equipment or who develops an elevation of temperature or any other general symptoms should be advised to contact his physician at once. The patient also should carry an identification card that states the following: type of pacemaker, rate, milliamperage, manufacturer and model number, and physician's phone number.

Sinus irregularity. In sinoatrial block the sinus node pauses momentarily, causing an interruption in the discharge of impulses over the atria and into the ventricles. This interruption is caused by increased activity of the vagus nerve and may be precipitated by quinidine, potassium salts, or digitalis.[6] It may also follow stimulation of an oversensitive carotid sinus by sudden turning of the head, pressure of a tight collar, or bending forward. The heartbeat will be irregular, and if no stimuli are discharged for several seconds, the patient may faint. This condition may be treated with such preparations as atropine sulfate, tincture of belladonna, ephedrine, and phenobarbital. Sometimes the carotid sinus must be denervated to relieve the symptoms.

Ventricular and atrial premature beats. When an atrial or ventricular beat occurs before the next expected excitation, it is called a premature beat (Fig. 17-13). The irregularity in rhythm of both the atria and the ventricles gives similar symptoms, but atrial premature beats occur more often in young persons, whereas ventricular premature beats occur more often in older persons. The patient is often aware of the irregularity, complaining of palpitation and "flutter." He may have a "catch" in his throat and a cough. This premature beat may occur only occasionally, it may occur in a regular pattern, or there may be several beats in sequence. Atrial and ventricular arrhythmias may be of no significance, or they may be associated with organic heart diseases such as mitral stenosis and coronary artery disease. Isolated premature atrial beats (PAB's) may occur in normal persons. Frequent PAB's indicate atrial irritability and may forewarn of a more serious arrhythmia such as atrial tachycardia or atrial fibrillation. The treatment may include sedation along with

quinidine or procainamide. Occasional premature ventricular beats (PVB's) are usually not clinically significant. Again, frequent PVB's indicate irritability and must be treated to avoid ventricular tachycardia or fibrillation, which may lead to cardiogenic shock and death from inadequate cardiac output. Quinidine, procainamide, diphenylhydantoin (Dilantin), and lidocaine (Xylocaine) are used to decrease myocardial irritability.[2,7]

Paroxysmal tachycardia. Paroxysmal tachycardia may be either atrial or ventricular in origin. Atrial paroxysmal tachycardia is seen more frequently in young people, and ventricular paroxysmal tachycar-

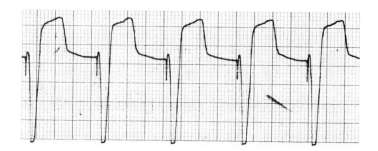

FIG. 17-11. Pacemaker ECG (lead V_1). Rate is 78, rhythm regular, QRS complex wide, no P waves visible, pacing stimulus (spike) precedes each QRS.

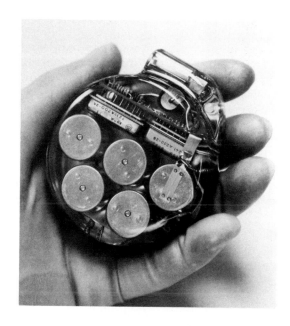

FIG. 17-12. Implantable pacemaker (pulse generator). The unit is implanted subcutaneously and then attached to electrode in contact with the myocardium. (Courtesy Cordis Corp., Miami, Fla.)

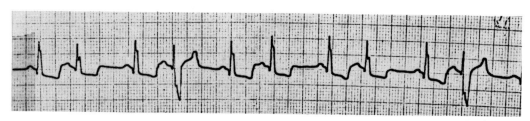

FIG. 17-13. Premature atrial beats (lead II). Rhythm is atrial bigeminy (normal sinus beat followed by a premature atrial beat), P-R interval normal. Note that P waves precede each premature atrial beat and that beats 4 and 10 are abnormally conducted in addition to being premature.

dia is seen more frequently in older persons. An attack is often precipitated by the consumption of large amounts of alcohol, by excessive smoking, by a gastrointestinal upset, or by an acute infection.[6] Both forms are characterized by a sudden onset of rapid, regular heartbeats. The rate frequently increases to over 150 beats/minute. The patient complains of palpitation and flutter of the heart, feels weak and faint, and is short of breath and apprehensive.

Patients often arrest attacks of atrial paroxysmal tachycardia by holding the breath, inducing vomiting, bending forward, or pressing on the carotid sinuses. The latter is dangerous and should be done only by a physician. He may suggest that the patient try the other measures himself. If the attack persists over an extended period of time, the patient is put to bed, and the physician may order digitalization and sedation. The treatment for ventricular paroxysmal tachycardia is bed rest and quinidine sulfate. This treatment terminates the tachycardia and restores normal rhythm. The physician may also order *procainamide hydrochloride* (Pronestyl hydrochloride), which decreases the irritability of the ventricular muscle and, when given orally, acts in 30 to 60 minutes. If given intravenously, it must be given very slowly, and the blood pressure must be taken as it is administered. If hypotension occurs, the rate of administration must be slowed down. The usual oral dose is 1 Gm. (15 grains), followed by 0.5 Gm. (7½ grains) every 4 to 6 hours. If untreated, this condition can lead to ventricular fibrillation and death.

Fibrillation. *Atrial fibrillation* is a common irregularity of cardiac rhythm (Fig. 17-14). It usually is associated with organic heart diseases such as rheumatic heart disease, mitral stenosis, and myocardial infarction, but it may follow the injudicious use of alcohol, excessive smoking, large meals, or anesthesia.[6]

The sinus node no longer controls the rhythm of the heart, the atria no longer contract in coordination, and there is a complete irregularity of the ventricular beats. The atria may receive as many as 400 to 600 stimuli/minute, but the ventricles rarely contract more than 130 to 150 times/minute, since not all the stimuli are carried through the A-V junction, and the ventricles do not respond to all the impulses that are sent through. When the ventricle contracts at a very rapid rate, there is little blood in the ventricle when systole occurs, and not enough blood is pumped into the aorta with each beat to produce radial pulsation. This accounts for the pulse deficit (the difference between the apical pulse and the radial pulse). The pulse deficit represents wasted cardiac energy.

The patient whose heart is in atrial fibrillation usually is put to bed and given either digitalis or quinidine sulfate. Digitalis acts by blocking the impulses that pass from the atria to the ventricles, increasing the interval between the heartbeats so that the ventricles will contain more blood before they contract. Quinidine sulfate restores the normal rhythm by increasing the rest period of the atrial muscles. The pulse is taken before quinidine sulfate is given. If there has been a marked slowing of the rate, the medication should be withheld and the physician consulted. The usual dose of quinidine is 0.2 to 0.4 Gm. (3 to 6 grains) by mouth. It may be repeated every 4 hours for 2 to 3 days. When quinidine is first given, the patient should be watched carefully for toxic signs since many persons are allergic to it. If he becomes flushed, complains of ringing in the ears, or becomes nauseated or faint or if the pulse rate increases, the medication should be withheld until the physician is consulted. In the patient with a diseased heart there is also the danger that the sudden return to a regular atrial heartbeat may cause emboli to break away from the atrial walls.

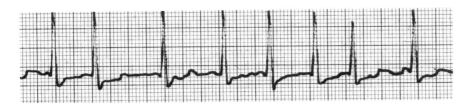

FIG. 17-14. Atrial fibrillation (lead II). Atrial rate is rapid with varying conduction to the ventricles, rhythm irregular, QRS complex normal, no definite P waves visible, P-R interval not measurable.

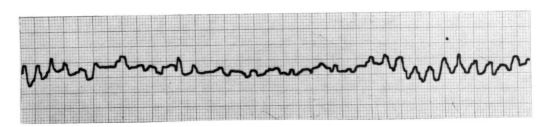

FIG. 17-15. Ventricular fibrillation (lead II). Rate is rapid, rhythm irregular, no QRS complexes, no definite P waves visible. This tracing shows electrical chaos in the myocardium.

Thrombi are likely to have formed there while the blood has been pumped inadequately.

The nurse often is asked to record the apical-radial pulse rate several times a day so that there will be an indication of how well the patient is responding to treatment. In taking an apical-radial pulse rate, one nurse counts the apical beats, using a stethoscope, while a second nurse simultaneously counts the radial rate. One must be responsible for indicating the beginning and ending count so that results will be accurate. As the patient improves, the apical beat should gradually decrease and strengthen until each beat is carried through to the radial artery and the two rates are the same.

In *ventricular fibrillation* the coordinated contraction of the ventricles is replaced by rapid, irregular twitching of the ventricular muscles[6] (Fig. 17-15). Ventricular fibrillation is one of the mechanisms of sudden cardiac death. This condition is known as *cardiac arrest* and requires immediate emergency measures. A sharp precordial blow with the fist is applied first. If this is not successful, cardiopulmonary resuscitation is begun and is continued until defibrillation is possible. The physician or specially prepared nurse will apply electric precordial shock to stop the fibrillation (Fig. 17-16). If this is not effective, cardiopulmonary resuscitation will be continued and precordial shock will be repeated. If the patient develops asystole, epinephrine is usually given intracardially.

Another mechanism of sudden cardiac death is *asystole.* A sharp precordial blow is also used in this situation, since it is often effective in stimulating a heartbeat. If it is not successful, cardiopulmonary resuscitation is begun and is continued until a transvenous pacemaker can be inserted.

■ CARDIOPULMONARY RESUSCITATION

External cardiac massage. External cardiac massage is the rhythmic compression of the heart between the lower sternum and the thoracic vertebral column. As pressure is applied, blood is forced out into the systemic and pulmonary circulation. With relaxation, the heart refills with venous blood. The physician or nurse either kneels or stands to one side of the patient and applies pressure with the heel of the hand to avoid pressing on a large area of the chest wall and possibly damaging or breaking the ribs (Fig. 17-17). The rate of compression and relaxation is usually 60 to 80 beats/minute. The patient's body should be supported by a firm mattress or board (floor when necessary) to provide the proper resistance when pressure is being applied to the sternum. While cardiac massage is being done, mouth-to-mouth breathing must also be maintained in order to oxygenate the blood being pumped through the circulatory system.

The nurse should keep the patient area clear of persons not helping with treatment. Usually two nurses working together can keep medications ready and assist in the observation of blood pressure and femoral pulse as well as obtain any additional equipment required. One nurse should check carefully for

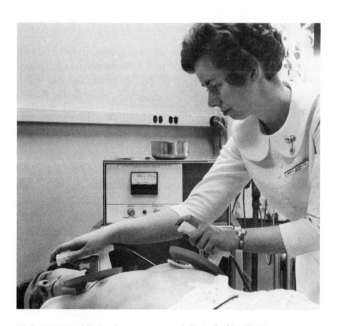

FIG. 17-16. Clinical nurse specialist defibrillating patient. Note placement of paddles across long axis of heart and saline-moistened pads under paddles.

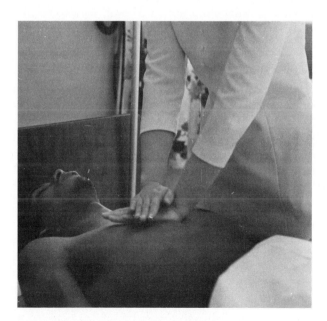

FIG. 17-17. Registered nurse performing external cardiac massage. Note position of hands on lower half of sternum with fingers extended away from ribs. Elbows should be straight and shoulders directly above patient's sternum. Cardiac board is under patient's chest.

signs of return of pulse in the carotid or femoral arteries. Constriction of pupils, occasional respiration, movement of the body, and improved color are signs of general improvement.

The most common complications of external cardiac massage are fracture or cracking of the ribs. If medications are injected into the heart, signs of pneumothorax or pericardial tamponade should be watched for carefully. They include chest pain and labored respirations. Other possible accidents are hepatic hematoma or rupture and fracture of the sternum.

Many hospitals have a prepared team of personnel, including physicians, nurses, anesthesiologists, and technicians who can be called on to give immediate and complete care when cardiac arrest occurs. Most hospital wards are equipped with a cardiac arrest tray or have access to a specially equipped cart on which all necessary items are available. Equipment needed includes an electrocardiograph, a defibrillator, a laryngoscope, a variety of endotracheal tubes, a venous cutdown set, fluids for intravenous use, a suction machine, oxygen, and a tracheotomy set. The drugs usually given are epinephrine (1:1,000) for direct intracardiac injection, sodium bicarbonate (44 mEq.) to combat acidosis, and calcium chloride (10% solution) to improve myocardial tone.

Cardiopulmonary resuscitation is now considered an emergency procedure. Formerly it was a medical procedure and could be performed by physicians only. Nurses and other persons who have received special preparation in this procedure may save a life by taking immediate action as well as summoning a physician. If nothing is done for the patient until the physician arrives, it may be too late to save the person's life, or extensive brain damage may have occurred. Very often nurses working in special cardiac units or intensive care units become very skilled in this procedure and are expected to use their own judgment in beginning cardiac massage. Nursing practice acts approved by the state or by individual hospital policy may prohibit nurses or other persons from taking the initial steps for cardiac massage. However, cardiopulmonary resuscitation is now an accepted part of first-aid training, and firemen and other lay persons have been trained in the necessary techniques.

Open cardiac massage. In this seldom used method of cardiac massage the chest cavity is surgically incised directly over the heart, the ribs are spread apart, and the heart is massaged with the hands or stimulated with an electric current. A 100-volt alternating current with an amperage of 1.5 is used. An electrically operated defibrillator and pacemaker may be used; the defibrillator stops the irregular heartbeat, and the pacemaker then restarts heart action. A combination machine, which acts as a defibrillator as well as a pacemaker and monitor, may be used.

Occasionally a patient is saved by the use of open cardiac massage, but it must be employed within 3 minutes after the cessation of cardiac function.[87]

■ CONGESTIVE HEART FAILURE

Heart failure is a state in which the cardiac output is inadequate to meet the peripheral needs of the body.[2] Failure may occur when there is inadequate ventricular filling (as in mitral stenosis, cardiac tamponade, pericarditis, or a shortened diastole in high ventricular rates), an increased blood volume, or a disease of the myocardium (including degenerative diseases, myocardial infarction, or arrhythmias). In these states the heart will initially try to compensate with an increased rate, dilatation, and hypertrophy. When this fails, the blood supply becomes inadequate and decompensation exists. With decreased cardiac output, homeostatic compensatory mechanisms come into play and the kidney works to retain salt and water. With continued low cardiac output, cardiogenic shock occurs. If allowed to persist, these conditions will lead to death. The amount of blood the heart pumps to all parts of the body varies with body activities. Under normal conditions the heart and blood vessels adjust the flow of blood to body needs, and usually the heart is not worked to capacity. Moderate activity such as sitting, standing, or walking places only nominal demand on the heart. However, when the pumping action of the heart is decreased because of some impairment, the heart may have to work to capacity to meet even modest demands.

In congestive heart failure the heart is unable to receive its normal flow of blood from the venous system and to pump out the required amount through the arterial circulation. The left ventricle does not empty completely into the aorta, and the blood that would normally enter the right atrium from the superior and inferior venae cavae cannot do so. Pressure rises in the venous circulation and the organs and tissues that are normally drained by the veins become congested with the blood that is flowing slowly against increased pressure. The left ventricle, meanwhile, tries to do extra work to pump this blood, and it becomes enlarged. This process is usually a gradual one, occurring over a period of months or years. Congestive heart failure is also known as *cardiac decompensation, cardiac insufficiency, heart failure,* and *cardiac incompetence.*

Congestive heart failure is often classified as right-sided or left-sided, according to the side of the heart at fault. Most often it begins in the left ventricle and later becomes a combination of left-sided and right-sided failure. Heart failure may temporarily disappear as soon as the mechanisms causing it are rectified. It may be present for the rest of the patient's life and require continuous care and medication, or despite treatment, it may quickly become worse and cause death.

Symptoms

The most common symptoms of heart failure are edema and dyspnea (shortness of breath). These symptoms are caused by the accumulation of fluid throughout the body and by an inadequate blood flow to body tissues. *Edema,* which is an excessive amount of fluid in the extracellular tissues and body cavities, is a common symptom of congestive failure. It may occur in the legs, the liver, the abdominal cavity, the lungs, the pleural spaces, or other parts of the body. When the heart becomes an inefficient pump, venous stasis occurs and venous pressure increases. Because of this, fluid remains in the venous system rather than circulating normally to the kidneys, where the excess sodium would be excreted. If the patient consumes more sodium in his diet than can be excreted, the excess is stored in the body. Sodium is a water-fixing ion; that is, it holds water to prevent body fluids from becoming too salty. Therefore the more salt in the body, the more water will be retained. Some of this fluid passes into the interstitial spaces and causes generalized edema.

In *right-sided heart failure* the right ventricle cannot effectively propel into the lungs the blood returning to it from the inferior and superior venae cavae through the right atrium. This causes the blood to dam back into the veins of the systemic circulation and leads to edema in the lower extremities. This edema is of the pitting type (can be depressed by pressure) and is nontender. It is known as dependent edema and almost always disappears at night, when the legs are not lower than the rest of the body. As the edema becomes more pronounced, it progresses up the legs into the thighs, external genitalia, and lower trunk. If the tissues become too engorged, the skin may crack, and fluid may "weep" from the tissues. The liver may also become engorged with blood, causing it to enlarge and producing tenderness in the right upper quadrant of the abdomen. As the venous stasis increases, increased pressure within the portal system often forces fluid through the blood vessels into the abdominal cavity. This is known as *ascites.* As much as 8,000 or 10,000 ml. (8 to 10 quarts) or more of serous fluid may accumulate in the abdominal cavity. The accumulation may cause severe respiratory distress as a result of elevation of the diaphragm, and a paracentesis may be necessary.

In *left-sided heart failure* the weakened left ventricle of the heart cannot effectively pump into the arterial circulation the oxygenated blood coming from the lungs through the pulmonary veins into the left atrium. This causes the blood to dam back into the pulmonary vessels so that serous fluid is pushed out into the pulmonary tissues, causing *pulmonary edema* and *pleural effusion.* The fluid may be present in the lower interstitial tissues of the lungs, in the alveoli of the lungs, in the bronchioles, or in the lower pleural cavity. *Dyspnea,* or shortness of breath, is an early symptom of left-sided congestive heart failure. It is caused by a decreased vital capacity because of the fluid level in the lungs. Dyspnea may occur or may become worse only on physical exertion such as climbing stairs, walking up an incline, or walking against a wind, since these activities require increased amounts of oxygen. Sometimes dyspnea occurs on lying down. This type is called *orthopnea.* When the patient is lying flat on his back, there is decreased vital capacity, and the blood volume to the pulmonary vessels is increased. Patients with orthopnea often must sleep propped upright in bed or in a chair. Although orthopnea may occur immediately after lying down, it often does not occur until several hours later, when it causes the patient to wake up with severe dyspnea and coughing. This condition is known as *paroxysmal nocturnal dyspnea* and is probably triggered by such things as a nightmare, a noise, or a full bladder, which causes the output of the right ventricle to be increased for a short time and increases the need for oxygen.[6]

In cardiac failure the patient may have alternating periods of apnea and *hyperpnea* (Cheyne-Stokes respirations). Often, because of respiratory insufficiency, an insufficient amount of oxygen is carried by the blood to the brain. Oxygen insufficiency makes the respiratory center in the brain insensitive to the normal amounts of carbon dioxide in the arterial blood, and respiration ceases until either the carbon dioxide content in the arterial blood increases enough to stimulate the respiratory center or until the oxygen level in the blood drops to a level that is low enough to stimulate the respiratory center. The carbon dioxide content of the arterial blood is also decreased by the periods of overbreathing. Periodic overbreathing often begins as the patient goes to sleep and decreases as sleep deepens and ventilation decreases.[6] Morphine sulfate may relieve Cheyne-Stokes respirations because it slows the respiratory rate. Usually the physician does not prescribe high concentrations of oxygen for this condition because this would prevent the reflex stimulus caused by low oxygen content in the blood, which is actually what stimulates the patient to start to breathe again.

Pulmonary edema caused by left-sided heart failure may be very severe, and moist rales (moist breath sounds) sometimes may be heard across the room. This condition is known as *acute pulmonary edema.* The patient is extremely dyspneic, is apprehensive and struggles for breath, has a persistent cough and may expectorate frothy or even blood-tinged sputum, is usually cyanotic, and his heart pounds rapidly. Acute pulmonary edema is a medical emergency, since, if it is not immediately treated, the patient may "drown" in his own secretions. Treatment will be discussed more fully later in this chapter.

A persistent hacking cough and expectoration of mucoid material are frequent symptoms of left-sided heart congestion. They are usually caused by the congestion of the lungs and bronchi. Cardiac pain is not common in congestive heart failure, although some patients develop discomfort in the chest on lying down. This discomfort is often described as a "heavy feeling" or a "feeling of pressure" and arises in patients with a diseased heart that is sensitive to a deficiency in the oxygen content in the coronary circulation because the blood is less completely oxygenated when the patient is lying flat than when he is sitting, standing, or even walking.

Fatigue is also a common sign of congestive failure and is one of the earliest signs to develop. The patient notices that he becomes tired following activities that ordinarily would not tire him. This fatigue results from the impaired circulation of blood to the tissues and from the consequent lack of sufficient oxygen and nutrients for the needs of the cells. In addition, the inadequate blood supply does not carry off wastes with sufficient speed to permit optimum muscle function.

Because of the edema, weight loss may not be noticed in patients with congestive heart failure. Often 5 to 10 kg. (11 to 22 pounds) of fluid may be retained. The patient, however, may have lost much muscle tissue because of inadequate nutrition. On reduction of the edema he may appear as emaciated as a patient with an advanced malignancy.[6]

Management

Medical authorities[6] state that the principles of treatment for congestive heart failure are to bring back into balance the demand for blood and the supply of blood and to remove and thereafter to prevent the accumulation of excess fluid and excess blood volume when the output of the heart cannot be made to meet normal requirements of the body. These objectives are accomplished by reducing the requirements of the body for oxygen, by increasing the cardiac output, and by eliminating the edema.

Rest. Physicians do not agree on the amount of rest the patient should have or the activity permitted. The body's oxygen requirements can best be reduced by providing the patient with both physical and mental rest. The patient with congestive heart failure is usually kept in a sitting or semisitting position in bed or in a chair until he is free from the signs and symptoms of the disease; that is, until the heart rate has been slowed, venous engorgement has disappeared, dyspnea and orthopnea have lessened, pleural effusion, ascites, and generalized tissue edema have decreased, and the liver has become smaller and is no longer tender. The time required

may be days, weeks, or months. If the attack is mild, with only edema of the legs or minimal signs of pulmonary edema, the patient may be treated on an ambulatory basis with only a regimen of less activity and more rest than usual. If the attack is severe, however, a program of strict bed rest may be maintained for some time.

Rest may be difficult to provide, and sometimes it takes the ingenuity of all persons concerned to obtain it for the patient. Providing rest is one of the major responsibilities of the nurse in caring for the patient who is acutely ill with congestive heart failure. A restless, anxious, disturbed patient cannot rest, and the nurse must employ measures that will help such a patient to relax.

The patient's environment is very important. In many hospitals where intensive care units or coronary units are available the patient who is seriously ill will be under the constant surveillance and attention of an especially skilled team of nurses and physicians. However, many institutions do not have special facilities, or the physician prefers that the patient be in a quieter environment, and the patient will receive care in the usual patient room accommodations. If possible, he should be in a room alone, where the atmosphere of quiet and relaxation can be maintained. Many patients relax better if a close family member stays with them.

Almost every patient in cardiac failure is extremely apprehensive and anxious, both about his own physical condition and about the welfare of his family. Many times the physician feels that it is best to tell the patient what he wishes to know, because an explanation will often quiet him. Visitors should be prohibited with the exception of close family members or significant others designated by the patient. However, if their presence disturbs the patient, the physician or nurse should explain the situation to the family and gain their cooperation. In any case the family should be kept well informed of the patient's condition. Members of the family should be encouraged not to worry him, but mention of daily problems should not be avoided since he may suspect that information is being withheld. No news often is worse than bad news, and the patient may imagine that conditions are much worse than they are.

The nurse should listen carefully to the patient to find out what concerns him and makes it difficult for him to rest. The acutely ill cardiac patient should be visited often in order to give him a chance to mention worries that are interfering with rest and sleep. Evening and night hours may be particularly stressful if the patient is worried. It may help if he can be in daily contact with a social worker to whom he can talk about his family, his job, and his plans for the future. Although the social worker will not make extensive plans with him at this time, immediate problems often can be taken care of, thus helping to relieve his mind. Visits from a spiritual adviser may be quieting to some patients. Visits from other patients who are progressing satisfactorily from the same condition sometimes give reassurance. Reading, watching television, and listening to the radio for short periods of time may be relaxing for some patients. Others find these activities very distracting, so that provisions for patients should be made on an individual basis. Occupational therapy that does not require extensive arm movements and that is not so intricate as to tire the patient may be a valuable pastime as the patient improves.

Weighing the patient. Although careful records of intake and output are kept on most patients with cardiac failure, the physician often relies more heavily on the patient's changes in weight to estimate his progress and his response to prescribed diet, medications, or other forms of treatment. The patient's weight should be carefully recorded on admission, after which time the physician orders how often he wishes the patient weighed and what procedure can be used. Some hospitals have large cart scales on which a stretcher has been placed; the patient may be moved to the stretcher by other persons without exertion on his part. Other hospitals have portable scales that can be brought to the bedside easily. The patient should be weighed at the same time each day with the same amount of clothing on.

Sedatives. The patient should have adequate sleep, and it is better for him to sleep at night and to be awake during the day. Cardiac patients are likely to be apprehensive. Phenobarbital, 30 to 60 mg. ($\frac{1}{2}$ to 1 grain), or diazepam (Valium), 2 to 10 mg. three times a day and at bedtime, may be ordered by the physician. Whiskey, 30 to 60 ml. (1 to 2 ounces), at bedtime may be ordered to increase the effectiveness of the barbiturates. For older patients and for patients with renal damage, paraldehyde by mouth, by rectum, or by intramuscular injection may be necessary. Chloral hydrate may also be used. If the patient is unable to sleep, time should be taken to talk with him, and nursing measures such as rubbing his back and straightening the bedclothes may help him to relax. It is usually impossible to give warm milk because of fluid and sodium restrictions, but if this measure seems desirable, it may be possible to plan with the dietitian to include warm milk in the patient's diet. Sometimes other warm fluids may be given when milk is not permitted.

If dyspnea under sedation is marked, if the patient complains of pain, or if he is very restless and anxious, the physician may order morphine sulfate, 10 mg. ($\frac{1}{6}$ grain). If necessary, it may be given as often as every 4 hours for 2 or 3 days. The nurse should give it before the patient becomes agitated, since worry and excitement normally cause constriction of the blood vessels, which increases the heart rate. Although a normal heart can accommodate to

an increase in pressure and activity, the diseased heart may be overburdened by it. Some patients are allergic to morphine sulfate and develop nausea and vomiting. The physician may then order meperidine hydrochloride (Demerol) or pantopium (Pantopon). Excessive sedation is to be avoided, especially in the elderly, since immobility increases the risk of venous thrombosis or embolism.[6]

Position in bed. A comfortable position in bed can best be determined by the patient. Since no two patients are alike, the nurse must be guided by the patient's habit patterns and his symptoms in finding a position that is most conducive to rest. Most patients with congestive heart failure are more comfortable and can breathe more easily with the head of the bed elevated in a high Fowler's position. A pillow may be placed lengthwise behind the shoulders and back in such a manner that full expansion of the rib cage is possible (Fig. 17-18). The patient who is in proper position for comfortable breathing will also be in correct body alignment. A foot block may help to prevent the patient from slipping toward the foot of the bed. Patients who must be in a high Fowler's position are usually more comfortable and have less pull on their shoulder muscles if pillows are used to support the lower arms. A small pillow slipped under the small of the back also may make the patient more comfortable. If the patient must remain upright all the time, his position may be changed occasionally

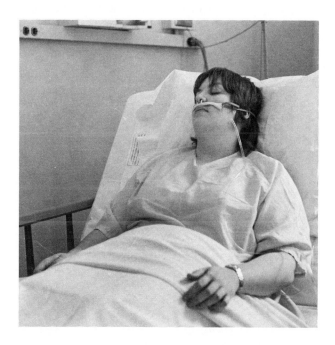

FIG. 17-18. A pillow placed under a patient's head and shoulders with the head of the bed in Fowler's position provides comfort and support for the patient with congestive heart failure. Pillows under the arms may provide additional comfort for some patients.

by allowing him to rest his head and arms on pillows placed on an overbed table pulled up close to him (Fig. 22-13). Both the pillows and the table should be tied to prevent them from slipping. Side rails should be kept on the bed to give the patient something firm on which to hold during changes of position and to prevent accidents.

Oxygen. The patient with congestive heart failure may be more comfortable and rest better when receiving oxygen, since it helps to relieve the dyspnea and cyanosis by providing a higher concentration of oxygen in the bloodstream. Oxygen is usually administered by nasal cannula at 4 to 6 L./minute. Whenever oxygen therapy is used, provision must be made for humidity to be added to the oxygen system, since oxygen is very drying and irritating to the mucous membrane. In cardiac failure the oxygen content of the bloodstream may be markedly reduced because of the less effective oxygenation of the blood as it passes through the congested lungs.

If acute pulmonary edema occurs, a high concentration of oxygen under pressure may be given by means of a positive pressure mask. This helps to prevent further transudation of serum from the pulmonary capillaries by exerting pressure on the pulmonary epithelium during expiration. The physician must determine the concentration of oxygen, the desired pressure, and the frequency of use. Oxygen concentrations of 50% to 100% are usually given at a pressure of 3 to 4 ml. of water, and later, although the oxygen is continued, the positive pressure may be used only every 1 to 4 hours for a short period of time. The patient receiving this treatment needs attention to the skin where pressure from the mask may cause irritation. The skin should be massaged, sponged, and powdered between treatments if they continue for some time. The nurse must protect the patient with pulmonary edema from *any* exertion since any activity increases the body's need for oxygen.

Activity. Restricted physical activity is necessary for the patient with congestive heart failure, and the nurse should find out from the physician how much activity the patient may be allowed. Some patients are not even permitted to turn or to feed themselves. Because dependence on nursing personnel for even these simple tasks is disturbing to some patients, the tasks should be carried out without apparent rush, and the patient's needs should be anticipated so that he will not have to ask for help. If it is evident that the patient simply cannot accept complete dependence on the nursing staff, the physician should be consulted. Occasionally it is better to let the patient do some things for himself.

Most patients with heart failure are not allowed to bathe themselves, and while they are acutely ill, they should not be disturbed more than is necessary for their safety and comfort. If special attention is given to the back and to bony prominences, a partial bath may suffice for several days. The patient's head often cannot be lowered to change bedclothes; thus, when the lower sheets need changing or tightening, he may need to be supported in an upright position while the head of the bed is lowered and made. The sheets are often more easily changed from the top to the bottom than from side to side. A recent study suggests that patients with cardiac disease consume more oxygen during bedmaking from top to bottom than when the head rest is at a 45-degree angle and the patient is turned from side to side as in the standard bedmaking procedure.[34] Since the study was done on a limited sample, further investigation is needed. However, this may be an example of a nursing procedure that needs changing to be in accord with the latest scientific evidence. The procedure to be used with a given patient should be based on an assessment of the patient's physiologic response to changes in position. These observations should be shared with the physican. If the patient is permitted to use a commode once a day, the bed can be changed at this time. Occasionally it seems best to have several people lift the patient to a stretcher and support him in a sitting position while the bed is completely changed. Some hospitals have special cardiac chairs that can be changed from a flat position, like that of a stretcher, to an upright position with a foot rest. These are very helpful in the care of the patient in heart failure, since the patient can be moved readily onto the flat surface and then the chair can be elevated to a comfortable upright position.

If the patient must remain on complete bed rest, he should move his legs about occasionally and tighten and relax his leg muscles to help prevent phlebitis and muscle wasting. While the patient is being bathed, the joints should be put through the complete range of motion (see Figs. 1-2 to 1-4). When the patient is acutely ill, this procedure should be done by the nurse while the patient remains passive. Later, when he is convalescing, he is taught to do the procedure without help. The patient also may be encouraged to breathe deeply 5 to 10 times every 1 or 2 hours to expand the lungs and help to prevent hypostatic pneumonia.

Skin care. Since there may be generalized edema, special skin care should be given to the patient. The patient may be thin, malnourished, or elderly. Bony prominences should be inspected carefully for any signs of irritation and should be massaged frequently. The elbows should be observed carefully, and a lubricant should be applied to the skin, since irritation often occurs, especially if the patient must be kept in high Fowler's position. Patients also easily develop decubiti in the sacral region because of continual pressure and the edema caused by the upright position. Only light, plastic, waterproof materials should be used for protecting the mattress. Soft tissue areas are not massaged without an order from the physician. It is best to use an alternating air-pressure mattress or a sponge-rubber mattress, but if neither type is available, pieces of sponge rubber, Gelfoam pads, or sheepskin are very helpful when placed under areas receiving pressure.

Nutrition. The nurse should try to make mealtime as pleasant an occasion as possible. Few people like to be fed, and the appetite of a patient with heart failure may be poor. During the acute stage of congestive failure, the diet should be soft or liquid, and the foods served should be easily digested. Edema is often effectively controlled in patients with heart failure by restriction of sodium intake. The degree of restriction depends on the severity of the failure. In mild failure, sodium may be restricted to 1 to 2 Gm./day.[130] The normal diet contains 3 to 6 Gm. of sodium/day. This diet is essentially normal except that no extra salt is added to prepared foods. If this measure does not control the edema, however, salt may be restricted to as little as 250 mg. of sodium chloride a day. Because it is difficult to maintain an adequate protein intake on a sodium-restricted diet, a very low-sodium milk such as Lanalac may be necessary to supplement the diet. Since the vitamin B intake may also be inadequate because of low protein in a sodium-restricted diet, vitamin supplements are usually ordered. A diet with a very low sodium content is unpalatable and expensive. If the patient does not have kidney involvement, the physician may permit the use of salt substitutes such as potassium chloride. (See p. 369 for suggestions for making sodium-restricted diets more palatable.) If the patient is on diuretic drugs, sodium may not be limited below 3 to 5 Gm. because of the danger of sodium chloride depletion in the blood (p. 115).

Fluids are often limited to 1,800 ml./day for patients with congestive heart failure. Such patients may have only about 6 glasses of fluid a day (including fluids used to administer oral medications) in addition to fluids contained in food. Canned soups are usually not served because they tend to be high in sodium content. Watery foods also must be restricted because they may appreciably increase the fluid intake. If the patient finds this degree of fluid restriction intolerable, the nurse should be sure that foods that might make him more thirsty are not being served, that fluids are spaced throughout the day, and that he is given frequent mouth care, using an iced mouthwash.

Some physicians feel that fluids need not be limited as long as the patient is on a restricted-sodium diet and is receiving diuretics and digitalis. They feel that under these circumstances fluids actually act as a diuretic and are beneficial in helping to remove fluids from the tissues. The nursing care would then be adjusted to this theory, and fluids would be urged.

The reason for diet and fluid restrictions should be explained to both the patient and his family so that the patient does not become unduly upset and so that the family does not bring him food or fluids that are unacceptable. The patient often must continue the diet and fluid restrictions after discharge from the hospital. Therefore, when he feels better, mealtime may be used to teach him about the type of foods he may include in his diet at home. If he does not eat well, efforts should be made to find food preparations that he will eat in order to maintain normal nutrition. Coffee, tea, and very hot or cold (iced) fluids are usually restricted because of their stimulating effects.

The work of the heart is increased during digestion, since blood is needed by the digestive tract for its functions. Several small meals a day may be better tolerated than three large meals. When the patient is allowed to feed himself, his appetite may improve as his morale improves with the feeling that he is making progress toward recovery.

Elimination. It is advisable for the patient with cardiac disease to avoid straining at defecation since it places an extra burden upon the heart. The feces are kept soft by giving daily a mild cathartic such as milk of magnesia, a mild bulk cathartic such as psyllium (Metamucil), or a stool-softening agent such as dioctyl sodium sulfosuccinate (Colace). If an oil enema is necessary, it should be given with a small rectal tube inserted only 3 to 4 inches. Most patients dislike using the bedpan, and the effort required to get onto the pan and to maintain a satisfactory position on it often puts a real strain on the heart. Some physicians prefer that the patient slide off the bed onto the commode to have a bowel evacuation. The desirability of using a commode depends on the size of the patient and his condition. Commodes raised to bed height, so that little moving is necessary to get the patient onto them, are now available. The patient with cardiac disease should not be left alone when on the commode or a bedpan, although the nurse or attendant may leave the room or step outside the curtain to give privacy. The patient should never be made to feel hurried.

Ambulation. Ambulation for the patient recovering from acute congestive heart failure is started slowly to avoid overburdening the heart and to determine how much activity the heart can tolerate without again showing signs of failure. The regimen varies according to each patient and according to the physician's orders. Even older patients who are acutely ill may be put on a modified schedule of bed rest after only a few days to prevent the development of circulatory or other complications.[98] The physician may wish them to be out of bed in a chair for several hours a day.

The usual procedure for ambulation is to have the patient dangle his legs from the side of the bed for

15 minutes twice a day. He then may progress to sitting in a chair at the side of the bed twice a day for gradually increasing periods of time. When dangling, the patient should have support at his back and a chair on which to place his feet if he so desires. If being up in a chair is tolerated well by the patient, walking is then permitted. It should also be increased very gradually and should be closely supervised. The patient may tolerate only a few steps around his room the first few times he walks. The activity permitted is increased slowly, and most patients are fairly self-sufficient before discharge from the hospital, usually having climbed stairs, taken a bath or shower, and performed all the activities of daily living.

The patient should be observed closely during his progress in ambulation. The nurse should be alert for signs of fatigue, increased pulse rate, and dyspnea. If at any point the patient shows that he cannot tolerate the activity, or if he shows signs of distress, he should return to bed. If he is at all dyspneic, the head of the bed should be elevated. The physician should be consulted before further ambulation is attempted. The plan for ambulation should be explained to both the patient and his family. They should understand that if activity tires the patient excessively, it may be curtailed. Overactivity can produce physical and mental setbacks that delay ultimate recovery. In the early stage of ambulation it is important to begin stressing to the patient the importance of rate of activity; that is, the demand on the heart is decreased when a normal activity is performed more slowly than before.

Digitalization. When digitalis, one of its derivatives, or a drug with similar action on the heart muscles is given to a patient with heart failure, the cardiac rate decreases and the contraction of the heart muscles become stronger, increasing the cardiac output and thereby producing improvement of all symptoms of heart failure. Over a period of 24 to 48 hours, the physician may order that the patient with congestive heart failure be given an amount of digitalis that will slow the ventricular rate to between 70 and 75 beats/minute. This amount of digitalis is called a *digitalizing dose,* or the *optimum therapeutic dose.* In some instances this amount of digitalis may approach the toxic level, and the nurse should watch the patient carefully for symptoms of toxicity. These include slowing of the pulse, irregular rhythm, loss of appetite, nausea and vomiting, mental confusion, and yellow discoloration of the conjunctivae and the skin. The nurse should be especially alert for these symptoms when the heart and circulation return to normal under treatment because the full effects of these drugs will then be realized. Since digitalis preparations have a cumulative effect and are slowly eliminated, early recognition of toxic symptoms and discontinuance of the drug will decrease their severity and duration.

After the optimum therapeutic dose has been determined, the patient is placed on a daily maintenance dose of digitalis. The selection of a particular preparation of this drug is determined by the rapidity of action desired, the route by which it is to be given, and the response of the patient.

Before a digitalis preparation is given, the pulse rate should be taken. If the radial rate is below 60, the apical rate should be taken. If this rate also is below 60, the medication should be withheld until the physician has been consulted. The pulse rate of patients with cardiac disease should always be taken for a full minute since the pulse may be irregular. The patient who is being digitalized usually is placed on recorded fluid intake and output, and, if possible, he is weighed before treatment is started and daily thereafter. A record of daily weight is a helpful guide to the physician in determining whether edema is being decreased. The weight should be taken at the same time each day, preferably early in the morning, since it is more accurate before the patient has eaten or has had a bowel movement. The patient's color, the amount of edema, and the amount of dyspnea should also be observed and recorded. When the color is otherwise normal, cyanosis may be noticeable in the nail beds, the earlobes, and the lips.

The nurse should be familiar with the usual dosage of the digitalis preparation being given. Since these preparations are very potent and thus are given in small units, an overdose is extremely serious. Many of the preparations have similar names, and some come in milligram doses whereas others come in gram doses. An error between 0.1 Gm. and 0.1 mg. might mean that the patient would be given 1,000 times the dose ordered.

Powdered digitalis, or the whole leaf digitalis, is a potent oral preparation to which many patients develop toxic reactions. Usually 1.5 Gm. (22 grains) of the medication is given in divided doses over a period of 24 to 48 hours in order to achieve initial digitalization. The usual maintenance dose is 0.1 Gm./day.

Several types of purified glycosides of digitalis have been developed for use when the patient cannot tolerate powdered digitalis. The effects are the same, but the speed of action and the rate of elimination are different. Although the toxic symptoms are the same, severe toxicity is less likely to occur.

Digitoxin is a glycoside of digitalis. It may be ordered under the following names: Purodigin, Digitaline nativelle, Crystodigin, and Unidigin. Digitoxin is excreted slowly. The usual digitalizing dose is 1.5 mg. ($^1/_{40}$ grain) given over a period of 24 to 48 hours. The maintenance dose is 0.1 or 0.2 mg. ($^1/_{600}$ to $^1/_{300}$ grain) a day. This preparation may be given either orally or intravenously.

Lanatoside C (Cedilanid) is also a purified glycoside of digitalis. It comes as an oral preparation only, and the usual maintenance dose is 0.5 mg. ($^1/_{120}$ grain) a day.

Deslanoside (desacetyl-lanatoside C; Cedilanid-D) is a glycoside of digitalis for intravenous use. An initial dose of 1.2 to 1.6 mg. ($^1/_{50}$ to $^1/_{40}$ grain) is usually given, followed by a maintenance dose of 0.2 to 0.6 mg. ($^1/_{300}$ to $^1/_{100}$ grain) each day.

Digoxin (Lanoxin) is a purified glycoside of digitalis that produces effects more rapidly than does digitoxin. It is also eliminated more rapidly. It may be given either orally or intravenously. The average digitalizing dose is 4 mg. ($^1/_{16}$ grain) orally or 0.5 to 1.5 mg. ($^1/_{120}$ to $^1/_{40}$ grain) intravenously. The maintenance dose both orally and intravenously is 0.25 to 0.75 mg. ($^1/_{250}$ to $^1/_{90}$ grain) daily. If any of the medication infiltrates into the tissues during intravenous injection, sloughing may occur since digoxin is a tissue irritant. Heat should be applied to the infiltrated area immediately to encourage absorption of the medication into the bloodstream.

Digalen is very similar to digitalis. It can be given both orally and intravenously. The usual maintenance dose is 0.5 to 1 U.S.P. unit three times a day.

Digilanid is a preparation that has an action similar to that of digitalis. It can be given orally, rectally, intramuscularly, and intravenously. Two to four tablets (0.67 to 1.33 mg.) are given by mouth daily until the patient is fully digitalized, and then one or two tablets are given daily as a maintenance dose.

Digifolin is also a form of digitalis leaf. It can be given orally and intravenously. Until the desired effects are obtained, 0.8 U.S.P. unit is given daily.

Gitalin (amorphous) (Gitaligin) is excreted more slowly than digoxin but more rapidly than digitoxin. It is given by mouth, and two or three tablets are given daily for 3 or 4 days or until 4 to 6.5 mg. ($^1/_{15}$ to $^1/_{10}$ grain) has been given. The daily maintenance dose is then usually 0.25 to 0.75 mg. ($^1/_{250}$ to $^1/_{90}$ grain).

Ouabain (g-strophanthin) is often used for emergency treatment of patients with congestive heart failure. It acts very rapidly when injected intravenously or intramuscularly, but it is quickly excreted. Therefore, it is not suitable for a maintenance medication and usually is used in conjunction with some other digitalis preparation. Usually no more than 0.5 mg. ($^1/_{120}$ grain) of this medication is given daily because of its potency.

Digitalis toxicity. The nurse must constantly be alert for signs and symptoms indicating digitalis toxicity. Anorexia, nausea and vomiting, diarrhea, headache, blurred or colored vision, restlessness, and irritability may be symptoms of digitalis toxicity. However, nausea and vomiting may be caused by gastric irritation from the digitalis preparation and will often subside after the patient becomes adjusted to the medication.[7] In addition to these less serious toxic effects, digitalis preparations can produce almost any type of cardiac arrhythmia. This is why the rate and rhythm of the pulse should be checked so carefully before each dose is administered.

Predisposing factors. There are several factors that predispose the patient to digitalis toxicity. One of the most common is hypokalemia, which potentiates the effects of digitalis. When potassium is depleted in the body or myocardium, the heart becomes more excitable and arrhythmias may occur.[7] Decrease in potassium levels below the normal range of 4.0 to 5.4 mEq./L. can occur whenever excess potassium is lost from the body, such as occurs in vomiting and diarrhea or induced diuresis. Most of the diuretics used to treat congestive heart failure result in the loss of potassium along with sodium and water. Therefore the nurse must be alert to changes in the patient's serum potassium blood levels. In order to replace the potassium loss through diuresis, patients are often placed on a supplemental form of potassium such as potassium chloride. Some diuretics have potassium added to them, but many physicians prefer to order the diuretics and potassium separately. In addition, foods such as orange juice or bananas, which are high in potassium and low in sodium content, may be ordered for the patient.

If digitalis toxicity occurs, the medication is stopped at once and other therapy instituted as necessary. This often includes administration of potassium chloride and procainamide.

Diuretic medications. If restrictions of sodium and fluids and the administration of digitalis do not appreciably relieve the tissue edema and the pulmonary edema, the physician may order diuretic medications. A diuretic also may be used to give prompt relief to the patient who is in acute distress because of severe edema of the tissues. Any patient who is receiving a diuretic should be weighed daily. If the patient is at home, arrangements will need to be made to provide scales, and the patient or his family must be taught to record the weight daily. Usually the medication is prescribed to be given during the early hours of the day so that the height of the diuretic effect does not fall within normal sleeping hours and disturb sleep unduly.

The organic mercurial diuretics are considered probably the most effective and are widely used, although chlorothiazide (Diuril) and its derivatives are now being used more often. Mercurial diuretics are available for use orally, intravenously, intramuscularly, and subcutaneously. The intramuscular route is usually preferred. Rare deaths due to ventricular fibrillation following intravenous injections of these medications have been reported.[7] The mercurial diuretic may be given every second or third day or weekly, depending on the individual patient. As much as 1 to 2 L. of fluid may be excreted during the day of the injection. The patient may complain of local discomfort at the site of the injection. Discomfort may be relieved by hot applications to the area, which hasten the absorption of the medication.

The patient who is receiving any mercurial diuretic over a long period should be watched for signs of toxic reactions to the mercury such as stomatitis, gingivitis, increased salivation, diarrhea, albuminuria, hematuria, and skin eruption. He may also complain of flushing and have febrile reactions to the medication. Toxic signs must be reported to the physician at once.

Some patients receiving mercurial diuretics may have toxic signs caused by sodium, calcium, or potassium depletion, since sodium, calcium, or potassium may also be lost in large amounts through the kidney while its reabsorptive powers are depressed by the mercurial diuretics. Nausea, vomiting, fever, and cramps in the calves of the legs and in the stomach can be due to sodium depletion. Potassium depletion causes extreme weakness and symptoms of paralytic ileus. The ECG may also reflect hypokalemia in S-T segment depression and prolongation of the P-R interval. Calcium depletion may cause the patient to develop tetany with muscle spasm. Skin rashes may also occur. The patient who is receiving both diuretic medications and digitalis needs to be watched closely for toxic reactions to digitalis, since toxicity occurs much sooner if the serum potassium is low. If a reaction to a mercurial preparation occurs, the physician will institute measures to replace the depleted electrolytes. Reactions often can be prevented by giving the patient a little more salt in his food (if medically approved) and by encouraging him to take food and fluids high in potassium and calcium. Another form of the medication often can be substituted later without untoward reactions.

Mercurial diuretics may be given in combination with *ammonium chloride,* which is a diuretic now seldom used alone. It has an acidifying effect that enhances the potency of the mercurial diuretics because, in an effort to prevent acidosis, the sodium from the tissues unites with the chloride to neutralize it, mobilizing both the salt and the water for excretion by the kidney.[6] Ammonium chloride in enteric-coated tablets may be given on the 2 or 3 days prior to, and on the day of, the administration of the mercurial preparation. For the best results it should then be omitted for a day or two. The usual dosage is 6 to 10 Gm./day given in four doses.[6] Ammonium chloride should be taken after meals or with food since it may cause gastric irritation. Neither the mercurial diuretics nor ammonium chloride are usually prescribed by the doctor if the patient has signs of kidney damage, since serious electrolyte imbalance may occur.

A widely used mercurial preparation is *meralluride injection* (Mercuhydrin injection). It contains organically combined mercury and theophylline and is given intramuscularly or intravenously. The addition of theophylline increases the diuretic effect by improving absorption and also decreases irritation at the site of injection.[7] The dosage is usually 1 to 2 ml. *Mercaptomerin sodium* (Thiomerin sodium) is a

mercurial preparation that can be given subcutaneously, and therefore the patient or his family members can learn to give the medication. It causes little pain on injection but may cause local reactions such as edema. The injection should be given quite deeply to avoid injection into subcutaneous fat. Since the medication deteriorates at room temperature, the patient receiving it at home must be cautioned to keep it in the refrigerator. Thiomerin is now available to be used in rectal suppository form. *Chlormerodrin* (Neohydrin) is a form of mercurial medication that can be taken orally, although it is seldom prescribed if edema is severe. The average dose is 55 to 110 mg. ($^3/_4$ to $1^1/_2$ grains) daily. Many other mercurial preparations are now available.

Chlorothiazide (Diuril) is a relatively new and effective oral diuretic. It inhibits the reabsorption of sodium from the glomerular filtrate by the kidney tubules and therefore causes less reabsorption of water and other electrolytes. It is often given in two doses of 0.5 to 1 Gm. ($7^1/_2$ to 15 grains) daily, although only one daily dose may be given. The medication is effective for about 12 hours.

Other preparations allied to chlorothiazide such as furosemide (Lasix) and ethacrynic acid (Edecrin) are now available and are most commonly prescribed when other diuretics have proved unsuccessful. They are also used intramuscularly to treat acute pulmonary edema.[6] Chlorothiazide and the related medications cause loss of potassium, and for this reason the physician may order that potassium be given parenterally or orally and that potassium in the diet be increased by having the patient take more high-potassium foods such as fresh fruit and fruit juice daily. Toxic signs are not common, but blurring of vision, dryness of the mouth, dizziness, muscle cramps, skin eruptions, and agranulocytosis have been reported. Large doses may lead to acidosis caused by excretion of bicarbonate and may be contraindicated if the patient has renal disease.

Acetazolamide (Diamox) is a preparation that depresses the renal tubules, promoting excretion of the bicarbonate ion rather than the chloride ion. It is given orally once a day in doses of 250 to 500 mg. and remains active for 6 to 8 hours. It often is given every other day, being alternated with a mercurial preparation. This medication may make the patient drowsy, and he may complain of numbness and tingling in the face and extremities.

Spironolactone (Aldactone) has a diuretic effect by blocking the action of aldosterone, a hormone that acts by increasing the retention of sodium and the excretion of potassium. Aldactone has been given in combination with other diuretics to lessen the excretion of potassium. This preparation is given orally in doses of 3 Gm. (45 grains) daily. It is slow in its action, and toxic signs have been reported, particularly in patients who have hepatic or renal damage.

Occasionally xanthine derivatives are used as diuretics. They act by increasing the rate of sodium elimination from the kidneys. *Theobromine calcium salicylate* and *theophylline ethylenediamine* (aminophylline) are the preparations most often used. Theobromine usually is given in doses of 0.5 Gm. (7$\frac{1}{2}$ grains), and 0.25 Gm. (4 grains) of aminophylline may be given. Aminophylline may be given orally, rectally, or intravenously. Xanthine derivatives given orally cause gastric irritation and therefore should be given with food. These drugs may be used if smooth muscle relaxation is also desired; for example, they are often prescribed for patients who have angina pectoris to help relax the smooth muscles of the coronary vessels.

To relieve ascites or pleural effusion, sometimes it is necessary for the physician to aspirate fluid. This is done through an abdominal paracentesis and a thoracentesis, respectively. (For the management of patients undergoing these procedures, see texts on fundamentals of nursing and pp. 580 and 720.)

Acute pulmonary edema. Acute pulmonary edema is a medical emergency in patients with heart disease. It is caused by additional or prolonged strain on an already damaged heart, with resultant failure. Either physical or emotional exertion can precipitate pulmonary edema. Cardiac output is decreased and serous fluid under pressure is pushed back through the pulmonary capillaries into the alveoli. Fluid rapidly reaches the bronchioles and bronchi, and the patient begins to drown in his own secretions. Acute pulmonary edema also may follow such conditions as inhalation of irritating gases, cerebrovascular accident, fractures of the skull, too rapid administration of plasma, serum albumin, whole blood, or other intravenous fluids, and barbiturate or opiate poison-

ing. Severe dyspnea, cyanosis, and restlessness are usual symptoms.

The goals in the treatment of acute pulmonary edema include the following: physical and mental relaxation, relief of hypoxia, retardation of venous return, and improvement of cardiovascular function. The patient with acute pulmonary edema should be placed in bed in a high Fowler's position, and the physician should be summoned immediately. He usually orders morphine sulfate, 15 mg. ($\frac{1}{4}$ grain), to be given at once to quiet breathing and to allay apprehension. It may be given intravenously since circulatory collapse may hinder its absorption from the tissues. To relieve hypoxia the physician may order intermittent positive pressure with oxygen and humidification and an airway pressure of 15 to 30 cm. of water. Rotating tourniquets are used to retard venous return; the tourniquets are placed on three of the extremities at a time, thus reducing the amount of blood that must be circulated by the overtaxed heart. (See Fig. 17-19.) Every 15 minutes, in clockwise or counterclockwise order, one tourniquet is removed and placed on the extremity that has had no tourniquet on it. In this way the vessels of each extremity are occluded for 45 minutes at a time, and then the tourniquet is released from the extremity for 15 minutes. The fourth tourniquet should be applied before one is removed. Care must be taken that no tourniquet is left on longer than 45 minutes lest the tissues be permanently damaged, and the tourniquet should not obliterate arterial pulses in the extremity. The use of a prepared diagram and time schedule kept at the patient's bedside helps ensure the proper changing of the tourniquets. This procedure may be done by either the physician or the nurse, and it is continued until the acute pulmonary

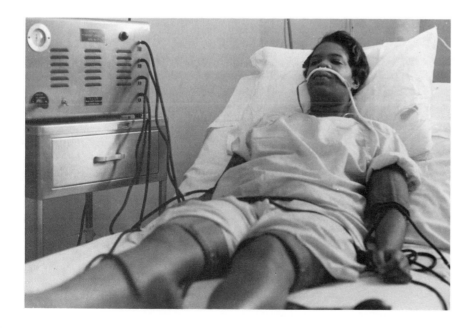

FIG. 17-19. Patient in acute pulmonary edema; rotating tourniquet machine is being used. Note that intravenous infusion is in a subclavian vein.

edema subsides. If the patient is alert, the procedure should be explained to him. He may need a narcotic to make him less conscious of the pressure of the tourniquets and of the uncomfortable sensation in the extremities caused by venous engorgement. If the procedure must be continued over a long period, the skin should be watched carefully for beginning signs of irritation from pressure. The tourniquet may be placed over the patient's gown or a towel to prevent damage to the skin. Blood pressure cuffs may be used in place of the rubber tourniquets, or an automatic rotating tourniquet machine that alternates the occluded extremities may be employed (Fig. 17-20). If an extremity does not readily return to normal color on release of a tourniquet, the physician should be informed. When treatment is to be discontinued, *one tourniquet is removed at a time, according to time intervals, until all tourniquets have been removed.* If all the tourniquets were released at the same time, the venous return would be substantially increased and pulmonary edema may reoccur. Some-

times, if the patient is not in shock, the physician will remove 500 to 800 ml. of blood by a *phlebotomy.* The decrease in the amount of circulating blood decreases pulmonary engorgement. This procedure is similar to that for taking blood from a blood donor.

Aminophylline usually is given because it helps to increase the cardiac output and to lower the venous pressure by relaxing the smooth muscles of the blood vessels. It also relieves bronchial spasm. Digitalization usually is started immediately. Either ouabain or deslanoside is given intravenously. Since it is dangerous to give either of these medications if the patient is routinely taking digitalis, the nurse should try to ascertain from the patient or his family whether he takes any heart medicines, and should inform the physician. Rapid-acting diuretics such as Edecrin or Lasix may also be used to help relieve the edema and decrease the circulating blood volume.

Home care. If possible, patients with acute pulmonary edema are hospitalized. However, if it is impossible to move them from their homes, improvisations

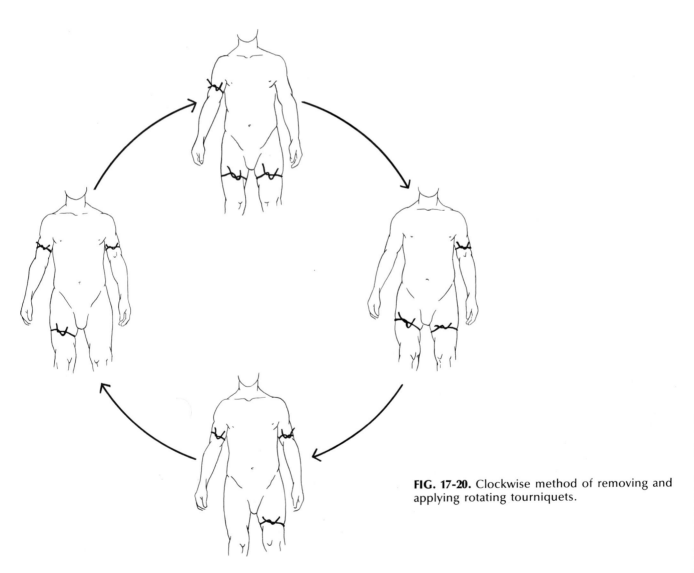

FIG. 17-20. Clockwise method of removing and applying rotating tourniquets.

can be made to care for them adequately. The principles of treatment are the same. Oxygen can be obtained from fire stations or ambulances for emergency use, and hospitals or medical supply houses will provide equipment for continued use. Other sickroom equipment usually can be borrowed from the local public health nursing agency. The local health department office often knows where equipment is available. The patient can be put in a high Fowler's position in the home by use of an inverted straight chair placed on the bed and padded with blankets and pillows. Six-inch blocks placed under the legs of the bed to raise the height make it easier to care for the patient, although side rails should then be used. The patient with acute pulmonary edema needs continuous nursing care. The nurse will need to assist the family in learning to provide parts of the patient's care, if possible, and may help them to secure a nurse who will remain in the home during the critical period. As the patient improves, his care will be that of any patient with heart failure. Continuing care can be planned by the patient's physician, the public health nurse, and the family.

■ MANAGEMENT OF THE SURGICAL PATIENT

Some cardiac diseases can be successfully treated by surgery. The majority of the operations on the heart are being performed with full visualization *(open technique)*. The heart is opened and the defect is inspected and repaired. Openings in the atrial or ventricular septa may be sutured or patched with plastic material. Valves may be opened or reconstructed, or they may be replaced with artifical cusps or ball valves. When the *closed technique* is used, the defect is not seen by the surgeon. He inserts his finger into the heart through a small incision and explores the obstructed valve digitally (Fig. 17-5). The surgeon may be able to open the obstructed valve with his finger, or he may have to guide a special knife or instrument into the area to release the adhesions. The closed technique is used most often to treat uncomplicated mitral stenosis. While the risks during and after surgery are greater with open heart surgery, the results generally are better than can be obtained using the closed technique. Operations such as repair of some congenital and acquired defects of the heart could not be performed unless direct visualization was possible.

The open heart approach can be used only if extracorporeal circulation is maintained by means of a heart-lung apparatus (pump oxygenator). In addition, hypothermia may be used to reduce the metabolic rate. This permits tissue tolerance of the somewhat lower blood flow rates with extracorporeal circulation (p. 209) and longer periods of total cardiac standstill than are tolerable at normal body temperatures.[26] Increased atmospheric pressure in spe-

cial chambers is occasionally used as a supplement to either hypothermia or extracorporeal circulation. The tissues appear to become so saturated with oxygen that they withstand temporary ischemia very well. An adequate amount of oxygen can be carried dissolved in the blood, with no need for hemoglobin.[26]

Surgery also is being used in the treatment of persons who have coronary artery disease of varying severity. The purpose of this surgery, called *coronary bypass* (jump graft), is to increase blood flow to the myocardium by using a segment of saphenous vein and/or an internal mammary artery to actually bypass the coronary artery obstruction or occlusion. Many patients show marked improvement after this surgery. The technique varies somewhat among surgeons, and some surgeons routinely use extracorporeal circulation during the operation while others do not. When the saphenous vein is used, one end is sutured to the aorta and the other is sutured to the coronary artery distal to the occlusion (Fig. 17-21). When an internal mammary artery is used, the distal end of this vessel is freed from the anterior chest wall and sutured in place distal to the occlusion in the coronary artery (Fig. 17-22). Presently coronary bypass surgery is performed on the right coronary, left anterior descending, and circumflex coronary arteries.

Preoperative period

Before a heart operation is scheduled, the patient's general health, and particularly the condition of the heart, is evaluated carefully, and he is built up to the best physical condition possible for him. He must undergo many tests, and although he probably has had previous experience in the hospital because of his heart condition, he should be given an adequate explanation of all procedures. When it has been decided that benefit can be derived from an operation, the physican or surgeon discusses the procedure with the patient and his family. He usually tells them why the operation must be done, what he hopes it will accomplish, and what will be done. If the patient is a child, the parents should explain the admission to the hospital and the operation to him as simply as possible. His age will determine the kind of explanation to be given. (See p. 194 for discussion of this preparation.)

In some instances patients or parents have read or heard about heart operations and have come to the surgeon and asked to have the procedure done. Some men and women, faced with increasing invalidism, decide that they would like to risk an operation in the hope of being able to live more normally.

Preoperative teaching. Although the surgeon has talked with the patient about the operation and the patient has prepared himself emotionally to some degree, he is still anxious and apprehensive and usual-

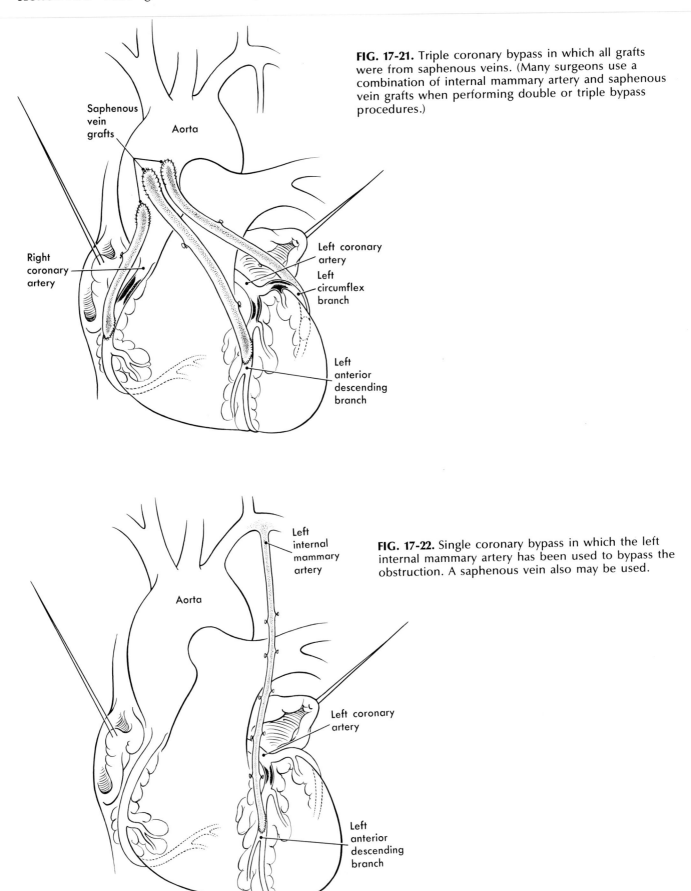

FIG. 17-21. Triple coronary bypass in which all grafts were from saphenous veins. (Many surgeons use a combination of internal mammary artery and saphenous vein grafts when performing double or triple bypass procedures.)

FIG. 17-22. Single coronary bypass in which the left internal mammary artery has been used to bypass the obstruction. A saphenous vein also may be used.

ly needs a great deal of reinforcement and emotional support from the nurse. Surgery on the heart carries a risk. The patient realizes that there is no substitute for the heart and that life without it is impossible. Provision should be made for him to visit with his family on the morning of surgery. Some patients may also desire to see their clergyman before surgery. Many patients may wish to prepare a will. The anesthesiologist's visit to the patient preoperatively may also provide some reassurance.

One of the most important contributions to the care of children can be made by the nurse through support, understanding, and teaching of the child's parents. Helping them to obtain the necessary examinations for the child and explaining necessary procedures can be tremendously saving of parents' worry and concern.

Accepting the fact that the child has a defect is sometimes the most difficult problem. Parents react in a variety of ways, but most wish to have all possible help given to the child. Helping parents to accept a "guarded" prognosis or a poor prognosis when operative procedures are recommended requires patient, careful guidance by physician, nurse, and social worker.

The preoperative care is similar to that discussed on p. 194. Most cardiac patients are very apprehensive about the surgery, and the nurse should learn to know the patient as well as possible in order to ascertain what he should be told.* For example, an

---

*See references 28, 36, 44, 65, 107, 125, and 127.

explanation of chest drainage is welcomed by some patients but greatly upsets others. Preoperatively the nurse should determine and record the amount of activity in which the patient is able to engage without becoming tired, because it will serve as a guide in determining his postoperative condition.

The physician orders a sedative so that the patient will sleep on the preoperative night. If necessary, the medication usually can be repeated. In the morning, before the patient leaves for the operating room, the physician usually will start an infusion. The infusion may also be started the afternoon before surgery. A *venesection* (cutdown) may be done to assure a patent large vein in the event of circulatory collapse. A narcotic usually is not ordered as a preoperative medication for the patient who will be undergoing cardiac surgery since it depresses respirations. Often phenobarbital sodium, 120 mg. (2 grains), is ordered, and only 0.2 mg. ($^1/_{300}$ grain) of atropine sulfate is given to decrease secretions, because a larger dose might block the vagus nerve, increasing the stimuli to the sinoatrial node and increasing the possibility of fibrillation.

Extracorporeal circulation and heart surgery

During open heart surgery the pump oxygenator is used as a temporary substitute for the patient's heart and lungs. The heart and lungs of the patient are bypassed so that the surgeon can work in a relatively bloodless field and can see the defect more clearly. Maintenance of body circulation by this artificial means also allows more time in which to correct the defect (Fig. 17-23).

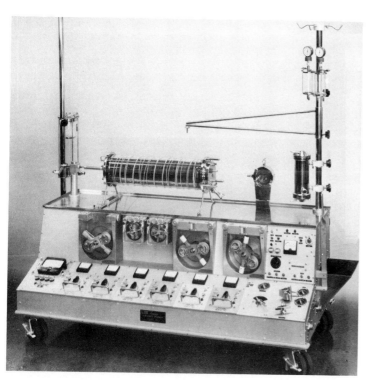

FIG. 17-23. Pump oxygenator used during open heart surgery. (Courtesy PEMCO, Inc., Cleveland, Ohio.)

There is a variety of extracorporeal oxygenator systems. The most widely used are the bubble method and the screen or rotating disk types. Immediately before the operation the machine is prepared or primed for use by filling it with 2,500 ml. (5 pints) of fresh blood that must match that of the patient. Donors are asked to report the morning of the operation to ensure freshness of the blood. Heparin is added to the blood to prevent clotting. Another method is to prime the pump oxygenator with glucose or lactated Ringer's solution. While amounts vary, one medical center primes the unit with 16 to 20 ml. of fluid/kg. body weight. Two thirds of the fluid consists of 5% dextrose in water and one third of 10% dextran 40 (Rheomacrodex) in saline solution. The use of solutions other than blood leads to a significant decrease in complications and also is much less costly for the patient. Also, an oxygenator primed with glucose can be used on short notice. This is not possible with blood priming.

The patient receives a general anesthetic via an endotracheal tube. The surgeon then makes a thoracotomy incision, transects the sternum, and enters the pericardium. The patient receives heparin intravenously, and catheters are inserted into the superior and inferior venae cavae. By means of a Y connecting tube, these catheters are attached to the machine, and through them will pass the venous flow of blood. Another catheter is inserted into the common femoral artery and attached to the pump, and through this catheter, blood that has been oxygenated will be returned to the systemic circulation.

When all catheters are inserted and attached, the machine is set into operation, the venae cavae are occluded, and correction of the defect is undertaken. Blood is returned to the patient's body at the rate of 50 to 60 ml./kg. of body weight/minute to maintain adequate peripheral blood pressure. Blood return does not determine rate, which will be slowed if hypothermia is used. A heating unit within the machine keeps the blood the same temperature at which the body is being maintained. Oxygenation of blood is accomplished by means of an oxygen inlet within the machine, and carbon dioxide is removed by a chemical bath process. Throughout the surgical procedure heart action, brain action, and blood pressure are monitored. These recordings allow the anesthesiologist and the surgeon to keep a constant check on the adequacy of circulation for the patient.

After the defect has been corrected, heart action is stabilized, air is vented from the cardiac chambers, the venae cavae are unclamped, the venous catheter sites are closed, and the pump is discontinued. Protamine sulfate is given to counteract the heparin and to restore the coagulation time of the blood to normal.

Postoperative period

Postoperative unit. Some medical centers have special units (cardiac recovery rooms) set aside to care for patients who have had cardiac surgery. Patients usually remain in these units longer than they do in regular recovery rooms.

While the patient is in the operating room, the nurse should prepare the unit for his return. It is preferable that he be in a room by himself since he will need constant observation for several days. Oxygen equipment should be prepared. Other inhalation therapy equipment such as ultrasonic nebulizers and intermittent positive pressure machines may be used depending on the practice of the individual surgeons. Chest suction apparatus should be ready to attach, and a thoracentesis set, equipment for cardiac massage, and emergency stimulants should be readily available in the event that air or fluid must be withdrawn from the chest cavity or cardiac massage done as emergency measures. Infusion poles, a sphygmomanometer, and a stethoscope should also be at the bedside. Suction apparatus should be available since the patient may need to be suctioned to maintain a patent airway. If the cardiac surgery was done while the temperature of the body was lowered (hypothermia), equipment to apply external heat or to maintain hypothermia will be needed (p. 209).

Postoperative care. The patient who has undergone heart surgery under either the closed or the open technique requires constant nursing care. The nurse must be alert for signs of hemorrhage, hypotension, fibrillation, arrhythmias, sudden chest pain, and pulmonary edema. Mortality is highest within the first 48 hours.

After open heart surgery the patient is usually maintained on continuous respiratory support for the first few hours. To accomplish this a respirator is connected to the endotracheal tube. Oxygen is administered to increase the efficiency of breathing and to minimize complications of hypoxia such as cardiac arrhythmias. The patient may be placed with his head elevated to facilitate movement of the diaphragm. The patient will be connected to a cardiac monitor to provide a continuous ECG. Central venous pressure and vital signs will be monitored frequently. When his blood pressure remains relatively stable, the patient is turned from his back to his operated side at least every 2 hours. Chest tubes are attached to closed drainage and to chest suction apparatus (Fig. 22-17) to drain air and fluid from the pleural space. The amount and color of the drainage should be checked at least hourly and the time and amount recorded. There will be some bleeding during the first 48 hours, and provision should be made for blood replacement. The dressings should be inspected frequently for blood and the chest tubes for patency. Because of the large amounts of heparin used when the pump oxygenator is used, bleeding may occur. Preparations of vitamin K and protamine sulfate are given to counteract the bleeding tendency caused by the heparin. The patient should be observed for any signs of shock, hemorrhage, spontaneous pneumothorax, mediastinal shift, cardiac arrhythmias, or congestive heart failure. Sudden hypotension with sharp pain would indicate a coronary occlusion. Blood-tinged or frothy sputum usually indicates pulmonary edema. The patient is urged to take deep breaths as soon as he awakens from anesthesia. Intermittent positive pressure may be used to facilitate deep breathing and coughing. Following heart surgery the patient needs constant attendance for 24 to 72 hours. If left alone, he may become extremely apprehensive, and mental stress increases the work of the heart.

Blood pressure and pulse rate measurements are taken every 15 minutes and the frequency is decreased gradually as the patient's condition stabilizes. The pulse should be checked carefully for rhythm, strength, and rapidity of beat; it may also be monitored electronically. The physician may order the apical-radial pulse rate taken since atrial fibrillation develops in patients who have had heart surgery. The patient may be aware of palpitation. Since it may frighten him, the patient should be told that it can be expected and controlled. When atrial fibrillation occurs, it is usually controlled by medication. Depending on the physician's findings, digitalis or quinidine sulfate may be prescribed, or procainamide hydrochloride (Pronestyl hydrochloride) may be given intravenously. A cardioverter or a pacemaker may be used to treat persistent atrial fibrillation or cardiac arrest. If the patient has been on digitalis, antiarrhythmic preparations, and/or diuretics preoperatively, these medications may be resumed.

Cardiac monitors may be used continuously for the first few days. The nurse observes the readings closely and reports abnormal rhythms to the physician at once. Radiographs of the chest taken with a portable machine and ECG's are made daily to evaluate lung expansion and heart function.

Although the patient usually is allowed clear fluids as soon as tolerated, supplementary intravenous fluids are given for 2 or 3 days to ensure prescribed intake and an intravenous route for medication. Depending on the postoperative cardiac condition, the physician determines the amount of fluids the patient may take. He usually is permitted to have from 1,500 to 1,800 ml./day. The patient, the nurse, and members of the auxiliary staff should be aware of this restriction and keep accurate measurement of the fluid intake, including that used to swallow oral medications. Intravenous fluids should be administered slowly to prevent overloading the circulatory system, thus placing additional strain on the heart. The prescribed diet usually does not exceed 2 or 3 Gm. of salt, and some restriction may be continued indefinitely to prevent fluid retention.

A self-retaining (Foley) catheter is commonly inserted into the bladder; urine is collected every hour and checked for specific gravity, color, and amount. Hourly urine volume should not be less than 15 to 30 ml. Frequent observation of urine output helps detect signs of hypovolemia, hemolysis, and kidney shutdown or failure. Disturbance of electrolyte balance with development of acidosis can occur following open heart surgery, particularly following a shunt repair. The nurse should anticipate that blood chemistries will be ordered and should have the needed equipment available.

A narcotic such as meperidine hydrochloride (Demerol) or morphine sulfate may be prescribed to relieve pain. Some surgeons order small doses given frequently because the pain is severe and larger doses may depress respirations. Severe pain usually persists for 2 or 3 days, caused in part by severance of the intercostal nerves and retraction of the ribs and sternum. The chest catheters may also irritate the pleura and cause pain. If pain in the incision persists over a long period of time, the physician may infiltrate the area above and below the incision with procaine. Since the pain is often made more severe by coughing, the patient may refuse to cough or take deep breaths. The pain experienced during an attempt to cough may frighten the patient so that he is afraid to try agin. He is able to cough best about half an hour after a narcotic is given. When assisting the patient to cough, the incision should be splinted manually on both sides or with a towel or drawsheet, with firm counterpressure applied on expiration (Fig. 22-16). IPPB treatments or carbon dioxide rebreathing devices may be used to stimulate coughing and deep breathing. If the patient does not cough productively, and if his breathing sounds moist or he has "rattles," endotracheal suctioning may be necessary to clear his airway. After the chest catheters have been removed, coughing and turning usually are less difficult. There is no definite day on which the chest catheters are removed, for it depends on the amount of drainage and air present in the pleural cavity and on the reexpansion of the lungs as seen on radiographs. Commonly, however, they are removed 2 or 3 days postoperatively. Antibiotics may be given routinely to prevent infection.

While the patient is in bed, the nurse should encourage him to do arm and leg exercises. They may be done passively by the nurse at first. However, as the patient becomes stronger, he is encouraged to tighten his leg muscles, move his feet up and down, and move his arms through the full range of motion. The patient usually will not use his left arm without being urged, since motion causes pain in the operative area. To prevent a stiff shoulder with limited function, however, exercises should be gradually instituted. The nurse should supervise the exercising of the left arm and shoulder until the patient has regained full range of motion.

Many patients have profuse diaphoresis after cardiac surgery, and it may be more pronounced at night. The exact reason is not known. The patient should be kept dry and comfortable and should be reassured that it is a fairly common occurrence and that it will gradually subside. The temperature may rise markedly and remain elevated for several days. In the immediate postoperative period this is attributed to postperfusion syndrome, a transfusion reaction, or atelectasis.

Some patients experience a period of depression or even disorientation after cardiac surgery, although this reaction does not generally last very long. [31a,36,66] The patient may become very excited and fearful or may have hallucinations (false visual perceptions). Other patients exhibit varying degrees of depression. This reaction often occurs about 3 days postoperatively, and the nurse should be aware of this possibility. The cause is unknown, but it is thought that it may be caused by medication, fear, or some sleep loss or sensory monotony. Panic may develop. The nurse should be alert for these changes in behavior and should reassure the patient and his family that these are common reactions and that the patient is not "losing his mind." The patient needs a calm environment, orientation as to time and place, and much support and understanding. Because sleep loss and sensory monotony are more likely to occur when the patient is kept in an intensive care unit, some cardiac surgeons are transferring their patients out of these units as early as 24 hours after surgery. This is only possible when the patients can be closely monitored in another setting.

Ambulation. Mobilization of the patient depends on the operation and the status of the heart. In general, patients who have had surgery for a coarctation of the aorta or any other surgery on the aorta are kept flat in bed for several days to prevent unnecessary strain on the vessel (the blood pressure is lower when the patient is flat). Some surgeons do not permit the patient to be turned for several days. Before getting out of bed, the patient must gradually become accustomed to having the head of the bed elevated. When this procedure is first attempted, he may complain of dizziness and faintness. If so, he is returned to a flat position, and elevation is attempted again later. Patients who have had surgery for patent ductus arteriosus and mitral stenosis may be kept in Fowler's position postoperatively and are encouraged to move their arms and legs. Backache from lying flat on the back is common.

The time of ambulation for each patient depends on his progress and condition, but (other than the above exceptions) it usually proceeds as follows: The first day he dangles his feet over the side of the bed for 15 minutes in the morning and afternoon. The second day he is allowed to sit in a chair at the side of the bed for 15 minutes in the morning and afternoon. The third day he walks around the room while he is up. The fourth day he is allowed to walk around the room and to sit in the chair for gradually increasing periods of time. By the fifth day he may walk longer distances. He should be closely supervised during ambulation, and no activity that causes excessive fatigue, dyspnea, or an increased pulse or respiratory rate should be continued. If any of these symptoms appear, he should return to bed, and the physician should be consulted before further activity is attempted. Definite instructions are left by the physician regarding when the patient may attempt to climb stairs. The activity should be done slowly under the supervision of a nurse. Only two or three steps should be attempted the first time, after which the number of steps is gradually increased, depending on the surgeon's evaluation of the patient's condition. The patient should rest two or three times while climbing one flight of stairs. For further information and explanations concerning postoperative cardiac care, the reader is referred to specialized articles and texts.*

Long-term postoperative care. The patient and his family need to be told that no marked improvement will be noticed immediately after the operation —that it will be at least 3 to 6 months before the full result of the surgery can be ascertained. It is essential that all patients be given this information so that they will not be depressed by dyspnea or pain that may still be present postoperatively.

In preparation for discharge from the hospital the patient is asked to make a list of activities usually carried out at home. This list is discussed with the physician to ascertain the activities he feels are appropriate. A woman usually will want to know if she may dust, make beds, wash dishes, and do other household chores. A man may wish to know exactly what he may do—how much he may walk, what he may do about his house and yard, and when he may report to work. Patients are usually advised to start slowly and progress gradually to more energy-consuming tasks. The physician will want a patient to return for frequent medical follow-up examinations, at which time he will advise him regarding additional activities. The patient should not think of himself as an invalid and should be allowed to do anything that does not tire him. On the other hand, he must be kept from attempting too much.

The family of the patient who has undergone cardiac surgery should be aware of his condition and how much he can do. Since the patient may have been an invalid preoperatively, the family may be as fearful as he is about his activity. They should un-

---

*See references 13a,14,17a,21a,22,37a,88,93,114, and 133.

derstand how important it is for him to continue to see his physician regularly and why he must continue to take his medication and remain on his diet. A public health nurse is often asked to supervise his care and activity at home.

If the patient is a child and has had congestive failure, his family will need help with medications and any diet restrictions. They should also be taught how to prepare a temperature chart, which they usually are asked to keep during the first month. After this time, the postoperative danger of infection or endocarditis usually is past.

The patient and his family should have ample time to review their questions and concerns, which often come out more easily during discussion of the more tangible parts of care. Most parents appreciate home visits from a nurse to be certain that what they are doing is right for their child.

Heart transplantation has received much publicity. The basic postoperative care is the same as that for the patient with open cardiac surgery. In addition, signs of tissue rejection are important clinical parameters to be evaluated. These signs may be as vague as fever and malaise or may include ECG and enzyme changes characteristic of myocardial ischemia.

■ REHABILITATION

To help patients with diseases of the heart and circulatory system learn to live within the limits of their cardiac capacity, the nurse needs to know as much about the patient's condition as possible. The nurse will need to know what the physician has told the patient and his family and what limitations he has set for the patient. This information should be shared with other persons such as the family, the social worker, the occupational therapist, the public health nurse, the industrial nurse, the employer, or the schoolteacher, who may assist in the patient's rehabilitation.

It is helpful to prepare a list of the activities in which the patient usually engages at home and at work so that the physician can check those he considers appropriate to resume. As the patient's condition improves, more of the activities may be added to the approved list. Such a list serves as a guide for the patient and his family, and it may help him strike a balance between too many and too few restrictions. The patient, however, must use judgment and discretion in carrying out these activities, especially the pace at which they are performed. If they cause him to be tired or out of breath, they are too strenuous. Moderation should be the guiding principle. All activities should be carried out at a slower pace, and extra rest periods should be taken. Walking against a high wind and exercising at a higher altitude than usual also cause additional strain on the heart.

Patients with cardiac disease should strive for equanimity. All removable burdens such as those imposed by fatigue, obesity, infections, and emotional upsets should be removed. It is often difficult for a patient to achieve this goal without the help of his family. Cardiac disease usually affects the lives of others as well as the life of the patient. The entire family's mode of living may have to be changed, responsibilities may need to be reapportioned, and another member of the family may even have to become the wage earner. The life of a child patient should be planned so that he is not continually frustrated by restrictions. Major adjustments cannot help but disturb the patient, especially if the patient is a mother or a father. The nurse should find opportunities to talk to the family while the patient is still in the hospital, since it is better if the family can begin to make adjustments at this time so that life will be smoother for the patient on his return home. The family members may be unaware of the changes that may be required in their lives, or if they are aware of the changes, they may need help in planning for them. They should realize that adjustments may be permanent rather than temporary. Their successful adjustment to a new way of life may have a direct effect on how long and how happily the cardiac patient will live.

The physician will prescribe the patient's diet. On discharge from the hospital some patients will be allowed to eat a regular diet but are told to eat in moderation because large meals increase the work of the heart during digestion. If the patient is overweight, a low-caloric diet will probably be ordered. A controlled fat diet, high in polyunsaturated fatty acids, may be ordered, especially if the patient has an elevated blood cholesterol level.[130] The most common diet restriction, however, is a mild sodium-restricted diet (2,000 to 3,000 mg./day) or a moderate sodium-restricted diet (600 to 1,200 mg./day). Occasionally a strict low-sodium diet (500 mg./day) is ordered. Both the nurse and the dietitian should work closely with the patient and the family to be sure that they understand the dietary restrictions, why they are essential, and how to prepare acceptable meals. Plans should be worked out with the homemaker so that special food will not need to be prepared for the patient. If salt is restricted, for instance, the simplest method is to cook the food for the entire family without salt, set aside the patient's portion, and season the remainder. If the patient is on restricted salt intake, he should be advised not to take medications or other substances containing salt or sodium, such as saline cathartics, sodium bicarbonate, or soft drinks containing soda water. The teaching program should be started well in advance of the patient's discharge from the hospital. Usually a public health nursing referral should be made, listing the specific problems to be checked.

Many patients with heart disease and their families can profit from regular health supervision visits by a public health nurse. If arrangements need to be made because the patient cannot climb stairs, for example, it may be helpful for the public health nurse to visit the patient's home before he is discharged. After seeing the situation, the nurse may be able to make suggestions that will make him more comfortable and will make his care easier. If the patient happens to be a housewife, minor changes, especially in the work area of the kitchen, may be possible so that she can carry out many of her housekeeping duties while seated (Fig. 17-24). After the patient has arrived home, problems and questions often arise with which the nurse can help. This additional help may reduce the patient's fear and the uncertainty of his family so that he will accept his restrictions more readily. If the patient cannot return to full activity, the family may need help in providing nursing care in the home. For instance, sometimes it is known that an elderly patient will be a semi-invalid. If one or more members of the family take a course in home nursing offered by the American Red Cross, it is easier for the family to give essential care. Sometimes it is possible to take the course while the patient is still hospitalized.

Provision for follow-up care should be made, and the patient should understand the importance of this care. The patient with heart disease should remain under medical supervision for the remainder of his life. In this way he may be kept in the best possible physical condition, which will cause the least burden on his heart. He should also avoid the danger of additional damage and burden on the heart imposed by infections. If possible, he should avoid colds and other upper respiratory infections. If he does develop an infection, he should go to bed and call a physician. The patient with cardiac disease will have a longer convalescence from any illness than the normal person and should return to full activity gradually.

When the patient with cardiac disease is ready to return to school or work, the health service, if one is provided, should know exactly what the patient can and cannot do. Most patients will be allowed to return to normal activity unless it is too strenuous or they have marked incapacity. If the nurse in the health service becomes aware that normal activity tires the patient, this fact should be reported to the medical adviser so that further medical follow-up can be given and necessary adjustments made. Although many patients may return to their former work, some must change their type of work

Because heart diseases do cause loss of time at work and because the financial strain placed on the family is great, every effort should be made to evaluate each patient's condition and to place him in a position where he will be gainfully employed within his physical limitations. Help in locating a suitable position for the cardiac patient may be obtained from the local branch of the American Heart Association, from the office of vocational rehabilitation in state employment services, and occasionally from adult cardiac clinics in hospitals. Using the functional and therapeutic classifications set up by the Criteria Committee of the American Heart Association, the

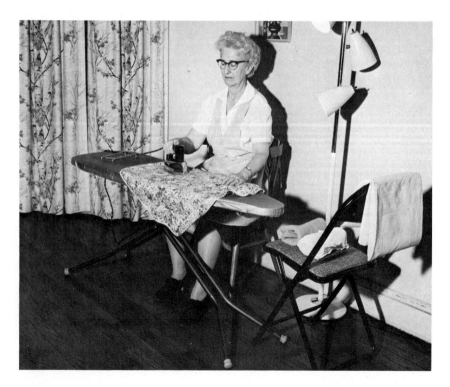

FIG. 17-24. The patient with cardiac disease can be helped to make household activities easier. Note the comfortable position and the placement within easy reach of articles to be ironed.

physician places the patient in the appropriate categories. There are four functional classifications and five therapeutic classifications.

Functional classification

Class I	No limitation of physical activity
Class II	Slight limitation of physical activity
Class III	Marked limitation of physical activity
Class IV	Unable to carry on any physical activity without discomfort

Therapeutic classification

Class A	Physical activity not restricted
Class B	Ordinary physical activity need not be restricted, but patient should be advised against unusually severe or competitive efforts
Class C	Ordinary physical activity should be moderately restricted, and more strenuous habitual efforts should be discontinued
Class D	Ordinary physical activity should be markedly restricted
Class E	Complete rest, confined to bed or chair

In some communities special sheltered workshops (such as the Altro Workshops in New York City) have a demonstration and research program for cardiac patients requiring rehabilitation.

The housewife with cardiac disease should also be considered, and some rehabilitation centers and hospitals have developed programs to help her adjust to her limitations and still be able to function in her usual role. Kitchen facilities similar to those found in most homes have been provided so that she may practice work-simplification measures and plan possible adjustments in the physical setup of her own kitchen. In a booklet entitled *Heart of the Home*, prepared by the American Heart Association, work simplification is discussed, and changes that can be made in the physical facilities are outlined so that the housewife with cardiac disease can manage with a minimum of effort.

Many communities now have rehabilitative help available, and no patient with heart disease should be without this type of assistance. Nurses and physicians can do much to help each patient, and this assistance may be more important than medication.

REFERENCES AND SELECTED READINGS*

1 Abdellah, F.: The physician-nurse team approach to coronary care, Nurs. Clin. North Am. 7:423-430, Sept. 1972.

1a American Academy of Pediatrics: Report of the Committee on Infectious Diseases, ed. 17, Evanston, Ill., 1974, The Academy.

2 Andreoli, K. G.: The cardiac monitor, Am. J. Nurs. 69:1238-1243, June 1969.

3 Andreoli, K. G., and others: Comprehensive cardiac care—a handbook for nurses and other paramedical personnel, ed. 2, St. Louis, 1971, The C. V. Mosby Co.

4 Baden, C.: Teaching the coronary patient and his family, Nurs. Clin. North Am. 7:563-571, Sept. 1972.

5 Barstow, R.: Nursing care of patients with pacemakers, Cardiovasc. Nurs. 8:7-10, March 1972.

6 Beeson, P. B., and McDermott, W., editors: Cecil-Loeb textbook of medicine, ed. 13, Philadelphia, 1971, W. B. Saunders Co.

7 Bergersen, B. S.: Pharmacology in nursing, ed. 12, St. Louis, 1973, The C. V. Mosby Co.

8 Berne, R. M., and Levy, M. N.: Cardiovascular physiology, ed. 2, St. Louis, 1972, The C. V. Mosby Co.

9 *Betson, C., and Ude, L.: Central venous pressure, Am. J. Nurs. 69:1466-1468, July 1969.

10 Bielski, M.: Continuity of care for the patient with coronary heart disease, Nurs. Clin. North Am. 7:413-421, Sept. 1972.

11 Blake, F. G.: Open heart surgery in children, a study of nursing care, Children's Bureau, Washington, D. C., 1964, U. S. Department of Health, Education and Welfare.

12 *Blakeslee, A.: How to live with heart trouble, New York, 1950, American Heart Association.

13 Blakeslee, A., and Stamler, J.: Your heart has nine lives, New York, 1966, Pocket Books, Inc.

13a *Bozorgi, S.: Postoperative care of the cardiac surgical patient, Heart & Lung 3:891-892, Nov.-Dec. 1974.

14 Braimbridge, M. V., and Ghadiali, P. E.: Post-operative cardiac care, Oxford, 1965, Blackwell Scientific Publications, Ltd.

15 *Breast, A. N., and others: Mechanisms of antihypertensive drug therapy, J.A.M.A. 211:480-484, Jan. 1970.

16 Brener, E.: Surgery for coronary artery disease, Am. J. Nurs. 72:469-473, March 1972.

17 Brogan, M.: Nursing care of the patient experiencing cardiac surgery for coronary artery disease, Nurs. Clin. North Am. 7:517-527, Sept. 1972.

17a *Calhoun, P. L., and Bozorgi, S.: Postoperative care following coronary surgery, Heart & Lung 3:912-915, Nov.-Dec. 1974.

18 Callard, G., and Jude, J.: Cardiopulmonary resuscitation in the cardiac care unit, Nurs. Clin. North Am. 7:573-585, Sept. 1972.

19 Chow, R.: Postoperative cardiac nursing research: a method for identifying and categorizing nursing action, Nurs. Res. 18:4-13, Jan.-Feb. 1969.

20 *Closed-chest method of cardiopulmonary resuscitation, Am. J. Nurs. 65:105, May 1965.

21 Cogen, R.: Cardiac catheterization: preparing the adult, Am. J. Nurs. 73:77-79, Jan. 1973.

21a *Collins, J. J., and Morgan, A. P.: Automated management of postoperative cardiac surgical care, Heart & Lung 3:929-932, Nov.-Dec. 1974.

22 *Creighton, H., and Hufnagle, C. A.: Aortic insufficiency and its surgical treatment, Am. J. Nurs. 58:547-550, April 1958.

23 *Cross, C. J.: Back to work after myocardial infarction, Am. J. Nurs. 62:58-61, Feb. 1962.

24 Culbert P., and Kos, B.: Teaching patients about pacemakers, Am. J. Nurs. 71:523-527, March 1971.

25 Curtin, B. C., and Reick, K. L.: Effects of bodily position on the systolic blood pressure response to Valsalva's maneuver, Nurs. Res. 18:119-123, March-April 1969.

26 Davis, L., editor: Christopher's textbook of surgery, ed. 10, Philadelphia, 1972, W. B. Saunders Co.

27 Dawber, T. R., and Thomas, H. E.: Risk factors in coronary heart disease, Cardiovasc. Nurs. 6:29, Feb. 1970.

*References preceded by an asterisk are particularly well suited for student reading.

28 *DeMeyer, J. A.: The environment of the intensive care unit, Nurs. Forum **6**(3):262-272, 1967.

29 *Dick, L. S., and Grant, M. D.: The nurse's role in rehabilitation of the child with rheumatic fever, Public Health Rep. **79**:533-536, June 1964.

30 Dietschy, J. M., and Weis, H. J.: Cholesterol synthesis by the gastrointestinal tract, Am. J. Clin. Nutr. **24**:70-76, Jan. 1971.

31 Douglas, G. W.: Rubella in pregnancy, Am. J. Nurs. **66**:2664-2666, Dec. 1966.

31a *Ellis, R.: Unusual sensory and thought disturbances after cardiac surgery, Am. J. Nurs. **72**:2021-2025, Nov. 1972.

31b Escher, D. J. W.: Types of pacemakers and their complications, Circulation **47**:1119-1130, May 1973.

32 Examination of the heart, parts 1-4, New York, 1970, American Heart Association.

33 Fletcher, A. P., and Sherry, S.: Thrombolytic (fibrinolytic) therapy for coronary heart disease, Circulation **22**:619-626, Oct. 1960.

34 Flores, A. M., and Zohman, L. R.: Energy cost of bedmaking to the cardiac patient and the nurse, Am. J. Nurs. **70**:1264-1267, June 1970.

35 *Foster, S.: Pump failure, Am. J. Nurs. **74**:1830-1834, Oct. 1974.

35a *Foster, S., and others: The postcoronary patient, Am. J. Nurs. **70**:2344-2352, Nov. 1970.

36 Fox, H. M., and others: Psychological observations of patients undergoing mitral surgery: a study of stress, Psychol. Med. **16**:186, 1954.

37 Frank, C. W., and others: Myocardial infarction in men, J.A.M.A. **198**:1241-1245, Dec. 1966.

37a Frater, R. W. M.: Postoperative care in the pediatric cardiac patient, Heart & Lung **3**:903-911, Nov.-Dec. 1974.

38 Fredrickson, D. S., and Lees, R. S.: Familial hyperlipoproteinemia. In Stanbury, J. B., Wyngaarden, J. B., and Fredrickson, D. S., editors: The metabolic basis of inherited disease, New York, 1966, McGraw-Hill Book Co.

39 Friedberg, C. K.: Diseases of the heart, ed. 3, Philadelphia, 1966, W. B. Saunders Co.

40 French, R. M.: Nurse's guide to diagnostic procedures, ed. 3, New York, 1971, McGraw-Hill Book Co.

41 Glenn, F., and others: The circulatory system and surgery, Surg. Clin. North Am. **41**:265-496, April 1961.

42 Goldman, M. J.: Principles of electrocardiography, ed. 8, Los Altos, Calif., 1973, Lange Medical Publications.

43 Grace, W. J., and others: Use of the permanent subcutaneous transvenous pacemaker in Adams-Stokes syndrome, Am. J. Cardiol. **18**:888-891, Dec. 1966.

44 *Graham, L. E.: Patient's perceptions in the CCU, Am. J. Nurs. **69**:1921-1922, Sept. 1969.

45 *Grollman, A.: Diuretics, Am. J. Nurs. **65**:84-89, Jan. 1965.

46 *Hanchett, E. S., and Johnson, R. A.: Early signs of congestive heart failure, Am. J. Nurs. **68**:1456-1461, July 1968.

46a *Harken, D. E.: Postoperative care following heart-valve surgery, Heart & Lung **3**:893-902, Nov.-Dec. 1974.

47 Harrison, T. R., and others, editors: Principles of internal medicine, ed. 7, New York, 1974, Blakiston Division, McGraw-Hill Book Co.

48 *Heller, A. F.: Nursing the patient with an artificial pacemaker, Am. J. Nurs. **64**:87-92, April 1964.

49 Hodges, L.: Systems and nursing care of the cardiac surgical patient, Nurs. Clin. North Am. **6**:415-424, Sept. 1971.

50 Humphries, J. O.: Treatment of heart block with artificial pacemakers, Mod. Concepts Cardiovasc. Dis. **33**:857-862, June 1964.

51 *Hunn, V. K.: Cardiac pacemakers, Am. J. Nurs. **69**:749-754, April 1969.

52 Hypertension and hypertensive heart disease in adults, United States 1960-1962. Vital and Health Statistics, National Center for Health Statistics, series 11, no. 3, Washington, D. C., May 1966, U. S. Department of Health, Education and Welfare.

53 Hurst, J. W., and Logue, R. B.: The heart, ed. 3, New York, 1970, McGraw-Hill Book Co.

54 *Imboden, C. A., Jr., and Wynn, J. E.: Machines in perspective, the coronary care area, Am. J. Nurs. **65**:72-76, Feb. 1965.

55 *Jarvis, D.: Open heart surgery: patients' perceptions of care, Am. J. Nurs. **70**:2591-2593, Dec. 1970.

56 Jenkins, A. C.: Successful cardiac monitoring, Nurs. Clin. North Am. **1**:537-547, Dec. 1966.

57 *Jenkins, A. C., and others: Symposium on care of the cardiac patient, Nurs. Clin. North Am. **1**:561-649, Dec. 1969.

58 *Johnson, J., and Kirby, C. K.: Surgery of the chest, Chicago, 1970, Year Book Medical Publishers, Inc.

59 *Jones, B.: Inside the coronary care unit—the patient and his responses, Am. J. Nurs. **67**:2313-2320, Nov. 1967.

60 Joyce, P.: The effectiveness of coronary-care units in reducing the mortality of acute myocardial infarction, Heart & Lung **1**:487-489, July 1972.

61 Jude, J. R., Kouwenhoven, W. B., and Knickerbocker, G. G.: Cardiac arrest, J.A.M.A. **178**:1063-1070, Dec. 1961.

62 Julian, O. C.: Cardiac pacemakers, Surg. Clin. North Am. **48**:155-162, Feb. 1968.

63 Kannel, W., and Dawber, T.: Contributors to coronary risk implications for prevention and public health: the Framingham study, Heart & Lung **1**:797-809, Nov. 1972.

64 *Kelly, A. E., and Gensini, G. G.: Coronary arteriography, Am. J. Nurs. **62**:86-90, Feb. 1962.

65 *Kennedy, M. J.: Coping with emotional stress in the patient awaiting heart surgery, Nurs. Clin. North Am. **1**:3, March 1966.

66 Kornfeld, D. S., and others: Psychiatric complications of open heart surgery, N. Engl. J. Med. **273**:287, Aug. 1965.

67 *Lamberton, M. M.: Cardiac catheterization: anticipatory nursing care, Am. J. Nurs. **71**:1718-1721, Sept. 1971.

68 Lane, C.: Intra-aortic phase-shift balloon pumping in cardiogenic shock, Am. J. Nurs. **69**:1654-1659, Aug. 1969.

69 *Larson, E. L.: The patient with acute pulmonary edema, Am. J. Nurs. **68**:1019-1021, May 1968.

70 Lawson, B.: Clinical assessment of cardiac patients in acute care facilities, Nurs. Clin. North Am. **7**:431-444, Sept. 1972.

71 *Lees, R. S., and Wilson, D. E.: The treatment of hyperlipidemia, N. Engl. J. Med. **284**:186-195, Jan. 1971.

72 Le Maitre, G. D., and Finnegan, J. M.: The patient in surgery; a guide for nurses, Philadelphia, 1970, W. B. Saunders Co.

73 *Long, B.: Sleep, Am. J. Nurs. **69**:1896-1899, Sept. 1969.

74 *Maclean, D. M., and Fowler, E. A.: Heart transplant: early postoperative care, Am. J. Nurs. **68**:2124-2127, Oct. 1968.

75 *MacVicar, J.: Exercises before and after thoracic surgery, Am. J. Nurs. **62**:61-63, Jan. 1962.

76 Malmros, H.: Dietary prevention of atherosclerosis (letter to editor), Lancet **1**:94-95, Jan. 1970.

77 Mansour, K. A., and others: Cardiac pacemakers: comparing epicardial and pervenous pacing, Geriatrics **28**:151-155, March 1973.

78 Marienfeld, C. J., and others: Rheumatic fever and rheumatic heart disease among U. S. college freshmen, 1956-1960, Public Health Rep. **79**:789-811, Sept. 1964.

79 Marriott, H. J. L.: Practical electrocardiography, ed. 6, Baltimore, 1972, The Williams & Wilkins Co.

80 Mattingly, T. W.: The clinical concept of primary myocardial disease, Circulation **32**:845-851, Nov. 1965.

81 *Meltzer, L. E.: Coronary care, electrocardiography, and the nurse, Am. J. Nurs. **65**:63-67, Dec. 1965.

82 Meltzer, L. E., Pinneo, R., and Kitchell, J. R.: Acute myocardial infarction. In Meltzer, L. E., Abdellah, F. G., and Kitchell, J. R., editors: Concepts and practices of intensive care for

nurse specialists, Philadelphia, 1969, The Charles Press, Publishers.

83 Merkel, R., and Sovie, M. D.: Electrocution hazards with transvenous pacemaker electrodes, Am. J. Nurs. **68:**2560-2563, Dec. 1968.

84 Meserko, V.: Preoperative classes for cardiac patients, Am. J. Nurs. **73:**665-669, April 1973.

85 Meyer, H. M., Jr., Parkman, P. D., and Hopps, H. E.: The control of rubella, Pediatrics **44:**5-23, July 1969.

86 Modell, W., and others: Handbook of cardiology for nurses, ed. 5, New York, 1966, Springer Publishing Co.

87 Modell, W.: Drugs of choice, 1974-1975, St. Louis, 1974, The C. V. Mosby Co.

88 Moffitt, E. A., Sessler, A. D., and Kirklin, J. W.: Postoperative care in open heart surgery, J.A.M.A. **199:**161-163, Jan. 1967.

89 *Moore, Sister Mary Consilium: Nursing care of a patient with an implanted artificial pacemaker, Cardiovasc. Nurs. **2:**19-23, Winter 1965.

90 Narrow, B. W.: Rest is . . . , Am. J. Nurs. **67:**1646-1649, Aug. 1967.

91 Nelson, W. E., and others: Textbook of pediatrics, ed. 9, Philadelphia, 1969, W. B. Saunders Co.

92 Netter, F. H.: Ciba collection of medical illustrations: the heart, 5, Summit, N. J., 1969, Ciba Pharmaceutical Co.

93 Norman, J. C., editor: Cardiac surgery, New York, 1967, Appleton-Century-Crofts.

94 *Nurse, A. G.: "But why can't I get up?" Am. J. Nurs. **53:**172-174, Feb. 1953.

95 Nursing and summary papers, Second National Conference on Cardiovascular Diseases, Division of Nursing, Washington, D. C., 1964, U. S. Department of Health, Education and Welfare.

96 *Nye, A. W., and others: Sixteen patients: postoperative nursing experience with heart transplantation, Am. J. Nurs. **69:**2630-2634, Dec. 1969.

97 Ochsner, J. L.: Surgery for myocardial revascularization, Postgrad. Med. **49:**127-130, April 1971.

98 *Olsen, E. V., and Johnson, B. J.: Hazards of immobility: effects on cardiovascular function, Am. J. Nurs. **67:**781-782, April 1967.

99 Perloff, J. K.: The cardiomyopathies—current perspectives, Circulation **44:**942-950, Nov. 1971.

100 Pinneo, R.: Cardiac monitoring, Nurs. Clin. North Am. **7:**457-467, Sept. 1972.

101 *Pitorak, E.: Open-ended care for the open heart patient, Am. J. Nurs. **67:**1452-1457, July 1967.

102 *Pitorak, E., and others: Nurses' guide to cardiac surgery and nursing care, New York, 1969, McGraw-Hill Book Co.

103 Pryor, R., editor: Heart disease in children, training program in cardiology, Division of Chronic Diseases, Heart Disease Control Program, Washington, D. C., Feb. 1966, U. S. Department of Health, Education and Welfare.

104 *Rawlings, M. S.: Heart disease today, Am. J. Nurs. **66:**303-307, Feb. 1966.

105 Riker, W. L.: Intracardiac surgery for common congenital heart lesions, Surg. Clin. North Am. **43:**133-145, Feb. 1963.

106 *Roberts, S. L.: The patients' adaptation to the coronary care unit, Nurs. Forum **9**(1):56-63, 1970.

107 *Ross, J.: The nurse and the patient with open heart surgery, J. Nurs. Ed. **1:**25-29, Sept. 1962.

108 Sanderson, R. G.: The cardiac patient, Philadelphia, 1972, W. B. Saunders Co.

109 Schamroth, L.: Some basic principles governing the electrophysiology and the diagnosis of heart rhythms, Heart & Lung **1:**45-50, Jan. 1972.

110 Schamroth, L., and Jaspan, J.: Variant angina pectoris: a typical Prinzmetal's angina pectoris, Heart & Lung **2:**431-433, May 1973.

111 Scheuer, R.: Cardiopulmonary resuscitation in seven community hospitals, Heart & Lung **1:**810-817, Nov. 1972.

112 *Schmitt, Y., Hood, W. B., Jr., and Lown, B.: Armchair treatment in the coronary care unit: effect on blood pressure and pulse, Nurs. Res. **18:**114-118, March-April, 1969.

113 Schrogie, J. J.: Cardiopulmonary resuscitation in practice, Public Health Rep. **81:**128-132, Feb. 1966.

114 Sirak, H. D.: Operable heart disease, St. Louis, 1966, The C. V. Mosby Co.

115 *Smith, C. A.: Body image changes after myocardial infarction, Nurs. Clin. North Am. **7:**663-667, Dec. 1972.

116 Sovie, M., and Fruehan, C.: Protecting the patient from electrical hazards, Nurs. Clin. North Am. **7:**469-480, Sept. 1972.

117 Spandau, M.: Insertion of temporary cardiac pacemakers without fluoroscopy, Am. J. Nurs. **70:**1011-1013, May 1970.

118 *Stamler, J., and others: Coronary proneness and approaches to preventing heart attacks, Am. J. Nurs. **66:**1788-1793, Aug. 1966.

119 Swan, H. J.: Complications of cardiac catheterization, Cardiovasc. Nurs. **4:**27-30, Nov. 1968.

120 Traught, E.: Equipment hazards, Am. J. Nurs. **73:**858-862, May 1973.

121 Turpeinen, O.: Diet and coronary events, J. Am. Diet. Assoc. **52:**209-213, March 1968.

122 *Turell, D. J.: The cardiac patient returns to work, Am. J. Nurs. **65:**115-117, Aug. 1965.

123 *Twerski, A. J.: Psychological considerations on the coronary care unit, Cardiovasc. Nurs. **7:**65-68, March-April 1971.

124 U. S. Department of Health, Education and Welfare, National Center for Health Statistics: Monthly Vital Statistics Report, Annual Summary for the United States, vol. 18, 1972, Aug. 1973.

125 *Varvaro, F. F.: Teaching the patient about open heart surgery, Am. J. Nurs. **65:**111-115, Oct. 1965.

126 *Vinsant, M., and others: Pacemakers in 1972, Heart & Lung **1:**362-373, May 1972.

127 *Weiler, Sister M. Cashel: Postoperative patients evaluate preoperative instruction, Am. J. Nurs. **68:**1465-1467, July 1968.

128 Whipple, G., and others: Acute coronary care, Boston, 1972, Little, Brown & Co.

129 *Williams, C.: The CCU nurse has a pacemaker, Am. J. Nurs. **72:**900-902, May 1972.

130 Williams, S. R.: Nutrition and diet therapy, ed. 2, St. Louis, 1973, The C. V. Mosby Co.

131 Willis, F. N., and Dunsmore, N. M.: Work orientation health attitudes and compliance with therapeutic advice, Nurs. Res. **16:**22-25, Winter 1967.

132 Wilson, S.: Aortocoronary saphenous vein bypass: a review of the literature, Heart & Lung **2:**90-103, Jan. 1973.

133 *Wolfer, J., and Davis, C. E.: Assessment of surgical patients' preoperative emotional condition and postoperative welfare, Nurs. Res. **19:**402-414, Sept.-Oct. 1970.

134 *Wood, E. C.: Understanding the patient with heart disease, Nurs. Outlook **7:**90-92, Feb. 1959.

135 Yokes, J.: The influence of bioengineering on the nurse and the cardiac patient. In Bergersen, B. S., and others, editors: Current concepts in clinical nursing, vol. 1, St. Louis, 1967, The C. V. Mosby Co.

136 Yokes, J. A., and Reed, W. A.: Heart surgery. In Meltzer, L. E., Abdellah, F. G., and Kitchell, J. R., editors: Concepts and practices of intensive care for nurse specialists, Philadelphia, 1969, The Charles Press Publishers.

137 *Yudkin, J., and Morland, J.: Sugar intake and myocardial infarction, Am. J. Clin. Nutr. **20:**503-506, May 1967.

18 Peripheral vascular diseases

Health education
Arterial disease
Venous disease
Lymphedema
Special surgical procedures

■ Peripheral vascular diseases are usually only part of a complex disease syndrome, cardiovascular-renal disease, that affects the entire body. It is rare for anyone to live to old age without undergoing some pathologic change in the cardiovascular system. It has been estimated that at least 60% of all persons in the United States who are 50 years of age or over will die of cardiovascular-renal disease. Because peripheral vascular disease of the extremities is so often associated with other cardiovascular diseases, it is difficult to determine statistically how many persons die primarily of the former condition. It is obvious, however, that this is one of the most important disease groups with which the nurse will work and one in which the greatest effort toward early control is well justified.

Peripheral vascular disease is a general term that refers to all disease of blood vessels outside the heart and to disease of the lymph vessels. It also includes all tissue changes caused by disease of these vessels. This chapter, however, will be concerned largely with peripheral vascular disease of the lower extremities. There are certain aspects of nursing care common to most patients with peripheral vascular disease. To avoid repetition, nursing intervention that applies to many patients with peripheral vascular diseases will be considered before individual disease conditions and related nursing responsibilities

are discussed. Only disease conditions that occur quite often are included. For information about other important, though less frequently occurring, diseases the reader is referred to specialized texts. Lower limb amputations are discussed in this chapter because, unfortunately, they are necessary for some patients who have peripheral vascular disease. Techniques of treatment and management are similar to those used for the patient who has had an amputation following trauma, although rehabilitation of the latter usually is less difficult because the amputation is less likely to accompany a chronic medical disease.

■ HEALTH EDUCATION

At present there is no specific way to prevent peripheral vascular disease. However, measures that help people avoid situations predisposing to impaired circulation, and thus to peripheral vascular diseases, should be taught. Much of the nursing care of persons with peripheral vascular disease is concerned with limiting the progress of the disease and with preventing complications so that patients can live out their lives with reasonable health and comfort. The patients often are cared for in the outpatient clinic, and thus it is important that a careful record be kept of the instructions given to the patient and his understanding of them. Such a plan will assure continuity of care on subsequent visits.

The nurse should teach health conservation measures to persons who have early signs of vascular disease. Indeed, any patient, especially one of middle age or over, can benefit from similar teaching. Since danger of peripheral vascular disease is greatest in

■ STUDY QUESTIONS

1 Review the anatomic structure of the arteries and veins. What are the major differences? What forces work to assist the return of blood from the veins to the heart?
2 What is meant by collateral circulation? Is it uniform throughout the body?
3 Review the major differences between arteriosclerosis and atherosclerosis. What vessels are primarily affected by these two conditions?
4 List the factors contributing to the development of arteriosclerosis and atherosclerosis. Explain the physiologic mechanisms through which each factor affects the disease process.
5 Review the basic procedures for warm soaks and for continuous warm packs. What are the general precautions to be taken in care of patients having these treatments?

dependent parts of the body, where adequate circulation is hardest to preserve, people should be taught measures to maintain and improve circulation in the lower extremities. In industry the nurse who helps the employees find chairs of a suitable height in order to prevent sharp knee flexion is contributing to prevention of disease. Sitting for long hours with the knees bent causes pressure on the arteries and veins of the legs, resulting in slight swelling and discomfort. The nurse may plan with supervisors in industry to provide short rest periods at frequent intervals for persons who must stand still or sit with knees bent while they work. Since walking and moving about improve circulation, such activities should be encouraged during these periods. The nurse caring for a patient hospitalized for acute peripheral vascular disease should use this opportunity to teach the patient general preventive measures. Any patient undergoing surgery or anyone who must be immobilized for a period of time should also be taught preventive measures. The nurse making an antepartal home visit is contributing to prevention of vascular disease when questioning the patient about her posture and the kind of girdle and shoes she wears and when the patient is reminded to take regular exercise such as walking and to rest periodically with her legs elevated above the heart level.

Psychologic and emotional problems

Peripheral vascular diseases are demoralizing for a variety of reasons. The nurse should understand these reasons because they vitally affect the patient's response to preventive teaching and his adjustment to hospital care and necessary treatment.

Age. The patient with peripheral vascular disease is often in the older age group. Although some relatively infrequent conditions such as Raynaud's disease and thromboangiitis obliterans (Buerger's disease) usually occur in younger persons and varicose veins are fairly common among persons who are young, the vast majority of patients who develop peripheral vascular disease are over 50 years of age. The person at this age faces many serious emotional problems in addition to illness. He may be adjusting to the idea that his children have grown up and established homes and families of their own and no longer are dependent on him. For the first time, he may be meeting younger workers whose decisions and judgments are taking precedence over his, or he may fear approaching retirement. He is at the age when some of his friends have died, causing him to become lonely and introspective. At this time of life other diseases often appear, so that the patient may have not just one but a number of physical ailments, leading to further discouragement. Thus, the patient may have many psychosocial and emotional concerns that will alter his response to the new illness

and make his adjustment to its restrictions difficult.

Chronicity of illness. Peripheral vascular diseases are chronic or lead to chronic illness. They are usually slow in onset, and much irreversible vascular damage may have occurred before symptoms are severe enough to bring the patient to a physician. Treatment is often long and tedious. The period of hospitalization is usually longer than for many other conditions that may require dramatic surgery or related treatment. For example, months of hospital or convalescent care may be necessary for the treatment of a small ulcer of the leg or some other seemingly trivial but extremely discouraging condition. During this time the patient may worry about finances, curtailment of normal social outlets, and innumerable other problems. Even if he is being treated on an ambulatory basis, he still faces a long period of medical treatment, probable loss of income from absence from work, and the possibility of becoming even more incapacitated and a burden to his family or to others as he grows older.

Discouraged by the chronic nature of his ailment and its attendant problems, the patient may seek a quick cure by following the advice of nonprofessional persons or by using patent remedies. Some of these remedies only waste the patient's money, and others are actually harmful. Mechanical devices are sometimes advertised as being successful in restoring normal circulation. Massage and other physical modalities may be recommended by persons who have no real evidence of their effectiveness. Thus the nurse should encourage the patient to remain under the supervision of one physician in whom both he and his family have confidence and should encourage him to take newspaper clippings describing miracle treatments to his physician for explanation. Well-meaning friends and relatives may do the patient harm by describing more rapid progress of someone with the same condition. The nurse can help by explaining that each patient is different and that the blood vessels of one person cannot be accurately compared with those of another. Again, the patient may be referred to his own physician for reassurance.

The patient's main worry may be the expense of hospitalization, although the 1965 federal hospital insurance and medical care law (Medicare) has decreased this problem for persons over 65 years of age. The data obtained in a nursing history should provide the nurse with the information necessary to determine whether or not the patient can be safely cared for at home. If a responsible relative or friend is willing to give the prescribed care and someone can run necessary errands so that the patient may remain off his feet, the patient will probably be happier being cared for in his own home. Even the person living in a rural area and the one living alone may be able to leave the hospital if community nursing service is available to give or to supervise care and to report changes to the physician.

Pain. Most peripheral vascular diseases cause pain, but the pain may vary as to kind. For example, it may be sudden and excruciating, as in embolic thrombosis; constant and gnawing, as in arteriosclerosis; "heavy" and burning, as in varicose veins; or steady and throbbing, as when gangrene threatens. The characteristic symptom of pain is doubly significant because of the chronicity of most vascular diseases. Having lived with pain for a long time, the patient has suffered from its demoralizing effects. His outlook on his surroundings, his attitudes regarding medical treatment, and his response to improvement and rehabilitation may be affected by constant pain. The patient is greatly in need of people who show a real interest in him as a person and who have a positive approach to his physical ailment. The nurse cannot expect a mental outlook developed over weeks or months to change in a day or two.

The patient who has a long history of continuous pain or who is in intense pain may be irritated easily. A tardy medication, sugar missing from the breakfast tray, or a neglected errand are incidents that may upset him unduly and increase his discouragement. Knowledge of the disease, of how it has affected the individual patient, and his response to pain will help the nurse understand the patient's behavior.

Physical care

Warmth. Warmth is advised for most patients with peripheral vascular disease because it causes vasodilation and thereby improves circulation to the affected part. However, warmth in the form of direct heat is seldom, if ever, applied to the affected part because it results in an increased demand for blood in the extremity already suffering from depleted circulation. Another reason for not applying local heat is that many patients with peripheral vascular disease also have peripheral nerve degeneration, which lessens sensitivity to heat, thus predisposing to burns. A safe rule to follow is never, under any circumstances, apply hot-water bottles, heating pads, or other forms of local heat to the legs or feet without a specific order. Soaking the feet in hot or even very warm water is seldom advised. The temperature of the water into which the individual places his feet should always be tested; it should not exceed 90° F. The patient must be cautioned not to attempt to warm his feet by placing them on a warm radiator or in an open oven. Warmth to the extremities can be increased by placing a hot-water bottle or heating pad on the abdomen. This causes reflex dilation of the blood vessels of the legs. Immersing the entire body in a warm bath also warms the extremities. Loose woolen bed socks can be worn at night.

The patient should be in a warm environment whenever possible. The temperature of the room should be at least 21° C. (70° F.), and hospitalized patients may need even more warmth for maximum comfort. The patient should be able to sense that he is rather warm but should not be warm enough to perspire more than usual.

It must be remembered that exposure of any part of the body to cold can cause chilling of the entire body. This in turn causes vasoconstriction and lessens circulation in a diseased extremity. In cold weather the patient with peripheral vascular disease should wear warm clothing such as long underwear, fleece-lined shoes, earmuffs, scarf, and extra-heavy coats, suits, or dresses. If chilling has been experienced, the patient should drink something hot and get to a warm room as soon as possible.

Cleanliness and avoidance of infection. Because resistance to infection is low when tissues are inadequately nourished and oxygenated, all patients with vascular disease need instruction in the care of their feet and in prevention of infection. A daily bath is recommended unless the patient is quite elderly, in which case two or three baths a week are sufficient. The patient should be advised to check the temperature of the bathwater carefully with his elbow before stepping into the tub, because sensation in his feet may be diminished. This simple practice would prevent many patients from being burned. A small amount of a mild soap or a superfatted soap should be used. The skin should be dried by gentle patting; vigorous rubbing should be avoided.

While bathing, the patient should look for any skin changes on his legs and feet. A dry scaling over the tibia may be the beginning of "bath itch," which is common in older people who have dry skin and who bathe too often and use harsh soaps. If it appears, fewer baths should be taken, superfatted soap should be used, and the skin should be lubricated with lanolin or a moisturizing agent. Blueness or swelling around varicosities, and hard, reddened, or painful areas, which may indicate phlebitis, should be reported to a physician at once. Trophic changes such as dryness, cracking, hardness, thickening, and brownish discolorations of the toenails indicate impairment of blood supply and should also be called to the physician's attention.

If the patient does not bathe each day, he should wash his feet in tepid water, dry them thoroughly, being particularly careful to dry between the toes, and inspect them for calluses, blisters, or any other abnormalities. If he is old and has failing vision, a member of the family should inspect his feet periodically. In the daily routine care of the feet, the skin and base of the nails should be gently massaged with lubricants or moisturizing agents. Alcohol is drying to the skin and should not be used. Each toe should be gently massaged from the distal end proximally to stimulate circulation. Powder may be used between the toes, with care being taken that it does not cake and that it is thoroughly removed at the next washing. Authorities maintain that epidermophytosis (athlete's foot), which is often a precursor of infection, ulceration, and gangrene in the feet of persons with arterial insufficiency, will seldom develop if the toes and feet are kept dry at all times. Therefore the patient who perspires profusely should powder between his toes more than once a day and should change his socks at least daily. Preparations advertised in drugstores should not be used, since they are usually too strong for feet with impaired circulation. Foot powders should only be used if prescribed by the physician. Directions should always be read carefully. Small pieces of lamb's wool or cotton can be placed between the toes to absorb the perspiration.

To prevent ingrown toenails, the nails should be cut carefully at regular intervals. Before the nails are cut, the feet should be soaked in tepid water. The nails should be cut straight across and slightly rounded at the sides with a file. They must never be cut down to the level of the tissue. Pocketknives, razor blades, or scissors should never be used. The patient should equip himself with a pair of toenail clippers. Files are usually considered safe. However, tissues can be traumatized by emery boards and files, particularly when the patient lacks normal sensation in the toes. Elderly persons with poor vision should not cut their own toenails. A member of the family or a podiatrist should do it for them.

With daily care a toenail that has a tendency to "curl under" at the side of the toe can be trained to grow more normally, but no efforts should be made to "straighten" the nail by vigorous treatment. With the rounded end of an ordinary toothpick, a small wisp of cotton should be inserted gently under the edge of the nail. The cotton must be changed daily. Although it may be weeks before any improvement is seen, with patience and persistence most nails that tend to grow under can be made to grow more normally unless there is aggravation by a condition such as pressure from shoes. Nails that are thickened or deformed should not be cut or filed. They should be treated only by a podiatrist or physician who knows of the individual's circulatory impairment.

Medical care should be sought for blisters and for corns, calluses, and areas of thickened skin that cannot be rubbed away with a washcloth and an emery board after having been soaked. Soap poultices made of any soft soap such as shaving cream may be used to soften corns and calluses before rubbing is attempted. The patient with circulatory disease of any kind should be advised to seek medical advise before going to a podiatrist.

Protection from trauma and pressure. The patient should be warned to avoid injury to his feet and legs and to watch carefully for infection following trauma. He should not walk barefoot for fear of splinters causing injury. It also is dangerous for him to scratch any minor skin lesions. Many stubborn ulcers of the leg have followed the vigorous scratching of mosquito or other insect bites. Venous stasis may cause itching that can be most annoying. This itching usually follows long periods of standing and will subside if the patient rests with the feet elevated for a few minutes every hour or two. The warning not to scratch the skin is hard to heed at times. Calamine lotion is sometimes prescribed by the physician when pruritus is troublesome. Any minor infection of the legs or the feet should be viewed as a major one by a patient with peripheral vascular disease. He should never attempt self-treatment when any signs of infection develop.

To avoid fungal infections of the feet, socks or stockings should be washed daily. If they are wool or have a tendency to shrink, they should be stretched over a dryer. Otherwise they may constrict circulation. Sock frames can be purchased at most notion counters, or a simple, inexpensive dryer can be made from a metal coat hanger.

The patient should have at least two pairs of shoes and should wear them on alternate days, thus giving each pair a chance to air. If shoes become wet, they should be dried slowly on shoe trees to help preserve their shape. New shoes should be broken in gradually. Leather shoes are best because they give good support to the feet. Canvas, linen, or perforated nylon shoes provide ventilation, are comfortable in warm weather, and are safe if they have leather soles. Rubber-soled shoes are not advised for persons who have any kind of vascular disease because they retard evaporation and thus may contribute to the development of fungal infection. Shoes should be carefully fitted by experienced persons. They should extend about $1/2$ inch beyond the longest toe and should be wide enough to avoid pressure anywhere on the foot and to allow fairly free movement of the toes within the shoe. The inner last of the shoe should be straight, and the longitudinal arch of the shoe should support that of the foot. Playshoes and ballet slippers, which afford little or no support, are not recommended for persons with peripheral vascular disease, although there is no objection to women wearing pumps with moderately high heels. In fact, pumps are good inasmuch as the feet can be slipped out of the shoes and the toes wiggled at intervals. However, the shoes should be roomy enough so that they can be put on again easily.

When sleeping, the person with peripheral vascular disease should have lightweight covers that are loose and do not permit any pressure on the toes, which often burn and are painful. The patient who lives at home should be taught how to improvise a board at the foot of his bed to keep the weight of

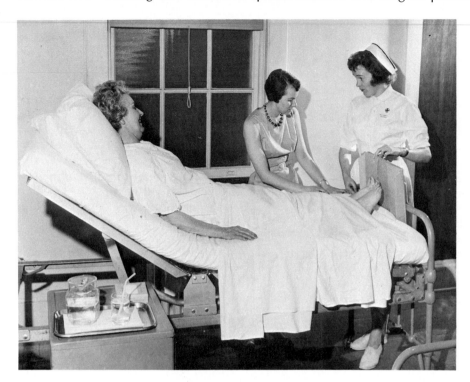

FIG. 18-1. The nurse instructs the patient's daughter how to improvise equipment to keep bed linen off the patient's sensitive feet.

covers from his feet (Fig. 18-1). The patient who is hospitalized also should have a padded board or box at the foot of the bed. These devices are preferable to a cradle, which may hamper freedom of movement and against which the patient may accidentally strike his foot. If a cradle must be used, it should be padded and bath blankets should be placed over the cradle and tucked securely under the mattress to prevent drafts on the feet.

Rest, exercise, and posture. A careful balance of rest and exercise is necessary for the patient with peripheral vascular disease. Exercise improves arterial circulation by promoting alternate muscle contraction and relaxation, thereby causing blood vessels to contract and dilate. Exercise not only improves return of venous blood from the extremities to the heart but also is one of the most important stimuli for the development of collateral circulation.[8] Too much exercise, however, increases metabolism, thereby increasing the demands placed on the circulation to take nutrients to the tissues and to remove the products of metabolism. Complete rest may be necessary in the presence of associated medical illnesses such as heart disease, thrombophlebitis, or gangrene. The nurse should check with the physician so that proper instruction can be given regarding balance between rest and activity. In regard to posture, the following is a safe guide for all patients with peripheral vascular disease (or, indeed, for anyone): Do not stay in *any* position too long. This is particularly important for the elderly person, who often has both arterial and venous disease.

Much emphasis has been placed on elevation of

the feet, and many persons believe that it will benefit them. However, it may cause damage when the patient has arterial insufficiency because it will interfere with adequate circulation through arteries in the lower extremities. The nurse must *clearly understand* the patient's condition and the physician's orders before giving instructions in this regard. The effect of position on circulation can be clearly understood by relating direction of blood flow to the effects of gravity. Arteries take oxygenated blood away from the heart; elevating the extremities tends to deliver blood back to the heart, hence it tends to hamper arterial function. Long periods of standing may result in venous congestion as the simple effects of gravity increase the work of the veins as they return deoxygenated blood to the heart. It is safe to assume that the flat position is best over an extended period of time unless otherwise ordered.

Long periods of standing still should be avoided by persons with either venous or arterial disease, and short periods should be alternated with exercise such as rapid walking. Those who have venous disease should alternate standing and walking with elevation of the affected limbs.

The importance of posture must be stressed in the care and teaching of patients with peripheral vascular disease. The patient should sleep on a firm mattress. A soft mattress may allow enough flexion of the trunk at the hips to impede circulation to the lower extremities. It may also permit the lower limbs to be higher than the heart, which is undesirable in arterial disease. The height of a chair should be such that the knees are not bent at more than a right angle, and the depth of the seat should permit two fingers between the chair seat and the popliteal spaces. Both of these provisions will help to prevent pressure on the popliteal vessels that would obstruct arterial flow to the limbs and interfere with venous return. Furthermore, the patient should never cross his legs at the knee, because this position also causes pressure on the popliteal vessels. He should develop the habit of rotating his foot at the ankle, bending the foot up and down, and straightening the knee at intervals. The patient should be taught to do these exercises while traveling also. The importance of frequent stops if traveling by car or getting out of one's seat and walking in the aisle for a few moments if traveling by plane, bus, or train should be emphasized. Attendance at movies or other satisfying diversion can sometimes be made safe and comfortable for patients with impaired circulation by the use of these simple measures to improve circulation.

Specific exercises (*Buerger-Allen*) to empty blood vessels and stimulate collateral circulation are rarely used. Instead, moderate exercise is recommended. One of the best exercises for stimulating the flow of blood to the legs is walking. The patient may be able to build up tolerance so that he can walk a mile or more a day. He should be instructed to stop and rest if pain develops and then to continue walking after it disappears.[8] Some physicians also recommend the use of a rocking chair because it helps to stimulate the muscles in the legs to contract and relax as the patient rocks.

Avoidance of constriction of circulation. The patient with peripheral vascular disease must not wear anything that constricts circulation. Rolled garters, knitted hose designed to stay up without garters, and girdles that cause constriction around the thighs and groin should not be worn. Some physicians also believe that tight waistbands should not be worn. Men may be advised to wear suspenders instead of belts, and women should select garter belts that do not constrict or light, full-length corsets instead of girdles. Socks that do not require garters should be worn by men. Shoelaces should be tied loosely. If edema of the feet occurs at the end of the day, the shoelaces should be loosened and relaced several times each day. Elastic shoelaces are preferred by some patients who have a moderate amount of edema of the feet or ankles.

Diet. The patient with peripheral vascular disease should avoid becoming overweight. Excess fat places an added burden on diseased arteries that already have difficulty in keeping up with tissue demands. Obesity in the patient with venous disease increases congestion and probably lessens the effectiveness of muscles in assisting with the return flow of blood. If the patient has limited cardiac capacity in addition to vascular disease, the heart and the entire vascular system are taxed to such an extent that distribution of blood to the extremities is curtailed. Reducing diets, however, must always be under medical supervision. Harm can be done, particularly to the elderly patient, by rapid loss of weight, which may alter pressure within sclerosed arteries and make it possible for a clot to form, causing further depletion of the nutrient supply to tissues supplied by the arteries.

When a reducing diet has been prescribed the nurse can be of real assistance in helping to plan meals that are satisfying to the patient and yet within his caloric restrictions and financial means. The patient with peripheral vascular disease is usually advised to have a diet high in protein but low in saturated fats because protein helps to prevent breakdown of tissues. If he has a lesion such as a varicose ulcer, a diet high in protein should help to promote healing. The diet should include foods high in B complex vitamins, which are important in maintaining normal health of blood vessels, and vitamin C, which is essential in healing and in the prevention of both internal and external hemorrhage.

It is generally recommended that patients with peripheral vascular disease take more fluids than the normal person. As many as 15 to 20 glasses of water or equivalent fluids are often recommended. This amount may improve the quality of the limited blood supply to the limbs by increasing elimination of waste products. It is also believed that it may lessen the viscosity of the blood and thus help to prevent the formation of thrombi.

As part of the nursing history, the nurse should learn about the patient's life-style and how this affects his ability to comply with the prescribed therapy. For example, does the patient have to walk a long distance or climb several flights of stairs to bring groceries home? Climbing may cause severe pain in the legs because of inadequate oxygenation of the tissues. Some arrangements, therefore, must be made to assist the patient with this chore. If he lives alone, it should be determined whether someone in his building or neighborhood can shop for him. A thorough nursing history would reveal that the young mother with a stubborn ulcer that complicated phlebitis before delivery is so harassed with feeding the baby, getting other children off to school, or otherwise attended to that she neglects her own breakfast and lunch. The nurse may discover that the elderly man with arteriosclerosis develops intermittent claudication when he walks from his rooming house to the nearest restaurant, causing him to skip one or two meals each day. The assistance of the family and/or social worker may be needed to solve particular problems.

Medications. In addition to medications for pain, the two important classes of drugs given to patients with peripheral vascular disease are vasodilators, which dilate blood vessels, and anticoagulants, which lessen the tendency of the blood to clot. These agents are used most commonly for patients receiving long-term medical therapy who are not candidates for surgery. Drugs such as fibrinolytic agents that are capable of dissolving thrombi that have already been formed have not been demonstrated as being completely safe for general use and are still experimental. Streptokinase and urokinase are such agents being studied. These drugs hold future promise in the field.[25]

Vasodilators may be given when the objective is to lessen vasospasm in the arterioles of the lower extremities, when arteriosclerosis has caused narrowing of the lumen of the vessel or neighboring vessels, or when a thrombus has formed and caused partial or total obstruction. If a clot is adherent to a blood vessel, an anticoagulant drug may be given with the vasodilator to prevent further clot formation. While several drugs are useful for vasodilation, the excellent vasodilatory effects of warm baths, heat to the abdomen, and hot fluids taken orally should not be overlooked.

Vasodilators. The drug *papaverine,* an alkaloid of opium, has long been known to have a relaxing effect on the smooth muscle of the blood vessels, especially if smasm occurs. It is not habit-forming. The usual dose is 30 to 60 mg. ($1/2$ to 1 grain) intramuscularly or intravenously, or 100 mg. ($1^1/2$ grains) orally.[9] This drug may be used in the treatment of acute arterial occlusion associated with arteriosclerosis obliterans.

Tolazoline hydrochloride (Priscoline), 25 to 50 mg. ($3/8$ to $3/4$ grain), given orally three to four times a day, is an adrenergic blocking agent (sympatholytic drug).[9] It also may be given intravenously. It prevents the transmission of impulses from the ends of the vasoconstrictor sympathetic fibers to the smooth muscle of the arterioles, and thus produces vasodilation. Some other drugs that have a similar effect and that are prescribed for vasodilation in peripheral vascular diseases are *azapetine phosphate* (Ilidar), *dibenzyl-β-chloroethylamine* (Dibenamine), and *phenoxybenzamine hydrochloride* (Dibenzyline). Toxic reactions to these drugs include palpitation, tachycardia, nausea and vomiting, pruritus and abnormal skin sensations, and drop in blood pressure. Toxic signs should be carefully watched for in any patient receiving these drugs and must be reported to the doctor at once. The patient who cannot tolerate one of these drugs may be able to take another without untoward reactions.

Besides the adrenergic blocking agents there are newer drugs that are used for their beneficial effect in peripheral vascular disease. *Isoxsuprine* (Vasodilan) and *nylidrin hydrochloride* (Arlidin) are sympathomimetic amines that are chemically similar to epinephrine. They possess vasodilating effects, particularly in the vessels in skeletal muscles. Favorable results have been reported with the use of these agents in the treatment of intermittent claudication. Isoxsuprine is usually given orally (10 to 20 mg. four times a day); an intramuscular form is also available. Nylidrin is administered orally (6 to 12 mg. three times a day) or intramuscularly (5 mg. once daily). Side effects include nervousness, palpitation, and nausea and vomiting. *Cyclandelate* (Cyclospasmol) and *nicotinyl tartrate* (Roniacol) produce direct vasodilation of the smooth muscle of the peripheral blood vessels. The usual dosage of cyclandelate is 100 to 200 mg. four times daily; the dose of nicotinyl is 50 to 150 mg. three times daily after meals. Both can produce dizziness, flushing, and nausea and vomiting. The latter is more likely to occur with nicotinyl because it acts like nicotinic acid.

Alcohol is a very useful drug in dilating the blood vessels. The usual dosage is 30 to 60 ml. three to four times a day. The alcohol preparation often ordered is whiskey and soda, but any of the common beverages containing alcohol can be used. Some physicians order a double dose at bedtime to produce maximum effect during the hours when muscle action is not assisting the flow of blood to the legs. *Caffeine* (contained in tea and coffee) and *theobromine* (found in chocolate) also are peripheral vasodilators, but these drugs are seldom given for their vasodilating effect. However, because they have this effect, there usually is no need to eliminate tea, coffee, and chocolate from the diet of the patient with peripheral vascular disease.

Anticoagulants. Two of the commonly used anticoagulant drugs are *heparin* and *bishydroxycoumarin* (Dicumarol), although there are many other prothrombin depressants now available.[51] These drugs are used widely in the treatment of both venous and arterial thrombosis and are used prophylactically for persons with a threatened thrombosis or threatened recurrence of conditions such as thrombophlebitis. They act therapeutically by prolonging the clotting time of the blood. They will not dissolve clots already formed but will prevent extension of a clot and inhibit formation of new ones.

Heparin antagonizes the activation of prothrombin to thrombin and in this way prolongs the clotting time of blood. It can be given only parenterally because it is destroyed by the gastric secretions of the stomach. Its effect is almost immediate, but its action ceases after 3 to 4 hours. Heparin dosage is expressed in units or milligrams and is calculated individually for each patient; 5,000 units (50 mg.) is an average dose and is administered through an intravenous line every 3 to 4 hours. This drug is often used to lower the prothrombin time until an oral anticoagulant that acts more slowly can take effect; frequent clotting time determinations must be done.

Planning of nursing care must emphasize the increased tendency for bleeding in these patients. (For further discussion of nursing responsibilities, see p. 344).

Bishydroxycoumarin acts by suppressing the activity of the liver in its formation of prothrombin. It takes 12 to 24 hours to take effect, and its action persists for 24 to 72 hours after the drug is discontinued. The usual maintenance dosage is 25 to 100 mg./day administered orally.[9] Frequent determinations of the prothrombin level must be obtained and the dose regulated accordingly. Daily prothrombin levels are important while the dose is being regulated. Most physicians believe that the prothrombin level should be kept between 10% and 30% of normal.

Warfarin sodium (Coumadin, Prothromadin) is now widely used. Ethyl biscoumacetate (Tromexan) is another synthetic drug that has an action similar to that of bishydroxycoumarin, although it acts more quickly and its effect lasts for a shorter time.

Any anticoagulant drug requires very careful regulation as to amount and continuity of dosage. If the dosage is too large, the patient's increased tendency to bleed reaches dangerous levels, and if given in combination with other drugs predisposing to bleeding such as acetylsalicylic acid preparations, the problem becomes aggravated. If the dosage is too small, the patient may have no relief from symptoms of thrombosis and may even have additional thrombus formation.

If bleeding results from too much heparin, *protamine sulfate,* a heparin antagonist, is given. Protamine acts almost immediately, and its effect persists for about 2 hours. The physician slowly injects a 1% solution intravenously. The total amount given depends on the amount of heparin that was given and on the patient's symptoms. If a patient taking bishydroxycoumarin should bleed from any body orifice such as the nose, mouth, or urinary tract, the physician should be notified before another dose is taken. Usually the drug is discontinued, and vitamin K (menadione sodium bisulfite) or vitamin K_1 (phytonadione) is given intravenously or orally. If the hemorrhage is excessive, transfusions are given. Nursing care includes reassurance of the patient and careful observation for signs of further hemorrhage.

Anticoagulant therapy undoubtedly has prolonged the lives of many persons and enabled them to live quite satisfactorily and productively. The patient who must remain on this drug indefinitely, however, needs encouragement and sympathetic medical and nursing care. Unfortunately the vein must be punctured at regular intervals to obtain blood for a prothrombin determination. If large doses are needed, this procedure must be done at least two to three times a week and sometimes daily. When smaller doses of anticoagulant are given over long periods, a prothrombin determination is done every 1 to 4 weeks. This experience is unpleasant for the patient, and its continuance over weeks and months may place a real restraint on the activities of the ambulatory patient. Vacations, for example, present real problems, and even short trips must be carefully planned.

Teaching is one of the most important nursing measures in caring for the patient treated with anticoagulants. The patient must be taught to recognize the signs of bleeding from any site and to report them immediately. He should carry an identification card stating that he takes anticoagulant drugs so that, in the event of accident, persons who give him medical care will know this fact. The identification card should also contain the name and telephone number of the physician prescribing the drug.

Patients should also be taught not to take any other medications while taking anticoagulants without consulting a physician first. Aspirin preparations and steroid preparations can be particularly dangerous in conjunction with heparin and coumadin.

Proteolytic enzymes. Streptokinase-streptodornase (Varidase), purified trypsin crystalline (Tryptar), and fibrinuclease (Elase) are proteolytic enzymes that will dissolve fibrinous material and purulent accumulations. They are valuable in removing necrotic tissue for debridement. These enzymes are frequently ordered in treatment of ulcers on the legs, which may occur as a complication of peripheral vascular disease resulting from inadequte circulation. The enzymes used in conjunction with antibiotics seem to promote more rapid healing. The drugs are usually applied topically in the form of wet dressings or are injected into cavities.

Smoking. Nicotine causes vasoconstriction and spasm of the peripheral arteries; therefore smoking is contraindicated in all vascular diseases. Damage comes from inhaling smoke; there is no evidence that chewing tobacco or using snuff contributes to vasospasm. The relationship between arteriospasm and smoking is so definite that many physicians feel it is useless to try to treat the patient unless he gives up smoking. Smoking should be immediately discontinued in any kind of arterial vascular disease and is also contraindicated in venous disease because the arteries surrounding a thrombosed vein often develop spasms. Gangrene has even been known to follow spasm from this cause.

Although difficult for the nonsmoker to understand, giving up cigarettes is almost impossible for some people. The dependency on cigarettes can be almost as strong for some as a dependency on narcotics. Many patients continue to smoke even after they have lost a toe or foot as a result of vascular disease and know that their smoking aggravates the condition.

Although there is no sure way to help the patient give up smoking, there are some measures that may be helpful. Gum or coffee sometimes helps or finding activities to keep the patient busy. Some find that cutting down to fewer and fewer cigarettes each day is easier than stopping suddenly. Constant reminders and strict discipline often do more harm than good. Patient understanding and reiteration of faith in the patient's ability to stop smoking are more helpful than disapproval of lapses.

Special beds. The *oscillating bed* (Sanders) may be used to improve circulation to the lower extremities. The electrically operated bed seesaws in a cycle that usually takes 1 to 2½ minutes but can be regulated according to need or preference. The foot of the bed rises 6 inches above the horizontal and descends 12 to 15 inches with a smooth transition from one motion to another (Fig. 18-2). The patient should be given an adequate explanation of why the bed is recommended and may need time to become adjusted to the motion. Dizziness, nausea, and headache are probably of psychic origin, but the patient is encouraged to stop the bed for a few minutes should these symptoms occur. He is given the control switch and is shown how to use it. The bed is usually stopped for meals and other necessary care, but otherwise the patient is encouraged to keep it operating both day and night. Since some patients tend to slide downward as the foot of the bed lowers, and pressure of the feet against the footboard causes pain, a padded footboard should be placed on the bed. The bed should be checked frequently by an electrician. It should work smoothly without disturbing sounds or vibration.

The *CircOlectric bed* may be used to change the patient's position at intervals and thus improve his circulation. This bed allows for more extreme changes in position than does the oscillating bed (Fig. 32-21). For example, the patient confined to bed can be placed in an erect position if desired. The bed does not move constantly but is changed from position to position by turning on an electric motor. Some patients are taught to change the tilt of the bed themselves. At first the patient may feel quite insecure when the bed is placed in tilted positions, and the nurse should stay with him until he becomes used to the position.

Care of ulcers. Ulcers occurring in any patient with vascular disease require meticulous care to prevent infection or to prevent further infection with new organisms. Since local tissue resistance to infection is lessened and the rate of healing is slowed because of impaired circulation to the area, a long period of healing must be anticipated. Wet-to-dry dressings are often used for debridement. These dressings are applied wet, using sterile saline solution, allowed to dry, and then removed, taking away necrotic and sloughed tissue that adheres to the dried dressing. Foot soaks may be used, although this procedure cannot be sterile because it is impossible to cleanse the entire foot sufficiently.

Preventing infection is one of the two most difficult problems confronting the nurse in caring for these patients. The second is providing for comfort. Although there is often diminished sensation in superficial tissue, when ulcers involve deep tissue layers, the patient may suffer a great deal of pain during dressing changes and wound soaks. Adminis-

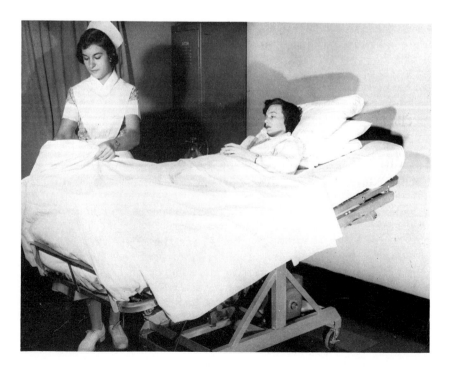

FIG. 18-2. The oscillating bed is used to improve circulation. Here the nursing student checks the temperature and color of the affected limb. Note that a cradle is being used to protect the feet from weight of the covers.

tering pain medication 15 to 30 minutes prior to wound care is of major importance.

The patient with an ulcer on his foot usually is urged to keep off his feet, although there is not complete agreement on the value of this restriction. Some physicians feel that, provided there is no direct weight bearing on the wound, the arterial circulation and healing are improved by a moderate amount by moving about and by keeping the limb in a dependent position for part of the day at least.

Light cradles are seldom used, but occasionally the physician may feel that dry warmth will improve healing of the ulcer. Using extreme caution, the nurse then leaves the wound exposed and places a cradle with a light in it over the ulcerated part. The bulb should never be larger than 25 watts, and there should be a definite order from the physician as to how long it should be left on and how far from the limb it should be placed. Too much heat will increase the metabolic needs of the tissues and thus will be injurious.

A wide variety of agents are used in the local treatment of ulcers. These include castor oil and zinc oxide, nitrofurazone (Furacin), and scarlet red ointment. The effects of antibiotic and antibacterial topical agents such as penicillin, nitrofurazone, bacitracin, and neomycin need to be carefully observed by the nurse, since local allergic reactions are common. Streptokinase-streptodornase is applied locally. Deep ulcers that do not heal properly often require skin grafting. (Special treatment of ulcers occurring in conjunction with varicose veins will be described in the section of this chapter dealing specifically with that condition.)

Since many patients who have chronic ulcers of the legs and feet are not hospitalized, they must be taught how to bathe and otherwise care for themselves without contaminating the ulcer. Many elderly patients have lived with a chronic ulcer for so long that they become careless about their technique in changing soiled or loosened dressings. The patient will often benefit from a periodic visit from a public health nurse, who can reemphasize essentials of care both to the patient and to members of his family.

Tests and examinations

Several specific procedures help the physician to diagnose vascular disease and to determine the progress in treatment. Most tests are relatively simple and require no particular preparation. The patient, however, usually is in pain and fears any procedure that he believes may even temporarily increase his pain. Nervousness sometimes causes spasm of blood vessels and sensations of chilliness that may interfere with the accuracy of a test by diminishing pulsations and altering circulation. The patient should be told that the tests are painless, and

the nurse should explain to him what is to be done if the physician has not already done so.

The room in which the tests are done should be kept warm, and if the patient has to be transported to another area for the tests, the nurse should check to see that he has sufficient covering to prevent chilling.

Test for intermittent claudication. Intermittent claudication is characterized by pain in the muscles caused by inadequate arterial circulation to the contracting muscles. Although this symptom usually occurs in the muscles of the lower extremities, it may occur also in the muscles of the forearm, wrists, or fingers. Except in rare instances, it is brought on only by continuous exercise and is relieved at once by resting. Knowing the amount of exercise that can be done before claudication occurs helps determine the severity of the condition and the improvement made. Unfortunately the severity of the condition is not easy to measure. One method is to have an attendant walk with the patient to count the number of steps taken and record the time lapse before pain occurs. Sometimes mechanical devices are used. The patient stands with his foot on a pedal which he presses down, thereby lifting a weight of 6.3 kg. (13.6 pounds). This is done at the rate of 120 times/ minute until the onset of pain. A normal person may continue for 5 to 10 minutes before he has severe fatigue, whereas one with vascular disease may be able to continue only for a few seconds. While this method of testing is not entirely accurate, it is more reliable than the patient's statement of the number of city blocks he can walk before the onset of pain.

Oscillometric readings. Oscillometric readings help determine the effectiveness of the larger arteries by measuring their pulsations. (Collateral vessels cannot be measured with an oscillometer.) Oscillometric readings are more useful in demonstrating relative differences between the deep pulses of two contralat-

Table 18-1 Generally accepted normal oscillometric readings

Extremity	Oscillometric reading
Lower extremity	
Midthigh	4 to 16
Upper third of leg	3 to 12
Above ankle	1 to 8
Foot	0.2 to 1
Upper extremity	
Upper arm	4 to 16
Elbow	3 to 12
Wrist	1 to 10
Hand	0.2 to 2

eral limbs than in measuring absolute deviations from normal.[8] An inflatable cuff is wrapped about the limb at the desired level and is connected to a delicate diaphragm that transmits arterial pressure to a needle moving across a dial that measures in units what is called the oscillometric index. The generally accepted normal oscillometric readings are given in Table 18-1.

Skin temperature studies. Attempts are made to record the skin temperature as a gauge to the effectiveness of the circulation to an extremity. These tests are not done too often because to be accurate they must be done in an environment with carefully controlled temperature and humidity. Normal skin temperature can be recorded by applying a thermocouple (a device for measuring skin temperature) to the skin. The temperature then is recorded on a potentiometer. With a humidity of 40%, the surface temperature of the skin usually varies from 24° to 35° C. (73° to 93° F.). Normal persons have a wider range of temperature difference in various parts of the body. For example, the forehead and the thorax are usually 5° to 8° warmer than the toes. People with arterial disease may have even greater temperature variations between the extremities and the rest of the body. The physician usually considers the skin temperature readings as only suggestive, because many factors (for example, a rise in metabolic rate) increase the temperature of the skin surface. The patient who is excited or upset by the anticipated test may have an increase in skin temperature. The test is usually done several hours after a meal since eating alters the skin temperature. Smoking also affects the accuracy of the readings.

A test for the efficiency of vasodilation in the extremities consists of immersing one of the limbs in water heated to 42° to 44° C. (107.6° to 112° F.) and then recording the skin temperature of the opposite limb. In the normal person with no vascular disease the temperature of the unimmersed limb will rise to a minimum of 34° C. (93° F.) within 35 minutes. A person with arterial disease may have little elevation in the skin temperature. The nurse may be asked to assist with this test. An accurate bath thermometer is needed to measure the water temperature, and sufficient blankets should be used to protect the patient from chilling during and after the test.

A simpler way to test the efficiency of vasodilation in a limb is to place a hot-water bottle or heating pad on the abdomen and then manually test both extremities for elevation in skin temperature. Many physicians rely on this test because it is simple, and the hands of the experienced person are quite skillful at judging skin temperature of each limb.

Arterial disease can be confirmed by the *cold pressure test.* The patient's blood pressure and pulse pressure are determined under normal conditions. He then immerses his hand in ice water and his blood pressure and pulse pressure are taken again. Normal subjects have an average blood pressure increase of 25 mm., with no change in pulse pressure; patients with internal occlusive disease have an average increase in blood pressure of 45 mm., with an increase in pulse pressure of 20 mm.

Angiography. Angiography is an x-ray procedure that permits visualization of the internal anatomy of the heart and blood vessels through the intravascular injection of radiopaque contrast material. By this method, calcification and other anomalies of the arteries may be demonstrated. Calcified atherosclerotic plaques at the site of an occlusion may be visualized, and calcification can sometimes be traced throughout the entire length of an artery and can even be seen as far distally as the great toe. The information revealed by such an examination is not, of itself, evidence of arterial insufficiency, for some patients who have extensive calcification of the small arteries evidently have sufficient collateral circulation to permit good blood supply and have no symptoms of arterial insufficiency.

Radiopaque substances such as Hypaque or Renografin are injected into an artery, and serial radiographs are taken during the last few seconds of the injection and immediately thereafter. Usually this test is done in the x-ray department, where occasionally a cutdown must be done on the vessel in order to inject the dye. When visualization of the arteries of a lower extremity is desired, the dye is injected into the femoral artery.

The substances used contain iodide, and the patient may have a severe allergic reaction to the dye, with dyspnea, nausea, vomiting, numbness of the extremities, diaphoresis, and tachycardia. Any signs of a reaction should be reported at once. Occasionally a delayed reaction occurs after the patient returns to his room. Antihistaminic drugs, epinephrine, and oxygen are used to combat reaction to the dye. The site of injection of the dye must be observed for signs of irritation or local thrombosis, which may occur if any of the irritating dye gets into the surrounding tissue. The area may have to be treated with massive warm moist packs.

The procedure is uncomfortable for the patient because, even without a reaction to the dye, he feels a flushing and burning sensation. One or more injections into deep arteries are made, and he must remain on the x-ray table for an hour or more. Afterward, he needs to be given water in generous amounts to hasten the excretion of the dye through the kidneys. He usually needs a back rub to relieve pressure areas resulting from lying on the hard table.

Of utmost importance after arteriography is assessment of the involved limb. The injection site must be closely observed for excessive bleeding. The patient will return from having the arteriogram with just a small dressing over the site and should have a 1- or 2-pound sandbag placed over the dressing for 3 or 4 hours. Peripheral pulses distal to the injection site should also be checked every hour for the first 4 to 8 hours after angiography.

A newer x-ray technique that is safer and less invasive involves the use of ultrasound. No injections or medications are necessary. Ultrasound, at this time, is used to confirm the presence of an aneurysm, which will be discussed later.

Plethysmography. Sometimes plethysmography is used as an aid to diagnosis. This is a graphic device that measures variations in the size of a part due to variations in the volume of blood passing through or contained in a limb.

Capillary fragility test. A test for capillary fragility is sometimes ordered for patients with peripheral vascular disease. Since it is more often ordered for patients with suspected disease of the blood or blood-forming organs, it is described on p. 409.

Lumbar sympathetic block. Paravertebral injection of the sympathetic rami of sympathetic ganglia may be used to diagnose peripheral vascular disease. Evidence of vasodilation following the block indicates that the circulation to the limbs may be improved by subsequent injections of procaine or by sympathectomy.

With the patient in a prone or semiprone position, the physician inserts a needle at the level of the second or third lumbar vertebra into the sympathetic tract within the spinal canal and injects 10 to 20 ml. of a 1% solution of procaine hydrochloride. If the procedure is successful, the sympathetic tracts will be blocked, causing a definite warming and drying of the skin surface of the limb on the same side as the injection. This response may be roughly measured by touch, or skin temperature studies may be done.

The patient should be told that there will be little pain associated with the test beyond the first needle prick and that there may be a sensation of tingling and warmth in the legs for several hours following the test. He should be observed carefully during and immediately following the procedure for signs of shock, which may result from the sudden shifting of so much blood into the peripheral circulation that the blood volume in the heart and vital vessels is depleted.

■ ARTERIAL DISEASE

Some arterial changes occur in almost all persons over 50 years of age, and some venous changes usually occur concurrently. For example, the elderly person suffering from arterial insufficiency often has varicosities of the veins as well. Persons who have diabetes mellitus usually develop vascular impairment more rapidly than others.

The function of the arteries is to transport blood from the heart to the tissues, utilizing the pressure pulses generated by the heart. Any disturbance in the structure of the arteries interferes with this function, resulting in diminished blood and thus oxygen supply to the tissues. The symptoms of arterial disease are not caused by the degree of obstruction or narrowing per se, but by the degree to which the involved body part is deprived of circulation. This, in turn, is affected by such factors as blood pressure and presence or absence of collateral circulation. For example, a 50% occlusion of one artery may cause severe symptoms, while a 50% occlusion of another artery will cause no symptoms if collateral circulation is sufficient to provide oxygenation.

The arteries are comprised of three layers: the innermost endothelium, the intima; the internal elastic membrane, the media, containing smooth muscle cells and elastic fibers; and the adventitia. The proportion of elastic tissue and muscle tissue varies with location in the body and age.

Arteriosclerosis is a general term that literally means hardening of the arteries. It primarily affects the medial layer and occurs as the result of senile changes and calcification. In time the arteries become less distensible and lose their elastic properties. The cerebral arteries and arteries of the lower extremities are the most commonly affected.

Atherosclerosis is another form of arteriosclerosis, affecting primarily the aorta and its large branches (mesenteric, renal, iliac-femoral) and the cerebral and coronary arteries. The basic process of this disease takes place in the intima and inner medial layers. The major event associated with atherosclerosis is the accumulation of lipids in the form of plaques in the cell walls, but a complex process involving many factors leads to the resultant obstruction.

The factor that has gained the most attention in the pathogenesis of atherosclerosis is the high association of dietary lipids and plaque formation. Triglycerides and cholesterol have been shown to be the two major types of lipoproteins involved.[13] A third type, phospholipids, is believed to be synthesized in the arterial cell wall itself as a local response to injury. Lipoproteins, generally measured and classified according to density by electrophoresis, may be elevated due to dietary excesses alone; may be genetically determined, as in type II hyperlipoproteinemia; or may be a combination of excessive intake of saturated fats in combination with inborn errors of carbohydrate metabolism, as in type IV hyperlipoproteinemia.

Atherosclerotic changes may begin to take place in early childhood. Although there is no way to reverse the changes that have taken place, substitution of polyunsaturated fats for saturated fats in the diet, reduction of total caloric intake, and weight loss are recommended to slow the process. This prescription involves a great deal of teaching on the nurse's part, which must begin with obtaining an accurate dietary history from the patient.

Other factors associated with atherosclerosis include hypertension, anoxia, shock, interruption of normal lymphatic drainage, sex, and race. It must be remembered that arteries are not merely elastic conduits for blood flow, but are composed of actively metabolizing cells. Shock, hypoxia, and the presence of toxins increase the permeability of cells to lipids and thereby favor the development of plaques. Hypertension also favors the deposition of lipids, although it is not known for certain if this is because of the increased pressure against the arterial wall or if hypertension causes some change within the wall itself such as increased rates of metabolism and lipid synthesis. Atherosclerosis is more common in males than females, and the incidence varies with geographic location, being more common in the United States, for example, than in Greece or Yugoslavia.

Arteriosclerosis obliterans

Arteriosclerosis obliterans is an obstructive, degenerative, arterial disorder representing a late stage of atherosclerosis. It is characterized by partial or complete occlusion of arteries by atheromata on the intima, often with superimposed thrombosis; it is segmental in nature, but changes are evident distal and proximal to the stenosis. It is the most common form of obstructive arterial disease after 30 years of age; the superficial femoral artery is the most commonly involved. It affects men more often than women, and the greatest incidence is between 60 to 70 years of age. The media, or middle layer, of the arterial wall loses its elasticity. As a result, the artery gradually becomes unable to transport the required amount of blood to the affected part. Symptoms appear when the blood vessels can no longer provide enough blood to supply oxygen and nutrients to the limbs and to remove the waste products of their metabolism.

Signs and symptoms. Early signs and symptoms of arteriosclerosis obliterans may include skin temperature changes, differences in color and size of the lower limbs, and altered arterial pulsations; intermittent claudication is the most common symptom. Later, the patient may complain of pain in the affected part even at rest; this is an indication of the severity of the disease if the artery cannot supply sufficient circulation to meet even minimal metabolic demands. Ulcers and gangrene may develop. Pain at rest often occurs at night, and the patient may report that it subsides with movement and particularly with walking. Very elderly patients may be awakened by excruciating cramplike pains in the muscles of the calf and the thighs that are believed to be due to lack of oxygen to the tissue (ischemia).

Tingling and numbness of the toes may be mentioned by the patient, and a very common complaint is difficulty in keeping the feet and hands warm enough for comfort. Occasionally the first sign of limited circulation is necrosis following mild trauma, such as cutting the skin when trimming the nails. The disease is usually present to some extent in both limbs, although symptoms may be grossly apparent in only one. They may follow an occlusion of a fairly large artery by a thrombus. This occlusion will cause numbness, marked coldness, and a chalky-white appearance to the part of the limb supplied by the obstructed vessel. An essential nursing function when caring for patients with peripheral vascular disease is the checking of the arterial pulses. Arterial pulsation can be checked at the femoral artery, popliteal artery, posterior tibial artery, or dorsalis pedis artery of the foot.[1,8]

Management. Treatment for arteriosclerosis obliterans includes provision for general warmth, use of drugs to produce vasodilation, specific exercises to stimulate collateral circulation, carefully prescribed general exercise to maintain circulation and yet not tax the arterial system, encouragement, and instruction in avoiding injury, preventing infection, and maintaining nutrition. Pain at rest may be treated by having the patient sleep with the head of the bed elevated on blocks 3 to 6 inches in height to aid gravity in carrying arterial blood to the legs and feet.[8] He should be advised not to walk about during the night unless he is warmly clothed and to avoid sitting with his legs over the side of the bed since he may become chilled and since right-angle knee flexion further hampers circulation. He should not rub the extremity because of the danger of trauma and of releasing an embolus into the circulation. Vigorous massage is always contraindicated in any patient with vascular disease.

Arteriosclerosis obliterans is a chronic progressive disease for which there is no cure, although there are measures to relieve symptoms.

Nursing intervention is directed toward helping the patient to live within his limitations and encouraging him and his family to carry out medical instructions so that the disease may be held in check for an indefinite time. All nursing measures discussed earlier in this chapter under health education may be necessary in caring for the patient. If the condition cannot be checked, gangrene of the extremity eventually may occur, making amputation necessary.

If the disease is rapidly progressive and the patient is in reasonably good health otherwise, surgery may be indicated to correct the obstruction. The most common procedure is a bypass of the obstructed arterial segment, using saphenous vein grafts or grafts made of synthetic materials such as Teflon or Dacron. A new procedure is also being perfected in which a silicone rod is implanted in the diseased artery and left in place for 6 to 8 weeks. The patient then has secondary surgery and the rod is removed; the fibrous tissue that has grown around the rod is used to bypass the diseased arterial segment.

Postoperative nursing intervention centers around assessment of circulation to the involved extremities. The nurse should be aware of the preoperative condition of the extremities in order to make meaningful postoperative comparisons. The color, temperature, sensation, and quality of pulses in the extremity must be checked hourly for the first 8 hours. Initially in this period, vasospasm may make it difficult or impossible to palpate the pedal or posterior tibial pulses and a Doppler machine, which magnifies the sound of the pulses, may be used. If adequate circulation has been restored, it will be evident from the color and temperature of the limb, which is often warmer than its counterpart. Obstruction is indicated by a marked coldness, sudden disappearance of a pulse that was palpable the hour before, or a progressive whitening, later changing to cyanosis, of the toes and foot. The surgeon should be notified immediately if these changes occur.

Patients are usually kept flat in bed for the first 12 to 24 hours and then are allowed out of bed, but must avoid sharp flexion in the areas of the grafts. The success of the surgery is dependent on the general health of the patient and the size of the vessels involved. The larger the vessel, the more effective the surgery, with aortic-iliac grafts having the highest success rate (90%).[6]

Thromboangiitis obliterans

Thromboangiitis obliterans (Buerger's disease) causes inflammation of the walls of the blood vessels, thrombus formation, and subsequent destruction of both arteries and veins. It is largely a disease of younger men; patients are often between 20 and 45 years of age when symptoms appear. About half of the patients are Jewish. Although the feet usually are affected first, vascular changes may occur in the hands and eventually throughout the entire body. The cause of inflammation is not known, but smoking definitely aggravates the condition and may even be the only cause in patients who are sensitive to inhaled smoke. As the inflammation subsides, there is partial or complete replacement of the affected blood vessels with scar tissue. The outcome of acute exacerbations, therefore, depends on the size of the area deprived of normal blood supply and the amount of collateral circulation that can be established. Collateral vessels attempt to keep pace with the destruction, but over a period of years they usually cannot do so without treatment, and gangrene develops.

Signs and symptoms. The signs and symptoms of thromboangiitis obliterans are due to peripheral is-

chemia. The most common complaint is persistent coldness of one or both lower extremities. Arterial pulses are either reduced or absent. Numbness, tingling, and aching pain may also be present. General chilling and exposure of the hands and feet to cold aggravate the symptoms. There may be hardened, red, and painful areas along the affected vessels, and the patient often reports that there is a burning or boring pain that is aggravated by chilling, smoking, and nervous tension. There is often edema about the areas of inflammation, and the entire limb, except where there is acute inflammation, may be cooler to the touch and whiter than normal. Cyanosis may occur when the feet are lowered.

Management. It is often possible to arrest thromboangiitis obliterans completely and indefinitely by merely having the patient stop smoking. This restriction is considered the most important aspect of treatment. Smoking must be given up immediately, completely, and forever. Other measures are prescribed to foster circulation and to help make use of limited resources. They may include warmth, use of vasodilating drugs such as alcohol and tolazoline (Priscoline), moderate exercise, use of an oscillating bed, and instruction to prevent infection and to avoid trauma and exposure to cold. Some physicians believe that bilateral preganglionic sympathectomy is helpful when the lower extremities are involved because it produces permanent vasodilation of the blood vessels. Sympathetic impulses may also be blocked by paravertebral injection of alcohol. Although pain may be severe, narcotics are rarely prescribed because of the real danger of drug addiction in young patients with a chronic disease such as thromboangiitis obliterans.

The nurse can often help by emphasizing to the patient the precautions he should take to prevent the onset of acute symptoms, including pain. He should be encouraged not to smoke, and he should be advised to wear warm gloves and footwear in cold weather. Both of these measures prevent extensive vasoconstriction. He should be taught to avoid any injury to his feet, especially when cutting toenails. Wounds heal slowly, and gangrene may develop.

Raynaud's disease

Raynaud's disease is a disease of unknown etiology that occurs most often in young women. There is some evidence that there is a familial incidence of the disease. Most of the women affected are underweight and asthenic in body build. Patients with Raynaud's disease have spasms of arteries in the extremities, which lessens the blood supply. Often the hands and arms are affected before the feet. The condition may lead to coldness, numbness, cyanosis, pain, dryness and atrophy of the nails, and eventually gangrene of the ends of the fingers. The symptoms are intensified by exposure to cold and by emotional excitement. Patients often respond well to a sympathectomy in which the nerve control of blood vessels to the hands is removed, leaving the blood vessels permanently dilated. Patients in whom the condition is mild may be treated with drugs that inhibit sympathetic nervous system activity, such as Dibenamine. The patient is advised to avoid smoking and to keep the hands and the rest of the body warm.

Raynaud's disease is often associated with rheumatoid arthritis and with scleroderma, a condition in which there is disturbance in the collagen content of the body and in which the skin becomes tightly stretched, firm, partially atrophied, and fibrosed (p. 952).

Aneurysm

An aneurysm is a localized or diffuse enlargement of an artery at some point along its course. A *saccular aneurysm* involves only a part of the circumference of the artery. It takes the form of a sac or pouchlike dilatation attached to the side of the artery. A *fusiform aneurysm* is spindle shaped and involves the entire circumference of the arterial wall (Fig. 18-3). Aneurysms may be due to trauma, congenital vascular disease, infection, and arteriosclerosis. The aorta is the most common site for the formation of aneurysms. Syphilitic aneurysms of the arch of the aorta are still found, but the vast majority of aneurysms, regardless of location, are due to arteriosclerosis.

Although the pathologic processes involved in the formation of an aneurysm are varied, certain factors are common to all. Once an aneurysm develops and the arterial tunica media (the middle coat composed of layers of smooth muscle and elastic tissue) is damaged, there is a tendency toward progressive dilatation, degeneration, and eventual rupture. The treatment of aneurysms is surgical.

Routine chest and abdominal x-ray films have proved to be very helpful in case finding and preliminary diagnosis. Such studies frequently reveal a ring of calcification outlining the aneurysm and displacement of surrounding structures. Angiographic studies are usually conducted to provide the surgeon with a definite diagnosis, accurate location, and delineation of the lesion. Numerous techniques are used for these studies, and selection of the particular angiographic procedure depends on a number of factors, including the clinical condition of the patient and the location of the lesion. Surgical intervention, treatment, and nursing care differ depending on the location of the aneurysm.

Surgical treatment of aneurysms that involve the ascending, transverse, and descending thoracic aorta is considered comparable to open heart surgery. Therefore a form of a total cardiopulmonary bypass is needed to maintain the patient's tissue oxygenation when the aorta is clamped. Hypothermia may be used to decrease the need of tissues for oxygen and thus decrease metabolic waste production (see p. 209). After the chest is opened, the aneurysm exposed, and an extracorporeal bypass instituted to produce a satisfactory flow of oxygenated blood, cross clamps are applied proximal and distal to the lesion (Fig. 18-4). The aneurysm is then resected and replaced with a Teflon or Dacron prosthesis. Preoperative and postoperative care of the patient with a thoracic aneurysm is the same as that described for the patient having heart surgery (p. 363).

Aneurysm of abdominal aorta. The most common site for the formation of aortic aneurysm is the abdominal aorta below the renal arteries. The patient

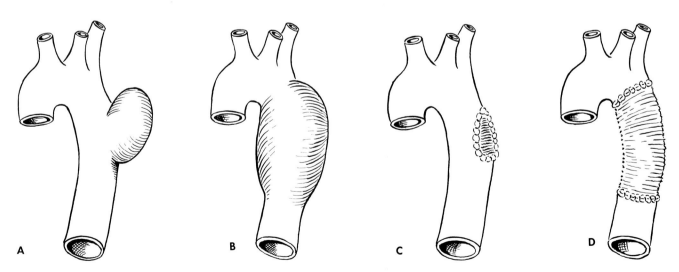

FIG. 18-3. Aneurysms of the thoracic artery. **A,** Saccular aneurysm. **B,** Fusiform aneurysm. **C,** Patch graft repair of saccular aneurysm. **D,** Replacement graft for fusiform aneurysm. (Redrawn from Bloodwell, R. D., and others: Surg. Clin. North Am. **46:**901-911, Aug. 1966.)

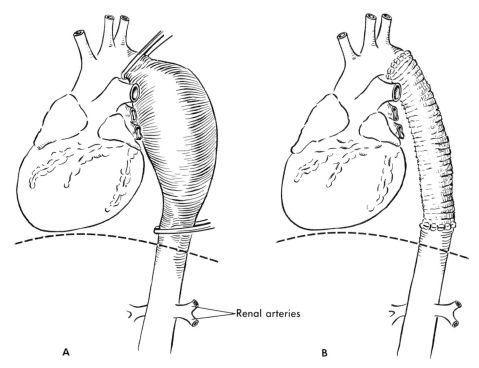

FIG. 18-4. Aneurysm of the descending thoracic artery. **A,** Resection of thoracic aorta with cardiovascular clamps in place. **B,** Permanent replacement graft after resection of aneurysm. (Redrawn from Bloodwell, R. D., and others: Surg. Clin. North Am. **46:**901-911, Aug. 1966.)

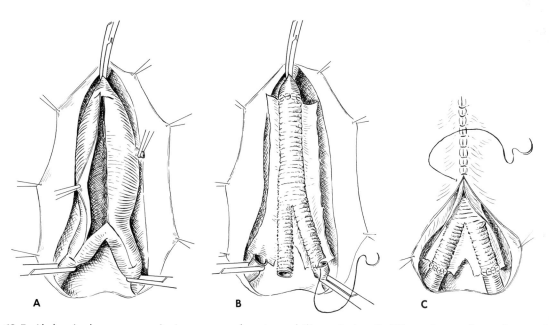

FIG. 18-5. Abdominal aneurysm. **A,** Aneurysm of aorta and iliac arteries. **B,** Bifurcation graft used to replace excised aneurysm. **C,** Closure of posterior peritoneum over graft and suture line. (Redrawn from Crawford, E. S., and others: Surg. Clin. North Am. **46:**963-978, Aug. 1966.)

may be asymptomatic, and the condition evident only as a pulsatile abdominal mass, which may be found on a routine physical examination. At other times the patient may have pain and/or tenderness in the mid or upper abdomen. Aneurysm of the abdominal aorta is a serious disease entity. Death from rupture and hemorrhage is not uncommon if surgical intervention is not instituted promptly. Treatment of an abdominal aneurysm is resection of the lesion and replacement with a graft. Extracorporeal perfusion (heart-lung bypass) is not necessary because arterial flow to the lower extremities can be interrupted safely for the time needed to complete the operation. The aneurysm is opened, the clots and debris are removed, the graft replacement is inserted, and the remaining arterial wall is closed over the graft (Fig. 18-5).

A dissecting aneurysm of the aorta may also occur (Fig. 18-6). It happens when there is a hemorrhage into a vessel wall that splits or dissects the wall, causing a widening of the vessel. Dissecting aneurysms are caused by a degenerative defect in the tunica media, probably a result of the great hemodynamic stresses to which it is subject. These aneurysms may be acute, with symptoms developing suddenly and with severity, or chronic. The most common symptom is chest pain, which is frequently mistaken for a myocardial infarction. If chronic, with no worsening of symptoms, the patient may be

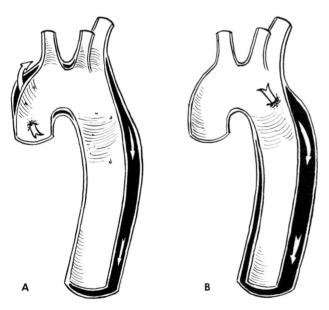

FIG. 18-6. Schematic representation of dissecting aneurysm of thoracic aorta. **A,** Typical site of tear in intima of proximal ascending aorta with dissection of the entire thoracic aorta. **B,** Dissection originating just distal to left subclavian artery. (Redrawn from Moyer, C. A., and others: Surgery: principles and practices, ed. 3, Philadelphia, 1965, J. B. Lippincott Co.)

treated medically with antihypertensives, pain medication, and negative inotropic agents (Inderal). Rupture of the aneurysm is almost always fatal. Operative mortality is highest in those patients who have an acute onset of symptoms and in whom the dissection begins in the ascending aortic arch and causes insufficiency of the aortic valve.

Postoperative nursing intervention. Immediate postoperative management of the patient who has had an abdominal aortic prosthesis replacement includes constant nursing observation in the recovery room or intensive care unit. Continual reassessment and monitoring of all parameters are essential in the first 24 to 48 hours. The blood pressure, pulse (radial and apical), and respirations are taken every 15 minutes until stabilized. The central venous pressure is also monitored. This measurement is used to evaluate the adequacy of total blood volume. "Overload" of venous circulation due to administration of too much blood or fluid replacement, inadequate cardiac function, or both is indicated by a rising or elevated central venous pressure (p. 326). The pulses of the distal arterial vessels of the extremities are taken hourly, as is done with peripheral arterial bypass grafts. These include the posterior tibial and dorsalis pedis pulses. It is customary for the physician to locate and mark these areas on the patient's skin before the operation. This procedure is done so their location can be easily determined postoperatively. Initial spasm or trapping of air bubbles may cause this pulse to be absent on the patient's return from the operating room.

If the pulses continue to be absent for more than 6 to 12 hours (even less if a prosthetic failure has occurred), it generally indicates an arterial occlusion. Signs of *poor* peripheral perfusion include a drop in the blood pressure and a weak and thready pulse. The patient may feel cool to the touch and be perspiring. Signs of *advanced* occlusion distal to the thrombus are pain, cramping, and/or numbness in one or both of the extremities. The leg or legs may be blanched (white or blue in appearance) and be cool or cold to the touch. The patient may appear anxious and the elderly patient may even be disoriented. The nurse must report any of these signs or symptoms to the physician immediately. The patient who has had an abdominal aneurysm resected must be observed for complaints of back pain, which may indicate a retroperitoneal hemorrhage or a thrombus at the graft site.

Renal failure may be a complication of abdominal aortic aneurysm resection. Maintenance of adequate urine output is essential. Accurate *hourly* intake and output records must be maintained. Anuria deserves immediate attention and must be reported to the physician. Oliguria (less than 30 to 50 ml./hour) may indicate poor hydration and should also be reported.

The patient usually is placed flat in bed, and sharp flexion of the hip is avoided because it causes pressure on the femoral artery. Flexion of the knee is also avoided because it causes pressure on the popliteal artery. The patient can be moved gently from side to side and should dorsiflex and extend his feet at regular intervals to prevent congestion of venous blood in the lower legs. Because the incision is a long one and pain may be pronounced, the patient is able to breathe more deeply, cough productively, and move more easily if a firm abdominal binder is used and if he is instructed to support his incision as he coughs or moves. Often the nurse must help him. Narcotics are given fairly liberally for pain during the first few days postoperatively. Since some handling of the viscera must occur during surgery, postoperative ileus and distention is sometimes a problem. Aspiration of flatus from the stomach with a nasogastric tube may be necessary. On about the second postoperative day the patient usually is permitted out of bed for a short time, and he often leaves the hospital in about 2 weeks.

Thrombophlebitis may also be a complication of abdominal aortic surgery. The use of elastic stockings and early ambulation are thought to be helpful in preventing venous stagnation and thrombus formation, but they do not eliminate the risk completely. Ambulatory patients who complain of a pain or cramp in the calf; tenderness at a particular site, regardless of location; redness along the course of a vein; or superficial venous dilatation are manifesting signs of thrombophlebitis. The patient should be restricted to bed, the leg elevated, and the physician notified.

Embolus

Emboli are blood clots floating in the circulating blood. These clots most commonly originate in the heart. They may be a fragment of an arteriosclerotic plaque loosened from the aorta or a thrombus released when inefficient heart pumping is suddenly corrected by digitalization. They usually lodge at the bifurcations, or divisions, of the arteries because of the diminishing caliber of the vessels beyond these points. An embolus lodging at the bifurcation of any artery is called a *saddle embolus.* As soon as an embolus lodges, thrombi (propagated emboli) form in the involved vessel.

The signs of sudden lodging or formation of a large thrombus in an artery are dramatic and vary with the part of the arterial system and associated organ system involved. There is severe pain at the site of the thrombus formation. Fainting, nausea, vomiting, and signs of pronounced shock may appear. Almost immediately, areas supplied by the vessel may become white, cold, and blotched, and they may tingle and feel numb. Cyanosis, followed by even greater darkening and gangrene, occurs if the

blood supply is completely obstructed and collateral circulation is inadequate. Vasodilating drugs are given to improve the collateral circulation, warmth is applied to the body, and a sympathetic block of the lumbar ganglia may be done in an attempt to produce vasodilation of other vessels. Oxygen may be administered to alleviate hypoxia and dyspnea. Vasopressors such as metaraminol bitartrate (Aramine) may be necessary if shock ensues. Heparin and bishydroxycoumarin may be administered to help prevent further thrombus formation. The patient who is suspected of, or who has, an acute embolic obstruction of a large artery needs constant nursing supervision. Pain is severe, and fear is pronounced.

If the patient does not respond to the medical treatment within a few hours, surgery may be performed. Surgical procedures that may be done include opening the vessel and removing the clot *(embolectomy),* removing the clot and also removing adherent substances and part of the lining of the vessel *(endarterectomy* or "reaming"), arterial resection with removal of the clot and the adherent diseased artery surrounding it with subsequent grafting, and bypassing the diseased portion of the vessel with a graft, as is sometimes done for an aneurysm. Various means are used in an endarterectomy. A long catheter with a balloon (Fogarty catheter) has been used. It can be passed distally from a larger vessel, and the balloon can be inflated and withdrawn, bringing with it long thrombi that are filling the vessel.[15] Embolectomy is usually the treatment of choice for aortic embolus and for an embolus of the common iliac artery.

Nursing care following embolectomy is similar to that needed by the patient who has had surgery for an aneurysm. Blood pressure must be carefully recorded preoperatively so that suitable comparisons can be made postoperatively. It is important that the blood pressure not vary too much from what it was preoperatively because variation would predispose to thrombus formation. A complication that must be carefully watched for is hemorrhage. Small arteries that may have been useless while the embolus was in the artery may not bleed freely during surgery and may therefore be missed in tying bleeding vessels. They may resume normal function after the operation and cause hemorrhage.

Aneurysm of the extremity and arteriovenous fistula

Aneurysms of the arteries of the lower extremities, particularly in the popliteal area, are quite common in persons over 60 years of age who have pronounced arteriosclerosis (Fig. 18-7). These aneurysms often are easily palpable. Thrombi form at the site of an aneurysm, and emboli may travel to obstruct more distal portions of the artery. This type of aneurysm is sometimes confused with an arterio-

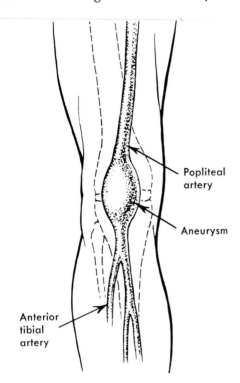

FIG. 18-7. Posterior view of the knee with aneurysm of the popliteal artery. (From Anderson, H. C.: Newton's geriatric nursing, ed. 5, St. Louis, 1971, The C. V. Mosby Co.)

venous fistula, which is an abnormal communication between an artery and a vein caused either by a congenital anomaly or by trauma. In arteriovenous fistulas the blood in the artery bypasses the capillary bed, which has a strong resistance to flow, and flows instead directly into the vein. Both lesions produce a characteristic sound called a *bruit,* which is heard on auscultation. If the cause is an aneurysm, the bruit may be interspersed with the arterial pulsations, whereas the bruit caused by a fistula is often a constant soft, purring sound. Both conditions impair the supply of blood to the portion of the limb supplied by the vessel, and various signs of poor blood supply such as atrophy, cyanosis, trophic changes, or even gangrene may occur.

Closure of the fistula or removal of a portion of the aneurysm is the preferred treatment. If one of these measures is not possible, the vessel may be ligated unless ligation is incompatible with the life of tissues distal to the lesion. Homografts (a section of the patient's vein) or Teflon or Dacron grafts can be used in larger blood vessels of the extremities either to replace portions of the artery that contain the aneurysm or to bypass the abnormality. In addition to general postoperative care, the patient who has had this surgical procedure may be treated with any or all of the medications and other means described in this chapter to augment circulation when arterial supply is limited or when thrombosis threatens.

■ VENOUS DISEASE

Thrombophlebitis

Thrombophlebitis is inflammation of a vein associated with clot formation. Many relatively simple circumstances contribute to the development of thrombophlebitis in persons who are perhaps particularly susceptible to congestion in the venous system. For example, thrombophlebitis of superficial leg veins may follow a trip during which long hours were spent sitting in a plane or car with the knees bent sharply. Flying at high altitudes in nonpressurized cabins seems to predispose to recurrence of thrombophlebitis in persons who have a tendency toward this condition. Pregnancy is often complicated by thombophlebitis due to interference with venous return in the lower abdomen. Thrombophlebitis may occur from inactivity following surgery, and before the days of early ambulation and emphasis on postoperative exercises, it was a dreaded complication of surgery. Despite early ambulation, patients still develop thrombophlebitis postoperatively, and occasional deaths from subsequent emboli are reported. (For prevention of postoperative thrombophlebitis, see p. 221). It is not understood why some patients develop thrombophlebitis while others do not. There are some factors, however, which increase a patient's risk. These are prolonged immobilization, preexisting venous disease, and hypercoagulability of blood. Thrombophlebitis is also caused by trauma to venous walls, with subsequent inflammation and congestion, and the irritating effects of certain drugs. Changes in blood pressure, blood volume, and abnormal substances in the blood such as bacteria may also contribute to development of the condition.

Signs and symptoms. Thrombophlebitis of superficial veins is easily apparent. On palpation the veins appear hard and thready and are sensitive to pressure. The entire limb may be swollen, pale, and cold, and the area along the vein may be reddened and feel warm to the touch. Deep veins in the legs may be affected, and the pain they cause when the patient dorsiflexes his foot in bed or walks is known as *Homan's sign.* Thrombophlebitis may be accompanied by reflected pain in the entire limb. Systemic reaction to the infection, which sets in rapidly in any blood vessel when free flow of blood is interrupted, may cause symptoms such as headache, malaise, and elevation of temperature. Sometimes a thrombus in a vessel may be "silent," giving no signs or symptoms until an *embolus* is released, floats in the bloodstream, and lodges in a vital structure such as the lungs, heart, or brain. An embolus lodged in a vital structure may cause death within a few seconds or an overwhelming shock reaction that is followed by death or by slow recovery.

Management. Superficial thrombophlebitis is usually treated by rest. However, physicians differ in regard to the amount of activity the patient can be allowed. Some believe that the clot is sufficiently adherent to the vein wall to make its release unlikely and that moving about helps to improve general circulation and to prevent further congestion of blood in the veins. Others believe that complete immobilization is necessary to prevent a part of the thrombus from breaking away and becoming an embolus. The patient who has thrombophlebitis of large and deep vessels, however, usually is kept quiet. Care must be taken that the patient is not frightened by being kept quiet, and the nurse may need to seek the physician's help in explaining to the patient why precautions are necessary. Occasionally the vein is ligated above the involvement (usually at the femoral juncture) to decrease the danger of embolism, but this procedure is not possible unless there is an adequate collateral circulation. The period of immobilization depends entirely on the response of the patient to treatment.

Continuous applications of warm moist heat are often used for both deep and superficial thrombophlebitis. Some physicians feel, however, the heat increases the risk that emboli will be released because it induces vasodilation. They order ice packs for their patients, especially for those with deep venous thrombosis. When warm packs are used, they are usually ordered to cover the entire extremity.[7] Heating pads permanently set on "low" may be used to keep the packs at a consistently safe temperature.

Many physicians prefer that the affected limb be elevated slightly to reduce edema and to prevent stasis distal to the thrombus. It may also relieve pain. Some physicians believe, however, that the danger of an embolus being released is greater if the limb is elevated. Therefore the nurse will need to check on the procedure to be followed in the care of each patient.

Heparin and bishydroxycoumarin are used for patients who have thrombophlebitis, and sometimes patients must remain on prophylactic doses of bishydroxycoumarin for an indefinite period to prevent recurrences of the disease. Vasodilating drugs are given to combat the arterial vessel spasm that occurs at the site of a venous thrombus and to impvove general circulation, thus increasing the rate of absorption of the thrombus.

All patients with thrombophlebitis should be observed closely for any signs of embolism, which must be reported at once. Pulmonary embolism (p. 581) is the most common type, but emboli may also lodge in the coronary vessels (p. 343) or elsewhere.

Following thrombophlebitis in a lower limb severe enough to require hospitalization or bed rest, the patient usually needs to wear an elastic stocking or elastic bandage when walking. The stocking or bandage is also often ordered for patients who have superficial thrombophlebitis, which tends to recur.

After 1 month to 6 weeks, if the patient is progressing favorably, the stocking or bandage may be removed for $\frac{1}{2}$ to 1 hour and the results noted. If there is no evidence of edema or discomfort, it may be removed for longer and longer periods until its use may be discontinued completely. Many patients wear the stockings indefinitely if their work necessitates standing for long periods of time or sitting with the knees bent. Two stockings or bandages are necessary for each affected limb so that they can be laundered as necessary.

The *elastic stocking,* accurately fitted to the patient's measurements, must be obtained before the patient gets out of bed for the first time. The stocking is used to compress superficial veins, increase flow through the deep veins, and prevent venous pooling. Stockings of various sizes and lengths are usually stocked by hospital supply stores, and many large department stores also carry them. The measurements that must be taken can be obtained by calling the store. The most satisfactory length is 1 inch below the bend of the knee joint. The patient must be taught how to put on the stocking. It should be rolled on evenly before he gets out of bed in the morning. It should be removed once during the day for a few moments and the skin very gently stroked and powdered as necessary. The stocking need not be worn during sleeping hours.

Elastic bandages may be used instead of an elastic stocking, but they are more conspicuous and are difficult to apply evenly. They may be used for short periods following surgery and are sometimes ordered for use on those occasions when the patient will be lifting heavy objects or standing still. If a bandage has been ordered for continuous use, it should be applied before the patient gets out of bed in the morning. The bandage is applied from the foot upward. Usually the entire foot, including the heel, is wrapped. The bandage will extend either to just below the knee or up to the groin, depending on the physician's orders. It should be smooth and snug but must not be so tight that it interferes with circulation.

Swimming and wading in water are among the best activities for prevention of recurrences of thrombophlebitis of the lower extremities and are highly recommended for patients with other venous diseases as well. Water, which is denser than air, exerts a smooth, even pressure on the skin, and wading is especially beneficial because the greater pressure (the deeper water) surrounds the distal portion of the extremity and helps in the return flow of venous blood.

Varicose veins

Varicose veins are abnormally dilated veins with incompetent valves, occurring most often in the lower extremities and the lower trunk. In the lower limbs the great and small saphenous veins are most often involved. At least 10% of the total population is affected by varicose veins. The highest incidence is in the third, fourth, and fifth decades of life.[43] There are several definite factors that predispose a person to the development of varicosities. Among them are congenitally defective valves and hereditary weakness of the vein walls and prolonged standing, which places strain on the valves because muscle action is not helping to return the blood. Man's upright position further aggravates the problem, and poor posture with sagging of abdominal organs causes additional pressure. Pregnancy and abdominal tumors that cause pressure on the large veins of the lower abdomen and interfere with good venous drainage predispose a person to the development of varicose veins. Chronic systemic disease such as heart disease and cirrhosis of the liver may interfere with adequate return of blood to the heart and contribute to varicosities. Infections and trauma to the veins with resultant thrombophlebitis may also lead to varicose veins, since the valves are destroyed as the acute inflammation subsides.

Signs and symptoms. Varicosities of superficial veins are often quite apparent through the skin even before they cause symptoms. They appear as darkened, tortuous, raised blood vessels that become more prominent when the patient stands and when he assumes positions that cause congestion such as sitting with the knees crossed. Sometimes the sclerosed valves can be seen as nodular protrusions. The varicosity is more pronounced just above the valve, which has become ineffective. The patient may have pain, fatigue, feeling of heaviness in the legs, muscular cramps, and emotional reactions of discouragement and depression. Discomfort is worse during hot weather and when the patient goes to higher altitudes. It is greatly increased by prolonged standing.

The simplest test for varicose veins is known as the *Trendelenburg test*. The patient lies down with the leg raised until the vein empties completely. He then stands, and the vein is observed as it fills. A normal vein fills from below; a varicose vein fills from above, because the valve fails to retain the blood that has drained into the portion of the vessel above it.

Conservative management. Mild discomfort from varicose veins may be treated conservatively by advising the patient to elevate his feet for a few minutes at regular 2- to 3-hour intervals throughout the day, to avoid constrictions about the legs, to avoid standing for long periods of time, and to wear an elastic stocking or elastic bandage. All of these measures help to reduce venous pooling and increase venous return. Improvement in posture sometimes helps to prevent further development of the varicosities, and the patient may be advised by his physician to lose weight.

Ligation and stripping of veins. Surgical treatment

for varicosities consists of ligation of the vein above the varicosity and removal of the varicosed vein distal to the ligation, provided, of course, that the deep veins are able to return the venous blood satisfactorily (Fig. 18-8). The great saphenous vein is ligated close to the femoral junction if possible, and the great and small saphenous veins are then stripped out through small incisions at the groin, above and below the knee, and at the ankle. Sterile dressings are used to cover the wounds, and an elastic bandage, extending from the foot to the groin, is applied firmly.

Ligation and stripping are usually done under general anesthesia since the procedure is very tiresome and painful. To prevent the development of thrombi in other veins, the patient usually walks about on the day of the operation and at frequent intervals during his remaining 2 or 3 days in the hospital. Unless the patient is elderly and also has arterial insufficiency, the foot of the bed is usually elevated on blocks for the first 24 hours to help in venous return of blood. Moving, walking, and bending are extremely difficult for the patient, and he may have more pain and discomfort following this surgical procedure than following much more serious sur-

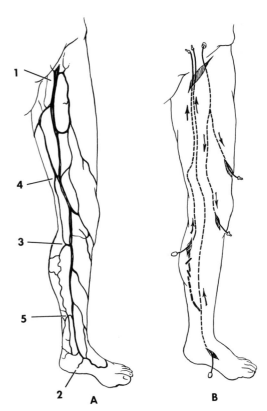

FIG. 18-8. A, Outline of incompetent great saphenous system, with numerals indicating main tributaries. **B,** Passing of strippers in preparation for removal of incompetent veins. (Redrawn from Allen, E. V., Barker, N. W., and Hines, E. A.: Peripheral vascular disease, Philadelphia, 1962, W. B. Saunders Co.)

gery. Analgesic drugs may be necessary for the first 24 to 48 hours.

Although the operation is considered a relatively minor one and the patient is out of bed at once, nursing care is important. The patient should be assisted when he walks on the first day and thereafter if he is receiving analgesic drugs. Throughout his hospitalization, he should be encouraged and assisted as necessary. The elastic bandage and the dressings should be checked several times a day because they may become loosened with walking and the wounds may be exposed. Hemorrhage from the wound may occur and should be watched for, especially on the operative day. If bleeding does occur, the leg should be elevated, pressure should be applied over the wound, and the surgeon should be notified. The patient has difficulty in handling himself because of the firm binding around his knees; therefore he must be protected from accidents.

A patient who has had surgery for varicose veins should know that the condition may recur since large superficial collateral vessels may develop and in turn become varicosed. Therefore he should take the general precautions of any patient with varicosities, since the operation cures his acute symptoms but does not remove his tendency to have varicose veins. Weight reduction, posture improvement, avoidance of pressure on blood vessels, and elevation of the lower limbs should be practiced postoperatively exactly as is recommended for the patient with mild varicosities who is receiving conservative treatment only. The booklet *Varicose Veins* is useful in teaching patients who have this condition and can be obtained from the American Heart Association.

Treatment by sclerosis. Sclerosing solutions are sometimes used in the treatment of varicosities in small and easily dilated tributaries of larger veins, and they may be used when, for some reason, varicose veins cannot be treated surgically. The solutions cause an irritation within the vein and cause a thrombus to form. As the inflammation subsides, the lumen of the vein is usually obliterated. Sodium tetradecyl sulfate (Sotradecol) in a 1% to 3% solution may be used. It can cause allergic reactions, and an antihistaminic preparation such as diphenhydramine hydrochloride (Benadryl) may be needed and should be readily available when this treatment is given. If severe reaction occurs, epinephrine and oxygen may be needed.

The injection of sclerosing solutions is usually done in the clinic or in the physician's office. The nurse must take the responsibility for seeing that emergency equipment for treating reactions is on hand and for preventing accidents to patients. Many patients are elderly, and some tend to become faint when standing for the treatment. Footstools can be equipped with side attachments and handlebars on which the patient may lean for comfort and security.

The site of injection is covered with a small dressing. The patient is urged not to scratch the skin over the site of injection, because scratching may lead to an infected excoriation and eventual ulceration. He also should be cautioned about bruising or otherwise traumatizing the veins, which also may lead to ulceration.

Management of varicose ulcers. Stasis of blood in tissues around marked varicosities, particularly when deep veins are also involved, leads to replacement of normal tissue with fibrous tissue that is firm to the touch and colored with pigment from extravasated blood cells. This condition often causes severe pruritus and general discomfort in the limb. It is called *stasis dermatitis.* Ulcers occur easily when stasis dermatitis has developed, and they are difficult to control. Ligation of varicose veins is usually necessary because the ulcer will not heal while marked varicosities persist in the vessels above it. Besides the general measures already mentioned for any ulcers of vascular origin, treatment of *varicose ulcers* includes grafting of skin to cover the wound and the use of pressure bandages. Grafting may not be successful if the arterial supply is also affected, since poor circulation to the fibrotic tissue surrounding the ulcer causes healing to be slow. (See p. 239 for care of a graft.)

Gelatin paste bandages applied to the entire lower limb, and known as "boots," are sometimes used in the treatment of varicose ulcers. This dressing, or boot, provides constant even pressure that supports the superficial veins, protects the ulcer from injury and infection, and fosters healing. *Unna's paste boot* is the best known. It contains zinc oxide, glycerin, gelatin, and water and must be melted before it is ready for application. It is applied with a brush, usually four layers of 3- or 4-inch bandage being alternated with layers of the paste. Many variations of this boot are now available in which the bandage comes already impregnated with the paste, sealed in a special airtight wrapping and ready for immediate use. They save time and obviate the danger of burning the patient when melted paste is used.

Before a paste bandage is applied, the patient should rest for $1/2$ hour with the feet elevated. Hair on the legs should be shaved, and a small, Telfa dressing should be placed over the ulcer. Adhesive tape should not be used to hold the dressing in place because it is irritating to the skin. The boot is evenly applied beginning with the instep and ending 2 inches below the knee (Fig. 18-9). It takes 15 to 20 minutes for the paste to set. The boot is then dusted with talcum powder and may be covered with a Surgitube dressing, although a stocking or a sock may be worn directly over the boot. Boots are usually changed every 10 days to 2 weeks, depending on the condition of the patient and the amount of drainage from the ulcer.

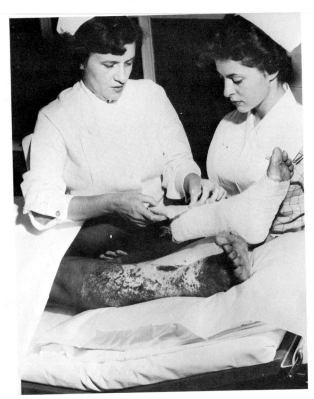

FIG. 18-9. The zinc oxide bandage can be applied easily to the ambulatory patient in the clinic. Note the skin discoloration around the leg ulcer.

While caring for the patient, the nurse should learn whether or not he has been able to follow the physician's instructions in regard to diet, rest, and exercise. The nurse may need to consult the dietitian, physician, and/or social worker in assisting the patient to follow the prescribed regimen.

LYMPHEDEMA

Lymphedema is a swelling of soft tissue and is a result of an increase in the quantity of lymph. It occurs most often in the lower extremities, but it can occur in the arms. Lymphedema is a relatively rare condition and is seen most often in young women. It may be of unknown cause (primary), or it may be due to infection or other disease of small veins and lymph vessels. Lymphedema of the arm may be a complication of mastectomy. (It is discussed on p. 813.) Congenital underdevelopment of the lymph vessels is believed to be the cause of primary lymphedema. Symptoms often appear at the time of puberty. Lymphedema of the lower extremities begins with mild swelling on the dorsum of the foot, usually at the end of the day, which gradually extends to involve the entire limb. It is aggravated by prolonged standing, pregnancy, obesity, warm weather, and the menstrual period. Exaggerated forms of this disease are known as *elephantiasis.*

One of the greatest problems in lymphedema is the emotional reaction of patients to disfigurement. The patient often attributes difficulties encountered in working in her chosen field or social rebuffs to her disfigurement and tends to become withdrawn and depressed. The emphasis on women's legs in our culture adds to her difficulties. One leg only may be involved, accentuating the abnormality even in fairly mild cases.

There is no cure for lymphedema, and the treatment is not too satisfactory. Therefore the patient needs help and encouragement in learning to live with an exasperating chronic condition. Treatment is conservative, making use of basic physiologic principles to improve the lymph drainage. Since gravity helps to drain lymph from the extremities, the patient may be advised to sleep with the foot of the bed elevated 4 to 8 inches. Very light massage in the direction of the lymph flow is recommended,[26] and the patient is advised to wear elastic stockings and to take moderate exercise regularly. Constricting clothing must not be worn, and avoiding salty or spicy foods that increase thirst and predispose to edema may be helpful. The thiazide diuretics relieve the edema in some patients.[2] Pneumatic cuffs or sleeves that help to exert a steady, gentle massage are being tried and appear to be helpful, although no spectacular results have been reported. Surgical removal of lymph nodes and vessels has been found beneficial for some patients with lymphedema due to filariasis (infection with tropical organisms that block the lymph channels). Operations also are sometimes performed to improve lymph drainage or to reduce the size of the extremity.

SPECIAL SURGICAL PROCEDURES
Sympathectomy

Vasospasm often accompanies arterial diseases, and a sympathectomy often is performed in an attempt to relieve it, although there is not full agreement as to its value. Occasionally the operation, which helps dilate the blood vessels, is done as an emergency when there is severe vasospasm from poisons such as ergot, when a limb has been frozen, or when an arterial embolism has lodged in a major vessel supplying the limb. Usually, however, before a sympathectomy is performed the ganglia are injected with procaine to determine whether or not the treatment will be of value for the particular patient (p. 385).

A *lumbar sympathectomy* deprives the leg and foot of sympathetic innervation and thereby dilates the vessels in the lower extremity. It is accomplished by making a small incision in the lower lateral aspect of the abdomen. The peritoneal cavity is not opened, but the sympathetic ganglia supplying the lumbar region are removed and their fibers are cut.

This operation may be unilateral or bilateral, depending on whether dilation of vessels is needed in both legs.

After a lumbar sympathectomy the patient should be placed on his side. Blood pressure must be taken every 15 minutes until it is stable. Pulse rate and respiratory rate are also checked, and the patient is watched closely for signs of shock, which may result from the sudden reallocation of the blood in the dilated vessels of the lower abdomen and legs. Distention may be troublesome after a lumbar sympathectomy, and a rectal tube or rectal irrigations may be used to expel the flatus. Hourly turning should be insisted on, and deep breathing should be encouraged. Following a lumbar sympathectomy the patient may notice a new feeling of warmth in his feet and legs. Very occasionally this warmth causes a slight discomfort and a feeling of fullness, which is relieved by wearing an elastic stocking.

To relieve vasospasm in the arms and hands, the thoracic ganglia of the sympathetic chain may be resected *(cervicothoracic sympathectomy)*. Because the ribs must be resected in this operation, nursing care is similar to that for any patient having chest surgery (p. 584). The problem of postoperative shock, which is encountered in the patient with a lumbar sympathectomy, also is present. In addition, the patient may become quite dizzy on assuming an upright position. Dizziness gradually subsides as the circulation becomes readjusted, but meantime the patient must be assisted when he is up. Elastic bandages may be ordered to prevent pooling of blood in the legs and thus lessen the circulatory problem.

Amputation

Although partial or complete amputations of either the legs or the arms may be necessary as a result of sarcoma and infections such as gas bacillus infection, the majority are necessitated by arteriosclerosis and by trauma. It is believed that amputations will increase each year because of the longer life span and the consequent increase in the number of elderly people in whom peripheral vascular disease is likely to develop, and because of an increasing number of automobile accidents. This later fact may no longer prove to be true in the United States if the number of automobile accidents continues to decrease as it has since the 55 mile/hour speed limit was imposed in an effort to conserve energy.

An amputation is a serious operation that is usually done as a lifesaving measure, and it may be necessary at any age. Occasionally a deformed leg or arm is amputated because it is believed that the patient can get along better with a prosthesis than with the deformed limb. Only simple amputations of the lower limb are considered here. Selected readings pertinent to amputations of the arms[49] and to disarticulation procedures[67] are given at the end of this chapter.

Emotional reaction to amputation. Because of the severe emotional reaction to the idea of an amputation, the news that amputation is necessary is usually withheld from the patient for as long as possible. Very occasionally a patient with severe pain such as occurs in thromboangiitis obliterans may welcome an amputation. However, to most patients the thought of losing a limb is almost intolerable.

Emotional reactions of distress are normal and to be expected. In ancient times the human body with perfect symmetry was glorified, as reflected in the remarkable sculpture that remains. In some ancient cultures only the physically perfect could perform certain religious rites because it was believed that only the physically perfect should appear before God. Even though one's personal faith may emphasize beauty of the spirit rather than of the body, some feeling of rejection at marring of the body is probably felt by each of us. This feeling must be faced by the patient who must have an amputation.

Loss of the power of locomotion means loss of the power of flight, which is one of the instinctive means of self-preservation. It may be for this reason that loss of a leg depresses the patient more than loss of an arm, even though the latter is a much greater handicap. Something about the loss of power to move about at will casts a shadow on the patient's spirit that can be relieved only by the most thoughtful and sensitive care. Even the patient who has suffered for a long time with a chronic disease that has hampered his freedom of motion feels the anticipated loss very keenly. Perhaps this is because there is such finality in an amputation. As long as the limb is there—imperfect though it may be—the patient usually retains the hope that normal or near-normal function will be restored. If amputation is necessary because of an accident, the suddenness of the changes in the patient's picture of himself may produce real shock.

Other emotional reactions to amputation are more tangible and more easily understood. The handicap is obvious (or at least the patient believes that it is), and he fears that he will be pitied. Young children, although they adjust to the physical limitations readily, actually may be taunted by their playmates for being different. Older children and adolescents also are handicapped in their social life and may develop serious emotional problems. To the wage earner, father, and husband, an amputation may mean that he must learn a new occupation or that he may lose his place as head of his household. To the older person, it may mean dependence on children or on the community.

Emotional reactions to an amputation have an enormous effect on the patient's rehabilitation. The reactions depend on the patient's emotional makeup and his response to other life crises as well as on circumstances leading to the amputation and on the care he receives. The most perfect surgical operation and the best-fitting prosthesis are useless if the patient remains a complete invalid and a burden to himself, his family, and the community. The nurse must think of the long-range plans for the patient from the time that it is learned that an amputation is necessary. It is at this time, when emotional reactions to the amputation and the idea of using a prosthesis are forming, that the nurse can make the greatest contribution to the patient's rehabilitation by helping him to realize that his problems are not insurmountable and by utilizing other members of the health team in planning for his care and rehabilitation.

Members of the patient's family can often be called on for help. They are usually told of the amputation before the patient, or at the same time, so that they can help him accept the news. When the patient does know that an amputation is necessary, he often benefits from a visit from someone who has undergone the same operation and has made a full recovery. With a positive mental outlook, most patients can return as functioning and useful members of society. The percentage is, of course, lower among aged persons, many of whom have other disabilities such as cardiac disease and osteoarthritis that slow their progress in learning to manage themselves independently.

The amputation. In amputating a limb the surgeon endeavors to remove all diseased tissue yet leave a stump that permits satisfactory use of a prosthesis. There is not full agreement among surgeons and limb makers as to the correct levels for amputations for best use of the stump. Most agree, however, that an amputation below the knee should be in the middle third of the leg, and that thigh amputations should be in the lower third of the thigh. Each inch of bone that must be removed from the femur above the lower third decreases the function of the limb.

Below-the-knee (BK) amputations are best for wearing a prosthesis and permit a more natural gait than thigh amputations because knee function remains. Unfortunately many patients with arterial disease require amputations above the knee (AK) because the poor circulation extends far up the limb.

For the best function of the limb, the stump should be long enough to permit sufficient leverage to move the artificial limb, but not long enough to interfere with the movement of the joint distal to the amputation. The end of the bone should be covered with skin and subcutaneous tissue and with muscle that is not adherent to the bone end. The stump should be healthy and firm, without creases, folds, and flabby parts. It should be painless, with no nerve endings remaining in the scar, and the scar should not fall over the weight-bearing end of the bone. The

stump should have a smooth, conical contour and should be freely movable by the patient in any normal range of motion.

There are two types of amputations. One, the guillotine or circular amputation, is done when there has been serious trauma, when gas bacilli are present in the wound, or when there is moist gangrene (gangrene with infection). The blood vessels and nerves are ligated, but the wound is left open. This operation is relatively simple and quick and can be done on patients who are quite poor operative risks. The disadvantage of this amputation is that usually another operation is necessary. Healing may take weeks or months unless a secondary closure operation is done. Because the wound is not sutured, there also may be muscle and skin retraction, which makes the fitting of a prosthesis difficult or impossible unless the stump is operated on again.

The flap type of amputation is by far the more satisfactory if it can be done. In this operation a long flap of full-thickness skin is loosened from the anterior of the portion of the limb about to be amputated. Following the amputation, the end of the flap is sutured to the skin edges of the stump so that the stump is covered and the suture line is along the back of the stump. This wound usually heals completely within 2 weeks.

In arterial disease it has been found that, if possible, surgery should be delayed until demarcation sets in, so that healthy tissue can be more accurately identified. Otherwise the stump may not heal because of an inadequate blood supply, and reamputation at a higher level may be necessary.

Preoperative management. If the operation is not an emergency one, the patient is told what to expect before and following the surgery. The surgeon explains the operation to him and usually mentions phantom limb sensation. He is also told whether it is expected that traction will be used. The nurse tells the patient that he will be turned or asked to turn and move about almost immediately following the operation, and explains why he must lie on his abdomen at intervals. If the condition of the diseased limb permits, he may be taught to do *push-up exercises* while lying on his abdomen. Simply by using his arms to raise his chest from the bed and repeating this exercise several times at regular intervals daily, the patient can substantially improve the muscle tone and muscle strength of his arms and shoulders. He will then be able to move more easily postoperatively.

The choice of anesthetic depends on the surgeon and the condition of the patient. General anesthesia (intravenous and inhalation) is the most frequently used. However, an amputation can be done under spinal anesthesia or with only the leg being cooled (refrigeration anesthesia), but the procedure is then very distressing to the patient since the sawing of bone can be heard despite large doses of sedation.

An intravenous infusion is usually started before the patient goes to the operating room, or it is started in the operating room before surgery begins so that fluid can be given immediately if shock or hemorrhage occur.

Postoperative management. When the patient returns from the operating room or the recovery room, vital signs should be checked and signs of hemorrhage from the stump should be watched for. If there is bright red drainage, an outline of the stain should be marked on the outside of the dressing with pencil so that the rate of bleeding can be determined easily.

Usually the stump is elevated on a plastic-covered pillow when the patient returns from the operating room, and it is left in this position for 12 to 24 hours to lessen edema and bleeding or serous oozing from the wound. However, the pillow must be removed after 24 hours at the most to prevent hip and knee contractures.

When a guillotine operation has been done, the patient usually returns to his room with traction applied to the stump to prevent retraction of skin and muscle away from the line of operation. Wide bands of adhesive tape are placed on the skin above the wound, a spreader is used, and weights are attached to provide traction. (See skin traction, p. 962.) Traction pulleys at the foot of the bed should be placed toward the center so that the patient can turn onto his abdomen. A Thomas splint sometimes is used for traction so that the patient can be moved more easily and can be out of bed without the traction's being released. (See p. 965 for care of the patient in traction.)

If the amputation is below the knee, the stump may be firmly bandaged on a padded board to prevent contracture at the knee joint. The nurse must check the padding carefully because muscle spasm that results in pulling of the limb against the board may be so great that a pressure sore develops. If spasm seems severe, a piece of sponge rubber can sometimes be slipped between the bandaged stump end and the padded board for additional protection. Sometimes, the surgeon removes the limb from the board for part of the day.

Rigid plaster dressings and immediate postsurgical fittings. Some surgeons utilize the techniques of rigid plaster dressings or immediate postsurgical fitting (IPSF). After surgery, while the patient is still in the operating room, the prosthetist applies plaster bandages to the bandaged and protected stump. Embedded in the base of the cast is a metal socket to which a metal pylon can be attached when the patient is to bear weight. This plaster mold or cast reduces postoperative edema, hastens desired stump shrinkage, and, if a foot attachment is to be used, allows for early standing and ambulation by the amputee. In fact, the plaster mold becomes the patient's

first or temporary prosthesis. IPSF procedures are also utilized for upper extremity amputees.

For the plaster mold to be effective, it must remain tight and snug. If the cast slips on the stump or comes completely off, the physician and prosthetist must be notified immediately so that a new cast can be applied. A heavy strap, attached proximally and on the anterior surface of the cast, is fastened to a waist band to help secure the cast and prevent it from slipping. This strap is loosened to a slight degree when the patient is in bed and tightened when he is out of bed. Any drainage coming through the cast should be marked (including the time) with indelible pencil. Hemovac drainage or a Penrose drain will have been inserted before the plaster is applied, so drainage should not be great. In 48 hours a window may be cut in the cast to permit removal of the drain. The opening in the plaster is then closed. This rigid dressing is kept in place for approximately 2 weeks when it is taken off for removal of sutures. A new cast is then applied. As the stump shrinks in size, the cast becomes too large and will have to be replaced by a tighter one. Usually after the application of the third plaster cast, the cast can be removed daily for stump hygiene and inspection for pressure areas.

Usually a foot-ankle attachment with a shoe is attached to the pylon when the patient is to stand. In this case the prosthetist will mark on the pylon the place where the attachment is to be placed. Most often the prosthetist and physician will be in attendance when the patient first bears weight. No weight is to be placed on the stump until the cast is completely dry. The exact amount of weight the patient should bear on the amputated side will be specifically ordered by the physician. Unless otherwise ordered by the physician, the prosthetic foot should always be removed whenever the patient is in bed, as it will produce harmful torque on remaining bone (for example, the anterior tibial crest in the below-knee amputee).

In IPSF, as with any cast prohibiting full view of the involved area, the nurse must be alert to the patient's complaints of pain under the cast, elevated temperature, or foul odor coming from the cast. Such signs or symptoms should, of course, be reported to the physician at once. Continued observation will be necessary to determine whether the cast is sufficiently snug.

Exercises. To prevent flexion contracture of the hip, unless there is a medical order to the contrary, the patient who has had a lower limb amputation should turn on his abdomen for a short time the day following surgery. Thereafter, he should lie on his abdomen for some time at least three times each day. Even the patient who has a limb in traction can turn on his abdomen with assistance. If the leg has been amputated below the knee, the patient can begin at once to hyperextend his thigh and leg as he lies on his abdomen. This exercise strengthens muscles in preparation for walking. If the amputation is above the knee, a medical order should be obtained before the patient hyperextends the thigh, because this exercise may cause strain on the suture line. While on his abdomen, the patient can practice the push-up exercises he started before the operation, strengthening his arm and shoulder muscles in preparation for crutch-walking.

While on his back, the patient with a recent midthigh amputation should be kept flat or in a low Fowler's position, except for short periods of time such as for meals. A firm trochanter roll (a sheet or bath blanket firmly rolled) should be placed along the outer side of the affected limb to prevent its outward rotation. If permitted, the patient should lie on the side of the amputation part of the time.

The patient with a below-the-knee amputation can be in a mid or high Fowler's position if he wishes, but special care must be taken to prevent flexion contracture of the knee. Usually the physician orders the stump removed from the padded arm board or splint several times a day and has the patient sit on the edge of the bed. While sitting, he should practice extending his knee and lower limb.

The nurse may be asked to press lightly against the lower limb to provide resistance.

The patient with either type of amputation should practice lifting the stump and buttocks off the bed while he is lying flat on his back. This exercise helps develop the abdominal muscles, which are necessary for stabilizing the pelvis when the patient stoops or bends.

The nurse must not become so occupied with the affected limb that she neglects the other leg and foot if the amputation involves only one limb. Supervision of regular exercises to strengthen leg muscles and care that drop foot and pronation deformities do not occur are nursing responsibilities. The patient should have a firm board or block of wood at the foot of the bed against which he can push and thereby receive essential active exercise.

When the patient is permitted out of bed, the nurse should begin to teach him self-care activities such as rising from a chair. To preserve his center of gravity and balance, the patient should keep his good leg well under him before he shifts his weight, as when rising from a chair. If a physical therapist is available, the nurse should consult him regarding exercise.

The patient who has had an amputation because

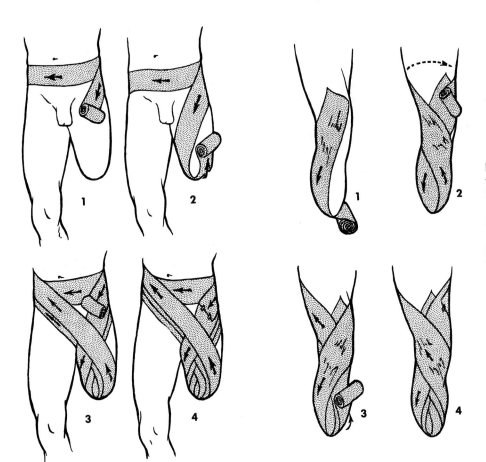

FIG. 18-10. The four sketches on the left side of the diagram illustrate the correct method for bandaging a midthigh amputation stump. Note that the bandage must be anchored around the patient's waist. The four sketches on the right side illustrate the correct method for bandaging a midcalf amputation stump. Note that the bandage need not be anchored about the waist.

of vascular disease must be reminded to take particular care of his remaining foot and leg. Exercises and other measures to keep the arterial supply as adequate as possible must be carried on while the patient is in the hospital, and he must be urged to follow his physician's instructions carefully when he leaves the hospital.

Stump care. If a prosthesis is to be worn comfortably, a healthy stump is necessary. Teaching the patient how to care for his stump is a nursing responsibility that may be carried out both in the hospital and in the patient's home. The patient may be discharged from the hospital within a few weeks but may not be fitted for a prosthesis for 6 weeks to 6 months after surgery, depending on the condition of the stump.

When the wound is completely healed, the patient is taught to wash the stump daily. Most surgeons advise their patients not to soak the stump because soaking may cause maceration of the skin. The skin should be massaged gently, directing the motion toward the suture line. No oils or creams should be applied to the stump, as these agents only increase the possibility of skin maceration. Usually the patient is instructed to push forcefully over the bone to toughen the limb for weight-bearing. Sometimes this process is begun by placing a pillow on a footstool, chair, or high stool (depending on the site of operation) and having the patient bear some weight on the stump while steadying himself on the bed or against the wall.

There should be no tenderness, redness, or other signs of skin irritation or abrasion at the end of the stump. The skin and underlying tissue should be firm and without flabbiness and should be without tautness over the bony end of the limb. The stump should be bandaged firmly both day and night. Some patients are taught to bandage the stump themselves. However, they need careful instruction and supervision. (See Fig. 18-10.) The bandage must not be tight enough to cause pain or numbness from hampered circulation. If it is too loose, it will defeat its purpose. If the patient is unable to apply a firm, even bandage, a member of his family may help him. The bandage should be removed and reapplied at least twice daily, and the skin should be washed, dried, powdered, and exposed to the air for a short time before the bandage is reapplied. The patient should have at least two bandages so that one may be washed daily; they should be laid flat to dry so as not to stretch.

When the prosthesis is used, the patient should have several pairs of stump socks of the right size. They should be made of cotton and wool and should be washed daily after use and dried over a mold to prevent shrinkage. Usually the patient wears out about one sock a month when he begins to use a prosthesis. A worn sock should not be mended be-

cause it may cause irritation to the stump. Routine care of the stump, including bathing, massage, and inspection, should be continued. If the weather is warm and the skin perspires freely, the limb should be removed from the socket, bathed and exposed to the air more often than during cooler weather. The patient who works may take an extra stump sock with him so that he can change during the day in hot weather. To prevent tension on the sock as the limb is placed in the socket, a string may be attached to the end of the sock and brought through a hole that is usually left in the prosthesis below the level of the stump. The patient should be instructed to report calluses or any abnormalities on the stump to his physician at once.

Phantom limb sensation. Phantom limb sensation is an unpleasant complication that sometimes follows amputation, and it is difficult to treat. It is a sensation that the limb is in its normal position. The sensation may disappear if the patient looks at the stump and recalls that the limb has been amputated. *Phantom limb pain* also occurs, but less often. The patient may have the sensation, for example, that something is burning his foot, or that someone is stepping on his toes. Phantom limb pain may disappear of its own accord, or it may lessen for a time and then recur with severity. When it is really troublesome to the patient, the nerve endings may be injected with alcohol to give temporary relief. Occasionally, when pain persists, an operation is done for removal of the nerve ends that may have developed to form a tuft on a weight-bearing part of the stump. A few patients are troubled with phantom limb pain for an indefinite time following amputation, and it may interfere seriously with their rehabilitation. Reamputation is sometimes done, but even this procedure does not always bring relief since the same sensations may be experienced at the end of the new stump.

Ambulation. Teaching the patient who has had an amputation to walk with crutches, with crutches and prosthesis, and then with the prosthesis alone is a complicated task that lies within the responsibility of physical medicine. In the past, teaching the patient to walk with a prosthesis often was left to the limb maker. However, learning to walk well with an artificial limb requires instruction by a skilled physical therapist. It is the responsibility of nurses working with the surgeon, the social worker, the physical therapist, the prosthetist, and other members of the professional health team to see that the patient receives continuous care, teaching, and encouragement until he is able to manage on his own.

Crutch-walking. The nurse has the responsibility to prepare every patient for crutch-walking and may have to teach the patient to use crutches if a physical therapist is not available. Therefore every nurse should know the essentials about using crutches and something about the gaits that can be used. Preparation for the use of crutches should include exercises to strengthen the triceps, which is a muscle used to extend the elbow and is therefore most important in the satisfactory use of crutches. These exercises can be started before the operation by teaching the patient to lie on his abdomen and do the push-up exercises described on p. 398. When lying on his back, he can hold bags of sand or other weights on his palms and straighten his elbows. In another exercise that strengthens the triceps muscles, the patient sits on the edge of the bed with his foot in a chair and, while pressing his palms against the mattress, lifts his hips off the bed. This procedure provides good exercise in extension of the elbow and helps the patient become accustomed to resting his weight on his hands. Use of an overbed trapeze bar postoperatively is helpful in that it enables the patient to handle himself much more independently than would otherwise be possible. Its use, however, strengthens primarily the biceps muscle, which is less essential in crutch-walking than is the triceps. Further preparation includes prevention of contractures and defor-

mities that will interfere with the use of crutches and with the use of a prosthesis. Exercises to prevent hip and/or knee contractures and to maintain the muscle tone and strength in the unaffected leg are described on p. 399. Even before the stump may be healed enough to permit use of a prosthesis, the patient can learn to do a good deal to help himself.

Crutches should be measured for each patient. In *method 1,* the patient lies on his back with his arms at his sides. The measurement is taken from the axilla to a point 6 inches out from the side of the heel. This is the length of the crutch minus $3/4$ inch for the crutch tips. In *method 2,* the patient is measured from 2 inches below the level of the axilla to the base of the heel. In *method 3,* 16 inches are subtracted from the patient's total height. Even with careful measurement, alterations may have to be made after the crutches are used. Posture, for example, may change, altering the length needed. The crutches should not cause pressure on the axillae, and the patient is taught not to rest his weight on the axillary bars more than a few minutes at a time. Pressure on the axillae causes pressure on the brachial

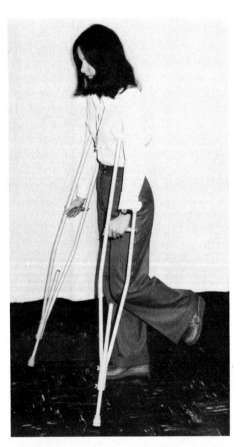

FIG. 18-11. Axillary crutches are ambulatory aids best used by young persons or persons with good motor ability, particularly if the patient is nonweight bearing on one leg. Here the patient has good balance and erect posture.

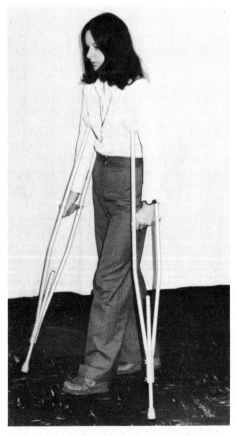

FIG. 18-12. A three-point gait is a more stable crutch gait and can be used by most patients who can use a walker. It provides for greater mobility than a walker so the patient may also negotiate stairs.

plexus, which can lead to severe and sometimes permanent paralysis of the arms ("crutch paralysis"). The patient is taught that weight should be borne on the palms of the hands.

Before the patient attempts to walk with crutches, he should be assisted out of bed and should stand with help by the bed to get the feel of normal balance. He may then use a walker or parallel bars until he is relatively secure. At this time he should begin to practice correct standing posture with head up, chest up, abdomen in, pelvis tilted inward, a 5-degree angle in the knee joint, and the foot straight (Fig. 18-11). Practice in front of a mirror is very helpful. The patient is encouraged not to look toward his foot. Next, the patient should practice standing while supported by his crutches so that he can get the "feel" of them. The nurse should be sure that he begins at this time to bear his weight on his palms and not his axillae. Before the patient begins to try to use crutches, he should be shown the proper hand and arm position and the gait he will use. This not only helps him to understand what he must do but, if he is worried about whether the crutches will support him, it may increase his confidence. In all crutch-walking the patient is taught to concentrate on a normal rhythmic gait (Fig. 18-12).

The first gait that he will use is the *swing-to* or *swing-through gait* that requires no carefully guided instruction, provided the patient knows how to bear his weight and has been taught to check posture, balance, and rhythm. In this gait the amputated limb and the crutches both advance either to or beyond the level of the normal limb and are followed by the normal leg. This is a simple fast gait that gives little leg exercise but is useful for rapid maneuvers such as are needed in crossing streets. The patient may use this gait when he begins to walk with one prosthesis, in which case both crutches and the prosthesis move forward, followed by the normal leg.

When the patient with double amputations has been fitted with prostheses, he may be taught the *four-point gait* (Fig. 18-13). This gait is taught to the count of four as follows: right crutch, left foot, left crutch, right foot. Some patients with bilateral amputations must always use this gait (which is also widely used by those with involved neuromuscular

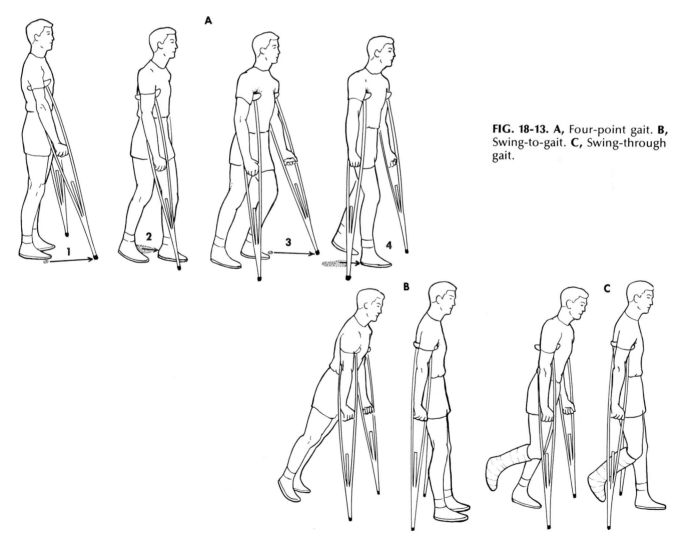

FIG. 18-13. A, Four-point gait. **B,** Swing-to-gait. **C,** Swing-through gait.

disabilities and poor balance). It is a safe gait because the patient always has three points of contact with the ground at any time. Most patients progress to the *two-point gait,* in which the foot and the opposite crutch move together and then the prosthesis and the opposite crutch. It is often taught to the count of two as follows: left crutch and right foot (one) and right crutch and left foot (two). The two-point gait produces a much faster gait and is easier to maintain in a rhythmic pattern than the four-point gait.

The patient with one prosthesis may progress to one crutch, and then to a cane, which should be abandoned eventually. The crutch or cane should be held in the hand on the side *opposite* the prosthesis because, as the patient normally walks, the arm on the opposite side of the body alternately swings forward. Holding the cane or crutch on the same side as the prosthesis results in an awkward, unrhythmic gait.

It is important for the nurse to know which gait the physical therapist is teaching the patient so that he may be reminded if, on leaving the physical therapy department, he reverts to a swing-to gait, for example. It is to be expected that the patient with a double amputation will learn to manage himself much more slowly than if only one limb were gone. Patients with amputations above the knee also take much longer to learn to walk and otherwise manage their movements.

The prosthesis. The physician prescribes the type of prosthesis that is best for the patient and usually refers him to a limb maker. After the limb is made, the patient returns to the amputee clinic, hospital department of physical medicine, physician's office, or rehabilitation center to learn the best use of the artificial limb (Fig. 18-14). The public health nurse, particularly if also trained in physical therapy, often gives care and supervision to the patient in his home.

The type of prosthesis is selected for the individual patient. Most prostheses are made of well-seasoned willow wood, although some are made of metal (duralumin and aluminum) and fiber materials. Metal prostheses are lighter in weight than wooden ones, but they tend to be noisy. Usually the below-the-knee prosthesis weighs about 5 pounds and the midthigh prosthesis about 7½ pounds, although the weight of the prosthesis is adapted to the size and weight of the patient and the kind of work he does.

The prosthesis has a socket, or "bucket," into which the limb fits. In the past, leather was the material most widely used, but plastic materials are now widely used as they are lighter, easier to keep clean, and odorless. The stump should fit snugly into the socket, and no more than two socks should be needed for a comfortable fit. If more are needed, the stump has shrunk, and the prosthesis needs adjusting. Shrinking may continue for as long as 10 years.

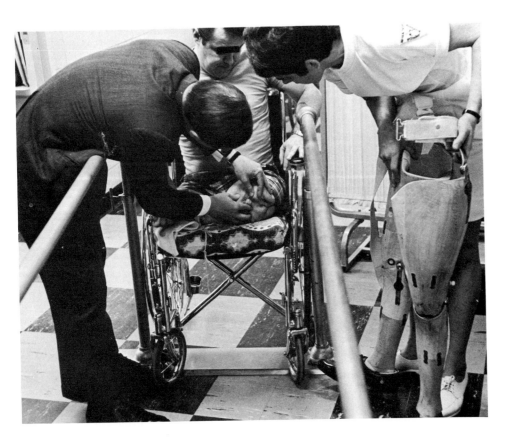

FIG. 18-14. Physician examining the stump of a patient with bilateral above-the-knee amputation while physical therapist holds the prostheses. (Courtesy Rehabilitation Institute of Chicago, Chicago, Ill.; photograph by Edwin Bonk.)

It is usually greater after amputation of the foreleg than after amputation of the thigh. Suction is now quite generally used to hold the stump in the socket and obviate wearing a heavy, laced belt about the waist, although patients with high, above-knee amputations may wear a pelvic band (Fig. 18-15). The patient needs constant encouragement to use the prosthesis, particularly in the beginning, when he is adjusting to all features of the device. He should start to use the prosthesis as soon as his stump has healed.

The nurse should learn whether or not the patient is using his prosthesis when at home. If he is not, the reason should be learned and reported to the physician. Often the nurse can help make the arrangements for more instruction. It is important that there be no delay, because the longer the patient puts off using the prosthesis, the less likely he is to use it satisfactorily. If crutches are used for too long, and if the patient depends on other forms of getting about, such as a wheelchair, he may have real difficulty in developing a normal rhythmic gait.

Care of the prosthesis should be reviewed with the patient. He should be taught to fasten the cuff above the stump from the bottom up, even though this method may seem more difficult at first. The cuff should be snug but not uncomfortable. If the cuff is leather, care should be taken that the stump sock is long enough to protect it from perspiration, and it should be rubbed with saddle soap at least

weekly. The inside of the stump socket should be washed frequently to ensure cleanliness. Shoes should be kept in good repair and should have rubber heels. Broken shoelaces should be replaced at once. If the limb has a joint, the patient should be taught to keep this free from lint and dust, to oil the joints and locks every few weeks, and to keep screws tightened. If he feels adjustments are needed, he should return to the limb maker.

The patient should be told that his artificial limb is a tool and that it will be most useful to him when he has mastered its use. With good care it will last him 3 to 10 years. Its value will depend on how well he can learn to balance himself, how much muscle strength he develops, and how smooth and rhythmic a gait he learns. Above all, its value will depend on his attitude toward the challenge that its use presents.

Long-term care. Most patients who have an amputation must remain under medical supervision for a long time, and it is safe to assume that any patient with an amputation needs nursing care and supervision long after the wound has healed. If possible, a public health nurse should visit the patient's home before he leaves the hospital and help the family make any structural changes necessary for facilitating the patient's ambulation. If it should happen that a patient is equipped with an artificial limb but is not taught how to use it, the community nurse should initiate steps toward his rehabilitation. Occa-

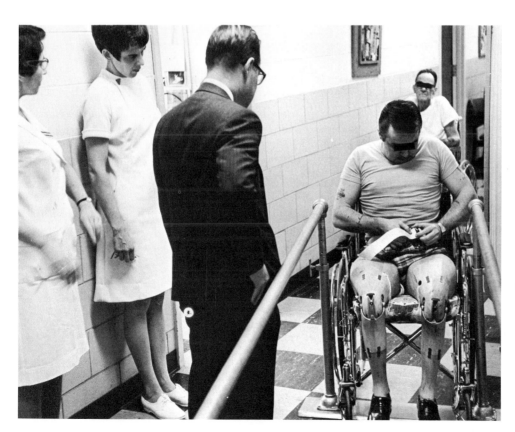

FIG. 18-15. The physician and physical therapist observing the patient with bilateral above-the-knee amputation fastening pelvic belt to secure prostheses. (Courtesy Rehabilitation Institute of Chicago, Chicago, Ill.; photograph by Edwin Bonk.)

sionally the limb maker believes that the hospital clinic personnel are taking responsibility for teaching the patient to walk, and the physician or the hospital clinic personnel believe that the limb maker is taking the responsibility. The patient may become discouraged and, after months of what appears to be a good adjustment, may lay the limb aside and return to a wheelchair or crutches. Sometimes he reports that the prosthesis is not comfortable and that he is reluctant to go back to the limb maker because of costs. If so, the nurse can help to find agencies in the community that can give appropriate assistance. It may be, however, that this statement is made by the patient to conceal a much more important and deep-seated rejection of his difficulties. This problem, of course, is much more difficult and should be reported to the physician, who will decide what steps should be taken.

Occasionally a patient, especially an elderly one, can use neither a prosthesis or crutches but must be confined to a wheelchair. The nurse should give special attention to the rehabilitation of this patient in an effort to make him as self-sufficient and happy as possible. Many patients can be taught to move themselves from the bed to the wheelchair, from the chair to the toilet, and even in and out of a car. The patient and family often need help in arranging facilities at home, and plans should be made with the family to let the patient do useful chores such as fixing vegetables, mending, or doing small repairs. He also should be encouraged to become interested in some hobby or pastime.

There are many rehabilitation centers in the United States, but most of them are located in the larger cities. The division of vocational rehabilitation of the department of education in every state is, however, available to all patients. Most communities, counties, and states have voluntary programs that are designed to help the physically handicapped, including the amputee. The nurse should consult the local health department for information on the resources available in the patient's own community. Some excellent pamphlets to use in teaching the amputee also are available: *Handbook for the Leg Amputee,** *Industrial Amputee Rehabilitation,*† and *Stump Hygiene.*‡

---

*Veterans Administration pamphlet 10-37, Washington, D. C., 1951, U. S. Government Printing Office.
†Published by Liberty Mutual Insurance Co., Boston, Mass.
‡Published by the Regents of the University of Calfornia, 1961.

REFERENCES AND SELECTED READINGS*

1 *Ajemian, S.: Bypass grafting for femoral artery occlusion, Am. J. Nurs. **67:**565-568, March 1967.
2 Allen, E. V., Barker, N. W., and Hines, E. A., Jr.: Peripheral vascular diseases, ed. 3, Philadelphia, 1962, W. B. Saunders Co.
3 Artificial Limbs 2(2):1-103, May 1955.
4 Artificial Limbs 5(2):1-172, Autumn 1958.
5 Barker, W. F., editor: Surgical treatment of peripheral vascular disease, ed. 2, New York, 1966, McGraw-Hill Book Co.
6 Beeson, P. B., and McDermott, W., editors: Cecil-Loeb textbook of medicine, ed. 13, Philadelphia, 1971, W. B. Saunders Co.
7 Bergan, J. J., and DeBoer, A.: Venous thrombosis and pulmonary embolism; total care, Surg. Clin. North Am. **50:**173-192, Feb. 1970.
8 *Bergersen, B. S.: Detection of peripheral arterial disease and instructions of patients. In Bergersen, B. S., and others, editors: Concepts in clinical nursing, vol. 1, St. Louis, 1967, The C. V. Mosby Co.
9 Bergersen, B. S., and Krug, E. E.: Pharmacology in nursing, ed. 12, St. Louis, 1973, The C. V. Mosby Co.
10 Block, M. A., and Whitehouse, F. W.: Below-knee amputation in patients with diabetes mellitus, Arch. Surg. **87:**682-689, Oct. 1963.
11 *Bosanko, L. A.: Immediate postoperative prosthesis, Am. J. Nurs. **71:**280-283, Feb. 1971.
12 *Breslau, R. C.: Intensive care following vascular surgery, Am. J. Nurs. **68:**1670-1676, Aug. 1968.

13 Brown, D. F.: Blood lipids and lipoproteins in atherogenesis, Am. J. Med. **46:**691-704, May 1969.
14 Burgess, E., and others: Immediate postsurgical prosthetics in the management of lower extremity amputees, Department of Medicine and Surgery, Veterans Administration, Washington, D. C., April 1967.
15 Chassin, J. L.: Improved management of acute embolism and thrombosis with an embolectomy catheter, J.A.M.A. **194:**845-850, Nov. 1965.
16 Childress, D., Hampton, F., Lambert, C., and others: Myoelectric immediate postsurgical procedure: a concept for fitting the upper extremity amputee, Artif. Limbs **13:**55-60, Autumn 1969.
17 *Cobey, J. C., and Cobey, J. H.: Chronic leg ulcers, Am. J. Nurs. **74:**258-259, Feb. 1974.
18 Committee on Prosthetics Research and Development: The geriatric amputee (conference held in Washington, D. C., April 13-14, 1961), Washington, D. C., National Academy of Sciences–National Research Council.
19 Conn, H. F., editor: Current therapy 1970, ed. 22, Philadelphia, 1970, W. B. Saunders Co.
20 Curtin, B. C., and Reick, K. L.: Effects of bodily position on the systolic blood pressure response to Valsalva's maneuver, Nurs. Res. **69:**119-123, March-April 1969.
21 Davies, M.: Streptokinase therapy for deep vein thrombosis, Nurs. Times **69:**211-212, Feb. 1973.
22 De Bakey, M. E., editor: Symposium on vascular surgery, Surg. Clin. North Am. **46:**825-1071, Aug. 1966.
23 De Bakey, M. E., and others: Basic biologic reactions to vascular grafts and prostheses, Surg. Clin. North Am. **45:**477-497, April 1965.
24 Ellis, H.: Arteriosclerotic disease of the lower limbs, Nurs. Times **69:**698-700, May 1973.

---

*References preceded by an asterisk are particularly well suited for student reading.

25 Fletcher, A.: Thrombolytic agents. In Sherry, S., and others, editors: Thrombosis, Washington, D. C., 1969, National Academy of Sciences.

26 Foley, W. T.: The medical management of lymphedema, Mod. Concepts Cardiovasc. Dis. 24:255-257, Jan. 1955.

27 *Fulcher, A. J.: The nurse and the patient with peripheral vascular disease, Nurs. Clin. North Am. 1:47-55, March 1966.

28 *Garrett, J. F., and Levine, E. S., editors: Psychological practices with the physically disabled, New York, 1962, Columbia University Press.

29 Getz, G. S., and others: A dynamic pathology of atherosclerosis, Am. J. Med. 46:657-673, May 1969.

30 Gordon, T., and Kennel, W. B.: Predisposition to atherosclerosis in the head, heart, and legs—the Framingham study, J.A.M.A. 221:661-666, Aug. 1972.

31 Greep, J. M., and others: A combined technique for arterial embolectomy, Arch. Surg. 105:869-874, Dec. 1972.

32 Guyton, A. C.: Textbook of medical physiology, ed. 4, Philadelphia, 1971, W. B. Saunders Co.

33 Hirschberg, G. G., and others: Rehabilitation: a manual for the care of the disabled and elderly, Philadelphia, 1964, J. B. Lippincott Co.

34 Hoerner, M. T.: The role of lumbar sympathectomy in the treatment of obliterative peripheral vascular disease, J. Am. Geriatr. Soc. 11:781-788, Aug. 1963.

35 Hopps, H. C.: Principles of pathology, ed. 2, New York, 1964, Appleton-Century-Crofts.

36 *Horvath, P. N., and Wilson, S.: Chronic leg ulcers, Am. J. Nurs. 67:94-99, Jan. 1967.

37 Hull, P. and Thomas, E.: Nursing regimen in the care of the amputee with contracture, A.N.A. Clinical Sessions, Dallas, Texas, 1968, American Nurses' Association.

38 Jackson, B. S.: Chronic peripheral arterial disease, Am. J. Nurs. 72:928-934, May 1972.

39 *Kessler, H. H., and Kiessling, E. A.: The pneumatic arm prosthesis, Am. J. Nurs. 65:114-117, June 1965.

40 *Kirkpatrick, S.: Battle casualty: amputee, Am. J. Nurs. 68:998-1005, May 1968.

41 Klopsteg, P. E., and Wilson, P. D.: Human limbs and their substitutes, New York, 1968, Hafner Press.

42 *Knocke, L.: Crutch walking, Am. J. Nurs. 61:70-73, Oct. 1961.

43 *Krause, G. L., and Vetter, F. C.: Varicose veins—diagnosis and treatment and nursing care, Am. J. Nurs. 53:70-72, Jan. 1953.

44 Kyllonen, R. R.: Body image and reaction to amputations, Conn. Med. 28:19-23, Jan. 1964.

45 Larson, C. B., and Gould, M. L.: Orthopedic nursing, ed. 8, St. Louis, 1974, The C. V. Mosby Co.

46 *Latham, H. C.: Thrombophlebitis, Am. J. Nurs. 63:122-126, Sept. 1963.

47 Laughlin, E., Stanford, J., and Phelps, M.: Immediate postsurgical prosthetics fitting of a bilateral, below-elbow amputee, a report, Artif. Limbs 12:17-19, 1968.

48 Lord, J. W., Jr.: Cigarette smoking and peripheral atherosclerotic occlusive disease, J.A.M.A. 191:249-251, Jan. 1965.

49 *Martin, N.: Rehabilitation of the upper extremity amputee, Nurs. Outlook 18:50-51, Feb. 1970.

50 *Moore, W. S., and others: Below the knee amputation for ischemic gangrene, Am. J. Surg. 124:127-134, Aug. 1972.

51 O'Reilly, R. A., and Aggeler, P. M.: Determinants of the response to oral anticoagulant drugs in man, Pharmacol. Rev. 22:35-96, March 1970.

52 *Plaisted, L. M., and Friz, B. R.: The nurse on the amputee clinic team, Nurs. Outlook 16(10):34-37, Oct. 1968.

53 *Rose, M. A.: Home care after peripheral vascular surgery, Am. J. Nurs. 74:260-262, Feb. 1974.

54 Rosenberg, H. L., and Muldar, D. G.: Dissecting thoracic aneurysms, Arch. Surg. 105:19-20, July 1972.

54a Sabiston, D. C., editor: Davis-Christopher's textbook of surgery, ed. 10, Philadelphia, 1972, W. B. Saunders Co.

55 *Sarmiento, A., and others: Immediate postsurgical prosthetics fitting in the management of upper-extremity amputees, Artif. Limbs 12(1):14-16, 1968.

56 *Sensenig, D. M., and Morson, B. J.: Buerger's disease, Am. J. Nurs. 57:337-340, March 1957.

57 *Sister Mary Elizabeth: Occlusion of the peripheral arteries—nursing observations and symptomatic care, Am. J. Nurs. 67:562-564, March 1967.

58 *Smith, L. A.: An orthotist, prosthetist—what are they? Nurs. Outlook 7:34-35, Jan. 1959.

59 Steele, S.: Children with amputations, Nurs. Forum 7(4):411-423, 1968.

60 Vultee, F.: Some problems in the management of upper extremity amputees, Artif. Limbs 2(2):36-46, May 1955.

61 Warren, R. and Recard, E.: Lower extremity amputations for arterial insufficiency, Boston, 1967, Little, Brown & Co.

62 *Wesseling, E.: The adolescent facing amputation, Am. J. Nurs. 65:90-94, Jan. 1965.

63 Williams, S. R.: Nutrition and diet therapy, ed. 2, St. Louis, 1973, The C. V. Mosby Co.

64 Wilson, A. B., Jr.: Limb prosthetics, Huntington, N. Y., 1972, R. E. Krieger Publishing Co., Inc.

65 Wintrobe, M. M., and others, editors: Harrison's principles of internal medicine, ed. 6, New York, 1970, McGraw-Hill Book Co.

66 Wright, I. S.: The treatment of occlusive arterial disease and the treatment of thrombophlebitis, J.A.M.A. 184:186-191, 194-198, Jan. 1963.

67 Young, E. L., and Barnes, W. A.: Hemipelvectomy, Am. J. Nurs. 58:361-364, March 1958.

19 Disorders of the blood

■ This chapter will include a discussion of the more important aspects of nursing care for patients with blood disorders and diseases of the blood-forming organs. Since detailed discussion of blood transfusions and nursing problems related to the taking and giving of blood can be found in fundamentals of nursing texts, they will not be included here. (See also p. 95.)

■ DIAGNOSTIC TESTS AND PROCEDURES

Blood studies. Of the many tests that may be done to help determine the patient's exact blood disease, the simplest and perhaps the most significant are hematocrit, hemoglobin, red blood cell count, white blood cell count, and blood smear. Platelet count and bleeding time may be ordered also. Blood for these tests is obtained from the patient's fingertip, earlobe, or vein. Other tests such as prothrombin time and clotting time require blood from a vein. Because many patients with a blood disorder have a tendency to bleed abnormally, prolonged bleeding from the puncture site or bleeding into surrounding tissues may occur. The nurse should inspect the site of venipuncture frequently to see that clotting does occur. Since frequent examinations of the blood are required to determine the patient's progress and are used as a guide for treatment, the patient with a blood dyscrasia should understand why they are necessary. Having blood samples taken is an unpleasant procedure, particularly when many have to be obtained.

Bone marrow studies. A bone marrow aspiration is done to obtain a sample of the cells active in blood cell production. It may be done when leukemia, aplastic anemia, or a number of other conditions are suspected. The aspiration is usually obtained from the sternum, iliac crest, vertebral body, or, in infants, the tibia. Most institutions require that signed permission from the patient be obtained before this procedure is performed. The procedure is upsetting to some patients, who fear that it will be painful and who dread the insertion of a needle "so near the heart" as is necessary for a sternal puncture or bone marrow aspiration. Actually, there is danger of puncturing the pericardium during this procedure, particularly if the sternum is abnormally thin. It is important that the patient be as relaxed and composed as possible. If he expresses extreme fear or apprehension, the nurse should report this fact to the physician, who may then order a sedative.

For a sternal puncture the patient lies on his back, and a small pillow may be placed lengthwise under the thoracic spine to bring the sternum forward. For punctures at other sites the patient is placed in a position that gives the physician good visualization and the patient maximum comfort. The skin over the aspiration site is cleansed and prepared with an antiseptic solution, and the area is anesthe-

■ STUDY QUESTIONS

1 What are the normal cellular constituents of blood? Where are blood cells formed? How are they destroyed? What are the normal red blood cell count, white blood cell count, hemoglobin, and hematocrit for men? For women?

2 Trace the successive processes that occur when blood clots. List the nursing responsibilities in preparing for and assisting with a blood transfusion. What observations should the nurse make while blood is being given?

3 From your understanding of physiology, explain why the patient who is anemic may have dyspnea and tachycardia.

4 Find out the price of vitamin B_{12} from your local druggist or from your hospital pharmacy. What would be the yearly expense for a patient requiring an injection of 100 μg every month?

tized with procaine. A few minutes are allowed for the drug to take effect on the periosteum before the sternal needle (a short, stout needle with a protecting hub to prevent its being inserted too far) is inserted into the center of the bone. The stylet is then withdrawn, a dry 5 or 10 ml. syringe is attached, and a small amount (0.2 to 0.3 ml.) of material is aspirated. At this time the patient may have a feeling of mild pain or discomfort. The specimen is deposited immediately into a specimen bottle in the laboratory. Several direct smears are made from the specimen. The patient may have slight soreness over the puncture site for several days, but the puncture should not cause real discomfort unless pressure is exerted.

If a solid piece of bone marrow is desired, a biopsy of bone marrow is performed. A needle somewhat larger than the aspiration needle is inserted in the iliac crest or vertebral body and a core of tissue is removed. Alternately, a piece of bone marrow could be removed surgically through an incision.

Capillary fragility test. This simple test helps to determine the status of small capillaries that become fragile and rupture easily in certain blood disorders. If a patient has one of these disorders, what is known as the *Rumpel-Leede phenomenon* appears. A blood pressure cuff is placed on the patient's arm and inflated, and pressure about midway between systolic and diastolic pressure is maintained for 5 minutes. When the skin is examined 5 minutes after removing the cuff, only one or two petechiae (small hemorrhagic spots) per square inch will normally be found. If the platelet count is low, numerous petechiae may appear. This test is painless, but it should be explained to the patient lest he become overly concerned with the results. It usually helps to tell him that every person will respond to this test with the appearance of some petechiae.

■ GENERAL PRINCIPLES OF MANAGEMENT

Chronicity of the disease. With the exception of a few conditions such as nutritional anemia and fulminating leukemia, diseases of the blood and the blood-forming organs are chronic. Patients with these diseases are seldom cured, and knowledge of this fact colors their attitude toward treatment and may alter their efforts in carrying on from day to day. Each patient is individual in his response to knowledge that he has a chronic disease. Some patients become depressed, discouraged, and resigned to invalidism, whereas others show magnificent courage in overcoming their problems and living productively from day to day.

The nurse can help the patient by listening to him when he becomes discouraged, giving him attention and care as needed, helping him determine realistic goals, discussing the need for and encouraging him to continue medical care and treatment, maintaining

a positive attitude about his progress and prognosis, and contributing to patient and family planning so that, within his limitations, he may remain a productive and contributing member of society. Individual family members may also turn to the nurse and may be in need of much the same help as the patient.

Acuity of the disease. When the patient suffers from an acute blood disease such as acute leukemia and has only a short life expectancy, the nurse's role is one of support for both the patient and the family. The family will need help in understanding the nature of the disease and in accepting the diagnosis. They will need encouragement, reassurance, and strengthening of faith in the medical care being given. Present treatment increases the length of life, controls symptoms, and may restore the patient to apparent health for periods of time. When the patient is to be at home during a remission, the nurse instructs the family in the care needed so that the patient will be protected from infection and injury but permitted to live as normally as possible. While the patient is hospitalized, the nurse should be aware of the concern of the patient's family and should try to give them necessary help by listening, observing, and answering questions. The patient is likely to be irritable, discouraged, and apprehensive. The nurse should accept his reaction and understand his need for the love and attention of his family. Vol-

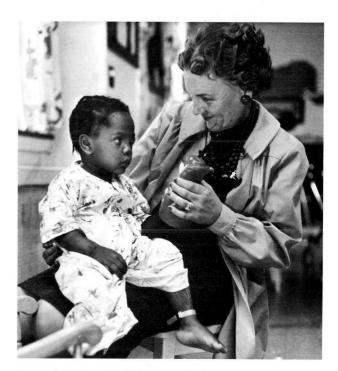

FIG. 19-1. The child who must have repeated hospitalizations for treatment of a blood dyscrasia benefits from motherly interest on the part of hospital personnel. (Courtesy Muhlenberg Hospital, Plainfield, N. J.; photo by Warren R. Vroom.)

unteers can often be helpful in providing for the patient some of the attention he needs (Fig. 19-1).

Fatigue. Most patients with diseases of the blood and the blood-forming organs suffer from fatigue that may be almost overwhelming. The patient may go to the doctor because he is "tired of being tired." Chronic fatigue adds to discouragement and influences the patient's emotional reaction to his symptoms.

Fatigue may be caused in part by a low red blood cell count and a low hemoglobin level since insufficient oxygen is being carried to the tissues. Insufficient blood supply may cause fainting, which is fairly common among persons who have severe anemia and which may lead to serious accidents. Some patients who do not really faint complain of feeling "light-headed"; this feeling, combined with general fatigue, also predisposes to accidents. Lying flat without a pillow for frequent short periods increases arterial supply to the brain and may help to prevent the light-headedness.

Fatigue may be lessened by specific medications and treatment such as transfusions. The nurse should question the ambulatory patient to be certain he is taking the medications as prescribed. Fatigue may decrease with better nutrition, and this fact should be emphasized to the patient. The patient should be encouraged to discuss the problem of fatigue frankly with his physician. The ambulatory patient may feel that this complaint will appear trivial to the busy physician and may therefore fail to mention it.

Temperature, pulse, and respirations. These three classic signs of sickness or health are particularly important when the patient has disease of the blood or the blood-forming organs. Temperature, pulse, and respirations are taken with such regularity and become so routine in hospitals that the tendency may be to regard them as not very important. This attitude is unfortunate because probably few complicated tests give clues that are as useful to the patient's progress as these simple ones give. If the temperature, pulse, and respirations are taken and recorded by auxiliary nursing personnel, the nurse has a responsibility to see that their findings are accurate and that they are correctly recorded.

Increases in pulse rate and respiratory rate are common in anemia, regardless of its cause. The heart beats faster in an effort to send the limited number of red blood cells more quickly on their way to the tissues or the lungs. The lungs work harder in response to the great need of the limited blood cells for oxygen. Increase in respiratory rate may also be a sign that a disease such as Hodgkin's disease, lymphosarcoma, or malignant lymphoma is causing pressure on the bronchi or the trachea, with resultant respiratory distress. Episodes of high temperature that last for several days and then disap-

pear for several weeks, only to recur, are characteristic of Hodgkin's disease and of some forms of leukemia. Finally, increase in these vital signs may mean that the patient—whose resistance to superimposed infection is very poor—may be developing an infection of some kind.

Hemorrhage. Bleeding from various body orifices is common in persons who have blood disorders. The nurse should be particularly alert for signs of bleeding from anywhere in the body. Stools should be examined at regular intervals for signs of fresh blood or for the tarry appearance characteristic of bleeding high in the gastrointestinal tract. The physician often orders examination of stools for occult, or hidden, blood, since it is possible for patients to lose small amounts of blood regularly from the intestinal tract and to become severely anemic without frank blood or tarry stools giving any warning. Red meat is sometimes restricted for 24 to 48 hours before the stool sample is collected, and the reason for this restriction must be explained to the patient.

Urine should be noted for evidence of blood. Bright blood in the urine is usually observed by the patient, but smoky urine, caused by lesser amounts of blood, may go unnoticed.

The patient should be protected from trauma that may cause bleeding into the tissues. The ambulatory patient is cautioned to avoid bumps and similar injuries. He should not, for example, walk in the dark. If the patient is critically ill and is disoriented, his fingernails should be cut short to prevent scratching the skin, and side rails should be used to prevent falling out of bed. Tight clothing should not be worn; for example, the patient's gown should be left untied at the neck if he is inclined to be restless. Medications are ordered to be given either by the oral or intravenous route, since intramuscular injection may cause bleeding into the muscle.

Bleeding from the mouth and gums is common in patients with blood disorders. Sometimes, awareness that gums bleed excessively after brushing the teeth is the first sign to the patient that anything is wrong. Mouth care for patients with an advanced blood disease such as leukemia becomes a major nursing problem. The lips may become cracked and bleed easily, and mouth odor follows the accumulation of old blood in the mouth. The patient is often reluctant to have care given for fear that it may start fresh bleeding. The teeth and gums should be carefully swabbed with large, soft cotton applicators. Petrolatum or a similar softening cream should be applied to the lips with an applicator. A weak solution of hydrogen peroxide (1%) seems particularly effective in cleansing old blood from the mouth. Sodium perborate is sometimes used if ordered by the physician. Carbonated beverages are sometimes a pleasant means of softening crusts of blood and exudate in the mouth. If the patient tires of sweet fluids, plain carbonated water may be tried. Zinc peroxide has been found effective for some patients. Flavored mouthwashes can be tried. Peppermint flavoring can also be used in solutions to cleanse the mouth. If the patient is alert and can be relied on not to inhale the solutions, oil solutions that can be sprayed into the mouth with an atomizer help to protect bleeding or oozing surfaces. Mineral oil flavored with peppermint, oil of cloves, or menthol may make the patient's mouth feel better. The nose needs the same kind of meticulous care as the mouth. Small wicks of cotton soaked in mineral oil are usually better than nose drops because they remain longer and seldom drain into the posterior nasopharynx. These wicks are sometimes placed in the nostrils alternately, or else very small ones may be used against oozing surfaces on the nares, permitting breathing through the nostrils.

Infections. Patients with diseases involving the white blood cells are especially prone to both local and systemic infections. Staphylococcal, gram-negative, tuberculosis, and fungal infections are common, and a variety of other organisms are likely to attack the patient who is receiving radiation treatment, antimetabolite drugs, and steroids and whose polymorphonuclear leukocyte response to infection is already limited by his disease.

Special care needs to be taken to prevent the exposure to infection of patients with diseases involving the tissues that form the white blood cells. Meticulous washing of the hands and strict asepsis are mandatory. The environment should be kept scrupulously clean and dustless, and no person with any type of infection should be allowed in contact with the patient. Occasionally isolation technique (reverse precautions) is ordered to protect the patient from hospital personnel and visitors (p. 80).

Since steroids and antibiotics may mask fever as a symptom of infection, the nurse needs to be particularly alert for any sign of infection such as local redness, cough, increased malaise, or anorexia. Any slight change or seemingly unimportant symptom should be called to the physician's attention.

Diet. Almost all patients with disease of the blood or the blood-forming organs should have a diet high in protein. If there is gastrointestinal bleeding and if the mucous membrane of the mouth is irritated, foods containing roughage should be avoided. Hemorrhage of the gums and of the mucous membrane anywhere along the gastrointestinal tract can follow the ingestion of rough food such as whole kernels of corn. Hot foods should also be avoided because the thin, irritated mucous membrane of the mouth is burned easily. Highly spiced foods are not given because they may cause irritation.

Seeing that the patient eats enough is a real nursing challenge in many instances. The patient may be too tired or too discouraged to be interested in food,

he may have a poor appetite, and he may have anorexia or even nausea from the constant presence of blood in his mouth. Companionship during meals, small, attractive servings of foods that he likes, and mouth care before meals often help to improve his appetite. The ambulatory patient or his family are often interested in suggestions for planning high-protein meals that are palatable yet within their means and for including enough nutrients yet avoiding high-roughage foods.

The patient's environment. The family of the critically or terminally ill patient should be given special consideration. If he is in a hospital, close relatives may appreciate opportunities to help in giving care. If he is at home, they may welcome assistance from the public health nurse so that they may continue to participate in care and prevent the need for hospitalization. Sometimes relatives may be overcome by their own feeling and want to avoid the sight of such things as bleeding or the patient's growing helplessness. The nurse needs to determine the family's feeling and plan care accordingly.

■ THE ANEMIAS

Anemia is an extremely common condition in which there is an abnormal reduction in the number of circulating red blood cells and/or an abnormality of the red blood cells with a reduction of hemoglobin. Asthenia, fatigue, and pallor are the classic signs of anemia. Its main causes are loss of blood, faulty blood cell production, and excessive destruction of red blood cells.

Anemia secondary to blood loss

Anemia resulting from frank hemorrhage such as may follow trauma, childbirth, surgery, or administration of drugs such as bishydroxycoumarin (Dicumarol) is usually apparent. It presents relatively simple medical problems provided that not too much blood is lost and the cause of hemorrhage can be corrected. The adult of average build has approximately 6,000 ml. of blood in the total circulating blood system. Usually he can lose 500 ml. without serious or lasting effects. If the loss reaches 1,000 ml. or more, serious consequences may result, and 1 to 2 months may be required for the hemoglobin concentration of the blood to return to normal. (Care of the patient who suffers from hemorrhage is discussed on p. 107.)

The body has remarkable adaptive powers and may adjust fairly well to a marked reduction in red blood cells and hemoglobin provided the condition develops gradually. The total red cell count may even drop to almost half of its normal figure of between $4\frac{1}{2}$ and 5 million/mm.^{3} of whole blood without the patient's experiencing the usual symptoms to a noticeable extent. Another example of the body's capacity is the increase in red blood cells that occurs when a person moves from a low to a high altitude (more cells are needed to carry oxygen from the rarefied atmosphere).

Chronic, unrecognized blood loss can also cause anemia. It may occur in the presence of an unsuspected gastrointestinal malignancy, a slowly bleeding peptic ulcer, or hemorrhoids that bleed without the patient's awareness. When blood loss is continuous and moderate in amount, the bone marrow may be able to keep up with the losses by increasing its production of red blood cells if enough protein and iron are supplied in food. Eventually, however, if the cause of chronic blood loss is not found and corrected, the bone marrow usually cannot keep pace with the loss, and symptoms of anemia appear.

Anemias caused by defective blood production

There are several reasons for defective and inadequate red blood cell production. A diet deficient in meat and green vegetables, which supply folic acid and protein (raw materials from which blood cells are manufactured), and poor absorption of food from the gastrointestinal tract can lead to anemia. Lack of production of substances within the body that are essential in blood cell formation, such as the intrinsic factor secreted by the stomach, may cause anemia. The bone marrow's capacity for manufacturing red blood cells may be depressed by drugs such as chloramphenicol or sulfonamides, by toxic chemicals such as benzene, by infection, by aplasia of unknown cause, and by hyperactivity of white blood cell production, which occurs in leukemia.

Nutritional anemia. Nutritional anemia is common and may be due to lack of knowledge of the foods necessary for building normal blood cells, lack of money to purchase essential foods, or fads or notions about diet. Occasionally a nutritional anemia follows lengthy adherence to a special diet, alcoholism, abdominal surgery, or gastrointestinal disease. To manufacture red blood cells, the body must ingest and use foods containing the essential substance (vitamin B_{12}) necessary in the manufacture of red blood cells as well as the protein and iron needed. Some foods containing these essentials are meat, eggs, yeast, and whole-grain cereals.

Nutritional anemia should be entirely preventable in a country such as ours. The nurse can help in prevention by teaching the importance of good nutrition. Emphasis should be on the essentials of good nutrition and on a wide selection of foods. When nutritional anemia has occurred, it is necessary for the patient to have more than the usual amounts of protein, minerals, and vitamins. Extra iron is also usually given. The simple form of ferrous sulfate usually is as effective as more elaborate trade preparations. To speed the absorption of oral preparations of iron, they can be given before meals or between meals when there is little or no food in the upper digestive tract; however, because of their irritating effect, they often must be given after meals.[7] The patient who is given iron should be told that the stools will be black, lest he worry about bleeding from the gastrointestinal tract. If iron is not tolerated orally, it may be given intramuscularly. The drug is more completely absorbed by this route than when it is taken orally. An iron preparation widely used for intramuscular injection is iron-dextran (Imferon). Iron-dextran must be given by deep intramuscular injection into the gluteal muscle using the Z (zigzag line) method.

Pernicious anemia. Pernicious anemia was first described by Thomas Addison in London in 1849, and the term "addisonian anemia" is still sometimes used. In this disease a substance called the *intrinsic factor,* normally produced by the stomach mucosa, is lacking. In normal function the intrinsic factor promotes the absorption of vitamin B_{12} (extrinsic factor) normally found in food. Without the intrinsic factor, the red blood cells become abnormal. They may be large (macrocytic) and assume peculiar shapes (poikilocytosis) and sizes (anisocytosis). A diet high in protein and iron does not correct these abnormalities, since the basic defect is not in the raw materials provided.

Pernicious anemia usually occurs after the age of 40 years. More people are affected in the temperate zones than in the far northern or southern hemispheres. In the United States the incidence is higher in the northern sections of the country, where there are many people of Nordic descent. There appears to be a hereditary influence in the development of pernicious anemia. Several members of the same family may have the disease. Many patients with pernicious anemia have characteristics in common. Many are of the Nordic race and have broad faces, blond hair that grays early, and wide-set blue eyes.

Pernicious anemia develops slowly. Fatigue is a common symptom, but it comes on so slowly that the patient seldom remembers its beginning. There may be anorexia and symptoms of poor digestion, yet little weight loss. Gastric analysis invariably reveals an absence of free hydrochloric acid in the stomach secretions (achlorhydria) due to the lack of the intrinsic factor. The tongue becomes smooth, and the patient may notice soreness, burning, or other signs of irritation in the mouth. They may disappear, only to reappear after a few weeks or months. There is usually a characteristic waxy pallor which, as the disease progresses untreated, will turn to a light lemon yellow, with mild jaundice noticeable in the sclera. Dyspnea and palpitation also occur.

Pernicious anemia affects the nervous system. Irritability and depression are signs of the disease, and occasionally the patient even develops a psychosis that usually responds almost immediately to treatment for the anemia. As neurologic involvement develops, there may be numbness, tingling, or a burning sensation in the hands and feet. Some patients have signs of peripheral neuritis with decreased or lost sense of vibration in the feet and legs. Sense of position becomes disturbed, and eventually incoordination develops. Some patients complain of a sensation of constricting bands around the lower limbs and the trunk. It is estimated that approximately 80% of persons with pernicious anemia have some neurologic involvement by the time they seek medical care. In those with advanced disease the rectal and urinary sphincters may function poorly. Although patients with far-advanced and permanent neurologic damage are now seldom seen in the United States, some patients still have neurologic symptoms for months before they seek medical advice. When the nurse sees a patient with signs of pernicious anemia who feels that his symptoms are not serious, he should be encouraged to seek medical aid at once.

There is no cure for pernicious anemia, since at the present time there is no way to help the stomach lining regain its capacity to produce the intrinsic factor. Fortunately, however, the anemia can be corrected by supplying cyanocobalamin (vitamin B_{12}). Although some neurologic damage may not be completely reversible, the patient may now live out his life with no serious increase in symptoms provided he continues treatment with this drug.

The preparation of vitamin B_{12} is extremely potent, and daily intramuscular injections of as little as 1 μg will cause production of normal blood cells. Vitamin B_{12} is marketed in 5 and 10 ml. vials and in four different strengths. Each milliliter may contain 10, 15, 30, or 50 μg. An initial dose of 50 to 100 μg is given and is repeated every day for 7 to 10 days. Dosage is then usually reduced to 15 to 30 μg once or twice a week, and after a few weeks the patient can often be maintained on a dosage of 50 to 100 μg at monthly intervals. Sometimes adequate treatment is maintained with injections given as infrequently as every 6 months.

Folic acid should never be used in the treatment of pernicious anemia, although it may be prescribed for certain forms of nutritional and related macrocytic anemias. For reasons not understood, folic acid enables the body to produce red blood cells of normal appearance. It may, however, accelerate the development of neurologic involvement in pernicious anemia.

Nursing care for the patient with pernicious anemia depends on the symptoms present at the time of treatment. Irritability, impatience, and apprehension should be expected and should be dealt with by showing the patient particular attention and by giving medications and other treatments on time and with as little confusion as possible. The patient may

need extra warmth, special mouth care, and a carefully selected diet until severe symptoms subside. However, with present treatment the more superficial symptoms usually disappear within 1 to 2 weeks. Neurologic symptoms may be much more persistent and may even be partially irreversible despite intensive treatment with vitamin B_{12} and physical therapy. The patient may be discouraged when he finds that the neurologic symptoms do not disappear as quickly as the others. In the presence of permanent nerve damage, patience and persistence are tremendous assets to the patient in learning to manage himself effectively.

The prospect of needing intramuscular injections at monthly intervals for the rest of one's life is not a happy one. The nurse can help the patient in his adjustment by developing skill in giving injections as quickly and as painlessly as possible. The patient may need to be reminded that although injections must certainly be continued, he may need them less often when symptoms completely subside. If he must receive medication frequently, the physician may wish the patient or a member of his family to learn to give the injections. Most patients receiving vitamin B_{12}, however, return to the physician's office or clinic for injections or may make arrangements through the physician to have the public health nurse give them. The patient and his family must be taught the absolute necessity of returning regularly, since symptoms will not reappear at once to remind them. The patient with residual neurologic involvement also needs help in learning safe and relatively simple methods of getting about without assistance. If a cane or a crutch is necessary, the patient needs to be encouraged to accept this aid.

A review should be made of the daily food intake of every patient who has pernicious anemia to be certain that he understands the essentials of a good diet. Cost may be a problem in the selection of suitable foods, particularly since vitamin B_{12} is expensive, and some of the money that the patient previously budgeted for food may be needed for its purchase. Usually the patient with pernicious anemia benefits from having a public health nurse visit his home to help plan low-cost, nutritious meals.

Folic acid deficiency anemia. Persons who have a deficiency in folic acid develop a macrocytic anemia associated with megaloblastic arrest in red blood cell production. The body can store only small amounts of folic acid, and without adequate dietary intake, this supply will be depleted within 3 to 4 months. The symptoms of folic acid anemia are similar to those of pernicious anemia. However, patients with folic acid deficiency anemia will not respond adequately to treatment with vitamin B_{12}.

Folic acid deficiency accompanies malnutrition such as occurs in the chronically malnourished, in alcoholic cirrhosis, in the last trimester of pregnancy when metabolic needs are increased, in intestinal malabsorption, and in infants who are fed exclusively a milk diet. Most patients respond promptly to oral doses of 0.1 to 0.2 mg. of folic acid daily for 1 to 2 weeks along with a well-balanced diet. However, women whose anemia developed during pregnancy should be treated for several months after delivery.[6] Most patients can remain well as long as they are on a normal diet adequate in meats and vegetables. Foods high in B complex vitamins are also good sources of folic acid.[28]

Aplastic anemia. Aplastic anemia is characterized by aplasia, depression, or cessation of activity of all blood-producing elements. There is a decrease in white blood cells (leukopenia), a decrease in platelets (thrombocytopenia), and a decrease in formation of red blood cells. The disease may occur in more than one member in a family. It may follow exposure to chloramphenicol, sulfonamides, phenylbutazone (Butazolidin), anticonvulsants such as mephenytoin (Mesantoin), DDT and other insecticides, benzene, thiazide diuretics, and gold. Disseminated tuberculosis may also produce symptoms similar to those of aplastic anemia.

Symptoms of aplastic anemia may appear suddenly, but they usually develop gradually over a period of weeks and months. They include pallor, weakness, dyspnea, anorexia, headache, fever, and bleeding of the mucous membranes, often first noticed in the mouth or the nose. Treatment consists of removing causative toxic agents if they are known and of giving transfusions to raise the hemoglobin level and to supply platelets so that bleeding may be controlled. Iron, vitamin B_{12}, and high-protein foods are not effective. Antibiotics may be given to prevent and control secondary infection. The mortality rate for aplastic anemia is high, and almost all patients with the disease die. Occasionally recovery occurs when the causative agent is found and removed. An inherited childhood form of the disease does, however, respond to treatment with anabolic steroids. Nursing care of the patient with aplastic anemia includes all the measures mentioned in the first part of this chapter.

Anemias caused by excessive destruction of red blood cells

Anemia in which there is an abnormal destruction of red blood cells is known as *hemolytic anemia*. Cells are destroyed at such a rate that the bone marrow is unable to make up the losses. Hemolytic anemia can be due to a congenital condition or to an acquired one.

Congenital hemolytic anemia. Congenital hemolytic or hereditary anemia is due to a defect resulting in formation of abnormal red blood cells. These cells are fragile and rupture easily, causing anemia and jaundice. The condition is usually chronic, but he-

molytic crisis similar to the acute episodes occurring in acquired hemolytic anemia occur. Frequently these episodes are precipitated by trauma, infections, or pregnancy; therefore the patient should be instructed to seek immediate medical attention in any of these situations.

Ten percent of black male Americans have a deficiency of glucose-6-phosphate dehydrogenase (G-6-PD), and these individuals will develop hemolysis when exposed to certain oxidant drugs such as the sulfa drugs or antimalarial compounds. These patients generally do not have anemia between exposure to these external agents. Other patients, particularly those with hereditary spherocytosis, have a chronic hemolytic anemia and develop difficulty when their bone marrow fails to keep up with their accelerated needs because of infection. The prognosis for inherited anemia is poorer when symptoms appear in childhood. Death occurs from inability to keep up with blood losses, steroid side effects, hepatitis, or secondary complications.

Sickle cell anemia. Sickle cell anemia is one of the inherited types of hemolytic anemias. It has its highest incidence in the United States among blacks, Puerto Ricans, and persons of Spanish, French, Italian, Greek, Turkish, North African, Middle Eastern, and Indian origin. The disease is attributed to a chemical defect within the hemoglobin of red blood cells. The characteristic sickle shape of red blood cells is due to a mutant gene that is responsible for the synthesis of hemoglobin that is different from normal hemoglobin.

The basic abnormality lies within the globin (protein) fraction of the hemoglobin, where a single amino acid is substituted for another in one of the polypeptide chains. This single amino acid substitution profoundly alters the properties of the hemoglobin molecule, changing its electric charge and making it less soluble and more prone to precipitate. Crystallization within the red blood cells distorts their shape and they take on the characteristic appearance of sickles. As a consequence of the intermolecular rearrangement, hemoglobin S is formed instead of normal hemoglobin (A). The tendency toward sickling is dependent on both the relative quantity of hemoglobin S in the red blood cells and the levels of oxygen tension within the tissues of the body.

The sickling phenomenon is seen in patients with sickle trait (SA), homozygous sickle cell disease (SS), sickle cell–hemoglobin C disease, and sickle cell–thalassemia. Sickle cell trait is present in those who are heterozygous for sickling and represents a combination of sickle hemoglobin (SA) and normal hemoglobin (AA). The red cells of such persons contain from 20% to 40% hemoglobin S but are not misshapen under normal living conditions. The sickle cell trait produces no clinical disorder and is compatible with a normal life span. The person may, however, suffer sickling if exposed to conditions causing hypoxia such as flying at high altitudes in nonpressurized airplanes, respiratory depression of deep anesthesia, or severe respiratory disease with extreme oxygen unsaturation. It is reported that 8% to 12% of the black population has sickle cell trait.

Unfortunately the most common form of sickle cell disease is homozygous sickle cell disease (SS), which occurs in a ratio of 1:400 to 1:500 of the black population in the United States.[6] Persons with this variant have inherited sickling genes from both parents and cannot form normal hemoglobin. The average age of onset of symptoms is 2 years. Sickling is present at all times and minor reductions in blood oxygen levels induce sickling crises. These individuals have full-blown anemia and their red blood cells contain 80% to 100% hemoglobin S. Few patients live beyond 40 years of age. Intercurrent infections, multiple pulmonary emboli, or thrombosis of a vessel to a vital organ may cause death.

Some persons inherit more than one genetic mutation and produce not only hemoglobin S but hemoglobin C, D, or one of the many other abnormal hemoglobins. Sickle cell–hemoglobin C disease is second in occurrence among black Americans. It is caused by the presence of the gene for sickle hemoglobin and the gene for hemoglobin C. Although the symptoms and course of the disease are milder than in homozygous sickle cell disease (SS), it nonetheless can cause marked discomfort and occasionally painful crises.

Sickle cell–thalassemia is a combination of sickle cell trait and beta-thalassemia trait. The defect in this variant is in the beta chain of the globin that produces defective hemoglobin. This disease is also known as Mediterranean anemia and occurs in most cases of sickle cell disease in nonblacks, particularly those persons of Greek or Italian ancestry. The clinical course and symptoms are less severe than in other forms of the disease and crises are not as common.

Persons with sickling disorders may experience increased sickling during the stress of pregnancy, surgery, or as a consequence of infection, dehydration, or trauma. Acidosis and conditions that lead to fluid and electrolyte imbalance such as vomiting, fever, or disturbed renal flow may promote sickling of the patient's red blood cells. The distorted shape of the cells, the changes in red cell membrane, and the presence of cells that will not unsickle even when oxygenated lead to thickening of the blood and predispose to sludging in the microcirculation. These disturbances can cause impaired blood flow and produce ischemic obstruction and infarction of vital organs. Because sickled cells are fragile, they are less able to survive the mechanical trauma caused by circulating in the blood. When they are released

into the free circulation, hemolysis occurs and repeated episodes lead to severe anemia. The clinical manifestations then are due to anemia, thrombosis, and infarction.[16]

The sudden exacerbation of sickling can bring about a condition known as "crises," which is serious and life-threatening. Crises are divided into the following three types: painful or thrombotic, aplastic, and hemolytic.[16] *Painful crisis* is the most common type and is due to occlusion of small arterioles and venules by the abnormally shaped cells. The pain is usually severe and may be confined to the abdomen, musculoskeletal systems, brain, lung, or heart. The patient will generally require pain medication, including narcotics to obtain relief from pain. In the treatment of painful crises it is important that dehydration and acidosis be corrected since they, in themselves, induce further sickling. Appropriate cultures and sensitivity studies are obtained and antibiotics administered when there is indication of infection. An attempt may be made to reverse sickling by the use of rapidly infused isotonic saline solution or with the phenothiazines, corticosteroids, or low molecular weight dextran. Limited exchange transfusion (replacing the patient's own blood with packed red cells unit for unit until the concentration of sickle cells is below 50% concentration of erythrocytes) may be used to reduce the number of circulating sickle cells. Urea and potassium cyanate have been used experimentally to impair the sickling process, but to date researchers remain cautious about the use of these two substances.[16]

Aplastic crisis occurs when the mechanism for erythroblast division or maturation is depressed, and a profound anemia results. Infection or drugs known to be toxic to hematopoiesis (for example, chloramphenicol) may be the cause. The diagnosis of aplastic sickle cell crises is made after bone marrow analysis. Since the anemia may progress rapidly, transfusions using packed cells may be used daily in volumes sufficient to maintain vital signs and function until erythropoiesis resumes.

Hemolytic crisis involves a rapid decrease in hematocrit, and this, too, may be due to infection or drug-induced destruction of red blood cells. Symptoms are those due primarily to increasing anemia together with severe jaundice. It is treated with infusion of packed red cells.

Since there is no cure for sickle cell disease, treatment is geared to alleviating symptoms and keeping the patient comfortable. Nursing care of the patient in crises involves managing the patient's activity, monitoring vital signs and infusion, observing his reaction to medication and transfusion, interpreting the plan of care to the patient, his family, and appropriate nursing personnel, as well as coordinating laboratory and treatment regimens. The patient and/or the family may need counseling to help them work through the many anxieties and fears associated with a chronic recurring disease. The nurse needs to assess the patient's response to the disease and provide appropriate emotional support and teaching.

Much more attention has been directed toward this disease in the past few years, and educational campaigns are being directed at helping those at high risk to seek genetic counseling.

Acquired hemolytic anemia. Acquired hemolytic anemia can be caused by burns, snake venom, certain heavy metals and organic compounds, and antibodies directed against either the red blood cells or against a number of different drugs. The use of incompatible blood for transfusions causes severe hemolysis of the red blood cells. Hemolysis can be associated with infections with *Plasmodium* (malaria), *Clostridia, Toxoplasma, Bartonella* (Oroya fever), the organism of primary atypical pneumonia, and *Streptococcus*. Hemolytic anemia also may be caused by pathologic processes involving the spleen and causing it to destroy red blood cells excessively. The treatment for the latter is splenectomy, which will be discussed later.

An acute episode of hemolytic anemia, with rapid destruction of red blood cells, usually causes chills and fever, headache, irritability, precordial spasm, and pain. There may be abdominal pain and nausea, vomiting, diarrhea, and red urine. Urinary output may be diminished. Shock and prostration may occur, and jaundice follows the destruction of red blood cells. In chronic forms of the disease there are varying degrees of weakness, pallor, dyspnea, and palpitation. Stones may form in the biliary tract.

The prognosis of patients with acquired hemolytic anemias depends on the cause, the severity of the hemolysis, and the promptness of treatment. Treatment is directed toward eliminating the cause and maintaining renal function and fluid and electrolyte balance. Corticosteroids are of significant benefit to many patients whose hemolytic anemia has an autoimmune basis. Transfusions are sometimes helpful for patients whose acquired hemolytic anemia is on another basis. Nursing care of the patient includes all the measures discussed in the first part of this chapter.

■ THE LEUKEMIAS AND LYMPHOMAS

Leukemia

Leukemia is a fatal disease of the blood-forming tissues characterized by an extensive and abnormal production of mature and immature forms of any of the white blood cells (granulocytes, lymphocytes, monocytes) that appear in the bloodstream, bone marrow, spleen, liver, and lymph nodes. Anemia is usually also present and is thought to be caused by the diminished production of erythrocytes in the bone marrow as the tissue-forming abnormal leukocytes

increase and spread throughout the marrow. Leukemia is a progressive malignant disease and for statistical purposes is now classified with cancer. It has increased in frequency and accounts for about 15,000 deaths annually in the United States. The cause is unknown. Any of the white blood cells involved may cause an acute or subacute form of the disease, with death occurring sometimes within a few weeks and usually within 1 year, or a chronic form, with an average course of 3 to 5 years.[6]

Treatment for both types of leukemia consists of supportive treatments such as giving blood transfusions to combat the anemia, antibiotics to treat infection, platelet transfusions to prevent bleeding, and supportive nursing care. Effort is made to control the abnormal cell production, and particularly in the acute leukemia of childhood, significant strides to this end have been made. Corticosteroids, antimetabolite drugs, the periwinkle alkaloids, alkylating agents, and radiation treatment have been effective in certain kinds of leukemia, particularly when used in combination. (See p. 301 for the care of the patient with cancer who is receiving drug therapy.) Total body irradiation followed by bone marrow transplantation is one of the newest treatments.

Acute leukemia. Acute leukemia occurs at all ages. The cell types of the leukemias are sometimes difficult to distinguish, but acute lymphocytic leukemia is more common in childhood, and myelocytic or monocytic leukemia is more common in adults. Symptoms include pallor; extreme fatigue; upper respiratory infection; fever; bleeding from the mucous membranes of the mouth, nose, or other body orifices; and petechiae or ecchymoses in the skin. The total number of leukocytes of various types is most often between 15,000 and 60,000, although occasionally they may go much higher. Sometimes a white count as low as 2,000 to 3,000/mm.[3] is present. A severe anemia almost always develops, with the red blood cell count falling as low as 1 million/mm.[3] and the platelet count falling also. The lymph nodes, spleen, and liver are frequently enlarged in acute childhood leukemia.

In adults the course is rapidly progressive, and even with a remission, death caused by hemorrhage, general debility, or infection usually occurs within 1 or 2 years. In children, optimal treatment apparently results in remissions extending, in some cases, to a median of 5 years. Indeed, very prolonged remissions in acute leukemia of childhood lasting 10 and 15 years have been achieved and the term "cure" is used in some of these instances.

Chronic lymphocytic leukemia. Chronic lymphocytic leukemia usually occurs in persons over 45 years of age. The onset is insidious, and the patient may complain of pallor and fatigue and may notice a painless lump in the neck, axilla, or groin. The lymph nodes, liver, and spleen are enlarged. The total white blood cell count is increased to between 30,000 and 200,000/mm.[3], with 60% to 90% of these cells resembling normal small lymphocytes. Abnormal bleeding usually occurs only during acute exacerbations of the disease and in the terminal phase. Average length of life after appearance of symptoms is 3 to 5 years. About one half of the patients have a normal life expectancy but many of the patients die of causes unrelated to their leukemia.

Chronic myelocytic leukemia. Chronic myelocytic (granulocytic and monocytic) leukemia occurs most often in persons between 35 and 55 years of age. The onset is insidious, and marked changes in the white blood cells have usually occurred before the patient has any specific complaint. Initial symptoms are usually weakness, pallor, palpitation, and dyspnea. Fever and chills often occur. There is marked enlargement of the spleen and liver and pronounced anemia. Complications occur in a variety of body organs as they become infiltrated with leukocytes. An abnormal tendency to bleed occurs during acute exacerbations and immediately preceding death. The average length of life is approximately 3 to 5 years after onset of the disease. Patients with chronic myelocytic leukemia frequently develop a form of acute leukemia (blastic crisis) as a terminal event.

Lymphomas

Lymphomas are tumors arising from lymphocytes or from the reticular cells of lymphatic tissues. They are considered malignant tumors and produce painless enlargement of lymph nodes throughout the body. Lymphosarcoma and Hodgkin's disease are two specific disorders classified as lymphomas. They cause about 15,000 deaths each year.

Hodgkin's disease produces painless enlargement of the lymph nodes. The first nodes to be involved usually are those in the cervical region, followed by the axillary nodes and those in the inguinal region. There is no known cause for this disease. It pursues a malignant course, although it has some features reminiscent of an infectious process. The highest incidence is in young adults, and men are affected more often than women. The clinical findings vary from mild lymph node enlargement without other symptoms to generalized disease with severe symptoms, including fever, excessive diaphoresis, anemia, anorexia, and weight loss. Twenty-five percent of patients with Hodgkin's disease have skin conditions such as pruritus.[18] Changes in the blood count are not of major diagnostic significance, although leukocytosis or anemia may occur and lymphopenia is common. Markedly enlarged nodes can cause severe symptoms from pressure. For example, respiration may be severely hampered by enlarged nodes in the mediastinum and neck. Death is usually caused by progressive neoplastic involvement or intercurrent infection but may be due to pressure of the enlarged lymph nodes on the bronchi and mediastinum.

In localized Hodgkin's disease (confined to one or two lymph node areas), x-ray therapy appears to produce prolonged remission and, in many instances, probable cure. Chemotherapeutic agents such as the mustards, corticosteroids, *Vinca* alkaloids, nitrosoureas, and procarbazine have been very effective in more disseminated forms of the disease. Very prolonged remissions have been achieved with these agents even when areas other than lymph nodes have been involved. Transfusions of whole blood or packed cells may be helpful both for the disease and for tiding the patient over the effects of therapy.

A *lymphosarcoma* is a malignant tumor arising in the lymph nodes or mucosal lymphatic tissue. Specific complaints vary with the location of the lesion. Mediastinal and retroperitoneal lymph node enlargement may cause symptoms of pressure on adjacent organs, gastric and intestinal masses may simulate gastrointestinal carcinoma, and large, hard lymph nodes may be adherent to the skin. Fever, excessive diaphoresis, weight loss, and weakness are common. Treatment with radiation therapy and with chemotherapy may be very helpful, and patients with localized disease may have extended survival following x-ray treatment. Although not as effective as in Hodgkin's disease, combination chemotherapy may provide extended remissions.

■ HEMORRHAGIC DISORDERS
Purpura

Purpura signifies platelet disorders that may be characterized by a reduced or an excessive number of platelets or disorders in which the platelets are normal in number but are functionally inadequate. In purpura the capillaries are exceedingly fragile and permeable. There is extravasation of blood into the tissues, under the skin, and through the mucous membranes. In the skin, areas of hemorrhage may be small (petechiae) or large and "black and blue" (ecchymoses). Purpura may be secondary to other disorders or it may be idiopathic.

Secondary purpura. Secondary purpura may occur with many acute and chronic illnesses in which the bleeding and clotting times are normal. For example, dark areas of hemorrhage into the skin are characteristic of a severe, fulminating form of meningitis that swept Europe in the fourteenth century and produced the Black Death (plague) so vividly described in medical annals of that time. Some forms of purpura occur with vitamin C deficiency (scurvy), and one form of purpura, with actual abnormality in the blood, occurs with liver disease and failure to utilize vitamin K. Purpura may also occur as an allergic reaction to certain drugs such as quinine. The treatment for secondary purpura is to remove the cause if possible.

Autoimmune reactions are believed to be responsible for purpura, and they cause bleeding by increasing the permeability of the capillaries, although the platelet count is not reduced. Occasionally they appear to follow infections. *Henoch's* purpura, associated with acute abdominal symptoms, and *Schönlein's* purpura, associated with joint pains, are two syndromes that occur most often in children.[32] The bleeding from these disorders is rarely excessive, and there is no specific treatment.

Idiopathic thrombocytopenic purpura. In idiopathic thrombocytopenic purpura there is a reduction of blood platelets, the cause of which is unknown. Evidence is becoming ever more convincing that platelet destruction in a great majority of patients is caused by an immune response to an unknown agent. The disease is usually seen in young people. Because of the low platelet count, petechiae appear on the skin and excessive bleeding occurs.

The treatment for this condition is corticosteroids, splenectomy, or immunosuppressive drugs such as azathioprine (Imuran). To lessen danger of severe hemorrhage during surgery, radiation treatment to the spleen may be given to decrease its activity and to make it less vascular before surgery is attempted.

Preparation for a splenectomy is similar to that for other major abdominal surgery. Usually a transfusion of fresh blood is given a very short time before surgery. The bleeding and clotting times are recorded, and the patient's blood is typed and cross matched preparatory to giving additional transfusions if necessary.

Following a splenectomy, the patient must be observed very carefully for signs of internal hemorrhage and thrombosis. Thrombosis occurs because of rebound in the number of platelets formed after splenectomy. As a rule the patient gets out of bed a day or two postoperatively to prevent thrombosis. If thrombosis does occur, its treatment is difficult because anticoagulants are contraindicated. Care must be taken that the patient does not bruise or otherwise injure himself when he first gets out of bed. A general diet high in iron and protein is given as soon as it can be tolerated. The patient with purpura and resultant anemia from blood loss responds very quickly to a diet high in protein and iron, together with supplementary iron. The patient should be advised to continue under medical supervision for an indefinite time and to report any signs of bleeding to his physician at once.

Hemophilia

Hemophilia is a rare hereditary coagulation disorder that is usually transmitted to the male by the female through a recessive sex-linked characteristic. The disease affects 1 in 20,000 persons. Most evidence suggests that the genetic abnormality alters the production of a single protein essential for the control of bleeding. Because of this deficiency of a single coagulation factor, clotting time is prolonged, and bleeding can occur at any time. The platelet count and prothrombin time, however, are normal. Hereditary coagulation disorders may be classified as hemophilia A, or classic hemophilia, in which there is a deficiency of factor VIII (antihemophilia globulin); hemophilia B, or Christmas disease, due to a deficiency of factor IX (plasma thromboplastin component); hemophilia C in which there is a deficiency in factor XI (plasma thromboplastin antecedent); and a related coagulation disorder known as von Willebrand's disease that is characterized by a reduction in factor VIII with prolonged bleeding and with lack of platelet adhesiveness. Von Willebrand's disease occurs about as frequently in females as in males and is not, therefore, sex linked. Although the relative incidence of these various forms depends on the population studied, hemophilia A appears to be the most common form of hemophilia and is the type diagnosed in 80% of the cases.

Since hemophilia is a congenital hereditary disease, it manifests itself early in life. The child must learn to avoid trauma of all kinds because the slightest bump may cause spontaneous bleeding into the tissues. Bleeding may occur in any organ or from any body orifice, but the most common sites for hemorrhage are the knees, elbows, and wrists. The patient may experience episodes of hematuria, epistaxis, hematemesis, and melena. Gums bleed easily and brushing the teeth must be done with care. Repeated injuries and bleeding into joints can cause bone destruction and deformity. Caution must be used in handling pins, nail files, scissors, and toys that have sharp edges. Because such care in ordinary activities is necessary, the patient and his family have serious psychologic handicaps, particularly because it is the active, growing child who is affected. Repeated episodes of bleeding are wearing and frightening, and the child may become sensitive and retiring or may attempt to defy his handicap. Social activities need to be planned to meet the patient's special needs. Minor medical problems that go almost unnoticed in the average household assume major proportions. For example, a simple tooth extraction requires hospitalization and transfusions.

Treatment consists of replacement of the deficient coagulation factor when bleeding episodes do not respond to local treatment (ice bags, manual pressure or dressings, immobilization, elevation, topical coagulants such as fibrin foam and thrombin). Because the deficient factors are contained in plasma, the treatment used for many years was fresh plasma and blood or fresh frozen plasma. In major hemorrhages, adequate blood levels were difficult to maintain without overloading the patient's circulation with large volumes of blood and plasma. The discovery of cryoprecipitate in 1964 led the way to the development of commercially prepared concentrated preparations such as fibrinogen, factor VIII, and a concentrate containing the four vitamin K–dependent factors (prothrombin and factors VII, IX, and X). Concentrates avoid the problem of circulatory overload and produce fewer adverse effects in some patients (urticarial or febrile reactions). High cost and contamination with the virus of serum hepatitis are drawbacks to their use, however.

In classic hemophilia the treatment of choice for an acute bleeding episode may be infusion of cryoprecipitated antihemophilic factor (factor VIII). This concentrate is made by slowly thawing previously frozen plasma at refrigerator temperature. Most of the factor VIII remains as a gel and can be separated from the rest of the plasma by centrifugation. The gel is reconstituted by the addition of saline solution to the bag. After the antihemophilic factor is extracted, the remaining plasma may be used for other purposes. This process results in a concentration of factor VIII as much as 15 to 40 times that of normal plasma. It can be produced and stored in any well-equipped blood bank at a cost well below that of other concentrates. Treatment with cryoprecipitate is being given in outpatient departments and clinics. Home infusion programs have gained interest and are seen as a way of more quickly controlling bleeding episodes, thereby decreasing the need for hospitalization and long absence from school or work.

Giving an injection requires that particular care be taken to use a small needle, to apply pressure at the site of injection, and to inspect it for bleeding frequently for some time thereafter. The patient should have a diet high in iron. One of nature's compensations for this condition is a remarkable capacity to regenerate red blood cells when bleeding has caused their loss. The patient who has hemophilia should carry a card on his person that includes his name, his blood type, his physician's name, and the fact that he has hemophilia, so that medical treatment will not be delayed if he should accidentally sustain injury and lose consciousness.

It is estimated that the average hemophiliac has between 10 and 18 bleeding episodes a year and will require 13 to 24 bags of frozen factor VIII (cryoprecipitate) to stop each bleeding episode. The cost of treatment is estimated at $4,000 to $5,000 a year. The impact of the hemophiliac patient population on national blood resources could also present a tremendous problem. A special program of the National Heart and Lung Institute (one of the National Institutes of Health) supports a broad range of research related to the nation's blood resources. This program, through research contracts to universities and private research groups, promotes improvements in the supply and use of blood and blood deviations and evalua-

tion of methods for treating clotting complications of cardiovascular disorders, hemorrhagic disorders, and other blood diseases.

The National Hemophilia Foundation* is an organization established for hemophiliacs and their families. There are 51 chapters scattered across the United States. The basic function of the national organization is hemophilia research. In addition, it establishes standards for chapters, publishes literature, produces films, and promotes health care legislation in Washington. Local chapter services include special camps for hemophiliacs; parent, child, and adult counseling; group therapy sessions for parents; and a printed newsletter that reports on advances in hemophilic care. A chapter may function as a liaison agent between hospitals and families with insurmountable blood bills.

The outlook for the patient with hemophilia has been greatly improved by the availability of transfusion therapy. In the past many persons with factor VIII deficiency died in infancy or in the first 5 years of life. Today patients with moderate or mild hemophilia may live rather normal lives, although they must be aware of the possibility of hemorrhage after dental extractions, injury, or surgery. Those with severe defect may require frequent admission to the hospital and may be incapacitated by joint deformities.

■ DISSEMINATED INTRAVASCULAR COAGULATION

Disseminated intravascular coagulation (DIC) is a recently recognized pathophysiologic response of a body's hemostatic mechanisms to disease or injury. DIC is a complicated and potentially fatal process that is characterized initially by clotting and secondarily by hemorrhage. It always occurs in response to a primary disease.

Many disease states may trigger the development of DIC. Some of the more common ones are septic shock, complications of pregnancy such as toxemia and abruptio placentae, surgical procedures involving extracorporeal circulation such as open-heart surgery, any condition involving extensive tissue damage such as massive trauma or burns, and metastatic carcinoma.[27a] All of these conditions in some way alter the balance of normal clotting factors in the blood and the coagulation process is initiated. For example, both gram-negative septicemia and extracorporeal circulation cause damage to platelets and initiate clotting by activating factor VII.[24a]

The initial phase of DIC, then, is characterized by the appearance of free thrombin in the blood and the activation of the coagulation system. The deposition of fibrin and the aggregation of platelets cause the

---

*25 West 39th St., New York, N. Y. 10018.

formation of microthrombi. The fibrin deposits cause red cell damage, and the microthrombi obstruct circulation in various organs. Ischemic renal failure, respiratory failure, and adrenal insufficiency are common sequelae. Often the first sign of DIC is the widespread appearance of purpura over the chest and abdomen, the result of numerous fibrin deposits in the capillary bed.

The second phase of DIC is one of hemorrhage. This paradox is caused by the depletion of clotting factors II, V, VIII, IX, X, and XII and platelets in the first phase and by the production of fibrin degradation products (FDP) through fibrinolysis. The thrombin that initially accelerated coagulation also converts plasminogen into plasmin, which then breaks fibrin and fibrinogen into fibrin degradation products. The fibrin degradation products act as anticoagulants, and bleeding from many sites ensues.[27a]

Laboratory determinations that confirm the diagnosis of DIC are the presence of thrombocytopenia, low levels of fibrinogen, and prolonged prothrombin and partial thromboplastin times. In addition, low levels of factors VIII and V are present, and abnormal red blood cells are found on peripheral smear.[24a]

The management of DIC must always begin with treatment of the primary disease. Once this has been initiated, the goal is to control the bleeding and restore normal levels of clotting factors. Heparin may be administered to inhibit the formation of thrombin and allow fibrinogen and platelet levels to increase; blood products such as platelet packs, cryoprecipitate, and fresh whole blood may be given to replace the depleted factors. Heparin, however, may increase bleeding while preventing clotting and therefore is not always used with surgical patients. The third aspect of management involves treatment of the sequelae, such as hemodialysis for renal failure.

Nursing intervention in the care of the patient with DIC is extremely challenging. The person who develops DIC is critically ill and frequently has numerous sites of bleeding before DIC becomes evident. Identification of the early signs may be made first by the observant nurse. The amount and nature of drainage from chest and nasogastric tubes, oozing from surgical incisions, or progressive discoloration of the skin should be noted and recorded.

Continual observation for new bleeding sites and for an increase or decrease in bleeding is an integral part of the nursing plan, especially if heparin therapy is being employed. The susceptibility of these patients to bleeding presents special problems; medications should be given intravenously if at all possible and small-gauge needles used when other injections are necessary. Toothbrushes must be used with caution and soft swabs are often more effective for mouth care. If scabs have formed over small bleeding sites, they should not be removed, as this will only initiate fresh bleeding. When bleeding occurs, pressure should be applied to both arterial and venous puncture sites for a minimum of 15 minutes.

Maintaining fluid balance is another aspect of nursing care that assumes great importance. Patients with DIC usually lose large quantities of blood and receive frequent transfusions and other fluid replacement. In addition to carefully monitoring blood infusion rates, the nurse must be alert to signs of fluid overload such as increasing pulse rate and central venous pressure. Hourly urine outputs should be recorded not only as another indication of cardiac function but also because of the possibility of renal thrombi formation and subsequent renal failure.

Emotional support of the person with DIC and his family is essential. Bleeding into joints may cause a great deal of pain, and the frequent venous and arterial punctures necessary for laboratory tests also may cause much distress. Frequently the patient is comatose and the presence of purpura, numerous intravenous lines, and drainage tubes makes his appearance especially upsetting to the family. Most of the primary conditions associated with DIC are of a sudden nature, and the family requires help in understanding this catastrophic occurrence and support during the long period of treatment.

■ POLYCYTHEMIA VERA

In polycythemia vera there is excessive production of red blood cells, white blood cells, and platelets. The red blood count may rise to 7 to 12 million. The hemoglobin is increased, and the patient characteristically has a reddish purple complexion, with reddening of the hands and feet. Headache, weakness, dyspnea, itching, and lacrimation may be other complaints. There may be bleeding from the skin and from the mucous membranes. This disease usually occurs in persons over 50 years of age, and the average age at death is approximately 60 years. Death is usually from thrombosis, progression to bone marrow fibrosis, or acute leukemia.

Phlebotomy is the main treatment and it may be necessary every 6 months or more often. Radioactive phosphorus, busulfan (Myleran), or triethylenemelamine (TEM) can often control the disease. The patient should have a diet not excessively high in iron, and the nurse can help him with the selection of foods. Other nursing care during an exacerbation consists of supportive care, with special attention to hemorrhage.

■ AGRANULOCYTOSIS

Agranulocytosis is a disease in which production of white blood cells is depressed, and the total number of white blood cells may be reduced to between 200 and 500/mm.[3] Exposure to drugs, chemicals, and physical agents about the home can cause the disease. Sulfonamides, coal-tar analgesics, tripelennamine (Pyribenzamine), thiouracil, chloramphenicol, and heavy metals such as gold are examples. The nurse has an important role in the prevention of this disease. In the community the nurse has frequent opportunity to advise against use of medications not therapeutically prescribed. In the hospital as well as in the home the nurse must constantly be aware of the possible toxic effects of various drugs. Many times good nursing care can reduce the period of necessary treatment with drugs. Also, nurses must be constantly alert for toxic signs of the drugs they administer.

Treatment consists of removing the offending agent. Sometimes the cause is difficult to determine, and a careful history is essential. With such a low white blood cell count, precautions must be taken to control infections. The first signs of the disease may be the onset of an acute infection, with chills, fever, sore throat, and prostration. There may be enlargement of cervical lymph nodes. Infection may occur anywhere in the body. The mortality in agranulocytosis is high, although antibiotics have been found extremely helpful in controlling the infection until the cause can be found and removed. Transfusions of fresh whole blood are often given.

■ INFECTIOUS MONONUCLEOSIS

Infectious mononucleosis is an acute disease apparently caused by a herpeslike virus, the Epstein-Barr virus. The disease is not new, having been described many years ago as acute "glandular fever" because of the enlargement of the lymph nodes. Infectious mononucleosis is more common in young persons, the largest number of cases occurring in those between 15 and 30 years of age. It sometimes occurs in more or less epidemic form among closely associated groups and yet may also be sporadic in its appearance. Hospital personnel seem to be affected often by the disease, although this apparently higher incidence is thought to be due to better reporting. The infection is believed to be transmitted from one person to another by means of the secretions of the mouth and throat, although repeated efforts to transmit it to man in this fashion have failed. The incubation period has not been definitely established, but it is believed that it may be several weeks in length.

Signs and symptoms of infectious mononucleosis are varied. Usually it is a benign disease with a good prognosis. Malaise is a frequent early complaint, and it is often accompanied by elevation of temperature, enlargement of the lymph nodes, sore throat, headache, increased nasal secretions, aches and pains resembling those of influenza, and moderate enlargement of the liver and spleen. Jaundice, rupture of the spleen, encephalitis, and even death may occur. Diagnosis can be conclusively established by means of a test of the blood—the heterophil agglutination test. This test makes use of the fact that a certain substance that is present in the patient's blood causes clumping, or agglutination, of the washed erythrocytes (antigen) of another animal (in this case, sheep cells are used). The test is almost always positive at the end of 10 to 14 days of the illness. Another conclusive laboratory finding is a marked increase in mononuclear leukocytes, which lends the name to the disease. At the height of the disease the white blood cell count usually ranges between 10,000 and 20,000 cells/mm.[3] of blood. So far, no modern antibiotic is effective in treating infectious mononucleosis, and no immunization is available.

Nursing care of the patient with infectious mononucleosis is purely symptomatic. If sore throat is severe, hot gargles may be ordered; glucose solutions often give greater relief than saline solution. Liquid and soft foods may have to constitute the patient's entire menu. An ice cap may be helpful if headache is severe. Acetylsalicylic acid is usually given for headache and generalized discomfort, and the patient is encouraged to remain in bed. If he is allowed to be up, he is advised to stay indoors and engage in little activity. The disease usually disappears within 2 weeks, but it may continue in a chronic form for several weeks and even months. Relapses do occur, and this fact explains the need for rest at the time of acute illness even though the patient does not feel ill and resents the time spent away from his work or regular activities.

REFERENCES AND SELECTED READINGS*

1 Aledort, L.: The management of hemophilia: a perspective, Drug Ther. **1:**55-59, March 1971.
2 *Alexander, M. M.: Physical examination. IV. The lymph system, Nursing '73 **3:**49-52, Oct. 1973.
3 American Cancer Society: 1975 cancer facts and figures, New York, 1974, American Cancer Society, Inc.
4 *Arnold, P.: Total-body irradiation and marrow transplantation, Am. J. Nurs. **63:**83-88, Feb. 1963.

*References preceded by an asterisk are particularly well suited for student reading.

5 *Baldy, C. M.: The lymphomas: concepts and current therapies, Nurs. Clin. North Am. **7:**763-775, Dec. 1972.
6 Beeson, P. B., and McDermott, W., editors: Cecil-Loeb textbook of medicine, ed. 13, Philadelphia, 1971, W. B. Saunders Co.
7 Bergersen, B. S.: Pharmacology in nursing, ed. 12, St. Louis, 1973, The C. V. Mosby Co.
8 Bouchard, R., and Owens, N. F.: Nursing care of the cancer patient, ed. 2, St. Louis, 1972, The C. V. Mosby Co.
9 *Child, J., and others: Blood transfusions, Am. J. Nurs. **72:**1602-1605, Sept. 1972.

10 Cohn, H. D.: Hemostasis and blood coagulation, Am. J. Nurs. **65:**116-119, Feb. 1965.

10a *Colman, R., and others: Disseminated intravascular coagulation (DIC): an approach, Am. J. Med. **52:**679-687, May 1972.

10b *Colman, R., and others: Disseminated intravascular coagulation: a problem in critical care medicine, Heart & Lung **3:**789-796, Sept.-Oct. 1974.

11 Crosby, W. H., editor: Hematologic disorders, Med. Clin. North Am. **50:**1485-1720, Nov. 1966.

12 *Drug update: Bleomycin—calusterone, Nursing '74 **3:**70-75, March 1974.

13 *Eisenhauer, L. A.: Drug-induced blood dyscrasias, Nurs. Clin. North Am. **7:**799-808, Dec. 1972.

14 *Franklin, F. I., and others: The many facets of hemophilia, J.A.M.A. **228:**85-92, April 1974.

15 Greenwald, E.: Cancer chemotherapy, New York, 1973, Medical Examination Publishing Co., Inc.

16 *Guy, R. B., and Rothenberg, S. P.: Sickle cell crisis, Med. Clin. North Am. **57:**1591-1598, Nov. 1973.

17 Guyton, A. C.: Textbook of medical physiology, ed. 4, Philadelphia, 1971, W. B. Saunders Co.

18 *Hynes, J. F., and Jansson, E. B.: Hodgkin's disease, Am. J. Nurs. **58:**371-372, March 1958.

19 *Isler, C.: Blood—the age of components, RN **36:**31-41, June 1973.

20 *Jackson, D. E.: Sickle cell disease: meeting a need, Nurs. Clin. North Am. **7:**727-741, Dec. 1972.

21 *Johnson, N. E.: Coping with complications of intravenous therapy, Nursing '72 **2:**5-8, Feb. 1972.

22 Lazerson, J.: The prophylactic approach to hemophilia A, Hosp. Practice **16:**99-102, 106-109, Feb. 1971.

22a *Mayer, G. C.: Disseminated intravascular coagulation, Am. J. Nurs. **73:**2067-2069, Dec. 1973.

23 Mengel, C. E., Frei, E., and Nachman, R. E.: Hematology principles and practice, Chicago, 1972, Year Book Medical Publishers, Inc.

24 *Patterson, P. C.: Hemophilia: the new look, Nurs. Clin. North Am. **7:**777-785, Dec. 1972.

24a Rapaport, S. I.: Defibrination syndromes. In Williams, W. J., editor: Hematology, New York, 1972, McGraw-Hill Book Co.

25 Robbins, S. L.: Pathologic basis of disease, Philadelphia, 1974, W. B. Saunders Co.

25a *Rocco, F. and others: DIC—disseminated intravascular coagulation, Nursing '74 **4:**66-71, Nov. 1974.

26 *Schumann, D., and Patterson, P. C.: The adult with acute leukemia, Nurs. Clin. North Am. **7:**743-761, Dec. 1972.

27 *Sergis, E., and Hilgartner, M. W.: Hemophilia, Am. J. Nurs. **72:**2011-2017, Nov. 1972.

27a Simpson, J. G., and Stalker, A. L.: Clin. Hematol. **2:**189-199, Feb. 1973.

28 Williams, S. R.: Nutrition and diet therapy, ed. 2, St. Louis, 1973, The C. V. Mosby Co.

29 Williams, W. J., and others: Hematology, New York, 1972, McGraw-Hill Book Co.

30 *Wilson, P.: Iron-deficiency anemia, Am. J. Nurs. **72:**502-504, March 1972.

31 Wintrobe, M. M.: Clinical hematology, Philadelphia, 1967, Lea & Febiger.

32 Wintrobe, M. M., and others, editors: Harrison's principles of internal medicine, ed. 7, New York, 1974, McGraw-Hill Book Co.

33 *Vaz, D. D. S.: The common anemias: nursing approaches, Nurs. Clin. North Am. **7:**711-725, Dec. 1972.

20 Diseases of the urinary system

The patient's emotional response
Urologic diagnosis

Diseases of the urinary system
Obstruction of the urinary system
Congenital malformations of and trauma
  to the urinary tract
Diseases of the kidney
Management of the patient with disease
  of the urinary system
Planning home care for the patient
  with urinary drainage

Renal failure
Acute renal failure
Chronic renal failure

■ In maintaining an internal environment compatible with life, the body must be able to regulate fluid volume and electrolyte composition and maintain a means for excreting metabolic wastes. Primary effectors of these regulative functions are the organs and structures of the urinary system. The kidneys control composition of body fluid, waste, and electrolytes and maintain these substances in the body within a narrow and critical range. The ureters, bladder, and urethra serve as the mechanism whereby waste that is filtered and secreted by the kidneys is eliminated from the body.

Disease of the urinary system is a major cause of morbidity in the United States; it also is a significant cause of mortality. In 1972 disease of the urinary system was reported as a causative factor in approximately 33,000 deaths.[103] Of these, 15,500 were from malignancy, 8,200 from nephritis and nephrosis, 7,000 from kidney infections, and 1,900 from hypertrophy of the prostate gland (a disease of the male reproductive system leading to kidney damage from urethral obstruction). These figures indicate that mortality from disease of the urinary system is generally associated with destruction of renal tissue. When disease involves the kidneys, renal function is directly threatened; when disease occurs in the lower urinary tract, it not only affects tissue locally but can threaten renal function through spread of infection and obstruction of urine flow. The primary objective for treatment of disease in any part of the urinary tract should be early detection and adequate therapy directed toward preserving or improving renal function. Without renal function, life can continue for only a few days.

During the past decade some of the most striking developments in treatment of individuals with disease of the urinary system have been in the area of prolonging life after renal function has ceased. Dialysis and renal transplantation have given hundreds of people each year a continued, though somewhat uncertain, life expectancy. Technical, physical, and

■ **STUDY QUESTIONS**

1 Review Chapter 5.
2 Review Chapter 9.
3 Review the physiology of urine formation. Identify the major parts of the nephron and the function of each. What are the normal ranges for urine specific gravity? Urine pH?
4 Identify signs and symptoms indicating loss of the kidneys' ability to regulate or influence the following body functions: electrolyte balance, fluid balance, excretion of metabolic wastes, acid-base balance, and erythropoiesis.
5 What foods are high in potassium? Sodium? What are complete protein foods?
6 What is the normal serum creatinine level? Blood urea nitrogen level? Where do these substances originate in the body?
7 Review principles involved in catheterization of the urinary bladder. What nursing actions help to decrease urinary tract infection from this procedure?
8 What is the relationship of output to intake in the normal person? What should be recorded on an accurate fluid balance record?
9 Review the physiology of voiding. What is the normal bladder capacity? At what point does one normally have the urge to void? What is retention of urine?

psychosocial components of the new life-style of these individuals demand the nurse's attention.

Nurses can assist in significantly reducing the morbidity from disease of the urinary system. This can be achieved through increasing public awareness of preventive measures, assisting in early detection of signs and symptoms of disease, and providing long-term care to the growing population of chronically ill individuals with urinary tract disease. This chapter will define common problems of the patient with disease of the urinary system and will identify requirements for nursing care in preventive, acute, and chronic phases of illness.

■ THE PATIENT'S EMOTIONAL RESPONSE

Although most laymen have only a vague understanding of the anatomy and physiology of the urinary system, they do know that the kidneys are necessary for life. They are also aware that urinary and sexual functions are performed by the same organ in the male and that in the female these organs exist in close proximity. Hence both fear and embarrassment are commonly exhibited emotional reactions to suspected or diagnosed disease in the urinary system.

At times these normal emotional reactions may lead to a delay in diagnosis and treatment of the urinary problem. The patient may hesitate to seek attention for his problem, or when he does, he may be unable to express his concerns. Fear and embarrassment may also be manifest as aggressive or even immodest behavior. Nursing care that is directed toward identifying the patient's concerns and feelings about his problem can increase the patient's ability to express his problem openly and assist the physician and nurse in dealing with the patient's health needs.

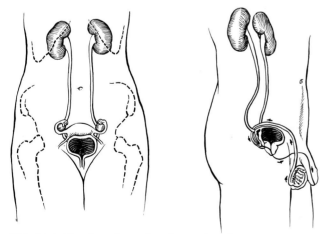

FIG. 20-1. The female and male genitourinary systems and reproductive systems. The arrows indicate the route by which seminal fluid passes from the testes to the urethra.

Embarrassment can be lessened through a candid approach on the part of the nurse. As the patient identifies the nurse's lead in frankly discussing his problem, he likely will show less self-consciousness. Value should also be placed on ensuring the patient's privacy during examination and testing procedures. Fear of diagnosis and treatment can result from lack of knowledge or from incorrect knowledge. Fears regarding loss of health, sexual function, or life are appropriate in some instances of urinary system disease. It is important first to identify the patient's understanding of the problem and the treatment he is receiving and then to proceed with teaching and giving directions. Simple diagrams are helpful (Fig. 20-1).

■ UROLOGIC DIAGNOSIS

Since impairment of renal function can threaten life, it is fortunate that disease in the urinary system can be diagnosed with a high degree of accuracy. The urologic examination usually begins with a complete medical history and physical examination, including pelvic and rectal examinations. Urinary symptoms may result from numerous systemic disorders as well as from primary renal or urologic disease. The nurse can be helpful to the patient undergoing general examination by interpreting to him the need for thoroughness. Special examinations of the urinary system are performed to further identify the location and nature of existing disease. The accuracy of findings in many of these tests is dependent on patient assistance (that is, remaining on special diets prior to testing and collecting specimens at designated time intervals). It is important for the nurse to explain to the patient his role in the testing procedure and to ascertain his understanding of and ability to follow the directions he has been given. Regardless of whether the patient will be examined in a hospital, physician's office, or clinic setting, written instructions are a valuable supplement to clear and precise verbal direction. Some tests are performed with the patient under sedation. If the patient is to return home after such a procedure, the nurse should advise that the patient be accompanied by someone who can ensure his safety.

The examinations and tests mentioned in this section are those most commonly performed in diagnosing disorders of the urinary system. Preparation of the patient, the test or examination procedure and its significance, aftercare of the patient, and precautions or special observations necessary for each test are described.

Examination of the urine

Urinalysis. A voided urine specimen is usually examined first. This analysis includes a description of the color and degree of cloudiness of the urine; determination of the pH (acidity or alkalinity), specific gravity, and amount of protein, glucose, and ketones; and examination of the sediment, which may contain any of the following elements: red blood cells, white blood cells, casts, tissue shreds, and bacteria. Analysis of the urine yields information about probable locations and causes of urinary disease. Findings may indicate need for further testing to confirm or refine the diagnosis. Urinalysis may also indicate disease of nonrenal or urologic origin.

For collecting the specimen the patient should be given a clean container in which to catch urine, three to four cotton balls soaked in a cleansing solution such as 1:1,000 benzalkonium chloride, and specific directions to be followed. Cleansing of the meatus prior to collection of the specimen decreases the likelihood of external contamination, especially in the female where there is great chance of vaginal cells and organisms entering the specimen. At least 50 to 100 ml. of urine is collected for the test; smaller amounts are acceptable for children. Urine from the first voiding of the day is preferred because it is concentrated and abnormal constituents are less likely to be missed. If analysis of the urine cannot

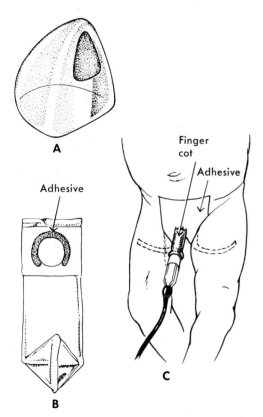

FIG. 20-2. Methods of collecting urine specimens from infants and small children. **A,** Birdcage feeder used for an infant girl. **B,** Plastic collecting device for boys and girls. **C,** Finger cot anchored with adhesive tape attached to drainage apparatus for collecting 24-hour specimen.

be performed immediately, the specimen should be refrigerated to retard bacterial growth.

A voided urine specimen is difficult to obtain from an infant or young child, and special techniques must be used. A plastic urine specimen collector treated with material that adheres readily to the skin is available commercially for both boys and girls (Fig. 20-2). All such collectors are applied after thoroughly cleansing the area about the urinary meatus. The open end of the 24-hour urine collector (Fig. 20-2, C) is attached to a drainage apparatus to prevent the collector from becoming distended with urine and possibly dislodged. A specimen of a single voiding from a male infant or a small boy can be obtained in a finger cot secured to the penis with adhesive. A single specimen can usually be collected from an infant girl by placing her on a small basin and, while holding her in an upright position, giving her fluids to drink. Another method is to separate the labia and place a Spicer infant urinal or birdcage feeder over the meatus. This apparatus is secured by using two long strips of adhesive tape running from the abdomen under the buttock. Before adhesive is used on a child's skin, the skin should be painted with tincture of benzoin to prevent irritation. Replacing the diaper prevents the child from pulling the apparatus off. Sometimes ankle and hand restraints may be needed.

Multiple glass test. This test is performed on a male patient when infection of the lower urinary tract is to be evaluated. The patient should have a full bladder for this test as a number of samples will be taken during a single voiding. The patient should cleanse the area about the meatus with an antiseptic solution prior to specimen collection, and care should be taken throughout the procedure to avoid introducing new bacteria to this area. The patient is asked to void about 100 ml. into the first container (the urethral "washings"). Without interruption of the urinary stream, another 100 ml. of urine is voided into a second container (the kidney and bladder "washings"). If prostatic "washings" are desired, the patient is instructed to stop voiding and the physician gently massages the prostate. The patient then finishes emptying the bladder; this specimen contains prostatic secretions.

Composite specimens. A specimen of all the urine excreted over a specific period of time is often needed. Time durations for urine collections may vary from 2 to 24 hours. Specimens are examined for such constituents as sugar, protein, sediment (blood cells and casts), tubercle bacilli, 17-ketosteroids, electrolytes, catecholamines, and breakdown products of protein metabolism.

The accuracy of findings in this type of test is in most instances wholly dependent on cooperation of the patient. Whether the specimen is to be obtained in the hospital or in the patient's home, the patient should be told exactly how to collect it. Again, written instructions are a good reinforcement of those verbally given. Points for the nurse to understand and discuss with the patient are as follows:

1. Reason for collection of the specimen.
2. Specified time interval for collection (12 hours, 24 hours, etc.).
3. Method of collecting the specimen. The collection should be started at the appointed time by having the patient empty his bladder and discard this urine. Urine from all subsequent voidings is saved, including that voided at the hour designated for closing the collection. It is important for the patient to understand that *all* urine must be saved. To prevent possible fecal contamination and loss of part of the specimen, the patient should be instructed to void into a separate receptacle before a defecation.
4. Preservation of the specimen. The specimen should be kept refrigerated to prevent bacterial growth that may alter its composition. Some urine collections require the addition of special preservatives to the collection container to prevent alterations in constituents of the urine.

In addition to these responsibilities, the nurse should ensure that the specimen is properly labeled and properly prepared for the laboratory. The entire specimen or, depending on the specific test and laboratory, only a 5 to 10 ml. sample of the total collection may be sent. If the whole specimen is not to be sent, it should be well mixed before the sample is taken, and information as to the total amount of urine collected in the allotted time should be recorded on the label.

Composite urine specimens are difficult to obtain from infants and young children. Restraints must sometimes be used. The most satisfactory method is to use an infant urine collector (previously described) connected to a collection bottle. For other procedures, see specialized texts.[111]

When a test involves the collection of total urine output, it is important that the urine be collected from all available sources. For instance, the patient may pass urine from his urethra and also have a nephrostomy tube from which urine drains. In such instances, specimens from each source should be collected in separate, well-labeled containers. Urine from a cystostomy tube and a urethral catheter may, however, be combined into one specimen because both specimens come from the bladder.

Urine culture. When infection appears to be present in the urinary system, a urine culture is often ordered. A 5 to 10 ml. specimen of urine is collected in a sterile tube under aseptic conditions. This is sent to the laboratory, where any organisms present are allowed to grow in culture media and then identified microscopically. The results of the culture and sensitivity test assist the physician in making the diagnosis and in ordering drug treatment.

Specimens for urine culture may be obtained either by catheterization or voiding. It should be made clear, however, that urethral catheterization should never be used routinely in collecting urine for culture because of the risk of introducing additional bacteria into the bladder. Catheterization may be necessary to obtain a sterile urine specimen when the patient is unable to void even after being adequately hydrated or if the patient is incontinent of urine. When a catheter is passed, meticulous attention is given to nontraumatic aseptic technique. After urine flow from the catheter is established, 5 to 10 ml. of urine should be collected directly into a sterile specimen container. Care must be taken to ensure that the rim and the inside of the container are not touched by the catheter or by the hands. If a culture tube with a cotton plug is used as a specimen container, care must be taken to keep the tube upright to prevent moistening the cotton and thereby contaminating the specimen. Cultures may also be ordered on the urine taken from the renal pelvis during ureteral catheterization or when ureterostomy or nephrostomy tubes are in place.

In collecting a voided specimen for culture, the nurse must decide if the patient is capable of independently obtaining the specimen or if nursing or medical personnel will need to collect the specimen. Remembering that the specimen must be free from contamination during collection should guide the nurse in this decision. Most ambulatory patients who are given precise and unhurried direction will be able to collect their own midstream urine specimen.

The directions given the female patient for collecting her own urine specimen should guide her in collecting a specimen that is free from contamination. Points to stress in accomplishing this are separating the labia, maintaining this separation throughout the procedure, cleansing the meatus with one front-to-back motion with each cleansing pad, collecting urine in the sterile container well after the urinary stream has been started, and touching only the outside of the urine container. The equipment she should be given includes a sterile container for the urine and four cotton or gauze sponges saturated with a cleansing solution. To collect a clean voided specimen from a female patient, the nurse should follow a similar procedure.

The directions given the male patient are similar to those given the female patient. Proper equipment is provided (same as that for the female patient) and directions are given that contain the following points: the foreskin is to be retracted if the patient is uncircumcised, and the glans cleansed with each of the cleansing pads; urine is to be caught in the sterile container once the stream has been well established; and precautions should be taken to touch only the outer surface of the urine container. To collect a specimen from a male patient, the same procedure is followed; it is usually performed by a male member of the nursing team or male physician.

To obtain a sterile voided specimen for culture from an infant or a young child, the nurse uses the procedures for collecting a single voided specimen of urine. The local area should be cleansed well and a sterile collecting apparatus should be used.

Two further general points regarding collection of urine for culture are that (1) the first voided specimen of the day is used when possible because bacteria will be more numerous and (2) if the specimen is not cultured immediately, refrigeration is mandatory to prevent growth of organisms in the specimen.

Evaluating bladder function

Normally the bladder contains little or no urine after voiding. However, certain disease states inhibit the bladder from emptying completely. Some common conditions in which incomplete emptying of the bladder occurs are benign prostatic hypertrophy, urethral strictures, and interruptions in bladder innervation. Urine retained in the bladder after voiding becomes a culture media for bacterial growth; stagnation of urine also encourages the formation of bladder stones. Inability to urinate properly may also predispose to the development of hydronephrosis, a condition in which urine backs up into the kidneys; this results in destruction of renal tissue. The need, then, for evaluation of bladder function can be appreciated when these problems are kept in mind.

Urine left in the bladder after voiding is called residual urine. One way to determine the amount of residual urine is to catheterize the patient immediately after voiding. This may be ordered by the physician on a one-time or a serial basis.

The urine obtained from the voiding may, if handled without contamination, be used for culture if such a specimen is needed. Prior to catheterizing the patient the nurse should consult with the physician as to the plan for establishing urinary drainage. If a large residual urine is suspected, the physician may wish the catheter to be left in place in the bladder. In such an instance a Foley catheter would be used for the procedure. Residual urine volumes of 50 ml. or less indicate near-normal or returning bladder function.

To avoid passing a catheter to measure residual urine volume, x-ray determination of retained urine may be done. In this procedure the patient is injected with a radiopaque substance excreted by the kidneys. As the dye is excreted in the urine, it passes into the bladder. A sufficient amount of urine containing the radiopaque material is allowed to accumulate in the bladder and the patient is instructed to void. Immediately after voiding a radiograph is taken. Any urine retained in the bladder will be visualized on the radiograph. An inherent danger in this procedure is that of allergic reaction to the injected radiopaque material. Precautions and treatment for this problem are discussed on p. 384.

Evaluating renal function

Tests of renal function are carried out when findings in the general physical evaluation of the patient and in the urinalysis suggest renal disease. The best overview of the patient's clinical condition is obtained when the results of a number of tests are compared.

Blood chemistry tests. A major function of the kidney is excretion of by-products of metabolism. The two most commonly ordered tests of renal function, serum creatinine and blood urea nitrogen (BUN) tests, are measures of the kidneys' ability to excrete metabolic wastes. Specifically, these tests measure serum concentrations of nitrogenous products derived from protein breakdown. In health, serum creatinine concentration approximates 0.9 to 1.5 mg./100 ml., and blood urea nitrogen ranges from 10 to 20 mg./100 ml. In the later stages of renal insufficiency, nitrogen products are retained and serum values are markedly elevated. No special preparation of the patient is required for these tests. In interpreting test results, however, it should be remembered that high-protein diets; rapid cellular destruction from trauma, infection, and fever; and strenuous, prolonged muscular activity increase nitrogen waste levels. Abnormally high laboratory values may result in these states and may not reflect the patient's true level of renal function.

Since the kidneys are also responsible for regulating the concentration of electrolytes in the extracellular fluid compartment, analysis of the levels of these electrolytes may yield information about kidney function. The electrolytes most frequently evaluated include potassium (3.5 to 5.0 mEq./L. of blood), sodium (138 to 148 mEq./L.), calcium (9.0 to 11.0 mg./100 ml.), chloride (100 to 106 mEq./L.), and phosphorus (3.0 to 4.5 mg./100 ml.). Levels of serum electrolytes in patients with renal disease are dependent on the location and severity of pathologic conditions of the kidneys and hence can be quite varied from patient to patient.

Urinary chemistry tests. In kidney disease involving the glomeruli, loss of plasma proteins may occur. It has been demonstrated that various types of glomerular lesions exist and that these lesions allow passage of different amounts and types of plasma proteins into the glomerular filtrate. Serum determinations of plasma protein fractions and total protein content can assist in evaluating the nature and extent of the renal disease.

Urea and creatinine excretion tests also provide information about glomerular function. The amount of creatinine normally excreted in the urine each day is approximately 1.0 to 1.5 Gm.; the amount of urea excreted in the urine each day is approximately 25 to 30 Gm. Excretion tests of these metabolic wastes are most useful clinically when test results are compared to those previously obtained. When comparing current with previous test results, both the amount and direction of change in glomerular filtration can be appreciated. In performing a urea or creatinine excretion test, a 24-hour composite urine specimen is collected, and the amount of urea or creatinine excreted in the sample is measured.

The sodium excretion test measures tubular function. Specifically, this test provides information as to the kidneys' ability to appropriately excrete or conserve this electrolyte; in chronic renal failure either inappropriate retention or excretion of sodium can occur. Knowledge of urinary excretion of this electrolyte is helpful in calculating sodium intake requirements of the patient. Again, in order to determine change in direction and degree of tubular functions, comparison of current and past sodium excretion studies should be made. The test is performed by analyzing the sodium content of a 24-hour urine collection.

Phenolsulfonphthalein test. The commonly used abbreviation for the phenolsulfonphthalein test is the PSP test. The test primarily measures renal blood flow and renal tubular function. PSP is a red dye that, when injected intravenously, is removed from the body primarily through secretion in the renal tubules. The test is performed as follows: the patient drinks 2 glasses of water prior to the test and takes extra fluid during the test to ensure a sufficient volume of urine for collection of necessary specimens. (Caution must be used when performing this test in individuals with renal insufficiency or failure as they may not tolerate fluid loading. Clarification with the physician of the amount of fluid to be allowed is needed prior to testing.) Then 6 mg. of dye is injected intravenously, and the time of injection is recorded. Urine specimens are collected 15 minutes, 30 minutes, 1 hour, and 2 hours after injection of the dye. The patient must be told to completely empty his bladder at each voiding; incomplete emptying of the bladder causes inaccuracy in test results as the amount of dye excreted by the kidneys in each time period cannot be determined. Each specimen must be correctly labeled with the exact time of collection. In the laboratory the amount of dye in each sample is measured and compared to a standard sample. With normal renal function, 25% to 50% of the dye is excreted in the first 15 minutes; as renal function declines, less dye is excreted in this time period.

The presence in the urine of blood or phenazopyridine hydrochloride (Pyridium), a urinary tract antiseptic that gives urine a red-orange color, will produce inaccurate test results. Prior to beginning the test the patient's urine should be checked for abnormal coloration.

Because the ability to void at precise time intervals during the test is necessary, the patient should be checked prior to the PSP test for any difficulty in emptying the bladder. The patient's state of hydration should also be adequate. If the patient is unable to void at the appropriate times during the testing procedure, the physician should be notified, and any deviations in the time schedule should be marked on the specimen labels so that adjustments may be made in interpreting the test.

The patient may have a light meal during the procedure. No inaccuracies in the test occur as the result of intake of food.

Drugs such as penicillin, aspirin, diuretics, and sulfonamides and high serum uric acid levels decrease excretion of the dye because they compete with PSP in the tubular cells for excretion. Information concerning drugs the patient has recently taken should be obtained prior to initiating the PSP test.

The patient who is not acutely ill can usually collect his own urine specimens if given a watch, properly labeled collection containers, and thorough instructions. Included in the instructions should be the need for calling the nurse if the specimen cannot be collected at the appointed times.

Clearance tests. Clearance can be defined as the amount of blood that can be "cleared" of a substance in a specified amount of time. Clearance is determined according to the following equation:

$$\text{Clearance (ml./min.)} = \frac{\text{Urine volume (ml./min.)} \times \text{Urine concentration (mg./ml.)}}{\text{Plasma concentration (mg./ml.)}}$$

Clearance tests are useful clinically in determining changes in glomerular filtration. Urea and creatinine are the substances most commonly used in measuring clearance. Because these substances are primarily removed from the blood through glomerular filtration, decreases in "clearance" of these substances can be equated with reduction in the glomerular filtration rate (GFR). The creatinine clearance test is a more accurate indicator of GFR than is the urea clearance test, and it is the more widely used of the two tests.

Urine for clearance testing is generally collected over a 24-hour period. However, in some instances, maintaining accurate urine collections over this length of time can be extremely difficult. Because analysis of the total urine volume for the test period is essential for accurate determination of renal function, a shorter time period for urine collections may be used (usually 2 hours).

Normal dietary intake is maintained during tests for creatinine clearance. Urinary excretion of creatinine remains fairly uniform throughout the day and is proportional to the muscle mass of the patient rather than to the day's dietary protein intake. When urea clearance is being tested, however, dietary protein intake significantly influences test results. Either a short urine collection period during which the patient fasts or a 24-hour collecting period in which dietary protein intake is calculated into test results is needed to maintain test validity.

Although it is important that the patient be adequately hydrated for determining both creatinine and urea clearance, it is crucial for the latter test. To promote a constant excretion of urea, an important factor in the test, urine flow rates of at least 2 ml./minute must be maintained. This is accomplished through administration of oral fluids when the patient's condition permits (absence of oliguric renal failure, congestive heart failure, etc.). Two glasses of water are taken at the beginning of the test, and additional water is taken during the test.

To begin the 2-hour test, the patient is asked to completely empty his bladder and to discard the urine. A notation of the time is made. One hour later the patient voids again and a blood sample for creatinine and/or urea determination is drawn. All urine obtained from this voiding is collected and labeled as the "first" urine specimen. The exact times at which the discarded urine and this specimen were voided should be indicated on the specimen label. The blood specimen should also be labeled by number and time of collection. One hour later another urine and blood sample are obtained. After proper labeling of the specimens, all samples are sent to the laboratory.

For the 24-hour test a 24-hour urine collection that runs from one morning to the next morning is obtained. (Refer to collection of composite urine on p. 425.) As urine collecting is completed, a blood specimen is drawn to determine the serum creatinine and/or serum urea level.

Normal clearance values for urea are approximately 75 ml./minute; normal clearance values for creatinine are approximately 95 to 140 ml./minute for males and 85 to 125 ml./minute for females. In individuals with depressed renal function these values will be decreased.

Urine concentration and dilution tests. The ability of the kidneys to concentrate urine permits simultaneous excretion of waste material and conservation of needed body fluid. This concentrating ability is lost early in renal disease, especially when damage occurs in the medullary portion of the kidneys and thus impairs tubular function.

The specific gravity of the urine is one indicator of concentrating ability, especially after periods of limited fluid intake such as occurs with the first voiding of the morning. In a healthy person the specific gravity of the first morning voiding will be toward the middle to higher end of a normal range of 1.010 to 1.026. As nephrons are destroyed, the specific

gravity of the urine falls. In severe renal disease, where a small remaining population of nephrons attempts to excrete proportionally larger volumes of waste materials, specific gravity falls to a 1.010 to 1.012 range and remains "fixed" at this level.

Concentration tests are more controlled efforts to determine the ability of the kidneys to conserve fluid. For these tests the *osmolality* rather than the specific gravity of urine is determined.

For the *Fishberg concentration test* the patient is instructed to eat his usual evening meal and then take no more food or fluid until after completing the test the following morning. Urine specimens are collected at 6 A.M., 7 A.M., and 8 A.M. In addition to withholding of fluid, morning specimens are collected to ensure maximum concentration in test results.

The *Addis concentration test* yields more reliable measurement of concentrating ability through a more vigorous dehydration of the patient prior to testing. In this test, fluids are restricted for a 24-hour period. During the last 12 hours of the test all urine is collected.

Determination of concentrating ability through withdrawal of fluids over extended time periods can (1) lead to severe dehydration and electrolyte imbalance in older individuals and children, (2) precipitate acute renal shutdown in patients with chronic but compensated renal disease, and (3) induce obstruction in patients with infections of the urinary tract. Thorough evaluation of the patient for possible risk factors should be carried out prior to starting either of the above tests.

The *Mosenthal concentration test* requires neither food nor fluid restriction. The test is carried out over a 24-hour period; total urinary output from 7 P.M. to 7 A.M. is collected, followed by collection of separate specimens at 2-hour intervals through 7 P.M.

Urine dilution tests are performed to measure the kidneys' ability to excrete fluid loads while conserving necessary electrolytes. The ability to dilute urine is a function of the tubular portion of the nephron. The potential danger inherent in this test is in its possible performance on a patient incapable of rapidly excreting extra fluid. A detailed history taken on the patient prior to initiation of the test should include details of any cardiac, liver, or kidney disease.

The *Fishberg dilution test* may be performed at any time of the day. During the test the patient should remain inactive to prevent production of extra fluid and waste through increased metabolism and to prevent excessive loss of fluid through perspiration and respiration. The patient should completely empty his bladder at the beginning of the test. The adult should drink 1,200 ml. of fluid within $1/2$ hour. The physician should determine the amount of fluid to be given a child. Urine specimens are then collected every half hour for 3 hours. A person with normal hydration and normal renal function will excrete almost the entire 1,200 ml. in the 3-hour period, and the urine will have a specific gravity of about 1.002. Because most patients will have difficulty in drinking 1,200 ml. of fluid in a $1/2$-hour period, it sometimes helps if water is mixed with fruit juice to make a weak fruit ade. Each specimen should include all urine voided and should be sent to the laboratory. The label on the specimen should include the exact time of each voiding.

Visualization of the urinary tract

Visualization tests measure both structure and function of organs and tissues in the urinary system. They are used both in initially diagnosing and in evaluating a patient's response to treatment over a period of time.

Several of these tests are dependent on radiographs for visualization of the urinary tract. Since the kidneys lie retroperitoneally, any accumulation of flatus or feces in the intestines could obstruct the view of the kidneys on a radiograph. To assure visualization, emptying of the bowel is carried out prior to examination. The patient's age and state of health are considered in determining the extensiveness of the bowel preparation. The preparation of an adult who is not severely debilitated would usually include a diet low in residue the day prior to examination, a generous dose of cathartic the night before the test, nothing by mouth after midnight, and a cleansing of the lower bowel on the morning of the examination. Cathartics that may be used include castor oil preparations, mineral oil, senna powder, and bisacodyl (Dulcolax) tablets. Lower bowel preparation may include enemas or bisacodyl suppositories. Infants, young children, elderly people, and physically debilitated individuals should not be subjected to vigorous bowel preparation as dehydration and serious electrolyte disturbances may ensue. Some instances of preexisting conditions in which bowel cleansing is especially hazardous are severe nutritional deficiencies, colitis, presence of an ileostomy, fluid and electrolyte disturbances, and renal insufficiency or failure. Bowel preparation for individuals with any of these conditions should be discussed with the physician.

The results of any efforts to evacuate the bowel should be determined and recorded clearly on the patient's chart. Ineffectiveness of these efforts should be communicated to the physician well before the time scheduled for the examination.

Physical safety of the patient must be assured when vigorous cathartics are employed. Urgency, fatigue, and weakness are common following bowel cleansing; falls and accidents easily occur in these states. Sedation, which slows reaction time and further unsteadies gait, should be withheld. Prior to sleep the patient should become familiar with his surroundings and with the location of his call light. The patient should be observed closely throughout the night with assistance provided as indicated.

Radiographs of the urinary tract may be ordered in conjunction with other abdominal studies. Problems may arise in visualizing the urinary system if barium studies have been recently carried out. This problem is prevented by scheduling tests so that examination of the urinary tract precedes barium swallows, gastrointestinal series, and barium enemas.

Radiologic examination of the abdomen (KUB). A flat plate film of the abdomen can reveal gross structural changes in the kidneys and urinary system. The size, shape, and placement of the kidneys can be determined, and calcifications or stones located in a kidney, pelvis, or ureter can be visualized. Bowel preparations may or may not be ordered for this examination.

Intravenous pyelography. In the intravenous pyelogram (IVP) a radiograph can demonstrate the size and location of the kidneys, cysts or tumors within the kidneys, filling of the renal pelves, and the outline of the ureters and bladder. This is accomplished through the excretion by the kidneys of a radiopaque dye that has been injected intravenously. The IVP tests kidney excretory function and the patency of the urinary tract. This test may be performed in a clinic or hospital setting.

Preparation of the patient includes bowel cleansing (p. 200) and withholding of fluids for up to 8 hours prior to testing to produce slight dehydration and greater concentration of dye in the kidneys and urinary system. Again, withholding of food and fluids prior to testing children and older individuals should be discussed with the physician. Included in the preparation of the patient is an explanation of the procedure, including the reasons for bowel cleansing and dietary restrictions. Before examination, an attempt is made to learn whether or not the patient is sensitive to iodine, as the radiopaque material injected intravenously contains this substance. The test should not be performed on individuals with known sensitivity to iodine because anaphylaxis can result. At times it is difficult to determine sensitivity prior to use. Two precautions are taken to prevent serious reactions to the dye during IVP examination: (1) most dye preparations contain antihistamine and (2) emergency drugs such as epinephrine are immediately available in the examination area.

For the radiograph the patient is placed on an x-ray table. A radiograph of the abdomen is taken first to identify size and position of the kidneys, the amount of gas in the bowel, and any radiopaque stones in the urinary tract. After this film is read, the radiopaque dye (Hypaque, Renografin) is given intravenously. The patient should know that he may experience a feeling of warmth, a flushing of the face, and a salty taste in the mouth as the physician slowly injects the dye. These sensations should abate within a few minutes; some relief may be obtained by taking deep breaths. The nurse should closely observe the patient for any signs of respiratory distress, sudden diaphoresis and clamminess, urticaria, instability in vital signs, or any unusual sensation; any of these may indicate a reaction to the contrast medium. Tripelennamine (Pyribenzamine), diphenhydramine hydrochloride (Benadryl), epinephrine (Adrenalin), and oxygen should be available for immediate use.

Sometimes a large plastic ball is strapped firmly on the abdomen to prevent dye from passing freely down the ureters until after radiographs of the kidneys have been taken. Radiographs are usually taken 2, 5, 10, and 15 minutes after the dye has been injected. If obstruction or poor renal function is present, additional films may be taken 1 and 2 hours later. When delayed films are necessary, the patient must either be returned to his bed or protected from discomfort on the x-ray table. If he remains on the table, a soft bath blanket should be placed under him, and his position should be changed at 15-minute intervals.

Radiorenography. Radiorenography tests involve scintillation scanning or photography techniques in visualizing the urinary tract. Diagnostically these tests can measure renal blood flow and renal tubular or excretory function. Therefore they are useful tests in (1) detecting obstructions in the upper urinary tract, (2) detecting renal vascular disease in hypertensive patients, (3) detecting acute renal failure within 48 hours of onset of oliguria, (4) monitoring the function of transplanted kidneys and detecting early signs of rejection, and (5) general follow-up of

patients with renal disease and evaluation of the effectiveness of their treatment.

In radiorenography a dye containing a radioactive isotope such as iodohippurate sodium tagged with ^{131}I or ^{125}I (Hippuran) is injected intravenously. No precautions need be taken against radioactivity, as only tracer doses of the isotope are used. When iodine isotopes are used, the patient need not be given Lugol's solution prior to examination to prevent thyroid damage because the isotopes used are bound to large molecules that prevent their uptake by the thyroid gland. There are no dietary or activity restrictions prior to testing. The test lasts only minutes and can be repeated a number of times.

In performing the test the patient is placed on an x-ray table and scintillating probes are placed over the kidney(s) being examined (Fig. 20-3). The radioisotope is injected and scanning or photographic recording is begun. The patient should feel no pain or discomfort as the test is being carried out.

Renal angiography. The renal angiogram provides an outline of the vascularization of the kidneys. The examination is particularly useful in attempting to evaluate the possibility of renal artery stenosis as a causative factor in hypertension and in demonstrating renal neoplasms and abnormal renal vessels.

Preparation of the patient is similar to that for the IVP. In addition, sedation of the patient is often carried out using secobarbital or similar medication. When sedation is used, attention must be given to patient safety.

In performing the test, a contrast material similar to that used in intravenous pyelography is injected. Precautions should be taken against iodine sensitiv-

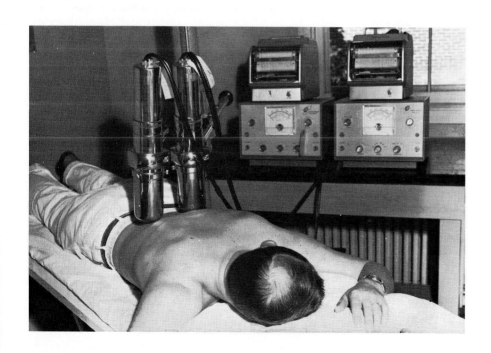

FIG. 20-3. Radiorenography. Scintillation probes are in place over both kidneys. (Courtesy Veterans Administration Center, Martinsburg, W. Va.; from Abt, A. F., and Balkus, V. A.: J. Urol. **85:**95, 1961.)

ity reactions. As the dye is injected and passes into the renal vasculature, radiographs are taken in rapid succession. The dye may be injected intravenously, and circulation time is calculated to ensure proper timing in taking the radiographs, or it may be injected intra-arterially. The latter technique is more widely performed and is termed aortography. In *translumbar aortography* the radiopaque dye is injected into the aorta by way of a long needle inserted through the soft tissue in the lumbar region. If a *femoral percutaneous aortogram* is performed, a catheter is threaded from a puncture of the femoral artery upward to the level of the renal arteries; dye is then injected through this catheter. After the radiographs have been taken and the catheter or needle removed, a pressure dressing is applied to the puncture site.

Care of the patient includes observing the site for bleeding, especially within the first 4 hours after the procedure. The dressing should be observed for fresh bleeding, the puncture area should be checked for swelling and increasing tenderness, vital signs should be monitored frequently, and distal pulses should be taken if femoral percutaneous aortography has been performed. The patient should remain on bed rest for at least 8 hours after the test, and the pressure dressing should be left in place until the following morning.

Venocavography. Venocavography determines patency in the venous system and can detect masses in the renal veins. A contrast medium is injected into the inferior vena cava via the femoral vein, and radiographs are taken. Preparation of the patient and precautions observed during and after the test are similar to those for angiography.

Retroperitoneal pneumography. The retroperitoneal pneumogram is an x-ray examination performed to diagnose adrenal or retroperitoneal tumors not visible on a flat plate examination. In this test the patient is placed in a side-lying position, and 1.0 to 1.5 L. of gas is injected in the retroperitoneal space as a contrast medium. Carbon dioxide is the gas most commonly used as it is rapidly absorbed into the bloodstream.

Preparation of the patient for this examination is similar to that carried out for the IVP. The patient is sedated, as discomfort, abdominal cramping, and nausea and vomiting may occur as the gas is injected. Following this test the patient should be kept in bed for a few hours and comfort maintained. Bleeding should not be precipitated by this procedure.

Cystoscopy and retrograde pyelography. Cystoscopy is the examination of the inside of the bladder through an instrument called a cystoscope (Fig. 20-4). The instrument is connected to an illuminating source, thus enabling direct visualization of the bladder wall. This procedure is indicated for all patients who have or have had hematuria. Although

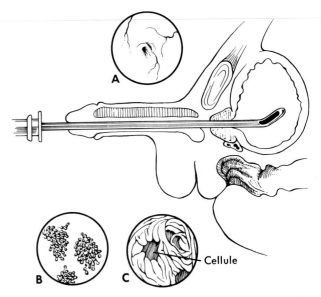

FIG. 20-4. Cystoscope inserted for examination of the bladder. **A,** Appearance of a normal ureteral orifice as seen through the cystoscope. **B,** Appearance of papillomas of the bladder as seen through the cystoscope. **C,** Appearance of a trabeculated bladder as seen through the cystoscope. Note the formation of cellules.

blood in the urine can result from numerous causes, it is one of the earliest signs of malignancy in the urinary system. Cystoscopic examination may be performed as part of a series of diagnostic tests or as an emergency measure in locating the source of and controlling heavy bleeding.

Nursing attention before and during a cystoscopic examination can contribute greatly to the success of the procedure and to lessening of the patient's discomfort. The patient should understand what he will experience in the cystoscopy room. Thorough explanations should be given before the procedure is begun, and if the patient is awake, someone should remain with him during the procedure to provide reassurance and to encourage relaxation. Much of the discomfort felt by the patient during this procedure is the result of contraction or spasm of the bladder sphincters; this can be decreased through deep breathing exercises and general relaxation on the part of the patient. To further assist the patient in relaxing a sedative such as phenobarbital and a narcotic such as morphine or meperidine hydrochloride (Demerol) are usually given an hour prior to the examination. General anesthesia is required for cystoscopy when the patient is quite apprehensive or when much manipulation is anticipated. In these instances, anesthesia reduces the possibility of trauma to the urethra or perforation of the bladder caused by sudden vigorous movement by the patient during the examination. Children are usually given a general anesthetic for this procedure.

Most hospitals require a signed permit prior to cystoscopy. The nurse should check to ascertain that it has been obtained.

Fluids are usually forced for several hours before the patient goes for the procedure. This ensures a continuous flow of urine in case specimens are to be collected and aids in preventing multiplication in slowly forming urine of bacteria that may be introduced during the procedure. If general anesthesia is to be used during the procedure, fluids may be administered intravenously. Food is usually withheld from all patients up to 8 hours prior to examination. If radiographs are to be taken during the procedure, cathartics and enemas may be ordered as for an IVP.

Clothing must be removed for the examination and replaced with a hospital gown and lithotomy boots. The patient is placed in a lithotomy position on the cystoscopy table and is draped so that only the perineum is exposed. In placing the patient in this position, care must be taken so that pressure is not exerted on the popliteal spaces, since this may lead to thrombosis in blood vessels. Because of arthritis and related disorders, some elderly patients are unable to rest comfortably in the stirrups; it may be necessary to use slings instead. If prolonged time on the table is necessary, the patient's legs should be removed from the stirrups at intervals and flexed and extended a few times to stimulate circulation. Extra pillows may be placed under the patient's head and shoulders for comfort.

If the patient is relatively comfortable, the cystoscope should be passed with little pain, provided there is no obstruction in the urethra. A local anesthetic such as procaine (usually 4%) may be instilled into the urethra prior to insertion of the cystoscope.

When the patient is awake, passing the instrument will be followed immediately by a strong desire to void. This occurs as a result of the pressure the instrument exerts against the internal sphincter. During the examination the bladder is distended with distilled water to make visualization more effective. As the bladder becomes increasingly distended, the urge to void will become increasingly strong.

During cystoscopy a number of tests may be performed on the urinary system. Cystography involves the injection of a radiopaque dye (Skiodan) or air as a contrast medium to visualize the bladder and determine its size, shape, and any irregularities. Bladder capacity may be measured through instillation of distilled water. A *voiding cystourethrogram* can reveal reflux of urine into the ureters on voiding, a bladder malfunction that can lead to pyelonephritis. *Ureteral catheterization* (with a nylon, radiopaque, size 4 or 6 Fr. catheter) can be performed through the cystoscope. The catheter is inserted into the ureteral opening in the bladder, into the ureter, and into the renal pelvis (Fig. 20-5). This procedure may involve one or both ureters. It is performed (1) when

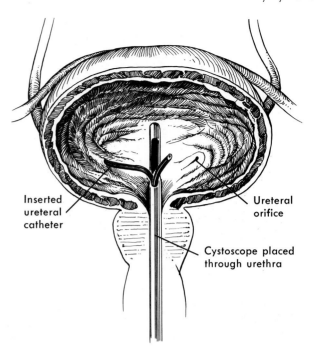

FIG. 20-5. Ureteral catheterization through the cystoscope. Note the ureteral catheter inserted into the right orifice. The left ureteral catheter is ready to be inserted.

culture and analysis of urine from individual kidneys is required, (2) when tests of renal function are to be performed on the kidneys separately, and (3) when visualization of the urinary tract is desired and IVP visualization has been inadequate, obstruction is present, or sensitivity to intravenous radiopaque material is noted.

Visualization of the urinary tract through ureteral catheterization is termed *retrograde pyelography*. This involves injecting 4 to 8 ml. of radiopaque material (Hypaque, Renografin) gently into the ureteral catheter. While the solution is being injected, the patient who is awake may feel slight discomfort in the kidney region. Pain should not be experienced unless too much of the solution is injected and the renal pelvis becomes overdistended. Radiographs are taken and demonstrate filling of the renal collecting structures. As the catheter is withdrawn, more of the contrast medium is injected, filling the ureter. Immediately another radiograph is made to outline the ureteral structure.

Urethrography involves instilling 20 ml. of radiopaque water-soluble lubricant into the urethra in order to visualize urethral irregularities of size and shape.

Care should be taken that the patient does not stand or walk alone immediately after cystoscopy. Blood that has drained from the legs while in the lithotomy position will flow back into the vessels of the feet and legs as the patient stands. Accidents caused by dizziness and fainting can occur from the sudden change in distribution of blood. (See Chapter 11 for further discussion.) On returning to his hospital room or home, the patient should remain in bed for a few hours. His urinary output should be observed for several hours; the urine may be pink-tinged, but more extensive bleeding should be reported to the physician. Frequent local and systemic reactions to a cystoscopic procedure include a full sensation and feeling of burning in the bladder, pain in the lower back, and a sensation of chilliness. Mild analgesics such as acetylsalicylic acid and codeine sulfate may be prescribed for discomfort. Usually, though, the greatest relief from discomfort is obtained from warmth, which produces relaxation and relieves muscle tension. A heating pad or hot-water bottle may be applied over the bladder region or to the lower back. Warm fluids should be offered at hourly intervals for at least 4 hours. When chilliness subsides, a warm tub bath may be taken. Generous amounts of fluid dilute the urine and thereby lessen irritation to the mucous membrane linings of the urinary tract.

Sharp abdominal pain should be reported to the physician, and analgesics should be withheld until the patient has been examined. Bladder or ureteral perforation may have occurred during the procedure, resulting in peritonitis. Pronounced chills with marked elevation of temperature sometimes follow cystoscopic examination. This is believed to result from a general systemic reaction to the foreign substances introduced, the instrumentation, and the pain. Usually these symptoms respond within a short time to extra warmth and to warm fluids by mouth. If these symptoms persist, the physician should be notified.

Renal biopsy. Renal biopsy is potentially the most accurate diagnostic test for determining both the type and the stage of progression of renal pathologic conditions. Specifically, this test aids in differentiating diagnoses, in following the progression of disease, in choosing therapy most beneficial to the patient, and in determining prognosis of the illness.

Inherent in biopsy of this vascular tissue is a potential threat of hemorrhage. Throughout the procedure, medical and nursing care is given to prevent and to detect early any loss of blood. Before biopsy is performed, the patient should have a thorough medical evaluation with particular attention being given to detection of any abnormality in bleeding or coagulation time. The patient's blood should be typed and cross matched with 2 units of blood; this should be held for the patient until any threat of bleeding has passed.

Preparation of the patient prior to biopsy also includes discussing the procedure with him, covering the necessity for the examination, the procedure itself, and care to be anticipated and identifying his concerns. The preparation of the patient is shared by the physician and the nurse. In most institutions it is necessary to have the patient sign a special permit prior to having the biopsy performed. The biopsy is carried out in the patient's room, in the x-ray department, or in the operating room.

The procedure for the biopsy is as follows: Prior to biopsy, the patient is taken to the x-ray department for localization of the kidney. This is accomplished with a plain film, a dye contrast film, or fluoroscopic location. The position of the kidney in relation to body landmarks is marked on the patient's skin in ink. The lower pole of the kidney is located, this being the site for biopsy since it contains the fewest number of large vessels. The patient is then transported to the area where the biopsy will be performed. Sedation is usually not required except for children or adults who are restless and unable to relax sufficiently to follow necessary instructions during the test. The patient is placed prone over a sandbag or firm pillow and an additional soft pillow. The body should be bent at the level of the diaphragm, with the shoulders on the bed and the spine in straight alignment. Blood pressure and pulse rate are determined at this point and are recorded. Preparation of the skin is carried out to remove as many surface contaminants as possible. The physician identifies the location for biopsy, and a local anesthetic agent is injected. As the biopsy is being taken, the patient is instructed to hold his breath. Pain may be felt in the kidney region as the tissue sample is taken. The needle is withdrawn immediately, and pressure is applied to the site for 20 minutes. A pressure bandage is then applied, and the patient is turned onto his back; he is kept flat (one small pillow may be used under the head) and motionless for the next 4 hours. Coughing and any activity that increases abdominal venous pressure is to be avoided during this time. Blood pressure and pulse should be taken each 15 minutes for 1 hour, every 30 minutes during the next hour, and every hour for an additional 2 to 3 hours. The patient should remain in bed for at least 24 hours. All urine is observed for hematuria, and bed rest is maintained until the urine is clear. Initially the patient's urine is likely to demonstrate blood, but this rarely continues after a 24-hour period. Once out of bed, the patient should be cautioned against any heavy lifting for a period of 10 days.

Diseases of the urinary system

One of the primary responsibilities of the nurse is to prevent disruption of the urinary system. Thus prevention may take the form of public education in personal hygiene and health, early detection of urinary diseases, encouragement of prompt and adequate medical treatment of systemic or upper respiratory diseases that may lead to urinary diseases, and sterile nontraumatic technique in catheterization procedures.

Diseases of the urinary system may be classified for convenience and understanding into three major categories, which are not necessarily mutually exclusive: (1) obstructive diseases, including calculi, benign prostatic hypertrophy, and neoplasms; (2) congenital malformations and trauma; and (3) diseases of the kidney, including glomerulonephritis, pyelonephritis, and autoimmune diseases. Diseases in each of these categories may be progressive and lead to renal failure, may be static and compatible with life, or may be controlled by medical or surgical intervention.

■ OBSTRUCTION OF THE URINARY SYSTEM

Obstruction of any part of the urinary system from the kidney to the urethra will generate pressure, which may cause functional and anatomic damage to the renal parenchyma. Partial obstruction may produce slow dilation of structures above the obstruction without functional impairment. As the obstruction increases, pressure builds up in the tubal system above the obstruction, eventually causing a reflux of urine as the bladder contracts to empty. With obstruction, urine flow is decreased even to the point of stagnation. This stagnant urine provides a good culture medium for bacterial growth, and rarely is obstruction seen without some infection. Obstruction may occur at the tubule level (in the form of casts or inflammation), in the pelvis (from calculi or polycystic disease), at the ureters (from trauma, calculi, or lymphomas), in the bladder (from neoplasms or diverticuli), at the urethra (from benign prostatic hypertrophy or calculi), and at the meatus (from stricture). No matter what has caused the obstruction, the symptoms are usually the same and stem from the pressure and urine backup, which lead to hydronephrosis, renal damage, and eventual renal failure.

Hydronephrosis

Obstruction of the upper urinary tract eventually causes hydronephrosis, or dilatation of the renal pelvis. Common symptoms of hydronephrosis are pain, nausea, vomiting, local tenderness, spasm of the abdominal muscles, and a mass in the kidney region. The patient may, however, have no symptoms. The pain is caused by the stretching of tissues and by hyperperistalsis. Since the amount of pain is proportionate to the rate of stretching, a slowly developing hydronephrosis may cause only a dull flank pain, whereas a sudden blockage of the ureter, such as may occur from a stone, causes a severe stabbing (colicky) pain in the flank or abdomen. The pain may radiate to the genitalia and thigh and is caused by the increased peristaltic action of the smooth muscle of the ureter in an effort to dislodge the obstruction and force urine past it. Narcotics such as morphine and meperidine and antispasmodic drugs such as propantheline bromide (Pro-Banthine) and belladonna preparations are usually used to relieve severe colicky pain.

The nausea and vomiting frequently associated with acute ureteral obstruction are caused by a reflex reaction to the pain and will usually be relieved as soon as pain is relieved. A markedly dilated kidney, however, may press on the stomach, causing continued gastrointestinal symptoms. If the renal function has been seriously impaired, nausea and vomiting may be symptoms of impending uremia. (See p. 462 for discussion of uremia and renal failure.)

When the upper urinary tract becomes infected, symptoms of pyelonephritis appear. If the infected kidney is completely obstructed, no pus or bacteria may be found in the bladder urine.

When obstruction occurs, the treatment consists of reestablishing adequate drainage from the urinary system. This may be temporarily accomplished by placing a catheter above the point of obstruction. Sometimes surgery must be performed to insert a catheter (for example, nephrostomy). Later, definitive treatment is dependent on the cause. The infection is treated with antibiotics, chemotherapy, fluids, and rest. Urinary antiseptics may also be given.

The patient is frequently acutely ill, but if he has severe colic, he may not be able to remain in bed until the pain has been relieved. It is not unusual to see a patient with acute renal colic walking the floor, "doubled-up" and vomiting. After narcotics have been given, such a patient must be protected from injury due to dizziness. As the pain eases, the patient can usually be made relatively comfortable in bed. As soon as the nausea subsides, large amounts of fluids should be urged.

Ureteral constriction and obstruction

Hydronephrosis may be caused by constriction of the ureteral lumen. The constriction may be due to trauma, to an enlarged lymph node (as in lymphosarcoma, reticulum cell sarcoma, or Hodgkin's disease) impinging on the ureter, to nephroptosis, or to a congenital anomaly. Symptoms may not appear for years. The constriction, however, finally increases and causes an acute obstruction. In a child or adult with undiagnosed recurrent attacks of acute pyelonephritis, the possibility of a congenital lesion is always considered.

A plastic repair of the ureter may be done to relieve ureteral strictures. In cases of chronic constriction where continuous artificial drainage is necessary, a segment of the ureter may be replaced by a segment of ileum. A flank or suprapubic incision is made, depending on the location of the stricture. If a ureteropelvic stricture has been repaired, the patient usually will return from the operating room with a nephrostomy tube in place and a splinting catheter in the ureter (Fig. 20-6), which prevents a new stricture from forming as the ureter heals. Some urologists do not use catheters because they believe they cause irritation and predispose to new strictures. The patient will require the routine care given anyone having renal surgery plus the special considerations mentioned here.

The splinting catheter is usually a small catheter that extends into the ureter to a point below the anastomosis. It is brought out through the wound beside the nephrostomy tube. No drainage should come through this catheter. If it does, it is likely that the nephrostomy tube is partially blocked or that the splinting catheter has slipped into the renal pelvis. The splinting catheter is incorporated into the dressing, not attached to drainage, and it usually is not removed until 2 or 3 weeks postoperatively.

The nephrostomy tube may be left in place for several months. Many patients go home with it and

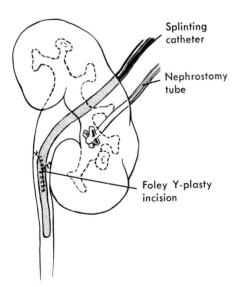

FIG. 20-6. Placement of a splinting catheter after repair of a ureteropelvic stricture. Note the use of a nephrostomy tube for drainage of urine during healing of the anastomosis.

Splinting catheter

Nephrostomy tube

Foley Y-plasty incision

return later for its removal. Before it is removed, evidence of ureteral patency is desirable. The evidence may be obtained by several methods. The patient may be taken to the x-ray department and radiopaque dye run by gravity into the nephrostomy tube. If the ureter is patent, the dye will pass through it into the bladder, and the radiographs will give evidence of the size of the lumen.

A *burette test* may be ordered to test the patency of the ureter. In this test the nephrostomy tube is attached to a calibrated burette, placed so that the center is at kidney level, and filled with a solution of methylene blue dye to a level equal to renal pressure. This procedure is done by the physician. The patient remains flat in bed during this test, which may last from 4 to 24 hours. A burette reading is taken every hour. Notation should be made of the activity of the patient at the time of the reading, since any activity that causes increased intra-abdominal pressure, such as turning, coughing, and straining, will give an elevated reading. If the ureter is patent and the patient is quiet, the reading will not fluctuate from the original reading by more than 2.5 to 5 cm. (1 to 2 inches). If the ureter is still obstructed, the urine will become stagnant in the renal pelvis, causing increased pressure. The burette readings will progressively increase, and the urine will be forced out through the top of the burette. If pressure increases, the test should be immediately discontinued and the nephrostomy tube reattached to straight drainage equipment. Otherwise infection is likely to occur. Before the nephrostomy tube is finally removed, it is usually clamped for a day or two. If fever or back pain occurs, the catheter will be reattached to drainage apparatus.

If the stricture is at the ureterovesical juncture, the surgery is done through a suprapubic incision. The ureter is partially resected as it enters the bladder and then reimplanted into the bladder a short distance from the original site. The splinting catheter may then be brought out through the urethra or through the ureterostomy onto the abdominal wall. This catheter is used for drainage and as a splint. The patient may or may not have a cystostomy incision with urinary drainage through a cystostomy tube.

If the strictures are bilateral, as often occurs in patients with congenital lesions, bilateral nephrostomies are performed, and later the ureters are resected and replaced by a graft such as a piece of ileum or are partially resected and reimplanted into the bladder.

Occlusion of the ureters by trauma may be treated in a similar manner. If the trauma has caused a constriction, nephrostomy tubes may be used to promote drainage and allow time for healing. If healing does not occur, the section of affected ureters may be resected and/or replaced by a graft. If the obstruction is caused by a lymphoma, surgical removal of the lymph tissue is attempted in the early stages of the disease. Radiation and chemotherapy are used to shrink the tissue. During this therapy and during the terminal stage of the disease, nephrostomy tubes may be used to promote urinary drainage, which would add to the patient's comfort and help to prevent renal failure.

Nephroptosis

Since the kidneys are not anchored in place by ligaments but are kept in normal position by blood vessels, the fatty pads surrounding them, and the pressure of the abdominal organs, they may drop slightly under certain circumstances, such as when a patient has lost a considerable amount of weight. This is known as nephroptosis, commonly called "dropped kidney" or "floating kidney" by the layman. The right kidney, which normally is lower than the left, is most frequently affected. The liver, a very large organ, lies directly above the right kidney.

Nephroptosis rarely causes severe symptoms. The patient may have a "dragging ache" in the flank that is usually relieved by bed rest. Occasionally the doctor suggests that the patient sleep in the Trendelenburg position. He may elevate his bed at home by placing 6-inch blocks under the foot of the bed. If higher elevation is desired, the footboard can be placed on the seat of a sturdy straight chair. A *kidney belt* may be ordered to help keep the kidneys in normal position. It should be applied before arising in the morning and fastened from the bottom up. A high-calorie diet may be ordered if the condition follows weight loss, because additional weight helps to restore the fatty pads around the kidneys.

Conservative treatment is usually effective, but rarely the kidney drops enough to cause the ureter to become kinked, impairing the flow of urine. In such cases, *nephropexy* is done. In this procedure the kidney is sutured to the adjacent structures in order to straighten the ureter and provide adequate drainage of the renal pelvis. The nursing care is similar to that given any patient undergoing surgery of the kidney.

Renal calculi

Renal calculi can develop at any age. Although the cause is not completely understood, it is known that the problem is essentially one of crystallization around a microprotein matrix, which may be pus, blood, devitalized tissue, crystals, tumors, or a foreign body such as a catheter. Stasis of urine is known to predispose to formation of some stones (phosphatic), especially if there is associated infection that makes the urine markedly alkaline.

Patients with fractures or other bedridden patients who cannot move about freely are prone to develop renal calculi. This probably is due to the excessive amount of calcium released from the bones in patients who remain in bed without normal activity and to stasis of urine in the lower calices of the kidneys when the erect posture is not assumed. To prevent the formation of renal calculi, patients usually are mobilized early or at least turned from side to side in bed every 1 to 2 hours. If a patient cannot walk, the physician may order him placed in a wheelchair or, if necessary, on a tilt table (board) twice a day for an hour or two or in a CircOlectric bed. If his legs are immobilized, he should be encouraged to exercise his arms. Using a trapeze also helps to prevent formation of renal calculi.

Hyperparathyroidism and gout are metabolic diseases that result in hyperexcretion of calcium and uric acid, respectively. These substances are excreted through the kidneys and may form stones.

Because recurrence of renal calculi is common, not only must the immediate problem be treated, but the reason for stone formation must also be discovered, if possible, and treated. Therefore intensive diagnostic studies may be done after the removal of stones.

The patient usually seeks medical care because of symptoms of obstruction and/or infection. He may have gross hematuria due to trauma from the jagged stone; although hematuria from stones is more often microscopic. Sometimes he complains of frequency and urgency—symptoms of cystitis. The bladder infection is probably a direct extension of an infection behind the stone. Any or all of these symptoms may occur. Often a stone is "silent," causing no symptoms for years. This is true especially of large renal stones.

Diagnostic procedures. The diagnosis of calculi is made from the history and by intravenous pyelography. Sometimes a cystoscopic examination is done, and a ureteral catheter with wax applied to the tip may be passed. This procedure is done if there is any suspicion that the defect in the ureter is a tumor rather than a stone. A stone may scratch the wax.

If it is impossible to pass a catheter beyond the stone so that a retrograde pyelogram is necessary, a perforated bulb tip may be placed on the ureteral catheter to block the ureter, and the pressure thus created forces some of the dye beyond the stone. This procedure is known as *Woodruff pyelography*.

Stones are usually sent for laboratory study to determine their composition. The results serve as a guide in further search for the cause and in determining suitable prophylactic treatment.

Urine specimens from a 24-hour period may be analyzed for their chemical content. Tests to determine blood uric acid levels are done if gout is suspected. Tests for calcium and phosphorus blood levels and the *Sulkowitch test* to determine the calcium content of the urine (a single urine specimen) may be ordered if hyperparathyroidism is suspected.

A parathyroid screening test may be done. Infections and obstructive lesions are sought (p. 435).

Management. Renal calculi may pass out through the urethra spontaneously. All patients with relatively small stones, therefore, should have the urine strained. Urine can be strained easily by placing two opened 4 by 8 inch gauze sponges over a funnel. The urine from each voiding should be strained, and one needs to watch closely for the stone because it may be no bigger than the head of a pin, and the patient may not realize it has passed. Stones larger than 0.5 cm. in diameter are rarely passed.

If there is no infection and if there is not a complete obstruction, the stone may be left in the ureter for several weeks. The patient is usually allowed to continue work, and the stone is closely observed by x-ray examination. A person who is up and about is more likely to pass a stone than is a person who is in bed. Therefore the patient should be urged to move about actively. Fluids should be taken freely to promote urine formation, which will possibly aid in the passage of a stone, and to prevent infection.

Patients frequently have two or three attacks of acute pain (renal colic) before the stone passes. This is probably because the stone gets lodged at a narrow point in the ureter, causing temporary obstruction. The ureters are normally narrower at the ureteropelvic and ureterovesical junctions and at the point where they pass over the iliac crest into the pelvis. If the stone is to pass along the ureter by peristaltic action, the patient must expect some pain. He should determine his tolerance to pain and anticipate when he needs medication to prevent colic. Drugs used include morphine sulfate and meperidine hydrochloride (Demerol) for direct pain and atropine, methantheline bromide (Banthine), and propantheline bromide (pro-Banthine) to depress the smooth muscles of the ureter and lessen pain from spasm.

If the stone fails to pass, one or two ureteral catheters may be passed through a cystoscope up the ureter and left in place for 24 hours. The catheters dilate the ureter, and when they are removed, the stone may pass into the bladder.

If the patient shows signs of infection, an attempt is made to pass a ureteral catheter past the stone into the renal pelvis. If such an attempt is successful, the catheter is left as a drain, since pyelonephritis will quickly follow if adequate urinary drainage is not reestablished.

The very small ureteral catheters may be most effectively attached to drainage equipment without encroaching on the catheter lumen by punching a small hole in the rubber top of a medicine dropper and threading the catheter through it. To make the hole, use a large, red-hot needle or pin. Hot metal permanently perforates rubber. The medicine dropper top is then attached to the glass connector of the drainage tubing. If there is a catheter in each ureter,

consult the physician to determine which is right and which is left. Label the catheters with adhesive tape. Check ureteral catheters frequently to see that they are draining. If the urine is purulent, the catheters may become obstructed. If there is no order for irrigation or if patency cannot be reestablished by irrigation the physician should be notified at once. Patients with ureteral catheters should be kept in bed and in a low Fowler's position to prevent pull on the catheters and their possible dislodgment.

If the stone has passed to the lower third of the ureter, it can sometimes be removed by *manipulation.* Special catheters with corkscrew tips, expanding baskets, and loops are passed through the cystoscope, and an attempt is made to "snare" the stone. This procedure is done under anesthesia, and the patient knows that if the manipulation is unsuccessful, he may have surgery immediately. The aftercare of a patient on whom manipulation has been carried out is the same as that following cystoscopy. Any signs suggestive of peritonitis or a decreased urinary output should be carefully watched for, since the ureter occasionally is perforated during manipulation.

The operation for removal of a stone from the ureter is a *ureterolithotomy.* A radiograph is taken immediately preceding surgery, since the stone may have moved, and it is desirable to make the incision

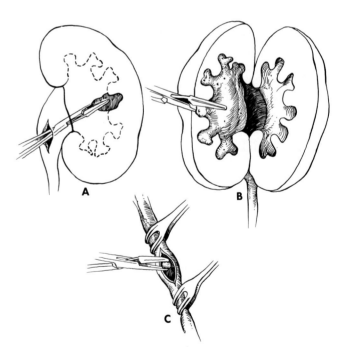

FIG. 20-7. Location and methods of removing renal calculi from the upper urinary tract. **A,** Pyelolithotomy, the removal of stone through the renal pelvis. **B,** Nephrolithotomy, the removal of a staghorn calculus from the renal parenchyma (kidney split). **C,** Ureterolithotomy, the removal of stone from the ureter.

into the ureter directly over the stone. If the stone is in the lower third of the ureter, a rectus incision is made. If it is in the upper two-thirds, a flank approach is used. If the patient has a ureteral stricture that causes stones to form, a plastic operation to relieve the stricture may be done as part of the operation.

Removal of a stone through or from the renal pelvis is known as a *pyelolithotomy.* Removal of a stone through the parenchyma is a *nephrolithotomy.* (See Fig. 20-7.) Occasionally the kidney may have to be split from end to end (a kidney split) to remove the stone. Patients in whom such a split is done may have severe hemorrhage following surgery.

Ureteral surgery. The patient who has had a ureterolithotomy through a rectus incision needs the routine postoperative care given any patient who has had abdominal surgery. The incision, however, will drain large amounts of urine for 2 or 3 weeks postoperatively because the ureter usually is not closed with sutures for fear that closure will cause strictures to form. A tissue drain is placed proximal to the ureteral incision and may be left in place for a week or more. (For special nursing measures that should be used to care for the draining urinary fistula, see p. 444.) Occasionally a ureteral catheter will be left in place for several days.

If the ureter has been approached through a flank incision, nursing care includes the general care given any patient with renal surgery and care of the urinary fistula.

Flank (kidney) incision. Whenever there has been a flank incision, there are special nursing responsibilities. Because the incision is directly below the diaphragm, deep breathing is painful and the patient is reluctant to take deep breaths or to move about. He tends to splint his chest and therefore is likely to develop atelectasis or other respiratory complications. He needs adequate medication for pain. Usually he will need a narcotic every 3 to 4 hours for 24 to 48 hours after surgery. After this time, medication may be slowly tapered off. After the patient has been given enough medication to relieve pain and mechanical support has been given to the incision, he should be encouraged to expand the rib cage fully and to cough at least every 2 hours. He should turn from side to side while he is in bed, and he should be encouraged to get up as soon as permitted. Most patients will be more comfortable turning themselves. After renal surgery the patient can turn to either side unless he has a nephrostomy tube inserted. Even then, he can be tilted to the affected side with pillows placed at his back for support. It must be ascertained that the tube is not kinked and that there is no traction on it.

Following surgery on the kidney, most patients have some abdominal distention, which may be due in part to pressure on the stomach and intestinal tract during surgery. Patients who have had renal colic prior to surgery frequently develop paralytic ileus postoperatively. This condition may be related to the reflex gastrointestinal symptoms caused by the pain. Because of the problem of abdominal distention following renal surgery, the patient is often given no food or fluids by mouth for 24 to 48 hours postoperatively. A nasogastric tube may be passed prophylactically. Fluids by mouth should be started slowly, and the nurse should watch for signs of distention. It is preferable to give warm fluids. Iced fluids, citrus fruit juice, and milk tend to cause flatus and gastric distress in some patients. By the fourth postoperative day most patients tolerate a regular diet. Fluids are usually forced to 3,000 ml./day, and the surgeon may believe it desirable for the patient to continue to take this amount of fluids throughout his life.

If distention occurs, a rectal tube and heating pad may be ordered. Neostigmine (Prostigmin) and carminative enemas may also be ordered. If neostigmine is given, a rectal tube usually is inserted for 20 minutes after its administration. In addition, the patient should be helped to turn frequently, since turning encourages the gas to pass along the bowel.

Hemorrhage may complicate renal surgery. It occurs more often when the highly vascular parenchyma of the kidney has been incised. (See p. 459 for a discussion of hemorrhage in urologic surgery.) The bleeding may occur on the day of surgery, or it may occur 8 to 12 days postoperatively, during the period when tissue sloughing normally occurs in healing. Because of the possibility of hemorrhage, some surgeons put the patient who has had extensive surgery of the parenchyma back to bed for 3 or 4 days after the eighth postoperative day. The nurse should observe the patient closely during this period for any signs of hemorrhage.

Following renal surgery, the patient frequently will have a nephrostomy or a pyelostomy tube inserted. He may have a moderate amount of urinary drainage on his dressing, but if the catheter drains adequately, this diminishes steadily.

Prophylaxis and home care. Since urinary calculi are likely to recur or to develop following surgery on the kidney, patients should understand the importance of following prescribed prophylactic measures. A patient who has had any renal pathologic condition should drink fluids freely for the remainder of his life providing that his kidneys are able to excrete this extra fluid. It is unwise for him to consume large amounts of high-calcium foods, although adequate nutrition should be maintained. Because toxins from infections are eliminated through the kidneys, and because infections may localize in the urinary tract and produce an alkalinity of the urine, he should avoid upper respiratory infections and any other infections. If he develops an infection, he should force fluids, take extra rest, and seek medical attention at the first sign of complications. He should return to his physician for examination as recommended.

Special medications and diets designated to eliminate conditions conducive to the formation of stones may be prescribed. Phosphatic calculi comprise about 21% of all calculi and develop in *alkaline* urine.[32] Their prevention depends on keeping the urine acid and preventing infection. Enteric coated ammonium chloride is often used to assure acidity of the urine.

The Shorr regimen has given beneficial results in the prevention of phosphatic calculi. A diet containing only 1,300 mg. of phosphorus daily is prescribed, and 40 ml. of aluminum hydroxide gel is taken after meals and at bedtime. The aluminum combines with the excess phosphorus, causing it to be excreted through the bowel instead of through the kidney, thus decreasing the possibility of stone formation. Patients who must have a catheter in use for long periods of time may be placed on this regimen prophylactically.

Aluminum hydroxide gel tends to constipate some persons. Usually this tendency can be counteracted by drinking a glass of prune juice or by eating a dish of prunes each morning. Additional fruits and vegetables may be recommended, but these foods produce an alkaline ash and, in quantities, may defeat the purpose of an acid ash diet (see Table 20-1). If necessary, a mild cathartic such as psyllium seed (Metamucil) may be prescribed. Patients should be advised not to take mineral oil routinely, because it may decrease absorption of the fat-soluble vitamins A, D, E, and K. Since a patient usually discontinues the regimen because of constipation, the nurse should anticipate this and tell him that bowel regularity can often be maintained by drinking plenty of fluids, by eating some fresh fruits and vegetables that will add bulk to the diet, and by defecating at a regular time each day.

Table 20-1 Acid and alkaline ash food groups*

Acid ash	Alkaline ash	Neutral
Meat	Milk	Sugars
Whole grains	Vegetables	Fats
Egg	Fruit (except cran-	Beverages (cof-
Cheese	berries, prunes,	fee and tea)
Cranberries	and plums)	
Prunes		
Plums		

*From Williams, S. R.: Nutrition and diet therapy, ed. 2, St. Louis, 1973, The C. V. Mosby Co.

Calcium oxalate crystallization accounts for over 50% of all urinary tract calculi.[32] These calculi occur in *acid* urine and in the absence of infection, obstruction, or hyperparathyroidism. Attempts are made to prevent recurrences by prescribing a diet high in phosphorus. Sodium or potassium phosphate, to be taken by mouth in dosages of 1 to 3 Gm. daily, may also be prescribed.

Sometimes stones are found to contain both oxalates and phosphates. The diet and drug therapy prescribed for these patients is highly individualized.

A small percentage of urinary tract calculi are composed of uric acid or cystine. Uric acid crystals may form in patients with gout or hyperuricemia (as occurs in the treatment of carcinomas when there is increased tissue breakdown). The diet often prescribed includes cereals, fruits, and most green vegetables. Meats high in purines (such as sweetbreads, liver, kidney, pork, and beefsteak) are to be avoided. Drugs frequently used include allopurinol (Zyloprim) and probenecid (Benemid). The physician may order an acid ash or alkaline ash diet, depending on the type of stones present in the urine.

Cysts and tumors of the kidney

Masses in the kidney may represent cysts or tumors. Either may eventually result in obstruction.

A *solitary cyst of the kidney* can usually be differentiated from a tumor by intravenous or retrograde pyelography. The solitary cyst may be aspirated with a needle because it often occurs in the renal cortex. However, it usually is explored surgically because it occasionally contains malignant cells. Fluid from a cyst is usually sent for cytologic examination. If there is no evidence of carcinoma, the renal capsule covering the cyst is removed (*decapsulation*).

Polycystic disease is a familial disease characterized by multiple cysts of both kidneys. The cysts press on the parenchyma and cause death from renal failure. There is no specific treatment, and the patient may die at a fairly early age. If the disease is diagnosed early and dietary control to prevent symptoms of uremia is instituted, the patient can be maintained for many years. As the disease progresses, however, or if it is initially quite severe, the patient may be admitted to a chronic dialysis program, often after removal of both diseased kidneys.

Tumors of the kidney are usually malignant. They grow insidiously, producing no symptoms for a long time, and finally the patient seeks medical care because of hematuria, dragging back pain, or weight loss. Unfortunately the hematuria is often intermittent, lessening the patient's concern and causing procrastination in seeking medical care. Any patient with hematuria should have a complete urologic examination, since it is only by immediate investigation of the first signs of hematuria that there is any hope of cure.

Wilms' tumor is an embryonal type of highly malignant growth occurring in children (usually under 7 years of age). It metastasizes early. A mass in the abdomen may be the first sign, and later, hematuria and anemia may occur. The treatment is nephrectomy and radiation treatment if there is no evidence of metastasis.

Tumors of the renal parenchyma, often called *hypernephromas,* are the most common tumors of the kidney. They rarely occur before the age of 30 years. A small tumor in the parenchyma may not be apparent in a routine pyelogram. Therefore special techniques that give pictures of sections of the kidney may be used. *Tomography, laminography, planigraphy, stratigraphy,* and *body section radiography* are plain radiographs of a section of the body taken with a rotating x-ray tube. No physical preparation of the patient is needed. A *nephrotomogram* is a tomogram taken after intravenous injection of a radiopaque dye. The patient is placed on an x-ray table, and a circulation time study (p. 327) is done to guide the timing of serial radiographs to be taken. A radiopaque dye such as sodium acetrizoate (Pyelokon R), with dehydrocholic acid (Decholin) added, is then given intravenously. The patient is instructed to indicate the moment that he tastes the dehydrocholic acid and the films are then taken. Physical preparation of the patient is the same as that for intravenous pyelography. He should be instructed to expect the same sensations when the dye is given, and he should be observed for the same drug reactions. Since the regulation of the time interval is dependent on the patient's cooperation, the nurse should explain the procedure carefully so that the patient will understand his role.

If a series of "metastatic" radiographs shows no signs of metastasis, and if there is good function of the unaffected kidney, the diseased kidney is removed. This operation is called a *nephrectomy* and may be done through a lumbar (flank), retroperitoneal, abdominal, thoracic, or thoracic abdominal approach.

The nursing care following nephrectomy is similar to that of any patient who has had renal surgery. The patient usually has less distention than patients who have had a nephrolithotomy or other operation performed on the kidney. There should be only a minimal amount of serosanguineous drainage on the dressing. Since the renal vessels, which are normally short, are often involved in the tumor mass, they may be difficult to ligate at operation. Therefore the patient should be carefully observed for signs of internal hemorrhage. If a suture should slip from a renal vessel, death from exsanguination may occur quickly. Blood is usually kept available for immediate emergency use, and the surgeon may request that an emergency hemostatic tray be kept at the bedside. The patient also should be observed closely

for symptoms of spontaneous pneumothorax (p. 582) since the pleura may be accidentally perforated during the operation. If the thoracic approach is used, a chest tube will be placed in the pleural space and connected to a water-seal drainage bottle. The nursing care will be similar to that for a patient having chest surgery (p. 586).

Following surgery for a malignant tumor that is radiosensitive, the patient is usually given a course of x-ray therapy. He will not necessarily be hospitalized during this time. Radiation also may be used over the metastatic sites as palliative treatment for the patient with an inoperable tumor.

Benign prostatic hypertrophy

Benign prostatic hypertrophy (prostatism), the cause of which is unknown, is a common urologic disease. The prostate is an encapsulated gland weighing about 25 grams. It encircles the male urethra directly below the bladder, and as it hypertrophies, it impinges on the bladder outlet.

More than half of all men over 50 years of age have some symptoms of prostatic enlargement. Although the patient's main complaint is inability to void, destruction of renal function is the most serious consequence of this disease. The patient first notices that the urinary stream is smaller and more difficult to start as the urethra becomes partially obstructed by the adenomatous growth. As time goes on he may develop frequency, urgency, and burning on urination. These are symptoms of cystitis, caused by prolonged incomplete emptying of the bladder. Stagnant urine is held in trabeculae or cellules formed by sagging of the atonic mucous membrane between overworked hypertrophied muscle bands in the bladder (Fig. 20-4). The patient complains of increasing frequency as the bladder fails to empty completely at each voiding and therefore refills more quickly to the amount that causes the urge to void (usually 250 to 500 ml.). Nocturia is used as a good index of frequency since it is not normal to awaken frequently to void.

The earlier treatment is instituted, the greater the likelihood of an uncomplicated course. Therefore, if any of the problems just mentioned come to the nurse's attention, an immediate urologic examination should be recommended in the hope that treatment can be given before renal damage occurs.

Management of the patient with acute retention. It is not uncommon for men with prostatic disease to be admitted to the hospital with acute retention of urine (inability to void). This condition occurs especially after drinking alcoholic beverages and after being exposed to cold. If the patient has acute retention, a urethral catheter will be inserted. When the residual urine is more than 1,000 to 1,500 ml., the catheter may be connected to a decompression drainage apparatus, since sudden emptying of an overdistended bladder may cause some of the problems described in the following discussion of decompression drainage.

Decompression drainage is an arrangement that encourages bladder muscles to maintain their tone since the urine must flow against gravity and the bladder does not empty completely. If the mechanical pressure caused by a markedly distended bladder is suddenly released from the large abdominal vessels and bladder mucosal capillaries, the patient may faint or develop hematuria. As blood rushes to fill the vessels, the blood supply to the brain is momentarily depleted, causing dizziness and faintness. The hematuria is caused by the rupture of some of the capillaries in the mucosa of the bladder.

The decompression may be high (5 to 8 inches above bladder level), medium (3 to 5 inches above bladder level), or low (at bladder level). A Y tube is attached to a standard at the desired level. The tubing from the catheter is connected to one arm of the Y, and the tubing to the drainage bottle is connected to another arm. The third arm of the Y tube is left open as an air outlet. Since changing the position of the bed, such as raising the bed to a high Fowler's position for meals, changes the bladder level of the patient, the Y tube must be adjusted accordingly.

The catheter will usually be attached to the high decompression drainage apparatus first and the level then lowered an inch at a time (usually every hour) until low decompression is reached. It may then be attached to straight drainage equipment.

Preoperative preparation. The treatment for prostatic enlargement is surgery. Some patients require catheter drainage prior to prostatic surgery. The results of the examinations with radiopaque media and of renal function tests are used to determine the need. If a catheter is inserted, it should be connected to drainage at all times since the purpose is to provide an empty bladder, which in turn provides for more complete emptying of the renal pelves. Some patients will have so much renal damage that a cystostomy tube is inserted, and they are sent home with the tube in place for several months until renal function can be restored to a satisfactory level and prostatic surgery can be performed. If no catheter is used, the patient should measure and record the time and amount of each voiding for 24 to 48 hours. Such a record gives a fairly accurate picture of the severity of his difficulties.

The usual diagnostic procedures are a blood urea nitrogen test or a blood nonprotein nitrogen test, intravenous pyelography (excretory urography), cystoscopy, and occasionally, urethrography. A fasting blood sugar determination is usually taken because diabetes mellitus is common in the age group affected by prostatic hypertrophy. An ECG and a radiograph of the chest also may be taken.

In caring for patients with prostatic disease, the nurse should apply principles of geriatric nursing. For example, elderly patients may need smaller doses of narcotics than younger ones, and sometimes no narcotic is given preoperatively. Elderly persons often have a low tolerance to sedatives, narcotics, and anesthetics and in some instances are less sensitive to pain.

Surgical treatment. In treating benign prostatic hypertrophy, the capsule of the prostate is left intact while the adenomatous soft tissue is removed by one of four surgical routes: transurethral, suprapubic, retropubic, or perineal.

A *transurethral resection of the prostate* is done when the major enlargement is in the medial lobe, directly surrounding the urethra. There must be a relatively small amount of hypertrophied tissue so that undue bleeding will not occur and so that the patient will not be under anesthesia for too long, because removal by this method is time consuming. The surgeon needs special training to use this technique.

A resectoscope (an instrument similar to a cystoscope but equipped with a cutting and cauterization loop attached to electric current) is passed through the urethra. The bladder is irrigated continuously during the procedure. The patient is grounded against electric shocks by a lubricated metal plate placed under his hips. Tiny pieces of tissue are cut away, and the bleeding points are sealed by cauterization (Fig. 20-8). A transurethral prostatectomy may be performed under general or spinal anesthesia.

Following a transurethral resection of the prostate, a large (24 Fr.) three-way Foley catheter with a 30 ml. inflation bag usually is inserted into the urethra. After the retention bag of the catheter has been inflated, the catheter is pulled down so that the

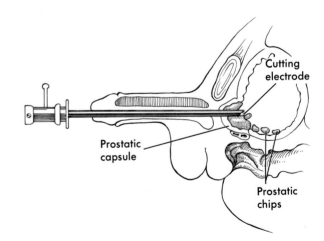

FIG. 20-8. Transurethral resection of the prostate by means of the resectoscope. Note the cutting and cauterizing loop of the instrument, the enlarged prostate surrounding the urethra, and the tiny pieces of prostatic tissue that have been cut away.

bag rests in the prostatic fossa and provides hemostasis. The bag puts pressure on the internal sphincter of the bladder, giving the patient a continual feeling of having to void. If the catheter is draining properly, this sensation usually passes momentarily. Trying to void around the catheter causes the bladder muscles to contract, causing a painful "bladder spasm."

The nurse should discuss the physiology of the "need to void" with the patient preoperatively. He will be less upset by the occurrence of spasms if he understands that they are expected. He can be told that the catheter is placed so that it gives the same sensation as a full bladder but that, because the bladder is empty and the urine is being continuously drained out by the catheter, he will have more pain if he tries to void around the catheter, causing the bladder mucosa to be irritated by the catheter. Drinking plenty of fluids helps since it ensures constant passage of fluid over the bladder mucosa, decreasing irritation. Narcotics should be given to the patient as ordered since they lessen the pain, although they do not decrease the contraction of the bladder muscle. Belladonna and opium suppositories are frequently prescribed to relieve bladder spasms and are usually quite effective. As the nerve endings become fatigued, the frequency and severity of the spasms will decrease. The length of time required for spasm to lessen varies. Most patients have less spasm by the end of 24 to 48 hours.

The bladder is constantly irrigated with normal saline solution or another solution prescribed by the surgeon. This is accomplished by attaching one opening of the Foley catheter to tubing connected to a bottle of irrigating solution hung on an intravenous pole. The other opening of the Foley catheter is attached to a collection receptacle. The purpose of constant irrigation is to keep the bladder free of clots. A full bladder tends to put pressure on the outside of the prostatic fossa, "milking" the bleeding vessels. For this reason the catheter must be kept open.

The patient should not strain to have a bowel movement because straining may cause prostatic hemorrhage. Stool softeners are usually prescribed and when necessary a laxative such as citrate of magnesia is given. Enemas are not given, and rectal tubes and rectal thermometers are not used for about a week postoperatively, since they may exert pressure on the resected prostatic capsule and may even cause perforation or hemorrhage. Hemorrhage is a potential complication for several days after surgery.

Persistent bladder discomfort, bladder spasm, or failure of a catheter to drain properly after transurethral prostatectomy usually signifies one of several serious complications, all of which require immediate medical attention. There may be excessive bleeding from the prostatic fossa with plugging of the catheter by clots. If the clots are not removed, they may cause overdistention of the bladder with the possibility of rupture of the bladder. The excessive bleeding can, of course, lead to shock. The catheter may be displaced, which will eventually lead to hemorrhage because of the pressure of the filling bladder "milking" bleeding vessels in the prostatic fossa. There may have been an unsuspected perforation of the bladder or prostatic capsule during surgery, and the drainage may be extravasating into local tissues or emptying into the peritoneal cavity, necessitating additional surgery. Complaints of abdominal or pelvic pain should be reported to the surgeon, and narcotics should be withheld until the patient has been examined.

Sometimes patients develop water intoxication, formerly known as TUR syndrome, as a result of too much irrigating solution being absorbed into the venous sinusoids during surgery. Cerebral edema may result, and the patient should be watched closely for confusion and agitation, which are the first signs of this condition.

Constant irrigation of the bladder is usually discontinued in 24 hours if there are no clots draining from the bladder. The catheter is then irrigated every 4 hours until it is removed.

The catheter may be removed from 4 to 7 days after a transurethral prostatectomy, depending on the extent of the resection. Following removal of the catheter, the patient should measure and record the time and amount of each voiding. The nurse should ascertain whether he has any incontinence. Since the external sphincter of the bladder lies directly below the prostate and the internal sphincter directly above it, damage to one or both sphincters occasionally is a complication of this type of surgery. The patient may not be able to void on removal of the catheter because of urethral edema. If he cannot void, the catheter may be reinserted for another day or two.

About 2 weeks after a transurethral prostatectomy, the patient may have a secondary hemorrhage as desiccated tissue is sloughed. He usually is at home by this time. Therefore he should be told before discharge to contact his surgeon at once if any bleeding occurs. Irrigation with silver nitrate solution (1:10,000) or reinsertion of a Foley catheter for a day or two usually controls the bleeding. Occasionally it is necessary to cauterize the bleeding points. Following irrigation with silver nitrate solution, the bladder is irrigated with normal saline solution to prevent burning of the mucosa by the silver nitrate.

The patient should not exercise vigorously or do any heavy lifting for about 3 weeks after discharge from the hospital. He is also usually advised not to drive a car. If he becomes constipated, a stool softener or mild cathartic may be ordered to obviate straining. Fluids should be taken freely for at least 3 weeks after discharge. After healing is complete, dilation of the urethra may be necessary because urethral mucosa in the prostatic area is destroyed by the operation, and strictures may have formed with healing.

A *suprapubic prostatectomy* is done if there is an extremely large mass of obstructing tissue. A low midline incision is made directly over the bladder, the bladder is opened, and, through an incision into the urethral mucosa, the adenomatous prostatic tissue is enucleated. (See Fig. 20-9.)

Following a suprapubic prostatectomy, various types of drainage and hemostatic measures may be used. There will be some type of hemostatic agent in the prostatic fossa (a hemostatic bag, Foley catheter, gauze packing, oxidized cellulose packing). Urine may be drained by a Foley type of catheter and a cystostomy tube, by only a Foley catheter with tissue drains into the cystostomy wound, or by only a cystostomy tube. If the latter is used, the prostatic fossa is packed or a hemostatic bag is used. Hemostatic bags may be inflated to contain 75 or 100 ml. of fluid and may be placed on traction to ensure constant steady pressure. Traction may be accomplished by placing a padded wire frame (known as a birdcage) between the patient's thighs and tying the catheter to it, or the catheter may be pulled taut and securely taped to the inner aspect of the thigh. Traction is used only for a few hours, and part of the fluid from the bag is removed after 4 to 6 hours to prevent damage to the sphincters of the bladder. Since so much pressure is placed on the internal sphincter, patients usually have severe bladder spasm and require narcotics for pain.

If gauze packing or a hemostatic bag has been used, it is usually removed in the operating room with the patient under anesthesia. Following its removal, a many-eyed Robinson catheter is usually inserted into the urethra to ensure drainage. Some urologists use no packing or catheters, or if they do use them, remove them within 24 to 72 hours. The bladder is sutured, and a Penrose drain is inserted through the abdominal incision. Some blood and serous fluid will drain through the incision for about 48 hours, and the dressing should be changed frequently (p. 459).

When a tissue drain is not used, there still may be a small amount of leakage around the cystostomy tube. If there is a large amount of drainage, the Foley catheter and cystostomy tube should be checked for blockage. The abdominal incision may take 2 to 4 weeks to heal completely. Cystostomy wounds easily become infected. *Bacillus pyocyaneus* often is the causative organism. Such infection can be recognized by the light bluish green drainage it causes. It is treated by irrigation and packing with an antiseptic solution. Infections with other organisms are treated with antibiotic drugs.

Hemorrhage is a possible complication following suprapubic prostatectomy. The precautions are the same as those taken following transurethral prostatectomy. Since there is usually some oozing of blood from the prostatic fossa, continuous bladder irrigations are usually ordered (as discussed on p. 443).

The cystostomy tube is usually removed 3 to 4 days postoperatively, but the urethral catheter may not be removed until the suprapubic wound is well healed. When the urethral catheter has been removed, the nursing care of the patient is the same as that for one who has had a transurethral resection of the prostate. The nurse should check to be sure

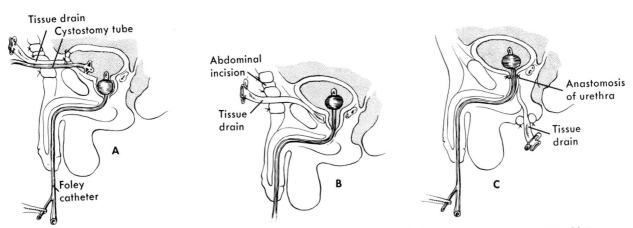

FIG. 20-9. Three methods of surgical removal of the prostate gland. **A,** Suprapubic prostatectomy. Note placement of the tissue drain, the cystostomy tube, and an inflated Foley catheter in the prostatic fossa. **B,** Retropubic prostatectomy. Note the intact bladder, the placement of tissue drain, and the retention catheter. **C,** Radical perineal prostatectomy. Note the placement of the tissue drain in the incision between the scrotum and the rectum and the anastomosis of the urethra made necessary by the excision of the prostate and its capsule.

that the suprapubic wound does not reopen and drain urine. If it does, a urethral catheter usually is reinserted. If oxidized cellulose gauze has been used, the urine may have a black discoloration caused by disintegration of the gauze.

The instructions for home care are the same as those after a transurethral operation except that the patient is less likely to have hemorrhage.

In a *retropubic prostatectomy* a low abdominal incision similar to that used for suprapubic prostatectomy is made, but the bladder is not opened. It is retracted, and the adenomatous prostatic tissue is removed through an incision into the anterior prostatic capsule (Fig. 20-9).

The sphincter muscles are seldom damaged by retropubic prostatectomy, and there is no urinary fistula. A large Foley catheter is inserted postoperatively, but bladder spasms are not usually very troublesome. On removal of the catheter the patient rarely has difficulty voiding. Hemorrhage from the prostatic fossa and wound infection may complicate the surgery. Therefore precautions to prevent bleeding similar to those discussed for transurethral prostatectomy should be taken. There should be no urinary drainage on the abdominal dressing. If urinary or purulent drainage, fever, or pain on walking occurs, the surgeon should be notified since such symptoms may be due to deep wound infection or pelvic abscess. Infection may appear after the patient has been discharged since he is usually hospitalized only a week. During his convalescence he should take the same precautions previously suggested for patients who have had other types of prostatectomy operations.

The adenomatous tissue of the prostate can also be enucleated through a perineal incision. This procedure is called *perineal prostatectomy.* The incision is made between the scrotum and the rectum. The posterior capsule of the prostate is incised, and all the adenomatous tissue is removed.

Preoperative and postoperative care following perineal prostatectomy is similar to that given a patient having radical perineal surgery (p. 533). The patient, however, will not be impotent, and he is no more likely to have urinary incontinence after a simple perineal prostatectomy than after any type of uncomplicated prostatectomy. Convalescent care is the same as for patients who have had other types of prostatectomies.

Bladder diverticula and bladder calculi

A diverticulum of the bladder is a large herniated sac of bladder mucosa that has sagged between the hypertrophied muscle fibers. Diverticula are usually seen in men and are often secondary to chronic prostatic obstruction. Since the diverticulum holds stagnant urine, infection often occurs, and calculi may form. Diverticula are excised surgically, and the bladder wall is repaired. The care is the same as that for a patient having a bladder resection.

Bladder stones may be removed through a suprapubic incision, or they may be crushed with a lithotrite (stone crusher) that is passed transurethrally. This procedure is known as a *litholapaxy.* Following bladder stone removal, the bladder may be irrigated (intermittently or constantly) with an acid solution such as magnesium and sodium citrate (G solution) or renacidin[26,111] to counteract the alkalinity caused by the infection and to help wash out the remaining particles of stone. If there has been a suprapubic incision, the care of the incision is similar to that following a suprapubic prostatectomy.

Tumors of the urinary bladder

Hematuria should always be investigated. Although it occurs in nonmalignant urinary tract diseases, painless hematuria is the first symptom in the majority of tumors of the bladder. It is usually intermittent, and patients may therefore fail to seek treatment. Cystitis (p. 449) may be the first symptom of a bladder tumor since the tumor may act as a foreign body in the bladder. Renal failure due to obstruction of the ureters sometimes is the reason the patient seeks medical care. Vesicovaginal fistulas may occur before other symptoms develop. The last two conditions indicate a poor prognosis because usually the tumor has infiltrated widely.

Management. Most bladder tumors start as *benign papillomas* or as *leukoplakia.* Although these conditions may be successfully treated by early fulguration, a new tumor may appear at any time. Any patient who has had a papilloma removed should have a cystoscopic examination every 3 months for 2 years and then at less frequent intervals if there is no evidence of a new lesion. Repeated cystoscopies may seem unacceptable to patients who dread them. The necessity for frequent examination should be fully explained by the urologist and the explanation reinforced by the nurse. Emphasis should be placed on the necessity for repeated cystoscopies, since papillomas tend to recur without symptoms until they are far-advanced tumors.

Carcinoma of the bladder occurs more frequently in men than in women (2.5 to 4 times as often). Multiple tumors are common, with about 25% of patients having more than one lesion at the time of diagnosis. This figure increases to about 50% in patients with papilloma, grade I carcinoma over a 5-year period. Approximately 40% of the tumors involve the trigone, and an additional 45% involve the posterior and lateral bladder walls. Known factors predisposing to bladder cancer are exposure to the chemicals beta-naphthylamine and xenylamine, infestation with *Schistoma haematobium,* and smoking.

Because gross hematuria is the presenting complaint in about 70% of patients with bladder neoplasm, it is imperative that all patients with hematuria seek immediate medical attention. This is especially so because microscopic hematuria may have been present for some time before the urine appeared bloody. Other symptoms may include urgency, frequency, and dysuria. The diagnosis is established by cystoscopic visualization of the bladder with biopsy. Clinical determination of the invasiveness of the tumor is important in establishing a therapeutic regimen and in predicting the prognosis, especially since some bladder tumors are more malignant than indicated by grading of the biopsy.

The treatment is dependent on the size of the lesion and the depth of the tissue involvement. Small tumors with minimal tissue layer involvement may be adequately treated with *transurethral fulguration* or excision. The patient may or may not have a Foley catheter inserted after surgery. The urine may be pink-tinged, but gross bleeding is unusual. Burning on urination may be relieved by forcing fluids and applying heat over the bladder region by means of a heating pad or a sitz bath. The patient is discharged within a few days after surgery.

If a cancerous lesion of the bladder is small and superficial, *radioisotopes* contained in a balloon of a Foley catheter may be inserted into the bladder. The catheter is attached to drainage, and all urine must be saved and sent to the radioisotope department for monitoring prior to disposal. Severe cystitis and proctitis usually result from this treatment, and the patient may be very uncomfortable for several days or weeks. Forcing fluids gives some relief from the symptoms, and urinary antiseptics and antispasmodic drugs are usually ordered. A low-residue diet and mineral oil may be ordered to keep the stools soft and lessen rectal discomfort.

Sometimes radioactive substances such as *radon seeds* are implanted around the base of a bladder tumor. This usually is done through a cystotomy but may also be done transurethrally through a cystoscope. If a cystotomy has been done, the patient may have a cystostomy tube inserted, but more often a urethral catheter will be used, and the cystotomy incision will be completely closed. (See p. 295 for precautions that should be taken when radiation treatment is used.) Radiation treatment usually causes a rather severe cystitis, which is treated by giving sedatives, antispasmodic drugs, fluids, and heat locally.

External radiation of tumors of the bladder with x-rays or cobalt teletherapy is used much more commonly now that improved equipment is available. Unless the urinary stream has been diverted prior to radiation, contraction of the bladder and serious cystitis often occur. If a urinary diversion procedure has been done, however, radiation of the bladder may decrease bleeding from the tumor and relieve pain.

Chemotherapy using purine antagonist drugs

such as 5-fluorouracil occasionally may be used to treat tumors of the bladder that have metastasized. The drugs may be given either orally or intravenously. (See p. 301 for dosages and for nursing care necessary when these drugs are given.)

Surgical procedures. If the tumor involves the dome of the bladder, a segmental resection of the bladder may be done. Over half of the bladder may be resected, and although the patient may have a capacity of no more than 60 ml. immediately postoperatively, the elastic tissue of the bladder will regenerate so that the patient is able to retain from 200 to 400 ml. or urine within several months.

The decreased size of the bladder, however, is of major importance in the postoperative period. The patient will return from surgery with catheters draining the bladder both from a cystostomy opening and from the urethra. This is to obviate the possibility of obstruction of drainage, since it would take only a very short time for the bladder to become distended and there would be danger of disrupting the suture line on the bladder. Because the bladder capacity is limited, the catheters usually cause severe bladder spasm. Usually the urethral catheter is not removed until 3 weeks postoperatively. Sometimes, if the cystostomy wound is not completely healed, the urethral catheter will have to be left in place longer.

As soon as the urethral catheter is removed, the patient becomes acutely aware of the small capacity of the bladder. He usually will need to void at least every 20 minutes. He needs to be reassured that the bladder capacity will gradually increase. Meanwhile, he should be urged to force fluids to 3,000 ml., but he should be advised to space the fluids so that time spent in the bathroom is not an inconvenience. He should thus take large quantities of fluids at one time, limit fluids for several hours before he plans to go out, and take no fluids after 6 P.M.

Cystectomy. A cystectomy, or complete removal of the bladder, usually is done only when the disease seems curable. Complete removal of the bladder requires permanent urinary diversion. This may be accomplished by various methods. The ureters may be transplanted into the intact bowel (*ureterointestinal anastomosis*). A sigmoidal colostomy may be performed to divert the fecal stream, and the ureters may then be transplanted into the lower bowel *(anal bladder)*. A section of the ileum may be resected with its blood supply and the remaining bowel segments anastomosed. One end of the resected ileum is sutured closed and the other end is brought to the skin as an ileostomy and the ureters are transplanted into it. This procedure, which is called an *ileobladder* or *ileal conduit,* is used most often at the present time (Fig. 20-10). The ureters may be brought directly onto the abdomen (ureterostomies), although this procedure is seldom done. A *colocysto-*

446

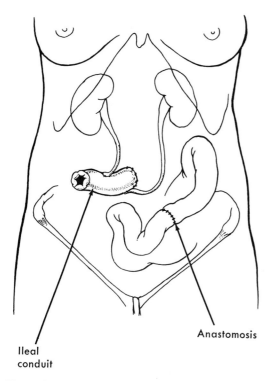

Ileal conduit

Anastomosis

FIG. 20-10. Ileal conduit or ileal bladder.

plasty has been used also. A portion of sigmoid is resected and fashioned into a bladder. The urethra and ureters are anastomosed to it in an anatomic position that is as nearly normal as possible. After healing, there is relatively normal physiologic bladder function. Whether or not this procedure is feasible depends partly on the extent of the cystectomy.

The patient whose ureters are transplanted into the normally functioning bowel is usually socially acceptable, but hydronephrosis and renal infection frequently occur. The kidneys may empty poorly because the rectum normally has a higher pressure than the bladder due to fecal contents and peristalsis. As the ureters and renal pelves dilate, bacterial organisms easily start an infection. The intestinal tract also has absorptive powers, and waste products in the urine may be reabsorbed, upsetting the electrolyte balance of the body. This has been found to be a serious disadvantage of anastomosis of the ureters to the bowel.

Recently, many urologists have come to feel that transplantation of the ureters into an ileobladder is the diversional procedure of choice since the patient seems able in most cases to cope with an ileostomy bag used for drainage, and the problem of reabsorption of substances from the urine through the segment of ileum does not seem to present serious problems.

Immediately after the cystectomy the patient is usually acutely ill. Since not only the bladder but also large amounts of surrounding tissue are re-

moved (the male patient also has a radical perineal prostatectomy), the patient may have a circulatory disturbance. This may be surgical shock, thrombosis, or cardiac decompensation. There is a long vertical or transverse abdominal incision, and there may be a perineal incision. The patient may be given nothing by mouth for several days, and a nasogastric tube may be inserted. The nursing care is the same as that given any patient after major abdominal surgery plus the routine care for a perineal wound and the care of the diverted urinary drainage.

Management of the patient with an ileal conduit. The most common method of urinary diversion is via the ileobladder. The nurse who encounters other, newer procedures should refer to recent periodicals.*

Preoperatively the patient who is to have an ileal conduit constructed is given a bowel preparation (usually cathartics, enemas, one of the sulfonamides such as sulfathalidine or neomycin, and a clear-liquid diet) for 3 days. If surgery is delayed for any reason, the surgeon should be consulted before continuing the regimen longer since vitamin B and K deficiencies may result, and sometimes fungous infections occur. Fluids, vitamins, and glucose may be given intravenously to supplement the diet.

Following an ileal conduit procedure, the patient usually returns from the operating room with a catheter inserted through the ileostomy opening to provide for urinary drainage. Since the ileum secretes mucus, the catheter usually needs to be irrigated gently every 2 to 4 hours. Sometimes no catheter is used, and an ileostomy bag (usually a plastic one) is secured over the opening to collect drainage. Regardless of what method is used, the nurse must watch carefully for, and report at once, any signs such as lower abdominal pain or decreased urinary output that indicate distention of the isolated segment of ileum with urine, since distention may cause the suture line to rupture, or it may cause back pressure on the kidneys. The collection bag should be emptied frequently so that it cannot contribute to back pressure and stop drainage. Special ileal conduit bags that can be attached to drainage apparatus are available, and they are preferable to a regular ileostomy bag. Swelling about the stoma may also prevent emptying of the conduit. Swelling about the uretero-ileal anastomoses or pressure of distended organs against the conduit may prevent drainage from the ureters.

Symptoms of peritonitis (fever, abdominal pain) should be watched for carefully and reported at once. After this type of surgery, the intestinal anastomosis may leak fecal material, or the ileal conduit may leak urine into the peritoneal cavity. If leakage occurs, an emergency operation is necessary to repair the weakened area.

*See references 10, 51, 81, and 106.

The patient usually has a nasogastric or intestinal tube inserted for several days after an ileal conduit procedure to prevent distention of the bowel with resultant pressure on the intestinal anastomosis. (Details of care relating to the intestinal anastomosis are discussed on p. 690.)

A temporary ileal conduit bag is used until the stoma has shrunk to its permanent size. The stoma should then be measured carefully, and a pattern of the exact size of the opening needed should be made. The cuff of the bag should exert no pressure on the stoma, and no skin surface should be exposed. Using the pattern, a surgical supply house will provide permanent bags. Usually at least two bags are ordered so that they can be cleaned and aired alternately.

Ileal conduit bags are applied by a method similar to that used for ileostomy bags (p. 680). Since the skin must be dry, it is easier to apply the bag when the patient has had nothing to drink for 3 or 4 hours. Placing a cotton ball over the ileal opening while the skin is prepared helps to prevent urine from draining onto it. Care of the skin and the equipment is the same as for the patient who has an ileostomy. Care should be taken that clothing does not constrict the bag. Depending on the placement of the ileostomy opening, it may be preferable for men to wear suspenders rather than a belt. Women should not wear garter belts since they tend to "ride" over the stoma. If a girdle is necessary, an opening should be cut in it over the bag.

A written procedure that includes a list of equipment and where to procure it, the steps of routine care, and management of problems that frequently are encountered is helpful for the patient learning to care for his own ileal conduit.[77]

The ileal conduit is placed in such a way that it should not act as a reservoir but only as a passageway from the ureters to the outside. Therefore patients with ileal conduits should have less difficulty with electrolyte imbalance than those in whom the bowel serves as a reservoir. Some problems do occur, however, and the patient should be advised to report signs of renal failure or electrolyte imbalance such as nausea, vomiting, diarrhea, or lethargy to the physician.

Management of patients with other types of urinary diversion. Patients who in the past have had other types of urinary diversional procedures may be admitted to the hospital or be seen in the home. Therefore the nurse must know how to cope with the problems presented by these patients.

After *ureterointestinal anastomosis,* the bowel adjusts to being a reservoir for urine. The stool will be soft, but the patient will be able to tell when he needs to void and when he needs to defecate. He will be able to retain about 200 ml. of urine. If the patient is incontinent or has symptoms of renal failure or electrolyte imbalance, a large rectal tube (28 Fr. attached to drainage) is left in the rectum. It often

is secured in the gluteal fold with a double-flap adhesive tape anchorage. Ethyl aminobenzoate ointment may be used to lubricate the tube because of its local anesthetic effect. The urinary output should be carefully measured and recorded. The tube must be removed for the patient to defecate and then reinserted.

Even if rectal tube drainage is not used during the day, patients with ureterointestinal anastomoses often are advised to insert a tube each night. When the tube is out, the patient should be urged to void every 4 hours to minimize the reabsorption of waste products and to improve emptying of the renal pelves. Any nausea, vomiting, diarrhea, or lethargy should be reported to the surgeon. These symptoms are suggestive of electrolyte imbalance, and alkalizing or acidifying drugs may be prescribed. The patient should not be given enemas, rectal suppositories such as bisacodyl, or strong cathartics such as castor oil or licorice powder because the increased peristalsis in the lower bowel may force contaminated urine up the ureters. Small doses of milk of magnesia may be ordered if a cathartic is necessary. The patient usually is encouraged to eat a regular diet and to drink approximately 3,000 ml. of fluid daily.

When an anal bladder has been constructed, urinary output is cared for in a manner similar to that used by patients with ureterointestinal anastomoses. Fecal discharge, however, is through a colostomy. (See p. 691 for care of the patient who has a colostomy.)

When the patient has cutaneous ureterostomies, the urine is drained either through ureterostomy cups or ureteral catheters inserted into the renal pelves. Catheters inserted into ureterostomies are cared for in a manner similar to that for any catheter draining the renal pelvis. *Ureterostomy cups* (Singer cups) are applied to the skin with skin paste or double-sided adhesive disks and may require changing only every 2 or 3 days. Patients are taught to care for these cups themselves, but the nurse should know the correct procedure to be able to assist them as necessary. Because few patients now use this method, it will not be described fully here.*

If the patient wearing a cup complains of back pain, the cup should be removed at once and the doctor notified unless, on removing it, the ureter drains. If it does, the drainage apparatus should be checked carefully for blockage before the cup is reapplied. Catheters may be necessary to provide drainage. Each time the cup is removed, the patient should take a warm bath. If this is not possible, the skin around the ureterostomy opening should be washed thoroughly and a warm compress placed over it for about 15 minutes. If the skin is irritated, a heat lamp

*For the details of the procedure see Winter, C. C., and Barker, M. R.: Sawyer's nursing care of patients with urologic disease, ed. 3, St. Louis, 1972, The C. V. Mosby Co.

(60-watt bulb placed 2 feet away from the abdomen) should be used for 20 minutes. The cup should be reapplied since the cement and the pressure exerted by the cup have healing properties. A ureteral catheter sometimes may have to be inserted until the skin heals. If the stoma swells, provision of an air outlet by inserting a no. 20 hypodermic needle with the hub uppermost into the tubing close to the cup may help. If the cup irritates the stoma, a plastic postoperative ileostomy appliance should be used until the swelling subsides (p. 680).

Inflammation and infection of the urinary bladder (cystitis)

Cystitis is an inflammation of the lining of the bladder. It is often secondary to infection or obstruction elsewhere in the urinary tract. As a primary condition, it is seen more frequently in women than in men and is usually associated with a nonspecific urethritis. It is sometimes caused by vaginal trauma and contamination of the urethra with organisms in the vagina and rectum. A urine culture, however, may yield no growth of organisms. Frequency, urgency, and severe burning on urination are the usual symptoms, but hematuria may occur.

Because cystitis may precede or accompany pyelonephritis, which is a serious disease, the person who has any signs of cystitis should seek medical care without delay. Treatment includes antibiotics, chemotherapy, and increased fluid intake. Hot sitz baths give relief, and tincture of hyoscyamus, an antispasmodic drug, and potassium citrate, a urinary alkalizer, may be prescribed. Irrigation of the bladder with a mild antiseptic solution such as potassium permanganate (1:8,000) or acetic acid (1:3,000) may be ordered, and is often followed by instilling a 5% solution of mild silver protein (Argyrol). Cystitis frequently becomes chronic and is then extremely difficult to cure. A wide variety of treatments may be tried. The urethra may be dilated to open the ducts of the periurethral glands and to allow them to drain. Dilation is followed by the instillation of an antiseptic solution such as silver nitrate 1:1,000 to 1:10,000. Adrenocortical steroids may be given systemically for their anti-inflammatory action. Partial cystectomy, irrigation, and even psychotherapy may be tried. Improvement of general health and the eradication of vaginal infection may help. Unless fluids are contraindicated by other disorders, the patient should drink 3 to 4 L. of fluid daily in order to dilute the urine and relieve the discomfort.

■ CONGENITAL MALFORMATIONS OF AND TRAUMA TO THE URINARY TRACT

Congenital malformations

Exstrophy of the bladder and epispadias (Fig. 20-11) are developmental anomalies that often occur together. They result from failure of the midline to

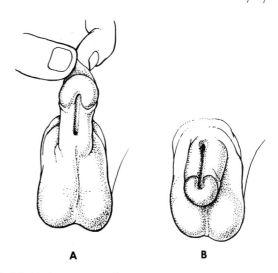

FIG. 20-11. A, Hypospadias. **B,** Epispadias.

close adequately during fetal development and may vary a great deal in their extent. *Exstrophy of the bladder* may consist of only a small fistula leading to the surface on the lower abdominal wall and draining urine, or it may be so extensive that most of the interior of the bladder is visible or is partially everted on the outer abdominal wall. Usually the sphincter muscles of the urethra are faulty, and other anomalies such as undescended testicles may be present. *Epispadias* is a failure of closure of the midline on the ventral surface of the penis and may extend from the glans to the perineum. Hypospadias is a defect of closure of the dorsal surface of the penis. It is almost always accompanied by *chordee,* a ventral curvature of the penis caused by abnormal fibrous tissue beneath the shaft of the penis distal to the urethral opening, and most easily noted when penile erection occurs. Both epispadias and hypospadias can usually be noted when the newborn infant is examined closely, even if the defect is only slight. Usually a defect that appears only minimal causes a urinary stream that is far from normal.

Operations for exstrophy of the bladder may include attempts to reconstruct the sphincter muscles of the urethra and to close the ectopic bladder opening. The surgery done depends on the degree of abnormality. Infection and bladder calculi are frequent if closure cannot be done and normal function cannot be restored soon after birth. Nephrostomies may be done prior to reconstructive surgery, and if satisfactory repair cannot be made, permanent diversion of urinary drainage may be necessary by means of a ureteroileostomy (ileal conduit) (Fig. 20-10) or other means.

The treatment for epispadias and hypospadias is surgical reconstruction of the urethra. Usually a cystostomy is done prior to surgery to ensure adequate urinary drainage. A problem postoperatively is incontinence, which may be treated with postoperative exercises. Treatment may consist of several operations in stages, so that hospitalization may be prolonged or have to be repeated. As growth occurs, scar tissue may fail to be absorbed sufficiently, and distortions may occur or interference with urinary flow may develop. For these reasons the doctor usually wishes to see the child at regular intervals for years. The nurse should impress on the child's family the importance of keeping medical appointments as advised and to report at once any difficulty the child may develop in voiding. (For further details in the care of the patient having surgical treatment for these conditions, see specialized nursing texts.[111])

Trauma

The urinary tract may be seriously damaged by external trauma. If the pelvis has been fractured, one should observe the patient for signs of a perforated bladder or urethra. There may be no urinary output, the urine may be bloody, or there may be symptoms of peritonitis. When the lower urinary tract is injured, provision must be made for urinary drainage at once. A cystostomy frequently is performed. Reparative surgery is undertaken when the patient's condition warrants it.

The kidney may be contused, torn, or completely ruptured by an external blow. Since spontaneous healing may occur, the patient is observed closely, and surgical intervention is usually necessary only if the kidney has been ruptured or if severe hemorrhage occurs.

■ DISEASES OF THE KIDNEY

Functions of the kidneys. The major functions of the kidneys include (1) controlling fluid balance, (2) regulating composition of electrolytes in the extracellular fluid, (3) excreting metabolic wastes, (4) assisting in regulating acid-base balance, (5) producing erythropoietin to stimulate red blood cell production, (6) assisting in regulating calcium-phosphorus balance, and (7) exerting influence on control of blood pressure.

Classification of renal disease

Reduction in urinary output can result from any factor that decreases blood supply to the kidneys, alters directly the structure and function of the kidneys, or obstructs the flow of urine in the urinary tract. The outline that follows lists specific pathologic states that illustrate each of these categories.

I Prerenal diseases
  A Hypovolemic states
    1 Hemorrhage
    2 Dehydration
  B Endotoxic shock
  C Cardiac failure
  D Vascular conditions

    1 Renal artery stenosis
    2 Thrombus or embolus
II Renal disease
  A Glomerular conditions
    1 Glomerulonephritis
    2 Hemolytic-uremic syndrome
    3 Lupus erythematosis
    4 Nephrotic syndrome
  B Vascular conditions
    1 Kimmelstiel-Wilson syndrome
    2 Nephrosclerosis
  C Tubular conditions
    1 Shock with hypovolemia
    2 Crush or trauma
    3 Transfusion reaction
    4 Analgesic intoxication
    5 Antibiotic drug toxicity
    6 Metal, carbon tetrachloride, or mushroom poisoning
  D Interstitial conditions
    1 Pyelonephritis
    2 Tuberculosis
    3 Tumor or cyst
III Postrenal disease
  A Tumor
  B Calculus
  C Other urinary tract stricture or stenosis

Prerenal disease. Prerenal disease includes any health problem that decreases the amount of blood delivered to the kidneys. Essentially, inadequate perfusion, not true damage to the kidney tissue, is the underlying problem. However, if not rapidly corrected, a decreased blood supply to the kidneys will lead to actual damage.

Renal disease. Usually renal disease alters the functioning ability of one of the major structural parts of the kidney: the glomeruli, the tubules, the vascular bed, or the interstitial tissue. If disease is persistent or severe in nature, all of the kidney structures may become affected, and the kidney becomes nonfunctional.

Disease that affects the glomeruli alters the filtration process in the capillary tufts. Large amounts of protein and red blood cells may be lost in the urine. Disease that affects the tubules destroys the ability of these structures to modify the fluid delivered to them from the glomeruli. Appropriate conservation of electrolytes and excretion of waste materials cannot be carried out. Vascular disease in the kidney leads to constriction or narrowing of the arterioles leading to the glomeruli and hence decreases the amount of blood supplied to these structures. Interstitial disease is generally cystic or infectious in nature. It destroys kidney tissue through pressure exerted on renal structures as cysts fill and scar tissue secondary to infection forms.

Postrenal disease. Reduction in urinary output also occurs as a result of obstruction in the urinary tract. If promptly removed, obstruction will not result in true renal damage. However, if it is untreated, increased back pressure of urine in the kidneys, stasis of urine, and infection result.

Common diseases of the kidney

Glomerulonephritis. Glomerulonephritis is a disease that affects the glomeruli of both kidneys. The disease may follow exposure to a variety of foreign protein substances, the most common of which are bacterial and viral infections. A common form of glomerulonephritis most frequently seen in children and young adults is acute poststreptococcal glomerulonephritis. It has received medical and public attention because it can be traced to a specific causative agent and can to some extent be prevented. This form of glomerulonephritis occurs after infection with group A *Streptococcus*. Commonly these infections include tonsillitis ("strep throat"), laryngitis, "colds," sinusitis, and scarlet fever. Glomerulonephritis appears to be the result of an antigen-antibody complex reacting with glomerular tissue to produce swelling and death of capillary cells.

The onset of illness in the patient may be either sudden or gradual. The patient may complain of any number of the following symptoms: shortness of breath, headache, blurred vision, oliguria, weakness, anorexia, and nausea and vomiting. Any of the following signs may be present: bloody urine, tachycardia, hypertension, puffiness about the face, generalized edema, and low-grade fever. Laboratory findings show evidence of nitrogen retention, proteinuria, casts in the urine, and increased antistreptolysin O titers in the serum.

Treatment consists of supportive care. The infection is promptly treated to help further decrease antigen-antibody complex formation. Penicillin treatment is begun when streptococcal organisms are identified and continued until negative cultures are obtained; this therapy may be continued prophylactically for months after the acute phase of illness. Potential foci for repeated streptococcal infections, such as diseased tonsils, may be removed after acute illness has subsided. Bed rest is essential until clinical signs disappear. The patient is allowed to begin progressive ambulation when blood sedimentation rates, blood urea nitrogen levels, and blood pressure become normal. If ambulation causes an increase in proteinuria or hematuria, bed rest is reinstituted. Since the period of bed rest may be long and the patient usually does not feel "ill," the nurse may need to continue to reinforce the importance of bed rest and assist the patient in planning constructive use of time. When bed rest is reinstituted after periods of ambulation, the patient may become depressed. Helping the patient to express his concerns and feelings can serve as a basis for helping him to plan realistically for his illness. Exposure to upper respiratory infections should be avoided since even mild infections may reactivate the disease. Dietary restrictions depend on the patient's signs and symptoms. When the blood urea nitrogen level is elevated and oliguria is present, protein intake is reduced. Sodium restriction depends on the severity of fluid retention. Fluids are ordered according to the kidneys' ability to excrete fluid. The nurse should be alert for signs of congestive failure, pulmonary edema, and cerebral edema, which may result from fluid overloading.

Acute glomerulonephritis is usually self-limiting and most patients recover completely within a few days to a year. Only about 5% of patients who develop acute glomerulonephritis die from the disease. Less than 25% of patients with acute glomerulonephritis develop chronic and latent forms of the disease. Little inference regarding prognosis for the patient can be made on the basis of the severity of an acute episode of glomerulonephritis. Patients with mild illness may develop chronic disease, and patients who are acutely ill may completely recover and have no further recurrence of the illness.

The term "subacute" (latent) glomerulonephritis refers to a state in which proteinuria, hematuria, and cellular debris exist in the urine but the patient may be feeling well. This state of illness may continue up to a year or two after an acute episode of glomerulonephritis. During latent stages of nephritis the patient may continue normal activities. He should, however, avoid fatigue, trauma, and infection as these conditions exacerbate illness.

Good general health measures should be stressed. Dietary protein may be restricted depending on blood urea nitrogen levels; fluid is encouraged if the patient is able to excrete it. Since the patient usually feels well, he must often be convinced of the need to continue prescribed treatment and to return for routine medical follow-up. If symptoms recur, the patient should be advised to seek immediate medical attention, even though he may have been thoroughly examined only a short time previously.

Although chronic glomerulonephritis may follow acute disease, the majority of patients with this disease give no history of acute glomerulonephritis. In most instances, no evidence of any predisposing infection can be found. Various symptoms of failing renal function, none of which may seem severe, may bring the patient to the physician. The patient may notice the slow onset of dependent edema that comes and goes. He may complain of headache, especially in the morning. Dyspnea on exertion or difficulty sleeping in a flat position may be noted. Blurring of vision may lead the patient to an ophthalmologist, who may be the first to suspect chronic glomerulonephritis because of retinal changes. Nocturia is a common complaint and is due to the kidneys' inability to properly concentrate urine so that waste products must be excreted in larger volumes of urine. Occasionally chronic nephritis is discovered during a routine physical examination or it may be discovered by a school nurse who observes marked visual changes and lassitude in a student. Weakness, fatigue, and weight loss are common, though nonspecific, symptoms of chronic glomerulonephritis. Early in the disease, urinalysis shows the presence of albumin, casts, and blood. At this point renal function tests may be normal. However, the ability of the kidneys to regulate the internal environment will begin to decrease as more and more glomeruli become scarred and the amount of functional renal tissue is reduced. Finally, when few intact nephrons remain, hematuria and proteinuria decrease, the specific gravity of the urine becomes fixed, and the nonprotein nitrogen level in the blood increases.

The course of chronic glomerulonephritis is unpredictable. Some patients with minimal impairment in renal function continue to feel well and show little progression in their disease. With other individuals, the progression of renal deterioration may be slow but steady and end in renal failure. In still other individuals the progression of disease is rapid. With any exacerbation of hematuria, hypertension, and edema, the patient is put to bed, and the treatment is similar to that for acute glomerulonephritis. Signs of pulmonary edema, congestive failure, and cerebral edema should be watched for when caring for these patients. Treatment is symptomatic and supportive.

Patients with chronic glomerulonephritis who become pregnant seem susceptible to toxemia and to spontaneous abortion. Occasionally it may be necessary to induce labor prematurely. The woman who has had nephritis of any nature should be urged to see a physician if she plans on pregnancy. When pregnancy does occur, she should remain under close health supervision.

Nephrotic syndrome (nephrosis). The term "nephrotic syndrome" designates a condition involving increased permeability of the glomeruli. It is associated with a variety of renal diseases. Characteristic manifestations of nephrotic syndrome include severe generalized edema that is particularly noticeable about the eyes and abdomen, pronounced albuminuria of 4 to 10 Gm./day or more, hypoproteinemia, and usually hyperlipemia. The blood pressure and blood urea nitrogen levels may or may not be elevated. The mechanism that alters the glomerular structures so that protein is lost in the urine is unknown. In adults particularly, the nephrotic syndrome seems correlated with some underlying kidney disease; in children the syndrome frequently appears with no evidence of a causative factor.

Treatment of the patient with nephrotic syndrome is aimed toward reducing albuminuria, controlling edema, and promoting general health. The diet should contain normal amounts of protein (1 Gm./kg. body weight/day) and be high in calories. Increasing dietary protein to allow for that lost in the urine has questionable benefit as it often only increases urinary protein loss and can be a considerable expense to the patient. Dietary sodium intake is limited to approximately 0.5 to 1 Gm./day. Diuretics are employed to decrease fluid retention. If diuretics are regularly administered and the patient has no signs of renal failure, hypokalemia usually results. Potassium should be supplemented in dietary and medication forms. Corticosteroids are often beneficial in decreasing proteinuria. Prednisone is the steroid preparation most frequently prescribed. Patients with nephrosis need particular attention directed toward preventing infection since edematous tissues are susceptible to trauma and infection and body defenses are impaired by protein losses. Bed rest is usually ordered for patients with severe edema or infection.

Nephrosis tends to be chronic in most adults and in about one half of the children who develop it. Normal activity should be encouraged as much as possible. Often patients do well for long periods of time before serious loss of renal function occurs. Development of hypertension, hyperkalemia, and nitrogen retention indicates further loss of renal function. Management of the patient with renal failure is described on p. 462.

Hypertensive renal disease. Hypertension is a major precipitating factor of renal failure. Regardless of origin (essential or renal), hypertension that is untreated over a period of time leads to sclerosing of renal arterioles. Gradually the blood supply to the kidneys decreases. Death and scarring of kidney tissue occurs, and signs of renal insufficiency develop after approximately four fifths of the kidney tissue has been destroyed. *"Nephrosclerosis"* is the term given to this destructive process.

Care for this health problem is directed toward early detection and treatment of hypertension. Renal hypertensive disease can be prevented. Yearly screening of blood pressure is an essential part of preventive health care. When hypertension is diagnosed, causative factors are sought, and treatment to lower blood pressure is begun.

Pyelonephritis. Pyelonephritis refers to bacterial infection of kidney tissue. Usually the infection begins in the lower urinary tract and ascends into the kidneys. Lower urinary tract infection may be asymptomatic, and kidney involvement can occur without awareness of the presence of infection. Common factors contributing to infection of the urinary tract include stasis of urine from benign prostatic hypertrophy, residual urine in the bladder, pregnancy, instrumentation of the urinary tract, and trauma to the genitourinary system. Pyelonephritis is commonly seen in young female and older male populations. It may occur in both acute and chronic forms of illness. Chronic pyelonephritis leads to scarring and death of kidney tissue. It has been estimated that it accounts for approximately one third of all deaths from renal failure. Usual symptoms of pyelonephritis are fever and chills, malaise, costoverte-bral tenderness, leukocytosis, and pyuria.

Optimal treatment includes early detection of the illness (in order to prevent or arrest death of kidney tissue) and administration of antibacterial medications. Anyone with symptoms of dysuria, cloudy urine, or frequent small voidings should be examined for urinary tract infection and appropriately treated. Individuals complaining of fever and costovertebral tenderness should be encouraged to seek medical attention. Therapy for pyelonephritis consists of antibiotics selected on the basis of urine cultures. The course of antibiotic therapy may extend over weeks, and the patient may need to be reminded of the necessity to continue taking the medication as his symptoms disappear and he begins to feel better. Continuing drug therapy to prevent relapse and eradication of all infection should be stressed. Treatment of any underlying obstruction or stasis of urine is also required. Increasing fluid intake to around 3 L./day in patients capable of excreting this amount of fluid is desirable to prevent stasis of urine and further bacterial growth.

Tuberculosis of the kidney and urinary tract. Most individuals who develop tuberculosis of the kidney relate in their history an episode of pulmonary tuberculosis or close contact with someone having this disease. Tubercle bacilli reach the kidneys through the bloodstream or lymphatic system. Signs of renal involvement may first occur several years after the primary tuberculosis infection and usually consist of frequency, pain on urination, and hematuria. In the kidney the tubercle bacilli spread to the papillae, and obstruction of entire kidney segments may result. Renal failure develops when the disease spreads throughout the kidney and scarring becomes widespread. Urinary tract tuberculosis is most common in males between 20 and 40 years of age. Involvement of genital organs is common if the disease is left untreated.

Urinary tract tuberculosis can be difficult to diagnose. Bacilli may not be readily found in the urine. Culture of the first morning voiding provides the best opportunity for identifying the organisms. Pyelography is indicated to assess the degree of tissue destruction; frequently the appearance of the calices is "moth-eaten."

Treatment is primarily medical and consists of antituberculosis drug therapy coupled with rest and good nutrition. Surgery may be required when severe damage of a kidney exists. Other foci of the bacillus in the body are always sought. Care of the patient should include explanations and answers to questions about the disease, its communicability, and probable rehabilitation course. Isolation of the patient need not be instituted if there is no evidence of active pulmonary disease. During the period when tubercle bacilli are present in the urine the patient should not engage in sexual intercourse, as the disease may be spread by genital contact. The question of fertility may be raised by patients who have involvement of the genital organs. Fertility is not impaired when treatment has been prompt and adequate. The patient should be taught to wash his hands well with soap and water after any contact with urine or the genitalia. Antituberculosis drug therapy generally continues for 1 to 2 years after the disease has been diagnosed. Tests of renal function determine the extent to which actual kidney damage has occurred and should be considered when discussing prognosis with the patient.

■ MANAGEMENT OF THE PATIENT WITH DISEASE OF THE URINARY SYSTEM

Although patients with urologic disease present many unique nursing problems, there exist some fundamental and common care requirements. Two of the major common needs for care of a patient with urologic disease are maintenance of normal fluid and electrolyte balance and provision for elimination.

Maintenance of fluid and electrolyte balance

Normal relationships of fluid intake to output and normal electrolyte composition may be disrupted when disease affects the urinary system. Alterations in sodium, potassium, calcium, phosphorus, hydrogen ion, and fluid balance occur with renal disease; alterations in sodium and fluid balance occur with disease of the lower urinary tract.

The nurse must not only maintain accuracy in fluid balance recording but should be able to appreciate the meaning of the information gathered. The significance of these nursing contributions to patient management cannot be overlooked; fluid balance records are often the first indicators of progressing disease or of recovery and indicate when further examinations and medications are needed. The status of an individual's fluid balance can be figured using the following equation:

Fluid intake + Water of oxidation =
a. Oral   (300-400 ml./day)
b. Parenteral

Urine output + Insensible losses + Other drainage
                  a. Skin   a. Wounds
                  b. GI tract   b. Vomitus
                  c. Respiratory tract c. Diarrhea
                    (800-1,000 ml./day) d. Hemorrhage
                                    e. Diaphoresis

The equation indicates that for the healthy individual who is neither retaining nor losing excessive fluid, intake will balance output, and the specific intake of fluid will be roughly equivalent to or slightly in excess of urinary output (400 to 500 ml./day). For the individual who is losing fluid through wound drainage, diarrhea, vomiting, diaphoresis, or severe blood loss, the amount of the loss must be balanced through either a decreased urinary output or an increased fluid intake. In addition to the sources of fluid intake and loss indicated in the equation, the temperature of a patient and his weight are helpful in determining whether a patient may need to limit or increase intake of fluid. As temperature rises, more fluid will be lost through the skin and lungs. Determination of weight helps detect changes in fluid balance when compared with measurements obtained on preceding days; large increases may be attributed to retention of fluid, and significant decreases in weight may reflect loss of body fluid. When the weight of a patient is used to predict fluid balance, determinations should be performed at the same time of day on the same scale with the patient wearing clothing of similar weight.

In patients with urinary disease, diminishing output can result from decreased intake or from inadequate excretion (that is, advancing renal disease or obstruction of the urinary tract). Increases in output over intake may be less commonly seen; this state results when damage occurs to the medullary portion of the kidneys and the ability to conserve needed fluid and electrolytes is lost. It is important that the nurse understand both actual and potential fluid and electrolyte complications so that pertinent observations will be made regarding the patient's response to his illness and therapy.

Provision for elimination

Obstruction of the urinary tract may result from tumors, blood clots, calculi, or sediment from infection. Any obstruction retards flow of urine and leads to infection and probable renal damage. Reestablishing the flow of urine is an immediate treatment goal, and various types of catheter drainage are used to achieve this.

Drainage of the kidney pelvis. If a ureter becomes obstructed, a catheter must be placed directly into the renal pelvis. This prevents renal damage that otherwise would occur as pressure in the kidney increases because of continuing urine formation. When there is complete obstruction of a ureter, a nephrostomy or pyelostomy tube may be inserted surgically into the renal pelvis. The surgical incision is located laterally and posteriorly in the kidney region. Catheters used as nephrostomy or pyelostomy tubes are usually of the Pezzer (mushroom) or Malecot (batwing) types (Fig. 20-12). An alternative form of drainage for an ureteral obstruction is the surgical placement of a ureterostomy tube (a whistle-tip or many-eyed Robinson catheter, size 6 to 18 Fr.), which is passed through an incision in the upper outer quadrant of the abdomen into the ureter above the obstruction. The catheter is then passed through the ureter to the renal pelvis.

Ureteral catheterization. Ureteral catheterization is performed prior to gynecologic and lower abdominal surgery when there is danger of not recognizing and injuring a ureter during the operation. Catheterization in these instances sharply defines the ureter. Ureteral catheterization is also performed to bypass an obstruction and drain the renal pelvis when a stone becomes lodged in a ureter. Insertion of a ureteral catheter is accomplished through a cystoscope; the catheters are 1 to 2 mm. in diameter.

Suprapubic bladder drainage. When the urethra is completely obstructed or when there is danger of infection of the male genital system because of extended urethral intubation, a *cystotomy* may be performed. In this procedure a catheter is placed into the bladder through a *suprapubic incision.* During some operative procedures both a cystostomy tube and a small urethral catheter will be inserted to drain the bladder. Both catheters must be monitored for patency. If patency is assured, it is not necessary to

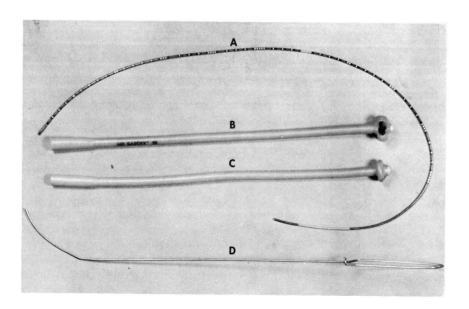

FIG. 20-12. A to **C,** Catheters used to drain the renal pelvis: **A,** ureteral catheter; **B,** Malecot (batwing) catheter; **C,** Pezzer (mushroom) catheter. **D,** Stylet used to insert urethral catheter into a male patient.

record separately the output from each catheter on the fluid balance record since both of these tubes drain the bladder. It should be noted that the catheters will not necessarily drain equal amounts of urine.

Urethral catheterization. The most common means of draining the bladder is through a urethral catheter. Several modifications of size and shape in catheters exist. Soft red rubber catheters are commonly used for one-time or nonindwelling procedures. Several of the more common catheter shapes are the coudé catheter, which has a curved tip and is used with older men or when hypertrophy of the prostate is suspected to avoid trauma to this gland; the whistle-tip catheter, which has a large end opening ideal for use when hematuria and blood clots are present; the many-eyed Robinson catheter, which may be used when an increase in drainage surface in the catheter is desired; and the filiform catheter, which is a stiff catheter used when urethral strictures are present (Fig. 20-13). Indwelling or continuous bladder drainage catheters are usually made of latex rubber as this material is more flexible and less irritating to tissues than the red rubber catheter. The Foley catheter or self-retaining catheter is usually employed when drainage of the bladder is necessary for a period of time. These catheters are constructed with either a 5 ml. (for normal use) or a 30 ml. (for use when hemostasis is required) balloon. The balloon should be inflated with either normal saline solution or sterile water after it has been placed well within the bladder. Straight catheters of the coudé, Robinson, and filiform type may also be used as indwelling

catheters in the male patient when transversing the urethra requires a stiffer catheter. The straight catheter can be anchored to the penis by the following method (Fig. 20-14): (1) cut two strips of adhesive tape $1\frac{1}{2}$ by 4 inches; (2) cut two pieces of twill tape 12 inches long; (3) apply one strip of the $1\frac{1}{2}$ by 4 inch adhesive tape, bringing the edges together beyond the penis (to permit easy removal and room for expansion in case of erection); (4) place one end of each piece of twill tape over the adhesive tape on either side of the penis and apply the second strip of the adhesive to hold the tape in place; and (5) wind the two pieces of twill tape in opposite directions around the catheter and tie them securely about 2 inches from the tip of the penis. Catheter size is measured according to the French scale; 1 Fr. equals $\frac{1}{3}$ mm. in external diameter of the catheter. Appropriate catheter sizes for males are 16 to 22 Fr.; for females, 14 to 20 Fr.; and for children, 6 to 10 Fr.

Catheterization is a major cause of urinary tract infections, and rigid asepsis should be practiced when carrying out this procedure and in assembling drainage equipment.[59,60] When a woman is to be catheterized, the procedure is generally performed by a female nurse. The patient may be prepared in either the dorsal or lateral position.[28] When a man is to be catheterized, a male member of the nursing team or a male physician should carry out the procedure. The male patient should be placed on his back. When any patient is being catheterized, he should be encouraged to take deep breaths during insertion of the catheter. This will help to divert attention from the procedure and increase relaxation of the bladder

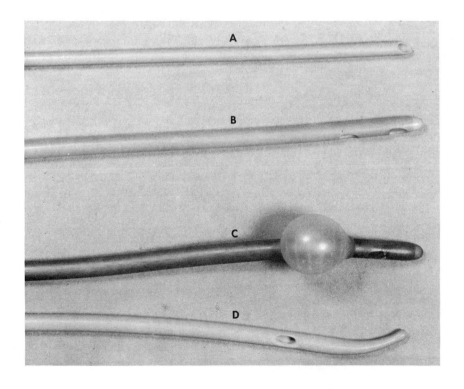

FIG. 20-13. Urethral catheters. **A,** Whistle-tip catheter. **B,** Many-eyed Robinson catheter. **C,** Foley catheter. **D,** Coudé catheter.

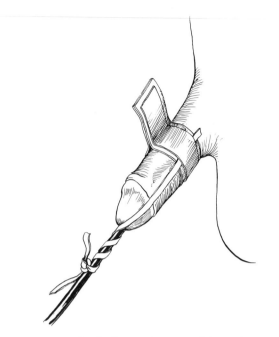

FIG. 20-14. Method of securing a straight catheter used as an indwelling catheter in a male patient.

sphincters, making the procedure less uncomfortable.

If in performing a catheterization the nurse finds it difficult to pass the catheter, the procedure should be discontinued and the physician notified. Traumatic catheterization predisposes to urinary tract infection and formation of urethral strictures. In patients who have urethral disorders it is not unusual to be unable to pass a standard catheter; special equipment such as catheter directors, filiform catheters, or sounds may be needed. The introduction of such equipment into the urinary tract is not a nursing procedure; neither is catheterization of a patient in the immediate postoperative period following surgery on the urethra or bladder. For specific information on the catheterization procedure, refer to a fundamentals of nursing or urologic nursing text.

It is important that catheters be adequately anchored to prevent accidental dislodgement and trauma to the tissues in which they lie. *Cystostomy, nephrostomy,* and *ureterostomy* tubes should have two points of anchorage to prevent their being dislodged. The openings made for the insertion of these tubes are essentially fistulas that rapidly decrease in size on removal of the catheter. Even half an hour after removal of this type of catheter it is often impossible to reinsert a similar sized tube. When a catheter is inserted during surgery, it is usually sutured in place. In this case, additional anchoring consists of affixing the tube to the skin with adhesive tape after the skin has been well cleansed. If the tube is not sutured in place, it should be anchored to the skin at two points using adhesive with some slack

in the tubing between the anchor points. Urethral catheters, including the self-retaining or indwelling type, should be secured to the inner thigh of the female patient and to the inner thigh or the abdomen of the male patient (Fig. 20-15).

Care of catheters. Since the purpose of the catheter is to promote drainage of urine, patency of the system must be ensured. The flow of urine from a catheter should be checked hourly when urine is bloody and at least three to four times each day when there is no evidence of disturbance in drainage. Common causes of obstruction of urine flow may be internal or external. Hemorrhage leads to formation of clots in the bladder that may plug the catheter, and infection increases sediment in the urine that may encrust and clog the drainage system. Any evidence of bleeding or change in amount of bleeding should be reported to the physician. To detect the buildup of sediment in the drainage system, the catheter may be rolled between the fingers to detect any gritty accumulation, and the drainage tubing should be visually inspected. External causes of obstruction in urine flow include kinking and dependent loops in the tubing. If these measures are unsuccessful in restoring urine flow, the catheter may be rotated slightly to ensure that it is not occluded by its position in the bladder. In the event that none of these measures restores the flow of urine the physician should be notified. Catheters should not be irrigated without a specific order.

Catheters should not be clamped or plugged; they should remain freely draining. The procedure of clamping drainage tubes is especially hazardous when the catheter leads directly into the kidney. The normal renal pelvis has a capacity of only 5 to 8 ml., and great back pressure can be exerted on renal structures when nephrostomy, pyelostomy, and ureterostomy tubes are clamped for periods of even a few minutes.

The color, clarity, and odor of the urine should be noted and recorded. Any changes in the nature of the urine should be brought to the attention of the physician.

In helping to prevent urinary tract infection, the meatal area should be cleansed with soap and water at least twice a day. A cleansing solution such as benzalkonium chloride may be used in place of soap and water. When cleaning the meatal area and the outside of the catheter, the cleaning should be done away from the genitalia. This motion prevents pushing bacteria on the outside of the catheter closer to the urinary meatus. Catheters should not be advanced in the urethra once they are in place; in-and-out motions of the catheter serve to introduce organisms into the urinary tract. Increasing the patient's fluid intake to 3 to 4 L./day unless contraindicated should help to control urinary infection. This measure increases urinary flow and thus decreases stasis and

FIG. 20-15. Disposable closed urinary drainage system. The tubing is attached at the top interior of the drainage bag.

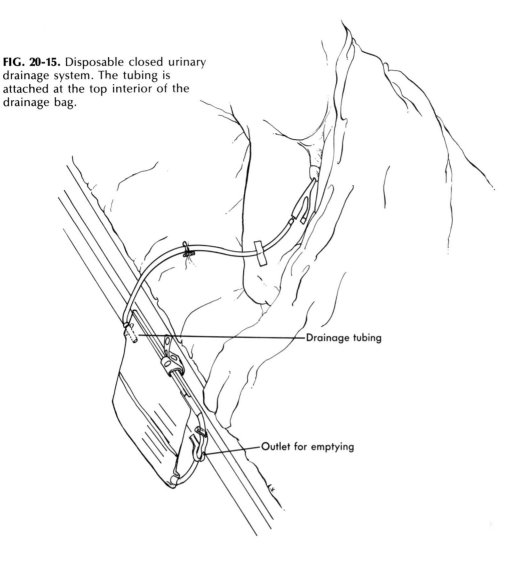

—Drainage tubing

—Outlet for emptying

possible growth of organisms in the urinary tract. Good handwashing technique is mandatory when caring for patients with catheters.

The drainage system. Catheters that have been placed in the urinary system usually are allowed to drain by gravity. The procedure of connecting a catheter to a collecting device and allowing drainage to flow by gravitational force is called *straight drainage. Closed drainage* refers to the design of the collection setup and indicates that the drainage tube is sealed to the collection container; this lessens the chance for contamination of the setup and decreases the likelihood of urinary tract infection. For drainage to occur in a system that is closed to the outside, some air must be introduced to break the vacuum that would otherwise exist. In the closed system an air vent that is filtered to lessen the danger of infection is provided. Most closed urinary drainage systems employ disposable plastic drainage bags and tubing (Fig. 20-15).

Proper maintenance of the drainage system is a nursing function. Attention to the following points

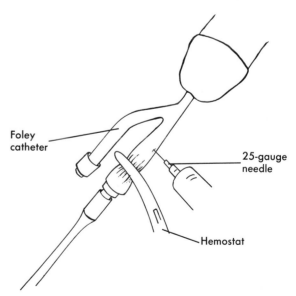

Foley
catheter

25-gauge
needle

Hemostat

FIG. 20-16. A needle and syringe are used to remove a sterile specimen from a Foley catheter in a closed drainage system.

will help to maintain drainage and decrease the entry of organisms into the system. (1) Once the catheter has been connected to the drainage system it should not be disconnected except when performing ordered irrigations. Samples of urine should be obtained by inserting a small-bore needle at a slant directly into the catheter at a point immediately above the connection with the drainage tubing (Fig. 20-16). (2) The drainage bag must not be elevated above the level of the patient's bladder or cavity being drained as reflux of urine will occur. Drainage bags should be suspended from the bed frame when the patient is recumbent, suspended from the frame of the cart when a patient is being transported, and from below the knee level when the patient is ambulatory. (3) Drainage bags and tubing should not be allowed to rest on the floor. (4) Kinks or loops of tubing below the level of the drainage container should not exist; to prevent interference with flow or urine, excess tubing may be clipped and coiled on the bed. The patency of all tubes should be checked when a patient is repositioned. (5) The drainage bag should not be allowed to become completely filled with urine as this leads to stasis of urine in the drainage tubing and wetting of the air filter in the drainage container. (6) The drainage container should not be held upside down when being emptied as this causes reflux of urine into the drainage tubing and bladder. (7) Cultures of the urine should be taken at frequent intervals when a patient has an indwelling drainage tube. (8) The collecting system should be checked daily for signs of sediment and leaks. Any of these findings indicates the need for a new collection system.

Catheter irrigation. The safest and most effective means of irrigating the urinary tract when there are notable amounts of sediment or clotted blood in the urine is through increasing the patient's oral intake. Approximately 3,000 ml./day should be encouraged when the patient's condition permits; the fluid may be administered orally or in a combination of oral and parenteral routes.

When the irrigation of a catheter is ordered, some threat to the patency of the drainage system is usually obvious. Potential sources of obstruction of the catheter include sediment from infection, blood clots or hematuria, and tissue shreds. The purpose of irrigation is to prevent obstruction of the catheter and not lavage of the organ that the tube drains.

Gentleness is mandatory in any irrigation procedure. Vigorous instillation of fluid into the bladder or kidney is likely to damage these organs and spread or initiate infection. All equipment used must be sterile, and attention to asepsis must be maintained throughout the procedure. Sterile normal saline solution is usually ordered for catheter irrigation because it is nonirritating to tissues and because its clarity makes for easy observation of abnormal constituents

in the urine. Acetic acid and neomycin solutions may also be ordered as irrigating substances.

When a catheter is to be irrigated, the size of the cavity into which the fluid is being instilled should be considered. The renal pelvis should never be irrigated with more than 5 to 10 ml. of fluid. Commonly 30 to 60 ml. of fluid is used to irrigate a urethral catheter. After instillation, the irrigating fluid should be allowed to return by gravity. If fluid can be easily instilled but fails to return, a clot or small plug may be acting as a valve over the catheter eye. If this occurs, the nurse should not continue adding fluid, but instead may try to dislodge a possible obstruction by "milking" the tubing. If after a 10- to 15-minute period the catheter is not draining properly, the physician should be notified.

When frequent irrigation of a urethral catheter appears necessary, intermittent irrigation should be considered. This setup can be incorporated into a closed drainage system and hence decreases the possibility of entrance of bacteria into the bladder. Intermittent irrigation involves alternately instilling fluid from a reservoir (usually suspended above patient level) into the bladder via the catheter and allowing the solution to return freely into the collecting bag. Intermittent irrigation is usually not employed for irrigation of the kidney because control of inflow in 5 to 10 ml. amounts is difficult, and instillation of larger amounts of fluid into the renal pelvis leads to tissue damage.

Another variation in irrigating the bladder involves the use of a three-way Foley catheter. Constant irrigation involves continuous and simultaneous inflow and outflow of irrigating solution from the bladder. This system is used most frequently after surgery of the bladder when bleeding is expected and clot formation with obstruction of the bladder outlet is an actual threat. In calculating the patient's output when either intermittent irrigation or constant irrigation of the bladder is employed, the amount of irrigating fluid used is subtracted from the total volume of urinary drainage obtained in the same time period. The difference between these two values is the patient's actual urinary output.

Management of the patient after removal of a catheter

It is normal to note some dribbling of urine for a few hours after a catheter has been removed because of dilation of the sphincter muscles by the catheter. However, dribbling of urine that persists longer than a few hours should be reported to the physician; this symptom may indicate damage to the sphincters. In determining the type of intervention necessary to reestablish bladder control, information about the nature of the incontinency should be gathered. Incontinence should be described as complete (constant dribbling) or occurring only on urgency or stress. Also, it should be observed whether the patient is incontinent in all positions (lying, sitting, standing). If muscular weakness of the sphincters is the major problem, the patient is least likely to have incontinence in a prone position and most difficulty with control of urination when walking or standing. (Refer to Chapter 9 for bladder retraining and muscle strengthening exercises.)

Another problem that may arise after removal of a catheter is inability to void. No patient with an adequate intake should go longer than 6 to 8 hours without voiding. It is not uncommon for a patient with edema of the bladder neck to require temporary reinsertion of a catheter to facilitate urinary output. It is the nurse's responsibility to accurately determine and record all spontaneous voiding of the patient until adequacy of output has been well established.

Color and consistency of the urine should be noted. *Cystitis* (inflammation of the bladder) may develop after catheter removal because of incomplete emptying of the bladder as muscle tone is being reestablished. Any abnormalities in color, odor, or sediment should be reported.

Education of the patient about signs and symptoms of urinary retention, changes in the color and consistency of the urine, and incontinence and dysuria should be undertaken when bladder drainage is discontinued. Often the first indicators of dysfunction are subjective judgments that the patient offers about himself. This information greatly increases the ability to detect early recurrence of urinary drainage problems and should be sought and clearly recorded.

Management of the patient requiring urologic surgery

The basic needs of patients requiring urologic surgery are the same as those of any other surgical patient. However, since urologic surgery may necessitate mutilation of normal anatomy, the patient may have to adjust to the problem of "being different," such as having to adjust to a new route of urine excretion.

Emotional support. The male patient may be made sterile, impotent, or both by some operative procedures. If a radical operative procedure is contemplated, the urologist usually discusses the implications in detail with the patient and his family. Many physicians feel that the patient should make the final decision to undergo such an operation. While attempting to reach a decision, the patient often is very depressed. If he accepts surgery, he usually has a second period of depression at the time active rehabilitation begins.

During these stages there is little that the nurse can do except to give moral support by providing for privacy, allowing extra family visits if they seem to help the patient, caring for his physical needs, and answering or channeling to appropriate persons the questions raised by either the patient or his family. The patient also is often helped by talking with his spiritual adviser, with understanding members of the family, and with patients who have made good adjustments following similar surgical procedures. The nurse should be alert for changes in mood or behavior that might indicate the need for psychiatric guidance.

Hemorrhage. Hemorrhage may follow such operative procedures as transurethral prostatectomy, suprapubic prostatectomy, nephrolithotomy (complete kidney split), and nephrectomy. If drainage tubes are used, the bleeding may be visible. After surgery involving the urinary system, urine is usually dark red or pink, but it should not be bright red or viscid or contain clots. The wounds often normally drain copious amounts of light red urine, but bright red blood on dressings indicates hemorrhage. Following surgery on the kidney, the nurse should look along the posterior edge of the dressing for blood draining over the sacral area. If the patient has a suprapubic incision, blood may be noted along the side of the dressing and in the inguinal region. The classic symptoms of hemorrhage, including pallor, skin clamminess, and apprehension will usually be present. The blood pressure drops, and the pulse becomes rapid and thready. Since many patients with urologic disease have hypertension, the blood pressure may be relatively high but still represent a marked drop for the individual. If hemorrhage occurs, the physician should be called at once. If the bleeding is external, a pressure dressing should be applied over the incision while awaiting the physician's arrival. If the patient is lying in a pool of blood, the nurse should slip some absorbent material under him until after the physician has examined him. His bed should then be changed if he can be moved at all. The patient should be protected from the sight of blood on his bedding or in the tubing and bottle.

Dressing materials and equipment for intravenous therapy should be at the bedside. If the patient has a catheter in place, materials for irrigation should be prepared. In addition, a suction syringe, several liter bottles of sterile physiologic saline solution, and several large waste basins should be available. The patient should be placed flat in bed, or the physician may order him to be placed in the position used for shock, with the lower extremities raised above the level of the heart.

Dressings. Since urine drains from many urologic incisions for several days and sometimes much longer, the nurse working with a urologic patient is more likely to have an order to change postoperative dressings as necessary than is the case in care of other surgical patients. Montgomery straps are often used to hold these dressings in place. It is not necessary, nor is it good practice, to allow dressings to become saturated with urine. Not only is the patient made very uncomfortable, but frequently he is also unable to rest, the skin becomes irritated, and there is an unpleasant odor.

There are many ways to prevent the patient from lying in wet dressings, and the nurse should seek an order to use appropriate procedures. If the wound must be kept sterile, incorporate a small sterile, many-eyed Robinson catheter inside a sterile 4 by 8 inch dressing and place it with the eyes directly over the drainage site. Fasten the catheter and gauze in place with a strip of adhesive tape, and attach the end of the catheter to a suction apparatus (Fig. 20-17). This method not only keeps the patient dry but it also permits the amount of drainage to be recorded. The patient may be out of bed but only within range of the suction.

Any suction used to drain closed cavities and affecting the mucous membrane or the skin surface should be limited to a specific, constant negative pressure; 5 cm. (2 inches) of negative pressure is often ordered. Suction may be used directly from the source if an electric pump on which the amount of negative pressure exerted can be regulated (Gomco or Emerson pump) is used. Tubing from the pump is attached to one arm of a drainage-bottle cap, and the catheter tubing is attached to the other arm.

When the amount of suction cannot be regulated at the source, methods to decrease it must be used. It can be decreased by placing a bottle containing water between the source of suction and the drainage apparatus. A glass tube with one end open to the air is inserted through a cork and immersed a specific number of inches under water placed in one bottle, the "water" bottle. The depth of immersion determines the amount of suction; for 5 cm. (2 inches) of negative pressure, the end of the tube must be under 2 inches of water. Since the water bubbles when the apparatus works smoothly, this method is called *bubble suction.*

Tubing from the source of suction may be connected to the drainage system by one of two methods:

Method 1. Using a three-holed cork in the water bottle, attach tubing from the source of suction to a glass connector inserted in one hole. Attach one end of a piece of tubing to a second connector and the other end to one arm of the drainage bottle cap. The long glass tube regulating the suction and open to the air is in the third hole. The other arm of the drainage bottle cap is attached to the drainage tubing. This setup is similar to that depicted for chest drainage in Fig. 22-17 except that the drainage tube is not immersed in water.

Method 2. Tubing should run from the source of suction to one arm of a Y connector. Tubing from a

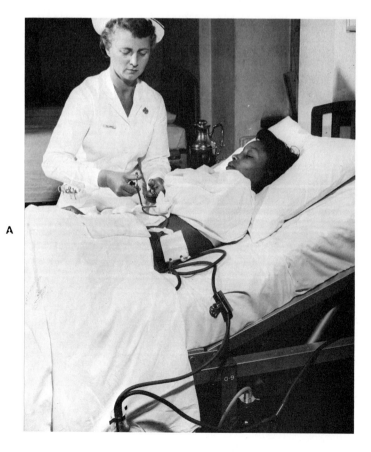

A

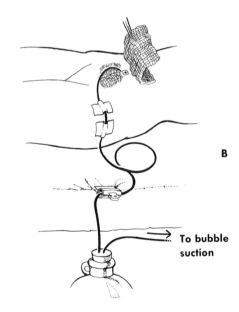

B

To bubble suction

FIG. 20-17. **A,** The nurse is incorporating a sterile catheter attached to bubble suction drainage into a gauze dressing. This apparatus will collect urine draining from a ureterolithotomy incision. **B,** Note that the catheter is anchored to the skin with two flaps of adhesive tape, that the drainage tubing is attached to the bedclothes with a clamp, and that the excess tubing is coiled on the mattress.

second arm of the Y connector is attached to a glass connector inserted into one hole of a two-holed water bottle cork. The long glass tube open to the air is inserted through the other hole. Tubing from the third arm of the Y connector is attached to one arm of the drainage bottle cap. The drainage tubing is attached to the other arm of the drainage bottle cap (Fig. 20-17).

Suprapubic wounds may sometimes be kept dry by the use of a piece of equipment known as a *suction cup*. A suction cup can be used only after the sutures have been removed. Before applying it, protect the skin around the area with tincture of benzoin and then place the cup so that the drainage spout is uppermost over the fistula. Be careful not to cover the air outlet in the top of the cup, since the increased suction that is produced may cause the skin under the cup to blister. Securely fasten the cup in place by a wide strip of adhesive tape, Montgomery straps pulled snugly together, or skin cement applied to the edges of the cup. Attach the cup to bubble suction. If the patient is to be out of bed or if gravity drainage is needed, a drainer cup may be substituted for the suction cup. It differs from the suction cup in that it has no collecting tube around the inner edge and will cause blistering of the skin if attached to suction drainage. It must be used only with gravity drainage.

If the urethral catheter is still in place and if there is leakage from the suprapubic wound, the catheter should be checked to ensure that it is draining and is properly placed. The urethral catheter should provide for draining of urine, and the suprapubic wound should be dry.

Another method sometimes used to drain urine from an abnormal opening is the application of a large-sized ureterostomy cup over the fistula, attaching it to straight drainage.

Disposable *plastic ileostomy bags* may be secured over the fistula with skin paste. Since the opening in these bags can be cut to the appropriate size, the skin can be completely protected from urine. The bag may be emptied as necessary, and no dressings are required. This method often works well following ureterolithotomy when the drain is still in place.

• • •

In still another method, a 12-inch square of rubber dam is used. An opening large enough to fit around the draining wound is cut in the center, and the rubber dam is pasted to the skin area immediately surrounding the fistula. Dressings are then placed over the drainage site, with the rubber dam folded over them in envelope style (Fig. 20-18). Montgomery straps will be needed to hold such a dressing in place. If this method is used, dressings still require frequent changing. Although the patient

may be dry externally, the urinary drainage lies in a pool over the incision. Unless the dressings are frequently changed, the wound will become infected from organisms growing in the stagnant urine. Patients can usually be taught to change their own dressings when necessary.

None of the methods described works well with every patient. The nurse must study the type of wound, the placement of the incision, and the contour of the surrounding tissue to determine the most satisfactory method for the particular patient.

Frequently, in changing a urologic dressing, a catheter must also be irrigated. If the wound opens into the cavity drained by the catheter, the same sterile field may be used for the irrigation and the dressing. Each kidney and the bladder are considered separate cavities, and care must be taken not to cause cross-contamination. Irrigation should be done before redressing the wound since some fluid may seep out through the incision.

■ PLANNING HOME CARE FOR THE PATIENT WITH URINARY DRAINAGE

Occasionally a patient may be discharged from the hospital with a catheter in place. The catheter may

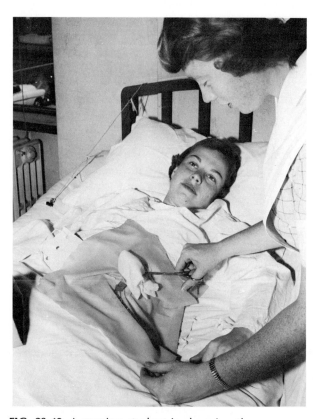

FIG. 20-18. A nursing student is changing the dressing over a drain that is inserted into a ureterolithotomy wound. Rubber dam has been pasted to the skin around the drain so that urine will not run over the skin.

be placed in the bladder or in the pelvis of the kidney and may be needed as a temporary or permanent means of urinary drainage. Every patient leaving the hospital with a catheter in place should be taught to care for the urinary drainage system so that introduction of organisms into the urinary tract can be minimized and patency of the system maintained. If an *ileal conduit* operation has been performed, the patient should learn to care for the stoma and the equipment that will be used in permanently altering urinary drainage. The same principles used in the hospital in caring for the patient's drainage equipment should be taught the patient, modifying procedures as necessary to fit the individual's home environment. If the patient will be unable to provide his own care, a member of the immediate family should be taught how to assume this responsibility. Anticipation of discharge needs should begin a number of days prior to the patient's leaving the hospital. This allows sufficient time to procure needed equipment for the patient and for him to use and familiarize himself with the equipment while supervision is still readily available. The nurse in the hospital should plan the content and approach for patient teaching after considering the specifics of care prescribed by the physician, general catheter care and principles of asepsis, the specific equipment the patient will be using, and the patient's ability and readiness to assume his care.

Care at home always requires further adjustment on the patient's part in developing security and manipulative skill with his equipment. Provision for continued home supervision of the patient by a public health nurse can immensely benefit the patient's adjustment. Visits with the family and the patient should be maintained at regular intervals until the patient's comfort in self-care is achieved.

Renal failure

Renal failure indicates a state of total or nearly total loss of the kidneys' ability to excrete waste products and to maintain fluid and electrolyte balance. Laboratory tests reflect the changes in the internal environment, and the patient appears clinically ill. The patient in renal failure cannot independently sustain life. Dietary adjustments, medications, and preventing additional illnesses can partially compensate for loss of kidney function in early stages of gradually progressing renal failure; with rigid adherence to the treatment program, the patient may be able to maintain some or many of his previous activities. As renal function continues to deteriorate, dialysis and/or transplantation becomes necessary for supporting life. When renal failure develops suddenly, internal changes are often dramatic and the patient has little time to adjust to these changes; he is usually quite ill, and hospitalization is necessary.

Renal insufficiency designates significant loss of renal function, but with enough function remaining to maintain an internal environment consistent with life, provided no additional stresses to health occur. The individual may appear and feel well, although laboratory data reflect a decreased level of renal function. Renal insufficiency occurs as a phase in gradually and chronically progressing renal disease.

When symptoms of renal failure appear (when the individual looks and feels ill), *uremia* is said to exist. Uremia is a complex of symptoms and laboratory findings resulting from disordered biochemical processes of the entire body.[85] *Azotemia* is one manifestation of uremia; it refers to the buildup of nitrogenous products in the blood.

◼ ACUTE RENAL FAILURE

Acute renal failure occurs as a sudden and frequently reversible decrease or cessation of kidney function. Either *oliguria* or *anuria* may be present, although oliguria is more frequent. Oliguria refers to a urine output below 400 ml./day; anuria refers to a urine output below 75 to 100 ml./day. Acute renal failure generally follows an identifiable trauma of either toxic or ischemic nature. The health of the individual prior to the insult is usually good to adequate.

Etiology

Ischemic injury. The kidneys receive approximately 25% of the cardiac output. To maintain filtration pressure in the glomeruli and perfusion of the kidneys with oxygen sufficient for cellular metabolism, the body must maintain an adequate circulating volume of blood at a systolic pressure over 60 mm. Hg. Several disease states leading to acute renal failure arise from reduced circulating volume and decreased cardiac output. The response of the normal kidney to either of these conditions is vasoconstriction, which compounds the problem of reduced renal blood flow and increases renal ischemia. When ischemia is prolonged, renal tubular tissue dies and frank renal failure develops. Inadequate perfusion of the kidneys occurs commonly in those states summarized in the following outline. These perfusion problems affect both kidneys.

I Hypovolemia
  A Blood loss (surgery, trauma)
  B Plasma loss (burns, surgery, acute pancreatitis)

C Sodium and water loss (prolonged diarrhea, prolonged vomiting, gastrointestinal drainage, sustained high fever)
II Cardiac failure
  A Myocardial infarction
  B Cardiac arrhythmias
  C Congestive failure
III Septic shock

Nephrotoxic injury. A variety of substances are toxic to the cells of the renal tubules. The kidney with its large blood flow, ability to concentrate solute inside the tubules, and ability to concentrate fluid in the medullary portion of the kidney (where the tubules are located) creates conditions where exposure of tubular cells to toxins is maximized. The kidneys are affected bilaterally. Substances that cause toxic injury to the kidneys are as follows:

I Solvents (carbon tetrachloride, methanol, chloroform)
II Heavy metals (lead, arsenic, mercury)
III Antibiotics (kanamycin, gentamicin, polymyxin B, amphotericin B, colistin, neomycin, phenazopyridine)
IV Pesticides
V Mushrooms
VI Glycols (ethylene glycol antifreeze)

Other injuries. Additionally, other conditions can precipitate acute renal failure. These conditions commonly include (1) acute glomerular disease (p. 451), (2) acute severe infection of kidney tissue, (3) bilateral occlusion of the renal arteries, and (4) mechanical obstructions in the urinary tract. All of these conditions lead to massive and rapid destruction of kidney tissue.

Prognosis

As previously mentioned, acute renal failure is frequently a reversible process. The prognosis for return of function is dependent on the underlying cause of the illness. In many instances of toxic injuries to the kidneys, regeneration of tissue occurs (usually by 3 to 6 weeks), and the individual is left with little or no residual damage from the illness. When *ischemia* causes acute renal failure, there exists a greater likelihood of permanent kidney damage. Return of renal function is determined by the extent of tissue necrosis, varying from minimal residual damage to no return of kidney function. Approximately one half of adults with glomerulonephritis develop significant to total loss of kidney function after the acute phase of illness. Overall, approximately 30% of individuals who develop acute renal failure show signs of permanently reduced renal function.[70] Some of these individuals remain clinically well and others develop a chronic form of renal failure.

Because of the suddenness with which acute renal failure develops, the body shows little tolerance to the rapidly changing internal environment. Mortality from acute renal failure results from rapid changes in fluid and electrolyte balance and from the body's inability to withstand additional illness. Mortality in acute renal failure is most frequently attributed to potassium intoxication, fluid overload, acidosis, and infection.

Prevention

The incidence of acute renal failure can be reduced. Significant factors in preventive care for the general population include nephrotoxic drug control measures, public education efforts, and increased case finding and treatment of individuals with bacteriuria and obstructive disease of the urinary system.

The Federal Drug Administration (FDA) attempts to control the distribution and identification of nephrotoxic drugs and chemicals to the public. Prescription dispensing of various drugs increases chances for medical supervision so that dosage of the drug and measures of renal function can be periodically evaluated. Labeling of toxic chemicals and inhibiting the use of lead in paint are further legislative attempts to reduce public contact with potentially destructive agents.

Public education measures can reduce the incidence of acute renal failure. Since glomerulonephritis has been demonstrated to follow streptococcal infections, general health education includes advising medical attention for sore throats and other upper respiratory infections. Pyelonephritis accounts for a small percentage of individuals who develop acute renal failure, but it is a population where preventive measures are significant. Over 95% of cases of pyelonephritis are caused by gram-negative enteric bacilli.[7] Cleansing from front to back after bowel evacuation will reduce the numbers of such organisms entering the urinary tract. Health education of the public should stress that symptoms of pain or difficulty on urination should be medically evaluated. Proper labeling and storage of all potentially toxic drugs and chemicals in the home can reduce the number of accidental ingestions of nephrotoxic substances.

Increased case finding and treatment of individuals with bacteriuria and obstructive disease relies greatly on public education but also on the availability of such services to the population. The taking of a health history is becoming more prevalent in well-child care and health maintenance care. Routine urinalysis and questioning regarding the urinary system should be carried out yearly as a minimum health check. Individuals in risk categories for developing urinary tract problems, such as older men and pregnant women, should be closely evaluated for evidence of disease.

Since acute renal failure is often precipitated by inadequate perfusion of the kidneys, detection of excessive losses of body fluid is crucial in preventing kidney damage. Postoperative patients should have vital signs monitored frequently, dressings checked frequently, and all drainage from the body accurately recorded. All sources of abnormal fluid and electrolyte loss must be identified. Accurate fluid balance records are essential for determining the relationship of intake to output. Urinary output itself should be monitored in all individuals prone to perfusion problems; the physician in charge of the patient's care should be notified when output reaches a level of 20 ml./hour or less.

Inadequate perfusion of the kidneys results from inability of the heart to circulate the blood adequately and from expansion of the vascular bed, which decreases cardiac output. Early detection of pump failure can prevent prolonged ischemia in the kidneys. The volume of urine excreted by patients suspected of developing cardiac problems should be monitored and, again, the physician should be notified when urine volume appears to be decreasing.

Signs and symptoms

Signs and symptoms indicating the onset of acute renal failure appear rapidly and are a direct result of retention of fluids, electrolytes, and waste materials. Classically, the patient's urinary output falls suddenly. *Proteinuria* and *hematuria* may be present. The specific gravity of the urine is low and is similar to that of plasma (1.010 to 1.014); it remains within this range and reflects damage to the renal tubules with loss of ability to concentrate urine. Retention of fluid is reflected through development of such problems as central nervous system irritability, which can progress to stupor, coma, and convulsions; signs of congestive failure; and development of edema, especially of the legs and sacral and periorbital areas. Hypertension accompanies acute renal failure when the patient is hypervolemic.

Prominent electrolyte alterations are likely to include continued sharp increases in serum potassium, decreases in serum sodium and chloride caused by dilution of the serum with accumulating fluid, and a rise in the serum phosphorus level. Carbon dioxide content of the blood decreases as acidosis develops.

Retention of metabolic wastes is reflected early in the course of acute renal failure and is marked by rapidly rising blood urea nitrogen and creatinine levels. The urea nitrogen level may rise as much as 20 mg.%/day and is usually accompanied by nausea and vomiting.

When oliguria is noted, the physician initially determines whether the decreased urinary output is the result of inadequate perfusion of the kidneys or actual death of kidney tissue. This distinction is vital in treatment of the patient. Rapid restoration of blood flow through the kidneys prevents death of renal tissue and hence development of renal failure; treatment includes giving fluids or otherwise increasing cardiac output. In contrast, frank renal failure occurs

when kidney tissue has been destroyed; treatment involves restricting fluid intake.

The mannitol provocation test frequently is used in distinguishing oliguria of low renal blood flow from that caused by frank renal damage. Mannitol is an osmotic diuretic; it increases glomerular filtration in the undamaged kidney. Fifty grams of mannitol is infused intravenously, and the patient is observed for increasing urinary output. If the patient does not respond by producing more urine, the test may be repeated. If there is still no response to the osmotic load, a diagnosis of renal failure or shutdown is made, and further fluid loading is contraindicated.

The patient with severe oliguria or anuria is also evaluated for obstruction of the urinary tract. Cystoscopy and various x-ray techniques aid in detecting the presence of obstructive urinary tract disease.

Management

The course of acute renal failure is usually characterized by an initial oliguric phase followed in a number of days to a few weeks by a diuretic period. Major patient care problems during the oliguric phase of illness include (1) inability to excrete metabolic wastes, (2) inability to regulate electrolytes, (3) inability to excrete fluid loads, (4) difficulty maintaining adequate nutrition, (5) increased potential for physical injury, and (6) discomfort. Major patient care problems arising during the diuretic portion of the illness include (1) inability to appropriately conserve fluid and (2) inability to appropriately conserve electrolytes.

Oliguric phase

Inability to excrete metabolic wastes. Because the patient's ability to excrete metabolic wastes (nonprotein nitrogen products and acids) cannot keep pace with production of these substances, nursing care should be centered around two major objectives: (1) decreasing the metabolic load by decreasing production of wastes and (2) promoting excretion of volatile acid by the lungs.

Decreasing production of wastes can be partially achieved through dietary control. For the patient in acute renal failure a diet of 2,000 calories/day in the form of fats and carbohydrates is ordered. No protein is given unless the patient can be treated with dialysis, in which case protein intake of 20 to 40 Gm./day may be allowed. Calories in the form of carbohydrates and fats provide energy and spare body protein stores, thus decreasing nonprotein nitrogen production. The body recycles urea to synthesize amino acids for protein building so that regeneration of tissues can occur even though protein intake is curtailed. The patient will lose about $\frac{1}{2}$ pound/day of body weight on this diet. If the patient is unable to take food orally, intravenous feedings consisting of hypertonic glucose solutions will be administered. Between 100 and 200

Gm. of carbohydrate/day is infused; a large vein is used for the infusion to prevent irritation of the vein by the hypertonic solutions. If the patient is able to tolerate oral feedings, foods in the form of concentrated sweets and fats are given. Butter balls, cream, oils, hard candies, and syrups are encouraged.

Preventing infections and tissue breakdown decreases production of nonprotein nitrogen products. Aseptic technique should be rigorously pursued in all treatments performed on the patient. Indwelling catheters are a common source of infection and should be avoided. Isolation of the patient from anyone with an infection, patient or staff, should be carried out. Detecting existent infections early so that treatment can be promptly instituted decreases tissue breakdown. When the patient is extremely weak and immobile, frequent turning and repositioning to prevent bed sores must be performed. Skin care in patients with edematous tissues should include observation and prevention of pressure and trauma as these tissues are especially susceptible to breakdown.

Activity encouraged within the tolerance of the patient will help arrest *catabolism* of body tissue. The patient can begin activity gradually through assisting with feeding and sitting for short periods of time. Passive exercises should be performed for the patient when he is unable to expend the energy himself.

Daily laboratory work to determine nonprotein nitrogen levels should be performed because of the potential for rapid increase of these substances in the blood and development of nausea and vomiting. Any change in the patient's appetite or ability to tolerate food is significant and should be reported to the physician. Severe nausea and vomiting compound the problem of fluid and electrolyte management.

Acidosis develops when hydrogen ion secretion and bicarbonate ion production diminish in the tubular cells. The pH of the blood decreases, the carbon dioxide content decreases, and central nervous system symptom of drowsiness progressing to stupor and coma may appear. The lungs attempt to assist in regulation of acid-base balance by excreting more carbon dioxide; the rate and depth of respirations increase. To maximize this pathway for excretion of metabolic acids, pulmonary hygiene should be carried out. Preventing atelectasis and maintaining maximal lung expansion are goals for nursing care. Good pulmonary hygiene helps prevent development of a reservoir for infection within the body and in this manner decreases tissue breakdown.

Inability to regulate electrolytes. Some common electrolyte disturbances occurring in acute renal failure are hyperkalemia, hyponatremia (usually indicative of overhydration), and increased body sodium content. The ability of the kidneys to properly eliminate or conserve electrolytes varies greatly in acute renal failure. Each patient must be managed individually. Daily or more frequent assessment of laboratory data and clinical signs and symptoms is needed to determine current electrolyte abnormalities and need for treatment.

Hyperkalemia. In the normal individual the potassium ion is exchanged in the distal convoluted tubule of the nephron for either sodium or hydrogen ions; for the healthy person there is no mechanism in the body to conserve the potassium ion. However, in the individual with acute renal failure in whom a large number of tubular cells are no longer functional, there exists no mechanism to remove potassium from the body. Hyperkalemia is said to exist when the serum concentration of this ion reaches a level of 5.5 mEq./L. or higher. Serum concentrations of 7 to 10 mEq./L. can be quickly reached in acute renal failure and are incompatible with normal cardiac function and life. In addition to laboratory data, signs that indicate hyperkalemia are muscle weakness and change in the regularity and rate of the heartbeat.

To assist in controlling the rise of potassium, the nurse should provide care that (1) decreases the intake of potassium, (2) decreases the liberation of potassium from body tissues, (3) assists in the removal of potassium from the body by nonrenal means, and (4) evaluates the patient for signs and symptoms of potassium toxicity. Decreasing the intake of potassium is achieved by administering intravenous feedings or a diet in which potassium content is very low or absent. All fluids and drugs that the patient receives intravenously should be checked for potassium content. Some medications (for example, most penicillin preparations) contain large amounts of this ion. Controlling the breakdown of body tissues is extremely important in preventing a rapid rise in serum potassium. Prevention of pressure sores, trauma, bleeding, and infections should be major goals for nursing care. To promote the excretion of potassium from the body when the kidneys are nonfunctional, an exchange resin such as polystyrene sodium sulfonate (Kayexalate) is likely to be ordered for the patient. This drug reduces serum potassium by exchanging sodium for potassium ions in the intestinal tract. It can be administered orally, through nasogastric tubes, or by enema. The medication is given orally when the patient's condition permits; oral daily doses range from 15 to 60 Gm./day. When Kayexalate is administered in enema form, the usual dose is 50 Gm. of exchange resin for each enema; it may be repeated daily or as necessary to lower serum potassium. The medication is a powder that, when mixed, becomes a thick paste in a matter of seconds; therefore preparation should take place at the bedside just prior to its administration. If the patient is constipated or has not produced spontaneous bowel movements, a cathartic or cleansing enema should be given to ensure the elimination of the potassium-containing substance from the bowel.

In monitoring the patient for signs of potassium

toxicity, electrocardiography and laboratory determinations of serum potassium are the most reliable indicators. Pulse changes and muscle weakness do indicate increased levels of serum potassium but are not reliable indicators of the degree of rise.

Hyponatremia. Hyponatremia in acute renal failure most commonly develops with overhydration of the patient. The oliguric patient cannot excrete large volumes of urine; when the administration of sodium-free or low-sodium intravenous or oral fluids continues in such an individual, the serum is diluted and the serum concentration of sodium falls. Signs and symptoms of hyponatremia include warm, moist, flushed skin, muscle weakness, muscle twitching, and behavioral changes involving confusion, delirium, coma, and convulsions. Serum sodium concentrations will be below 130 mEq./L. The hematocrit value suddenly falls without evidence of bleeding; this is caused by hemodilution.

Nursing care is directed toward carefully controlling and monitoring all fluids given the patient. Intravenous administration sets must be regularly and frequently observed for correct flow rate. Devices that allow 50 to 150 ml. of fluid to be isolated from the main intravenous solution container and drip chambers that allow precise control of fluids through administration of smaller drops of fluid are added safety measures when giving fluids to anuric or oliguric individuals. Accuracy in fluid balance records is essential. For the patient who is unable to take medications with small amounts of fluid, medications may be given in soft foods such as applesauce. The patient should be monitored for signs or symptoms of a low serum sodium concentration. If the patient develops generalized continuous muscle twitching, convulsions may appear. Precautions to protect the patient from injury should be taken. Side rails on the bed should be padded, and an airway should be kept at the bedside. If the patient is irritable or confused, feelings of restraint may initiate agitation. Placing the bed so that the patient is able to see his surroundings and individuals entering his room may lessen feelings of confinement. A calm, positive approach to the confused or irritable patient is least likely to add additional stimuli.

Increased body sodium content. Increases in total body content of sodium also occur in acute renal failure. Commonly this occurs when the patient is receiving medications high in sodium content and excess sodium in the diet. Edema and increasing blood pressure indicate retention of sodium and fluids even though the serum sodium concentration may appear normal. Observations that the nurse should make in relation to retention of sodium and fluids are described in the section dealing with retention of fluids.

Inability to excrete fluid loads. The oliguric or anuric patient is unable to excrete more than minimal amounts of fluid. Nursing care should be directed toward three broad objectives: (1) monitoring the patient for signs of fluid overload, (2) maintaining the patient's energy expenditure at a level compatible with his state of health, and (3) controlling or helping the patient to control fluid intake.

Numerous observations should be made regarding the patient's state of hydration. All observations should be prominently recorded so that hour-to-hour and day-to-day comparisons can be made. Any finding indicating retention of fluids should be reported to the physician. Development of peripheral edema, pulmonary edema, and congestive heart failure occur with fluid overloading. Approximately 6 to 10 pounds of excess fluid must be present before signs of peripheral edema occur. Edema, or accumulation of fluid in the tissues, can first be noted in the feet and legs, the presacral area, and around the eyes. The patient may be questioned as to whether he notices that his rings, shoes, pants, and other clothing are more snug. The patient and family members may be able to note changes in facial appearance when puffiness exists when compared to premorbid states. When edema is massive, fingers pressed into the skin may leave indentations; this is termed *pitting edema.* Pulmonary congestion may be identified through such complaints as shortness of breath with minimal or no exertion, inability to sleep flat in bed, awakening at night with a cough, and a cough that is productive when none previously existed. Signs that are observed in a patient with severe fluid overload include rales (especially in the lung bases), distention of the neck veins when the patient is elevated at a 30-degree angle, hypertension (with or without headaches, visual changes, and nosebleeds), tachycardia, development of an S_3 heart sound, and increasing venous pressure.

Increasing fluid in the body also may be detected through daily weighing of the patient and accurate recording of fluid intake and output. The importance of these two measures in both nursing and medical management of the patient cannot be underestimated. These assessment tools allow day-to-day comparison of the patient's overall state of hydration and his response to treatment.

The patient who is severely dyspneic, who has tachycardia, or who has breakdown of his skin is expending much energy just maintaining his current functional status. Each patient must be individually assessed as to tolerance for activities of daily living and for ability to adequately ventilate and circulate oxygen and nutrients to the cells of his body. The patient who is dyspneic and has tachycardia may be most comfortable in a sitting position with his arms supported on an overbed table (Fig. 22-13). Elevation of the arms on the table and lowering of the abdominal organs by gravity through sitting will increase the area for lung expansion. Care is provided for the patient whenever his attempts to care for himself result in increased shortness of breath, increased pulse rate, and increased fatigue. For care of the patient in congestive heart failure and pulmonary edema, refer to p. 353. Edematous tissues are especially susceptible to injury. Frequent observation of the skin, a smooth bed without wrinkles and foreign objects, and good hygiene are necessary nursing measures.

Controlling fluid intake is essential when the ability to excrete fluid is limited. All fluid that the patient receives parenterally and orally with medications, meals, and snacks must total only slightly more than his output each day if severe overhydration is to be avoided (p. 113). Thirst is a problem that can defy control of fluid intake. Fortunately, when the patient's sodium intake is controlled, extreme thirst does not develop. Control of sodium seems the key to control of oral fluid intake. For the patient who is thirsty, ice chips may be given. Ice contains approximately three-fourths the amount of fluid, volume for volume, as water. Also, ice chips are usually retained in the mouth longer than a sip of water and therefore may be more satisfying. Suggestions for controlling parenteral administration of fluids are given on p. 124.

Difficulty in maintaining adequate nutrition. Dietary restrictions of protein, potassium, and sodium will be ordered for the patient in acute renal failure.

Two major problems exist in maintaining intake of calories for the patient with acute renal failure. The diet prescribed for the patient is generally not considered a palatable one. Some measures that can increase the acceptance of the diet include allowing the patient some choice in menu planning so that he may select those foods most acceptable to him, increasing the number of feedings and snacks per day to increase quantity of intake, and attractively arranging food on the patient's tray to increase the aesthetic value of the meal. Butter balls and high-fat foods are best taken when cold.

A second problem encountered in maintaining intake of calories is combating the anorexia usually experienced by the patient in acute renal failure. Gastrointestinal irritation, a common accompaniment of uremia, may be alleviated by evenly spaced administration of aluminum hydroxide antacids. General comfort of the patient should be assured prior to meals as pain and other discomfort decrease ability to eat. If the patient continually experiences nausea, oral feeding may not be possible. When sporadic nausea and vomiting are present, the patient may be able to take oral feedings if they are given $1/2$ to 1 hour after emesis. Prochlorperazine (Compazine) can be used to control vomiting; it should be given about $1/2$ hour prior to meals. Attention to oral care is imperative. Patients in uremia develop a strong odor of the breath and strong taste in the mouth that produce or exaggerate anorexia. Adherence to the diet itself improves anorexia; as the production of waste lessens and uremia becomes controlled, anorexia lessens also.

Increased potential for physical injury. Monitoring the safety of the patient is a major nursing responsibility. Specific care should include preventing falls and physical trauma, preventing infection, and preventing drug toxicity through monitoring drug therapy.

The patient in acute renal failure is weak, may be confused, and may have visual changes. The amount of supervision the patient should have in daily care must be continually assessed. Falls from bed, chairs, and when ambulating and transferring can be prevented by judiciously acting on observations of the patient's behavior and capabilities.

Infection is a leading cause of mortality in patients with acute renal failure. Nosocomial infections are readily contracted by patients whose ability to resist invading organisms is low. *Protective isolation* of the patient is used in some medical centers, while in others it is not felt to be necessary. However, the patient must avoid contact with known sources of infection, and strict attention to aseptic technique in all nursing procedures must be maintained.

Monitoring prescribed medications is a nursing responsibility. The route of excretion and signs of toxicity should be known for all medications that the patient receives. The potential for drug toxicity exists when medications normally excreted by the kidneys are retained in the body as a result of renal damage. Drugs should also be monitored for potassium and sodium content; large increases in daily intake of these ions can result from drug therapy.

Discomfort. Major discomforts that the patient in acute renal failure is likely to experience are headache, nausea, pain (if surgery or trauma is involved in the illness), thirst, and itching. Control of headaches is best achieved through control of blood pressure and fluid volume. Mild analgesics such as acetaminophen (Tylenol) or dextropropoxyphene (Darvon) may be used to provide temporary relief. Acetylsalicylic acid (aspirin) should not be used as it is a gastrointestinal irritant and may precipitate bleeding because the uremic patient's gastrointestinal tract is already inflamed and susceptible to ulceration. The development of nausea and vomiting occurs when waste products accumulate in the blood; when waste production can be controlled and waste can be excreted, nausea will be reduced. Symptomatic relief with antiemetics can be provided.

Pain can be safely managed for the uremic patient by administering analgesics such as meperidine (Demerol) and morphine. In giving these medications, the nurse should be aware that the central nervous system depression produced by them can compound that already present in the acidotic uremic patient. The synergistic effect of the patient's metabolic state and pain medications could lead to unconsciousness and death. When morphine and meperidine are administered to the patient, the frequency and amount of medication given should be reduced. The patient's level of awareness should be closely and accurately observed.

Thirst is best controlled by restricting sodium intake. Gum and hard candies are beneficial to some individuals. Fluids that are allowed the patient provide greater relief of thirst if spaced evenly throughout the day and if given between rather than with meals. Oral care to prevent dryness of the mouth helps to reduce the desire for fluids.

Since waste products are not being eliminated adequately by the kidneys, the gastrointestinal tract and the skin have an increased excretory function. As more wastes are accumulating and being eliminated by the skin, itching occurs. Total relief of itching comes about only when uremia is controlled. However, a few comfort measures offer some relief from the generalized pruritus that uremic patients experience. Dilute vinegar baths, a cool environmental temperature, antipruritic lotions, oatmeal baths, and preventing dryness of the skin help to temporarily control itching. Medications with antihistaminic properties may be ordered to control severe itching.

Diuretic phase

After the period of oliguria or anuria, which may last a few days to a week, most patients with acute renal failure pass into another distinct phase of illness. This phase is characterized by increasing urinary output. Increased output indicates that the damaged nephrons are healing and are able to begin excreting urine. At first, daily urine volume increases slowly and progresses in some instances to a diuresis of up to 4 to 5 L./day. Although fluid can be excreted, the kidneys are not yet healed. Often the patient is unable to excrete proportional amounts of waste materials, and serum concentrations of urea nitrogen and potassium may rise or remain elevated as urine volume increases. At times, excessive excretion of sodium occurs during diuresis. Complete recovery of renal function is slow and requires anywhere from days to a few weeks. Return of renal function to normal or near-normal levels is evidenced when the kidney can both conserve and dilute urine and when serum electrolytes and nonprotein nitrogen levels become normal.

Nursing care during the diuretic phase is directed toward detecting fluid losses and electrolyte imbalances. Most of the fluid excreted during diuresis in excess of an amount proportional to the patient's intake is fluid that has accumulated in the body during the oliguric phase of illness. However, serious fluid and electrolyte depletion can occur. In addition to detecting fluid and electrolyte imbalances, several nursing care objectives established during the oliguric phase should be continued. These include maintaining nutritional intake, maintaining safety of the patient, and preventing infection.

Nursing observations and records that are needed in judging the adequacy of hydration and serum sodium of the patient include (1) changes in mental awareness and activity, (2) degree of thirst, (3) moistness of mucous membranes, (4) development of skin turgor, (5) development of tachycardia and hypotension, and (6) accurate daily weight, fluid balance, and vital sign records.

■ CHRONIC RENAL FAILURE

Chronic renal failure exists when the kidneys are no longer capable of maintaining an internal environment consistent with life and when return of function is not anticipated. For the majority of individuals the transition from health to a state of chronic or permanent disease is a slow one extending over a number of years. Recurrent infections and exacerbations of nephritis, obstruction of the urinary tract, and destruction of vessels from diabetes and longstanding hypertension lead to scarring of kidney tissue and progressive loss of renal function. Some individuals, however, develop total irreversible loss of renal function acutely; such loss of renal function usually develops in a matter of a few hours or days and follows a direct traumatic insult to the kidneys.

Although the clinical course and picture of chronic renal disease does vary from individual to individual, there are common features of the illness. Azotemia, anemia, and acidosis are always present. Potassium and hydrogen ion excretion is impaired. Fluid and sodium balance is abnormal, although this may involve either abnormal retention or secretion of sodium and water. Consequently, urinary volume can be decreased, normal, or increased. Signs and symptoms of uremia usually develop so slowly that the patient and his family often do not recall the time of onset of the illness. Symptoms generally noticed as uremia develops include lethargy, headaches, physical and mental fatigue, weight loss, irritability, and depression. Anorexia, persistent nausea and vomiting, shortness of breath on either mild or no exertion, and pitting edema are symptomatic of severe loss of renal function.

Prognosis

The individual with chronic renal failure can to some extent control and manage the symptoms of his disease. Although renal function that has been lost due to destruction of kidney tissue cannot be recovered, the life of the patient can be maintained by limiting the intake of substances that require excretion and by providing alternative routes of excretion from the body for waste and electrolytes. By adhering to a prescribed management routine, albeit quite strict and demanding on the patient, life may be sustained indefinitely. For some individuals, medication and diet therapy alone may control uremic symptoms; other individuals may require, in addition, dialysis and/or transplantation to control the symptoms of their disease.

Prevention

Obstruction and infection of the urinary tract and hypertensive disease are common and often asymptomatic causes of renal damage and renal failure. A significant reduction in the incidence of renal failure can be effected through increasing attention to general health promotion. Yearly physical examinations in which blood pressure is determined, urinalysis is performed, and the patient is questioned about dysuria or pain in the urinary tract assist in early detection of disease that may lead to renal failure.

General health maintenance can reduce the number of individuals progressing from renal insufficiency into frank renal failure. Care is aimed toward adequately treating medical problems and closely supervising the patient's health status in times of stress (infection, pregnancy).

Management

Major problems for the patient in chronic renal failure include (1) inability to appropriately control fluid balance, (2) inability to regulate electrolyte balance, (3) inability to excrete metabolic wastes, (4) inability to transport oxygen to cells, (5) inability to maintain normal rest and sleep patterns, (6) difficulty in maintaining adequate nutrition, (7) increased potential for physical injury, (8) discomfort, (9) alterations in fertility, and (10) changes in lifestyle, group membership, and feelings regarding the self.

Inability to appropriately control fluid balance. The ability to excrete sodium and water in the urine varies considerably in chronic renal failure. Although volume problems for most patients with chronic renal failure involve hypervolemia resulting from a marked inability to excrete sodium and water, some patients are unable to conserve these substances and are subject to hypovolemic states. With either marked inability to excrete or conserve body fluid, the patient can develop severe fluid imbalances in a relatively short period of time. Care is directed toward identifying fluid imbalances and in providing an intake of sodium and water equivalent to the amounts of these substances excreted. The desired effect of this care is to maintain the patient in a normotensive, normovolemic state.

When the patient is unable to conserve sodium and fluid as the result of tubular damage, hypovolemia can result. Laboratory data reveal a rising he-

matocrit level that correlates with the patient's loss of intravascular volume. His cardiac output decreases, his pulse rate increases, and his blood pressure may drop. Behavioral changes are often the first symptoms of hypovolemia. Confusion, hallucinations, and delirium can be seen when volume depletion is severe. Nursing care involves monitoring the patient for signs of adequacy of fluid volume and replacing or helping the patient to replace the sodium and fluid lost in the urine.

When the patient is unable to excrete sodium and fluid, hypervolemia results. Signs and symptoms that arise with this problem relate to development of peripheral and pulmonary edema, hypertension, congestive heart failure, pericarditis, and effusion. Nursing care involves controlling or helping the patient to control sodium and fluid ingestion and monitoring the patient for signs and symptoms of overhydration. Observations indicating overhydration of the patient are described in the section on care of the patient with acute renal failure (p. 466). Controlling sodium intake can be an extremely challenging problem for both the nurse and the patient. Any sudden increase in weight indicates accumulating fluid, and the source of this fluid must be sought with the patient. Often when the patient is not acutely ill and is responsible for control of his intake, the problem can be traced to excess sodium ingestion, which produces thirst. In helping to avoid this cycle of thirst leading to increased fluid ingestion and overhydration, the patient should be carefully taught the allowances of sodium and fluid in his diet and what restrictions he is to observe in purchasing commercially prepared foods. The words "sodium" and "salt" should be sought on food labels when the patient is on a severely sodium-restricted diet, and these foods should be avoided. At times the patient is unable to offer explanation for increasing thirst and sodium ingestion. At this point the question of home self-medication (for example, sodium bicarbonate for indigestion) should be raised with the patient. After failure to uncover increased intake of either sodium or fluid to explain hypervolemia, the patient can be asked to list for a period of 3 consecutive days all food and fluids ingested. This list can then be reviewed with the patient and used, not only to uncover instances of dietary indiscretion but also as a teaching tool.

Inability to regulate electrolyte balance. Potassium and phosphorus retention occur in chronic renal failure. Nursing care is aimed toward identifying signs and symptoms of hyperkalemia and hyperphosphatemia and toward reducing intake and providing alternative routes of excretion for these substances from the body.

Signs of potassium intoxication and the role of cation exchange resins in utilizing the intestinal tract as an alternative route of excretion are discussed on p. 465. Serum potassium can be at least partially controlled for the patient with chronic renal failure by decreasing dietary and drug intake. Thorough diet teaching of the patient and all persons responsible for food preparation is essential. This teaching should help the patient identify the foods that are high in potassium and the methods of cooking that can reduce the potassium content of the diet. Salt substitutes should be avoided by all patients with chronic renal disease as they contain large amounts of potassium. Medications that are prescribed for the patient should be reviewed for potassium content.

Significant rises in serum potassium can be averted by preventing tissue breakdown. Potassium is largely an intracellular cation, and extensive tissue damage can liberate a lethal amount of this ion into the system of the patient with chronic renal failure. Patients should be advised to seek medical attention when symptoms of infection or other problems first appear. For the patient who is acutely ill, prevention of pressure sores is mandatory if control of potassium is to be achieved.

When the kidneys fail, the ability to excrete phosphorus decreases. A vicious cycle of ionized serum calcium depletion and bone demineralization can begin. The problem is identified by laboratory determinations of serum calcium and phosphorus levels and through radiographs of the hands, feet, and skull to show demineralized areas of bone. Treatment involves administering an aluminum hydroxide preparation. This medication binds phosphorus in the intestinal tract, thus providing an alternative route for phosphorus excretion. Usual doses of aluminum hydroxide range from 1 to 5 Gm./day. Since constipation is an expected side effect of aluminum hydroxide administration, patients should be placed on prophylactic laxative therapy.

Inability to excrete metabolic wastes. *Azotemia* and *acidosis* occur in all patients with chronic renal failure, although the severity of the problems and the degree to which the patient has developed tolerance to his altered internal environment vary considerably. Nursing care should be directed toward (1) decreasing the production of metabolic wastes, (2) promoting excretion of volatile acids by the lungs, and (3) detecting increasing acidosis and its clinical effect on the patient.

Metabolic waste production can be significantly reduced by controlling dietary protein intake and by preventing catabolism of existing protein stores. The amount of protein allowed in the diet for a patient with chronic renal failure can vary from 20 to 80 Gm./day. The specific level of protein intake prescribed for the patient depends on the presence of some means for clearing the products of protein breakdown from the patient's system. Dietary protein intake is more liberal for patients who have some ability to excrete wastes in their urine and for patients being treated with dialysis. When restricting dietary protein, the quality of that allowed must be high. The patient must be taught to select foods that contain all of the essential amino acids. When calories are provided in the form of carbohydrate and fat for immediate energy needs, smaller amounts of protein can suffice for cellular growth and repair. Catabolism of existing protein stores liberates nitrogenous wastes. For this reason sources of potential infection such as indwelling catheters are avoided, and when infection is noted, it is immediately treated.

In chronic renal failure the kidneys are unable to excrete hydrogen ions and to manufacture bicarbonate. Metabolic acidosis results. On the basis of laboratory data acidosis may appear to be severe; however, patients with chronic renal failure adjust to lowered serum bicarbonate levels and often do not become acutely symptomatic even when bicarbonate levels reach values of 14 to 16 mEq./L. Because of this adjustment, treatment of the patient with bicarbonate is often not carried out. The lungs assume a prominent role in regulating acid-base balance, and helping the patient to maintain pulmonary function becomes an important objective for nursing care. Nursing measures to prevent pulmonary congestion and maintain maximal lung expansion are discussed on p. 568.

Determining patient tolerance of a state of acidosis that can fluctuate from moderate to critical levels (as additional stresses to the patient occur such as infection and blood loss) is important in the nursing care given the patient. Severe acidosis results in central nervous system depression. In assessing the level of mental function of the patient, the nurse should note any changes in the individual's ability to carry on a conversation. Deteriorating ability to carry on a conversation may be a first sign of increasing acidosis. Often the family of the patient may be helpful in assessing his behavior. Family members are often acutely aware of increasing irritability and lethargy in the patient. When acidosis is severe, central nervous system depression can be manifested by stupor and coma. Respirations increase in rate and depth. Laboratory data reveal a lowered carbon dioxide content and bicarbonate level.

Inability to transport oxygen to cells. Anemia is universally present in patients with chronic renal disease. Hematocrit values of 16% to 22% are not abnormal for these individuals. Anemia results from both a decreased production in red blood cells and a decrease in longevity of the cells in circulation. Although oral iron supplements may be tried, iron is not well absorbed by the gastrointestinal tract in chronic renal failure, and in some individuals it may cause nausea and vomiting. Since dietary sources of folate (folic acid) may be restricted in chronic renal failure, and food preparation may further decrease the amount of folate ingested, this vitamin may be given as a medication. A sufficient dose is 1 mg./day. Transfusions are not generally given unless the hematocrit level becomes extremely low. The reason for this is that when transfusions are frequently given, the patient's own stimulus to red cell production is decreased.

The severely anemic patient complains of extreme fatigue and shortness of breath. Because of a lack of red cells, the patient is unable to transport sufficient oxygen to his cells for energy production. Milder complaints of the anemic patient include an inability to work or play without extended rest periods. Nursing activities can be directed toward helping the patient identify activities essential to his daily living and helping him to modify these activities according to his energy level. Preventing the accumulation of excess fluid in a patient with a very low hematocrit level can allow the patient to use the energy he produces for activities of daily living rather than for carrying extra fluid. Other important nursing activities include helping the patient to control blood losses. A soft toothbrush is recommended for oral care. Antacids taken at regular and frequent intervals can reduce gastrointestinal tract bleeding. The patient should be instructed to observe for melena and to report this finding to the physician without delay.

Inability to maintain normal rest and sleep patterns. Insomnia and chronic daytime fatigue are common complaints of patients with chronic renal failure. This reversal of normal sleep patterns has been attributed to a variety of causes. These include (1) recurring occupation with thoughts concerning the disease state and changes in life-style required by the illness, (2) pruritus, and (3) the state of uremia itself. Reduction of high serum levels of urea nitrogen and creatinine through decreasing dietary intake of protein and/or dialysis may bring sleep patterns more toward normal. When control of uremia fails to cure insomnia, central nervous system depressants such as barbiturates and ethanol may be ordered. Barbiturates are primarily metabolized by the liver and can be safely administered in normal doses. Ethanol is also metabolized by the liver and can be used to induce sleep and calm the patient.

General comfort at bedtime is needed to induce sleep at any time and is especially important whenever sleeping problems arise. Comfort measures can include warm baths, pursuing quiet activities an hour or two before bedtime, controlling itching, or anything the patient finds calming and soothing.

The individual who is awake a significant portion of the night may need to plan for rest periods during the day. These rest periods should be taken far enough ahead of bedtime to prevent compounding sleeplessness.

Difficulty maintaining adequate nutrition. Maintaining a good nutritional intake can be difficult for patients with chronic renal failure. Anorexia, nausea, and vomiting frequently occur, and diets can be so severely restricted that they bear little resemblance to the normal dietary patterns of the patient. In uremia, disturbances in fluid, electrolyte, and waste composition of body fluids occur and produce changes in osmotic gradients in all cells. When these changes occur in the cells of the gastrointestinal tract and the central nervous system, anorexia, nausea, and vomiting result. Uremic patients are prone to bleeding of the gastrointestinal tract and the oral cavity. Urea is broken down to ammonia by the action of intestinal bacteria. Since ammonia is a mucosal irritant, ulceration and bleeding can occur. In addition to the gastrointestinal tract problems that lead to anorexia, nausea, and vomiting, there is a decreased salivary flow in patients with chronic renal disease. An ammonia smell and taste can accumulate in the mouth quickly and can further compound anorexia. Treatment includes administering antacids every 2 to 4 hours. Dietary control of uremia, perhaps augmented by dialysis, should help to control disturbances in fluid, electrolyte, and waste composition of body fluids and thus help to control nausea and vomiting. Oral hygiene, especially before meals, is important to combat anorexia.

Modifying the diet as possible to the preferences of the patient can also help to maintain intake of food. Dietary teaching and meal planning can be approached according to an exchange system similar to that used for individuals having diabetes. With this approach, patients have greater ability to modify the diet according to personal preferences. The pattern of meals during the day is also a matter of personal preference. Some patients may prefer a number of small feedings; others may prefer two or three meals a day. When the patient's eating patterns are known and used in dietary instruction and meal planning, intake of food is likely to increase.

Actual eating of prepared food can be promoted through attempting to decrease emotional tension at the dinner table. Periods other than mealtime should be used to discuss family and individual problems. Food that is attractively arranged and well flavored is likely to be more acceptable to the patient. Spices and other flavorings can add variety to foods that are prepared without sodium. Interestingly, most patients relate that their taste for salt disappears once they have adhered to a low-sodium diet for a few weeks. When the patient's gastrointestinal tract is ulcerated, bland foods may be tried in an attempt to increase ingestion of food.

Increased potential for physical injury. Common injuries to the patient in chronic renal failure include infection, accidents due to decrease in mental and visual awareness of the environment, and improper usage of medications. In chronic renal failure the patient's resistance to infection is decreased. Control of infection is essentially similar to that described in the section on care of the patient in acute renal failure. In addition, the patient should be counseled to avoid exposure to individuals with known infections and to avoid extreme fatigue, which lowers body resistance.

The buildup of osmotically active particles and fluid in the body that occurs in uremia produces changes in the cells of the brain that may lead to confusion and impairment in decision-making ability. In some instances, convulsions and coma may result from the changed internal environment. Fluid accumulation and hypertension can produce visual changes. Nursing care should involve assessing and helping the family to assess the safety of the decisions that the patient makes and his awareness of the environment. At times the patient may need to be helped in limiting activities to a level commensurate with his mental processes and level of awareness. For instance, blurred vision and delayed reaction time should contraindicate driving an automobile. Convulsions and coma may result from severe fluid, electrolyte, and waste imbalances. In most instances when the patient is subject to developing these complications, he will be hospitalized. Individuals caring for the patient need to be aware of the possibility of seizure activity and take appropriate precautions. Correcting abnormal body chemistry is the most important measure for preventing coma or convulsions.

Education about medications should be carried out with the patient in the areas of both medications that have been prescribed for him and "over-the-counter" or "folk" medicines. The use of common popular medications that are sold without prescription must be discouraged. All medications should be prescribed by the patient's physician. Aspirin is dangerous because it is normally excreted by the kidneys and may rapidly build to toxic levels. Ingestion of sodium bicarbonate (baking soda) to treat indigestion can result in extremely large intakes of sodium. Many cold preparations also contain large amounts of sodium. Remembering to take prescribed medications can be a problem for the patient who may have to take over 2 dozen pills each day. Correlating pill-taking times with major activities of the day is often helpful. Medications that are frequently given to patients with chronic renal failure include vitamins, antihypertensives, antibiotics, diuretics, cation exchange resins, aluminum hydroxide preparations, laxatives, and miscellaneous drugs such as oral calcium, oral iron, and allopurinol.

Discomfort. Rarely should the patient with chronic renal failure have acute sharp pain; however, these individuals are subject to a wide variety of chronic discomforts. Most commonly these discomforts include pruritus, muscle cramping, numbness and tingling in the hands and feet, thirst, headaches, and irritation of the eyes. Most patients with end-stage renal disease develop pruritus. Patients relate that the itching is of a deep sensation. A variety of theories have been postulated as to the origin of the itching. However, the exact cause of this problem has not yet been identified. Factors that seem to exacerbate the itching that the patient experiences include increasing levels of serum phosphorus, dry skin, warm moist heat, and emotional stress. Itching is largely symptomatic and measures that are effective in controlling it vary from individual to individual. Reducing levels of serum phosphorus with aluminum hydroxide preparations decreases itching for most patients. Keeping the skin moist and supple through use of lotions and bath oils, controlling the room temperature during sleep to prevent excessive warmth, emollient baths, and bathing with a vinegar solution are measures alone or in combination that may provide some relief from itching. Medications such as trimeprazine tartrate (Temaril) are also prescribed on a p.r.n. basis and for some individuals provide much relief from itching. Since emotional stress seems to increase the itching, helping the patient discuss his feelings to provide for some resolution of conflict may help decrease these manifestations of psychologic stress. The urge to scratch the skin is acute in some patients. Because scratching is often vigorous, injury to the skin with subsequent infection can result. Patients should be encouraged to keep their fingernails trimmed closely. In preference to fingernails, a soft cloth should be used to "scratch" the skin.

Muscle cramping in the lower extremities and the hands is common in renal failure. Often cramping can be correlated with sodium depletion in the patient; however, it frequently occurs when electrolyte abnormalities are not present. Primary treatment for muscle cramping involves controlling the state of uremia. Temporary measures of heat and massage are effective for some patients.

Some degree of peripheral neuropathy occurs in almost all patients with chronic renal failure. Numbness, tingling, and burning of the extremities are common complaints. Treatment that is effective in controlling these symptoms consists of more intensive management of the uremic state.

Thirst occurs in the patient whose sodium intake has been proportionately greater than his fluid intake. The key to controlling thirst lies in controlling the patient's sodium intake. When fluid intake is severely restricted, the patient may also need some assistance in planning how to allocate fluids during the day so that he will not use his entire fluid allotment early in the day.

Headaches in chronic renal failure result from a variety of causes. These include increasing blood pressure, progressing uremia, and rapid changes in osmotic gradients between cellular, interstitial, and intravascular compartments. Treatment of these problems has been discussed previously.

Ocular irritation in chronic renal failure is caused by calcium deposits in the conjunctiva. The patient complains of burning and watering in his eyes. Treatment involves controlling the plasma phosphate level through administration of oral aluminum hydroxide preparations. "Artificial tears" (methylcellulose) placed in the conjunctival sac every few hours can reduce irritation for the patient.

Alterations in fertility. As end-stage renal failure develops, most women note changes in their menstrual cycle. Bleeding may occur at more widely spaced intervals, may be heavier or lighter in flow than normal, or may cease all together. This obvious change in reproductive cycle is usually accompanied by changes in fertility. Ovulation may occur normally or may only occur a few times a year. Pregnancy in uremic women is of much lower incidence than in the normal population. In males, impotence may occur as chronic renal failure progresses toward end-stage disease. Dialysis or more vigorous treatment of uremia is indicated to return or maximize reproductive function. It should be stressed that sexual activity of some patients with chronic renal failure may remain quite normal, even though changes in reproductive ability are present.

Changes in life-style, group membership, and feelings regarding self. Numerous alterations in life-style, group membership, and feelings regarding the self occur for the patient with chronic renal failure. The numerous physical changes that occur often make it difficult to carry on activities that were once normally pursued. Chronic fatigue may make it impossible for the patient to continue with his former occupation. Because the patient is often tired and not feeling well, it may be difficult for him to plan in advance for social events. The former roles of the sick member of the family must often be taken on by another. When roles cannot easily be changed or additionally assumed by other members of the family, serious threats to the organization of the family group occur. Physical appearance also changes and is of much concern to most patients. As uremia progresses, the patient often becomes thin and weaker and appears sallow. Thoughts concerning death and the quality of this changed life are common.

Denial often becomes a chief defense mechanism for the patient. With it the individual can periodically forget the constant threat to his life and his family. The use of this mental mechanism for the patient with chronic renal failure can be quite appropriate as long as it is not manifested by maladaptive or harmful behavior. Inappropriate uses of denial involve continuous dietary indiscretion and failure to take prescribed medications.

The patient with chronic renal failure needs the hope and encouragement that with treatment he will be able to live with a lessening of discomfort and will have a continued existence to pursue what seems most productive and important to him. Hope should not be focused on cure but on learning to manage a new style of life. In managing the changes that occur as a result of chronic renal failure, the patient should be encouraged to be as independent and as active as possible. He should be taught to manage his treatment and should be given the responsibility of doing so. Nursing care should be provided as part of the team approach that assists the patient in identifying problems and resources and helps the patient and his family adjust to the changing style of life.

Management of the terminally ill patient

At times nursing care must be provided for the patient who is dying from renal failure. Major objectives should be maintaining the comfort and the safety of the patient and providing opportunity for the patient and his family to vent feelings and arrive at some degree of emotional comfort. In providing physical comfort to the patient, diets may be liberalized. Frequent turning and repositioning are necessary to prevent skin excoriation and breakdown. Oral care is extremely important since sores in the mouth, once developed, are almost impossible to cure. Mineral oil is an acceptable protective lubricant for the alert patient. A water-soluble lubricant with a vegetable base (such as KY jelly) is preferable for the stuporous patient. Hydrogen peroxide is helpful in removing blood from the mouth and the nose.

As death approaches, the patient often becomes severely confused or comatose. As his level of awareness and ability to control the environment decrease, it becomes the responsibility of the nursing staff to provide safety for the patient. The specific care required for a comatose patient is described on p. 187.

Providing an opportunity for the patient and family to ventilate feelings is one of the more important aspects of nursing care for a patient with either acute or chronic onset of uremia. Thoughts concerning death and alarm over treatments produce considerable anxiety. The wishes of the patient and family regarding spiritual counseling should be determined. Through demonstrating interest in the patient's needs and attending to his comfort, the nurse can do a great deal to help the patient and his family accept the patient's ultimate death.

Dialysis and renal transplantation

Dialysis. Dialysis involves the movement of fluid and particles across a semipermeable membrane. It is a treatment that can help restore normal fluid and electrolyte balance, control acid-base balance, and remove waste and toxic material from the body. It is a treatment that can sustain life successfully in

OSMOSIS   DIFFUSION

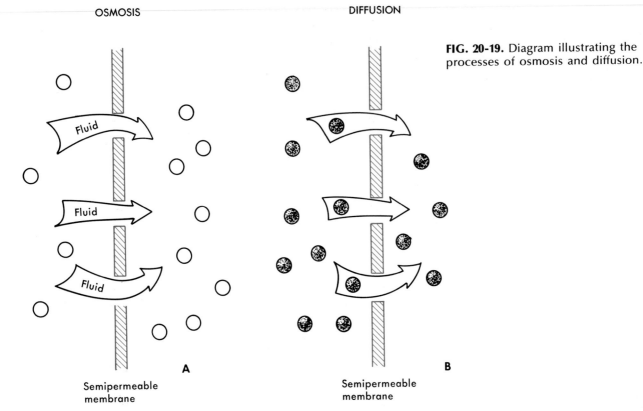

FIG. 20-19. Diagram illustrating the processes of osmosis and diffusion.

A

Semipermeable
membrane

B

Semipermeable
membrane

both acute and chronic situations where substitution for or augmentation of normal renal function is needed. Specifically, dialysis is used to remove excessive amounts of drugs and toxins in poisonings of both an intentional and accidental nature, to correct serious electrolyte and acid-base imbalances, to maintain kidney function when renal shutdown occurs as a result of transfusion reactions, to temporarily replace renal function in patients with acute renal failure of various origins, and to permanently substitute for loss of renal function in patients with chronic end-stage kidney disease.

Dialysis is based on two principles: osmosis and diffusion (Fig. 20-19). Osmosis involves the movement of fluid across a semipermeable membrane from an area of lesser to an area of greater concentration of particles. Diffusion involves the movement of particles from an area of greater to an area of lesser concentration. In the body this usually occurs across a semipermeable membrane.

During dialysis, osmosis and diffusion occur simultaneously (Fig. 20-20). Dialysis occurs when the patient's blood is brought in contact with a solution called the dialysate. This solution contains none or little of the particles that must be removed from the patient's bloodstream; it does contain substances that should be added to the patient's blood. Generally, the dialysate is slightly higher in total particle concentration than is the body fluid of the patient. The dialysate is separated from the patient's blood by a thin semipermeable membrane.

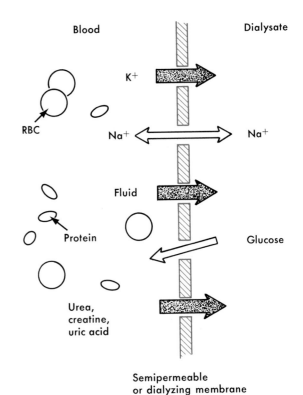

FIG. 20-20. Osmosis and diffusion in dialysis. Net movement of major particles and fluid are illustrated.

474

The principle of osmosis is demonstrated in dialysis when fluid is removed from a patient. In Fig. 22-20, glucose has been added to the dialysate to make its particle concentration greater than that of the patient's blood. Fluid will then move through the pores of the semipermeable membrane from the patient's blood to the dialysate.

The principle of diffusion is illustrated by the movement of urea, creatinine, and uric acid from the patient's blood to the dialysate. Since the dialysate contains no particles of this nature, the concentration of these protein waste products in the patient's blood will decrease because of random movement of the particles across the semipermeable membrane into the dialysate. The same principle applies to the movement of potassium ions. Although the concentration of red blood cells and protein is high in the patient's blood, these molecules are quite large and do not diffuse through the pores of the seimipermeable membrane. Hence they are not lost from the blood.

Hemodialysis. Hemodialysis has been a practical life-saving treatment for patients with impaired renal function for approximately 15 years. The major limitations in providing this treatment to all individuals who could benefit from it are the expense of equipment and the necessity of highly trained personnel. The availability of hemodialysis, especially for the chronically ill patient, still lags behind need. Home dialysis, established in the last few years, is an attempt to bridge this gap.

Hemodialysis involves shunting the patient's blood from the body through a machine in which diffusion and osmosis occur and back into the patient's circulation. In order to perform hemodialysis there must be an access to the patient's blood, a mechanism to transport the blood to and from the dialyzer, and a dialyzer, or area in which the exchange of fluid electrolytes and waste products occurs.

Presently, two major means exist for gaining access to the patient's bloodstream. These are the external shunt and arterial venous fistula. The external shunt (Fig. 20-21, A) is constructed by placing a cannula through a skin incision into a large vein and a large artery that lie close to each other. When dialysis is not occurring, the cannulas are connected to each other so that blood continually flows through the tubes, and patency of the system is maintained. For dialysis the cannulas are separated. The arterial cannula is connected to a line that delivers the patient's blood to the dialyzer; the venous cannula is attached to a line that returns blood to the patient's body. Infection, clotting of the shunt, and erosion of the skin around the insertion area of the cannulae are problems that occur with enough frequency to limit general use of the external shunt to situations that are acute and temporary.

The other common method of access to the pa-

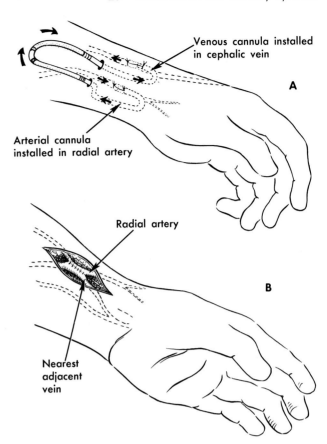

FIG. 20-21. Two common forms of venous access for hemodialysis. **A,** External shunt. **B,** Arteriovenous fistula.

tient's blood supply is the arteriovenous fistula (Fig. 20-21, B). Here a large artery and vein are sewn together below the surface of the skin. Access to the patient's blood is established during dialysis by inserting needles of large diameter into the fistula. The fistula, like the shunt, is generally located in an upper extremity, although the legs may also be used.

Precautions must be taken to maintain the patency of a shunt or fistula. During the patient's hospitalization it is the nurse who is the most consistent observer of the shunt or fistula, and the individual most able to see that precautionary measures are followed by all individuals dealing with the patient. To ensure proper maintenance of the shunt or fistula in the home, the same care that the nurse provides in the hospital must be taught to the patient and/or his family.

Decreasing the flow of blood through the shunt or fistula for even short periods of time can result in clotting. Decreased blood flow results from (1) systemic hypotension, (2) compression of the shunt or fistula, (3) inflation of the blood pressure cuff when taking the blood pressure, (4) tight bandages or restrictive clothing, (5) phlebitis from punctures of the involved veins, and (6) infection of the shunt or fistula. All of the above must be avoided.

Because the external shunt involves a break in the surface of the skin, special attention is given to preventing infection. A dry, sterile dressing that is changed daily should cover the shunt. The cannula insertion sites should be observed for any signs of infection. Any redness, tenderness, swelling, or excessive warmth of the skin in these areas should be reported at once to the physician.

Clotting of the shunt or fistula can be detected by an absence of the palpable or audible *bruit* along the venous portion of the shunt or fistula. Since blood can be observed as it flows through a shunt, clotting may also be detected by the presence of dark or separated blood in the tubing. When it is suspected that a shunt has clotted, the physician should be notified immediately, as it may be possible to clear the shunt.

Several types of hemodialyzers are currently in use (Fig. 20-22). Although quite different in appearance, all artificial kidneys function similarly.

Prior to the procedure, the patient should have an opportunity to familiarize himself with the dialysis unit. He should be given an explanation of what will happen to him and what will be expected of him during the treatment. The patient often wants to know (1) what types of pain he will experience during the treatment, (2) how long and how often the dialysis will be, (3) what he should feel like after the treatment, (4) what he will be allowed to do and to eat during dialysis, and (5) if his family may be present during the therapy.

When the patient has an external shunt, no pain should be experienced during initiation of dialysis. However, pain of a moderate degree may be present when venipuncture is performed in an arterial venous fistula. A local anesthetic is used in most dialysis centers prior to insertion of the needles.

The patient should be told that he may experience some nausea and headache during the treatment and for a few hours afterward. Headache and nausea result from changes in fluid, electrolyte, and waste balance during dialysis. The patient should be assured that these symptoms will abate and that his condition will be frequently monitored to control the degree of change that occurs in his body and hence the development of these symptoms.

A dialysis treatment lasts from 3 to 10 hours, depending on the type of dialyzer used and the time necessary to correct the fluid, electrolyte, acid-base, and waste problems that are present. Dialysis for an acute problem may be carried out daily or every few days as the condition of the patient warrants. Chronic hemodialysis is usually performed two or three times a week.

Many patients expect to leave the dialysis treatment with a feeling of well-being. Few patients feel this way; most experience some minor discomfort that diminishes a few hours after dialysis. The greatest feeling of well-being seems to occur the day after dialysis.

Eating and activity during dialysis are largely a matter of patient preference. Some patients sleep throughout their treatment; others may read and carry on various activities. The patient's ability to eat while being dialyzed must be individually determined. Some individuals may become quite hungry, while for others the smell of food causes nausea. Patients may ask that they be allowed to eat anything they wish during dialysis. This practice may be discouraged for two reasons: (1) dietary indiscretion adds extra waste that must be cleared from the patient's system and (2) the entire dialysis situation should be used to help the patient understand and adhere to his therapeutic plan.

Nursing care of the patient on hemodialysis should center around (1) monitoring the physical status of the patient prior to and during dialysis for evidence of physiologic imbalance and change, (2) comfort and safety needs of the patient, and (3) helping the patient to understand and adjust to the care and changes in life-style that he is experiencing. This latter objective involves educating the patient as to the specifics of his treatment program (diet and medications in particular) and how these relate to his altered kidney function. The patient should be encouraged to express his concerns and feelings, and attempts must be made to help the patient work through his feelings (Fig. 20-23).

Prior to dialysis the patient is weighed, his temperature and vital signs are taken, a sample of blood

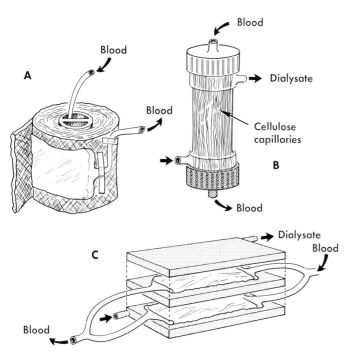

FIG. 20-22. Examples of commonly used dialyzers. **A,** Coil dialyzer. **B,** Hollow fiber dialyzer. **C,** Kiil (flat plate) dialyzer.

is usually drawn to determine the level of serum electrolytes and waste products, and the patient's physical status is assessed.

Most physical problems that occur for patients during dialysis are related to hypotension from excessive removal of fluid, disequilibrium from a rapid reduction in extracellular electrolytes and wastes, and bleeding due to the heparinization needed to prevent blood from clotting while passing through the dialyzer. Hypovolemia and shock can occur during dialysis as a result of rapid removal of fluid from the intravascular compartment. Since this can occur faster than reequilibration of intracellular and intravascular volume relationships, the patient may appear edematous and yet exhibit signs of shock. Signs and symptoms that indicate that the intravascular volume is being rapidly depleted are anxiety, restlessness, dizziness, nausea and vomiting, diaphoresis, hypotension, and tachycardia.

To avoid depleting the patient's intravascular space and producing shock, the blood pressure and pulse rates are checked every 30 minutes, more frequently when the patient shows any of the previously mentioned signs and symptoms. Blood pressure readings should show only a slight gradual drop during the course of dialysis. Because the rate and pressure at which blood flows through the dialyzer are proportional to the rate and amount of fluid removed, blood flow is carefully monitored. (A flow rate of 200 ml. of blood/minute or more can be obtained in dialysis.) Unless the patient is severely hypertensive, rapid-acting antihypertensive medications are usually withheld the morning of dialysis and until after the treatment has been completed.

In treating a patient who shows signs of hypovolemia, initial nursing measures include determining the blood pressure and pulse, placing the head of the bed in a flat position, and raising the patient's feet. Administration of normal saline solution may be necessary to restore blood pressure. Throughout a hypotensive episode, the patient's vital signs, his level of consciousness, and any complaints offered should be closely monitored. It is important for the nurse to know that vomiting frequently accompanies hypotension. Because an upper extremity of the patient must be maintained fairly immobile during the dialysis, it may be awkward for the patient to clear his mouth if vomiting should occur. The patient should be helped to a safe position so that aspiration will be avoided.

The patient is weighed before and after dialysis to determine the amount of fluid loss during treatment. When the weight losses of several dialysis treatments are correlated with the patient's blood pressure, pulse, and other indications of hypovolemia, an individual pattern of the patient's tolerance to fluid removal can be determined. This trend or pattern can be used to help adjust the rate and overall effect of the dialysis in keeping with the patient's physiologic tolerance.

A *disequilibrium phenomena* occurs for many dialysis patients. This syndrome occurs toward the end or after dialysis. It results when excess electrolytes and waste are cleared from the blood more rapidly than they can diffuse from the central nervous system into the vascular compartment. Hence the disequilibrium exists in the concentration of particles inside and outside of the cells of the central nervous system. Because particle content is greater inside the cells of the central nervous system, water is taken into the cells and edema results. Signs and symptoms of disequilibrium include headache, restlessness, mental confusion, and nausea and vomiting. Severe disequilibrium may result in convulsions, especially in children when blood urea nitrogen levels exceed the concentration of 100 mg./ml.

Treatment includes keeping the patient quiet, reducing environmental discomfort such as tempera-

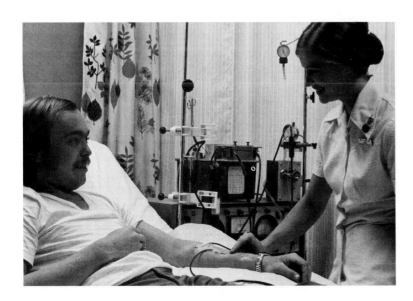

FIG. 20-23. A professional nurse must provide physical and emotional support to the patient receiving hemodialysis.

477

ture extremes and bright lights, and remaining with the patient to ensure his physical safety. Mild analgesics may help to relieve headache. If disequilibrium becomes severe and the patient is still on dialysis, the therapy may be discontinued. Disequilibrium reactions are more likely to occur during the first few dialysis treatments.

Care of the patient on dialysis should also include preventing blood loss. To prevent the patient's blood from clotting as it flows through the dialyzer, heparin is administered. Protamine sulfate may or may not be given to the patient to counteract the effect of heparin. The patient should be watched for signs of bleeding anywhere in the body. At the end of the treatment when dialysis needles are removed from the fistula, pressure dressings are applied to the puncture sites. They must be observed at frequent intervals to detect hemorrhage. During and shortly after dialysis, treatments that cause tissue trauma should not be performed. These commonly include venipuncture and intramuscular injections. The patient who has had recent surgery, dental extractions, or recent trauma to soft tissues will be given protamine sulfate during dialysis to prevent hemorrhage.

These patients need to be closely observed for signs of bleeding.

Nursing care should also include measures to increase the patient's physical comfort. Lying relatively immobile for a period of 4 to 8 hours can produce pressure over bony prominences and general restlessness. Massaging of pressure areas and changing the patient's position increase tolerance to limited movement. Mouth care is required if the patient is nauseated and vomiting. Because an upper extremity is generally kept immobile during dialysis, the patient will need help at mealtimes.

Peritoneal dialysis. In peritoneal dialysis the dialyzing fluid is instilled into the peritoneal cavity and the peritoneum becomes the dialyzing membrane (Fig. 20-24). In comparison to hemodialysis treatments, which last 3 to 8 hours, peritoneal dialysis is maintained continuously for up to 36 hours. The procedure, once instituted, becomes largely a nursing responsibility.

Prior to starting the treatment, the nurse should check the patient's understanding of what is to happen to him and should report any serious apprehensions of the patient to the physician. Mild sedation

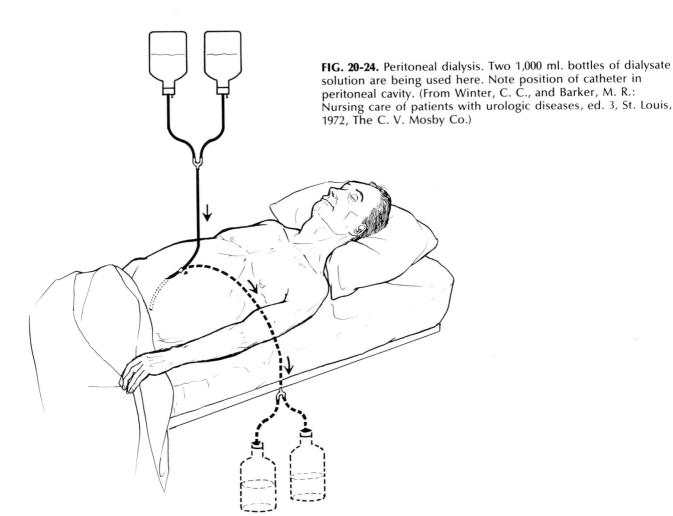

FIG. 20-24. Peritoneal dialysis. Two 1,000 ml. bottles of dialysate solution are being used here. Note position of catheter in peritoneal cavity. (From Winter, C. C., and Barker, M. R.: Nursing care of patients with urologic diseases, ed. 3, St. Louis, 1972, The C. V. Mosby Co.)

may help the severely anxious patient to better tolerate the insertion of the catheter. The patient's weight, blood pressure, and pulse should be recorded. These values serve as baseline information to use in assessing changes in the patient's condition. The patient should void just prior to start of the dialysis; this will decompress the bladder and prevent accidental puncture during catheter insertion. To insert the peritoneal catheter, the physician cleanses the abdomen and anesthetizes a small area in the midline of the abdomen below the umbilicus. He then makes a small incision and inserts a many-eyed, semirigid nylon catheter into the peritoneal cavity (Fig. 20-25). During insertion, the catheter is supported by a metal guide. The metal guide is then removed and a dressing is placed around the protruding catheter. Two liters of sterile dialysate (similar to that used in the artificial kidney) warmed to body temperature are attached by tubing to the catheter and allowed to run into the peritoneal cavity as rapidly as possible. This usually takes about 10 minutes. The tubing is then clamped, and 10 to 30 minutes are allowed for osmosis of fluid and diffusion of particles into the dialyzing solution. At the end of the dwell time the tubing is unclamped and the fluid is allowed to flow freely from the patient's abdomen. Fluid should drain in a steady stream. Drainage time should average about 10 to 15 minutes. The first drainage may be pink tinged as a result of the trauma of catheter insertion; however, this should clear with the second or third drainage. At no time should fluid draining from the abdomen appear grossly bloody. After fluid has drained from the abdomen, another cycle is started immediately. After the dialysis has been completed, the physician removes the catheter and covers the incision with a dry, sterile dressing. The small abdominal wound should heal completely in 1 to 2 days.

Hypotension is a frequent complication of peritoneal dialysis. As with hemodialysis, it results from rapid removal of fluid from the patient's intravascular space. In addition to checking vital signs and observing the patient's behavior, records of fluid balance are crucial in determining the amount of fluid that has been removed. The net gain or loss of fluid from the abdomen should be determined at the completion of each cycle. To decrease the amount of fluid that is being removed from the patient's vascular space, the physician may decrease the hypertonicity of the dialysate and may increase the rate at which fluid is running through an intravenous line.

Drainage of fluid from the abdomen can be slow or impossible to start. Generally this problem results when the tip of the catheter has become lodged against abdominal tissues. It may also result from plugging of the catheter with blood or fibrin that has accumulated as a result of tissue trauma. A small amount of heparin may be added to the dialysate to decrease the chance of a clot forming in the catheter. When the dialysate does not drain freely from the abdomen, the patient should be turned from side to side in an attempt to reposition the catheter in the peritoneal cavity. In addition, firm pressure may be applied to the abdomen with both hands, and the head of the bed may be raised. If the flow of the dialysate does not increase, the physician should be called to alter the position of the catheter.

Severe pain should not be experienced during peritoneal dialysis. Moderate levels of pain are often experienced as fluid is instilled and withdrawn from the peritoneal cavity. Procaine hydrochloride may be instilled with the dialysate in an attempt to control the patient's discomfort. Analgesics may be ordered for administration at 3- to 4-hour intervals during the procedure.

When the patient is markedly overhydrated and shows evidence of congestive failure and pulmonary edema, respiratory difficulty may be encountered as the dialyzing fluid infuses. The quality and rate of respiration should be closely observed. The head of the bed can be raised to decrease the pressure of the dialysate on the diaphragm. The patient, although encouraged to eat while being dialyzed, may find that this increases respiratory difficulty. To help overcome additional pressure created by a full stomach, frequent, small meals may be provided. The amount of dialyzing fluid used for each cycle may be decreased when respiratory distress becomes prolonged and severe.

Peritonitis is an ever-present threat during peritoneal dialysis. Aseptic technique must be rigidly maintained during insertion of the catheter and throughout the procedure. Care should be taken to avoid contaminating the solution or the tubing when new bottles of dialysate are hung. Cultures of the dialysate fluid and of the catheter tip are performed routinely to ensure continued attention to asepsis and to identify organisms if peritonitis should develop subsequently. The patient should be observed for signs of peritonitis. These include an elevated

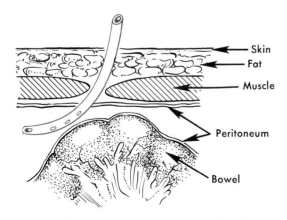

FIG. 20-25. Catheter in place in peritoneal cavity.

temperature and tenderness or pain of the abdomen.

Although the patient is confined to bed for the length of the dialysis, comfort and diversion can be provided. The patient may turn from side to side and move about in bed as he wishes as long as the catheter remains undisturbed. The patient may be provided assistance with oral care and bathing as needed. Visiting and other diversional activity should be encouraged when the patient's physical condition permits.

Kidney transplantation

Kidney transplants are being performed with increasing frequency in an effort to prolong the lives of patients with chronic renal failure. At present the ability to completely overcome the body's tendency to reject the grafted kidney has not been achieved. The patient undergoing kidney transplantation in essence exchanges a program of chronic hemodialysis and its limitations for a new problem. Unless the kidney has been donated by an identical twin, the body senses the graft as a foreign tissue and attempts to destroy it. Immunosuppressive medications such as azathioprine (Imuran) and prednisone are given to suppress rejection.

Nursing care of the patient in the preoperative phase includes physical and emotional preparation for the surgery. The patient and his family should understand the outcomes expected from the surgery and the follow-up care that will be required. They should be prepared for the possibility of the kidney not functioning after transplantation. The nature of the surgery and location of the kidney, the possible need for postoperative dialysis, the use of immunosuppressive drugs, and the need for infection prevention after surgery should be explained to them. As any surgical patient, the individual should know of any drainage tubes that will be inserted during surgery, that he will be given medication for relief of pain, and that after only a few hours he will be asked to move about and to cough and breathe deeply.

Throughout the period from the patient's acceptance as a transplant candidate to the time of surgery, the concerns and anxieties of the patient and his family regarding transplantation should be identified. As appropriate, the nurse and other members of the health team should be called to help them in dealing with these concerns and anxieties.

The patient must be in optimal physical condition for transplantation. Dialysis may be required prior to transplantation to assure optimal fluid and electrolyte balance, acid-base balance, and removal of wastes from the patient. A thorough medical evaluation will be performed prior to surgery.

During surgery the transplanted kidney is placed in the iliac fossa. Generally the peritoneal cavity is not entered. The patient's own kidneys may not be disturbed unless they are infected or are the cause of significant hypertension. A sump is placed in the wound to promote drainage of accumulating fluid.

Immediate postoperative care includes maintaining drainage of the urinary bladder, assessing the adequacy of fluid and electrolyte balance, protecting the patient from infection, observing for signs and symptoms of rejection, and identifying the effects of medications that have been administered throughout the entire care cycle. A free flow of communication must be maintained with the patient and his family regarding the individual's progress.

During surgery a Foley catheter is inserted into the bladder to promote drainage of urine and to prevent bladder distention and pressure on the newly anastomosed ureter. If gross hematuria or clots are noted in the drainage system, the physician should be notified immediately.

As with any surgical patient, the possibility of hemorrhage and hypovolemia exists. Blood pressure and pulse are determined frequently. Because the patient may have little or no urinary output for a number of hours to weeks after transplantation, fluid and electrolyte balance must be monitored carefully. Parameters indicating disturbed fluid and electrolyte balance are listed in the discussion of care of the patient with chronic renal failure (p. 469). Any drainage from dressing or tubes should be carefully calculated into the patient's fluid balance record.

Since the patient has been on immunosuppressive therapy, it is imperative to protect him from infection. In many institutions these patients are placed in reverse isolation (p. 80). A system of closed drainage should be meticulously maintained for the catheter draining the bladder. Cleansing of the perineum should be performed once each shift to help prevent bacteria entering the meatus and bladder. Turning, coughing, and deep breathing coupled with early activity help to prevent stasis of secretions in the tracheal bronchial tree.

If the patient has little or no function in the transplanted kidney, signs of increasing fluid retention and increasing urea nitrogen, creatinine, and potassium levels cannot be used as indicators of graft rejection. However, when some renal function does exist in the new kidney, these signs are indicative of decreasing function and possible rejection. Symptoms of rejection that are present in both functioning and nonfunctioning kidneys include low-grade fever and tenderness or pain over the graft site.

Side effects of the therapy with immunosuppressive steroids and azathioprine include depression and psychosis, hypertension, leukopenia, increased bleeding time, and decreased wound healing. Any of these side effects can be noted within the first few days of administration. Some white cell and platelet depression are expected; however, severe depression may result in the patient's death. Often the patient is aware of changes in his behavior; he may hallucinate or feel depressed and lack ambition. These changes in mental status may frighten the patient. He needs to know that the medications he is taking are capable of producing these changes. The physician also must be informed of the patient's emotional state.

The integrity of the patient's fistula or shunt must be maintained. Prior to surgery the extremity containing the fistula or shunt may be wrapped to draw attention to it and identify it as containing a fistula or shunt. This identification will help all individuals caring for the patient to avoid using the affected extremity for blood pressure determinations, drawing of blood, or an intravenous infusion.

Early in the postoperative course the patient should begin to become involved in learning to manage his own care. By the time the patient is discharged from the hospital, he should know (1) his dietary limitation, (2) his medications, their dosage, and effects, (3) how to care for his wound, (4) any precautions he should take in regard to activity and preventing trauma to the graft site, (5) how to measure his own intake and output and record daily weights, (6) how to take his temperature, and (7) how to collect a 24-hour urine specimen. The impor-

tance of regular follow-up visits and close medical supervision should be stressed. If at any time the patient should note tenderness over the transplant site, fever, a decrease in urinary output, pain on urination, pulmonary congestion, general malaise, nausea or vomiting, or gastric pain or bleeding, he should notify his physician immediately. Concerns that the patient may raise during subsequent visits include changes in physical appearance resulting from steroid administration and changes in family roles and social relationships. The patient should be given the opportunity to express his concerns and receive help from appropriate members of the health team in working through his feelings.

The National Kidney Foundation* supported establishment of a nationwide program to increase the number of kidneys available for transplantation. As a result, legislation known as the Uniform Donor Act was passed. The act allows an individual to legally donate his kidneys and other body parts in the event of his accidental death. A signed and witnessed card carried in a purse or wallet identifies the individual as a potential organ donor.

---

*116 East 27th St., New York, N. Y. 10016.

REFERENCES AND SELECTED READINGS*

1 *Abram, H.: The psychiatrist, the treatment of CRF and the prolongation of life. II, Am. J. Psychiatry 126:157-167, Aug. 1969.

2 Albers, J.: Evaluation of blood volume in patients on hemodialysis, Am. J. Nurs. 68:1677-1679, Aug. 1968.

3 Anderson, H. C.: Newton's geriatric nursing, ed. 5, St. Louis, 1971, The C. V. Mosby Co.

4 Avery, D., and Wagenhals, D.: Hypertension secondary to renal artery stenosis, Am. J. Nurs. 66:2685-2689, Dec. 1966.

5 Bailey, G. L., editor: Hemodialysis principles and practice, New York, 1972, Academic Press, Inc.

6 *Beaumont, E.: Urinary drainage system, Nursing '74 4:52-60, Jan. 1974.

7 Beeson, P. B., and McDermott, W., editors: Cecil-Loeb textbook of medicine, ed. 13, Philadelphia, 1971, W. B. Saunders Co.

8 *Bennett, W. M., Singer, I., and Coggins, C. H.: A practical guide to drug usage in adult patients with impaired renal function, J.A.M.A. 214:1468-1475, Nov. 1970.

9 Bergersen, B.: Pharmacology in nursing, ed. 12, St. Louis, 1973, The C. V. Mosby Co.

10 Berman, H. I.: Urinary diversion in treatment of carcinoma of the bladder, Surg. Clin. North Am. 45:1495-1508, Dec. 1965.

11 Black, D. A. K.: The measurement of renal function, Am. Heart J. 85:147-152, Feb. 1973.

12 Black, D. A. K., editor: Renal disease, ed. 2, Philadelphia, 1972, F. A. Davis Co.

12a *Blount, M., and Kinney, A. B.: Chronic steroid therapy, Am. J. Nurs. 74:1626-1631, Sept. 1974.

13 Bois, M. S., and others: Renal transplantation, Am. J. Nurs. 68:1238-1239, June 1968.

14 *Borum, L., and Zimmerman, D.: Catheter plugs as a source of infection, Am. J. Nurs. 71:2150-2152, Nov. 1971.

14a Burge, J.: Vitamin requirements of hemodialysis patients, Dialysis & Transplantation 3:61-64, Oct.-Nov. 1974.

15 Campbell, M. F., and Harrison, J. H., editors: Urology, ed. 3, vols. 1-3, Philadelphia, 1970, W. B. Saunders Co.

16 Castelnuovo-Tedesco, P., editor: Psychiatric aspects of organ transplantation, New York, 1971, Grune & Stratton, Inc.

17 *Ceccarelli, F. E., and Smith, P. C.: Studies on fluid and electrolyte alterations during transurethral prostatectomy, J. Urol. 86:434-441, Oct. 1961.

18 Chapman, W., and others, editors: The urinary system, Philadelphia, 1973, W. B. Saunders Co.

19 Charghi, A., and others: A method of urinary diversion by anastomosis of the ureters into a sigmoid pouch, J. Urol. 94:376-379, Oct. 1965.

19a Clark, E. A., and others: Cadaver-kidney transplant failures at one month, N. Engl. J. Med. 291:1099-1102, Nov. 1974.

20 *Cleland, V., and others: Prevention of bacteriuria in female patients with indwelling catheters, Nurs. Res. 20:309-318, July-Aug. 1971.

21 Cohen, S., and Persky, L.: A ten year experience with ureteroileostomy, Arch. Surg. 95:78-283, Aug. 1967.

22 Cooper, H., and Robinson, E.: Treatment of genitourinary tuberculosis: report after 24 years, J. Urol. 108:136-142, July 1972.

23 *Creevy, C. D., and Tollefson, D. M.: Ileac diversion of the urine and nursing care of the patient with an ileac diversion of the urine, Am. J. Nurs. 59:530-536, April 1959.

24 Cummings, J. W., Foy, A. L., and Schlotter, L.: Hemodialysis—feelings, facts, fantasies, Am. J. Nurs. 70:70-83, Jan. 1970.

---

*References preceded by an asterisk are particularly well suited for student reading.

25 *David, D. S., and others: Dietary management in renal failure, Lancet **2**:34-37, July 1972.

26 *Davis, J. E.: Drugs for urologic disorders, Am. J. Nurs. **65**:107-112, Aug. 1965.

27 *deGreco, F., and Krumlovsky, F.: Chronic renal failure: clinical and therapeutic considerations, Postgrad. Med. **52**:176-183, Sept. 1972.

27a DeFronzo, R., and others: CHO metabolism in uremia: a review, Medicine **52**:469-481, 1973.

28 *Dobbins, J., and Aleit, C.: Experience with the lateral position for catheterization, Nurs. Clin. North Am. **6**:373-379, June 1971.

29 Downing, S. R.: Nursing support in early renal failure, Am. J. Nurs. **69**:1212-1216, June 1969.

30 Downing, S. R., and Watkins, F. L.: The patient who has peritoneal dialysis, Am. J. Nurs. **66**:1573-1577, July 1966.

31 Dutcher, I. E., and Hardenburg, H. C.: Water and electrolyte imbalances. In Meltzer, L. E., Abdellah, F. G., and Kitchell, J. R., editors: Concepts and practices of intensive care for nurse specialists, Philadelphia, 1969, The Charles Press, Publishers.

32 Elliot, J. S.: Urinary calculus disease, Surg. Clin. North Am. **45**:1393-1404, Dec. 1965.

33 Everett, H. S., and Ridley, J. H.: Female urology, New York, 1968, Hoeber Medical Division, Harper & Row, Publishers.

34 *Faigel, H.: Peritoneal dialysis—indications and application, Clin. Pediatr. **5**:459-461, Aug. 1966.

35 Fellows, B. J., Blagg, C. R., and Scribner, B. H.: Acute renal failure and renal dialysis. In Meltzer, L. E., Abdellah, F. G., and Kitchell, J. R., editors: Concepts and practices of intensive care for nurse specialists, Philadelphia, 1969, The Charles Press, Publishers.

36 Flamenbaum, W.: Pathophysiology of acute renal failure, Arch. Intern. Med. **131**:911-928, June 1973.

37 Fournet, K.: Patients discharged on diuretics: prime candidates for individualized teaching, Heart & Lung **3**:108-116, Jan.-Feb. 1974.

38 Franklin, S., and others: Use of a balanced low protein diet in CRF, J.A.M.A. **202**:141-148, Nov. 1967.

39 Fraser, Sir Kenneth: Hypospadias, Surg. Clin. North Am. **64**:1551-1570, Dec. 1964.

40 Frenay, Sister M. Agnes Clare: A dynamic approach to the ileal conduit patient, Am. J. Nurs. **64**:80-84, Jan. 1964.

41 French, R. M.: Nurses' guide to diagnostic procedures, ed. 3, New York, 1971, McGraw-Hill Book Co.

42 Garb, S.: Laboratory tests in common use, ed. 5, New York, 1971, Springer Publishing Co., Inc.

43 Glenn, J. F., editor: Urologic surgery, New York, 1969, Hoeber Medical Division, Harper & Row, Publishers.

44 Goldberger, E.: A primer of water, electrolyte and acid-base syndromes, ed. 4, Philadelphia, 1970, Lea & Febiger.

45 Goodman, L. S., and Gilman, A., editors: The pharmacological basis of therapeutics, ed. 4, New York, 1970, Macmillan Publishing Co., Inc.

46 Grollman, A.: Diuretics, Am. J. Nurs. **65**:84-89, Jan. 1965.

47 Gutch, C., and Stoner, M.: Review of hemodialysis for nurses and dialysis personnel, St. Louis, 1971, The C. V. Mosby Co.

47a Hansen, F.: Caring for patients with chronic renal disease, Philadelphia, 1974, J. B. Lippincott Co.

48 Harrison, T. R., and others, editors: Principles of internal medicine, ed. 6, New York, 1970, McGraw-Hill Book Co.

49 Hassett, M.: Teaching dialysis to the family unit, Nurs. Clin. North Am. **7**:349-362, June 1972.

50 *Hedger, R. W.: The conservative management of acute renal failure, Med. Clin. North Am. **55**:121-135, Jan. 1971.

51 Hradec, E. A.: Bladder substitution, indications and results in 114 operations, J. Urol. **94**:406-417, Oct. 1965.

52 Jaffee, B. M., and others: Surgical complication of ileal segmented urinary diversion, Ann. Surg. **167**:367-376, March 1968.

53 Kark, R. M.: Symposium on diseases of the kidney, Med. Clin. North Am. **55**:1-241, Jan. 1971.

54 *Kasselman, M. J.: Nursing care of the patient with benign prostatic hypertrophy, Am. J. Nurs. **66**:1026-1030, May 1966.

55 *Katz, A. I.: Kidney transplantation: patient selection and management, Med. Clin. North Am. **54**:75-94, Jan. 1970.

56 *Kelly, A. E., and Gensini, G. G.: Renal arteriography, Am. J. Nurs. **64**:97-99, Feb. 1964.

57 Keuhmelian, J., and Sanders, V.: Urologic nursing, New York, 1970, Macmillan Publishing Co., Inc.

57a Kopple, J., and Coburn, J.: Metabolic studies of low protein diets in uremia, Medicine **52**:583-595, 1973.

58 *Kossoris, P.: Family therapy: an adjunct to hemodialysis and transplantation, Am. J. Nurs. **70**:1730-1733, Aug. 1970.

59 Kunin, C.: Detection, prevention and managements of urinary tract infections, Philadelphia, 1972, Lea & Febiger.

60 *Kunin, C.: Prevention of catheter-induced urinary tract infections, N. Engl. J. Med. **274**:1155-1161, May 1966.

61 Kuruvila, K. C., and Beven, E. G.: Arteriovenous shunts and fistulas for hemodialysis, Surg. Clin. North Am. **51**:1219-1234, Oct. 1971.

62 *Lange, K.: Nutritional management of kidney disorder, Med. Clin. North Am. **55**:513-520, 1971.

63 *Langford, T.: Nursing problem: bacteriuria and indwelling catheter, Am. J. Nurs. **72**:113-115, Jan. 1972.

64 LeBlanc, G. A., and Richardson, J. F.: Elimination of catheters, tubes and packs in suprapubic prostatectomy, J. Urol. **86**:431-433, Oct. 1961.

65 Lennon, E. M.: The surgical dialysis patient, Nurs. Clin. North Am. **4**:443-450, Sept. 1969.

66 *Lombardo, L. J., Jr., Heyman, A. M., and Barnes, R. W.: Injuries of the urinary tract due to external trauma, J.A.M.A. **172**:1618-1622, April 1960.

67 Magnusson, M. O., and Kiser, W. S.: Human kidney preservation for transplantation, Surg. Clin. North Am. **51**:1235-1242, Oct. 1971.

68 Marshall, V. F.: Fiber optics in urology, J. Urol. **91**:110-114, Jan. 1964.

69 *Martin, A. J., Jr.: Renal transplantation: surgical technique and complications, Am. J. Nurs. **68**:1240-1247, June 1968.

70 Maxwell, M. H., and Kleeman, C. R.: Clinical disorders of fluid and electrolyte metabolism, ed. 2, New York, 1972, McGraw-Hill Book Co.

71 Miller, R., and Tassistro, C.: Peritoneal dialysis, N. Engl. J. Med. **281**:945-949, Oct. 1969.

72 *Mohammed, M. R. B.: Urinalysis, Am. J. Nurs. **64**:87-89, June 1964.

73 *Monroe, J. M., and Komorita, N. I.: Problems with nephrosis in adolescence, Am. J. Nurs. **67**:336-340, Feb. 1967.

74 *Morel, A.: The urologic nurse specialist, Nurs. Clin. North Am. **4**:475-482, Sept. 1969.

75 *Mossholder, I. B.: When the patient has a radical retropubic prostatectomy, Am. J. Nurs. **62**:101-104, July 1962.

76 Mueller, C. B.: The mechanism of acute renal failure after injury and transfusion reaction and its prevention by solute diuresis, Surg. Clin. North Am. **45**:499-508, April 1965.

77 *Murray, B., and others: The patient has an ileal conduit, Am. J. Nurs. **71**:1560-1565, Aug. 1971.

78 Najarian, J. S., and Simmons, R. L., editors: Transplantation, Philadelphia, 1972, Lea & Febiger.

79 *O'Neill, M.: Peritoneal dialysis, Nurs. Clin. North Am. **1**:309-321, June 1966.

80 Papper, S.: Renal failure, Med. Clin. North Am. **55**:335-357, March 1971.

81 Perlmutter, A. D., and Tank, E. S.: Ileal conduit stasis in children: recognition and treatment, J. Urol. **101**:688-691, May 1969.

82 *Peterson, M.: Understanding defense mechanisms, Am. J. Nurs. **72**:1651-1674, Sept. 1972.

83 *Peterson, R. D.: Tissue immunity and tissue typing, Med. Clin. North Am. **54**:43-58, Jan. 1970.

84 *Pillay, V.: Clinical testing of renal function, Med. Clin. North Am. **55**:231-241, Jan. 1971.

85 Pitts, R. F.: Physiology of the kidney and body fluids, ed. 2, Chicago, 1968, Year Book Medical Publishers, Inc.

86 *Programmed instruction: potassium imbalance, Am. J. Nurs. **67**:343-366, Feb. 1967.

86a Pullman, T., and Coe, F.: Chronic renal failure, Clin. Symp. **25**:1-32, 1973.

87 Rapaport, F. T., and Dausset, J., editors: Human transplantation, New York, 1968, Grune & Stratton, Inc.

88 Reidenburg, M. M.: Renal function and drug action, Philadelphia, 1971, W. B. Saunders Co.

89 *Rodriguez, D. B.: Moral issues in hemodialysis and renal transplantation, Nurs. Forum **10**:201-220, March 1971.

90 Schlotter, L., editor: Nursing and the nephrology patient. A symposium on current trends and issues, Flushing, N. Y., 1973, Medical Examination Publishing Co., Inc.

91 *Schneider, W. J., and Boyce, B. A.: Complications of diuretic therapy, Am. J. Nurs. **68**:1903-1907, Sept. 1968.

92 *Schumann, D.: The renal donor, Am. J. Nurs. **74**:105-110, Jan. 1974.

93 *Sieggreen, M.: The closed urinary drainage system, New York, 1970, Educational Services Division, The American Journal of Nursing Co.

94 *Snively, W. D., and Roberts, K. T.: The clinical picture as an aid to understanding body fluid disturbances, Nurs. Forum **12**:133-159, 1973.

95 *Spence, H. M., and Littlepage, S.: Genitourinary injuries and nursing care, Am. J. Nurs. **55**:970-974, Aug. 1955.

96 *Steele, B. W.: Interpretation of renal function tests, Geriatrics **29**:63-66, 69-71, Jan. 1974.

97 *Stewart, B. H.: Surgery of renal transplantation, Surg. Clin. North Am. **51**:1123-1131, Oct. 1971

98 Strauss, M. B., and Welt, C. G., editors: Diseases of the kidney, ed. 2, Boston, 1971, Little, Brown & Co.

99 Streiff, R.: Disorders of folate metabolism, Disease-a-Month pp. 1-32, April 1972.

100 *Takacs, F. J.: Nephrologic emergencies: acute renal failure, Med. Clin. North Am. **53**:397-405, March 1969.

101 *Topor, M. A.: Nursing the renal transplantation patient, Nurs. Clin. North Am. **4**:461-473, Sept. 1969.

102 *Trusk, C. W.: Hemodialysis for acute renal failure, Am. J. Nurs. **65**:80-85, Feb. 1965.

103 U. S. Department of Health, Education and Welfare: Monthly vital statistics report, provisional statistics, annual summary for United States, 1972, vol. 21, no. 13, Washington, D. C., June 1973, U. S. Government Printing Office.

104 *Walsh, M. A., Ebner, M., and Casey, J. W.: Neo-bladder, Am. J. Nurs. **63**:107-110, April 1963.

105 *Wang, T.: Conservative management of CRF, Med. Clin. North Am. **55**:137-154, Jan. 1971.

106 Watt, R.: Urinary diversion, Am. J. Nurs. **74**:1806-1811, Oct. 1974.

107 Weld, L. G., editor: Symposium on uremia, Am. J. Med. **44**:653-802, May 1968.

108 Whitehead, S. L.: Nursing care of the adult urology patient, New York, 1970, Appleton-Century-Croft.

108a Williams, H.: Nephrolithiasis, N. Engl. J. Med. **290**:33-38, Jan. 1974.

109 Williams, S. R.: Nutrition and diet therapy, ed. 2, St. Louis, 1973, The C. V. Mosby Co.

109a Wilson, M.: The influence of the diet prescription and the educational approach on patient adherence to sodium-restricted intake, Med. Times **94**:1514-1522, Dec. 1966.

110 Winter, C. C.: Practical urology, St. Louis, 1969, The C. V. Mosby Co.

111 Winter, C. C., and Barker, M. R.: Nursing care of patients with urologic disease, ed. 3, St. Louis, 1972, The C. V. Mosby Co.

21 Diseases of the reproductive system

Health education
Examination of the reproductive tract

Diseases of the female reproductive system
Common gynecologic disorders

Diseases of the male reproductive system

Venereal disease
Gonorrhea
Syphilis
Follow-up of contacts and prevention of venereal disease
Venereal lesions of the external genitalia

■ Conditions affecting healthful functioning of the reproductive systems take a high toll in terms of loss of life and acute and chronic physical and emotional stress. The nurse has a responsibility to assist in general health education, to direct patients to good medical care, and to understand the treatment available and the nursing care needed when disease has developed.

■ HEALTH EDUCATION

Although present-day society in general is much more open than in the past regarding the discussion of sexual matters, many people still find it difficult to ask questions about sex or to discuss sexual problems. When this occurs, they often act on the basis of misinformation received from uninformed sources. Therefore, if nurses are to assist persons in asking questions about reproduction, functioning of the reproductive system, sexual activity, and birth

■ STUDY QUESTIONS

1 Review the anatomy of the male and female reproductive systems.
2 Review the menstrual cycle. During which period does ovulation occur? What is the relationship of estrogen and progesterone to the cycle?
3 Review the methods of draping a patient for a pelvic examination and of assisting the physician with this examination.
4 What physical, hormonal, and psychologic changes occur at puberty in girls? In boys?
5 List the male hormones. What physiologic changes do they stimulate? List the female hormones. What physiologic changes do they stimulate?
6 Review the following basic nursing procedures: catheterization, insertion of retention catheters, use of T binder and methods of securing perineal dressings, measurement of drainage and care of drainage equipment, and use of cold applications.
7 What are the main purposes of a douche? Review the procedure. What solutions are most often used?
8 What are the purposes of using heat lamps and sitz baths? What is the physiologic principle for these therapeutic actions? Review both procedures.
9 What is the incidence of venereal disease in your community? What services are available for the detection and treatment of venereal disease? Are human sexuality and venereal disease taught in the local schools? Who teaches the content? Are there similar programs for adults?
10 Are birth control and family planning programs and services available in your community? Are there any constraints attached to the nurse's role? What methods are most often used?
11 What are the abortion laws in your state? Under what circumstances can an abortion be performed medically and legally? What services are available for people seeking an abortion? What methods are most commonly used in your community? Do nurses function in a counseling role?
12 Has there been an increase in the number of sterilizations performed (men and women) in your community during the past 10 years? Does your state have laws governing sterilization? What reasons do people in your community give for favoring or opposing sterilization as a method of birth control?

control, they must be knowledgeable in this area and comfortable in imparting information to others. To do this the nurse needs sound knowledge of the normal reproductive system and how it functions. The nurse must be able to recognize deviations from normal that require medical assistance and must also understand psychosexual growth and development. The nurse also needs to be able to put people at ease so that they will feel free to ask questions openly. Oftentimes the nurse can indicate to the patient a willingness to discuss sexual matters with them by giving appropriate cues or raising certain subjects.

In many instances, people are more comfortable in discussing sexual matters with someone of their own sex. The women's movement, in particular, has emphasized the need for women to understand their own bodies better and has raised questions about the insensitivity of some male physicians to female problems.* For this reason female nurses and physicians may be preferred sources of information for some women's groups.

Preparation for puberty

Sex education. Sex education begins when a child is born. From that moment on the infant begins to experience himself as a sexual being, responding to and absorbing the attitudes of those around him. From the way he is touched and handled, he senses the importance of all parts of his body. He touches himself and feels and learns from his own exploration and from the responses of others to his exploration. He learns from the way he is bathed. Therefore the genitalia should be bathed as carefully and tenderly as the rest of the body, for bathing is perhaps the most important introduction to sex education that the infant receives.

Sex education involves more than teaching the facts of life, for sexuality is the sum total of the self and the experiences of the self. Thus sex education teaches one how to be a responsible human being. As a child grows, he experiences attitudes and relationships and begins to interact with those around him and with his environment. During these early years he quite naturally incorporates the attitudes of those who surround him and also starts to behave like them. Since parents are usually the most influential persons to the very young child, it is necessary that they have healthy attitudes to accompany the facts that are needed for teaching children how to live.

Parents often ask the nurse questions about sex, and frequently they want to know how and what to teach their children. The nurse cannot only help parents understand the anatomy and physiology of the reproductive system but also can help them see the importance of their own attitudes and the importance of how they behave toward each other and how they relate to their children. For example, parents need to understand that young children do not want lengthy explanations, but that they do need direct and truthful answers to specific questions.

Although many schools have added sex education to their curricula, the subject has aroused much controversy among parents and educators. Careful planning with parents about course content will hopefully avoid misunderstandings, and it may help parents to learn facts that they need to know before they can teach children themselves. Thus in addition to teaching parents individually, the nurse can work with various community groups. The school nurse and the public health nurse are most likely to have this opportunity, but in small communities any nurse may be asked to help with sex education. The nurse may participate in parent-teacher programs and, by using drawings, filmstrips, and films, can explain anatomy and the reproductive processes. Church groups as well as organizations such as the Girl Scouts that include courses in sex education and personal hygiene as a part of their programs provide nurses with opportunities to participate in community programs. The school nurse may be asked to help physical education teachers cover course content and sometimes teach, or help teach, classes in hygiene for children.

The nurse should evaluate articles in daily papers and popular magazines so that she may advise parents on the use of this information. Often books for parents can be recommended to help them answer children's questions about sex. Books specifically for children can also be recommended. There are many pamphlets and books on sex education, but only a few can be mentioned here. Most state departments of health supply material. The following five books* on reproduction cover all age levels: *Facts Aren't Enough,* 1970, is written for adults to help them be better prepared to answer children's questions on sex; *Parents' Responsibility,* 1967, is for parents of preschool and early school-age children; *A Story About You,* 1966, is for children in fourth, fifth, and sixth grades; *Finding Yourself,* 1968, is for junior high boys and girls; and *Approaching Adulthood,* 1969, is for young people, ages 16 to 20. Another book for parents is *What to Tell Your Children About Sex.*† *Sex Education and the Teenager*‡ is also good. A highly recommended book for young children is *A Baby Is Born: The Story of How Life Begins,*§ and the authors of this book, a pedia-

---

*Boston Women's Health Book Collective: Our bodies, ourselves, a book by and for women, Boston, 1973, Simon & Schuster, Inc.

*Lerrigo, M. O., and Southard, H.: Sex education series, American Medical Association, 535 N. Dearborn, Chicago, Ill. 60610.
†Child Study Association of America: New York, 1968, Meredith Corp.
‡Farber, S. M., editor: Berkeley, Calif., 1967, Diablo Press.
§Levine, M. I., and Seligmann, J. H.: New York, 1949, Golden Press.

trician and a teacher, also wrote *The Wonder of Life** for preadolescent boys and girls. *Love and the Facts of Life†* is for teenagers.

Menstruation. Girls and young women ask questions regarding menstruation. Their understanding may be limited or inaccurate because of word of mouth information passed along by peers, parents, and others who are poorly informed. On the other hand, the nurse may find women who know about the entire menstrual cycle but have difficulty in accepting it as a normal process. Therefore, before engaging in education about menstruation, the nurse must first assess the current knowledge and understanding of the individual. Once this is done, a teaching plan can be designed to meet the specific learning needs of the individual to prevent fear and shock arising from the unknown and unexpected. To encourage healthful attitudes, instruction about menstruation should precede its onset, properly called the menarche.

The average age of the menarche has gradually decreased over the past 100 years. The decrease in the average age is attributed to improved nutritional status. In the northern hemisphere the average age of the menarche is 13 years with the normal age range between 10 and 17 years. The onset of menstruation usually occurs at an earlier age in countries in the Southern hemisphere.

Menstruation is a manifestation of normal functioning of the female body and should be treated as such. The "period" and "monthly period" are sensible and accurate terms to use if the individual does not wish to say "I am menstruating." Because of negative connotations engendered by such terms as "being sick" or "having the curse," girls and women should be encouraged to avoid using them. The girl should know how menstrual flow comes about, what its purpose is, and any special care that she should give herself during this time. She will probably have little discomfort if she has adequate rest, maintains good posture, eats a balanced diet, and participates in regular, moderate exercise. There may be slight discomfort in the lower back, legs, and pelvis, particularly on the day of the onset, and a slight tendency to fatigue. Some adolescent girls are concerned about circles that appear under their eyes during menstruation, which they fear are obvious; additional rest will usually control this problem. Girls should know that breast changes may occur either preceding the period or at various times throughout the monthly cycle; in some instances, rather marked tenderness and enlargement of the breasts occur. For those girls who have experienced some breast development, beginning to wear a bra or adjusting it for maximum support may help relieve the discomfort. Mild mood swings also occur in the normal menstrual cycle and should be understood and accepted, but excessive emphasis should not be placed on them. The preceding statements about health counseling in relation to menstruation apply not only to young girls but to older females as well, since many of them can benefit from accurate information.

Normally there is a loss of from 30 to 180 ml. of menstrual fluid during the period, which usually lasts from 3 to 7 days. One half to three fourths of the fluid is blood and the remainder is mucus, fragments of endometrial cells, and desquamated vaginal epithelium.[57] The average woman needs approximately a dozen napkins for the entire period. Tampons can be used safely instead of napkins; they do not block the flow nor do they cause irritation. They are comfortable when properly inserted and the right size is used. Tampons should be changed as frequently as any other type of protection, especially during the height of menstrual flow. Sexually inactive girls and women may have questions about whether they can use tampons and physicians agree that not all can use them. The size of the hymenal opening and the size of the tampon determine whether tampons can be worn comfortably. There should be no pain when the tampon is inserted, although at first there might be slight discomfort.* If a girl wishes to use this kind of protection and the tampon is not easily inserted at first, she should consult a gynecologist.

There is considerable individual variation in speed of onset, in duration, and in regularity of menstrual flow. Some irregularity is usual in the first few months and may continue for a few years or even indefinitely in some women. By the age of 18 to 20 years, the menstrual cycle usually assumes a rhythmic pattern with minor variations. However, there is considerable normal variation among women in the intervals between menstrual periods. Menstruation occurs on an average of every 28 days; but most cycles occur within a normal range of 26 to 34 days. The pattern of the menstrual cycle may be upset by such things as changes in climate, changes in working hours, emotional trauma, and acute or chronic illness. Any of these factors may alter the life-style temporarily and produce change in the nerve centers in the hypothalamus. This upset causes a change in the rate and timing of the secretion of the pituitary hormones, which probably maintain the normal menstrual cycle. An early menstrual period or absence of the period is not significant if it occurs only one month, but if either condition continues, a gyne-

---

*Levine, M. I., and Seligmann, J. H.: New York, 1940, Simon & Schuster, Inc.
†Duvall, E. M.: New York, 1967, Association Press.

*Dodge, E. F.: The doctor talks about menstruation, Tampax Educational Material on Menstruation, Palmer, Mass., 1967, Tampax, Inc.

cologist should be consulted. Any marked change in amount or duration of flow as well as consistent irregularity requires medical attention.

Clots should be reported since normally the menstrual fluid does not clot unless retained in the vagina for a prolonged period of time. It is believed that the endometrium produces a lytic or anticoagulant agent that prevents clotting in the uterus. There is no alteration in the coagulability of blood during menstruation.[57] In order to become knowledgeable about the patterns of their menstrual cycles, girls and women need to be encouraged to keep a written record. Establishing this habit assists with learning to predict the onset of the next menstrual period and to eventually determine the range of cycles. Should it be necessary to seek medical attention for any reason, the date of the onset of the last menstrual period (LMP) would be known. Women who are unable to remember the date of the first day of the last menstrual period can be assisted to recall it by being asked if they can associate the last period with a specific significant event.

Many young girls have marked discomfort during menstruation and take a variety of medications to relieve the symptoms. They should be encouraged to treat minor discomforts with rest, warmth, and small amounts of acetylsalicylic acid and to avoid the use of patent medicines and other unprescribed remedies.

During menstruation a bath should be taken daily. A warm tub bath often allays slight pelvic discomfort, although many women prefer to take showers during their menstrual period. Cold baths and showers may increase discomfort, but many women use tampons and go swimming during their period with no ill effects.

Sexual activity

In most social organizations the family is the basic unit of society. The family continues to serve the same basic human needs although its structure may vary across cultures and between generations.

Like the family, the institution of marriage is timeless and complex. Traditional monogamous marriages remain the norm, although different forms of marriage and family life-styles are practiced by some people. The communal living group in which people pool their resources and share the responsibilities of family life is one example. Single couples living together as husband and wife is another. Still a different notion is that of renewable marriages in which marriage is on a limited term contract with an option to renew the contract by mutual consent at the end of a specified time.

Single young people are experiencing a new sense of sexual freedom, and this has led to frequent sexual intercourse for its own sake rather than in association with love and marriage. While studies indicate that sexual behavior patterns are changing, they also show that the behavior is not in the direction of increased promiscuity.[63] An increasing number of unmarried couples no longer consider marriage as a prerequisite for sexual relationships. There is, among these couples, however, a mutual commitment to a love relationship before sexual intercourse. Among many of them there is, also, contemplation of marriage.

It is advisable for couples planning sexual relationships, marriage, and childbearing to have complete physical examinations, including a serologic test for syphilis (now compulsory in all except five states). Women should have a pelvic examination. At this time a tight hymenal ring, which could make intercourse difficult, can be dilated or incised, provided this procedure is psychologically and culturally acceptable to both the woman and her prospective husband.

Prior to marriage the couple should talk freely with their physician, their religious adviser, and particularly with each other concerning the physical, psychologic, and religious implications of sex. It is important that cultural differences be considered and that questions or differences about intercourse and size and spacing of the prospective family be discussed at this time. *Sexual Freedom in Marriage,** *A Marriage Manual,*† and *Sex Life in Marriage*‡ are books often suggested for reading either shortly prior to or immediately following marriage. Couples may also want to read *Birth Control and Love.*§ Roman Catholic couples may want to read *Marriage Manual for Catholics* ‖ or *Marriage Is for Grownups.*¶

Women often ask female nurses about intercourse. Tremendous variation exists in the sexual activity of married couples. With adequate knowledge, patience, and understanding, a couple can usually work out a plan that is satisfactory to both. Frequency of intercourse may vary from one or more times a day to once a month or less. The frequency normally drops considerably after the first year or two of marriage.

From 25% to 50% of married couples have some difficulty in intercourse because of emotional maladjustment. This is often due to worry or guilt feelings related to sex, inability to meet cultural standards

---

*Rubin, E., editor: New York, 1969, The New American Library, Inc.
†Revised by Aitken, G. S., and Sobrero, A. J.: New York, 1968, Simon & Schuster, Inc.
‡Butterfield, O. M.: New York, 1962, Emerson Books, Inc.
§Guttmacher, A. F.: New York, 1969, Macmillan Publishing Co., Inc.
‖ Lynch, W. A.: New York, 1964, Trident Press (also available in paperback, New York, 1968, Pocket Books).
¶ Bird, J., and Bird, L.: New York, 1969, Doubleday & Co., Inc.

for satisfactory intercourse, or fear of an unplanned or unwanted pregnancy. This may result in frigidity in women and impotence in men. The couple should be urged to discuss these problems frankly with their physician or spiritual adviser, since reassurance and additional sex education may relieve the situation. A few persons may need psychiatric help.

Absence of menstruation (amenorrhea) in the sexually active female who is not practicing effective conception prevention and who has a history of normal menstrual cycles usually indicates pregnancy. It is important to note that conception occurs approximately 14 to 16 days before a woman misses her first period. By this time, the fertilized ovum has become implanted in the uterus. From the standpoint of healthful embryonic development and the changing health needs of the pregnant woman, it is essential that women become knowledgeable about the importance of medical care as soon as pregnancy is suspected. Regardless of the cause of amenorrhea, medical assistance should be sought at once.

Some women may have a slight vaginal discharge following intercourse. If it is irritating, a douche with plain water or with a tablespoon of white vinegar to a quart of water may be used from 1 to 3 hours after intercourse. For marked discharge not alleviated by this means, medical advice should be sought. Normally, douches are not needed for cleanliness, and it is inadvisable to douche routinely because excessive douching alters the pH of the vagina and predisposes to acute and chronic infections. Some normal women have a troublesome odor, especially in warm weather and following the menstrual period, that can be relieved by an occasional douche with warm water or vinegar in water. Also, vaginal deodorants in powder, spray, and suppository form have become increasingly popular and are available without prescription.

Contraception and family planning

Overpopulation has become a worldwide problem of such magnitude that it affects every living being as explained in Chapter 3. Ecologic insights force us to look at life and our environment in an entirely new way. We now know that we have few choices left if we are to survive on this planet. Paul Ehrlich points out that one choice is either to lower the birth rate or to raise the death rate. Thus birth control becomes not only a personal concern, but a consideration of the rights of others and the rights of the unborn as well as a concern for that integrated life-system which is planet earth. For the first time in the history of man it is now possible to regulate conception with a high degree of reliability.

Contraception remains a controversial issue despite improved methods of conception control. The incentives and imperatives for separating sexual and reproductive functions have been widely discussed from the standpoint of medical care, sociology, psychology, demography, economics, theology, and the law. Alleviation of unchecked population growth, prevention of the birth of unwanted children, and prevention of illness are the major themes addressed pro and con. Regardless of the issues involved, couples are required more than ever before to examine the consequences of their own actions and to select from among the alternatives those actions most consistent with their beliefs and needs.

One of the greatest responsibilities of nurses is to assist sexually active couples in making decisions regarding contraception, childbearing, and spacing of children in a well-informed manner. Experience has shown that the best method of contraception (on an individual basis) is one that is acceptable to both sex partners, readily available, convenient to use, effective and safe in action, and inexpensive. Regardless of the method selected, it must be well understood and used consistently.

Current methods of conception control are summarized in Table 21-1. In addition to these methods, experimentation with newer types of contraceptives is in progress. The postcoital ("morning after") pill has enjoyed wide publication but is not widely prescribed. These preparations, taken by the woman after she has had intercourse, contain potent synthetic estrogens that probably prevent implantation of the ovum. Nausea commonly accompanies such high doses of estrogen. Additional studies are needed to determine short- and long-term effects.

Long-term preparations that could be administered orally or by injection are now being studied. Irregular uterine bleeding and an unpredictable interval between cessation of use and resumption of ovulation have been encountered.

Another area for study is the development of birth control pills and injections for males that would produce temporary infertility. One difficulty encountered with oral contraceptives for men is that the sperm produced in the seminiferous tubules take 2 to 3 months to reach the ejaculate, that is, residual fertility. Another problem encountered is that reduced fertility in males seems to be accompanied by decreased libido.

The range of contraceptive techniques available is wide and varied. It provides for couples in which one partner is seen to have or wishes to take the major responsibility for contraception; it provides for couples who wish to share responsibility jointly; and it provides for couples who wish to share responsibility by alternating use of their preferred methods. Although the failure rates of the methods available vary, each method seems to have convinced advocates. This is because, for most couples, effectiveness of method is influenced by social and psychologic factors that render one method acceptable over all others. However, the reliability of a method

Table 21-1 Summary of methods of conception control

Method	Action	Safety/Effectiveness	Effects	Contraindications
Oral contraceptive ("The Pill"): 1. Combination pill—each pill contains progestin and estrogen; schedule: one pill daily for 21 days, then discontinue for 7 days; placebo may be advised for last 7 days; pill cycle started and repeated on fifth day after onset of menstrual flow 2. Sequential pill—one pill containing estrogen alone daily for 16 days, then one pill containing estrogen and progestogen daily for 5 days; may be advised to take placebo last 7 days of cycle; pill cycle started and repeated on fifth day after menstrual flow begins	Both types: 1. Inhibit ovulation by suppression of pituitary gonadotropin 2. Produce cervical mucus that is hostile to sperm 3. Modify tubal transport of ovum 4. May have effect on endometrium to make implantation unlikely	1. 100% effective if taken accurately 2. Failure results from failure to take pill regularly 3. If woman forgets to take pill one day, she can "make up" by taking two pills next day 4. Chances of pregnancy increased if pill is missed for 2 days or more 5. Highly acceptable to users; easy to take 6. Linked with mortality due to thromboembolus phenomena 7. Does not alter fertility	Useful 1. Relief of dysmenorrhea in 60%-90% of cases 2. Relief of premenstrual tension 3. Regulation of menstrual cycles 4. Relief of acne in 80%-90% of cases 5. Improved feeling of well-being Minor (side effects usually decrease after third cycle) 1. Weight gain 2. Breast tenderness 3. Headaches 4. Corneal edema 5. Nausea 6. Breakthrough bleeding 7. Hypertension Major side effects 1. Thromboembolus disorders 2. May also decrease lactation in breast-feeding women	1. Undiagnosed vaginal bleeding 2. Breast or pelvis cancer 3. Liver disease 4. Cardiovascular disease 5. Renal disease 6. Thyroid disease 7. Diabetes Use with caution if history of: 1. Epilepsy 2. Multiple sclerosis 3. Porphyria 4. Otosclerosis 5. Asthma
Intrauterine contraceptive device (IUD or IUCD): Small objects of various shapes made of plastic, nylon, or steel inserted into uterus; most have nylon string attached that protrudes from cervix into vagina; inserted using aseptic technique; follow-up visits in 1 month, then individualized EXAMPLES: 1. Lippes loop 2. Saf-T-Coil 3. Birnberg bow 4. Margulies coil 5. Hall-Stone ring	Unknown 1. Probably modifies endometrium or myometrium to prevent inflammation 2. Probably hastens tubal transport of ovum	1. Easily inserted, highly effective: 97%-99% 2. Can be inserted any time during cycle; presence of menstrual flow rules out early pregnancy 3. Can be inserted immediately postpartum but expulsion rate is higher 4. Can be left in place indefinitely 5. Effectiveness highly dependent on knowing IUD remains in place; women need to be taught to feel for string after each period 6. Spontaneous expulsion occurs most often during menstruation (expulsion rates: 10%-20%)	1. Uterine cramping 2. Heavy menstrual flow 3. Irregular menses NOTE: Usually disappear in 2-3 months Problems 1. Infection—usually minor and occurs soon after insertion 2. Perforation of uterus—varies with types of device; highest rates in first 6 weeks postpartum; usually occurs at time of insertion	1. Current infection of reproductive tract 2. Uterine fibroids

Continued.

Table 21-1 Summary of methods of conception control—cont'd

Method	Action	Safety/Effectiveness	Effects	Contraindications
IUD—cont'd		7. Failure rate (pregnancy) 1.5%-3% during first year of use; rate declines thereafter 8. Does not alter fertility		
Diaphragm (with spermicidal foam, cream, jelly): Rubber dome attached to flexible metal ring; inserted into vagina to cover cervix; available in various sizes (require careful fitting); self-inserted by user; inner surface of diaphragm coated with spermicide before insertion; inserted at least 2 hours before intercourse and left in place at least 6 hours after intercourse	1. Provides mechanical barrier to sperm 2. Spermicidal preparation destroys large number of sperm	1. 97%-98% effective if fitted properly and used correctly 2. Requires sustained motivation for repeated insertion and removal 3. Refitting necessary after childbirth, abortion, or surgery of cervix and vagina; weight change of 10 lb. or more	None	1. Severe uterine prolapse
Condom ("rubber," "safes," "prophylactics"): Thin, flexible plastic worn over penis; available without prescription; does not require medical supervision	1. Provides mechanical barrier to prevent sperm from entering vagina 2. Also prevents spread of venereal diseases	1. Effectiveness increased with use of diaphragm by female 2. Effectiveness decreased by tearing or slipping of condom during intercourse 3. Failure rate 10%-15%	None	None
Rhythm ("safe period"): Periodic abstinence from intercourse during fertile periods of menstrual cycle; days 12-16 before expected date of menstruation are possible ovulating days; since sperm can survive up to 48 hours, days 11, 17, and 18 added to fertile period	1. Sexual abstinence around time of ovulation	1. Safe 2. 65%-85% effective 3. Fertile period varies; precise time of ovulation not known 4. Effectiveness increased with calculation of fertile period, high motivation to prevent pregnancy, determination of basal body temperature	1. Frustration 2. Lack of sexual gratification during period of abstinence	1. Irregular menstrual cycles 2. Medical contraindications to pregnancy
Chemical contraceptive (jellies, creams, foams, suppositories): Applied inside vagina by means of plunger-type applicator or aerosol spray	1. Contains spermicidal ingredients 2. Partial barrier to entrance of sperm into cervix	1. Effectiveness increased when used with diaphragm or condom 2. Easily available without prescription	None	None

Table 21-1 Summary of methods of conception control—cont'd

Method	Action	Safety/Effectiveness	Effects	Contraindications
Chemical contraceptive—cont'd		3. Effectiveness depends on dispersion of substance within vagina 4. Low effectiveness rate: 20% failure rate for foams, creams, jellies; 30% failure rate for suppositories		
Postcoital douche	1. Removes sperm from vagina by washing	1. Safe 2. 30%-35% failure rate 3. Some sperm have entered uterus 1-10 minutes after ejaculation	None	None unless douching is medically contraindicated

becomes more important for couples when the limit of intended family size is reached.

Because of the wide range of variables operating, there is no one "perfect" contraceptive. The counseling and teaching functions of the nurse assisting couples to make decisions related to conception control and family planning assumes a greater significance when seen in this light.

Counseling individuals or couples regarding "birth control" goes beyond teaching them how to use a method correctly. If couples are to accept responsibility for conception control, the nurse needs to assess the extent to which misunderstanding, superstition, and fear exist and to take action by presenting facts about reproduction as well as facts about contraceptive methods. For example, lay people sometimes confuse contraception, which is temporary and reversible, with sterilization, and the differences need to be pointed out to them.

People may have many questions about contraception, and the nurse can anticipate some that are frequently asked.

1. What methods are most effective in preventing pregnancy?
2. How safe are the available methods? Will they harm the couple, the individual, or a future child?
3. Will contraception interfere with sexual intercourse in any way?
4. Do the methods hamper or prevent later desired pregnancies?
5. How convenient are the different methods?
6. What do the different methods cost?

7. Where are contraceptive services provided?*

Utilization of contraception has increased in recent years. This is probably due to the greater motivation individuals have to prevent pregnancy for some reason, that is, actively seeking out services. It is also probably due to a greater effort on the part of professionals to refer individuals and couples for conception control. In this latter area, nurses can take greater initiative than in the past by seeking out opportunities to counsel regarding conception control.

For example, waiting for a patient who has been advised by a physician to refrain from becoming pregnant to ask about contraception may mean the question will not be raised. Likewise, waiting for a patient to give a cue about interest in contraception does not necessarily mean the cue will be picked up. Many women seem quite relieved that the nurse has posed questions about their plans for birth control.

Depending on the nurse's assessment of the type of approach that is most appropriate, direct or indirect questions can be used to determine a patient's interest or need for information about conception control.

Questions may be more direct; that is, "Would you like help in planning your family?" "Do you want

*Many communities are served by family planning clinics under various names as well as by outpatient services in hospitals. These can usually be found listed in telephone directories under "Planned Parenthood." Literature about family planning services can be obtained directly from Planned Parenthood World Population, 810 Seventh Ave., New York, N. Y. 10019.

help in preventing pregnancy before you are ready for another child?" "Do you want information about birth control?"

Also, questions can be posed more indirectly and individualized for the patients' circumstances. For example, new mothers and fathers often respond to the childbirth experience by remarking, "I don't want to go through that again for a while." This provides an opportunity for the nurse to raise the question of how they plan to prevent pregnancy until they are ready for another child. Another opportunity may arise when nurses are in contact with parents of an acute or chronically ill child. A statement such as "Your child is going to keep you busy for some time; how will you manage if a baby comes along?" can provoke discussion of contraception. A couple or family having economic problems might welcome such a comment as, "I've noticed you are having a hard time. How will things be if you find you are expecting a child?"

Pamphlets can be placed where patients have access to them and this often gives a cue to the nurse indicating the patient's interest. To verify this, the nurse might say, "I noticed you looking at this pamphlet. What information or help can I give you?"

If individuals and couples are to be assisted to make the best decision and choices about contraception, they need to be well-informed. This requires information about all the methods, presented factually and completely in easily understood terms. Therefore the nurse must be well-informed about all methods of contraception available; how they prevent conception, their advantages and disadvantages, and their cost and convenience (Fig. 21-1). Table 21-2 may be helpful in counseling women who are utilizing the rhythm method. In order to be used with reliability, however, the woman must be certain of the length of her menstrual cycles and the shortest and longest ranges of her cycles. The nurse must be prepared to discuss with individuals or couples their contemplated or usual sexual activity. For example, a woman who engages in sexual intercourse only occasionally is not necessarily a good candidate for birth control pills. For her, an alternative method may be more suitable.

Fears about a particular method may be expressed by the potential user. At first, many women seem hesitant about having an intrauterine device (IUD) inserted and may express fear that it will "get lost inside me." Utilizing pictures or a model can help the woman to understand that the uterus is a self-contained organ; showing the woman the IUD with the strings attached often eliminates this fear. Informing the woman that the strings become soft with body heat and that her sexual partner should not be aware of them during intercourse is usually

Table 21-2 Ovulation and the menstrual cycle

Shortest cycle (in days)	First unsafe day	Longest cycle (in days)	Last unsafe day
20	2nd	20	9th
21	3rd	21	10th
22	4th	22	11th
23	5th	23	12th
24	6th	24	13th
25	7th	25	14th
26	8th	26	15th
27	9th	27	16th
28*	10th*	28	17th
29	11th	29	18th
30	12th	30*	19th*
31	13th	31	20th
32	14th	32	21st
33	15th	33	22nd
34	16th	34	23rd
35	17th	35	24th
36	18th	36	25th

*EXAMPLE: A woman whose cycles range from 28 to 30 days has her first "unsafe" day on the tenth day after the start of any period and her last "unsafe" day on the nineteenth day after the start of any period.

reassuring. Many women also welcome hearing that tampons can be used during the menstrual period when an IUD is in place.

Some individuals and couples seem to have greater difficulty in making a choice from among the methods available. They may need repeated information and statements may need to be rephrased to increase their understanding and to encourage freedom of expression. However, information given in an accepting, nonjudgmental manner and approaches that convey a sincere desire to be of service usually are helpful.

In addition to the conception control methods mentioned, voluntary surgical sterilization has become increasingly acceptable to both men and women as a permanent method of preventing conception. It has been estimated that 1,500,000 American women have already been sterilized and that approximately 100,000 women elect sterilization every year.[49] In addition, it has been estimated that about 700,000 men elected to have vasectomies in 1971.[27]

Sterilization of women. The most common surgical procedure for elective sterilization of women is tubal sterilization. Hysterectomy, bilateral salpingectomy, bilateral oophorectomy, and pelvic radiation in large doses also bring about cessation of childbearing; however, the primary purposes of these procedures is not sterilization.

Tubal sterilization is accomplished by tubal ligation with or without bilateral partial salpingectomy. Excision of a small piece of each fallopian tube in addition to ligation of both tubes produces greater effectiveness.

Tubal sterilization is accomplished by way of a small incision through the abdominal wall. The fallopian tubes are located and a loop of the midportion is elevated. The loop is then ligated at the base. If bilateral salpingectomy is to be performed, the ligated segment is excised. Hospitalization for 2 to 4 days is required and includes the usual pre- and postoperative care. Tubal sterilization is often performed in the early postpartal period or at the time of cesarean section.

New approaches to simplifying tubal sterilization are emerging. The goals are to reduce physical and emotional stress and decrease the length of hospitalization required. For example, tubal ligation can be accomplished transvaginally through the cul-de-sac, and this approach may be preferable for women who have not recently undergone childbirth. This method results in less postoperative pain and a shorter period of hospitalization; long-term effectiveness is currently under study.

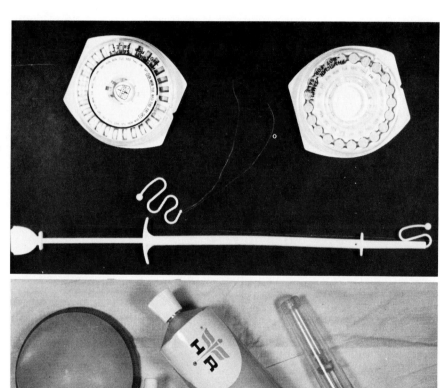

FIG. 21-1. **A,** Two types of oral contraceptives and Lippes loop with applicator. **B,** Left to right: Diaphragm, contraceptive foam for vaginal application, contraceptive jelly and vaginal applicator, and condom.

A newer technique for accomplishing tubal sterilization by means of a laparoscope is being developed. A small incision, about 2 cm. is made in the midline of the abdomen below the umbilicus. The laparoscope is inserted through the incision into the peritoneal cavity. A segment of each tube is grasped with forceps and an electric current is passed through the forceps to bring about coagulation of the tubes. Patients undergoing this type of sterilization have minimal discomfort and can be discharged within a few hours after the surgery. Because of the low incidence and minor nature of complications, it has been suggested that this method of tubal sterilization can be done on an outpatient basis.[121]

In healthy women, elective tubal ligation carries minimal risk. Death is rare; the major risks are hemorrhage, infection, pulmonary embolism, and subsequent pregnancy.

Successful sterilization (conception prevented) seems to be partly dependent on the specific technique used. The main causes for failure are recanalization of the tube, erroneous ligation, and pregnancy resulting because of tuboperitoneal fistula. The failure rates reported vary from 1 in 57 to 1 in 340 patients.[104]

While tubal sterilization terminates a woman's ability to bear children, ovarian hormones and menstrual functioning are not altered, and an artificial menopause is not induced. Attempts to reconstruct the fallopian tubes have met with poor results. Since the chances of reversibility are remote, patients should clearly understand and accept the fact that tubal sterilization is irreversible.

The laws governing sterilization vary from state to state; some states have laws that are unclear, while others have no laws at all. In general, if the surgery does not violate specific state provisions and if written, informed consent is given by a woman legally capable of giving permission, the surgery can be performed by the physician. The need for medical consultation may be regulated, however, by hospital policy.

Sterilization of men. Change in attitudes toward sterilization of men is reflected in the gradually increasing numbers of vasectomies performed during recent years. Spurred by movements toward equality between the sexes, knowledge that a man's sexuality will not be affected, a greater desire to separate sex and reproduction, contraceptive failures, and dissatisfaction with current contraceptive methods have all contributed to the increasing numbers of men seeking voluntary sterilization.

Bilateral vasectomy is the surgical procedure by which men are rendered infertile. It is considered to be a highly safe, simple operation and is most often performed on an outpatient basis in a physician's office or clinic.

A small incision is made, under local anesthesia, in the sheath of the vas. The sheath is opened, exposing the vas deferens. The vas deferens is then clipped and $1/4$ to $1/2$ inch removed. The segmented ends of the vas are then ligated. Some physicians prefer to coagulate the severed ends of the vas to ensure success. The incision is closed by suturing (Fig. 21-2). Complications are few and minor. Pain and swelling are minimal, readily relieved by mild analgesics, and rarely last more than 1 week. No deaths have been reported that can be attributed to the procedure itself.[99] Failure because of recanalization of the vas deferens is reported to be around 1% and may be even lower.[26] There is a postoperative residual fertility following vasectomy that extends through 8 weeks following surgery.[91] Since most men are advised they can resume intercourse as soon as there is no discomfort from the surgery, other contraceptive methods must be used for 8 weeks. Follow-up laboratory examination of the semen for presence of sperm is usually done at the end of 8 weeks.

Reversibility of vasectomy is undergoing intensive study. Surgical attempts to restore continuity of the vas deferens is successful only 50% of the time, and, of the successes, only 20% to 25% result in sperm that are capable of fertilizing an ovum.[27] Voluntary vasectomy is considered a legal operation in all states except Utah and may be performed for any reason in single or married men over the age of 21 or in an emancipated minor.

Psychologic aspects of sterilization. Liberalization of attitudes toward male and female sterilization as a method of contraception raises questions concerning previous findings about the psychologic effects of sterilization on one or both partners. Research in the area is ongoing, but additional studies of sterilized persons over a long-term period are needed.

Men and women who elect sterilization seem to have little or no regret after the surgery. One study reports that over 90% of women having tubal sterilization expressed no regret but that some women were disturbed emotionally by having been sterilized.[73] From psychologic studies it is suggested that women who regretted having the surgery had preexisting emotional problems.[91] Several studies indicate that 95% to 99% of men are satisfied with the results of vasectomy and that, like women, some men had increased emotional difficulties after the sterilization.[27] In a follow-up study of men having vasectomies, it was found that 70% stated they were happier than before the operation and that frequency of intercourse had increased.[35]

Women who are dissatisfied after sterilization have described themselves as having feelings of inferiority, weakness, emptiness, being torn up inside, being a damaged, changed person, and having less desire for and gratification from sexual intercourse. Regret is less likely if a woman requests sterilization and it is

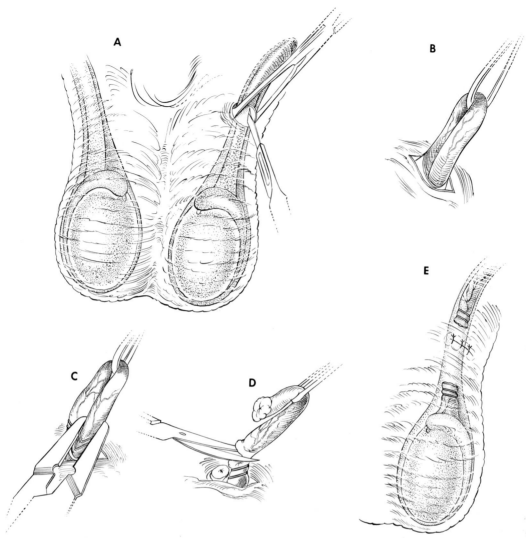

FIG. 21-2. Vasectomy procedure. **A,** Bilateral incision used to expose sheath. **B** and **C,** Vas exposed and occluded. **D,** Segment is excised. **E,** Vas is replaced in sheath and skin sutured. (Modified from Davis, J. E.: Am. J. Nurs. **72:**510, March 1972.)

done for reasons of family size rather than organic disease or previous cesarean section.[115]

Clearly, the findings of these studies make it imperative to identify men and women prior to surgery who may later have great regrets and therefore severe emotional problems. Counseling should be aimed toward confirming that the decision to have a sterilization is made as objectively as possible. Previous experience with other methods of contraception should be explored, and the reason for dissatisfaction with the method determined. It may be that a couple has very little knowledge of contraceptive methods and with adequate information might choose something other than sterilization. Care must be taken, however, that couples who are knowledgeable and have made a firm, objective decision are not made to feel that their decision is a poor one or is unacceptable.

The nature and consequences of the surgery must be explained to the patient. Many individuals want to know if the operation will change them and, if so, how. It is common for lay people to equate sterilization with castration and loss of femininity or masculinity. Even those patients who know the two are different need reassurance. Visual aids or models may be very helpful. Explaining that the ovaries and testes are left in place and that these produce hormones responsible for sexual behavior can be reassuring. If it is possible, having the patient meet someone of the same sex who has been sterilized may be helpful. Men and women may want to know what happens to the sperm and ova they will continue to produce following sterilization. Also, it is desirable to see the couple together at a preoperative interview. Group counseling in a special setting such as a clinic may have particular advantages. Use of films such as *Freedom from Pregnancy** and pamphlets such as *Voluntary Sterilization for Men and Women*† can be used to increase understanding.

Finally, there is a need to recognize that tubal sterilization affects men as well as women, and that vasectomies affect women as well as men when there is mutual caring and concern between them. This concern may be best illustrated by a woman who described her feelings when she and her husband selected vasectomy as their method of contraception: "The worst part of the experience was that I had not anticipated the range of my reactions. Now it seems that these transitions may have been natural. Perhaps if I had known the experiences of others, I would have passed more easily through these feelings. We try to prepare husbands for childbirth; we should recognize the need to prepare wives for vasectomy."[55]

The reproductive system and the aging process

In terms of increased scientific knowledge, as compared with other topics, little new knowledge has evolved concerning the reproductive system and the aging process.

Again, health education should precede the onset of the climacteric and should be presented objectively using facts. Understanding human behavior and the emotional impact of cessation of reproductive ability and skill in using direct and indirect approaches assists in establishing a climate that permits open, honest discussion.

As with all areas of health teaching, the nurse should first assess the learning needs, that is, the status of present knowledge, ability to understand, what has been done by others to assist with learning, and how the person has utilized the knowledge presented.

The climacteric, which usually lasts from 1 year to 18 months, is a period in which there is a gradual decline in ovarian function. It leads to the cessation of menstruation, or the *menopause.* During this time the interval between menstrual periods becomes increasingly longer or irregular, and the flow usually decreases in amount. Many women go through this interval of life with little awareness of its occurrence.

Approximately 10% of all women have pronounced symptoms of the climacteric. Vasomotor reactions producing hot flushes and excessive perspiration may occur and are caused by lack of stimulating hormones to or in the ovaries. Headaches, nervousness, heart palpitation, and sleeplessness may occur, and depression and other emotional reactions such as feelings of futility or uselessness may appear. Unfortunately the climacteric often comes at the very time when children are moving away from home and emancipating themselves. This fact in itself may make the woman feel that the better part of her life is over. Keeping busy, developing new interests, and recognizing her emotional reactions as an expected adjustment to a new hormonal environment help the woman to maintain a normal outlook. Most women's symptoms are relieved by a sedative such as phenobarbital or one of the ataractic (tranquilizing) drugs. Estrogen is widely prescribed during the menopause to combat psychologic difficulties, osteoporosis, arteriosclerosis, mucous membrane deterioration, and disorders of the skin that often appear. New evidence questions the wisdom of routinely prescribing estrogens for menopausal women. The risk factors associated with oral contraceptives and studies linking vaginal neoplasms in the female offspring of women treated with estrogen during their pregnancies have introduced the need to carefully evaluate complaints of women before prescribing estrogen during the menopause.[61] Prolonged estrogen stimulation without the balancing effect of progesterone is considered a high-risk factor in endometrial cancer.[105] It is believed that progesterone along with estrogen assists in periodic shedding of the endometrium and prevents hyperplasia. It is generally agreed that estrogen therapy should not be continued indefinitely. If there is a history of cancer of the reproductive system, including the breast, hormones are never given because it is believed that their use may stimulate growth of cancer cells that may remain in the body.

Men may also have a climacteric. However, it is usually less severe than in women and occurs at a much older age, or it may never occur. At this time men also suffer from feelings of depression and uselessness as the sexual drive diminishes. They, too, frequently have vasomotor instability. These changes may tempt some men to be promiscuous in an effort to prove to themselves that the aging process has not affected their virility. Because it is known that some chronic medical conditions such as diabetes mellitus and atherosclerosis can reduce the normal sexual drive, men who experience sudden reduction of this drive should be advised to consult a physician and have a complete physical examination.

It is an erroneous assumption that sexual activity must end with the climacteric. The frequency simply is decreased. Many women have a capacity to enjoy normal intercourse up to 65 years of age and beyond. This may be true even when the actual cessation of menstruation has occurred at a relatively early age. Men, too, often continue a fairly active sexual life after many signs of normal aging such as hypertrophy of the prostate have developed.

Many women have heard of "change of life"

---

*Allend'or Productions, Inc., 3449 Cahuenga West, Hollywood, Calif. 90068.

†Planned Parenthood World Population, 810 Seventh Ave. New York, N. Y. 10019.

babies and fear they may become pregnant. They require counseling about prevention of conception as do younger women. Women currently in this age group are of a generation reared at a time when such topics as reproduction, sexuality, and birth control were not as openly and freely discussed as today. Unless they have experienced changes in their attitudes, they may feel very hesitant about asking for help and information. Therefore it seems important that the nurse offer information and advice without waiting for the woman to ask.

In regard to prevention of conception, it is necessary to remember that the menstrual cycles and ovulation are irregular and that, if pregnancy is to be avoided, a highly reliable method is indicated. For example, the rhythm method would be inadvisable. There are some advantages to oral contraceptives during the menopause. They give complete protection at an age when pregnancy is usually not desired, when pregnancy is more dangerous from an obstetric viewpoint, and when some types of fetal abnormalities are more likely to occur. On the other hand, malignancies of the reproductive system are more common in menopausal women and these might be hormone stimulated or dependent. Also, oral contraceptives carry a greater mortality rate from thromboembolus problems in older women. Therefore it is necessary to assess the chances of pregnancy occurring, the risks pregnancy might carry, alternatives should pregnancy occur, and the chances of the woman being able to use an alternative method effectively.

Women may have pain with intercourse (dyspareunia) after the menopause because of shrinkage or adhesions of the vaginal canal caused by tissue atrophy. This condition occasionally is treated by a plastic repair of the vagina, but usually estrogenic hormones are given. Treatment is determined by the physician after reviewing the wishes and living pattern of the patient. A low-grade vaginal infection may also follow atrophy of the cells lining the vagina. It sometimes responds to vinegar-and-water douches, but if it continues, estrogen hormones may be prescribed. The older woman with such an infection should be advised to bathe frequently in a tub of warm water and to soak for 15 to 20 minutes at each bath.

With the onset of the climacteric, the predisposition to cancer of the sex organs, which are at this time undergoing involutional changes, seems to increase for both sexes. Every woman should have a yearly pelvic examination, including cytologic studies of the cervix and endometrium, since regular examination is the best way to diagnose early cancer of the female reproductive system. Women who have had children are more prone to cancer of the cervix than women who have had no children, but cancer of any part of the reproductive system is quite common in all women. Since cancer of the cervix has an unusually good prognosis if diagnosed and treated early, any delay in diagnosis by failure to have regular examinations is deplorable.

After the age of 40 years, the prostate gland also becomes unusually prone to carcinoma. Every man over 40 years of age should have a yearly rectal examination, since by this simple means many carcinomas of the prostate may be diagnosed early enough for treatment to be satisfactory.

The menopause may be artificially induced by such procedures as irradiation of the ovaries, surgical removal of both ovaries, or hysterectomy. Each of these have one common consequence, namely, cessation of menstruation. Beyond this, however, differences occur. Menstruation ceases if a hysterectomy is performed, but the ovaries continue to function when left intact provided the age of climacteric is not reached. If the ovaries are irradiated or removed, abrupt withdrawal of ovarian hormones results, and symptoms associated with the climacteric, including menopausal symptoms, appear regardless of the woman's age.

■ EXAMINATION OF THE REPRODUCTIVE TRACT

Both men and women often put off medical examinations of the reproductive system, since this type of examination may cause intense emotional reactions. Fear, embarrassment, and cultural background play an important part in this emotional distress. In our culture, people frequently are afraid that their anxieties concerning carcinoma, venereal disease, sterility, or the climacteric will be verified. Many people are embarrassed to discuss problems concerning their sexual life, such as inability to perform in the culturally accepted pattern during intercourse. Many are embarrassed by the necessary exposure of the external genitalia during the medical examination. A person may also be fearful that some condition will be discovered that will require surgery resulting in sterility or impotence. The nurse who is sensitive to the many thoughts and fears that may trouble patients will be better prepared to help them accept the necessary medical examination.

It often reassures patients to know that medical information will be given only to the physician and that this information goes no farther. They should know that complete, frank answers to all questions will help considerably in determining the cause of any difficulty and in planning suitable treatment. Patients should be encouraged to discuss any other related problems that may be of concern to them but about which the physician may fail to ask specifically. The woman should be prepared for the questions she will be asked. If she is told before the physician examines her that she will be asked about her monthly periods and about her pregnancies and deliveries, she is given a chance to think through her answers under less pressure and thus can give more accurate information. It is desirable to advise women scheduled for pelvic examination to avoid douching and application of any preparations (medicinal or deodorant) to the vagina for at least 24 hours prior to the examination. The presence of these substances may influence the findings of the examination, especially those obtained by inspection and smear or culture.

It is necessary to explain to the patient the procedures that will be performed during the examination, what he or she will be expected to do, and what the physician will do. Any likelihood of a cramping discomfort (which will occur if *anything* is introduced into the cervical canal) should be explained to the patient. A calm, thoughtful, interested, yet matter-of-fact manner often helps put patients at ease. The nurse should appraise each patient and adjust her approach accordingly. Some patients, particularly those who are very fearful, may need either a much more personalized or perhaps a more detached approach. Women, especially young girls, are often reassured by a female nurse's presence during the examination, whereas men or boys may need to know that they will be left alone with the physician after the nurse has made necessary preparations for the examination.

Examination and diagnostic measures used for female patients

Pelvic examination. The pelvic examination is relatively simple. However, if the patient is extremely upset and unable to relax sufficiently for satisfactory palpation or if any undue pain is anticipated, it may occasionally be done under anesthesia. An anesthetic usually is necessary if a complete examination of a young girl must be done.

The following equipment should be available:
1. Bivalve vaginal specula (various sizes)
2. Uterine tenaculum forceps
3. Sponge forceps
4. Biopsy forceps (sterile)
5. Cautery unit with tips
6. Uterine sounds and probes (sterile)
7. Gloves (disposable rubber or plastic)
8. Lubricant (water soluble, vegetable base)
9. Aspirator or wooden blade for Pap smear
10. Cotton applicators
11. Cotton balls
12. Gauze sponges
13. Topical antiseptic solution
14. Specimen bottles with fixative solution
15. Glass microscope slides
16. Test tubes and culture tubes

Good light is important for a pelvic examination. Probably the best lighting is obtained with a head

mirror. Gooseneck lights also are used frequently.

The patient should void immediately prior to the examination, since an empty bladder makes palpation easier, eliminates any possible distortion of the position of the pelvic organs caused by a full bladder, and obviates the danger of incontinence during the examination. The urine should be saved for laboratory examination if necessary.

Ambulatory patients should always be told what clothing must be removed, since panties or girdles interfere with the examination, waste time, and cause unnecessary embarrassment to both the patient and the physician.

The woman should know that the examination may be somewhat uncomfortable. It probably will not be painful unless disease makes it so. She can help most in making the examination effective and brief by relaxing as completely as possible. Breathing through the mouth often helps to relax the abdominal muscles. She should be assured that her modesty will be maintained. While on the table she will be draped, the door will be kept closed, and the nurse will be present during the entire procedure.

Several positions may be used (Fig. 21-3). The physician will indicate the one in which he wishes the patient placed. The nurse should check to see that the patient does not have arthritis or any other condition that may limit position or movement and will interfere with her assuming the desired position.

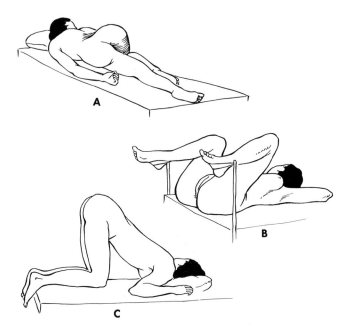

FIG. 21-3. Various positions that can be assumed for examination of the rectum and the vagina. **A,** Sims' (lateral) position; note position of the left arm and right leg. **B,** Lithotomy position; note position of the buttocks on the edge of the examining table and support of feet. **C,** Knee-chest (genupectoral) position; note placement of the shoulders and head.

Some positions such as the knee-chest position are uncomfortable and embarrassing for patients of almost any age or physical condition. As the nurse places the patient in the position desired, it should be explained why the position is necessary for an adequate examination.

1. *Dorsal recumbent position (also known as lithotomy position)* (Fig. 21-3, *B*). The lower leaf of the examining table should be dropped before the patient gets onto the table, since dropping it may be frightening to her after her feet have been placed in the stirrups. There should be a footstool handy so that she can be guided to step on the stool, sit down on the edge of the table, and then lie back. Most patients are able to place their own legs in the stirrups; they should be told to raise both legs and put them in the stirrups simultaneously. When a patient needs help, two persons may assist—one on each side of the patient so that both can hold one leg and simultaneously place them in position without abruptly lifting the lower extremities. Gentleness and gradual positioning are essential in order to prevent strain or twisting of the hip joint. Metal stirrups are the most satisfactory. However, if they are being used, the patient should wear her shoes because the heels help to hold the feet in the stirrups.

Care must be taken to see that there is no pressure on the legs when sling stirrups are used, since nerve damage and impairment of circulation can occur. The buttocks need to be moved down so that they are even with the end of the table. The nurse should see that the pillow under the head is pulled down at the same time to assure comfort for the patient. The patient is then draped in such a manner that only the perineum is exposed. The triangular drape is most often used since it provides a flap that can be brought down for protection if a few moments should intervene between draping and examination.

If this examination must be done in bed, the patient is placed across the bed with her feet resting on the seats of two straight chairs. This method can be used in the home if necessary.

2. *Sims' position (used also for rectal examination)* (Fig. 21-3, *A*). For this position the patient is placed on her left side, with her left arm and hand placed behind her. The left thigh should be only slightly flexed, and the right knee should be flexed sharply on the abdomen. She should be draped so as to expose only the perineum.

3. *Knee-chest position* (Fig. 21-3, *C*). After dropping the lower end of the examining table, have the patient get on her hands and knees on the table. The buttocks will be uppermost, and the thighs should be sharply flexed on the trunk. The patient's head should be turned to one side and should rest on the table. The arms should be flexed and resting well forward (often above the patient's head), and the knees should be apart. The feet should extend over the lower edge

of the table to prevent pressure on the toes. Drape so as to expose only the perineum. If this examination must be done in bed, place the patient crosswise on the bed.

The pelvic examination consists first of inspection of the external genitalia for signs of inflammation, bleeding, discharge, swelling, erosions, or other local skin changes. If the patient is a virgin, a very small speculum may be used, or examination with the speculum may be omitted. Using the speculum, the physician inspects the vaginal walls and cervix, thus making it possible to note any unusual signs such as alteration in the normal size or color, tears, erosion, or bleeding. The nurse should see that the light is adjusted so that the vaginal canal and cervix are well illuminated. If no other light is available, the nurse may hold a flashlight to provide suitable lighting. While the speculum is in place, smears and cultures are taken.

A digital examination then follows; for this the physician will need gloves and lubricating jelly. Placing one or two fingers in the vagina, he palpates the abdomen with his other hand. He concludes with a rectal examination, using one finger. (See Fig. 21-4.) By digital examination he can usually detect abnormalities in the placement, contour, motility, and tissue consistency of the base of the bladder and the uterus and its adjacent structures, including the ovaries, the fallopian tubes, and the rectum.

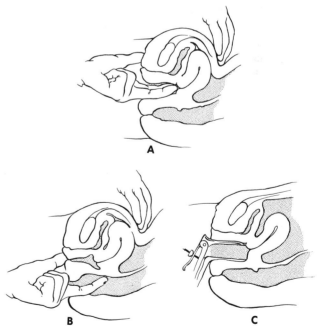

FIG. 21-4. Methods of pelvic examination. **A,** Digital examination of the vagina with abdominal palpation to determine size and position of uterus. **B,** Digital rectal examination with abdominal palpation. **C,** Examination of the vagina and cervix using a bivalve vaginal speculum.

Responsibilities of the nurse during the examination include being present during the entire procedure for the protection of both the patient and the physician, encouraging the patient to relax, and assisting as necessary. Equipment that may be needed should be available in the room so that the nurse will not have to leave the patient unattended.

Following the examination, the nurse should quickly remove any lubricating jelly or discharge that may be on the genitalia and should assist the patient from the table, taking both legs out of the stirrups simultaneously. In elderly patients, unnatural positions such as the knee-chest and lithotomy positions may alter the normal circulation of blood sufficiently to cause faintness. Extreme care must be taken not to leave an elderly patient sitting on the table. With the aid of a footstool, the nurse should assist her from the table and help her to a chair where she may wish to rest for a moment before beginning to dress. If necessary, the nurse should help the patient dress and during this time explain any statements made by the physician that are not clear to the patient. The patient is informed that after she is dressed the physician will talk to her again.

Equipment should be rinsed with cold water, washed well with soap and water, rinsed, and sterilized. The linen or other protective covering on the table should be changed. Often a protective waterproof square covered with a treatment towel or paper towel or napkin is placed under the buttocks to prevent cross contamination of linen. The protective square must be thoroughly washed with soap and water if it has become moistened. Disposable protective sheets are now available to facilitate easy preparation of the examining table for the next patient and also to prevent cross contamination of linen.

After the patient has completed her interview with the physician, the nurse is responsible for follow-up teaching as necessary. It may be necessary to further explain information or orders given by the physician such as the technique of douching, provide general health education, discuss the time and importance of her next appointment, and explain any referrals to a special department or physician.

Schiller's test. This test reveals the presence of atypical cervical cells. A solution of 3.5% iodine or Lugol's solution is applied to the cervix. Atypical cells, both malignant and benign, do not contain glycogen and will fail to stain. Early cancerous lesions and also benign lesions such as areas of cervicitis may show up as glistening areas of a lighter color than surrounding tissue. This simple test helps the physician decide whether or not other diagnostic procedures should be performed. For example, it helps identify the area of the cervix from which a biopsy should be taken. Because iodine stains clothing, the patient usually is advised to wear a pad for several hours after the test.

Cytologic test for cancer (Papanicolaou smear test). Tumor cells as well as normal cells of such structures as the fallopian tubes, the uterus, and the vagina exfoliate and pass into the cervical and vaginal secretions. When these secretions are aspirated and smears made, cellular changes may be seen and lesions of the cervix, the lining of the fallopian tubes, or the uterus may be detected in their early stages. The recently learned fact that malignant cells tend to separate more readily and clump together less than normal cells helps to explain the high rate of success in detection of early cancer by this means. Malignant lesions in the ovaries and in the outer structures such as the outer layers of the uterus do not, of course, exfoliate cells that are available for study in this manner. The death rate from cervical cancer has been reduced by 50% in the past 15 years, and this fact has led the World Health Organization to classify cancer of the cervix as a preventable disease. This is true provided women have Pap tests performed regularly.

Any positive Pap smear indicates a pathologic condition, most often but not exclusively cancer. A tissue biopsy (cone biopsy) must be done to make a definite diagnosis. The test is extremely valuable in leading the physician to suspect cancer of the cervix while there is yet no visible or palpable evidence of tumor growth. Cancer of the cervix, one of the most common forms of cancer in women, may thus be treated much earlier than was previously possible, and the rate of cure is relatively high. The patient should understand, however, that the smear test is not necessarily conclusive and that biopsy or even surgery may be necessary to verify the diagnosis. It is also used to screen patients needing further examination as well as to measure the effectiveness of radiation and surgical treatment. Many patients are familiar with the vaginal smear test from descriptions given in popular magazines. It is not painful, and some patients are taught to take smears themselves daily, especially when the physician is interested in determining the pattern of endometrial growth in women with sterility problems or in those receiving estrogen therapy.

Pap test kits of the "do-it-yourself" variety have been available for several years. These can be used by women who are reluctant or unable to visit a physician for examination. The reliability of self-taken smears is influenced by the woman's understanding of the correct procedure. It is imperative that the aspirator or wooden spatula be inserted deeply enough to reach the area around the cervix and the specimen must be fixed rapidly to prevent drying (Fig. 21-5). While this approach has value for mass screening and early detection, it is not a substitute for the more complete history and examination essential for preventive care.

Smears for cytologic study may be taken from the

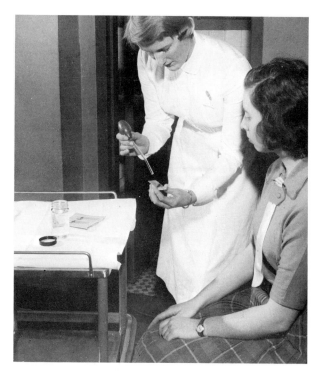

FIG. 21-5. The nurse shows the patient how to fix the slide after taking a vaginal smear, a necessary procedure if the patient must take daily smears at home.

vagina or, under sterile precautions, from within the cervix. In order to ensure obtaining an adequate and accurate specimen, certain precautions should be taken. The woman should not douche or take a tub bath for at least 48 hours before the smear is taken, nor should the smear be taken if she is menstruating. These precautions apply to all Pap smears regardless of whether they are taken by a physician, nurse, or the woman herself.

Cauterization of the cervix produces distortion of the cells of the cervix, and this may persist for 6 weeks. Radiation produces distortion of cells for a much longer period. The Pap smear should be delayed for at least 1 month after use of topical antibiotics because they produce rapid, heavy shedding of cells.[105] Systemic antibiotics do not produce this effect.

If the equipment must be sterilized with moist sterilization and if it is needed for use before it has thoroughly dried, it should be rinsed in equal parts of 95% alcohol and ether to hasten drying.

The equipment needed for taking a vaginal cytologic smear includes a vaginal pipette with a rubber bulb, an applicator for obtaining secretions from the external mouth of the cervix, a spatula for scraping around the cervix in order to obtain cells loosened but not yet exfoliated, slides, a widemouthed bottle containing equal parts of 95% alcohol and ether, labels, and laboratory slips.

With the patient in the lithotomy position, the physician takes the smears before beginning the vaginal examination. Dry, clean, unlubricated equipment is used, and the label on the slide is checked to be sure that it contains the name of the patient, the date, and the source of the specimen. After air is expressed from the bulb of the vaginal pipette, the pipette is inserted with an upward and backward motion so that the specimen will be obtained from the posterior fornix, which is most likely to contain cells from the endometrium, the cervix, and the vagina. A specimen of the secretion is aspirated, and the pipette is withdrawn. The secretion is then expressed thinly and evenly on the prepared slide, and the slide is placed in the solution of ether and alcohol. The secretion must not be permitted to become dry, since the cells will be distorted in appearance if drying occurs. Patients who take their own smears often do the aspiration while standing with one foot on a low stool or chair.

Obtaining an endocervical smear is a sterile procedure that is done only by the physician. If two specimens are obtained, one from the cervix and one from the vagina, the two specimens must be carefully placed into the solution so that the unsmeared sides are back to back with each other, thereby preventing any mixing of vaginal secretions with those of the cervix. This technique assists the pathologist or cytologist in determining the source of abnormal cells. The preparation is the same as for a vaginal smear except that a sterile metal cannula with a bulb or syringe attached is needed. The patient having this test will have some discomfort due to the dilation of the cervical canal, but there should be no real pain. There may be some cramping pain from uterine contractions after the procedure. Usually heat applied to the lower abdomen and the administration of acetylsalicylic acid will give relief.

Screening for endometrial cancer. With the decline in mortality due to cervical cancer, greater attention has been directed toward developing mass screening techniques to detect early cancer of the endometrium. Recent advances in cytologic screening for endometrial cancer now make it possible for such screening to become part of every woman's health care program.

Since women over the age of 50 are more likely to develop endometrial cancer, screening of postmenopausal women assumes greater significance.

The Pap test picks up only occasional cases of cancer of the endometrium. Until recently, dilatation and curettage was required to obtain adequate cell samples from the endometrium, and this procedure requires hospitalization and anesthesia. Probably the most adequate alternative method for screening endometrial cells involves irrigating the uterine cavity with normal saline solution. A disposable, suction-type irrigating device called the Gravlee Jet Washer

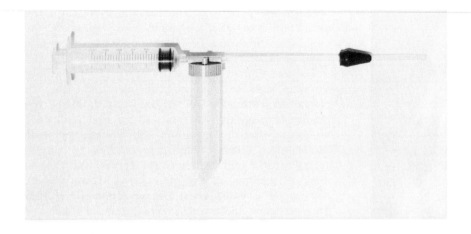

FIG. 21-6. Gravlee Jet Washer used to obtain endometrial cells for microscopic study by irrigation of the uterine cavity. (Courtesy The Upjohn Co., Kalamazoo, Mich.)

is used (Fig. 21-6). This method is safe, simple, and painless except for mild cramping. It does not require hospitalization and can performed on an outpatient basis. The irrigating device is inserted into the uterus and the uterine cavity is irrigated with about 30 ml. of normal saline solution. The normal saline solution containing cells from the entire uterine lining is returned by suction into a collecting chamber. The cells are then centrifuged out, stained, and examined microscopically.

Tests for pregnancy. Tests for pregnancy are based on the fact that a hormone, human chorionic gonadotropin (HCG), is produced by the placenta and is present in the urine by the tenth to fourteenth day after the first missed menstrual period. Some biologic tests that can be performed are the *Aschheim-Zondek* test, *Friedman* test, and *Hogben* test. Each of these requires injection of the woman's urine into a laboratory animal. If human chorionic gonadotropin is present in the urine, the test is positive as indicated by rapid maturational changes in the ovaries of the laboratory animal. These tests require up to 48 hours to obtain the results.

More recently, immunologic tests have gained in popularity because the test can be carried out within a few minutes. For some women the time element may be very important. Some clinics, for example, have pregnancy testing services and these are popular among women who may not wish to continue a pregnancy and seek therapeutic abortion.

The immunologic tests are based on the fact that human chorionic gonadotropin is an antigen that has the ability to produce specific antibodies when injected into an animal. The serum of the animal will therefore contain antibodies specific for human chorionic gonadotropin and can be used to detect the presence of human chorionic gonadotropin in the woman's urine.

When carried out correctly, the pregnancy tests are reliable 95% of the time. Two conditions, hydatidiform mole and choriocarcinoma, produce false positive pregnancy tests because of the presence of active chorionic villi.

Culdoscopy and related procedures. A culdoscopy is an examination in which the physician attempts to see the cause of disease in the pelvis by inserting an instrument (culdoscope) through the posterior fornix into the cul-de-sac of Douglas (Fig. 21-7). A tubal pregnancy, for example, can sometimes be observed by this means. Usually the patient is hospitalized for the procedure, which is done in the operating room under sterile conditions and with the patient under anesthesia. Occasionally sedation and only local anesthesia are used. *Peritoneoscopy* and *laparoscopy* are similar procedures through which pelvic structures may be observed by approaching through the abdomen rather than through the vagina. Air may be injected and radiographs taken to outline pelvic structures more fully, and a radiopaque, aqueous medium may be injected into the uterus and the fallopian tubes (p. 507). Following these procedures, air in the abdominal cavity may cause discomfort similar to that following the Rubin test for patency of the fallopian tubes.

After procedures in which air enters the abdominal cavity, the patient is placed in a face-lying position with a pillow under the abdomen. Occasionally a tight abdominal binder and pressure on the abdomen are prescribed.[68] The knee-chest position should be avoided for several days since the unhealed wound may permit air to enter the abdominal cavity. The patient should not take a douche or have sexual intercourse for a week. Hemorrhage occurs very occasionally. Since infection could develop, the patient should be observed for signs of infection such as elevation of temperature and pain or discomfort in the lower abdomen.

A *culdocentesis* is a procedure in which a needle is inserted through the posterior fornix of the vagina into the cul-de-sac of Douglas for the purpose of removing, for study, pus or other abnormal fluids that may be present. Usually this procedure is done in the

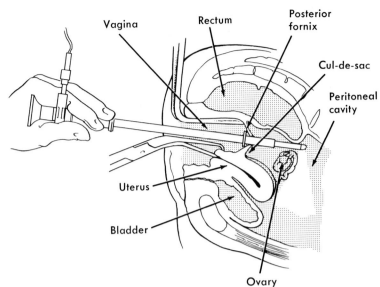

FIG. 21-7. With patient in the knee-chest position, the culdoscope is inserted through the posterior fornix of the vagina into the cul-de-sac of Douglas. Note that the ovaries can be seen.

physician's office and does not require hospitalization. Surgical aseptic precautions are used so that infection will not be introduced into the pelvis.

Cervical biopsy and cautery. Sometimes the physician wishes to send a piece of cervical tissue to the laboratory for pathologic examination. The biopsy procedure will usually be scheduled for a week after the end of the menstrual period, since the cervix is more vascular immediately before and after menstruation. The patient should know what is to be done and why. She should know that there may be momentary discomfort, but that no actual pain will be felt because the cervix does not contain pain fibers. If a cautery is to be used to treat erosion, to remove small polyps from the mouth of the cervix, or for other reasons, she should be told that a small, lubricated sheet of lead will be placed against the skin under the lumbar area as a safety device for grounding electrical charges and that there will be slight bleeding which will be controlled by a tampon or packing that will be inserted by the physician. The odor of burning tissue when a cautery is used nauseates some patients. They should be told that the odor may be noticed but that it actually is insignificant and that the procedure usually is over quickly.

In addition to the equipment needed for a pelvic examination, the nurse should have the following items available:

1. Biopsy forceps
2. Uterine tenaculum forceps
3. Specimen bottle containing 10% formalin or, if specimen can be delivered to pathology laboratory immediately following procedure, wet saline sponge and waxed paper may be used (specimens should be labeled with patient's name, date, source of specimen, and physician's name)

4. Cautery unit and cautery tips
5. Gauze packing or tampon

Following the procedure, the nurse should be certain that the patient understands the physician's instructions. Sometimes the main points are written out. Instructions will vary, but they usually include the following:

1. Rest more than usual for the next 24 hours. Avoid lifting and marked exertion.
2. Leave the tampon or packing in place as long as the physician advises (usually 8 to 24 hours).
3. Report to the hospital or physician's office if bleeding is excessive. (Usually more than occurs during a normal menses is considered excessive.)
4. Do not use an internal douche or have sexual relations until the next visit to the physician unless specific instructions have been given as to when intercourse can be safely resumed.
5. If cauterization has been done, an unpleasant discharge caused by sloughing of destroyed cells may appear 4 to 5 days following the treatment. A warm bath several times each day will help this condition, which should not last more than a few days.

A douche may be suggested if there is a vaginal discharge. Usually vinegar (2 tablespoons of white vinegar to 2 quarts of water) is ordered. The nurse should make sure that the patient knows how to take a douche. The temperature should be 40° C. (105° F.) unless otherwise ordered. Most physicians prefer that patients douche while lying in the bathtub rather than while sitting on the toilet seat (Fig. 21-8). A douche pan may be placed in the tub if so desired. A bath should be taken first to lessen the chance of contamination. The douche tip should be inserted

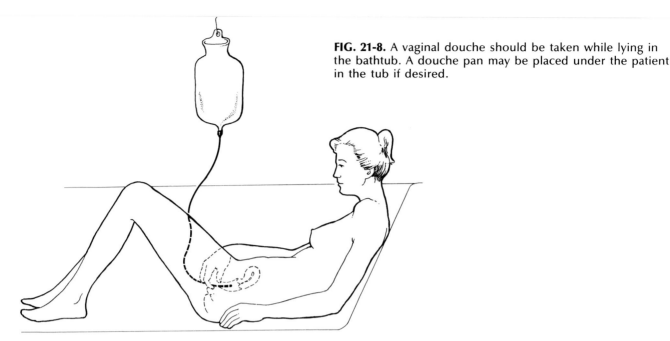

FIG. 21-8. A vaginal douche should be taken while lying in the bathtub. A douche pan may be placed under the patient in the tub if desired.

upward and backward and moved about to prevent fluid from being forced into the mouth of the cervix and to ensure flushing of the posterior fornix. If a medicated or hot douche is to be taken, the labia should be held together for a few moments to allow the vagina to fill up and thus benefit all areas. Douches prescribed to provide local heat should be continued for about a half hour. Petroleum jelly may be used to prevent burning the sensitive tissues of the labia. Following douching, the tub should be well cleansed with soap and warm water.

Dilatation and curettage (D and C). Dilatation of the cervix and curettage (scraping) of the endometrial lining of the uterus are minor surgical procedures usually done at the same time either to diagnose disease of the uterus or to correct excessive and prolonged bleeding. Occasionally dilatation of the cervix alone is done to treat dysmenorrhea or to treat sterility caused by stricture or stenosis of the cervical canal. Because the procedure is carried out under general anesthesia, the patient needs physical and emotional preparation and care similar to that given any patient undergoing general anesthesia. In addition, the patient should be told preoperatively that the pubic and perineal area will be shaved if this will be done. Some physicians now believe that shaving is not necessary and that the discomfort during regrowth of pubic hair can be avoided.[82] The patient should know that a nurse will be present with her during the entire procedure, and that she will not be exposed any more than during a pelvic examination. Sometimes the perineal shave and entire preparation is done in the operating room after the patient has been anesthetized and placed in the lithotomy position. If this procedure is followed, the patient should know what is planned. Otherwise she may worry because the

preparation is not done in her room or be upset when she awakens from anesthesia to find that it has been done. As in all surgery involving the perineum and lower abdomen, the lower bowel and bladder must be empty so that they will not interfere with the operation or be damaged.

At the conclusion of the operation, packing may be placed in the cervical canal and vagina. A sterile pad is placed over the perineum. When the patient returns to her room, the nurse should check the pad for amount of bleeding every 15 minutes for 2 hours and then every 1 to 2 hours for 8 hours. A blood loss of at least 60 ml. is required to saturate a perineal pad. The blood loss should always be recorded in estimated milliliters. It is important to record each pad change as well as blood loss. Usually the pad is only slightly stained. Any excessive bleeding should be reported to the physician. For the comfort of the patient, the pad should be anchored with a sanitary belt and changed as necessary. Sterile perineal pads are used until the packing is removed, usually within 24 hours after surgery.

Packing in the cervical canal may cause cramps similar to moderately severe menstrual cramps, since a dilated cervical canal stimulates uterine contractions. Mild analgesics such as codeine sulfate and acetylsalicylic acid are ordered to relieve cramps and are given every 4 hours for the first 24 to 48 hours as necessary. Abdominal pain that is not relieved by analgesics should be reported at once. An uncommon but serious complication of curettage is accidental perforation of the uterus during the procedure, with resultant peritonitis.

Voiding may be difficult following a dilatation and curettage because of the pressure of the packing against the urethra or because of local trauma and irritation from the procedure. Usually, however, the patient is permitted to be up almost as soon as she reacts from the anesthetic, and she can void if permitted to use the bathroom. Any packing that extends beyond the vagina should be kept dry during voiding if possible, and the patient should be instructed to protect the vaginal orifice from fecal contamination by cleansing with a backward motion.

Patients often go home the day after a dilatation and curettage. They can resume most of their normal daily activities, increasing to normal activity in about a week. Vigorous exercise such as horseback riding, tennis, and dancing is usually discouraged, since these activities may tend to increase pelvic congestion. The patient should abstain from sexual intercourse until her return visit to the physician, at which time he will advise her as to when intercourse may safely be resumed. The menstrual cycle usually is not upset by a dilatation and curettage, but a vaginal discharge may appear during the healing period. A vinegar-and-water douche may be prescribed for this (p. 503).

Examination of the female infant and young girl. At birth the female infant should be examined for evidence of any abnormalities of the external genitalia. *Gynatresia* (imperforate hymen) is a relatively minor abnormality that can usually be noted at an early age. It should be corrected before the onset of the menses. The nurse in the hospital and the public health nurse should observe the newborn infant and should be certain that the mother knows what is normal. Some mothers actually do not know what the external genitalia of a small girl should look like. Diagrams and pictures often help to clarify points for them. Infants born to women who have taken the hormone progesterone to maintain their pregnancy should be observed particularly carefully because large doses of this hormone causes abnormalities of various kinds. Some of the changes produced by this hormone are reversible with puberty. Without alarming the mother, the nurse should urge that any abnormality noted be brought to the physician's attention.

Unless there are definite indications making examination necessary, detailed examination of the internal genital system usually is not done until after puberty. When examination is necessary, it may be done under general anesthesia. A urethroscope may be used to visualize the cervix when a speculum cannot be used. Atresia of the vagina, absence of the vagina or the uterus (agenesis), double vagina, double uterus, or anomalies of the ovaries are some of the abnormalities that may be found.

Examination and diagnostic measures used for male patients

Examination of the male genitalia. Physical examination of the reproductive system in the male patient

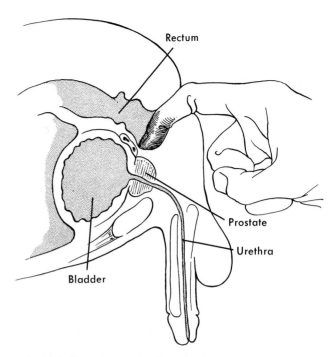

FIG. 21-9. Digital examination via the rectum to determine the size and consistency of the prostate gland. Note location of the gland in relation to other structures.

consists of careful inspection and palpation of the scrotum, noting skin lesions, differences in size and contour of the scrotum, and any evidence of swelling. Transillumination of the scrotum is done to detect absence of testicles and any unusual density of the structures contained within the scrotal sac. By means of a rectal examination, the physician can detect enlargement and general consistency of the prostate gland (Fig. 21-9) and any nodules in the adjacent tissues. The penis, foreskin, and meatus are inspected for signs of lesions or other abnormalities. By means of cystoscopic examination, the physician can detect prostatic encroachment on the urethra and observe the condition of the urethral and bladder mucosa. This procedure is not a part of routine examination, however. X-ray visualization and catheterization of the seminal vesicles to obtain specimens are also sometimes done.

The nurse should see that the patient is draped and that he understands what the physician will do and what will be expected of him, such as giving a specimen of urine and breathing deeply to make palpation easier for the physician. He should not empty his bladder immediately before examination because the physician may, by watching him void, be able to identify signs of possible urethral obstruction. Necessary equipment is prepared, and the nurse then leaves the patient alone with the physician.

After the examination, the patient may have questions to ask the nurse. If he is to have special examinations or treatments later, the nurse is responsible for explaining the preparation and the procedure to him.

Prostatic smears. If cancer or tuberculosis of the prostate is suspected, a prostatic smear may be desired. The physician first massages the prostate via the rectum. The next voided urine specimen is collected in an appropriate container (a sterile bottle for acid-fast [tubercle] bacilli; a bottle containing alcohol, 95%, or a commercial fixative for Pap or cytologic examination) and sent to the laboratory.

Testicular and prostatic biopsies. Testicular and prostatic biopsies may be obtained either by aspiration of cells through a needle or by obtaining a specimen of tissue through a surgical incision. Both of these procedures are carried out under sterile conditions using local or general anesthesia. If a general anesthetic is to be used, the preoperative and postoperative care is similar to that given any surgical patient. The incision used to obtain a testicular biopsy is a small one in the scrotum, usually about 1 inch in length. The only dressing is usually a sterile 4 by 8 inch gauze sponge inside a firm scrotal support. The patient may go home the evening of the operation, returning to have the sutures removed or to be prepared for further treatment if the biopsy shows that it is necessary.

To obtain a prostatic biopsy, a small incision is made in the perineum between the anus and scrotum. The dressing is usually held in place by a two-tailed binder. The patient must be instructed to be careful not to contaminate the incision while cleansing himself following defecation. If the incision is accidentally contaminated, the area should be carefully cleansed. Irrigation of the perineum by pouring sterile water over it or by washing with sterile sponges and antiseptic solution is sometimes ordered following defecation. A heat lamp with a 60-watt bulb placed 12 inches from the perineum is often used two or three times a day to encourage healing. The patient must be in a position in which the scrotum is elevated so that the heat strikes the incision. The best method is to allow the scrotum to rest on a wide piece of adhesive tape extending from thigh to thigh. Occasionally an exaggerated Sims' position gives satisfactory wound exposure. When the sutures have been removed, sitz baths are used instead of the lamp treatment, and they add a great deal to the general comfort of the patient. Usually following a prostatic biopsy the patient remains in the hospital until the laboratory findings are reported. A patient who has had a needle (aspiration) biopsy will not usually require hospitalization and has no dressings.

Frequently patients, both men and women, show signs of anxiety and depression following diagnostic procedures that necessitate waiting for pathologic reports. The nurse should reassure them by emphasizing their intelligence in seeking medical advice and, without undue discussion, should let them know that results of the examination will be available soon.

Evaluation of infertility problems

It has been estimated that 10% to 15% of married couples in the United States are unwillingly childless. Although infertility is most often attributed to females, approximately 40% of infertile marriages result from sterility of the male.

It is important that couples who wish to have children and are unsuccessful after about a year of trying to achieve pregnancy seek medical advice. Either one or both partners may contribute to the problem. Infertility studies are often time-consuming, and the emotional toll of feelings of inadequacy is great. Improved methods of treating infertility continue to become available, and about 30% of infertile marriages can be rendered fertile.

Evaluation of male fertility. Some physicians prefer to carry out a complete examination of the man first, as it is more easily accomplished and less time-consuming. Following a thorough physical examination, the first special test will be *multiple semen examinations* to determine the presence, number, maturity, and motility of the sperm. The man is instructed to bring a specimen of semen to the physician immediately after emission because sperm cells quickly deteriorate. The date of the last emission and the time of this specimen should be recorded. The absence of sperm in the semen may indicate a stricture somewhere along the vas deferens or absence of sperm production. A normal sperm count is approximately 60 million/ml. of semen, at least 75% of which have normal motility and are normal in shape. A sperm count below 20 million/ml. of semen and a motility rate of under 40% with over 25% of misshapen forms are known to lower the chance of fertilization of an ovum.

A *biopsy of the testicle* will show sperm production if the absence of sperm in the semen (azoospermia) is due to stricture of the tubal systems beyond the testes. Occasionally strictures may be repaired by a plastic surgery procedure (vasoepididymal or vasovasal anastomosis), but the results are often poor. Bilateral cryptorchism, or undescended testicles, even though corrected, may be the cause of sterility because of failure of the testicles to develop their sperm-producing function. This is particularly true if the correction is not done before puberty. Men sometimes will have no further sperm production following orchitis as a complication of mumps or following x-ray exposure of the testicles. A lack of vitamins A and E in the diet may also cause some atrophy of the spermatogenic tissue.

When the male is completely aspermatic, conception is impossible, and the couple should consider adoption of children if they really want a family. If the sperm count and the motility rate of the sperm cells are low, the physician usually prescribes thyroid extract and vitamins and treats any low-grade infections. Testosterone may be prescribed. It is important for the patient to eat a well-balanced diet, to maintain normal weight, to obtain adequate rest, and to participate in moderate exercise (preferably outdoors). The physician will suggest that the couple have frequent intercourse during the fertile period (14 to 16 days after the beginning of the menstrual period). Several days of continence should be practiced just prior to this period. If these methods are unsuccessful, the injection of several drops of the male's semen into the upper portion of the cervical canal may produce a pregnancy.

Evaluation of female fertility. The woman should also have a thorough physical examination, including a pelvic examination. In addition, a systematic check is made of each organ that might affect the reproductive system and each gland influencing it (Fig. 27-1).

In order for the ovum to be fertilized, the vagina, cervix, and uterus must be completely patent and have mucosal secretions that are not hostile to the sperm. Normally semen is alkaline in reaction, cervical secretions are alkaline, and vaginal secretions are acid. The Huhner test and vaginal and endometrial smears give necessary information about the secretions.

In the *Huhner test* the physician aspirates cervical secretions within 1 hour after intercourse and examines them for the presence and viability of the sperm cells. The woman should be instructed not to void, douche, or bathe between intercourse and the examination. She should use a perineal pad and go immediately to the physician's office. If the sperm are being killed by the secretions, vaginal smears are examined, and an appropriate antibiotic may be given to change the flora in the woman's vagina and cervix, timing its administration so that the secretions are most favorable to the sperm at the time of ovulation. If the secretions are too acid or too alkaline, medicated douches may be ordered. A douche using sodium bicarbonate (1 tablespoon to 1 quart of water) taken just before intercourse has been found to increase the motility of the sperm cells in many cases.[113] If the sperm cells do not reach the uterus, dilatation of the cervix may be tried.

The ovary must be producing ova, estrogen, and progesterone for an ovum to be fertilized and implanted and retained in the uterus. *Endometrial biopsy* and *vaginal smears* taken premenstrually give some of this information, but a *complete endocrine workup* may also be indicated. Urine studies to determine the amount of gonadotropin in the urine are used to study function of the pituitary gland. Hypothyroidism or general health that is below par may prevent an otherwise normal woman from conceiving. (See p. 736 for studies done.) Thyroid hormones sometimes are given, and vitamins C and E and extra rest may also be prescribed.

If the woman has an irregular menstrual cycle, it is important that she keep a temperature chart for several months to help determine her exact period of ovulation. The temperature will usually be lower at ovulation (the time at which conception most likely will take place) and then will rise abruptly as the corpus luteum begins to produce progesterone. It will drop to a lower level again a day or two before the start of the menstrual period. The temperature should be taken rectally before arising each morning. The temperature chart should be interpreted by the physician because there may be individual variations.

If the ovum is to reach the uterus, the fallopian tubes must be mechanically patent and not in spasm. The *Rubin test* (uterotubal insufflation) will provide information concerning patency of the tubes. In this test the patient is prepared as for a pelvic examination, and then compressed air or carbon dioxide is forced into the uterus under sterile conditions. If the fallopian tubes are open, the physician will be able to hear free air in the peritoneum on auscultation. The patient will feel pain under the scapula on the same side as the patent tube. If considerable pressure is required to force air into the tubes, there may be spasticity or partial stricture. Radiographs of the uterus and fallopian tubes *(hysterosalpingograms)* may be taken by forcing a sterile, aqueous, radiopaque substance through the uterus into the tubes. This examination is usually not carried out more than 7 days after the end of the menstrual period, since ovulation may be taking place.

The patient should prepare for these tests by taking a laxative the night before the examination and an enema or a bisacodyl suppository (Dulcolax) in the morning so that distention of the bowel will not obstruct the fallopian tubes and the radiographs will not be distorted by gas shadows in the intestine. Soluble phenobarbital and an analgesic are usually given since there will be some discomfort during and after this examination. Low abdominal pain, cramps, nausea, vomiting, and faintness occur occasionally. After the examination is over, the patient usually has "gas pains"; they may be relieved by lying on the abdomen, with the head lower than the feet, for 1 to 2 hours, since this position allows the gas to rise into the lower pelvis. Since the x-ray medium may stain the patient's clothing, she should wear a perineal pad for several hours, or the physician may insert a tampon and give instructions as to when it should be removed.

Tubal strictures may be the result of acute or chronic infections involving the fallopian tubes. Although they sometimes can be repaired by plastic surgery, the results are successful in only a few instances. Tubal insufflation is often therapeutic in itself, opening the fallopian tube(s) enough to allow the free passage of the fertilized ovum into the uterus.

A displaced uterus may occasionally be the only known cause of the infertility. Treatment usually consists of pelvic exercises, such as the knee-chest position, the monkey trot, or other exercises as described in specialized texts, and/or the use of a pessary.

The couple should not be disappointed if, even with medical treatment, pregnancy does not occur immediately, since many normal couples must wait many months and even years before pregnancy occurs. Pregnancy has been known to occur after years of childless marriage, perhaps because the couple begin to accept the situation and thus become more relaxed. Sometimes no physical cause for sterility can be found in either the man or the woman. Many couples will benefit simply from reassurance of normality. Others may need marriage counseling or psychiatric help to gain insight into psychologic and emotional problems that may be preventing conception.

Diseases of the female reproductive system

Advances in medical science have made it possible to treat effectively many diseases of the female reproductive system, but for optimum benefit from treatment an early diagnosis is essential. As the layman becomes better informed about normal reproductive functions throughout life, he or she could be able to recognize and report symptoms indicative of early disease. Since the female nurse is often the first member of the health team consulted by a woman with symptoms related to the reproductive system, she needs to know those for which she may safely suggest conservative hygienic measures and those for which the patient should seek medical advice. If disease is found, the nurse may also play an important part in helping the patient accept the prescribed treatment as well as in providing nursing care that is coordinated with the efforts of other disciplines to return the patient to a normal productive life.

■ COMMON GYNECOLOGIC DISORDERS

Abnormal menses

Dysmenorrhea. Pain with menstruation is known as dysmenorrhea. Although studies and estimates vary enormously,[57] it is generally believed that at least one third of all women suffer from dysmenorrhea in varying degrees. Studies in industry have shown dysmenorrhea to be one of the most important causes of absenteeism among working women, resulting in loss of 2 or more days a month for many employees. Present wide use of the antiovulatory drugs has compounded problems in analyzing and treating this condition.

The nurse frequently is asked for practical suggestions to relieve dysmenorrhea. Since dysmenorrhea occurs more frequently in individuals who have poor posture, take little exercise, and have poor eating habits, the nurse should encourage good general health practices. In helping with the immediate problem, an assessment is made to determine if the period is in any way abnormal. If it is not, rest in bed for an hour or two or the application of heat to the lower abdomen can be suggested. A woman who is busy, either mentally or physically, doing something she enjoys is less likely to notice discomfort. These measures will suffice in most instances, but anyone with further difficulty or consistent dysmenorrhea should be urged to seek medical attention. There are many causes that are not obvious, and curative treatment can be given only when the cause of the difficulty is known.

When the patient visits the physician, a pelvic examination is usually performed, and health practices are analyzed. Congestion of blood in the pelvic cavity or intrapelvic pressure resulting from constipation, a full bladder, or a tumor often causes menstrual pain. Frequently no definite cause can be determined, and the patient may again be urged to try such health measures as securing adequate rest, improving posture, participating in moderate exercise, eating a nonconstipating diet, and taking warm, rather than cool, baths during the menstrual period. The female nurse who by her own attitude shows that she considers menstruation to be a normal function and who augments the patient's understanding of normal sexual functions by giving explanations whenever possible may help some women make a better adjustment to the menstrual cycle.

If premenstrual fluid retention causes slight swelling of the abdomen and ankles, limiting salt and fluids during the week prior to the onset of menstruation may help. Tenderness of the breasts, either immediately preceding the onset of menstruation or at any other time during the cycle, headache, and mood swings are due to hormonal influences. The patient in whom these difficulties are marked should consult a gynecologist, since they may be due to hormonal dysfunction or other causes. For marked fluid retention the physician may order a low-sodium diet.

Displacement of the uterus may cause dysmenorrhea, although many women with known displacements have no difficulty. Some patients with displacement complain of chronic backache, pelvic pressure, easy fatigue, and leukorrhea in addition to painful menstruation.

Common kinds of displacement are *anteflexion, retroflexion,* and *retroversion* of the uterus caused by congenitally weak uterine ligaments, adhesions following infections or surgery in the pelvic region, or the strain of pregnancy on the ligaments. A space-filling lesion in this region or even a full bladder or rectum may also displace the uterus enough to cause symptoms. Normally the body of the uterus flexes forward at a 45-degree angle at the cervix. In retroflexion this angle is increased. In anteflexion it is decreased. In retroversion the whole uterus is tipped backward. (See Fig. 21-10.)

If the displacement is not due to some coexistent pelvic disease, various pelvic exercises may be recommended in an attempt to return the uterus to a normal position. These exercises, employing the principles of gravity, stretch or strengthen the uterine ligaments. Some exercises used are knee-chest exercises, the monkey trot, lying on the abdo-

men 2 hours a day, and premenstrual exercises. Corrective exercises for poor posture may also be prescribed.

In doing *knee-chest exercises,* the patient is instructed to assume a knee-chest position (Fig. 21-4) and to separate the labia to allow air to enter the vagina, since this helps to produce normal position of the uterus. This position should be maintained for 5 minutes two or three times a day.

In doing the *monkey trot,* the patient is instructed to walk about on her hands and feet, keeping the knees straight. This should be done for 5 minutes two or three times a day.

Premenstrual exercises as described in specialized texts are believed by some gynecologists to be helpful in selected patients with dysmenorrhea. Other gynecologists believe that equally good results are obtained by attention to posture and general exercise to improve muscle tone throughout the body.

The nurse may be responsible for teaching the patient how to do prescribed exercises. The patient should begin exercising gradually; for example, the knee-chest position should be maintained only 1 minute the first time, 2 minutes the second time, with gradual progression up to 5 minutes. Results from a

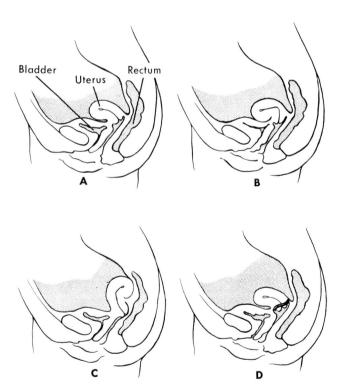

FIG. 21-10. Normal and abnormal positions of the uterus. **A,** Normal anatomic position of the uterus in relation to adjacent structures. **B,** Anterior displacement of the uterus. **C,** Retroversion, or backward displacement of the uterus. **D,** Normal anatomic position of the uterus maintained by use of a rubber S-shaped pessary.

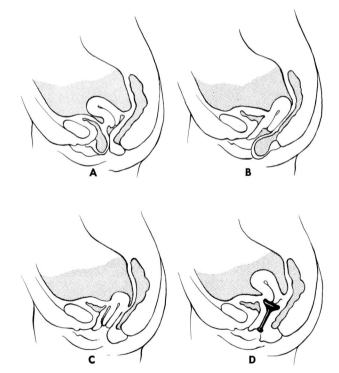

FIG. 21-11. Abnormalities of the vagina. **A,** Cystocele—downward displacement of the bladder toward the vaginal orifice. **B,** Rectocele—pouching of the rectum into the posterior wall of the vagina. **C,** Prolapse of uterus into vaginal canal. **D,** Stem pessary in place to maintain normal anatomic position of the uterus.

program of exercising will not be noticed immediately. The patient should be told this and should be encouraged to exercise regularly over a period of months. Performance of exercises should be reviewed each time the nurse sees the patient.

If the uterus can be manually returned to a normal position, a *Smith-Hodges pessary* may be inserted for a trial period to learn whether malposition causes the dysmenorrhea (Fig. 21-11). The pessary is an appliance introduced into the vagina for the purpose of supporting the uterus in a normal position. Sometimes, after the removal of the pessary, the uterus will remain in normal position. If, after about a 6-month trial, the uterus still returns to its displaced position on removal of the pessary, and if the pessary has relieved the symptoms, the ligaments may be shortened surgically through an abdominal incision. While the pessary is in use, the patient usually is instructed to take a daily cleansing douche with warm tap water to remove extra vaginal secretions caused by its use. The pessary is usually changed every 3 to 6 weeks. If it is left in place indefinitely, it may cause erosion of the cervix and become adherent to the mucosa.

A *stricture of the cervical canal* may cause dysmenorrhea. If so, dilatation of the cervical canal may relieve the discomfort. Dysmenorrhea may be due to endocrine disorders, but extensive diagnostic tests of hormone function are done only when there seems to be no other possible cause. In some instances, psychiatric therapy may be needed to attempt to relieve symptoms. The nurse may be helpful in making this treatment acceptable to the patient.

If dysmenorrhea is incapacitating and unrelieved by conservative therapy or hormone treatment, a *presacral neurectomy* may be performed. In this procedure the pain (sensory) fibers from the uterus are interrupted surgically through an abdominal incision. If a pregnant woman has had this operation, she will not feel uterine contractions during early labor, and contractions must be palpated carefully to prevent precipitate birth of the baby.

Amenorrhea. Amenorrhea is the absence of menstruation. Before the seriousness of this symptom can be ascertained, one needs to know if there has ever been menstruation and if there has been any recent change in the normal life pattern or in the general state of health of the patient. It is not unusual for a woman to miss one period, especially if she is adjusting to a change in her life pattern. If menses continue to be absent, medical consultation should be advised.

The most common cause of amenorrhea, aside from the menopause, is pregnancy. Some women, however, continue to menstruate during the first months of pregnancy. Menses are also usually absent at least until 6 weeks after delivery of the baby, and sometimes throughout the period of lactation. If a girl is over 14 years of age and has not started to menstruate, she should be examined by a gynecologist to rule out a congenital deformity such as imperforate hymen or absence of the vagina, uterus, or ovaries. If there is no apparent cause for the failure to menstruate regularly, endocrine studies may be done. Sometimes thyroid and ovarian hormones need to be supplemented. Nutritional anemia, wasting chronic illness such as tuberculosis, and psychogenic factors such as fear of pregnancy or desire for pregnancy may cause amenorrhea. A certain type of ovarian tumor (arrhenoblastoma) also causes amenorrhea.

Abnormal menstruation. Abnormal bleeding from the vagina requires immediate medical attention. There are two types: *menorrhagia*, or prolonged profuse menstrual flow during the regular period, and *metrorrhagia*, or bleeding between periods.

Menorrhagia in an adolescent girl may be due to a blood dyscrasia or to an endocrine disturbance. This is called *functional bleeding*. Menorrhagia in adult women is likely to be a symptom of an ovarian tumor, a uterine myoma, or pelvic inflammatory disease.

Any bleeding, even slight spotting, between periods is significant. Metrorrhagia may be a symptom of many disorders, including benign or malignant uterine tumors; pelvic inflammatory disease; abnormal conditions of pregnancy such as a threatened abortion, ectopic pregnancy, or hydatid mole; blood dyscrasias; senile vaginitis; and bleeding at ovulation caused by the withdrawal of estrogen. The wide use of combined ovarian hormones such as norethindrone to suppress ovulation sometimes causes bleeding at irregular times. When metrorrhagia is present, however, prompt medical examination is indicated even though the cause may not be serious. The cause, not the symptom, must be treated, and the nurse has a responsibility to help disseminate this information to all women. Early diagnosis and treatment increase the possibility of cure even when the cause is a malignancy.

Vaginal infection

Many women complain of *leukorrhea,* a white vaginal discharge. It is normal to have a slight white vaginal discharge the month prior to the menarche and then monthly around the period of ovulation and just prior to the onset of menstruation. Ordinarily the vagina is protected from infection by its acid secretion and by the presence of Döderlein's bacilli. Occasionally, if the invading organisms such as the colon bacillus are very numerous or if the resistance of the woman is lowered by malnutrition, aging, disease, or emotional disturbances, *vaginitis* may develop. Profuse discharge, yellow discharge, and mucoid discharge are abnormal and are signs of vaginitis, inflammation, or infection. Urethritis usually occurs simultaneously because the mucous membranes of the vagina and urethra are contiguous. The discharge may be irritating and cause redness, edema, burning, and itching. The burning and pruritus may be aggravated by voiding and by defecation.

Medicated vaginal jellies and vaginal suppositories are frequently prescribed for patients with vaginitis. The nurse will need to instruct the patient in the procedures for their use. Vaginal jelly is dispensed in a tube to which is attached an applicator. The applicator is inserted into the vagina in a manner similar to the way a pipette is inserted when obtaining a vaginal smear. The medication is then expressed into the vagina and the applicator is withdrawn. A vaginal suppository may be inserted directly into the vagina. It is dissolved by body heat, and the medication may be absorbed through the vaginal mucosa. Because some medications stain and soil clothing, a pad may be worn, or the patient may be advised to wear old clothing.

Simple vaginitis. Simple vaginitis is caused by contamination of the vagina with organisms from the rectum such as *Escherichia coli* or with other common pyogenic organisms such as staphylococci and streptococci. The organisms are usually introduced from outside sources such as clothing or a douche nozzle. Simple vaginitis is treated with warm douches of a weak acid solution such as vinegar (1 tablespoon to 1 quart of water). This solution increases the acidity of the bacterial environment within the vagina. To help control the infection, beta-lactose, a sugar that stimulates the growth of Döderlein's bacilli, may be prescribed as a vaginal suppository, and sulfonamide cream may be prescribed as an intravaginal application. The sulfonamide cream should be applied after douching. Sitz baths, taken two or three times a day to help relieve local irritation, and thorough gentle cleansing of the perineum with water after voiding and defecating are recommended.

Trichomonas vaginitis. Trichomonas vaginitis is one of the most common forms of vaginal infection and is often found in combination with other infecting organisms. A protozoan, *Trichomonas vaginalis,* is probably the causative agent. Symptoms include a frothy, white or yellowish vaginal discharge, itching, and irritation of the vulva. Inflammation of varying degrees may be present. The infection is diagnosed by examining a drop of vaginal secretion microscopically. When this test is to be made, a dry speculum should be used. The slide should be dry and warm, and as soon as the drop of vaginal secretion is placed on the slide, a drop or two of normal saline solution should be added.

A synthetic drug, metronidazole (Flagyl) is remarkably effective in treatment of trichomonas vaginitis. Treatment consists of 250 mg. tablets taken orally three times a day for 10 days. Other specific local treatment includes vinegar douches, insertion of diiodohydroxyquin (Floraquin) tablets in the vagina to restore glycogen and the acidity that characterizes normal vaginal tissue, and more recently, the high vaginal insertion of gelatin capsules of chlortetracycline every other night for a period of 2 weeks to destroy infective protozoa. Other local treatments include cleansing of the infected area by the physician using green soap and water and cotton balls on a Kelly clamp followed by insertion of a vaginal jelly or suppository. Tampons may be used to absorb vaginal discharge. A sulfonamide cream may also be administered intravaginally to combat streptococcal or staphylococcal infection. Carbarsone, an arsenic compound, may also be ordered for vaginal and rectal infections. Sunshine, rest, good nutrition, and treatment of any focal infections may help to improve the patient's general resistance. There is a good possibility that the patient has infected her sexual partner and the physician may wish to examine him also. Otherwise the couple will reinfect each other. If the man is found to have the infection, he is usually treated with metronidazole given orally in higher doses than those ordinarily prescribed for women.

Trichomonas sometimes attack the cervix, bladder, or rectum. If the cervix is involved, the infected portion may need to be surgically removed (conization of the cervix). When the bladder is infected, instillations of mild silver protein (Argyrol) or sulfonamide solutions are used, and carbarsone suppositories may be used to clear up persistent rectal involvement. Trichomonas vaginitis often resists treatment and may persist for months and years despite extensive treatment. It is discouraging and distressing to the patient. If she is to be encouraged to continue the treatment and not "shop around" in her effort to be cured, she needs to be treated with much patience and understanding.

Monilial vaginitis. Monilial vaginitis is a yeast infection caused by *Candida albicans.* It is commonly seen in patients with uncontrolled diabetes and in pregnant women. The fungi thrive on sugar. The infection is characterized by the presence of thick, white patches on the vaginal mucosa and a thick, cheeselike discharge that is highly irritating. If the infection is due to untreated diabetes mellitus, it usually responds to better control of the blood sugar level. Local treatment consists of gentian violet vaginal suppositories inserted twice a day and nystatin (Mycostatin), an antibiotic fungicide given orally and in the form of vaginal suppositories, one at bedtime for 15 nights. The application of nystatin ointment locally three times a day to a badly irritated perineum is also very effective. Douches should not be taken during the period of treatment. Since gentian violet stains clothing, a perineal pad should be worn. Monilial infection is sometimes resistant to treatment and tends to recur just when it is believed that treatment has been successful. Total recovery may be aided by attention to the improvement of general health.

Senile vaginitis. Senile (atrophic) vaginitis is caused by the invasion of the thin, atrophied, postmenopausal vaginal mucosa by pyogenic bacteria. The main symptom is an irritating vaginal discharge that is sometimes accompanied by pruritus and burning. The treatment is the same as that for simple vaginitis. Estrogenic hormones, given orally or applied locally as ointment, will help to restore the epithelium to normal and are often prescribed.

Perineal pruritus

Perineal pruritus, or excessive itching of the perineum, is a very common and very aggravating affliction that may be due to a variety of causes. It may be due to senile changes in the skin of the perineum, vitamin A deficiency, or the irritation from a chronic vaginal discharge or from the high sugar content of urine in persons with uncontrolled diabetes mellitus. Pediculosis pubis, allergies, cancer of the vulva, scabies, and superficial skin infections such as *tinea cruris* (a fungal infection) may be the cause. Sometimes the cause of the itching cannot be found. The pruritus is made worse by scratching and rubbing; edema, redness, excoriation of the skin, and infection may complicate the original condition.

Perineal pruritus is treated by correcting the aggravating cause if it can be found. Because perineal pruritus, like pruritus in any location of the body, is increased by nervous tension, small doses of sedatives such as phenobarbital or chloral hydrate may be given when symptoms are severe. Frequent bathing, sitz baths, and soothing lotions such as calamine lotion are helpful. The patient is urged not to scratch or further irritate the condition, and to avoid fecal contamination by careful cleansing from the front backward following defecation. Hydrocortisone ointment has been found to be extremely effective in controlling perineal pruritus and is now widely used.

Cervicitis

Cervical erosion is the mildest form of cervicitis. A small, reddened, irritated area appears about the external mouth of the cervix; the cause is obscure. Inflammation of the cervix may be due to an acute pyogenic infection such as sometimes follows abortion and childbirth, or it may be due to lodging of the gonococcus in a cervical erosion or laceration. This is known as *acute* cervicitis. If inadequately treated, it may become chronic.

In some instances the erosion may be diagnosed as *congenital* erosion. The erosion appears similar to acute cervicitis, but distinction is made because it occurs in girls before puberty and in virgins, in which case trauma and infection from external sources do not appear to be related to the cause.

In untreated cervicitis the local tissues are constantly irritated, and there is some evidence that this irritation predisposes to cancer. Since leukorrhea, the only symptom of cervicitis, does not appear unless there is severe irritation, the presence of unrecognized cervicitis must be determined by pelvic examination, including visualization of the cervix. If the practice of a careful examination 6 weeks postpartum was adhered to, much chronic cervicitis could be prevented. The cervix is frequently lacerated as it stretches and thins out to allow the baby to pass through the birth canal, and the torn surfaces do not always heal properly. At the examination made 6 weeks following delivery, improperly healed lacerations of the cervix can be cauterized so that the everted portion of the mucosa is turned back into the cervical canal. This minor procedure can be done in the physician's office or the clinic, and it will prevent chronic inflammation. Cervical erosions are often discovered during routine pelvic examinations. A biopsy is taken, and the erosion is then cauterized with silver nitrate.

Acute cervicitis can usually be adequately treated with hot douches and the local application of antibiotics. Antibiotics also may be given both orally and parenterally.

In *chronic* cervicitis the infection has extended deeper into the tissues, and the patient must be hospitalized for at least 1 day for *conization* of the cervix. This is the removal of a cone-shaped portion of the cervix containing the infected tissue. The nursing care is the same as that required after a dilatation and curettage. In addition, hemorrhage, which may occur from the operative site, is treated by such means as packing the vagina, raising the foot of the bed, and keeping the patient absolutely quiet for several hours. Occasionally the patient must be returned to the operating room for resuturing or cauterization of the site of hemorrhage. Untreated chronic cervical infections eventually may extend into the uterine cavity and into the pelvic cavity, causing endometritis (inflammation of the uterine lining) and pelvic inflammatory disease.

Bartholinitis

The Bartholin glands, located at the base of the labia majora and secreting a lubricating mucus through an opening between the labia minora and the hymen, may become infected with a variety of organisms, including *Gonococcus, Staphylococcus, Streptococcus,* or *Escherichia coli.* With infection, the duct from the gland may become obstructed, and severe redness, edema, and tenderness ensue, making even walking difficult. Sometimes the abscess that forms ruptures spontaneously, but surgical incision for drainage is often required. Usually the woman with this condition is treated on an ambulatory basis. Before rupture of the abscess, hot sitz baths and/or local heat in the form of compresses is prescribed. Antibiotics are given systemically, and a gauze packing may be inserted at the time of incision. Careful instruction in perineal care is needed to avoid further contamination after defecation.

Occasionally the acute inflammation subsides, leaving fibrotic or scar tissue. When this occurs, the gland develops a cystic dilation or a *Bartholin's cyst.* The cyst may vary in size from a few centimeters in diameter to the size of a hen's egg. The cyst is mobile and is not tender. If it grows to be of sufficient size to cause difficulty in walking or during intercourse or if it shows signs of inflammation, it may be excised surgically.

Pelvic inflammatory disease

Pelvic inflammatory disease (PID) is an inflammatory process within the pelvic cavity that may involve the fallopian tubes, the ovaries, pelvic peritoneum, pelvic veins, or pelvic connective tissue. Inflammation of the fallopian tube is known as *salpingitis,* and inflammation of the ovary is known as *oophoritis.*

Pelvic inflammatory disease frequently is a complication of acute infectious processes such as gonorrhea or puerperal infection and tuberculosis. The rupture of any adjacent structure may spill organisms into the pelvic cavity, producing secondary inflammation; for example, when the appendix perforates, pelvic peritonitis usually follows. Prevention or early and adequate treatment of the original infection should decrease the incidence of this problem.

Pathogenic organisms such as gonococci and staphylococci are usually introduced from the outside and pass up the cervical canal into the uterus. They seem to cause little trouble in the uterus but pass into the pelvis either through thrombosed uterine veins, through the lymphatics of the uterine wall, or by way of the fallopian tubes. Here they cause an inflammation. Before the discovery of penicillin, the *Gonococcus* was the most common organism causing pelvic inflammatory disease. This organism typically invades the pelvis through the fallopian tubes. Pus forms in the tubes, and adhesions develop so that sterility often follows. Although a generalized peritonitis can occur, the infection usually is localized in the lower abdomen, causing abscess formation and adhesions of the pelvic viscera. An abscess of the cul-de-sac of Douglas is common. In this location the abscess may rupture spontaneously into the vagina or may require surgical incision through the vagina for drainage.

Signs and symptoms of pelvic inflammatory disease include severe abdominal and pelvic pain, malaise, nausea and vomiting, and elevation of temperature, with leukocytosis. Often there is a foul-smelling, purulent vaginal discharge. The patient is usually hospitalized and placed on bed rest in a mid-Fowler's position to provide dependent drainage so that abscesses will not form high in the abdomen, where they might rupture and cause generalized peritonitis. The sulfonamide and antibiotic drugs are almost always given. Heat applied to the abdomen, either a hot-water bottle or an electric heating pad, or a hot vaginal douche twice a day may be ordered. Heat improves circulation to the involved parts and thereby allays the discomfort caused by stasis of blood and enhances the effectiveness of the body's natural defenses—leukocytes. If there is a vaginal discharge, tampons should not be used, since the drainage may be coming from the vaginal wall and a tampon would obstruct it. If the patient is hospitalized, the nurse should instruct her and ancillary personnel to report any change in the amount, appearance, or odor of vaginal discharge. If the patient is ambulatory, she should be advised to watch for these changes and to abstain from sexual intercourse during the acute stage of the disease.

Pelvic inflammatory disease becomes chronic unless it is quite vigorously treated at its onset. Chronic pelvic discomfort, disturbances of menstruation, constipation, and periodic exacerbation of acute symptoms sometimes occur. Occasionally the patient may be considered neurotic because of the repeated and nonspecific nature of her complaints. The most serious of the complications of pelvic inflammatory disease is *sterility,* which is caused by scar tissue that closes the fallopian tubes. Strictures of the salpinges may cause an *ectopic pregnancy,* since the fertilized egg may not be able to reach the uterus even though the smaller sperm has been able to pass the stricture and produce conception. Adhesions form as a result of chronic inflammation, and the ovaries, fallopian tubes, and uterus may have to be completely removed.

Puerperal infection

Puerperal infection is a uterine infection following interruption of pregnancy or a normal delivery. It usually is caused by streptococci, and the usual route of infection is through the vagina and the cervical canal. With improved obstetric care, puerperal infection now occurs most frequently in women who have had criminally induced abortions. Puerperal infections may occur, however, if the membranes have been ruptured for several days before delivery, if the removal of the placenta has been incomplete, or if clots or edema prevent normal drainage from the uterus following delivery. When the baby is delivered at home or elsewhere where it is impossible to use aseptic technique, there is increased danger of infection. If contamination has occurred, or if any symptoms of infection appear after a delivery, antibiotics are given. If pieces of the placenta have been retained, a dilatation and curettage of the uterus will be performed because the retained tissue not only causes continued bleeding but also serves as a culture medium for organisms. Uterine cramps, continued vaginal bleeding, or scanty normal uterine drainage *(lochia)* following delivery should be noted and reported so that appropriate treatment may be started if necessary.

Abortion

The obstetric and legal definition of abortion is termination of a pregnancy before the twenty-eighth week of gestation (viability). There is consensus that viability means that a state of development exists that, theoretically, is compatible with survival outside of the uterus. Argument prevails, however, as to when viability actually occurs. The definition used in reporting perinatal statistics is that fetal weight of 400 grams or less constitutes an abortion.[37] There are several types of abortions.

Spontaneous abortion. Spontaneous abortions result from "natural" causes, that is, without the aid of mechanical or medicinal intervention. Estimates of the incidence of spontaneous abortions range from 10% to 20% of all pregnancies. The wide range of estimate is partially due to the belief that many women may experience a spontaneous abortion without ever being aware conception had occurred. These women probably have very minor symptoms that they do not recognize as signs of abortion and that do not require hospitalization.

There is evidence from chromosomal studies that about one third of the embryos spontaneously aborted in the first 12 weeks of pregnancy are abnormal.[114] In addition to defective embryos, an intrauterine environment that is not adequate for sustaining embryonic and fetal development may result from injuries or abnormalities of the reproductive tract, endocrine disorders, and acute and chronic health problems. There is some evidence that emotional trauma may be a contributing factor in some cases.

Spontaneous abortions are classified according to a sequence of progression of severity of symptoms. Medical or surgical intervention at any point in the sequence may alter the progression. In *threatened abortion* the process has presumably started, as evidenced by vaginal bleeding or spotting, minor cramping from uterine contractions, and mild backache. The cervix has not started to dilate and the process may or may not respond to treatment. Management consists of bed rest and evaluation of the effects of blood loss. Mild sedatives and progesterone may be prescribed in an attempt to conserve the pregnancy.

In an *inevitable abortion* the process has progressed so far that it is impossible to salvage the pregnancy. The symptoms include copious vaginal bleeding, rupture of the amniotic sac, severe abdominal cramping, and dilatation of the cervix. Supportive treatment consists of bed rest, monitoring for effects of blood loss, blood transfusion as indicated, and medications for relief of pain. Medical intervention may take a variety of forms, depending on the patient's general condition. The process may be permitted to terminate spontaneously and be followed by a dilatation and curettage. Oxytocin may be administered to hasten the process and to decrease blood loss, and this may be followed by a dilatation and curettage, or a dilatation and curettage may be performed first with oxytocin administered concomitantly.

An *incomplete abortion* is one in which part of the products of conception (usually the embryo) is expelled and part is retained. There is abdominal pain from uterine contractions. Vaginal bleeding is usually moderate to heavy and continues until all the retained products are passed spontaneously or removed by dilatation and curettage. Oxytocic drugs are administered to control blood loss and transfusion may be required.

When all of the products of conception are expelled spontaneously, a *complete abortion* has occurred. Bleeding is usually minimal, but oxytocics may be given and a dilatation and curettage performed as precautionary management.

A *missed abortion* is one in which the products of conception are not spontaneously expelled after embryonic death occurs. The term is usually applied when at least 2 months elapse between embryonic death and expulsion. The uterus fails to increase in size and the changes anticipated with advancing normal pregnancy do not appear. There is some difference of opinion regarding management of the patient when the diagnosis is made. Some physicians feel that is is better to wait for spontaneous abortion to follow. Infection and hemorrhage are rare, but the idea of "carrying a dead baby" is distressing to many women. Occasionally hypofibrinogenemia may occur as a consequence of entry into the maternal circulation of thromboplastin from the uterus and placenta. For this reason as well as for the emotional stress resulting, many physicians believe the uterus should be evacuated as soon as possible. This may be accomplished by different methods, depending on the period of gestation reached when embryonic death occurs. If it is less than 12 weeks a dilatation and curettage may be performed, or the abortion process may be induced with oxytocin. Induction with oxytocin may be carried out after the twelfth week.

Habitual abortion refers to a condition in which spontaneous abortion occurs in three or more consecutive pregnancies. The causes are similar to those stated for spontaneous abortion. Treatment is dependent on the point in the abortive process reached and on determining the causative factors.

Habitual abortions that occur during the second trimester (usually 14 to 16 weeks) seem to be related to a condition called "incompetent cervix." Apparently, there is diminished resistance of the cervix to the increasing weight of the embryo, and this may be sufficient to cause cervical dilatation. The cervix dilates without the patient experiencing or being aware of labor, and this is usually followed by rupture of the membranes and expulsion of the embryo. Surgical intervention is possible for identified high-risk patients and in patients who are diagnosed before symptoms progress to the inevitable point.

The surgery consists of closing the internal os of the cervix by suturing in a purse-string (drawstring) fashion. Shirodkar's procedure, MacDonald's procedure, and Barker's procedure refer to the surgery performed; these are very similar to one another.

These patients must be closely observed in the postoperative period for signs of labor, rupture of the membranes, and vaginal bleeding. If labor ensues, it is necessary that the sutures be released in order to prevent trauma to the cervix. If the procedure is successful, pregnancy continues. The sutures, then, may be either left in place and delivery accomplished by cesarean section near full term, or the sutures may be released near full term and the woman is allowed to go into labor and deliver vaginally.

Induced abortions. The topics of therapeutic and criminal abortions have received great attention for hundreds of years. Volumes have been written on these topics, ranging from medical aspects to legal, sociologic, psychologic, moral, and economic aspects.

Criminal abortion refers to termination of pregnancy without legal justification. Usually such abortions are either self-induced or performed by nonphysicians outside of hospitals and clinics. Estimations of the number of criminal abortions in the United States range from 500,000 to 1,500,000/year.

Attempts to bring about abortion are generally made by ingestion of castor oil or quinine, douching with soap and water, or inserting lye or potassium permanganate crystals into the vagina. These rarely act as abortifacients. Instead, they can cause serious toxicity, local trauma, and may even result in death.

Insertion of foreign bodies such as catheters, knitting needles, and metal coat hangers is another common method by which abortions are attempted. While these are more effective, they are attended by highly serious consequences. Perforation of the uterus, hemorrhage, infection, permanent infertility resulting from infection, and death from blood loss or infection may occur.

In the United States the legality of abortions and the circumstances under which they might be justifiably performed by physicians became a major area of controversy by 1968, and by 1972 the legality and morality of abortions had assumed extremely unclear aspects.

On January 22, 1973, the United States Supreme Court, in an unprecedented action, reached a decision regarding legalization of abortions. It ruled that a state could not intervene in the abortion decision between a woman and her physician during the first 12 weeks of pregnancy.[100] Although the Supreme Court did not take the position that a woman has an absolute right to abortion regardless of period of gestation or individual circumstances, its decision regarding the first trimester renders all previous original and reform laws unconstitutional.

The major ground for the Supreme Court decision is based on personal liberty provided by the Fourteenth Amendment to the Constitution. In essence this means the woman has a right to privacy and includes the right to decide whether or not to terminate her pregnancy.

Not all the issues, however, were settled by the Supreme Court's action. After the end of the first trimester, the states reserve rights to enact legislation and other regulations to protect maternal health. The states are now required to adopt statutes specifying the circumstances under which abortions can be legally performed.

Despite the Supreme Court ruling, arguments continue pro and con. Many states have not revised laws to provide for second- and third-trimester abortions, and the laws vary greatly. Various attitudes, beliefs, and values are evident in the variety of terms used today. "Therapeutic" abortion no longer simply means an abortion performed by a physician when the mother's life is threatened by serious physiopathologic conditions. The term has gradually been broadened to include threats to health, both physical and emotional. However, some state laws have not clearly defined what constitutes a threat to health. "Abortion on demand," "legalized abortion," "abortion on request," "elective abortion," and "social abortion" are some of the terms in common usage today.

Therapeutic abortions for purely medical reasons (the presence of serious physiopathologic conditions) have become more rare as the science of obstetrics has developed. Severe heart disease, pulmonary hypertension, pulmonary tuberculosis, chronic nephritis, diabetes, and malignancy are listed as medically sound reasons for terminating pregnancy by abortion. With increased effectiveness of conception control and availability of sterilization, fewer women who are at risk of developing life-threatening conditions during pregnancy are becoming pregnant.

Today, many induced legal abortions are performed for "social" reasons. Social and economic pressures for small families are strong. There is an increased tendency among people to see abortion as an alternative method of birth control. Such factors as financial strain, life goals, desired life-styles, marital status, and desired number of children operate to motivate women and couples to seek abortion. The increased demand for abortion is viewed by some people as a reflection of inadequate sex education and conception control programs, and there is some consensus that it is not desirable to encourage abortion as a method of family planning and conception control.[100]

"Medically sound" reasons for performing abortions have been expanded to include such aspects as the fate of the unwanted child after birth, psychologic stress, history of genetic abnormalities, the effects of teratogens, maternal and fetal blood incompatibility, rape, and incest.

Several methods are available for inducing abortion. The particular method selected for a patient is highly dependent on the length of gestation at the time a woman seeks an abortion. As the pregnancy progresses, the methods required to be effective increase in complexity, are attended by greater risks to the woman, are more time-consuming in terms of length of hospitalization, are more expensive, and are perhaps more emotionally traumatic.

In the first trimester, abortion is performed in special clinics, as an outpatient procedure or in acute care settings. Many special abortion clinics have opened as a result of the demand for abortion in the early weeks of pregnancy. Some clinics provide counseling and referral services, others have facilities in which abortions can be performed. If admitted to an acute care setting, the woman may be admitted and discharged on the same day or remain only one night.

Vacuum aspiration. Vacuum aspiration (suction curettage) has become the method of choice for early termination of pregnancy in clinics and hospitals providing abortions for large numbers of patients.[50] This procedure can be performed under local anesthesia, although general anesthesia may be used. Vacuum aspiration is preferred in early pregnancy (12 to 14 weeks) because the risk of perforation of the uterus is low, there is minimal blood loss, and less physical trauma.

Using this method, the cervix is dilated as in a dilatation and curettage, and the uterus is evacuated by means of a vacuum suction machine.

Dilatation and curettage. Dilatation and curettage is an alternative method for accomplishing abortion in the first 12 to 14 weeks. The cervix is dilated with a series of instruments of graduated sizes to allow insertion of a curet into the uterus. The products of conception and superficial layer of the endometrium are then scraped from the walls of the uterus. A paracervical block or general anesthesia is used. Oxytocin is usually administered intramuscularly or in an intravenous infusion after the procedure is completed. Blood loss is usually minimal, and physical care is similar to that for any patient having a dilatation and curettage.

Intra-amniotic injection. Intra-amniotic injection (saline injection, "salting out") is the method most often used after the sixteenth week of gestation. Occasionally it may be attempted as early as the fourteenth week, but the chances of failure are greater since the amniotic sac is not well distended.

Since the patient must be responsive to detect adverse effects, general anesthesia is not used. Sedatives, analgesics, and tranquilizing agents are usually administered prior to the procedure and a local anesthetic is used. The procedure is performed under aseptic conditions. The local anesthetic is injected into the skin and abdominal wall in the midline below the umbilicus. A 17- or 18-gauge spinal length needle is introduced through the abdominal and uterine walls into the amniotic sac. The stylet is removed and the physician observes for the flow of amniotic fluid from the needle. When the amniotic fluid appears, a syringe is attached to the needle and the amniotic fluid is aspirated. An alternative method of using a size 14 trocar and cannula to which a short length of rubber or plastic tubing is attached may be preferred by the physician. The total amount of amniotic fluid aspirated averages 200 ml. for this period of gestation but may vary by about 50 ml. The amniotic fluid is replaced by 20% sodium chloride solution and the amount injected is at least equivalent to the amount of amniotic fluid aspirated. Some physicians prefer to inject an additional 50 ml. over the amount of amniotic fluid withdrawn, since there is some evidence that the additional fluid injected has a distending effect on the uterus. Most physicians elect to alternately withdraw and inject 15 to 20 ml. of fluid and sodium chloride solution to prevent collapse of the amniotic sac that might result from withdrawal of all of the amniotic fluid.

During introduction of the needle the injection is made slowly and care is taken to avoid insertion into the placenta or a blood vessel. The patient is closely observed during the procedure and for at least 1 hour afterward for untoward effects. These include shocklike symptoms or vascular collapse and abdominal pain resulting from injection into a blood vessel or the placenta.

The action of hypertonic solutions in inducing labor is not completely clear. The hypertonic solution disrupts the placenta and this result alone produces an intrauterine environment incompatible with life. Disruption of the placenta may also release the progesterone block, causing uterine contractions to result. The volume of fluid in the uterus may be significant in that the body attempts to balance the effects of the hypertonic solution. In doing so the volume of intra-amniotic fluid is increased. This expands the uterus beyond its normal size for gestation and probably triggers stretch receptors and pacemakers within the uterine muscles.

The abortive process (labor) begins 12 to 36 hours after the injection of sodium chloride solution. The patient is hospitalized throughout this time and observed for late untoward effects as well as the onset of the abortion. The products of conception are most often expelled as in a spontaneous, complete abortion. Once the symptoms of abortion appear (abdominal pain, vaginal bleeding, rupture of the amniotic sac), oxytocin may be administered by infusion to hasten the process and minimize blood loss. A dilatation and curettage may be performed after the abortion is completed as a precaution against excessive blood loss. If labor does not ensue within 36 to 48 hours following the injection, oxytocin by infusion is usually administered to initiate contractions of the uterus.

The thirteenth to sixteenth week of pregnancy poses difficulties for patients seeking an abortion. Most physicians consider this time to be too late for safe curettage and too early for intra-amniotic injection.

Hysterotomy. An abortion may also be performed by hysterotomy. This method is usually selected for terminating pregnancies that have advanced to 16 weeks or more, or when a tubal sterilization is to be carried out at the same time. Hysterotomy involves incision through the abdominal wall and uterus to remove the products of conception. A general or spinal anesthesia is administered and the patient has a longer period of hospitalization because of the surgical procedure. The postoperative complications that might occur are similar to those occurring after any abdominal surgery.

Experimental drugs. While an abortion pill, abortion injection, or uterine insert has not been developed as yet, it is quite likely that much simpler methods of inducing abortions will evolve if the current trend of increasing numbers of abortions continues.

One group of drugs, the prostaglandins, is currently undergoing research. Early studies indicate that prostaglandins stimulate contraction of the uterus. However, the amount required to induce first-trimester abortion produces nausea, vomiting, and diarrhea and the success rate is only 25%.[27]

Summary. Almost universally, when abortion is liberalized and legalized and made available, the maternal mortality rate drops and the incidence of septic and incomplete abortions decreases.[100]

Statistics document that mortality with legal abortions induced in the first trimester has dropped to such low levels that the risk of having an abortion is much less than the risk of carrying a pregnancy to full term. To point out the low risk to life associated with induced abortions, comparisons have been made with other causes of mortality[116] (Table 21-3).

Both the physical and psychologic long-term ef-

Table 21-3 Comparison of mortality rates

Causes of mortality	Mortality rate
Maternal mortality from childbirth	20/100,000 pregnancies
Criminal abortion	100/100,000 abortions
Legal abortion	3/100,000 abortions
Thromboembolic disorders from use of oral contraceptives	3/100,000 users

fects of induced abortions require continued study. It has been found that there is an increased tendency toward premature labor and development of incompetent cervix in succeeding pregnancies when an abortion requiring cervical dilatation has been performed. Except for hysterotomy, cervical dilation occurs with all currently used methods.

Psychologic studies indicate that adverse reactions to an abortion experience are influenced by legal, moral, and social antiabortion climates in that such a climate is punitive to the woman. Cultural attitudes have a pervasive effect and are likely to influence the way a woman reacts to an abortion. Attitudes of health care professionals influence the woman's feeling about herself and the abortion experience.

Counseling women regarding abortion is an appropriate function for nurses to assume, provided the nurse has the knowledge, skills, and abilities to assist individual women to cope with a situation that may have both immediate and long-term effects.

Preabortion counseling includes assisting the patient to make a decision regarding her state of pregnancy. This requires that the patient be helped with identifying the alternatives available to her, the consequences of the various alternatives, and selecting the alternative that is best for her in her circumstances. If this process is employed, the patient is more likely to arrive at a decision she feels is the best one she could make and less likely to experience excessive emotional distress. Therefore it is important in the counseling process to avoid telling the patient what to do or expressing opinions about what is best for her. For those women who seem unable to reach a decision, the nurse may arrange for referral to a counselor or social worker for further assistance.

For patients who decide to have an abortion, it is necessary that the nurse be able to explain the methods that will most likely be used, where an abortion may be obtained, and what will be required in terms of finances and time. It may be important that other health team members become involved in assisting the patient with planning. Preabortion counseling may also involve beginning explorations with the woman about conception control and family planning. Depending on her readiness to pursue these topics, the patient may be given information about the availability of services and methods. Otherwise she can be reassured the topic can be discussed at a later time.

In counseling the nurse will usually find that an objective approach, utilizing facts and terms the woman can understand and conveying an attitude of willingness and readiness to assist her, will encourage the woman to remain as objective as possible. Continuity in care seems to be particularly important to people in stressful situations and it may be helpful to inform the patient about the personnel she is likely to encounter. Nursing care plans should be prepared and available to other nurses who will be participating in the patient's care whenever this is possible.

When hospitalized for an abortion, patients feel some degree of anxiety, and their behaviors must be interpreted with great care. If a patient begins to ask questions or verbalize feelings, it does not necessarily mean she has "changed her mind." It might mean that, under anxiety, she cannot recall what she was told would be done and needs to have this information repeated. The nurse should not assume that the patient was not informed of the procedure and its consequences or that the patient has made a poor decision. Those patients who seem to be expressing "second thoughts" or seem to be doubtful about whether their decision should be carried out usually find it helpful to review how they initially reached the decision.

In the postabortion period a variety of emotional responses may be seen. Relief that the problem has been solved might be mingled with some minor feelings of guilt. Those patients who express regret and guilt can be helped by again reviewing with them their decision-making process. They may need to be aware that such feelings may recur from time to time and that remembering how and why they reached the decision to have an abortion may help. Postabortion patients are candidates for conception control information. Many of these patients wish to learn more about reproduction and prevention of pregnancy. The approaches and methods described previously will be of assistance to the nurse engaged in counseling about conception control.

Ectopic pregnancy

An ectopic pregnancy is one in which the fertilized ovum becomes embedded outside the body of the uterus. Since it is almost always located in the fallopian tube, the term *"tubal pregnancy"* is often used.

This condition occurs most often in women who have a narrowed fallopian tube caused either by inflammation or by a congenital stricture. The sperm may be small enough to pass through the stricture, but the larger fertilized ovum may be unable to do so. It may then attach itself to the tubal wall and develop into an embryo. As the embryo grows, the fallopian tube stretches and finally ruptures. This rupture usually occurs within the first 6 weeks of pregnancy. The patient experiences a sudden severe pain on one side of the abdomen and has a history of amenorrhea and often of suspected pregnancy. She may go into shock quickly after the onset of pain because of massive hemorrhage into the peritoneal cavity.

Emergency treatment for shock and hemorrhage is given. Early treatment of a ruptured ectopic pregnancy is imperative to prevent death from hemorrhage. Immediately on diagnosis the patient is prepared for a salpingectomy. If there has been prolonged bleeding preoperatively, the postoperative course may be complicated by peritonitis since the blood in the abdomen becomes infected with organisms.

The nursing care combines the aspects of emergency treatment of a patient who has sustained a severe hemorrhage, general care of a patient who has had major abdominal surgery and who may have peritonitis, and care of a woman whose pregnancy has been terminated prematurely. The patient needs reassurance regarding future pregnancies. She needs to understand that since ova are produced from alternate ovaries, she still has a good chance to become pregnant and have a normal baby.

Uterine displacement caused by relaxation of the pelvic musculature

Downward displacement of the uterus is caused by a relaxation of the muscles of the pelvic floor. It usually results from unrepaired lacerations due to childbirth and ill-advised bearing down during labor. With better obstetric care, use of episiotomies to prevent tearing of the pelvic muscles, immediate repair of all tears, and the trend toward fewer pregnancies and births per woman, fewer women should require vaginal wall repairs late in life. Perineal exercises practiced following delivery help to prevent relaxation. Apparently relaxation may also be caused by a congenital weakness of the muscles of the pelvis because it occurs occasionally in women who have had no children.

As the uterus begins to drop, the vaginal walls become relaxed, and a fold of vaginal mucosa may protrude outside the vaginal orifice. This is known as a *colpocele*. With the relaxation of the vaginal walls, the bladder may herniate into the vagina (a *cystocele*), or the rectal wall may herniate into the vagina (a *rectocele*). (See Fig. 21-11.) Both conditions may occur simultaneously.

A sign of relaxation of the pelvic musculature is a dragging pain in the back and in the pelvis. It is made worse by standing or walking. The patient who has a cystocele may complain of urinary incontinence accompanying activity that increases intra-abdominal pressure such as coughing, laughing, walking, or lifting (stress incontinence). The cystocele may become so pronounced that, in order for the patient to void, the bladder must be pushed back into place by holding the finger against the anterior vaginal wall. If the patient has a rectocele, she may complain of constipation and resultant hemorrhoids.

Older women may have suffered from these conditions for years and yet may not have sought medical attention. They may remember that their mothers had a similar condition and think that it is to be expected in women who have borne children. Since they are not incapacitated, some decide not to spend money to have reparative surgery that they know is available. Some delay seeking treatment because they dread surgery. However, untreated displacements of the uterus may cause complications such as cervical ulceration and infection, cystitis, and hemorrhoids.

Vaginal repair. Cystoceles and rectoceles are treated by plastic operations designed to tighten the vaginal wall. The operation is done through the vagina. The repair for a cystocele is called an *anterior colporrhaphy;* that for a rectocele, a *posterior colporrhaphy.* Old tears of the pelvic floor, usually caused by childbearing, may also be repaired. Such repair is called a *perineorrhaphy.*

As part of the preoperative preparation, a cleansing douche is frequently ordered the morning of surgery. When surgery involving the vagina is performed, postoperative nursing care includes prevention of pressure on the vaginal suture line and prevention of wound infection. Perineal dressings are seldom used. *Perineal care* is given at least twice a day and after each voiding or defecation. Sterile cotton balls moistened with benzalkonium chloride, bichloride of mercury, or normal saline solution may be used, or the patient may be placed on a douche pan and the solution poured over the perineum. Cleansing is always done away from the vagina toward the rectum so that contamination is avoided. An indwelling catheter may be inserted and attached to continuous drainage for 24 to 48 hours. After removal, the usual methods to encourage voiding can be employed. A heat lamp may be used for 15 to 20 minutes two or three times a day to encourage healing of the perineum. The heat lamp should be used after perineal care to help dry the area and thereby prevent sloughing of tissue. If the patient complains of perineal discomfort, an ice pack applied locally helps to reduce swelling and gives relief. A plastic bag or disposable glove filled with ice, firmly tied and covered, makes an adaptable pack. When sutures have been removed, sitz baths are usually ordered. Beginning on the tenth postoperative day, a daily vaginal douche with normal saline solution is usual-

ly prescribed. Occasionally douches are ordered during the immediate postoperative period. Sterile equipment and sterile solution should then be used. The douche nozzle should be very gently inserted and very carefully rotated.

After discharge the patient who has had a vaginal repair should continue to take a daily douche and a daily tub bath. The physician may also prescribe a laxative to be taken each night to prevent constipation and excessive stress on the surgical site. When she returns to the clinic or to the physician's office, the woman is told to discontinue the douches and laxative. The physician also tells her when it is safe for her to resume sexual intercourse. Patients who have had vaginal repair procedures, like other patients having gynecologic surgery, need to avoid jarring activities and heavy lifting for at least 6 weeks postoperatively.

If a posterior colporrhaphy is scheduled, a cathartic may be given approximately 24 hours before surgery, and several enemas usually are given preoperatively to help assure an empty bowel at the time of surgery and immediately thereafter. Up to 24 hours preoperatively the patient may be permitted only clear liquids orally to further reduce bowel contents. Postoperatively the patient may be kept flat in bed or in a low Fowler's position to prevent increased intra-abdominal pressure or strain on the wound. Special attention must be given to exercise for the patient's legs, to having her turn frequently, and to having her cough deeply. For 5 days, only liquids are permitted orally, and camphorated tincture of opium (paregoric) is also given to inhibit bowel function. At the end of this time, mineral oil is given each night, and an oil retention enema is given the morning after the first laxative is given. Only a soft rectal tube and small amounts of oil (200 ml.) should be used. The nurse should discourage straining to produce a bowel movement. Enemas for relieving flatus and for cleansing the bowel usually are not given until at least a week postoperatively.

After an anterior colporrhaphy, an indwelling catheter is usually left in the bladder for about 4 days. The catheter should keep the bladder completely empty. If a catheter is not used and if the patient is taking sufficient fluids, voiding should be checked at least every 4 hours. No more than 150 ml. of urine should be allowed to accumulate in the bladder. It is usually very difficult to catheterize a patient following a vaginal repair since the urethral orifice may be distorted and edematous. Having the patient take deep breaths may help in locating the orifice because it dilates slightly with each breath. A soft rubber catheter should be used. The patient is usually allowed out of bed immediately after surgery. A regular diet is given, and mineral oil is taken each night to lessen need to strain on defecation.

Sometimes a vaginal plastic procedure does not

relieve the *stress incontinence* caused by a cystocele and by general relaxation of the pelvic floor. When this happens, the ligaments about the bladder neck may be shortened in such a way that the bladder drops less easily into the vagina. The degree of incontinence may be tested by filling the bladder to various levels with sterile normal saline solution and then having the patient cough or strain while standing. If the incontinence is marked, the patient may be placed in a lithotomy position while the physician fills the bladder with normal saline solution and supports the bladder neck with a finger or with a clamp in the vagina to test the effectiveness of the bladder with this support. If the patient can cough and strain down without being incontinent, she is considered a good candidate for the operation. The surgery is done through a suprapubic incision, and it is usually combined with further vaginal repair. A urethral catheter is inserted, and the nursing care is similar to that following a vaginal repair. If the catheter does not drain freely or if the patient without a catheter does not void within 4 to 6 hours, the physician should be notified. Pressure from a full bladder may disrupt the repair.

Prolapse of the uterus. Prolapse of the uterus, or *procidentia uteri,* is a marked downward displacement of the uterus. The severity of the displacement is designated as first, second, or third degree. In a first-degree prolapse the cervix is still within the vagina. In a second-degree prolapse the cervix protrudes from the vaginal orifice. In a third-degree prolapse the entire uterus, suspended by its stretched ligaments, hangs below the vaginal orifice. In both second-degree and third-degree prolapses the cervix becomes irritated from clothing, the circulation becomes impaired, and ulceration often follows.

The usual treatment for a uterine prolapse is hysterectomy. This procedure may sometimes be done by the vaginal route. If any operation is contraindicated because of the age or general condition of the patient, a *Gellhorn* or *stem pessary* may be inserted to hold the uterus up in the pelvis (Fig. 21-11). A string should be attached to the pessary, and after its insertion the patient pins the string to her underclothing. This type of pessary occasionally becomes displaced and might cause the patient embarrassment.

Fistulas

Fistulas can occur in several locations (Fig. 21-12). They may occur when a malignant lesion has spread or when radiation treatment has been used for a malignancy, or they may be caused by trauma at surgery.

Ureterovaginal fistulas complicate gynecologic treatment rather frequently. In treating cancer of the uterus, either by radiation or surgery, or occasionally when a hysterectomy is done, the blood sup-

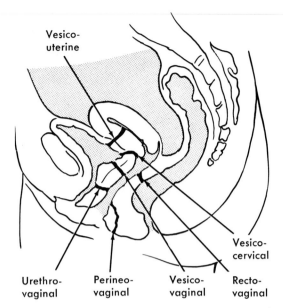

FIG. 21-12. Types of fistulas that may develop in the vagina and uterus.

ply to the ureter may be impaired or other damage may occur. The ureteral wall sloughs, and a fistula opens from the ureter to the vagina. This causes a constant drip of urine through the vagina. A ureterovaginal fistula usually heals spontaneously after a period of time. If it does not, repair procedures may be attempted, and occasionally an ileobladder must be made (p. 447).

Vesicovaginal fistulas, or fistulas between the bladder and the vagina, and *urethrovaginal fistulas,* between the urethra and the vagina, may follow radiation of the cervix, gynecologic surgery, or trauma during delivery. It is impossible to perform surgery to repair the fistula until the inflammation and induration have subsided. This may take 3 to 4 months. A suprapubic incision is made into the bladder, the fistula tract is dissected out, and the defect is closed by primary closure or by using a graft from the bladder or adjacent mucosal wall.

Postoperatively the patient usually has both a suprapubic tube and a urethral catheter inserted to drain the bladder. These tubes are sometimes attached to a "bubble" suction drainage apparatus in order to assure that the bladder is kept empty. Bladder drainage is maintained for about 3 weeks or until the wound is completely healed. The catheters should not be irrigated unless it is absolutely necessary, and only very gentle pressure should be used when irrigating them. Signs of urinary drainage from the vagina should be noted. There is normally a small amount of serosanguineous drainage from the vagina for a few days postoperatively. Vaginal douches may be ordered and should be given gently and with very little pressure from the fluid. The patient is kept on bed rest for several days and then is usually allowed to sit at the side of the bed. She will need to remain in her room and beside her bed if bubble suction is being used. Such confinement is tiring since she is not acutely uncomfortable. Visitors, television, radio, reading materials, and a variety of occupational therapy activities may help her to pass the time satisfactorily.

The results of repair operations for fistulas are not always successful. The patient must sometimes have several operations, and each successive hospitalization increases her anxiety about the outcome of surgery and lessens her ability to accept the discomforts and inconveniences entailed. All possible nursing measures should be taken to prevent infection and to be certain that free drainage of urine is assured. Obstruction of drainage tubes may place pressure against the newly repaired vesicovaginal wall and cause healing tissue to break down, resulting in return of the fistula.

Rectovaginal fistulas are less common than vesicovaginal fistulas. The constant escape of flatus and fecal material through the vagina is particularly distressing to the patient, especially so because rectovaginal fistulas are quite resistant to satisfactory surgical treatment. They may be due to the same causes as vesicovaginal fistulas. Surgical repair is usually done through the rectum. It may not be satisfactory, and operations may have to be repeated. The nursing care is similar to that needed by patients following surgery for other types of rectal fistulas (p. 701). In addition, the patient will need sympathetic understanding and encouragement since the emotional reactions are much more severe.

If there is dribbling of fecal material into the vagina it may be temporarily lessened by giving a high enema, and the patient who is at home is encouraged to do this before going out. After surgery, of course, enemas are never permitted until healing is complete. They may be given during the preoperative period. A soft rubber catheter should be used and should be directed carefully on the side of the rectum opposite the fistula. The catheter must go beyond the fistulous opening, or the fluid will return through the vagina and no benefit will be derived from the treatment. While a constipating diet will temporarily prevent fecal material from going into the vagina, it eventually will cause pressure and may aggravate the condition and increase the size of the fistula. The patient, therefore, is advised against restricting diet and fluids in an effort to control bowel action.

Most patients with vesicovaginal and rectovaginal fistulas tend to become withdrawn. Occasionally, however, a patient becomes immune to the odors, and this presents a serious problem to her family. It puts a strain on family relationships at a time when the patient is desperately in need of approval and acceptance. Often it is better for the physician or nurse

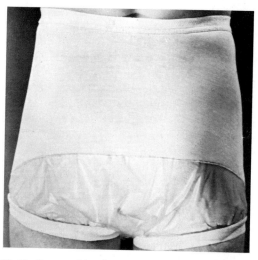

FIG. 21-13. Pants with plastic reinforcement of the crotch. They usually give adequate protection to the woman with stress incontinence. (Courtesy Ferguson Manufacturing Co., Grand Rapids, Mich.)

to bring the problem to the patient's attention than to have it mentioned by a member of the family, but the nurse should consult the physician before discussing this matter with the patient. The nurse can then help the patient to devise means of caring for herself so that she can be assured that she is free of odor. Chlorine solution (for example, 1 teaspoon of chlorine household bleach to 1 quart of water) makes a satisfactory deodorizing douche, and this solution is also excellent for external perineal irrigation. Sitz baths and thorough cleansing of the surrounding skin with mild soap and water are helpful. Deodorizing powders such as sodium borate can be used. Care is time-consuming and must be repeated at regular intervals to ensure cleanliness. Protective pants can be worn. Some large department stores now stock plastic pants for women that button at the side to avoid bulkiness (Fig. 21-13). A protective apron worn backward under other clothing or a petticoat with a posterior lining of plastic waterproof material also protects the patient from embarrassment of soiling clothing or furniture when she is seated.

The patient needs encouragement from the medical and nursing staff, and she needs assurance that they understand her problem. When fistulas persist, couples have special problems that require patience and understanding. Husband and wife should be encouraged to plan together a recreational and activity schedule that will help to minimize tensions until normal sexual relations can be resumed.

Malignant tumors

As stated earlier, the death rate from cancer of the cervix has been reduced by 50% in the past 15 years, and this reduction is largely attributed to early diagnosis by use of the Pap smear. The incidence of cancer of the endometrium is rising. This is partly due to the fact that women are living longer and this form of cancer is most prevalent among women of postmenopausal age. Mass screening of women in this age group is required if the incidence of endometrial cancer is to be reversed. Cancer ranks second among all causes of death in the United States and the mortality rate could be reduced dramatically if women availed themselves of detection and treatment services.

Cancer of the cervix. Despite the reduction in mortality due to cervical cancer, this form of malignancy has long been recognized as second only to cancer of the breast in its frequency of occurrence in women. If detected in the preinvasive stage, cancer of the cervix is 100% curable. Cancer of the cervix occurs most often in women between 30 and 50 years of age.

Early marriage and frequent intercourse have been implicated. First pregnancy at an early age, coitus before the age of 20 years and menarche before the age of 13 seems to increase the chances of developing cervical cancer. The carcinogenic effects of intrauterine devices and birth control pills are currently under investigation. In 1929 the Cancer Committee of the League of Nations developed for statistical study an international classification for cancer of the cervix (Table 21-4). This classification originally ranged from stages I to IV. However, since the discovery of the Pap smear technique, stage 0 has been added.

One of the most important functions of nurses is to actively participate in programs of preventive health care. For women, this includes encouragement to have a yearly pelvic examination, including a Pap smear test, and to be aware of the warning signs of cancer of the cervix. It is important to seek out candidates for education regarding cancer of the reproductive system and to offer them information. Hospitalized women, women in ambulatory care settings, and women seen in their homes provide opportunities for nurses to inform women about cancer detection and to teach them the warning signs of cancer. If there is early diagnosis, the prognosis is

excellent because the preclinical stage (stage 0 of cancer frequently exists 5 to 10 years before the visible stage I lesion appears. In the early stages the symptoms are a slight watery vaginal discharge, lengthening of the menstrual period, or occasional spotting of blood between periods. Spotting is often noticed following intercourse, after taking a douche, after defecating, or after heavy lifting.

If treatment is not instituted, the disease will advance progressively, with the vaginal discharge becoming dark, bloody, and foul smelling due to infection and necrosis of tissue. Bladder or rectal symptoms such as fistulas or symptoms of pressure may appear. As lymph glands anterior to the sacrum become involved, back and leg pains occur from pressure on the nerves. Emaciation, anemia, and irregular fever, secondary to the local infection and tissue necrosis, may then follow. The woman with untreated cancer of the cervix has a life expectancy of from 2 to 4 years following the appearance of the cervical lesion.

Cancer of the uterus. It is believed that 30% to 40% of all postmenopausal bleeding is due to cancer of the body of the uterus.[2] It occurs more often in women who have never been pregnant and is frequently associated with obesity, diabetes, and hypertension.[65]

Cancer of the endometrium is a slow-growing form of cancer and is very amenable to treatment if detected early. Regular screening methods for early detection are now more available than ever before and it is hoped that these methods will be used as part of regular physical examinations of women.

The early signs of endometrial cancer are unexpected or irregular vaginal bleeding. If these signs are heeded and medical attention is sought, the chance for cure is good. Since these tumors often arise from a polyp, anyone who has *uterine polyps* or who has had polyps removed from the uterus should have periodic pelvic examinations.

Cancer of the fundus may be treated by total hysterectomy (excision of the uterus including the cervix uteri) or by irradiation therapy (intrauterine radiation and deep x-ray therapy to the pelvis).

Table 21-4 Cancer of the cervix

Stage	0	I	II	III	IV
Involvement	Confined within epithelium of cervix	Completely confined to cervix	Extends outside cervix but does not involve pelvic wall or lower third of uterus	Involves pelvic wall and lower third of vagina	Extends beyond stage III; involves (1) bladder or (2) rectum or (3) metastatic spread

Often intrauterine irradiation is used preoperatively to shrink the tumor and to decrease the amount of local infection so that the operation will be safer and more easily performed. Since tumors of the fundus of the uterus occur later in life, the surgical course is frequently complicated by other conditions commonly seen in geriatric patients such as hypertension, diabetes mellitus, poor circulation, and malnutrition.

Cancer of the ovary. Cancer of the ovary appears to be increasing in the United States, and so far it has defied all attempts at early diagnosis. Over one half of all patients having this condition are inoperable when the disease is discovered, and the 5-year survival rate is only 15% to 20%.[110] Most gynecologists believe that the only hope for the patient lies in early and vigorous treatment of ovarian cysts, which may be precursors of malignant disease. They believe that all patients suspected of having tumors of the ovary should have an exploratory abdominal operation because malignant tumors of the ovary usually give no symptoms until local metastasis occurs and there is ascites from increased pressure within the portal system, edema of the legs from pressure on veins passing through the pelvic cavity, or pain in the back or the legs from pressure on nerves, or until there are symptoms of distant metastasis. The silent onset and growth of ovarian tumors almost surely doom the patient in whom diagnosis is not made prior to onset of symptoms. The only effective means of assuring early diagnosis is a pelvic examination every 6 months, including careful ovarian palpation, and surgical exploration of any questionable ovarian growth. If possible, the ovary and the tumor are completely removed at operation. If the tumor is malignant, the operation often is followed by deep x-ray therapy. Chemotherapy has prolonged the lives of some patients; nitrogen mustard and TEM are drugs often used, and the alkylating agent chlorambucil has been found to produce a favorable response in approximately 25% of all patients. (For the nursing care of patients receiving these drugs, see p. 301.)

Hydatidiform mole. Although a hydatidiform mole is usually benign, it may be malignant and for this reason is included with malignant tumors. A hydatidiform mole is a tumor mass of chorionic cells in the uterus that masquerades as a pregnancy. The cause is unknown, although a defective ovum is assumed to be involved. The uterus rapidly increases in size because of enlargement of the ovarian follicles. There is also an increase in the level of chorionic gonadotropin in the blood and urine. Treatment consists of the administration of Syntocinon (synthetic oxytocin), which causes evacuation of the mole from the uterus. After the mole is expelled, curettage is done. On rare occasions hysterectomy may be necessary. Bleeding following curettage is often quite ex-

tensive and several units of whole blood replacement may be necessary.[28]

Because approximately 10% of hydatidiform moles are malignant, it is recommended that a chemotherapeutic drug such as methotrexate (Amethopterin) be given before or immediately following the evacuation of the uterus. Therapy usually consists of 25 mg. of methotrexate intramuscularly for 5 days.[28] The chorionic gonadotropin levels should be checked periodically (usually monthly). Levels that fail to return to normal indicate that there may be a malignant component, which will need to be vigorously treated.[28] Since some spontaneous abortions actually may be the expulsion of hydatidiform moles, all aborted tissue should be sent for pathologic examination.

Chorioepithelioma (choriocarcinoma). Chorioepithelioma is a highly malignant neoplasm derived from chorionic epithelium. It may occur after a full-term delivery, miscarriage, or hydatidiform mole, although the previous pregnancy is not always recognized. The tumor appears as a dark, hemorrhagic grumose mass either on the uterine wall or in the substance of the uterine wall (the intramural cavity). The surface of the wall later becomes extremely ulcerated and there is spreading and penetration of the uterine musculature. The chief symptom is bleeding with offensive odor and profuse discharge. There may be early metastases involving the lung, brain, liver, bone, and even the skin as well as the vagina and vulva. Cough or hemoptysis is a sign indicative of pulmonary involvement and such involvement should be ruled out by x-ray examination.

As the disease advances, there is increasing emaciation and weakness with anemia from frequent, profuse hemorrhage. Treatment may be medical or surgical. Surgical removal of the involved organs such as a lobectomy (removal of a lobe of the lung) may be done. Medical treatment involves giving massive doses of nitrogen mustard or hormones such as estrogens or androgens.

A recent and more successful treatment is the use of the folic acid antagonist, methotrexate (Amethopterin), which is patently toxic to the decidua. A dose of 2.5 mg. orally is administered four times a day for 10 days and a similar course of therapy is repeated 2 weeks later. Complications of this drug (stomatitis, nausea, vomiting) sometimes interfere with the patient's treatment.

Benign tumors

Fibroid tumors of the uterus. Approximately 20% of all women over 30 years of age develop myomas or fibroid tumors of the uterus.[28] These benign tumors are more prevalent in black women and in women who have not had children. They are benign lesions and very rarely become malignant. With the advent of the menopause, they tend to disappear spontaneously because their growth is stimulated by ovarian hormones.

Menorrhagia is the most common symptom of myomas. If the tumor is very large, it may cause pelvic circulatory congestion and may press on surrounding viscera. The patient may complain of low abdominal pressure, backache, constipation, or dysmenorrhea. If a ureter is compressed by the tumor, there may be signs and symptoms of ureteral obstruction. Sometimes the pedicle on which a myoma is growing becomes twisted, causing severe pain. Large tumors growing into the opening of the fallopian tubes may cause sterility, those in the body of the uterus may cause spontaneous abortions, and those near the cervical opening may make the delivery of a baby difficult and may contribute to hemorrhage postpartally.

The treatment of fibroid tumors depends on the symptoms and the age of the patient and on whether she wants more children and how near she is to the menopause. If the symptoms are not severe, the patient may simply need close medical supervision. If the tumor is near the outer wall of the uterus, a *myomectomy* (surgical removal of the tumor) may be perfomed. This operation leaves the muscle walls of the uterus relatively intact. If there is severe bleeding or obstruction, a hysterectomy is usually necessary. Occasionally, if surgery is contraindicated or if the patient is approaching the menopause, x-ray therapy or radiation is used to reduce the size of the tumor and to stop vaginal bleeding.

Benign tumors of the ovary. There are many benign tumors of the ovary. These include *polycystic ovaries,* otherwise known as the Stein-Leventhal syndrome; *ovarian fibromas; Brenner's tumors;* and *pseudomucinous cystadenomas.* More information about these tumors can be obtained from specialized texts.

Ovarian cysts. The most common ovarian growth is a cyst of the graafian follicle or corpus luteum. This usually reabsorbs spontaneously. There are, however, other types of ovarian cysts arising from various types of tissue. Some are partly solid, such as the *dermoid cyst,* which may contain skin, hair, teeth, and bone. Others grow very large and cause distortion of the abdomen. Ovarian cysts are surgically removed. This usually includes an *oophorectomy* (removal of the ovary).

Sometimes an ovarian cyst twists on the pedicle that carries its blood supply, causing sudden, sharp pain and shock. An emergency oophorectomy is done since without blood supply the tissues rapidly become necrotic.

Endometriosis

Endometriosis is a condition in which endometrial cells that normally line the uterus are seeded throughout the pelvis and occasionally extend to as distant a location as the umbilicus (Fig. 21-14). The

524

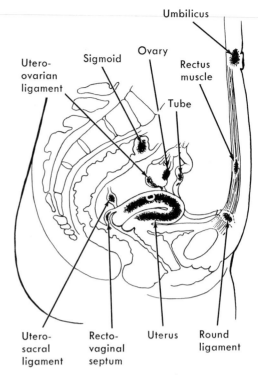

FIG. 21-14. Sites of endometrial implants.

disease appears to be increasing, although the increased incidence may be due to better diagnosis and recognition of the condition. It is not known how endometriosis first develops. Theories include congenital presence of endometrial cells out of their normal location, their transfer by means of blood vessels or the lymphatic system, and reflux of menstrual fluid containing endometrial cells up the fallopian tubes and into the pelvic cavity. None of these theories has been proved. With each menstrual period, the endometrial cells are stimulated by the ovarian hormones and bleed into the surrounding areas, causing an inflammation. Subsequent adhesions may be so severe that pelvic organs may become fused together, occasionally causing a stricture of the bowel or interference with bladder function. Encased blood may lead to palpable tumor masses, which often occur on the ovary and are known as *chocolate cysts.* Occasionally these cysts rupture and spread endometrial cells still farther throughout the pelvis.

Usually endometriosis progresses very gradually and does not produce symptoms until the patient is in her thirties or forties. Occasionally, however, symptoms appear when the patient is in her teens. The characteristic symptom of endometriosis is pain and general discomfort accompanying menstruation that becomes progressively worse and that was not present at the onset of the menses. This one characteristic feature should alert the nurse to urge that the patient see a gynecologist at once. Many women with severe pain related to menstruation have been judged to be neurotic when in reality they were suffering from endometriosis. Other symptoms of endometriosis are a feeling of fullness in the lower abdomen, dyspareunia, and general poor health. Sometimes the disease is far advanced and yet has caused no symptoms at all. Approximately 40% to 50% of women are infertile, and endometriosis is sometimes first detected when a woman presents herself with the complaint of inability to conceive.

Although a great deal of study of endometriosis is under way at present, its response to treatment is still variable and poorly understood. For this reason treatment is highly individualized. If the woman is young and wants to have children, the treatment for endometriosis is usually as conservative as possible. Pregnancy is beneficial because menstruation ceases during this time. If a young woman has endometriosis, the couple usually is advised to have their family without delay because fertility rate is low and sterility due to adhesions may occur and because a hysterectomy may have to be done within a reasonable period of time. Nursing the infant is also recommended because it delays the onset of menstruation following delivery. Because they imitate the state of pregnancy by inducing the ovaries to become unovulatory, antiovulatory drugs are frequently prescribed. Oral progestational drugs used over a period of 4 to 6 months are not uncommon. The starting dose is usually 5 to 10 mg. daily and the dose is increased by 10 mg. every 2 weeks until a therapeutic level is reached or until the maximum dose of 40 mg./day is reached. This dosage produces a situation known as pseudopregnancy and causes the errant endometrial cells to be temporarily quiescent. The disadvantages of this treatment are that irregular bleeding may occur and that the symptoms of early pregnancy, including nausea, vomiting, depression, and fatigue, may be troublesome. It is not believed that such drugs should be given indefinitely. Androgens are also given occasionally, but their masculinizing effects limit their usefulness.

When the involvement is severe and does not respond to hormonal treatment, surgery may be necessary. A total hysterectomy, oophorectomy, and salpingectomy may be done. Removal of the ovaries prevents further bleeding of endometrial implants that cannot be removed, and it has been found that removal of the uterus alone has lead to prolonged regression of the implants in some instances.[103] If the patient is premenopausal and the ovaries must be removed, she may be given very small amounts of estrogen to preserve secondary sexual characteristics and permit more normal living. The menopause stops the progress of this condition.

Disease of the vulva

Cancer of the vulva is seen most often in women over 60 years of age who have *chronic leukoplakia of the vulva*. The skin appears white and thickened, itches, and is easily fissured. If leukoplakia in women approaching 60 years of age does not respond to more conservative treatment, some physicians recommend a *vulvectomy,* surgical excision of the vulva, to prevent the development of cancer. If cancer is already present, the treatment is radical vulvectomy. This involves not only vulvectomy but also dissection of bilateral inguinal nodes; the mons pubis; terminal portions of the urethra, vagina, and other vulvular organs; portions of the round ligaments and the saphenous veins; and reconstruction of the vaginal walls and the pelvic floor.[5] Patients with cancer of the vulva are often poor surgical risks because of concurrent medical conditions related to age.

Kraurosis vulvae. Another condition seen in older women, kraurosis vulvae, causes a shrinking of the skin of the vulva. The skin is shiny and thin and itches severely. Kraurosis vulvae is not a precancerous condition, but it sometimes requires surgery because adhesions may interfere with voiding and with sexual intercourse. Cortisone ointment is often helpful. Occasionally female hormones are given, and local injections of alcohol may be tried to relieve the pruritus.

Management of the patient requiring a vulvectomy and inguinal node dissection

The patient requiring a vulvectomy has some special nursing needs in addition to routine preoperative and postoperative care. Preoperatively she is given enemas, and postoperatively she is given a low-residue diet. These measures obviate the need for straining to defecate and help prevent contamination of the vulval wound. A Foley catheter usually is employed to provide urinary drainage. When the catheter is removed, the patient may be unable to void because of difficulty in relaxing the perineum. Sitz baths may help. If the inguinal nodes have been dissected, a heat lamp may be directed to the groins. After all the sutures are removed, sitz baths may be substituted for the heat lamp. Large amounts of tissue are removed from the vulva and the groins during the operation, and the sutures are usually quite taut, leading to severe discomfort. The patient will usually need analgesic medication at frequent intervals during the 2 or 3 weeks before sutures can be removed. Following an inguinal node dissection, pillows need to be arranged to prevent undue pulling on the taut inguinal sutures when the patient moves. If the patient is lying on her side, she will be more comfortable if her upper leg is supported by a pillow. If she is lying on her back, a low Fowler's position puts less tension on the sutures. Wound hemorrhage is a possible complication.

The vulval wound is frequently left exposed, but if a dressing is used, it should be held in place with a T binder. The wound is cleansed twice a day with solutions such as hydrogen peroxide, normal saline solution, benzalkonium chloride, or other antiseptic solutions. Following this, a heat lamp is used to dry the area. The heat also improves local circulation, thus stimulating healing.

The wounds following a vulvectomy or an inguinal node dissection also heal slowly, and the patient may become quite discouraged. Diversional activities and socializing with other patients may help to keep the patient from thinking too much about herself and help her to pass the time. Privacy should be assured, and women should be encouraged to express their feelings concerning this disfiguring surgery. Some women feel that their femininity has been irreparably damaged or that the disfigurement may end their sexual life. Actually, by the time the patient is discharged, the wounds are usually healed, and the convalescence will be similar to that following any surgical procedure. Sexual intercourse can usually be resumed.

Management of the patient receiving radiation therapy

Internal radiation is used to treat cancer of the cervix and cancer of the body of the uterus because of the accessibility of these body parts and because of their generally favorable response to this form of treatment. The radioactive materials most often used are radium and cobalt (^{60}Co) or iridium (^{192}Ir), which have been made radioactive by artificial means. (For discussion of radiation treatment and the general nursing care and precautions involved, see p. 292.)

It is important that all normal tissues remain in their natural position and do not come nearer to the radioactive substance than is anticipated and provided for by the protective materials used. The patient is usually given a cleansing enema before the treat-

ment starts and is given a low-residue diet to prevent distention of the bowel, and a catheter may be inserted to prevent distention of the bladder. Gauze packing is usually inserted into the vagina to push both the rectum and the bladder away from the area being irradiated. Cleansing enemas are not given during the treatment. To prevent any displacement of the radioactive substance, the patient is kept flat in bed and is allowed to turn only from side to side. A radiograph is taken after the radioactive substance is inserted to determine its exact location.

The colpostat and tandem incorporating radioactive cobalt and intrauterine applicators or needles containing radium or radioactive iridium are most often used (Fig. 21-15). The amount of radioactive substance used and the number of hours it is left in place are determined by the amount of radiation needed to kill the less resistant cancer cells without damaging normal cells. Radioactive materials used for internal treatment must be removed at exactly the indicated time and the nurse is often responsible for reminding the physician to do this. If possible, the time of insertion should be planned so that removal will be at a convenient hour; for example, not in the middle of the night or during visiting hours.

Since the presence of *anything* in the cervix stimulates uterine contractions, the patient who has a colpostat or intrauterine applicator in place may have severe uterine contractions as a result of dilation of the cervix. The patient should know that they will occur. Often a narcotic is given at regular intervals while the applicator is in place. There will be foul-smelling vaginal discharge from destruction of cells. Good perineal care is essential, and it must be remembered that since the patient must lie on her back, she will need assistance. A deodorizer is helpful.

Patients may develop radiation sickness, with nausea, vomiting, diarrhea, malaise, and fever. This probably is a systemic reaction to the breakdown and reabsorption of cell proteins. (See p. 297 for discussion of care.) Local reaction may include cystitis and proctitis. Camphorated tincture of opium (paregoric) helps relieve the diarrhea. If it is severe, a cornstarch enema (1 tablespoon of cornstarch to 250 ml. of lukewarm water) may be ordered. Oil retention enemas are also sometimes given. The patient is urged to drink at least 3,000 ml. of fluid a day to help relieve any irritation of the urinary system.

Since the woman who is receiving radiation treatment usually either knows or suspects the diagnosis, she is likely to be depressed. The nurse should spend some time talking with her but should remain at the distance that is safe (p. 293). The reason for this precaution should be explained to the patient. Close members of the family should be encouraged to visit when it is considered safe for them to do so (p. 298).

Following the removal of the radioactive agent,

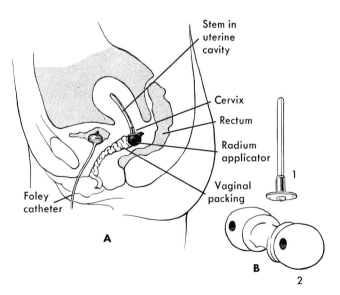

FIG. 21-15. A, Radium applicator in place in the uterus. Note the Foley catheter to decompress the bladder and that vaginal packing is used. **B,** *1,* Intrauterine applicator; *2,* colpostat.

the catheter is removed, a cleansing enema is given, and the patient is allowed out of bed. Vaginal discharge will continue for some time, and the patient may need to take douches for as long as the odor and vaginal discharge persist. Usually douches are ordered twice a day. The patient who is returning home needs detailed instruction in how to give herself douches and what solutions to use. Some vaginal bleeding may occur for 1 to 3 months after irradiation of the cervix or the body of the uterus. The patient who is at home should report persistent rectal irritation to the physician. Emollient enemas may be prescribed to be taken at home. The patient is usually discharged from the hospital within a day or two after the applicators are removed but may return for another course of radiation.

Complications to watch for following radiation of the uterus are vesicovaginal fistulas, ureterovaginal fistulas, cystitis, phlebitis, and hemorrhage. Each is due to irritation and destruction of adjacent tissue either by the radiation or by extension of the disease process. The patient is urged to report even minor symptoms or complaints to her physician.

If the patient is treated by x-ray therapy for a lesion of the reproductive system, the care is the same as that given a patient receiving this treatment elsewhere in the body (p. 295). However, one important point should be emphasized: the patient should always void immediately before the treatment to prevent damage to the bladder.

Management of the patient requiring partial or complete removal of the female reproductive system

Surgery such as a bilateral oophorectomy or a hysterectomy upsets most women emotionally. All women worry about the effect it will have on their femininity and wonder about possible changes in secondary sex characteristics. Young women may feel bitterly disappointed because they can no longer have children. Some women worry about gaining weight, although weight gain is more often due to overeating than to hormonal changes. It is true that the childbearing function will be terminated, but usually the vagina is intact so that several weeks following surgery women can resume normal sexual intercourse.

Older patients are usually less upset by the prospects of surgery of this kind than are those who have not reached the menopause. Postoperatively, however, almost all patients feel depressed for several days. This apparently is due to a change in hormonal balance and to psychologic reaction. The patient often is unable to explain why she is depressed and crying. Grieflike responses to loss of a body part may appear as they do following surgery in other cases. Feelings of guilt, shame, and remorse are not uncommon. Encouraging the patient to continue activities asso-

ciated with being female such as using makeup, arranging her hair, and wearing her own clothing often helps the woman to regain her perspective of being feminine. During this period, she needs understanding and sympathetic care since she may appear somewhat unreasonable at times. Families need to be helped to accept these responses calmly, and a husband may need help in understanding the patient's need for reassurance of his continued love and affection.

Hysterectomy. If a hysterectomy is to be performed, the preoperative physical preparation is the same as that for any other abdominal surgery, except that the perineum is completely shaved. A vaginal douche may be given. Postoperatively the patient has an abdominal dressing and wears a perineal pad. If a vaginal hysterectomy is performed, there will be no abdominal incision, but sterile perineal pads will need changing frequently. The dressings should be observed for any sign of bleeding every 15 minutes for 2 hours and then at least every hour for 8 hours.

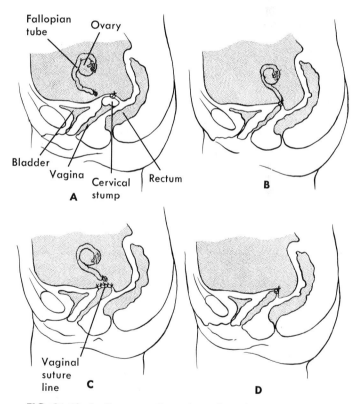

FIG. 21-16. **A,** Cross section of a subtotal hysterectomy. Note that the cervical stump, fallopian tubes, and ovaries remain. **B,** Cross section of a total hysterectomy. Note that the fallopian tubes and ovaries remain. **C,** Cross section of a vaginal hysterectomy. Note that the fallopian tubes and ovaries remain. **D,** Total hysterectomy, salpingectomy, and oophorectomy. Note that the uterus, fallopian tubes, and ovaries are completely removed.

There is normally a moderate amount of serosanguineous drainage. The perineal pad should be held in place with a T binder, and some physicians prefer that a snug scultetus binder be applied to the abdomen, especially if there has been a *radical hysterectomy* (removal of the ovaries, tubes, uterus with the cervix, and parametrial tissue) and extensive node dissection. (See Fig. 21-16.)

Following a hysterectomy, especially one in which there has been extensive node and parametrial resection, the bladder may be temporarily atonic as a result of nerve trauma, and a Foley catheter is used to maintain constant drainage of the bladder. If no catheter is used and if the patient is unable to void within 8 hours, she is usually catheterized. The catheter (if used) is removed on the third or fourth postoperative day, and the patient may be catheterized if abnormal residual urine is suspected.

Abdominal distention may complicate a hysterectomy. It is caused by nerve damage, by handling of the viscera during operation, or by sudden release of pressure on the intestines such as occurs on removal of a large myoma. Some physicians insert a nasogastric tube prophylactically following surgery, and most physicians restrict food and fluids orally for 24 to 48 hours. There is usually an order for a rectal tube and for a heating pad to the abdomen to be used as necessary. If the surgery has been extensive, a soft rectal tube should be selected to prevent trauma to the bowel. A Fleet's enema is usually given on the second or third postoperative day. When peristalsis returns, the patient is started slowly on fluids and food.

There may be interference with circulation during hysterectomy, and thrombophlebitis of the vessels of the pelvis and upper thigh is a rather common complication. The patient should never rest with the knees bent or with the thighs sharply flexed. The knee gatch should not be used, and the bed should not be raised at the head to more than a mid-Fowler's position. The patient should exercise her feet and legs every hour, and she should move about in bed, turning from her side to her back and to a partial face-lying position. A pillow can be used to support the abdominal wound. The head of the bed should be put completely flat for a short time every 2 hours during the first 24 hours postoperatively and then at least every 4 hours until the patient is ambulatory. These precautions help prevent stasis of blood in the pelvic vessels. If the patient has varicosities, the physician may order elevation of the legs for a few minutes every 2 or 3 hours to permit blood to drain from the legs. The nurse should be very careful that there is no undue pressure on the calves of the legs, that the elevation is uniform, and that there is no flexing at the popliteal region in order to lessen the possibility of thrombus formation. Ace bandages may be ordered to be applied from the toes to just below the knee,

excluding the popliteal region. Recent research on thrombophlebitis has indicated that improperly applied Ace bandages are a major cause of postoperative thrombus formation. The bandages should be reapplied twice a day to assure a snug, even pressure. The patient often is permitted out of bed the day following surgery. Other nursing care is the same as that following any abdominal surgery. Special attention should be given to any complaint of low back pain or to lessened urinary output since it is possible that a ureter could have been accidentally ligated. Occasionally the ureter, the bladder, or the rectum is traumatized.

The patient should know what surgery has been done, what changes in herself she should expect, and what care she needs when she leaves the hospital. If a *total hysterectomy* has been done, the premenopausal patient will not menstruate. A *subtotal hysterectomy,* however, permits menses to continue, since a portion of the uterus with its endometrial lining is left. She should not have sexual intercourse until told by the physician that it may be safely resumed. Most patients are more comfortable if they wear a girdle. Heavy lifting should be avoided for about 2 months. Activities such as riding over rough roads, walking swiftly, and dancing tend to cause congestion of blood in the pelvis and should be avoided for several months. Physical activity that does not cause strain, such as swimming, may be engaged in since it is helpful both for the physical and mental well-being of the patient.

Unilateral salpingectomy and oophorectomy. The patient who has a unilateral salpingectomy (removal of one fallopian tube) or a unilateral oophorectomy (removal of one ovary) usually requires postoperative nursing care similar to that given any patient having abdominal surgery. If the surgery is done to remove a large ovarian cyst, however, the patient may have considerable abdominal distention due to the sudden release of pressure on the intestines. The care is similar to that given for distention following a hysterectomy. If the surgery is done to remove a tumor that has caused changes in sex characteristics, the patient is usually quite sensitive and needs much understanding and encouragement from the nurse. She may shun others prior to surgery, and it is wise to let her have privacy if she so desires. She may be reassured that following surgery the abnormal sexual changes will gradually disappear. If the patient seems to withdraw from contact with others, the nurse should spend extra time with her provided she seems receptive to the nurse's interest.

Bilateral oophorectomy and radiation of the ovaries. The patient who has a bilateral oophorectomy or radiation treatment of the ovaries has specific problems. Although immediate preoperative and postoperative nursing needs are no different from those of the patient with other abdominal surgery, she will have an emotional reaction to being sterile that will need consideration. The extent of this reaction depends on her age, whether or not she already has or wants children, and her emotional makeup. She also will have symptoms of the climacteric. When the menopause is artificially induced, the symptoms are often more severe than in the normal climacteric. Therefore at least a portion of an ovary is left unless this is detrimental to the patient's prognosis. Estrogens relieve the symptoms and may be given to most patients unless surgery has been done for a malignancy. A bilateral oophorectomy may have been done primarily to remove the hormonal supply. This procedure is now used quite frequently in conjunction with radical mastectomy for cancer of the breast. The period of adjustment after a bilateral oophorectomy is long and is often trying not only for the patient but also for her family.

Pelvic exenteration. In a pelvic exenteration all reproductive organs and adjacent tissues are removed. Nursing care includes the care given the patient having a hysterectomy, the care given the patient having an abdominal perineal resection of the bowel, and the care given the patient having an ileobladder with transplantation of the ureters. Since this operation includes a radical hysterectomy, pelvic node dissection, cystectomy, vaginectomy, and a rectal resection, it requires unusual physical, social, and emotional adjustments on the part of the patient. Since it has not been found to help patients with cancer of the uterus more than less extensive operations and radiation treatment, it is not widely performed at this time.

The patient who has had a pelvic exenteration will have both urine and feces passing from the body through openings in the abdominal wall. She cannot contemplate having children, cannot have sexual intercourse, and will have symptoms of the menopause. Until she is able to accept her situation realistically, her rehabilitation will progress very slowly. This acceptance cannot be forced on the patient, but she must be encouraged gradually to resume self-care. She will undoubtedly have recurring periods of depression and discouragement. She should be helped to express her feelings and be given ample time and consideration by the nurse in order to do so. The family should understand what the surgery will entail, and they too, need encouragement. Acceptance

of the situation by the patient's husband is a very important factor in giving her the reassurance and courage necessary to face her future, and he may need to talk about his feelings with the nurse or others.

Care of the patient with incurable disease of the female reproductive system

The patient with incurable disease of the female reproductive system frequently has a lingering terminal illness. Most carcinomas of the female reproductive system do not metastasize to vital areas such as the liver. By direct spread they eventually cause death from carcinomatosis and from kidney failure that results from obstruction of both ureters by the tumor.

The nursing care is the same as for any patient with a terminal cancer elsewhere (p. 304), but there are some special measures that help to make the patient more comfortable. Frequent changes of position help relieve abdominal and pelvic pressure, and alternate hot and cold applications to the abdomen may bring some relief from pain. Often the use of these measures and the prescription of mild analgesics such as acetylsalicylic acid keep the patient comfortable for an indeterminate time and delay the need for narcotics. Most physicians believe that the patient should be kept relatively comfortable by the use of medications to relieve pain. Now that synthetic narcotics are available, there is less danger of the patient's developing addiction or tolerance to drugs since it is possible to change from one to another. A chordotomy is sometimes done to relieve severe pain (p. 881).

As cells die and are expelled, vaginal discharge may be profuse and have a foul odor. This is upsetting to the patient, her family, and her friends. The most effective means of decreasing the odor is to give the patient perineal care every 4 hours and to give a cleansing douche at least twice daily. Copious amounts of water should be used. Solutions containing chlorine are useful in destroying odors, and aromatic preparations added to the water may make the patient feel cleaner and more acceptable.

Meticulous care must be given to the skin since the patient is usually emaciated and may develop pitting edema. If the patient has ascites, she may rest better if the head of the bed is elevated.

Diseases of the male reproductive system

The female nurse must be particularly sensitive to the reactions and feelings of male patients who have disease of the reproductive system. The patient may

feel more comfortable discussing his problems with a male nurse or male physician, and the female nurse should respect his wishes.

Infections

Nonspecific pyogenic organisms as well as specific organisms such as gonococci and tubercle bacilli may cause stubborn infections of the male reproductive system. Urethritis, prostatitis, seminal vesiculitis, and epididymitis are the most common infections. Infecting organisms may reach the genital organs by direct spread through the urethra or they may be borne by blood or lymph.

Because urethral infection spreads so readily to the genital organs, men should not be catheterized unless it is absolutely necessary. Every means should be used to help them void normally. They are often allowed to stand to void even when they are to be on bed rest otherwise. Because of the length and curvature of the male urethra, some trauma to the urethral mucosa is likely to accompany catheterization or the passage of instruments such as a cystoscope. The distal part of the urethra is not sterile, and trauma makes the area susceptible to attack from the bacteria present. Fluids should be given liberally following passage of instruments through the urethra.

Nonspecific urethritis. Nonspecific urethritis is an inflammation of the urethra caused by such organisms as staphylococci, *Escherichia coli, Pseudomonas,* and streptococci. Although the symptoms and complications are essentially the same as those of gonorrheal urethritis, this infection is rarely caused by sexual contact. The patient complains of urgency, frequency, and burning on urination. There may be a purulent urethral discharge. (See p. 536 for discussion of gonorrheal urethritis.)

Treatment of nonspecific urethritis consists of antibiotics and chemotherapy, hot sitz baths, and increased fluid intake. To drain periurethral glands, the urethra may be dilated with sounds (Fig. 21-17). Dilation is followed by the instillation of a mild antiseptic such as 1:10,000 silver nitrate solution. Physical rest, improvement of general health, and decreased sexual activity are usually suggested. Nonspecific urethritis is difficult to cure and may become a chronic problem that ultimately results in chronic prostatitis.

Prostatitis. The patient with prostatitis usually has acute symptoms of urinary obstruction. He suddenly has difficulty in voiding, perineal tenderness and pain, and elevation of temperature. There may be hematuria. Treatment is usually conservative, consisting of antibiotics and chemotherapy, forcing fluids, physical rest, and local application of heat by sitz baths and/or low rectal irrigations.

Before having a rectal irrigation, the patient should have a cleansing enema. Then, by means of a Y connector on the rectal rube, tap water is allowed to flow alternately in and out of the rectum. The use of 2,000 ml. of water 46° C. (115° F.) and the insertion of the tube only 3 to 4 inches into the rectum will concentrate heat in the area of the prostate gland.

Prompt treatment of prostatitis may obviate the need for an indwelling catheter by preventing edema of the prostate and resultant obstruction of the urethra. Occasionally *prostatic abscesses* complicate the clinical course and may have to be drained surgically. Recurrent episodes of acute prostatitis may cause fibrotic tissue to form, and a prostatectomy may be necessary to relieve the resultant obstruction (p. 442).

Epididymitis. Epididymitis, one of the most common infections of the male reproductive system, may be caused by any pyogenic organism, but it frequently is a complication of gonorrhea or of tuberculosis of the urinary system. The patient complains of severe tenderness, pain, and swelling of the scrotum, which is hot to the touch. His temperature may be markedly elevated, and he has general malaise. He often walks with a characteristic "duck waddle" in an attempt to protect the affected part. This walk may first disclose difficulty in the patient who is too embarrassed to describe his trouble.

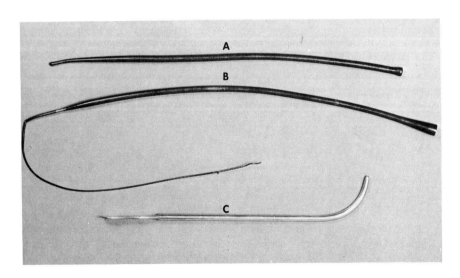

FIG. 21-17. A, Bougie for urethral dilation. **B,** Filiform. Note the long, fine, flexible tip. **C,** Metal sound for urethral dilation.

The patient with epididymitis is usually put to bed and the scrotum elevated either on towel rolls or with adhesive strapping known as a Bellevue bridge (Fig. 21-18). Ice is used to help reduce the swelling and to relieve the pain and discomfort. Heat is usually contraindicated because the normal temperature of the scrotal contents is below normal body temperature, and excessive exposure to heat may cause destruction of sperm cells. If an ice cap is used, it should be placed under the scrotum and should be removed for short intervals every hour to prevent ice burns. Antibiotic therapy is given. At least 3 quarts of fluid should be taken daily. When the patient is allowed out of bed, he should wear a scrotal support.

Since bilateral epididymitis usually causes sterility, special attention is given to the prevention of this infection. Untreated epididymitis leads rather rapidly to necrosis of testicular tissue and septicemia. When bladder drainage over a long period of time is necessary, a cystotomy is done so that a urethral catheter is avoided. An older patient who must have surgery of the prostate such as a transurethral resection that will require leaving a urethral catheter in place for a long time may be advised to have a *bilateral vasectomy* to prevent any infection from descending via the vas deferens to the epididymis. Often the operation is done prior to any cystoscopic examination. Since bilateral vasectomy causes sterility, permission must be granted by the patient. The vasectomies are done through two very small incisions in the scrotum or in the groins. Local anesthesia is used. Postoperatively the patient should still be watched for symptoms of epididymitis, since the organisms may have invaded the epididymis prior to the vasectomy.

Paraphimosis. Paraphimosis is a condition in which the prepuce is retracted over the glans and forms a constriction that is sometimes impossible to reduce as edema develops in the glans (Fig. 21-19). Cool compresses are applied to the penis and it is elevated for a short time before a gentle attempt is made to reduce the prepuce. If this measure fails, emergency surgery must be done. A dorsal slit is made in the prepuce to prevent necrosis of the glans due to impairment of its blood supply. A circumcision usually is done later to prevent recurrences.

Circumcision, or surgical excision of the prepuce, is widely recommended for all male infants in the immediate newborn period. The reasons are that it makes cleansing of the area so much simpler and that cancer of the glans penis is almost unknown among men who were circumcised soon after birth. If the operation is performed a few days after birth, no general anesthetic is needed. Older patients, even if they need anesthesia, are not hospitalized for more than a few hours for this operation. The wound is covered with gauze generously impregnated with petroleum jelly. Bleeding usually is controlled by applying a pressure dressing that may be bulky and that sometimes must be removed before the patient can void. It should be removed cautiously and replaced after voiding with a petroleum jelly dressing. If the patient goes home, he or his mother, if the patient is a child, is taught to change the dressing at each voiding for a few days and to try, if possible, to avoid fecal contamination of the area. Instruction is also given to be alert for signs of bleeding. If severe bleeding occurs, a firm dressing should be applied to the penis and the patient should go at once to the physician's office or the hospital emergency room. Very occasionally, if bleeding persists, it is necessary to resuture the wound. Frequently an estrogen preparation is prescribed for adult patients for several days after surgery to prevent penile erections, which are painful.

Orchitis. An infection of the testicle is known as orchitis. It may be caused by pyogenic bacteria, the

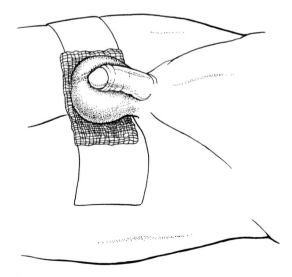

FIG. 21-18. Bellevue bridge.

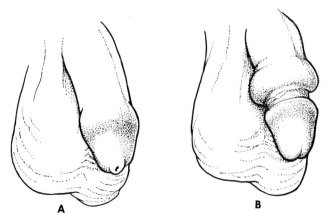

FIG. 21-19. A, Phimosis. Note pinpoint opening of foreskin. **B,** Paraphimosis. Note foreskin is retracted but has become a constricting band around penis.

Gonococcus, or the tubercle bacillus, or it may be a complication of mumps contracted after puberty. Although the latter occurs in a relatively small percentage of cases, if bilateral, it usually causes sterility. Any boy after puberty or man who is exposed to mumps usually is given gamma globulin immediately unless he has already had the disease. If there is any doubt, globulin usually is given. Although it may not prevent mumps, the disease is likely to be less severe with less likelihood of complications.

The symptoms and the treatment of orchitis are the same as those of epididymitis. Stilbestrol, which inhibits normal function, cortisone, and antibiotics may be given. Sometimes the tunica albuginea must be excised surgically to improve circulation to the testicle.

Scrotal and testicular enlargement

Immediate medical attention should be sought for any swelling of the scrotum or the testicles within it. Scrotal enlargements should be diagnosed—not treated symptomatically with suspensories, which give relief and encourage procrastination.

Hydrocele. A hydrocele is a benign, painless collection of fluid within the tunica vaginalis that leads to swelling of the scrotum. It occurs fairly often in infant boys as well as in adults. The cause is usually unknown. Occasionally hydrocele is treated by aspirating the fluid and injecting a sclerosing drug such as urea hydrochloride into the scrotal sac, but excision of the tunica vaginalis (hydrocelectomy) is the preferred treatment. Postoperatively a pressure dressing is applied on the scrotum, which is elevated. The patient should be observed carefully for any symptoms of hemorrhage. Bleeding may not be external. The patient needs a scrotal support when he is up and about and may still require one after he is discharged from the hospital. He should have two scrotal suspensories since they should be washed each day. Immediately after surgery or following an infection, most patients require an extra large suspensory or perhaps an athletic support (jockstrap).

Testicular neoplasm. Cancer of the testicle is usually painless, but it may be accompanied by an aching or dragging sensation in the groin and by swelling of the testicle. The swelling is frequently first discovered by the patient following trauma, but it usually is not caused by the trauma. Testicular swelling should always make one suspicious of neoplasm of the testicle. This condition is usually seen in men between 25 and 35 years of age, and it accounts for about 3% of all malignant tumors of the male reproductive system.[38]

An *undescended testicle* is much more likely to become malignant than one that is in the scrotum at birth or descends shortly thereafter. This is an important reason for encouraging parents to consent to surgical intervention to bring the undescended testicle of a young boy to a normal position. This does not eliminate the possibility of a neoplasm developing, but the testicle is located in a position where it may be examined carefully and regularly.

Men with suspicious testicular swelling are asked to collect a first-voided morning urine specimen. This is sent for an Aschheim-Zondek test, the same test used to detect pregnancy in women. One type of testicular tumor, the one with the poorest prognosis, gives a positive Aschheim-Zondek reaction. For all types of testicular tumors the testicle is removed surgically (orchiectomy) and the adjacent area is explored for metastatic node involvement. Metastasis often has occurred before the initial lesion is discovered.

The patient with cancer of the testicle is usually given a course of radiation therapy, and a *radical node dissection* may be done. This dissection may be unilateral or bilateral.

Following a radical node dissection, there is danger of hemorrhage. Active movement may be contraindicated since nodes may have been resected from around many large abdominal vessels, but gentle passive turning and leg and arm movement are essential to prevent postoperative pneumonia and thrombosis. Deep breathing should be encouraged at hourly intervals. A turning sheet and a chest support are usually helpful. The patient is extremely uncomfortable and needs frequent and large doses of narcotics and sedative drugs.

When a radical node dissection is performed, the patient may be placed in a Trendelenburg position for 2 weeks to allow the kidney to become fixed in place, since frequently all the fatty tissue supporting it must be removed. The patient may need to be fed and bathed during this period. He may have difficulty voiding in this position. For defecation, permission from the physician may have to be obtained to lower the foot of the bed. Occupational and diversional therapy should be provided. Since many patients find it impossible even to read in the Trendelenburg position, they may appreciate being read to, having the use of books that can be projected on the ceiling, or having access to "talking books" used by blind persons.

Since radiation therapy often is begun the day after surgery, the patient may develop radiation sickness during his hospital stay or during continued treatment as an outpatient. Hormones and chemotherapy are not effective in slowing the progress of cancer in this organ.

Patients and their families are extremely upset by the diagnosis of neoplasm of the testicle. The physician frequently is quite frank with the family and with the patient because he believes the man needs to be able to make necessary arrangements to provide for his family. The patient's prognosis may be measured in only months or in several years. Some patients are openly depressed. Others may seem to be taking the news too well. The nurse should listen carefully to both the patient and his family and sometimes suggest that help be obtained from others such as the social worker or the spiritual adviser. (For further discussion, see p. 291.)

Spermatocele. A spermatocele is a nontender cystic mass containing sperm. It is attached to the epididymis. Since the lesion is benign and usually there are few symptoms, excision is rarely necessary. If the patient is uncomfortable, he is usually advised to wear a scrotal support to prevent undue discomfort until after he has a family. Large masses may then be excised.

Varicocele. A varicocele is a dilation of the spermatic vein and is commonly seen on the left side only, probably because the left spermatic vein is much longer than the right. A varicocele on the right side only is suggestive of an abdominal tumor. The use of a scrotal support is usually all that is necessary to relieve any dragging sensation, but the spermatic vein may be ligated.

Torsion of the testicle. Torsion of the testicle or kinking of the spermatic artery causes severe pain, tenderness, and swelling of the testicle. It often follows activity that puts a sudden pull on the cremasteric muscle such as may occur from jumping into cold water. Operative intervention may be indicated and must be done within a few hours because interruption of blood supply to the testicle causes necrosis of the organ.

Cancer of the prostate gland

On autopsy examination, from 15% to 20% of all men past 55 years of age have been found to have microscopic carcinoma of the prostate gland. Although many of these men did not have clinical symptoms, it is known that the incidence of clinical cancer of the prostate gland increases with increasing age. It is believed that probably 25% of men in the seventh and eighth decades of life have cancer of the prostate gland.[42]

Cancer of the prostate gland is most often diagnosed when the patient seeks medical advice because of symptoms of urethral obstruction or because of sciatica (low back, hip, and leg pain). The pain is caused by metastasis of the cancer to the bones. This form of cancer frequently occurs concurrently with benign prostatic hypertrophy that causes the urethral obstruction. However, the cancer itself may be so far advanced as to cause obstruction.

Most carcinomas of the prostate gland are adjacent to the rectal wall and can be detected by rectal examination before symptoms appear. Since cancer of the prostate gland that causes obstruction of the urethra or back and leg pains may be too far advanced for curative treatment, one can readily understand the need for men past 40 years of age to

have routine rectal examinations. It is usually the lesions that are detected prior to symptoms that can be cured. A biopsy of any suspicious mass is taken.

An elevated acid phosphatase in the blood serum suggests cancer of the prostate gland, but since the acid phosphatase produced by prostatic cancer is not absorbed by the blood until the lesion has extended beyond the prostatic capsule, it is not a useful technique for early diagnosis.

In patients in whom a diagnosis is made prior to local extension of the cancer or distant metastasis, a *radical resection of the prostate gland* usually is curative. The entire prostate gland, including the capsule and the adjacent tissue, is removed. The remaining urethra is then anastomosed to the bladder neck. Since the internal and external sphincters of the bladder lie in close approximation to the prostate gland, it is not unusual for the patient to have urinary incontinence following this type of surgery. He also will be both impotent and sterile. The perineal approach is most often used, but the procedure may be accomplished by the retropubic route (Fig. 20-9).

If the patient is to have a perineal approach in surgery, he is given a bowel preparation, which includes enemas, cathartics, and phthalylsulfathiazole (Sulfathalidine) or neomycin preoperatively and only clear fluids the day before surgery to prevent fecal contamination of the operative site. Postoperatively he may be permitted nothing orally, clear liquids, or a low-residue diet until wound healing is well advanced. He may also be given camphorated tincture of opium to inhibit bowel action. If the retropubic approach is used, the preoperative care is similar to that of any patient having major surgery.

Regardless of the surgical approach, the patient returns from surgery with a urethral catheter inserted. A large amount of urinary drainage on the dressing for a number of hours is not unusual. It should decrease rapidly, however. There should not be the amount of bleeding that follows other prostatic surgery and, since the catheter is not being used for hemostasis, the patient usually has little bladder spasm. The catheter is used both for urinary drainage and as a splint for the urethral anastomosis. Therefore care should be taken that it does not become dislodged or blocked. The catheter is usually left in the bladder for 2 or 3 weeks.

The care of the perineal wound is the same as that following a perineal biopsy except that healing is usually slower. If there has been a retropubic surgical approach, the wound and possible wound complications are the same as for a simple retropubic prostatectomy (p. 445).

Since perineal surgery causes relaxation of the perineal musculature, the patient may suddenly have fecal incontinence. It is disturbing to the patient and sometimes can be avoided by starting perineal exercises within a day or two after surgery. Control of the rectal sphincter usually returns readily. Perineal exercises should be continued even after rectal sphincter control returns since they also strengthen the bladder sphincters, and unless the bladder sphincters have been permanently damaged, the patient will regain urinary control more readily on removal of the catheter. (See p. 180 for perineal exercises.)

The patient with carcinoma of the prostate gland is often very depressed after surgery because he suddenly realizes the implications of being impotent and perhaps permanently incontinent. He usually has been told by the physician before the operation that these consequences are possible, but he may not have fully comprehended their meaning. He needs to be encouraged, and provision should be made to keep him dry so that he will feel able to be up and to socialize with others without fear of having obvious incontinence. (See p. 180 for ways to manage incontinence.) Until the physician has ascertained that return of urinary sphincter control is unlikely, a method that gives only partial protection, such as the use of a bathing cap, is preferable since the patient is more likely to attempt to regain voluntary control.

When cancer of the prostate gland is inoperable, or when signs of metastasis occur following surgery, medical treatment is given. Relief from conservative treatment is quite dramatic in many patients and may last for 10 years or more in some instances. Usually the response is quite good for about a year and then the patient's condition begins to deteriorate.

The Huggins treatment may be used for inoperable cancer of the prostate gland to cause atrophy of the local lesion, control metastases, and relieve pain. It is based on the elimination of androgens by removal of the testicles and/or the giving of estrogenic hormones. The estrogen given is usually stilbestrol, 3 mg./day for 1 to 2 weeks. The dosage is then reduced to 1.5 to 3 mg./day. This measure frequently will relieve the pain. Stilbestrol causes engorgement and tenderness of the male breasts. It may also cause nausea. Severe side effects should be reported to the physician so that the dosage or type of estrogenic preparation may be adjusted. If a large tumor does not diminish in size with this treatment, some of the prostate gland may be resected to relieve obstruction. This procedure is most often done transurethrally (p. 442).

When symptoms begin to recur, or if the patient is very uncomfortable and needs immediate relief when the diagnosis of cancer is first made, a *bilateral orchiectomy (castration)* may be done. This operative procedure is technically minor and is often done under local anesthesia, but it may cause the patient considerable psychologic distress. The patient's permission for sterilization must be obtained. If he is married, he is usually urged to discuss the operation with his wife. This surgery eliminates the testicular source of male hormones and seems to cause regression or at least slows the cancer growth. Very occasionally a hypophysectomy may be done to further reduce hormonal stimulation.

Lesions of the external genitalia

Any lesion of the external genitalia requires medical attention, and no ulcer of the genitalia should be treated by the patient before seeking the physician lest the diagnosis be obscured. Although lesions are present in a wide variety of conditions, they should always be considered infectious until proved otherwise, since each of the venereal diseases, with the exception of gonorrhea, produces a genital lesion or ulceration. These lesions will be discussed in the section to follow, which deals with the venereal diseases.

Cancer of the penis. Cancer of the penis is far less common than formerly, but it still accounts for almost 3% of all cancers in males. Apparently it could be eliminated completely since carcinoma practically never develops in men who have been circumcised as infants. Usually the patient is over 50 years of age, but the condition has developed in men in their twenties. Most often the glans is the site of the initial malignant lesion.

Treatment for carcinoma of the penis is surgery with partial or total amputation of the penis. Removal of adjacent tissues and inguinal lymph nodes may be necessary, and this treatment may be followed by radiation therapy. Occasionally radiation therapy is used before surgery is done. Radiation therapy may be given externally, or needles, seeds, or plaques containing radioactive substances may be used. The physical nursing care is similar to that needed by women who have had a vulvectomy with inguinal node dissection (p. 525). Since the treatment causes such serious changes in a man's total life, the emotional reactions are profound, and very specialized care is needed. For further discussion of the treatment and the nursing care involved, see specialized nursing texts.[126]

Venereal disease

Venereal disease (VD) is the most common communicable disease in the United States today. Of the various types of venereal disease, gonorrhea and syphilis are the most prevalent (Fig. 21-20). Among

all of the reportable diseases, gonorrhea ranks first in this country. It has been estimated that over 2 million patients with gonorrhea were treated in 1970.[6] This represents an incidence of 308 cases

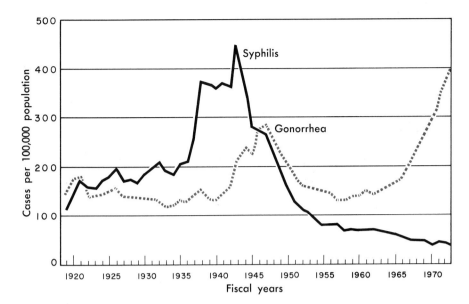

FIG. 21-20. Cases of reported syphilis and gonorrhea per 100,000 population in the United States—fiscal years 1919-1973. Note peak during period of World War II and increase in gonorrhea in recent years. (Data from VD fact sheet, ed. 30, 1973, Department of Health, Education and Welfare, Center for Disease Control, Atlanta, Ga.)

treated/100,000 total population. Since the early 1960's, the numbers of visits for treatment of gonorrhea have increased by 59%, and over 50% of all venereal disease visits made are currently made by teenagers and young adults.[119] Syphilis is also on the increase, with estimates of 20,000 to 85,000 new cases diagnosed and treated each year.[6]

Although these figures are staggering, they probably do not reflect the true incidence of sexually transmitted diseases. The accuracy of statistics requires reliable reporting of diagnosed cases and this in turn requires that medical advice be sought and all cases diagnosed be reported.

The increase in venereal diseases is not confined to the United States alone. It has become an international health problem. The World Health Organization estimates there are 100 million new gonorrheal infections each year throughout the world.[118] There has been a yearly increase in the venereal disease rate in Canada.[36] In Sweden the case rate is 514/100,000 population; in Denmark, 319; in Great Britain, 118; and in France, 30.[119]

Social factors

It is a common belief that sexual promiscuity within a community is reflected in the incidence of venereal disease. While statistics seem to indicate some relationship, the common belief may or may not be true. The highest incidence of venereal disease is reported by Sweden, a country that has had an openly permissive attitude about sexual behavior for many years. On the other hand, China, with its restrictive beliefs about sexual promiscuity and prostitution, is the only country in which the reported venereal disease rate is down appreciably.[119]

Sexual patterns and practices throughout the world have been influenced by increased availability of contraceptives, especially the contraceptive pill. In addition to reducing the worry over pregnancy, it has

permitted men and women more freedom and control by providing a wider range of alternatives for sexual behavior. Among younger people especially, oral contraceptives have influenced the value systems and beliefs about sexual behavior. Because of their different ideologies about sex, it is often said of younger people that they are morally lax and sexually promiscuous. Some studies indicate, however, that this is not so; in fact, those young people who are sexually active tend to keep to one sex partner even if sexual intercourse is premarital.[89]

Liberalization of attitudes toward sexual behavior and widespread use of contraceptives are incomplete explanations of the rising incidence of venereal disease. Greater mobility of people, increased job turnover, and changing ideologies have all had effects. Evidently, one important factor must be that people with venereal disease do not know they have the disease and may spread it unknowingly.

Education

Reluctance to permit and present programs about human sexuality and venereal diseases in the schools is in conflict with our highly sex-oriented society. Those who are in a position to present the facts and information hesitate to do so for a variety of reasons. Parental disapproval seems to stem from beliefs that their children are too young and innocent to learn about such things as sexuality and venereal disease. Another prevalent belief seems to be that to teach the facts or give information about these topics implies approval and encouragement of premarital sex at an early age. There seems to be fear that giving information increases curiosity and experimentation, and this might be a risk if facts are not presented completely and consequences are not included.

Sex education can be separated to some extent from venereal disease education by including venereal disease in general health courses. Even so, edu-

535

cators might remain hesitant. Inadequate instruction and inappropriate approaches can have negative consequences. If dealt with too lightly, young people may feel that venereal disease is no more serious than any other infection and that it is easily and simply cured by a shot of penicillin. They may not become aware of the immediate problems of infecting others or of the long-term effects of repeated or chronic infections. If presented in such a way that shame is associated with sexual activity and venereal disease, young people may be ashamed or afraid to believe they have venereal disease and delay seeking medical attention.

Physiologic factors

Certain biologic and physiologic factors have also influenced the increasing incidence of venereal disease. The normal acid environment of the vagina is changed to a more alkaline environment by contraceptive pills. Therefore women taking oral contraceptives are more vulnerable to venereal disease as well as other infections. The role of intrauterine contraceptive devices in the incidence and spread of venereal disease has not been clearly determined.

Some strains of venereal disease organisms, especially gonococci, are becoming increasingly resistant to the antibiotics used to effect treatment and cure. In order to be effective these infections require everincreasing doses, raising the risk of problems related to human tolerance. It is clear that new antibiotics and other forms of treatment are needed.

Sexual transmission

The venereal diseases are contagious diseases spread almost exclusively by contact during sexual intercourse, that is, when mucous membrane surfaces come in contact during genital, oral, or anal sex activity. Since the causative organisms survive only very briefly outside a warm, moist environment, there is almost no way to contract venereal disease from toilet seats, towels, or bed linens. There are some notable exceptions to sexual transmission. During pregnancy the fetus may become infected in utero by placental transmission or infection of the uterus and may be stillborn or infected at birth. Congenital syphilis is especially linked with placental transfer of the disease. Infants of mothers with gonorrhea may contract infections of the eyes (ophthalmia neonatorum) during birth, and unless treated, this can lead to permanent blindness.

■ GONORRHEA

Gonorrhea, often referred to as "GC" or "the clap" by lay people, is caused by *Neisseria gonorrhoeae*. The infection is usually confined to the genitourinary system in both males and females. However, fever and arthritis can occur if the disease is not treated.

If the hands are contaminated with the organism, the infection can be spread to the eyes. Anal intercourse, most often practiced by male homosexuals, can lead to infection of the anus and rectum.

The incubation period for gonorrhea is usually 2 to 5 days, although symptoms may be delayed as long as 3 months. Burning on urination and purulent discharge from the penis are the first symptoms to occur in men. As the infection spreads, the urinary bladder and prostate gland become involved, and increased frequency, burning, and urgency of urination result. Inflammation of the urethra makes the penis become red, sore, and painful. If the inflammation is severe, urethral scarring with narrowing of the tubules or obstruction of urine and semen can result. The scrotum may also become enlarged, inflamed, and painful. If scar tissue forms as a result of inflammatory processes in both epididymides, the man can become permanently sterile.

Only about 15% of women have early distressing signs of gonorrhea, that is, before the infection reaches the stage of acute pelvic inflammatory disease. The early signs include a slight purulent discharge, a vague feeling of fullness in the pelvis, and discomfort or aching in the abdomen. Since these symptoms are not perceived as severe, women may disregard them. If the bladder is involved, there is burning, frequency, and urgency of urination, and women are more likely to seek medical assistance because of the discomfort. The Bartholin's glands can become infected, resulting in distention and swelling that makes it painful for the woman to walk or sit. These symptoms may also lead the woman to see a physician.

Upward spread of the infection results in acute or chronic salpingitis. If an acute episode occurs, the woman experiences severe lower abdominal pain resembling ectopic pregnancy or appendicitis. The abdominal pain is often accompanied by fever and vomiting. The symptoms may subside if the woman does not consult a physician, and "dormant" chronic infection may result with or without periodic acute episodes. If chronic gonorrheal salpingitis results, the symptoms include abnormal menstrual periods, low back pain, and pain during intercourse. Scar tissue from inflammation and adhesions can obstruct the fallopian tubes, leading to permanent infertility. About 3% of women with gonorrhea become sterile.[18]

In men the diagnosis is made by gram-stained smear of the discharge from the penis. The diagnosis in women is most commonly made by cultures from the cervix, urethra, and anus. Fluorescent-tagged antibody methods are usually used since normal vaginal flora can resemble *Neisseria* when the gram-stain method is used.

Despite emergence of resistant strains of gonococci, the drug of choice for treatment is still penicillin. Careful history taking and observation for signs of reactions following administration of penicillin are important because of the large number of people who have become allergic to the drug. A single intramuscular injection of 2.4 million units of fortified procaine penicillin results in a cure in 80% to 90% of men having uncomplicated gonorrhea. For women with uncomplicated gonorrhea, the treatment most often used is aqueous penicillin G or PAM, 1.8 million units, intramuscularly in two injection sites at one visit. Because of the seriousness of complications that may result from gonorrhea, some physicians believe women should receive more treatment. In this event, three daily injections of 2.4 million units of aqueous penicillin G are given.

For patients whose organisms are penicillin-resistant or who are allergic to penicillin, tetracycline, chloramphenicol, streptomycin, or kanamycin may be prescribed.

■ SYPHILIS

Syphilis is caused by a spirochete, *Treponema pallidum,* that gains entry into the body through breaks in the mucous membrane or skin during intercourse.

The incubation period is usually 3 weeks. However, symptoms can appear as early as 9 days or as long as 3 months after exposure. If untreated, the disease progresses through four identifiable stages. Table 21-5 summarizes the outstanding features of each stage.

Syphilis is most often diagnosed by serologic testing. The test most often used for routine screening (premarital and prenatal) is the VDRL (Venereal Disease Research Laboratory) test. Positive reactions should be confirmed by an alternative serologic test. The test of choice for confirmation is the fluorescent treponemal antibody absorption (FTA-ABS) test because it is the most sensitive and specific. Serologic testing is dependent on the presence of specific antibodies (commonly called reagin) in the serum of the infected person. Because antibodies are not present in the serum until the organisms gain entry, the test may be negative and the individual may still be infectious. Once antibodies develop, the serologic tests may remain positive despite effective therapy. If therapy is given before the antibodies develop, these tests may never be positive.

Darkfield microscopic examination of tissue

Table 21-5 Stages of syphilis

	Primary	Secondary	Latent	Late
Duration	2-8 weeks	Appears 2-4 weeks after chancre appears; extends over 2-4 years	5-20 years	Terminal if not treated
Clinical signs	Hard sore or pimple on vulva or penis that breaks and forms painless, draining chancre; may be a single chancre or groups of more than one; may be present also on lips, tongue, hands, rectum, or nipples; chancre heals leaving almost invisible scar	Depends on site; low-grade fever, headache, anorexia, weight loss, anemia, sore throat, hoarseness, reddened and sore eyes, jaundice with/without hepatitis, aching of joints, muscles, long bones; sores on body or generalized fine rash; condylomata lata (venereal warts) on rectum or genitalia	No clinical signs	Tumorlike masses, gumma, on any area of body; damage to heart valves and blood vessels; meningitis, paralysis, lack of coordination, paresis, insomnia, confusion, delusions, impaired judgment, slurred speech
Communicability	Exudates from lesions and chancre are highly contagious	Exudates from lesions highly contagious; blood contains organisms	Contagious for about 2 years; not contagious to others after that; blood contains organisms	Noncontagious; spinal fluid may contain organisms

scrapings from lesions or material obtained by aspiration of regional lymph nodes may also reveal the presence of the spirochete, especially during the primary and secondary stages.

The spirochete causing syphilis can be destroyed at any stage of the disease, although treatment may have to be more prolonged in latent and late syphilis. While syphilis can be cured in late stages, the damage to the body produced is much less easily managed.

Penicillin is the drug that continues to bring about the highest cure rate. Treatment consists of intramuscular injection of 2.4 million units of benzathine penicillin in both buttocks. For patients who are allergic to penicillin, tetracycline or erythromycin can be used successfully. Patients who have been exposed to syphilis can be treated prophylactically.

■ FOLLOW-UP OF CONTACTS AND PREVENTION OF VENEREAL DISEASE

Both prevention of venereal disease and locating people who have been exposed to venereal disease are necessary if the trend in venereal diseases is to be reversed. Tracing of contacts and treating them for prevention and cure is very difficult. Because of fear, shame, and embarrassment and out of a sense of protection for themselves and others, some people are reluctant to divulge the names of their contacts. The attitudes of people in general, both lay and professional, may be a major obstacle to controlling the spread of venereal disease. Most people focus on how these diseases are spread rather than on the consequences of having the disease. For single people, especially, contracting venereal disease and securing help means they must admit to having sexual relations, and this means some of them, at least, may feel guilty about moral wrongdoing.

People treated for venereal disease can and must be given explanations of the importance of identifying contacts. They can and should be encouraged to inform their own contacts so that they in turn will seek medical attention. Because it is evident that people will not necessarily inform their own contacts when they are advised to do so, the department of health requires that all known cases of venereal disease be reported. Many lay people are aware of this and are very hesitant to give the names of their contacts. Every effort must be made in counseling patients with venereal disease to encourage them to participate in detection and treatment. Privacy, support, and reassurance are essential. Presentation of facts in an objective way and involving the patient in decision making reduce the possibilities of distrust, suspicion, and fear.

The nurse's role

The nurse's responsibilities include assisting in programs for the prevention of the disease, case finding, assisting with education and treatment of infected persons, interviewing patients for contacts (persons who have been exposed sexually to the patient and who may have the disease also), helping to secure medical care for contacts if necessary, and giving nursing care to patients who have not had adequate treatment and are in advanced stages of the disease.

Before nurses can be effective in working with patients with syphilis, they must face their own emotional reactions squarely. The patient is often young, fearful of pain, and unaccustomed to his surroundings in the clinic or the physician's office. Above all, he fears that his family and friends will learn of his predicament and that they will think less of him because of it. He must be certain that information he gives will be kept in strict confidence. The nurse who is successful in working with these patients is one who can create an atmosphere in which the patient feels free to discuss all aspects of the problem.

The patient should know that syphilis is a reportable disease and that he as well as the persons he names as contacts (if they are shown to have the disease) must be reported to the department of health. He should know that numbers instead of names are used in public places such as clinic waiting rooms so that there is little danger of others learning the nature of his disease unless he chooses to tell them. He should recognize the importance of reporting at intervals for checkups as recommended by his physician, because a few persons either are resistant to the drugs or have only slight resistance to the disease. Serologic tests made at intervals, as specified by the physician, reveal whether or not a relapse of active infection has occurred.

The nurse should make use of every opportunity to educate the public. Group meetings of citizens or patients, association with less-informed colleagues, and face-to-face relationships with patients all afford opportunities. All young people should know about the disease. In educational programs conducted in venereal disease clinics, patients themselves have stated that they wished they had known more about syphilis at an earlier age.* Health counseling, including sex education, is important in the prevention of syphilis. The *Social Health News,*† a monthly publication, is helpful in keeping the nurse informed in the field of venereal disease. The dangers of reinfection by spirochetes should be stressed in all health teaching. The effectiveness of penicillin in treatment of syphilis has produced mixed results. It has been a boon in making treatment easier, cheaper, safer, and more convenient and in rendering the patient

---

*Information on literature and programs is available from the Venereal Disease Program, Center for Disease Control, Atlanta, Ga. 30333.
†Published by the American Social Health Association.

noninfectious much more quickly than with any other treatment. However, according to some authorities, treatment has become so simple that patients tend to take the disease too lightly, to believe that they are immune to reinfection, or to believe that they need not worry about reinfection since they can again be easily cured. The incidence of reinfection in patients treated early is quite high, again demonstrating that not only must the spirochete be killed but also that the source of the disease must be controlled if the disease is to disappear.

Contact investigation. The nurse often interviews the patient and reviews with him his understanding of the disease. Success in obtaining the names of contacts and in securing the patient's confidence and cooperation in treatment depends largely on demonstrated objectivity, sincerity, and discretion. With the appropriate outlook and attitude, the nurse is often surprisingly successful in obtaining information that is difficult for the patient to impart to anyone. If the nurse is to win the patient's confidence, he must feel that the nurse is concerned about the disease and what it is doing to him as a person and to his associates. The patient should be given the opportunity to inform his contacts of the urgency to seek medical care voluntarily. Many situations in contact investigation become exceedingly complex and difficult (in the case, for instance, of a married patient who has contracted the disease extramaritally). Although the real burden of contact investigation in many clinics rests with the nurse, occasionally a patient may be referred to the social worker, to a community agency, back to his physician, or to his spiritual advisor, depending on the particular circumstances.

In contact investigation it is necessary to identify and bring under medical supervision all sexual contacts of the past 3 months if the person has a primary lesion, all contacts for the past 6 months if secondary manifestations are evident, and all contacts for the past year if the disease is in the latent stage of syphilis. In late latent syphilis, effort is made to determine the contacts at the time the disease was probably acquired, since such persons may also be suffering from latent syphilis that should be treated in the hope of preventing cardiovascular, neurologic, and other late complications. In latent and congenital syphilis, all members of the immediate family should be considered. It is not always necessary to examine the children of the patient, since the likelihood of congenital syphilis may already have been ruled out by routine blood tests done premaritally, on induction to the armed services, or at the time of a hospital admission. Because the problem of syphilis is such a personal one, most clinics designate one nurse to receive phone calls, make appointments, and provide further information requested by the patient's contacts. This nurse's extension number is also given to the patient for distribution to his contacts in the event

he notifies them first. Form letters and individual letters are sent out to patients who fail to report to the clinic as arranged. Telegrams have been effectively used by some clinics and health departments. In the event that contacts fail to report or patients with infectious disease fail to report for follow-up, law requires that the names be submitted to the local health department, which assumes the legal responsibility for the control of communicable disease.

Chronic disease. The nursing care of patients with chronic organic pathology from syphilis is similar to nursing in other conditions except that it is given within the framework of the patient's and his family's guilt feelings about the original cause of his trouble. *Gastric* crisis is one late manifestation that is most distressing to the patient. He has severe abdominal pain and nausea and vomiting. The pathology is in the nervous system, not in the stomach. *Optic atrophy* is sometimes treated by fever therapy, usually induced by giving a foreign protein such as milk intramuscularly or by placing the patient in a fever cabinet. *General paresis* occurs when there has been extensive and permanent damage to the brain. Patients with this condition occupy a large number of beds in mental hospitals throughout the country.

■ VENEREAL LESIONS OF THE EXTERNAL GENITALIA

Chancroid. Chancroid is a venereal disease seen in both men and women and is caused by *Ducrey's bacillus.* It is characterized by a raised lesion on the external genitalia 1 to 5 days after the contact. This lesion becomes a pustule and then develops into a painful ulcer, with extensive local inflammation and spread. It is treated with streptomycin and sulfonamides. One of the broad-spectrum antibiotics such as tetracycline, 1 Gm. daily in divided doses, is usually effective if response to sulfonamides is inadequate.

Lymphogranuloma venereum (lymphogranuloma inguinale). Lymphogranuloma venereum is a venereal disease caused by an agent intermediate between a virus and a rickettsia carried via the lymph stream. It is believed at this time that a bacterial organism may also be involved in the development of the disease. It is diagnosed by skin testing with the Frei antigen or by a complement-fixation test. The disease is widespread throughout the world and is endemic in tropical and subtropical areas and the southern United States. At any time from 6 to 60 days after contact the inguinal nodes in men and the perirectal nodes in women become very swollen and tender and sometimes ulcerate. These nodes are known as *buboes.* Rectal strictures and fistulas and urethral strictures develop, and superficial painless ulceration may occur also. There may be complete destruction of the bladder or bowel sphincter muscles, with resultant incontinence. If there is interference with lymph channels, elephantiasis, a hard lymphatic swelling of the lower trunk and legs that completely distorts their size and shape, may also develop and

may make walking about impossible. Until the advent of chlortetracycline, which has proved quite effective, the treatment was unsatisfactory. Some patients also respond to the sulfonamide drugs.

REFERENCES AND SELECTED READINGS*

1 Advisory Committee on Obstetrics and Gynecology, Food and Drug Administration: Report on intrauterine contraceptive devices, 1968, Washington, D. C., U. S. Government Printing Office.

2 American Cancer Society, Inc.: A cancer source book for nurses, New York, 1963, The Society.

3 American Social Health Association: Summary report: national survey of VD incidence, Washington, D. C., 1968, Public Health Service, U. S. Department of Health, Education and Welfare.

4 Arnold, E.: Individualizing nursing care in family planning, Nurs. Outlook 15:26-27, Dec. 1967.

5 Ballinger, W. F., Treybal, J. C., and Vose, A. B.: Alexander's care of the patient in surgery, ed. 5, St. Louis, 1972, The C. V. Mosby Co.

6 Barton, F. W.: Venereal disease, J.A.M.A. 216:1472-1473, May 1971.

7 Beeson, P. B., and McDermott, W., editors: Cecil-Loeb textbook of medicine, ed. 13, Philadelphia, 1971, W. B. Saunders Co.

8 *Behrman, S. J.: Management of infertility, Am. J. Nurs. 66:552-555, March 1966.

9 *Bergstrom, S. E., and others: Prostaglandins in fertility control, Science 175:1280-1287, March 1972.

10 Bernard, J.: The future of marriage, New York, 1972, World Publishing Co.

11 Borell, U.: Contraceptive methods—their safety, efficacy and acceptability, Acta Obstet. Gynecol. Scand. 45:5-64, 1966.

12 Boston Women's Health Book Collective: Our bodies, ourselves, a book by and for women, Boston, 1973, Simon & Schuster, Inc.

13 Brendler, H.: Therapy with orchiectomy or estrogens or both, J.A.M.A. 210:1074-1075, Nov. 1969.

14 *Brooks, S. M.: The VD story, New York, 1971, A. S. Barnes & Co., Inc.

15 Calderone, M. S., editor: Manual of contraceptive practice, ed. 2, Baltimore, 1970, The Williams & Wilkins Co.

16 Callahan, D.: Abortion: law, choice and morality, New York, 1970, Macmillan Publishing Co., Inc.

17 Campbell, M. F., and Harrison, J. H., editors: Urology, ed. 3, vols. 1 and 2, Philadelphia, 1970, W. B. Saunders Co.

18 Catterall, R. D.: Advances in the treatment of sexually transmitted diseases, Practitioner 207:516-523, Oct. 1971.

19 *Celano, P. J., and Sawyer, J. R.: Vaginal fistulas, Am. J. Nurs. 70:2131-2134, Oct. 1970.

20 *Char, W. J.: Abortion and acute identity crisis in nurses, Am. J. Psychiatry 128:66-71, Feb. 1972.

21 *Cianfrani, T., and Conway, M. K.: Ectopic pregnancy, Am. J. Nurs. 63:93-95, April 1963.

22 Copenhaver, E. H., and Iliya, F. A.: Treatment of urinary stress incontinence—a current appraisal, Surg. Clin. North Am. 45:765-773, June 1965.

23 *Cronenwett, L. R., and Choyce, J. M.: Saline abortion, Am. J. Nurs. 71:1754-1757, Sept. 1971.

24 Cutler, J. C.: Prophylaxis in the venereal diseases, Med. Clin. North Am. 56:1211-1216, Sept. 1972.

25 Dauber, B., and others: Abortion counseling and behavioral change, Fam. Plann. Perspect. 4:23-27, April 1972.

26 Davis, H. J.: Intrauterine devices for contraception, Baltimore, 1971, The Williams & Wilkins Co.

27 *Davis, J. E.: Vasectomy, Am. J. Nurs. 72:509-513, March 1972.

28 Davis, L., editor: Christopher's textbook of surgery, ed. 10, Philadelphia, 1972, W. B. Saunders Co.

29 Demers, L. M.: The morning-after pill, N. Engl. J. Med. 284:1034-1036, May 1971.

30 *Deschin, C. S.: VD and the adolescent personality, Am. J. Nurs. 63:58-62, Nov. 1963.

31 Duvall, E. M.: Family development, ed. 4, Philadelphia, 1971, J. B. Lippincott Co.

32 Ehrlich, P. R.: The population bomb, New York, 1968, Ballantine Books, Inc.

33 Erikson, E.: Identity, youth and crisis, New York, 1968, W. W. Norton & Co., Inc.

34 Fearl, C. L., and Keizur, L. W.: Optimum time interval from occurrence to repair of vesico-vaginal fistula, Am. J. Obstet. Gynecol. 104:205-208, May 1969.

35 Ferber, A. S., Tietz, C., and Lewit, C.: Men with vasectomies—a study of medical, sexual and psycho-social changes, Psychsom. Med. 29:354-366, July-Aug. 1967.

36 Ferrari, H. E.: The nurse and VD control, Can. Nurse 67:28-30, July 1971.

37 Fitzpatrick, E., Reeder, S., and Mastroianni, L.: Maternity nursing, ed. 12, Philadelphia, 1973, J. B. Lippincott Co.

38 Fletcher, E. C.: Essential urology, ed. 4, Baltimore, 1961, The Williams & Wilkins Co.

39 *Foreman, J.: Vasectomy clinic, Am. J. Nurs. 73:819-821, May 1973.

40 *Funnell, J. W., and Roof, B.: Before and after hysterectomy, Am. J. Nurs. 64:120-122, Oct. 1964.

41 Garcia, C., editor: Oral contraception, Clin. Obstet. Gynecol. 2:632-752, Sept. 1968.

42 Garvey, F. K.: Diseases of the genitourinary organs in the male and the urinary organs in the female. In Johnson, W. M., editor: The older patient, New York, 1960, Paul B. Hoeber, Inc.

43 Glynn, R.: Vaginal pH and the effect of douching, Obstet. Gynecol. 20:369-372, Sept. 1962.

44 *Gonzales, B.: Voluntary sterilization, Am. J. Nurs. 70:2581-2583, Dec. 1970.

45 Green, T. H., editor: Symposium on endometriosis, Clin. Obstet. Gynecol. 9:269-421, June 1966.

46 Green, T. H.: Gynecology, ed. 2, Boston, 1971, Little, Brown & Co.

47 *Guttmacher, A. F.: Family planning: the needs and the methods, Am. J. Nurs. 69:1229-1234, June 1969.

48 Hall, R. E.: Therapeutic abortion, sterilization and contraception, Am. J. Obstet. Gynecol. 91:518-532, Feb. 1965.

49 *Hall, R. E.: The supreme court decision on abortion, Am. J. Obstet. Gynecol. 116:1-8, May 1973.

50 Harting, D., and Hunter, H. J.: Abortion techniques and services, a review and critique, Am. J. Public Health 61:2085-2105, Oct. 1971.

*References preceded by an asterisk are particularly well suited for student reading.

51 Harting, D., and others: Family planning policies and activities of state health and welfare departments, Public Health Rep. **84:**127-134, Feb. 1969.

52 *Harvard, B. M.: Ureteral injuries in routine pelvic surgery, Med. Clin. North Am. **43:**1713-1729, Nov. 1959.

53 *Hodgkinson, C. P., and Hodari, A. A.: Trocar suprapubic cystostomy for postoperative bladder drainage in the female, Am. J. Obstet. Gynecol. **96:**773-783, Nov. 1966.

54 *Hofmeister, F. J., Reik, R. P., and Anderson, N. J.: Vulvectomy—surgical treatment and nursing care, Am. J. Nurs. **60:**666-668, May 1960.

55 Houghton, B.: Vasectomies affect women, too, Am. J. Nurs. **73:**821, May 1973.

56 Hreshchyshyn, M. M., editor: Symposium on chemotherapy of gynecologic cancer, Clin. Obstet. Gynecol. **11:**333-456, June 1968.

57 Israel, S. L.: Menstrual disorders and sterility, ed. 5, New York, 1967, Paul B. Hoeber, Inc.

58 Judge, R. A., and Zuidema, G. J., editors: Physical diagnosis: a physiologic approach to the clinical examination, ed. 2, Boston, 1968, Little, Brown & Co.

59 *Kane, F. J., and others: Motivational factors affecting contraceptive use, Am. J. Obstet. Gynecol. **110:**1050-1054, Aug. 1971.

60 *Kane, F. J., and others: Motivational factors in abortion patients, Am. J. Psychiatry **130:**290-293, March 1973.

61 *Kase, N.: Estrogens and the menopause, J.A.M.A. **227:**318-319, Jan. 1974.

62 Kasselman, M. J.: Nursing care of the patient with benign prostatic hypertrophy, Am. J. Nurs. **66:**1026-1030, May 1966.

63 *Katchadourian, H. A., and Lunde, D. T.: Fundamentals of human sexuality, New York, 1972, Holt, Rinehart & Winston, Inc.

64 *Keller, C., and Copeland, P.: Counseling the abortion patient is more than talk, Am. J. Nurs. **72:**102-106, Jan. 1972.

65 Kistner, R., and others: Endometrial cancers, rising incidence, detection and treatment, J. Reprod. Med. **10:**53-74, Feb. 1973.

66 *Lammert, A. C.: The menopause—a physiologic process, Am. J. Nurs. **62:**56-57, Feb. 1962.

67 Laros, R. K., Work, B. A., and Witting, W. C.: Prostaglandins, Am. J. Nurs. **73:**1001-1003, June 1973.

68 Lee, R. A., Welch, J. S., and Spraitz, A. F.: Use of posterior culdotomy in pelvic operation, Am. J. Obstet. Gynecol. **95:**777-780, July 1966.

69 Lefson, E., Lentz, J., and Gilbertson, E.: Contact interviews and the nurse interviewer, Nurs. Outlook **10:**728-730, Nov. 1962.

70 *Leroux, R., and others: Abortion, Am. J. Nurs. **70:**1919-1925, Sept. 1970.

71 *Lewis, S. C.: Vacuum termination of pregnancy, Br. Med. J. **4:**365, Nov. 1971.

72 Lorincz, A. B.: Septic abortion, Postgrad. Med. **49:**148-153, June 1971.

73 Lu, T., and Chun, D.: A long-term follow-up of 1,055 cases of postpartum tubal ligation, J. Obstet. Gynaecol. Br. Commonw. **74:**875-880, Dec. 1967.

74 Manfredonia, G.: Radiation therapy for cancer of the cervix, Am. J. Nurs. **59:**513-515, April 1959.

75 *Manisoff, M. T.: Intrauterine devices, Am. J. Nurs. **73:**1188-1192, July 1973.

76 Margolis, C. N., and others: Second trimester abortions after vaginal termination of pregnancy, Lancet **2:**431-432, Aug. 1972.

77 Marshall, M. H., and Caillouette, J. C.: Septic abortion, Am. J. Nurs. **66:**1042-1048, May 1966.

78 Martin, W. J.: Infections of the urinary tract, Clin. Obstet. Gynecol. **10:**166-184, March 1967.

79 McArthur, J. W., and others: Common menstrual disorders in the adolescent girl, Clin. Pediatr. **3:**663-670, Nov. 1964.

80 McCalister, D. V., Thiessen, V., and McDermott, M.: Readings in family planning, St. Louis, 1973, The C. V. Mosby Co.

81 McCammon, R. W.: Are boys and girls maturing physically at earlier ages? Am. J. Public Health **55:**103-106, Jan. 1965.

82 *McGowan, L.: New ideas about patient care before and after vaginal surgery, Am. J. Nurs. **64:**73-75, Feb. 1964.

83 Moore, A. J.: The young adult generation, New York, 1969, Abingdon Press.

84 *Mossholder, I. B.: When the patient has a radical retropubic prostatectomy, Am. J. Nurs. **62:**101-104, July 1962.

85 Mozden, P.: The management of patients with advanced cancer, Cancer J. Clin. **19:**211, July-Aug. 1969.

86 Nagesha, C. N., and others: Clinical and laboratory study of monilial vaginitis, Am. J. Obstet. Gynecol. **107:**1267-1268, Aug. 1970.

87 Naqvi, R. H., and others: Interceptives: drugs interrupting pregnancy after implantation, Steroids **18:**731-739, Dec. 1971.

88 Neuwirth, R. S.: Hysteroscopy: present and potential application, Hosp. Pract. **8:**141-142, 144-145, April 1973.

89 Nicol, C. S.: The sexually transmitted diseases, Practitioner **206:**277-279, Feb. 1971.

90 *Novak, E. R.: Benign ovarian tumors, Am. J. Nurs. **64:**104-109, Nov. 1964.

91 *Peel, J., and Potts, M.: Textbook of contraceptive practice, New York, 1969, Cambridge University Press.

92 *Pond, D. O.: Psychological aspects of sterilization, Nurs. Times **67:**1435-1437, Nov. 1971.

93 Potts, M., and Wood, C.: New concepts in contraception, Baltimore, 1972, University Park Press.

94 Presser, H. B.: Voluntary sterilization: a world view, Rep. Popul. Fam. Plann. **5:**1-36, July 1970.

95 Pugh, R., and Shettles, L. B.: From conception to birth: the drama of life's beginnings, New York, 1971, Harper & Row, Publishers.

96 *Reiterman, C., editor: Abortion and the unwanted child, New York, 1971, Springer Publishing Co., Inc.

97 Rubin, E., editor: Sexual freedom in marriage, New York, 1969, The New American Library, Inc.

98 Rubin, I.: Sex life after sixty, New York, 1965, Basic Books, Inc.

99 Rubin, P.: Cancer of the urogenital tract: prostate, J.A.M.A. **210:**1072, Nov. 1969.

100 *Sarvis, B., and Rodman, H.: The abortion controversy, New York, 1973, Columbia University Press.

101 Schwartz, B.: Clinical venereology for nurses and students, New York, 1966, Pergamon Press, Inc.

102 Semmens, J. P.: Sex education of the prepubescent and pubescent female, Clin. Obstet. Gynecol. **2:**757-768, Sept. 1968.

103 Sheets, J. L., Symmonds, R. E., and Banner, E. A.: Conservative surgical management of endometriosis, Obstet. Gynecol. **23:**625-628, April 1964.

104 *Siegler, A. M.: Tubal sterilization, Am. J. Nurs. **72:**1624-1629, Sept. 1972.

105 *Soika, C. V.: Gynecologic cytology, Am. J. Nurs. **73:**2092-2094, Dec. 1973.

106 *Sood, S. V.: Complications of hysterotomy, Br. Med. J. **4:**495-496, Nov. 1970.

107 Southard, H. F.: Sex before twenty, New York, 1967, E. P. Dutton & Co., Inc.

108 *Stephens, G. J.: Mind-body continuum in human sexuality, Am. J. Nurs. **70:**1468-1471, July 1970.

109 Stewart, G. K., and others: Medical and surgical complications of abortions, Obstet. Gynecol. **40:**539-550, Oct. 1972.

110 Sturgis, S. H.: Treatment of ovarian insufficiency, Am. J. Nurs. **64:**113-116, Jan. 1964.

111 Tanner, L. M., and others: Preabortion evaluation: decision-making preparation and referral, Clin. Obstet. Gynecol. **14:**1273-1277, Dec. 1971.

112 Taylor, H. C., Jr.: Responsibility of the obstetrician—gynecologist for lay education, Am. J. Obstet. Gynecol. **104:**301-309, June 1969.

112a *Taylor, S. D.: Clinic for adolescents with venereal disease, Am. J. Nurs. **63:**63-66, Nov. 1963.

113 TeLinde, R. W., and Mattingly, R. F.: Operative gynecology, ed. 4, Philadelphia, 1970, J. B. Lippincott Co.

114 Thiede, H. A., Creasman, W. T., and Metcalfe, S.: Antenatal analysis of human chromosomes, Am. J. Obstet. Gynecol. **94:**589-590, Feb. 1966.

115 Thompson, B., and Baird, D.: Follow-up of 186 sterilized women, Lancet **1:**1023-1027, May 1968.

116 Tietz, C.: Mortality with contraception and induced abortion, Stud. Fam. Plann. **45:**6-8, Sept. 1969.

117 *Valk, W. L., and Foret, J. D.: The problem of vesicovaginal and ureterovaginal fistulas, Med. Clin. North Am. **43:**1769-1777, Nov. 1959.

118 Venereal disease, Lancet **1:**691-692, April 1971.

119 Venereal disease rampant, J.A.M.A. **218:**731, Nov. 1971.

120 *Wallach, J.: Interpretation of diagnostic tests, Boston, 1970, Little, Brown & Co.

121 Wheeless, C. R.: Outpatient tubal sterilization, Obstet. Gynecol. **361:**208-211, Aug. 1970.

122 Williams, S. R.: Nutrition and diet therapy, ed. 2, St. Louis, 1973, The C. V. Mosby Co.

123 Wilson, R. A.: The roles of estrogen and progesterone in breast and genital cancer, J.A.M.A. **182:**327-331, Oct. 1962.

124 Wilson, R. A., and Wilson, T. A.: The fate of the non-treated post-menopausal woman: a plea for the maintenance of adequate estrogen from puberty to the grave, J. Am. Geriatr. Soc. **11:**347-362, Nov. 1963.

125 Winter, C. C.: Practical urology, St. Louis, 1969, The C. V. Mosby Co.

126 Winter, C. C., and Roehm, M. M.: Nursing care of patients with urologic diseases, ed. 3, St. Louis, 1972, The C. V. Mosby Co.

22 Pulmonary diseases

■ There are numerous diseases that affect the respiratory system. They include both acute (short-term) and chronic (long-term) diseases. Substantial changes in the relative incidence of diseases affecting the respiratory system have occurred in the past few decades. While chronic infectious disorders such as tuberculosis, lung abscess, and bronchiectasis have decreased, patients with chronic bronchitis and emphysema now survive longer and constitute an increasing number of patients with chronic respiratory disease, along with those with environmental lung disease. In addition, modern intercontinental travel has increased the incidence of parasitic lung infestations in the western world, and the reduction of immunologic competence that occurs in the treatment of patients with various malignancies and following organ transplantation has resulted in an increasing incidence of opportunistic infections of the lungs with a variety of microorganisms rarely pathogenic in the past.

The most significant pulmonary diseases are those that are chronic. According to the *National Health Survey Reports* for 1970, approximately 47 million persons in the United States had asthma, chronic bronchitis, chronic sinusitis, or other chronic respiratory conditions, including emphysema.

Since most diseases of the respiratory tract are not reportable, the full extent of both acute and chronic illness is difficult to estimate. However, known facts about disability caused by chronic respiratory diseases indicate clearly that they are a serious health problem and that they cause tremendous loss in the nation's productivity. Disability benefits reported by the Social Security Administration show that emphysema is the fourth most frequent single condition for which disability claims are made and that tuberculosis is eleventh. Disability benefits for emphysema and other chronic respiratory diseases were estimated at more than $400 million a year in 1970. Between 1962 and 1972, the mortality rate from asthma and tuberculosis was noted to decline slightly, while the rates from bronchitis, emphysema, and malignant neoplasms of the respiratory system continued to increase.[108]

The objectives of health education in relation to pulmonary diseases are the same as for other diseases. Prevention, early diagnosis, prompt and often continued treatment, limitation of disability, and re-

■ STUDY QUESTIONS

1 Review the anatomy and physiology of the lungs and diaphragm. How does an inadequate diaphragmatic excursion affect respiration?
2 Which muscles can be used as accessory muscles in breathing? What is meant by residual air?
3 Explain the exchange of oxygen and carbon dioxide in normal respiration. What is the normal respiratory rate? What is the normal carbon dioxide level in the bloodstream? How does carbon dioxide content affect respiration and general body function? What is meant by the hypoxic stimulus to the chemoreceptors?
4 Review the medications that facilitate the raising of sputum.
5 How many diseases can you name that begin with symptoms of the common cold?
6 What is the tuberculosis case rate in the area in which you live or where you go to school? If the rate in your community is below the national average, how do you explain this? If it is above the national average, what factors do you feel contribute to this?

habilitation should be emphasized for all persons. Early symptoms of respiratory diseases are probably those most often ignored by the general population. Perhaps this is because, with the exception of influenza and some types of pneumonia such as that caused by Friedländer's bacillus, respiratory diseases often develop slowly and progress without the individual's awareness. Nurses should encourage individuals and families to get proper medical attention if they have symptoms such as cough, difficulty in breathing, production of sputum, shortness of breath, and nose and throat irritation that does not subside within 2 weeks. These symptoms are suggestive of respiratory disease and should be investigated.

With increased study and new knowledge about the respiratory diseases, methods of treating patients with these diseases are changing rapidly. The American Thoracic Society, the medical section of the American Lung Association (ALA), publishes a jour-

nal* that is an excellent source of current information on all acute and chronic respiratory diseases. The ALA also publishes the *Bulletin,* many booklets and pamphlets, and newsletters that are useful to nurses in education of the public and in teaching patients.

■ PHYSICAL ASSESSMENT OF THE LUNGS AND THORAX

Physical assessment of the lungs and thorax requires knowledge of the anatomic structures located in the chest and the location of the lobes of the lung in relation to overlying ribs (for example, the lower border of the right upper lobe is normally between the third and fourth ribs and extends above the clavicle) (Fig. 22-1). Knowledge of appropriate methods

---

*American Review of Respiratory Diseases, published by the American Lung Association, New York, N. Y.

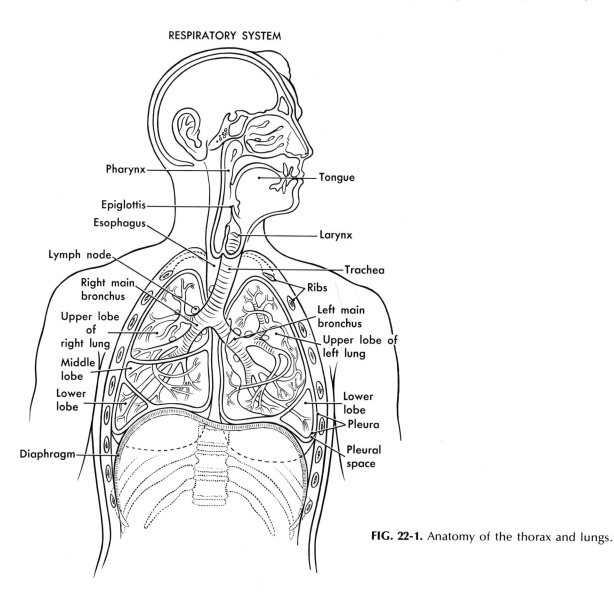

RESPIRATORY SYSTEM

FIG. 22-1. Anatomy of the thorax and lungs.

for examination are required for initial assessment of the patient and the subsequent detection of changes in the patient's condition. Interviews and nursing histories regarding such data as smoking habits, exercise tolerance, medications, allergies, recent respiratory problems, and sputum production aid the examiner in utilizing the skills of assessment.*

The methods for physical examination are performed in this order: inspection, palpation, percussion, and auscultation.

Inspection

If possible, the patient should be sitting upright. The examiner observes the following factors:

1. Posture and any variations from normal structure of the thorax such as scoliosis, kyphosis, funnel or barrel chest, and pigeon breast.

2. Rate, rhythm, and depth of respiratory excursions and uniform expansion of the chest wall. Diminished chest expansion may occur in pulmonary embolus, pneumonia, pleural effusion, and pneumothorax or the pain caused by fractured ribs. The examiner compares respiratory excursion of both sides of the posterior thorax by placing the hands so that the thumbs meet at the midline as the hands extend over the chest wall. The entire thorax should move as one unit as the thumbs move away from each other.

3. Any deviation of the trachea from the midline. Deviation occurs in pleural effusion, pneumothorax with mediastinal shift, and atelectasis.

Palpation

Palpation of the chest is performed with the palmar surface of the hand flat against the chest to determine the presence of vocal fremitus when the patient is asked to say "ninety-nine." Normally a vibration is felt over the exterior chest wall when the patient speaks. The examiner uses the same hand to palpate all areas of the chest. Diminished or absent fremitus may occur in pleural effusion, pneumothorax, and atelectasis. One may also detect areas of pain or masses of the thorax with this examining technique.

Percussion

Percussing the chest is performed by placing the middle finger flat against the chest at an interspace and striking the knuckle sharply with the end of the middle finger of the other hand. Percussion is done from apex to base with the patient in the supine position for examination of the anterior thorax and in a sitting position for examination of the posterior thorax. Normally percussion elicits a resonant

---

*See references 12a, 22, and 105 for further information on assessment.

sound. The examiner compares the sound of each area with the sound of the opposite side as percussion proceeds. During percussion of the posterior bases, the patient is asked to hold his breath at the end of inspiration and then at the end of an expiration. This maneuver allows the examiner to determine the amount of diaphragmatic descent during inspiration. Normally the diaphragm moves downward 5 to 6 cm.

Dull or flat percussion is heard in the presence of atelectasis, pneumonia, pleural effusion, or a tumor mass. The same dull sound is heard over the heart and liver.

Auscultation

Auscultation consists of listening to the chest to determine the presence of normal breath and voice sounds and to detect the presence of any abnormal sounds. If possible, the patient should be sitting upright. With the diaphragm of the stethoscope, the examiner begins auscultation of the anterior and posterior thorax at the positions shown in Figs. 22-2 and 22-3. The patient is instructed to take slow, deep breaths through the mouth. When listening to the posterior chest, the examiner has the patient bring his shoulder forward to abduct the scapula so that a greater lung surface can be auscultated. The examiner auscultates the anterior and posterior thorax from apices to bases, comparing one side with the other.

Breath sounds. The three types of breath sounds are vesicular, bronchial, and bronchovesicular (Fig. 22-4). *Vesicular breath sounds* are heard in the periphery of the lungs, are of a low pitch, and have a soft rustling or swishing quality (Fig. 22-2, *4* to *7*). The sound of the inspiratory phase is longer and higher in pitch than that of the expiratory phase, which is a short, soft, low-pitched, almost inaudible sound. *Bronchial breath sounds* are heard over the trachea and the main bronchi and are the opposite of the vesicular breath sounds (Fig. 22-2, *1*). Bronchial sounds are high pitched and loud; during the expiratory phase they increase in duration, pitch, and intensity. Bronchial breath sounds heard in other areas of the lung indicate the presence of consolidation from pneumonia, pleural effusion, or compression of the lung. *Bronchovesicular breath sounds* may be heard in the major airways of the lungs such as the anterior second interspaces (Fig. 22-2, *2* and *3*) and in the posterior interscapular area (Fig. 22-3, *3* and *4*). Inspiration and expiration are loud and nearly equal in duration and intensity.

Voice sounds. Auscultation for voice sounds aids in detecting changes indicating such conditions as atelectasis and consolidation. Whispers, normally indistinct, are heard over areas of compression or consolidation. In the presence of bronchial breathing in an area of consolidation, other changes occur. They

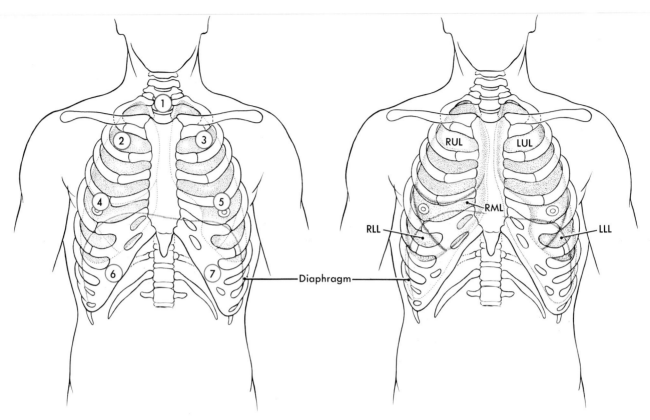

FIG. 22-2. Anterior thorax showing placement of stethoscope when listening to breath sounds and position of lobes of the lung.

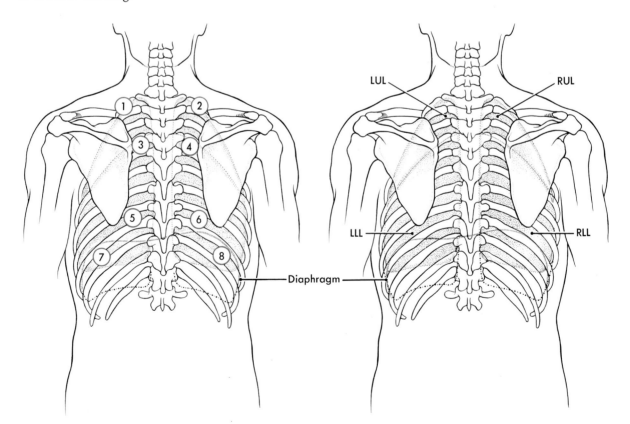

FIG. 22-3. Posterior thorax showing placement of stethoscope when listening to breath sounds and position of lobes of the lung.

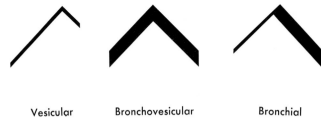

| Vesicular | Bronchovesicular | Bronchial |

FIG. 22-4. Schematic representation of the three types of breath sounds.

are egophony and whispered pectoriloquy. *Egophony* is an "E" to "A" change in which the patient says "E" and the examiner hears "A." *Whispered pectoriloquy* is the loud transmission of the patient's whispered voice. These changes are heard when there is consolidation or compression of the alveoli or replacement of air by fluid in the alveoli.

Abnormal sounds or extra sounds. These sounds are superimposed on the normal breath sounds and include rales, rhonchi, wheezes, and friction rub. *Rales* are divided into *fine, medium,* and *coarse.* Fine rales produced in the small airways, as in pneumonia or heart failure, are heard at the end of inspiration and likened to the sounds of several hairs rubbed together between the fingertips. Medium rales produced in the medium airways occur in the later stages of pneumonia, heart failure, and pulmonary edema. The medium rales have been compared to the fizzling of a carbonated drink. They are heard about midway through the inspiratory phase. Coarse rales are heard at the beginning of inspiration and produce a rough, gurgling sound; they often can be cleared with a cough, as they are produced by secretions in the larger airways. *Rhonchi* and *wheezes* are continuous sounds, although they may be more prominent in expiration. They are produced by air flowing through passages narrowed by secretions, mucosal swelling, tumors, or other obstructions; like coarse rales, they may be cleared with coughing. They are classified as high-pitched, sibilant rhonchi, which have a musical quality and originate in smaller air passages, and low-pitched, sonorous rhonchi, which originate in larger air passages and have a snoring sound. *Friction rubs* are crackling, grating sounds that originate in inflamed pleura. They are usually, but not always, heard on both inspiration and expiration and are not affected by coughing.

■ DIAGNOSTIC EXAMINATIONS AND RELATED NURSING CARE

Radiologic examination of the chest

X-ray examination is probably familiar to most patients and the general public. Radiology has had extensive use as a screening test and as a diagnostic

measure. When chest disease is suspected, a radiograph is almost always ordered to help identify the disease and to visualize the extent of the disease process. Various types of radiographs may be ordered. For survey purposes a *microfilm* may be used. If the history and physical examination or survey film indicate possible pulmonary pathology, full-size chest films are obtained. These include posteroanterior (PA) and lateral views.

When the patient goes to the x-ray department, the nurse should be sure that he is wearing an open-backed gown and that he has removed or will remove all metal objects above the waist, since metal restricts passage of the x-rays and will cause a shadow on the film. Care should be taken that such articles are not misplaced or lost. If the patient is acutely ill, a portable x-ray machine is brought to his bedside, and the nurse assists him into correct position and protects him from exposure. The x-ray plate is covered and then placed flat on the bed. If the patient can sit up, the plate is put in place, he leans back on it, and the bed is lowered as far as can be tolerated; or he may sit on the side of the bed holding the x-ray plate against his anterior chest, resting it on a pillow in his lap. If he is unable to sit up, he is turned on his side, the plate is correctly placed on the bed, and he is rolled onto it. When the x-ray is taken, the nurse should step out of the room to avoid being exposed to unnecessary radiation. If the patient requires nursing assistance during the procedure, the nurse should wear a lead-lined apron.

Fluoroscopic examination

Physicians vary in their recommendation of fluoroscopy as the initial x-ray examination. Some believe that it should be a routine examination, while others believe that it exposes the patient and physician to unnecessary radiation and that standard chest films offer better records. For certain types of information in which visualization of thoracic contents in a dynamic rather than static manner is helpful (such as diaphragmatic movement and size and contour of the heart), fluoroscopy is the preferred examination.

Whether fluoroscopic examination is done in the physician's office or in the hospital, the patient must go to a room where the fluoroscope is installed. He may need assistance in rising to a sitting or standing position or in remaining still during the examination. If he is in a wheelchair, he is helped to a stool in front of the machine. Prior to the examination, the physician wears dark red goggles to aid his adaptation to the darkened fluoroscopy room. During the examination the physician wears an apron and gloves containing lead to protect him from the x-rays. Fluoroscopic examination is done with the lights off, and the machine is operated with a foot pedal. The patient needs a careful explanation of the procedure and should be told that he will be in darkness and that he may be asked to hold his breath for a few seconds during the examination. He should be assured that there will be no pain.

Special radiologic examinations

Special views of the lungs may be obtained by placing the patient in various positions. The most common are the *right* and *left anterior obliques,* the *recumbent lateral (decubitus),* and the *lordotic.* The oblique positions allow better visualization of the mediastinum and areas of the lung often hidden or obscured by normal thoracic structures in the PA position. The decubitus film is used to locate fluid in the pleural space and the lordotic to better visualize the apices. *Laminography (tomography, planography)* is a technique whereby the level of the lung that is in focus changes. It is used to study cavities, neoplasms, and densities of the lung.

Examination of sputum

Examinations of sputum are usually required when chest disease is suspected. The mucous membrane of the respiratory tract responds to inflammation by an increased flow of secretions that often contain offending organisms. The nurse should always examine and record the volume, consistency, color, and odor of the sputum. These observations are helpful both in diagnosis and evaluation of therapy. For example, thick, tenacious mucoid sputum is characteristic of asthma; green, musty-smelling sputum, *Pseudomonas* pneumonia; and rusty sputum, pneumococcal pneumonia. A *smear of sputum* gives information about the morphology and staining characteristics of organisms. The presence of neutrophils and eosinophils is also noted. These data are helpful in making a diagnosis. A *culture of the sputum* is also ordered. On culture the specific organism can be identified. *Sensitivity studies* done on the culture serve as a guide to the selection of antimicrobial therapy. A *cytologic* examination of the sputum is ordered if carcinoma is suspected.

Tests to be done on sputum should be explained to the patient so that he will understand the need for obtaining a suitable specimen. He should be instructed to collect only sputum that has come from deep in the chest. When instructed inadequately, patients often expectorate saliva rather than sputum. They are likely to exhaust themselves unnecessarily by shallow, frequent coughing that yields no sputum suitable for study and that affords them little relief from discomfort. *The first sputum raised in the morning is usually the most productive of organisms.* During the night, secretions accumulate in the bronchi, and only a few deep coughs will bring them to the back of the throat. If the patient does not know this fact, on awakening he may almost unconsciously cough, clear his throat, and swallow or expectorate before attempting to procure a specimen.

The patient should be supplied with a wide-mouthed container and instructed to expectorate directly into it. Because the sight of sputum is often objectionable to the patient, and particularly to persons about him, the outside of a glass container should be covered with paper or other suitable covering. Usually 4 ml. of sputum is sufficient for necessary laboratory tests and examinations. Initial specimens for culture and sensitivity should be collected before antibiotic therapy is started. Occasionally, however, all sputum collected over a period of 24 to 72 hours is needed. If there is any delay in sending the specimen to the laboratory, it should be placed in the refrigerator.

Sputum collection using saline inhalation. Inhalation of a heated saline solution is being used to help patients raise sputum for specimens. A 10% solution of saline in distilled water is placed in a heated nebulizer, and a fine spray is produced by attaching the nebulizer to compressed air or oxygen. When inhaled, the heated vapor condenses on the surface of the tracheobronchial mucosa and stimulates production of secretions.

Patients who have difficulty raising sputum for specimens can learn this procedure readily. The patient should be taught how to deep breathe and cough before the procedure. He should place his mouth over, but not sealed around, the nebulizer and inhale. Inhalation of the vapor should be repeated for a few minutes or until coughing is stimulated. Some patients begin to cough after the first inhalation. The patient should have a supply of tissues in his hand to cover the cough and should expectorate sputum into the collection container.

The patient should be asked to rest for a few seconds between periods of inhaling and coughing so that he does not become overtired. If the patient complains of lightheadedness or dizziness due to hyperventilation, he should be encouraged to sit quietly and to breathe normally for a few minutes. If he complains of nausea, the inhalations should be discontinued. The patient usually feels nauseated for only a few minutes, and it may be associated with factors other than inhalation. The advantage of this method of raising sputum is that the patient can do the procedure at any time of the day and needs no special preparation. Many hospitals and outpatient facilities are now using this method in preference to gastric lavage.

If the patient is suspected of having tuberculosis and specimens are being collected for screening purposes, the hospital or outpatient personnel should use some precautions. The room should be well ventilated so that there are frequent changes of air. If the patient is known to have sputum positive for tubercle bacilli, the extra precaution of wearing a high-filtration mask may be taken. Special ultraviolet lights may be installed to rid the rising circulating air of infectious droplets. They are installed high enough to protect the patient and the personnel from direct exposure to the light.

Gastric washings. Gastric aspiration is done infrequently to collect gastric contents, which may contain swallowed sputum. It is usually done when the diagnosis or suspected diagnosis is tuberculosis. Since most patients swallow sputum when coughing in the morning and during sleep, an examination of gastric contents may reveal causative organisms. Breakfast is withheld for gastric aspiration. (The procedure for passing the nasogastric tube is the same as that discussed on p. 654.) Once the tube is passed, a large syringe is attached to the end, and by gentle suction a specimen of stomach contents is withdrawn. The specimen is placed in a covered bottle, and the tube is withdrawn. The specimen is examined microscopically on slides, and culture media are inoculated as is done with other sputum samples. For the patient the disadvantages of this method of sputum collection are the discomforts of going without food and the passage of the nasogastric tube.

Pulmonary function tests

Pulmonary function tests are done to assess lung function, to rule out nonorganic types of dyspnea such as that caused by psychoneurotic disorders, and to differentiate diseases of the lungs. They also may be used to evaluate the disability caused by diseases of the lungs. Localized disease of the lung such as carcinoma, tuberculosis, or lung abscess may have little effect on pulmonary function, whereas generalized disease such as emphysema or fibrosis may produce a significant alteration of pulmonary function. Physiologic tests cannot be used to diagnose *diseases,* but rather provide information regarding abnormalities in *function.* Based on this information regarding function the disorder may then be classified in one of a number of patterns, and the physician can then determine the specific disease.

The physiologic tests of pulmonary function are of two general kinds. One tests the bellows action of the chest and lungs for movement of air in and out of the alveoli (ventilation) and the distribution of inspired gas to the alveoli. The second is concerned with the *diffusion* of a gas across the alveolar capillary membrane to and from the blood *perfusing* the pulmonary capillaries of the lungs. In order for the lung to perform its respiratory function of gas exchange, the ventilation-perfusion ratio ($\dot{V}/\dot{Q}$ ratio) must be balanced. Although in the normal lung with its many millions of gas exchange units some imbalance in ventilation and perfusion exists, this has little effect on overall gas exchange function. In fact, adaptive mechanisms appear to exist that divert blood flow to the best ventilated regions of the lungs or redirect ventilation away from nonperfused areas

in order to maintain a normal ratio in the range of 0.8 to 1.0.[13] However, even though overall amounts for each of these two values (ventilation and perfusion) may be adequate, normal exchange of oxygen and carbon dioxide will not occur if areas of the lung that are well ventilated are not also well perfused. The reverse situation, in which well-perfused areas are underventilated, will also result in impairment of respiratory function with inadequate gas exchange caused by changes in the $\dot{V}/\dot{Q}$ ratio. In fact, $\dot{V}/\dot{Q}$ mismatch, or alteration in ventilation-perfusion relationships, is largely responsible for the *hypoxemia* and *hypercarbia* seen in clinical practice. (For a more detailed explanation, see specialized texts.[100,113]) The nurse should be familiar with the most commonly used tests to be able to explain them to the patient and tell him what is expected of him.

Measurement of pulmonary volumes and capacities. To determine the functional capacity of the lungs, basic ventilation studies are performed by using a spirometer. Some measurements such as the *residual volume* cannot be measured directly and are calculated mathematically. The total gas content of the lungs can be subdivided into volumes and capacities as defined below.

Definitions of lung volumes

Tidal volume (TV)	Volume of gas inspired and expired with a normal breath
Inspiratory reserve volume (IRV)	Maximal volume that can be inspired from the end of a normal inspiration
Expiratory reserve volume (ERV)	Maximal volume that can be exhaled by forced expiration after a normal expiration
Residual volume (RV)	Volume of gas left in lung after maximal expiration
Minute volume (MV)	Volume inspired and expired in 1 minute of normal breathing

Definitions of lung capacities

Vital capacity (VC)	Maximal amount of air that can be expired after a maximal inspiration (TV + IRV + ERV)
Forced vital capacity (FVC)	Maximal amount of air that can be expelled with a maximal effort after a maximal inspiration
Maximal midexpiratory flow (MMEF)	Average rate of flow during middle half of forced vital capacity
Forced expiratory volume in 1 second (FEV_1)	Amount of air expelled in the first second of the forced vital capacity maneuver
FEV_1/VC ratio	Amount of air forcefully expelled in 1 second compared to total amount forcefully expelled
Maximal voluntary ventilation (MVV), also	Amount of air exchanged per minute with maximal

termed maximal breathing capacity (MBC) — rate and depth of respiration

Inspiratory capacity (IC) — Maximal amount of air that can be inspired after a normal expiration (TV + IRV)

Functional residual capacity (FRC) — Amount of air left in lungs after a normal expiration (ERV + RV)

Total lung capacity (TLC) — Total amount of air in lungs after maximal inspiration (TV + IRV + ERV + RV)

These volumes and capacities vary with age, sex, weight, and height. Two ventilatory studies are of particular clinical significance. They are the *forced expiratory volume* (FEV), or *timed vital capacity,* and the *maximal voluntary ventilation* (MVV), or *maximum breathing capacity* (MBC). The FEV measures the volume expired forcefully at 1, 2, and 3 seconds after a full inspiration. The FEV at *1 second* is the most useful of the three values, particularly when it is compared with the vital capacity (FEV_1/VC ratio). The MVV measures the volume of air exchanged per minute with maximal rate and depth of respiration. Other tests and techniques of studying pulmonary function are described in specialized texts.[11,16,46,64,85,100]

The patient is usually instructed in how to participate in the tests by the physician or the technician in the testing laboratory. For all these tests the patient is asked to breathe only through his mouth. A recording device and a spirometer are used. When the patient breathes through the mouthpiece and connecting tube, a noseclip is usually used so that the patient cannot breathe through his nose. Although a noseclip may seem like a small, harmless piece of equipment, the patient often becomes apprehensive about it. He should be allowed time to adjust to the clip. Fear of cutting off the air supply, particularly when a person has a breathing limitation, may cause anxiety. As these tests are dependent on patient effort and can also be very exhausting to a patient with respiratory disease, the nurse should provide for rest both before and after the testing is carried out. If the patient is receiving bronchodilator treatments, he should not have these for 4 hours prior to testing if a part of the examination is to include measurements taken before and after the use of nebulized bronchodilators. Nurses can allay some of the patient's apprehension by giving him clear and confident explanations.

Blood gas studies. Recently arterial blood gas studies have become a common tool to aid in physiologic diagnosis and therapeutic management of patients. These studies determine blood pH, carbon dioxide tension (pCO_2), oxygen tension (pO_2), and percent of oxyhemoglobin saturation (SaO_2). Gas tensions refer to partial pressure, or that part of the total pressure exerted by a specific gas. For example, pressure exerted by the atmosphere at sea level is 760 mm. Hg.

The amount of oxygen in air at sea level is 21%; that is, 21% of the total pressure is exerted by oxygen. Since 21% of 760 is approximately 159, the pO_2 of air at sea level is 159 mm Hg. Definitions of gas exchange functions and their normal values are as follows:

Definitions and normal values of gas exchange functions

pH	Acidity of the blood	7.38 to 7.42
pCO_2	Partial pressure of carbon dioxide in the blood	38 to 42 mm. Hg
pO_2	Partial pressure of oxygen in the blood	80 to 100 mm. Hg
SaO_2	Percentage of the available hemoglobin that is saturated with oxygen	95% to 98%

The measurement of oxygen values includes both the pO_2 and SaO_2. The pO_2 measures oxygen dissolved in the blood; however, the amount of oxygen carried in the blood in this form is small, with most oxygen transported in chemical combination with hemoglobin. Oxyhemoglobin saturation refers to that percentage of the hemoglobin that is combined with oxygen. More than 90% of the oxygen-carrying capacity of the blood is accounted for by oxyhemoglobin, with the partial pressure of oxygen acting as the driving force for this chemical combination. Therefore both pO_2 and SaO_2 levels must be examined in order to determine the adequacy of oxygenation.

The pCO_2 is utilized as a measurement to determine the adequacy of ventilation and is dependent on the amount of carbon dioxide produced by the body and the ability of the lungs to eliminate it. *Hypoventilation,* therefore, is shown by an elevated pCO_2, while *hyperventilation* is indicated by a decrease in pCO_2 below normal levels.

The pH refers to the acidity of the blood and is an expression of the hydrogen ion concentration. Because pH is expressed as a negative logarithm, as hydrogen ion concentration increases and blood becomes more acid, the pH value falls. When hydrogen ion concentration decreases, the blood becomes more alkaline and the pH value rises.

The pCO_2 is related to the pH because of the chemical reaction of carbon dioxide and water in the blood, which results in the formation of carbonic acid. Carbonic acid, in turn, dissociates to form hydrogen and bicarbonate ions, as illustrated in the following equation:

$$CO_2 + H_2O \leftrightarrow H_2CO_2 \leftrightarrow H^+ + HCO_3$$

The maintenance of a normal pH is dependent on a ratio of 20 bicarbonate ions to 1 hydrogen ion. It can be seen from the equation that the presence of an elevated pCO_2 will result in an excess of hydrogen ions. When this occurs, the pH falls and the patient is said to be in *respiratory acidosis.* Conversely, when pCO_2 is decreased, the pH increases and the result is termed *respiratory alkalosis.* (For a more detailed explanation, see references 15, 30, and 113.)

Bronchospirometry. Bronchospirometry measures the ventilation and oxygen consumption of each lung separately. For this procedure a specially constructed double-lumen catheter with two balloons is used. When the catheter is in place, one balloon is inflated to seal off the contralateral lung. After measuring the ventilation of one lung, that balloon is deflated; the other balloon is inflated, and the procedure is repeated on the opposite side. This test aids the surgeon in determining whether the ventilatory capacity of the unaffected lung is sufficient to maintain the patient after pulmonary resection. This determination is most crucial prior to pneumonectomy.

Bronchography and bronchoscopy

Examinations by bronchography and bronchoscopy are somewhat complicated diagnostic procedures that may be ordered. Both are unpleasant and uncomfortable for the patient. A thorough explanation of what will happen and what will be expected of him during these examinations can do much to allay his anxiety. Since instruments are passed through one nostril or the mouth and pharynx, making the patient apprehensive about being able to breathe, he should practice breathing in and out through the nose with the mouth open. He can also practice consciously relaxing the shoulders and hands while lying on his back. Clenching the fists causes neck muscles to tense, interfering with the procedure.

A *bronchogram* enables the physician to visualize the bronchial tree by x-ray film after the introduction of an iodized radiopaque liquid. To lessen the number of bacteria introduced from the mouth into the bronchi, the patient should pay particular attention to oral hygiene on the night before and on the morning of the procedure. No food or fluids are allowed for 8 hours preceding the examination. Since, if the smaller bronchi contain secretions, the radiopaque liquid will not reach them, postural drainage may be ordered for the morning the bronchogram is made (Fig. 22-14). The patient should be asked about any loose or capped teeth or dental bridges. Dental prostheses should be removed, and loose teeth should be brought to the physician's attention. Bronchograms are *contraindicated* during acute infections and in individuals sensitive to iodine.

Approximately 1 hour before the examination, the patient is given a short-acting barbiturate to minimize the stimulating effects of the anesthetic agent and to sedate him. To lessen the patient's discomfort during the procedure, a local topical anesthetic agent is administered. Usually 0.5% tetracaine (Pontocaine) or cocaine is used. These drugs can cause toxic reactions in some patients. Thus the patient should be observed closely for signs of central nervous system stimulation. Rapid pulse rate, excitation, headache, and palpitation are some of the signs of toxicity. When these occur, the physician should be notified at once. Usually a short-acting barbiturate such as secobarbital (Seconal) is given intravenously. Oxygen may also be administered. If the patient is not treated promptly, the central nervous system can become depressed and the patient may die from respiratory failure.

The pharynx, larynx, and major bronchi are anesthetized immediately before the radiopaque substance is introduced. The patient should be told that the local anesthetic will taste bitter and that he should not swallow it but expectorate into the emesis basin or tissues provided. When the gag reflex disappears, a metal laryngeal cannula is passed into the trachea, and then a catheter is passed through the nose into the cannula and into the trachea. The radiopaque substance is then introduced, and the patient is tilted into various positions to distribute it to the bronchi and bronchioles. These positions are the reverse of those used in postural drainage. A series of radiographs is then taken. Following this procedure, postural drainage is usually ordered to help remove the radiopaque substance from the lungs. Follow-up films may also be taken to ascertain how much dye remains in the tracheobronchial tree. No permanent damage results, however, if some of it remains for an indefinite period. Food and fluid should be withheld until the gag reflex returns, which can be tested by gently tickling the posterior pharynx with a cotton swab.

A *bronchoscopic examination* is performed by passing a bronchoscope into the trachea and bronchi (Fig. 22-5). Preparation of the patient for a bronchoscopic examination is similar to that for bronchography except that postural drainage is less often ordered. In addition to a spray anesthetic, cocaine may be applied locally by holding small cotton pledgets soaked in solution in the posterior fossa of the pharynx. If the patient is very apprehensive or if a sponge biopsy (abrasion of the lesion with a sponge) is to be done or a tissue biopsy obtained, intravenous anesthesia may be used. A bronchoscope is a long, rigid, slender, hollow instrument through which light can be reflected and visual examination of the trachea and major bronchi with their branchings can be made. In recent years the *fiberoptic bronchoscope,* which is a flexible instrument allowing greater visualization with passage into segmental and subsegmental bronchi, has been employed with increasing frequency, particularly for diagnostic examination. The use of this instrument is also associated with less discomfort for the patient as compared to the larger, rigid instrument (Fig. 22-6). Bronchoscopy may be done to remove a foreign body, to facilitate free air passage by removal of mucus plugs with suction, to obtain a biopsy and samples of secretions for examination, and to observe the air passages for signs of disease.

Following bronchoscopy, the patient is given no food or fluids until the gag reflex returns. Some physicians prefer that the patient lie flat after this proce-

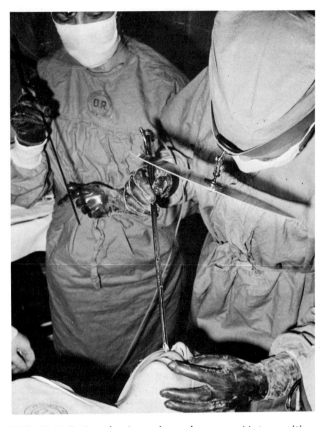

FIG. 22-5. Patient having a bronchoscopy. Note position of head and neck. The nurse is prepared to aspirate after the bronchoscope is passed. (From Horowicz, C.: Am. J. Nurs. **63:**107, May 1963.)

dure, while others prefer a semi-Fowler's position. Unless intravenous anesthesia is used, the patient is awake and conscious, although drowsy from sedation. Rather than attempt to swallow saliva, he should lie on his side and let mucus from the mouth flow into disposable tissues or a small emesis basin conveniently placed. The patient usually produces large amounts of sputum. All sputum is saved for culture and cytologic studies because the postbronchoscopy specimens are often positive diagnostically. However, if the patient has had bronchograms, the sputum is often not helpful for cytologic examination, as the base of the dye makes fixation of the cells difficult.

The patient frequently complains of a sore throat and may have hoarseness after the procedure. Lidocaine (Xylocaine) is often helpful in reducing discomfort. In some instances, laryngeal edema follows bronchoscopy and can cause airway obstruction. The nurse should be alert to increasing shortness of breath and laryngeal stridor. If laryngeal edema occurs, the physician should be notified immediately. Warm mist is often given prophylactically to prevent the development of this complication. When cocaine is used for local anesthesia, the patient is watched for the signs of central nervous system stimulation described previously.

If a biopsy is taken during bronchoscopy, the patient is kept under close surveillance until clotting occurs—usually in 5 to 7 minutes. His sputum should be observed carefully for a few hours after the procedure for signs of hemorrhage. The patient should not smoke for several hours because smoking may cause coughing and start bleeding. Although normally the sputum may be streaked with blood for a few days after a biopsy, any pronounced bleeding must be reported at once to the physician.

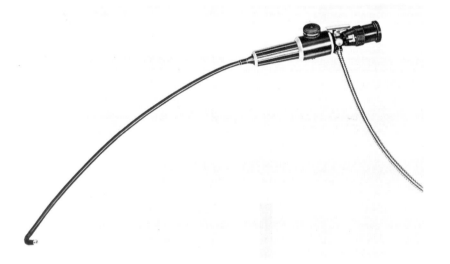

FIG. 22-6. Fiberoptic bronchoscope. Because of its flexibility, it allows better visualization of the bronchi. (Courtesy American Cystoscope Makers, Inc., Pelham, N. Y.)

Mediastinoscopy

In this examination a *mediastinoscope*, which is an instrument much like a bronchoscope, is inserted through a small incision in the suprasternal notch and advanced into the mediastinum where inspection and biopsy of the lymph nodes can then be carried out. Consult the article by Klause[61a] for further information.

Lung scan (pulmonary scintiphotography)

Lung scan procedures involve the use of a scanning device that records the pattern of pulmonary radioactivity after the inhalation and/or intravenous injection of gamma ray–emitting radionuclides, thus providing a visual image of the distribution of ventilation and/or blood flow in the lungs. These studies provide valuable information regarding *ventilation-perfusion patterns* and aid in the diagnosis of parenchymal lung diseases and vascular disorders such as pulmonary embolism.

Pulmonary angiography

Pulmonary angiography is used to detect pulmonary emboli and a variety of congenital and acquired lesions of the pulmonary vessels. A radiopaque material is injected via a catheter into a systemic vein, the right chambers of the heart, or the pulmonary artery, and the distribution of this material is recorded on film. Following this procedure, the nurse should observe the site of insertion of the catheter and report any adverse signs and symptoms such as inflammation, formation of a hematoma, absence of peripheral pulses, or complaint of numbness, tingling, or pain in the extremity involved.

Thoracentesis

Thoracentesis involves the insertion of a needle into the pleural space and aspiration of fluid for either diagnostic or therapeutic purposes. Biopsy specimens of the pleura may also be obtained by the use of needles specially constructed with a cutting edge and a mechanism for retaining the biopsy specimen. When thoracentesis is done for diagnostic purposes, the fluid may be examined for specific gravity, white blood cell count, differential cell count, red blood cell count, protein, glucose, and amylase concentrations. The fluid may also be cultured and checked for the presence of abnormal or malignant cells. The gross appearance of the fluid, the quantity obtained, and the location of the site of the thoracentesis should be recorded.

When a thoracentesis is to be done, the procedure should be explained to the patient. It is important that he be instructed not to move when the needle is inserted lest damage to the lung or pleura occur. Usually a local anesthetic such as procaine or lidocaine is used to eliminate pain at the site of insertion of the needle. However, when the pleura is entered, a sensation of pain or pressure may occur. Whenever possible, the patient should be in an upright position, either sitting on the side of the bed with his feet supported and arms and head on a padded overbed table or straddling a chair with his arms and head resting on the back of the chair. This position with arms and shoulders raised elevates the ribs and makes it easier for the physician to carry out the procedure. If the patient is unable to assume a sitting position, he may lie on his unaffected side.

The patient's pulse and respiratory rate should be taken several times during the procedure, and he must be watched for any changes in color and respiration and for excessive diaphoresis. The needle and syringe should be carefully checked to see that they fit snugly so that no air is permitted to enter the pleural space. Fluid may be aspirated directly into the syringe, or a three-way adaptor may be used with one end attached to tubing leading to a receptacle into which the fluid is drained. Specimens are placed in the appropriate containers and labeled according to the examinations ordered by the physician. Following a thoracentesis, the patient is watched for signs of coughing or expectoration of blood, since these signs might indicate that the lung was traumatized inadvertently. (For details on the equipment needed, see texts on fundamentals of nursing.)

■ ACUTE PULMONARY DISEASES

Viral infections

Many respiratory diseases are probably caused by viral infections. Presently, over 30 have been found to be directly related to viral infections, and there are probably many more.[53] Some diseases may be caused by one virus, or different viruses may cause the same symptoms.

If specific signs are not evident, the clinical illness is termed a common cold, viral infection, fever of unknown origin, acute respiratory illness, or the grippe. The most common specific respiratory illnesses caused by the various viruses are epidemic pleurodynia (Bornholm's disease), acute laryngotracheobronchitis, viral pneumonia, and influenza. Most adults have developed antibodies for the more common viruses, and most viral infections are relatively mild. However, they are frequently complicated by secondary bacterial infections. When new strains of the Asian flu virus develop, severe epidemics may ensue, and many people may die from secondary infections such as pneumonia.

The common cold

Few persons escape having a "cold." The average among the general population is three colds per person each year.[15] Respiratory diseases, primarily virus infections, are responsible for 30% to 50% of time lost from work by adults and from 60% to 80%

of time lost by children from school. The frequency of their occurrence, the number of people affected, the resulting economic loss, and the possibility that a cold may lead to more serious disease are reasons why colds merit serious attention.

Since persons with colds are rarely hospitalized, the nurse will encounter them at work, in public places, or in their homes. It is important to note the symptoms at the onset of the cold. Many other more serious diseases begin with a cold or with symptoms resembling those of the common cold. Because a cold is considered a minor but bothersome condition and because the person has possibly had many colds, he, rather than a physician, makes the diagnosis. Helping persons to realize the importance of an illness that may appear slight but that may have serious consequences is an integral part of the nurse's role.

Although the specific agent causing the common cold is unknown, it can be stated that it is a syndrome that is produced by a variety of viral infections. Viral studies do not yield the causative agent, nor is there usually any immunologic evidence of infection. Symptoms of a cold usually appear suddenly, and the infection may be full-blown within 48 hours. The acute inflammation usually begins in the pharynx, and there is a sensation of dryness or soreness of the throat. This is followed by nasal congestion with a thin, watery, profuse discharge and frequent sneezing. The eyes may water, the voice may become husky, breathing may be obstructed, and sense of smell and taste may diminish. Often a cough develops, and it may become productive of sputum.

The patient with a cold may have various complaints. At times he may feel lethargic and have vague, aching pains in the back and limbs. Most adults are afebrile, but those with a tendency toward developing complications, such as persons with chronic illness and lowered resistance, may have a temperature elevation. The course of the cold is variable, but ordinarily it lasts from 7 to 14 days. It is difficult to determine when the cold ends and when complications appear. Laryngitis and tracheitis may be part of the cold, while tracheobronchitis is a complication usually caused by secondary bacterial infection. Acute sinusitis and otitis media may also follow the common cold.

Prevention. The common cold is a communicable disease spread by droplet nuclei. The only known way to prevent spread of a cold from one individual to another is to isolate the infected person, and this is extremely difficult in our society. However, there are measures that help to prevent the development of a cold, its complications, and transfer to other persons. Good general hygiene, adequate rest, adequate diet, sufficient exercise, and fresh air presumably help maintain resistance to colds. Most persons can go through the usual course of a common cold without difficulty if they obtain enough rest.

The nurse should emphasize to the person the importance of not spreading his cold. Crowded places such as theaters should be avoided by persons with colds. The individual should particularly avoid contact with, and therefore exposing, infants and young children, persons who have chronic lung diseases such as bronchitis and emphysema, those who have recently had an anesthetic, and elderly people. He should remember to cover his nose and mouth when sneezing, coughing, and clearing his throat. Frequent washing of hands, covering of coughs and sneezes, and careful disposal of waste tissue are protective health measures that are advisable for everyone, but they become increasingly important when known respiratory infection exists. Since the common cold is a communicable disease, the principles for protection of oneself as well as others should be practiced.

Management. All treatment of colds is directed toward relief of symptoms and control of complications. If the patient has an elevated temperature and complains of headache and muscular aching, he should seek the advice of a physician. Acetylsalicylic acid may be prescribed for mild aches and discomfort. Salicylates, however, do not influence the course of the common cold and lack specific action in this disorder.

If the patient has *nasal congestion,* the physician may recommend nose drops. Ephedrine, 0.5% to 2% aqueous solution, with isotonic sodium chloride solution is used frequently. (See p. 604 for method of administration.) This medication shrinks swollen nasal tissues and allows for free passage of air. Many physicians advise against the use of nose drops, maintaining that constriction of the blood supply to the tissues lowers resistance. In general, oily solutions are not recommended because of the danger of inhaling oil droplets, which might cause lipid pneumonia. Nasal sprays containing antihistamine may be ordered. They should be given with the patient sitting upright. The nurse should emphasize to patients and their families the importance of using only prescribed solutions and only those that are fresh, since old solutions frequently become more concentrated. Nose drops should be prescribed by a physician, and only the specified amount should be used; excessive use may aggravate symptoms. Many persons prefer a medicated nasal inhaler since it can be carried easily in a pocket and is more pleasant to use. Benzedrex containing propylhexedrine is one that is widely used. Propylhexedrine is a volatile drug with a minimum stimulating effect on the central nervous system.[17] Soft disposable paper tissues or old, soft cotton handkerchiefs should be used to help prevent dryness, redness, and irritation about the nose. Some dryness can be prevented by treating the skin early with mild, soothing creams such as cold cream.

The *dryness, cough,* and *"tickling sensation"* in the throat so often associated with a cold can be

554

relieved in a variety of ways. There are many cough drops and lozenges on the market. Lozenges relieve irritation and are pleasant to use. Patients should be advised not to use them just before dozing off to sleep since they may be accidentally aspirated into the trachea during sleep. A mixture of honey and lemon may be preferred to cough medications by some patients. This mixture increases mucous secretions and thereby softens exudate and facilitates its expectoration. It also relieves dryness that predisposes to coughing. Some people report that undiluted lemon or orange juice is helpful. A section of the fruit with the rind may be placed at the bedside for easy accessibility during the night. Hot fluids often relieve coughing. The patient may be advised to keep a small vacuum bottle of hot water or other liquid at the bedside. If cough medication has been taken, it should not be followed by water because the effect will be dissipated. Patients should keep prescribed cough medications within reach to avoid chilling from getting out of bed during the night. If the cough associated with a common cold persists or does not yield to the simple home remedies mentioned or to specific medication that may have been ordered, the patient should be urged to consult his physician.

Pneumonia

Acute bacterial pneumonias are responsible for 10% of hospital admissions in the United States.[120] Pneumonia can occur in any season, but it is most common during winter and early spring. Persons of any age are susceptible, but pneumonia is more common among infants and the elderly. Pneumonia is often caused by aspiration of infected materials into the distal bronchioles and alveoli. Certain individuals are especially susceptible. This includes persons whose normal respiratory defense mechanisms are damaged or altered (those with chronic obstructive pulmonary disease, influenza, and tracheostomy, and those who have recently had anesthesia); persons who have a disease affecting antibody response (those with multiple myeloma, hypogammaglobulinemia, etc.); and alcoholics in whom there is increased danger of aspiration and persons with delayed white blood cell response to infection. Pneumonia is a communicable disease; the mode of transmission is dependent on the infecting organism.

Most patients with *pneumococcal pneumonia* complain of an upper respiratory infection several days before involvement of the lower respiratory tract. The spread of infection to the lower respiratory tract is usually very acute and is often what brings the patient to the physician. The patient is febrile; he has chills, chest pain, and cough with sputum production and possibly hemoptysis. Culture and sensitivity studies of sputum are obtained. Penicillin is the drug of choice for treating pneumococcal pneumonia.

Staphylococcal and *gram-negative pneumonias* have received a great deal of attention in recent years. These are not diseases of otherwise healthy individuals, but they occur as complications of other diseases. They are therefore seen frequently in hospitalized patients and are often caused by organisms that are resistant to commonly used antibiotics. Many times a patient has been on antibiotics prior to the development of pneumonia. Antibiotic therapy destroys the normal flora of the respiratory tract, and an infection caused by a resistant organism develops. Symptoms of staphylococcal and gram-negative pneumonias are similar to those of pneumococcal pneumonia. *Pseudomonas pneumonia* is often caused by contaminated aerosols that pass upper airway defenses.[119a] Culture and sensitivity studies of sputum are done to determine the causative agent and to select appropriate antimicrobial therapy.

Prevention. Pneumonia can often be prevented in susceptible patients by meticulous nursing care. Frequent turning or changing position of persons confined to bed will lessen the possibility of pulmonary stasis. Prompt suctioning of secretions in patients who cannot cough and expectorate forcibly will reduce the chances of aspiration and atelectasis. These patients need special attention when they are being given medication, food, or drink by mouth. An apprehensive patient with swallowing difficulties needs time to learn to swallow with expiration. He needs constant encouragement in his efforts to relax and continue to swallow safely.

Strict medical asepsis will decrease transmission of organisms from one patient to another via the nurse. Nursing personnel who have colds should not be in direct contact with patients. Good ventilation systems (transfer with fresh air rather than recirculated air) will decrease transmission of airborne infections between patients. The best way to prevent airborne transmission is to be sure that an infected individual covers his mouth and nose when coughing or sneezing.

Management. The patient with pneumonia has a temperature elevation and may have shaking chills and a cough. Thick purulent sputum is common in *staphylococcal pneumonia.* Increased temperature and pulse are indications that body defenses are mobilized and additional stress will be detrimental. The nurse can help prevent additional stress for the patient by helping him with personal hygiene, by keeping the environment generally quiet, by allaying fears and apprehension, and by arranging regular rest periods during the day. Activity necessary to maintain good general circulation and good tracheobronchial hygiene must be encouraged.

When the temperature is elevated, both fluids and salt are lost. Fluids are encouraged and additional salt may be given either in food or in intravenous fluids. If the patient is nauseated or otherwise unable to take fluids by mouth, infusions may be given. If the patient's temperature becomes extremely high, hypothermia may be used (p. 209).

Oxygen therapy is often necessary. Secretions may partially or totally obstruct the airway and the alveoli may be filled with exudative material. All of these changes decrease the surface area available for gas exchange. The oxygen may be given by cannula (nasal prongs), catheter, or mask. Tents may be used, but because the oxygen concentration is difficult to control in them, they are used primarily for humidity control. (For care of patients receiving oxygen, see texts on fundamentals of nursing.)

Since the treatment and prognosis of pneumonia depend on the causative organism, sputum smears are examined and cultures obtained. A sputum specimen for examination should be obtained *before* administration of an antibiotic is started, and it is a nursing responsibility to help obtain this specimen as quickly as possible. If antibiotic therapy is begun before cultures can be collected, it may be impossible to grow the causative organism.

Pneumonia is now classified according to the offending organism rather than the anatomic location (lobar or bronchial) as was previously the practice. The type of organism determines the antimicrobial agent that is given. Antibiotics must be carefully given as ordered to ensure that an adequate blood level is maintained. The patient should be observed carefully for any untoward reaction to the antibiotics he is receiving, and such a reaction should be reported to the physician at once. If antimicrobial therapy can be instituted promptly, the temperature drops markedly in 24 hours, the pulse rate may become normal, and the patient may feel generally much better.

Because of high temperature, dehydration, and mouth breathing, the patient needs frequent mouth care. Maintenance of cleanliness of the mouth may also inhibit extension of infection to the ears. Herpetic blisters about the mouth are common and are a source of much discomfort to the patient. Tincture of benzoin can be applied, and sometimes camphor ice is beneficial. Cold cream can be used to soften the crusted areas. If the nostrils are dry or are crusted with exudate, swabs moistened with water or hydrogen peroxide can be used, and cold cream can be applied to the external nares.

Chest pain in pneumonia is caused by inflammation of the pleura and usually is confined to the affected side. Involvement of the pleura and empyema often complicate staphylococcal pneumonia.[15,120] Pain may be severe and stabbing in nature and may be exaggerated by coughing and by deep breathing. Respirations are often described as "grunting." Close observation of the chest may show that there is limitation of movement of the affected side. The patient may use accessory muscles to aid in breathing in-

stead of expanding the lower chest fully. The patient with severe chest pain usually needs help and encouragement in changing his position at intervals. Measures to splint the patient's chest, such as applying a chest binder or turning the patient on the affected side, may help to reduce pain. Raising the head of the bed will often make it easier for the patient to breathe, but he may need pillows to support his arms, since otherwise the weight of the arms dropping forward puts a strain on the shoulder girdle and increases fatigue. Occasionally pain is severe enough to require regional block of the intercostal nerves (p. 208). If narcotics are used, codeine is usually the drug prescribed since it is less likely to inhibit productive coughing than stronger narcotic agents.

Severe cough and blood-tinged ("rusty") sputum are characteristic of *pneumococcal pneumonia*. The patient must be encouraged and helped to cough deeply to produce sputum from the lungs and not expend needed energy in raising secretions from the upper trachea and posterior pharynx only. The nurse can help the patient cough without too much pain by giving prescribed medications and by helping splint the chest as the patient coughs.

In severe pneumonia, peristaltic action may be decreased. The nurse should report failure to have a bowel movement and any distention, rigidity, or tenderness in the upper abdominal quadrants since these conditions are signs of paralytic ileus (p. 229). If peristalsis becomes suppressed or absent, there is respiratory distress due to elevation of the diaphragm by the accumulation of gas and fluid in the gastrointestinal tract, and vomiting may occur. Enemas are seldom given in the absence of peristalsis because they will be retained unless siphoned back, and they may increase distention and discomfort. Bisacodyl suppositories may be effective. Insertion of a rectal tube or the administration of neostigmine (Prostigmin) may help to relieve distention. A nasogastric tube may be inserted and intravenous fluids containing electrolytes given, since electrolyte imbalance will be made worse by continuous removal of stomach secretions, and potassium loss will contribute to the development of paralytic ileus. Peristalsis seems to be encouraged by exercise. If the patient's condition permits, sitting up in bed or even walking a little often helps. Eating solid food also appears to prevent the occurrence of paralytic ileus in some instances. For this reason, if patients are able to take this kind of nourishment, some physicians order food for those who are quite ill. However, the patient who has had paralytic ileus or in whom the condition has threatened should not be given foods that are gas forming. Excessive fatigue may severely limit appetite; in these instances, provision of high-calorie fluid or soft foods may encourage sufficient intake to meet the body's increased demand for energy.

Prevention of complications. With the advent of antibiotics and better diagnostic measures such as x-ray procedures, complications during or following pneumonia are rare in otherwise normal persons. Atelectasis, delayed resolution, lung abscess, pleural effusion, empyema, pericarditis, meningitis, and relapse are complications that were common in the past. The fact that pneumonia and influenza rank fifth as a cause of death in the United States is an impressive reason for strict adherence to the prescribed medical treatment. Careful and accurate observation as well as sufficient time for convalescence will also help to ensure the average patient a smooth recovery. Aged persons and those with chronic illness are likely to have a relatively long course of convalescence from pneumonia, and there is a great possibility of their developing complications. There has been an increase in the incidence of staphylococcal pneumonia subsequent to influenza. Consolidation of lung tissue, pleural effusion, and empyema frequently occur soon after the onset of this type of pneumonia and may cause death.

Acute bronchitis

Bronchitis can be acute or chronic. Acute bronchitis is an inflammation of the bronchi and sometimes the trachea (tracheobronchitis). It is often caused by an extension of an upper respiratory tract infection such as the common cold and is therefore communicable. It also may be caused by physical or chemical agents such as dust, smoke, or volatile fumes. As air pollution increases, the incidence of acute bronchitis increases.

The patient with acute bronchitis usually complains of chilliness, malaise, muscular aches, headaches, a dry, scratchy throat, hoarseness, and a cough. The temperature may be elevated. The patient may be confined to bed at home or in the hospital. In either case, exposure to others should be kept to a minimum. Early in the disease the patient's main complaints are the dry, irritating cough and the feeling of tightness and soreness in the chest that follows coughing. The patient may obtain relief by the same means as those described for the common cold. Cough may be relieved by cough mixtures or aerosol drugs. Humidifying the air eases breathing and lessens irritation. Tincture of benzoin, menthol, or oil of eucalyptus may be ordered for the steam vaporizor for its soothing and aromatic effect. Some physicians prefer that cool humidification be used. As the disease progresses, secretions usually increase. Congestion and dryness of the bronchial mucous membrane are then relieved.

Treatment of acute tracheobronchitis is usually conservative in an attempt to prevent extension of infection to the smaller bronchi, the bronchioles, and the alveoli of the lungs. Measures that maintain good drainage of tracheobronchial secretions are prescribed. (See details in section on chronic obstructive pulmonary disease.) The patient should be protected from drafts and should take from 3,000 to 4,000 ml. of fluid daily. A simple bland diet is usually most easily eaten. Often antibiotics are given if the patient has an elevation of temperature.

Most persons need a period of convalescence following an attack of acute bronchitis. Patients usually complain of weakness and fatigue. The nurse should caution the patient to guard against overexertion, including return to work without medical approval. He should be encouraged to take extra rest, to eat a well-balanced diet, and to avoid conditions that might expose him to further infection or predispose him to possible relapse.

■ TUBERCULOSIS

In 1900 tuberculosis was the leading cause of death in the United States. It remained a major cause of death until the introduction of antituberculosis drug therapy in the late 1940's and early 1950's. The most effective of these agents is isoniazid, which first became available clinically in 1952. The use of isoniazid in combination with two agents introduced earlier, streptomycin and para-aminosalicylic acid, resulted in a striking decrease in tuberculosis death rates. It also made it possible for patients with tuberculosis to be treated on an outpatient basis. However, some patients still have to be hospitalized at some time in their illness, and most all nurses will care for a patient with tuberculosis at some time in their careers. At one time patients with tuberculosis were hospitalized in specialized hospitals called sanitoria. Today these sanatoria are being used for patients with other illnesses, and the patient with tuberculosis is being admitted to the general hospital. Because many persons in our society, including medical personnel, are afraid of tuberculosis, it is important that nurses learn as much as possible about the disease so that they can give effective care to the patient with tuberculosis. Unfortunately some persons still associate tuberculosis with lack of cleanliness and careless living. This may make both the patient and his family unwilling to speak openly about the disease, making treatment of the disease difficult.

Although tuberculosis is now considered a preventable and curable disease, it still is a disease requiring public health attention. In 1972, 80,000 persons in the United States were reported to have active tuberculosis. This figure includes 44,000 cases in tuberculosis registeries as of January 1, 3,500 reactivated cases, and 32,882 new cases that developed within that year. These new cases were not evenly distributed throughout the population, however, and some differences bear mentioning.[109]

In the past few years the greatest numbers of tuberculosis cases have been found in the counties with the largest populations, especially when the county encompasses a major city. Nearly one half of the tuberculosis cases are found in cities, and rates are highest in the largest metropolitan areas. Other regions where the case rates are higher than the average are counties close to the Mexican border and a few areas where there is a large population of American Indians. Tuberculosis rates are also higher than the average in areas of the United States where there are large numbers of immigrants from countries where tuberculosis is far more prevalent than in this country. For example, in Hawaii a large portion of the new cases is among persons who have lived in Hawaii for 1 year or less. Other places where similar situations are reported are San Francisco, Dade County, Florida, and Boston. Canada reports a similar finding. These figures point out that with a few exceptions most countries of the world have much higher tuberculosis morbidity and mortality rates than does the United States. In general, Latin America, Africa, Asia, and Oceania have considerably higher case rates than do the United States and the English-speaking and Western European countries. Thus Americans residing for prolonged periods of time in countries where the tuberculosis rates are very high run an increased risk of becoming infected with tubercle bacilli.[109]

As had been true for several years preceding and including 1972, the new active case rate for men was double that for women. The nonwhite population has a case rate over four times as high as that of the white population (Fig. 22-7), but almost half of all new active cases occurred among white men. The highest case rate was among persons 65 years and over, and the second highest was in the 45 to 64 age group. The case rates for children under 5 and those 5 to 14 have shown a decline every year since 1964. The rates for nonwhite children under 15 are several times those for white children and are a reflection of the high case rates of nonwhite adults.

As was pointed out earlier, there has been a steady decline in deaths due to tuberculosis in the United States since the introduction of effective chemotherapeutic agents. Today the tuberculosis death rate is around 2.0/100,000 people. However, the tuberculosis death rate for males is more than double that for females, and the death rate for nonwhites is three times that for the white population.[109]

In an attempt to eliminate tuberculosis from the United States, concerted effort must be made to prevent persons from becoming infected with the tubercle bacillus. Measures to do this are discussed next.

Prevention and control

In order to eliminate tuberculosis, the following priorities must be met: (1) All persons with active tuberculosis must be identified and placed on uninterrupted antituberculosis therapy. (2) Persons who are *household contacts* or otherwise have *close contact* (as in work or school) with persons identified as having active tuberculosis must be identified and examined. (3) Contacts must be followed medically and placed on preventive treatment as appropriate. This will be discussed in more detail later.

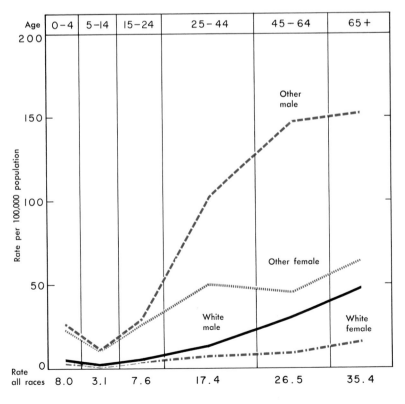

FIG. 22-7. New active tuberculosis case rates by age, race, and sex in the United States. (From Department of Health, Education and Welfare, Public Health Service: Tuberculosis programs 1972, Atlanta, 1974, Center for Disease Control.)

Tuberculin testing of contacts will indicate presence of infection (p. 560). A chest radiograph and a general physical examination will show any signs of clinical pulmonary tuberculosis. Findings on a chest radiograph suggestive of disease and a positive tuberculin test identify persons who are *suspect.* All persons suspected of having the disease need repeated chest x-ray and physical examinations to be certain that active disease is not present.

In addition to these control measures, persons in the community who are at special risk of developing tuberculosis should be identified. These *high-risk* groups include persons who have converted from a negative to positive tuberculin test within the last year; persons living in the same household or in close contact with an individual newly diagnosed as having tuberculosis; individuals with large tuberculin reactions (12 mm. or more induration); individuals who had active tuberculosis in the past without adequate chemotherapy; and persons with positive tuberculin tests who have diabetes mellitus, silicosis, sarcoidosis, gastrectomy, reticuloendothelial diseases such as leukemia and Hodgkin's disease, or who are receiving prolonged steroid therapy. Every effort should be made to identify these persons and to follow them medically to prevent their developing active disease.

Daily preventive therapy with isoniazid for 1 year is now recommended for persons under age 35 in high-risk groups. Any child under 5 who has a positive tuberculin test is considered a recent convertor. Preschool associates of children who are positive reactors should receive preventive therapy even if they are tuberculin negative. Persons on preventive therapy should be under medical supervision.

The Center for Disease Control (CDC) recommended early in 1974 that "in positive tuberculin reactors 35 years and over, the risk of hepatitis precludes the routine use of preventive therapy." However, the presence of additional risk factors may warrant the use of preventive therapy regardless of age. The CDC also recommended that pregnancy be included as a contraindication for the administration of isoniazid.[110]

In 1963 the Surgeon General of the United States appointed a task force to study the tuberculosis problem. One recommendation of the task force was that all children should be tuberculin tested when they enter school and at age 14 to determine those who are positive reactors. Since that time the recommendation has been modified because reactor rates have been found to be so low. It is now recommended that tuberculin testing efforts be concentrated in areas where the reactor rate is 1% or more. In general, this would be in large population centers where the tuberculosis rates are the highest. In addition, school personnel should be tuberculin tested periodically if they are nonreactors or have x-ray examinations if they are reactors, because they are in a position to infect many children if they develop active tuberculosis. Tuberculin skin testing is discussed in more detail later in this chapter.

Vaccination

Efforts continue in search of a more satisfactory tuberculosis vaccine. Presently, BCG (bacillus Calmette-Guerin) vaccine is in use in some parts of the United States and in many countries throughout the world. This vaccine contains attenuated tubercle bacilli, which have lost their ability to produce disease. The vaccine should be given only by persons who have had careful instruction in the proper technique. A multiple-puncture disk is used. When there is a positive reaction to skin testing with tuberculin, when acute infectious disease is present, or when there is any skin disease, BCG vaccine is not given. Possible complications following vaccination are local ulcers, which occur in a relatively high percentage of persons vaccinated, and abscesses or suppuration of lymph nodes, which occur in a small percentage.

In countries where living conditions are such that transmission of the disease is to be expected, BCG vaccine is given early in life and then repeated after 12 to 15 years. The intradermal method is used to administer the vaccine so that a uniform controlled dose can be given. BCG vaccine is not generally recommended for use in the United States, although some highly susceptible groups such as migrant workers may be immunized.

Infection

Tuberculosis is caused by a bacillus, the *Mycobacterium tuberculosis,* or tubercle bacillus, a gram-positive and acid-fast organism. If microscopic study of a slide prepared from the sputum of an individual reveals tubercle bacilli, the individual is said to have positive sputum, and this confirms the diagnosis of tuberculosis. Some persons with tuberculosis will not have positive sputum on smear, however, and a positive sputum culture will be necessary to confirm the diagnosis. Patients who have a positive culture and negative smear are less infectious than are those with both a positive smear and culture.

Transmission

When a person with tuberculosis coughs, sneezes, or laughs, minute droplets of moisture are expelled into the air around him. The larger droplets fall to the ground, while the smaller ones evaporate, leaving *droplet nuclei* that remain suspended indefinitely in the air and are carried on air currents. Droplet nuclei are 1 to 5 microns in size and are small enough to be inhaled into the alveoli. Thus it is by inhalation of tubercle-laden droplet nuclei that tuberculosis is transmitted.

When an individual with no previous exposure to tuberculosis (negative tuberculin reactor) inhales a sufficient number of tubercle bacilli into the alveoli, tuberculosis *infection* occurs. The body's reaction to the tubercle bacilli depends on the susceptibility of the individual, the size of the dose, and the virulence of the organisms. Inflammation occurs within the alveoli (parenchyma) of the lungs, and natural body defenses attempt to counteract the infection. Lymph nodes in the hilar region of the lung may be involved as they filter drainage from the infected site. The inflammatory process and cellular reaction produce a small, firm, white nodule called the *primary tubercle.* The center of the nodule contains tubercle bacilli. Cells gather around the center, and usually the outer portion becomes fibrosed. Thus blood vessels are compressed, nutrition of the tubercle is interfered with, and necrosis occurs at the center. The area becomes walled off by fibrotic tissue around the outside, and the center gradually becomes soft and cheesy in consistency. This latter process is known as *caseation.* This material may become calcified (calcium deposits), or it may liquefy. The first infection is usually successfully overcome, and the calcified nodule is known as the *Ghon tubercle.* The evidence on x-ray film of the calcified lymph nodes and Ghon tubercle is sometimes referred to as the *primary complex.*

Persons who have been exposed to the tubercle bacillus become sensitized to it, and this is confirmed by a positive tuberculin test. Sensitization, once developed, remains throughout life. A positive tuberculin test does not mean that one has tuberculosis, however, and nurses should explain this fact to persons who are having the test.

Tuberculosis infection is unlike other infections. Usually other infections disappear completely when overcome by the body's defenses and leave no living organisms and generally no signs of infection. However, a person who has been infected with tubercle bacilli harbors the organism for the remainder of his life. Tubercle bacilli remain in the lungs in a dormant, walled-off, or so-called resting stage. Under physical or emotional stress, these bacilli may become active and begin to multiply. If body defenses are low, active tuberculosis may develop. Most persons who have active tuberculosis developed it in this manner. However, it is generally accepted that only 1 out of 20 persons with a positive tuberculin test will ever develop active tuberculosis, and the incidence is expected to be much lower among those who receive preventive therapy with isoniazid.

Diagnosis

Tuberculin skin testing. Tuberculin skin testing provides evidence of whether the individual tested has been infected by tubercle bacilli. A negative tuberculin skin test usually rules out disease and past infec-

tion. A positive test indicates that infection has occurred.

Two substances are used in tuberculin skin testing: OT (old tuberculin), which is prepared from dead tubercle bacilli and contains their related impurities, and PPD (purified protein derivative), which is a highly purified product containing protein from the tubercle bacilli.

The tuberculin test that gives the most accurate results is the *Mantoux test,* or intracutaneous injection of either PPD or OT. A tuberculin syringe and a short ($1/_2$-inch), sharp, 24- to 26-gauge needle are used. With the skin (usually the inner forearm is used) held taut, the injection of 0.1 ml. of PPD or OT is made into the superficial layers, and it produces a sharply raised white wheal. Weak dilutions are used first. If the reaction is negative, stronger dilutions are used. This precaution prevents severe local reactions that might occur in highly sensitive individuals if the higher dilutions were used initially. If old tuberculin is used, tests are begun with a dilution of 1:10,000 or 0.001 mg. of OT. If this test is negative, successive tests with stronger dilutions are made. The most frequently used strength of PPD is an intermediate strength of 0.0001 mg./dose, or 5 tuberculin units (5 Tu). PPD is also available in first and second strength dilutions. For broad screening and case finding purposes, a single test of intermediate strength is recommended. Interpretations of the tests are made after 48 hours. A positive reaction may begin after 12 to 24 hours with an area of redness and a central area of induration, but it reaches its peak in 48 hours. The area of induration (not the erythema) indicates how positive the test is. Induration should be examined in a good light and palpated gently. Tuberculin reactions should always be measured and recorded in millimeters at the largest diameter of the induration. When successive dilutions are being used, it is advisable to have tests read by the same person so that individual variation in interpretation can be prevented. If the test is negative, there may be no visible reaction or there may be only slight redness with no induration.

One of the most important steps in tuberculin testing is the accurate measurement of reaction. A reaction is considered to be positive when it is 10 mm. or more in diameter. Reactions between 5 and 9 mm. are considered to be doubtful reactions and are more likely to indicate infection with atypical acid-fast bacilli (p. 565) than with *M. tuberculosis.* A reaction of 4 mm. or less is considered to be a negative reaction.

Other diagnostic studies. Results of radiographs and sputum examinations will either rule out the possibility or confirm a diagnosis of tuberculosis. Both tests have been described (pp. 547 and 548). Bacteriologic confirmation of the presence of *M. tuberculosis* is necessary to establish the diagnosis of tuberculosis. Because it is impossible to differentiate between typical and atypical acid-fast bacilli by a sputum smear, cultures are obtained on all persons. Cultures are also used for antimicrobial susceptibility (sensitivity) studies. *Despite the recent introduction of improved culture media, the tubercle bacillus grows slowly on artificial media, and culture reports will not be available for 3 to 6 weeks.*

Blood-streaked sputum in the absence of pronounced coughing may be the first indication to the patient that anything is wrong. Pathologic changes may have occurred in the lungs, but sputum examination may not show tubercle bacilli. However, if the nodules produced in the parenchyma of the lung become soft in the center and then caseated and liquefied, the liquefied material may break through and empty into the bronchi and be raised as sputum. Cavities in the lung may appear on x-ray film and may be present in more than one lobe of the lung.

Classification

A new classification of tuberculosis was recently developed, and as of January 1, 1975, it is to be used by states and territories of the United States when reporting morbidity statistics to the Communicable Disease Center of the Public Health Service. Now there are four basic classifications that cover the total child and adult population—unexposed, uninfected, infected, and diseased.*

0   No tuberculosis exposure, not infected—no history of exposure, negative tuberculin skin test

I   Tuberculosis exposure, no evidence of infection—history of exposure, negative tuberculin skin test

II   Tuberculosis infection, without disease—positive tuberculin skin test, negative bacteriologic studies (if done), no x-ray findings compatible with tuberculosis, no symptoms due to tuberculosis

III   Tuberculosis: infected, with disease—current status of patient's tuberculosis described by three characteristics: location of the disease, bacteriologic status, and chemotherapy status (For some patients, additional characteristics such as x-ray findings and tuberculin skin test reaction would be included.)

Preventing transmission

Once the diagnosis of "tuberculosis: infected, with disease" is made, steps are taken to prevent the patient from contaminating the air with tubercle bacilli. This is accomplished by (1) *treatment of the patient with antituberculosis drugs* and (2) *preventing contamination of air with tubercle bacilli.* Each of these measures will be discussed in detail.

Chemotherapy. Whether the patient with tuberculosis is being treated at home or in the hospital, the same drugs are given. Isoniazid (INH), streptomycin, para-aminosalicylic acid (PAS), and ethambutol,

*From Ogasawara, F. R.: A totally new classification of tuberculosis, Bull. Am. Lung Assoc. pp. 13-14, Jan.-Feb. 1975.

are the drugs in common use. These four drugs are considered to be the "first-line," or *primary,* medications in the treatment of tuberculosis. If they prove to be ineffective or if the patient develops resistant tubercle bacilli, the "second-line," or *secondary,* drugs are used—cycloserine (Seromycin), pyrazinoic acid amide (Pyrazinamide), viomycin (Viocin), kanamycin (Kantrex), and ethionamide (Trecator).

Previously untreated pulmonary tuberculosis can nearly always be controlled bacteriologically with drugs alone. Most failures of antimicrobial therapy are due to errors in choice of drug, inadequate dosage, or failure of the patient to take the drugs regularly as prescribed.[76] Choices of drugs are made with the objective of both effective treatment of disease and minimizing the development of drug-resistant organisms.

Susceptibility testing. Prescriptions for antituberculosis drugs are made according to the susceptibility of the organisms isolated from the patient's sputum to the primary drugs—isoniazid, PAS, ethambutol, and streptomycin. Susceptibility testing indicates the effectiveness of a specific drug in inhibiting the growth of the organism or the organism's resistance to the drug. Until testing can be completed, the physician will start the patients on the drugs to which it is believed the bacilli are most likely to be susceptible.

Testing is done by growing cultures of the organisms in special media. The culture plate is divided into sections so that the organisms, if present in the patient's sputum, will grow on one section. Each of the other sections contains a medium plus one of the primary drugs. Thus, if the organisms multiply on one section of medium but do not appear on other sections of the medium, the organisms are susceptible to those drugs that inhibit their growth. Testing usually takes about 3 weeks, about half the time formerly required to grow cultures of tubercle bacilli.

Although it is the physician's responsibility to make susceptibility tests, the nurse should understand the basis on which drugs are prescribed and help the patient understand the various changes in drugs that may be prescribed for him and why he may be receiving drugs that are different from those received by other patients.

Recently it has been recognized that there are naturally occurring drug-resistant tubercle bacilli. It is estimated that in every group of 100,000 bacilli there is one naturally occurring isoniazid-resistant organism, while for each group of 1 million bacilli there is one streptomycin-resistant organism.[60] Therefore, antituberculosis drugs are always given in combination. Usually two of the drugs are combined, but patients with far-advanced cavitary disease often receive three drugs (isoniazid, PAS, streptomycin).

Drugs frequently used. Isoniazid and PAS or

isoniazid and ethambutol are by far the most common combinations given. The daily dose of isoniazid for an adult is usually 5 mg./kg. body weight (about 300 mg. daily) given orally. Higher doses are given to some patients who have severe or acute disease. The daily dose of PAS in adults is 8 to 12 Gm. orally (200 mg./kg. body weight), usually in three divided doses and taken with or following meals. The daily dosage of ethambutol is 15 mg./kg. of body weight and it is given in a single dose.

PAS commonly causes gastrointestinal symptoms, especially early in treatment. Some physicians reduce the dosage temporarily to 4 to 6 Gm. daily and then increase the dosage when the intolerance to the drug has subsided. Nausea, vomiting, and poor appetite are the usual symptoms. Taking the drug following meals or with milk helps most patients. Some who receive PAS in powder form prefer to have the medication mixed in a glass of milk, which produces a consistency similar to that of a milkshake. Other signs of intolerance to the drug are skin rash, fever, headache, malaise, and sore throat. The nurse should observe the patient closely during the first 6 weeks of therapy for signs of hypersensitivity so that the dosage can be reduced if necessary.

Ethambutol is a newer chemotherapeutic agent and is beginning to replace PAS because it is better tolerated. Ethambutol is contraindicated in patients with known optic neuritis. It is recommended that any patient receiving ethambutol have periodic checks of his visual acuity, as optic neuritis may occur.

Isoniazid causes little toxicity. Occasionally, however, symmetric peripheral neuritis may develop, particularly in patients who are malnourished or who are receiving large doses of the drug. To prevent neuritis, the physician usually orders pyridoxine, 50 to 100 mg. daily. Occasionally isoniazid may affect memory and the ability to concentrate, and rarely it may cause psychosis. Recently there has been some evidence that isoniazid can cause transient changes in liver enzymes and may rarely cause hepatitis. However, the reported instances are too few to warrant any change in the use of the drug.

Streptomycin is often given as part of an initial program of *triple drug therapy*. It is given intramuscularly in 1 Gm. doses daily or three times a week for 6 to 12 weeks or more, depending on the patient's improvement. Smaller doses may be prescribed for elderly patients or for patients who have hearing impairment or renal damage. The most important untoward reaction to streptomycin is labyrinth damage with resulting vertigo and staggering. Skin rash, itching, and fever can occur. Although renal damage is uncommon, urinalyses and blood urea nitrogen determinations usually are ordered at periodic intervals. (For chemotherapy programs and toxicities of the secondary drugs, see pharmacology texts.)

Patients' problems with chemotherapy. It is *imperative* that the patient who has tuberculosis *take the prescribed medications regularly and without interruption.* Because the patient usually must take drugs daily for 18 to 24 months, he may become discouraged and stop taking the drugs. If symptoms of intolerance to a drug such as those produced by PAS occur, he may simply stop taking the one drug and continue with the other. The patient may feel quite well, work regularly, yet must continue the therapy. Because he feels well, he may be tempted to discontinue the drugs altogether or perhaps take the one drug that bothers him the least. All patients must be taught that the discontinuance of even one drug will allow drug-resistant organisms to flourish and will make the disease more difficult to treat. The nurse should help all patients develop a daily routine for taking the drugs. For those who have difficulty remembering to take their medications, pill calendars that have each day's medications in a plastic bag stapled to a large cardboard calendar may be helpful.

Some patients stop taking drugs and then restart them. Because they may feel guilty about this interruption in therapy, they do not tell the physician or nurse, and it may not be evident until their condition fails to improve. The nurse can help by allowing time for patients to talk about themselves, their families, and their treatment. This may be done when the patient visits a health department clinic to receive his new supply of drugs, when he comes for his periodic medical examination, or when the nurse visits him in his home. Patients may be asked to collect a urine specimen periodically for examination. Since the metabolic products of some of the drugs are excreted in the urine, a urinalysis will indicate whether the patient is following his therapy. The best indication, of course, is the progress of the patient. If he improves, therapy is effective and the medications probably have been taken as prescribed.

Preventing contamination of the air. As soon as the diagnosis of tuberculosis is established, the patient is taught to cover his nose and mouth with disposable tissues when he coughs, sneezes, or laughs. This stops the organisms at the source and prevents them from becoming droplet nuclei capable of transmitting disease (p. 559). Soiled tissues are collected in a paper bag for subsequent burning, or they may be discarded in the toilet. The patient should wash his hands after expectorating or handling the sputum container.

The most effective way to kill the tubercle bacillus in moist sputum is by burning. All tissues and disposable receptacles for collection of sputum should be burned. Direct sunlight destroys the bacillus in 1 to 2 hours. Five minutes at boiling temperature and 30 minutes at pasteurizing temperature (61.7° C., 143° F.) kill the bacillus. Autoclaving also destroys the bacillus. Disposable articles may be used if desired.

The natural movement of air in a room carries droplet nuclei containing the tubercle bacillus, and if windows are kept open or air is circulated mechanically, changes of air dilute the contaminated air below the level where infection can take place. If the patient who has positive sputum has been taught to cover his coughs and sneezes, air contamination in his room is even lower.

Tubercle bacilli in droplet nuclei are highly susceptible to sterilization by sunlight. *Ultraviolet light* also kills tubercle bacilli in droplet nuclei. Lights installed in air ducts through which room air passes or mounted high on side walls of the room are effective.

It is important that nurses understand how tubercle bacilli are transmitted through air so that they can teach the patient how to protect others and also allay fears that family members and others may have about contracting the disease. It has been well documented that the patient who is taking antituberculosis drugs is not likely to transmit the infection even when his organisms are resistant to treatment. Because only droplet nuclei are capable of transmitting tubercle bacilli, there is no need for those caring for the patient with active tuberculosis to wear either a mask or a gown. Droplet nuclei are so small (1 to 5 microns) that they readily pass through conventional masks or are breathed in around the edges of them. Chemotherapeutic treatment of the patient and adequate air changes in the patient's room offer all the protection that is needed. In a situation in which the patient is unable to cover his mouth when he coughs, it is more effective for him to wear a mask than for personnel to do so. Newer type high-filtration masks such as the Ultra-Filter have proved to be effective filters. If a mask is deemed necessary, this type should be used.

Since many patients with active tuberculosis are cared for in their homes, the nurse should help patients and their families to understand the communicability of tuberculosis and the precautions that must be taken. Family members and friends may be frightened at the thought of contact with the patient and with articles he has touched. On the other hand, they have often had long, intimate contact with the patient without developing the disease. Careful observation of the family will help the nurse determine how many and what kind of explanations are needed regarding spread of infection. If the family is overly cautious in handling the patient's personal articles, the nurse may need to advise against discarding articles that are costly to replace. In contrast, if the family is too casual about spread of the disease, the nurse should urge more caution in care of sputum and in exposure to the patient's cough. If possible, the patient should occupy a room alone, but if he is allowed to stay at home, he usually does not need to be strictly isolated from the rest of the family. Careful planning with the family often helps ensure that he will not infect others yet can be located so that he and his family are as happy as possible under such circumstances. The susceptibility of babies and very small children must be emphasized in all teaching.

Management of the patient with tuberculosis

Acceptance of the diagnosis. Acceptance of a diagnosis of tuberculosis and of its many implications for the future is difficult for anyone. The patient and/or his family should be referred to a public health nurse immediately after the diagnosis of tuberculosis is made so that initial explanations can be given and essential teaching begun. It is important that any problems that might interfere with acceptance of the disease be identified early since the earlier efforts are made to solve them, the less difficult they may be to overcome.

Real acceptance of the disease, however, may come only after months of illness and after steady help and support from the family, the physician, the social worker, and the nurse. The acceptance of facts and realities varies according to each patient's basic personality and his lifelong pattern of behavior in stress situations. The nurse should realize that for some time after the diagnosis is made the patient may deny that he has tuberculosis or be very angry that it has happened to him. Some patients may become depressed and may have periods of withdrawal as they work through their feelings about their diagnosis. Many of their feelings about the diagnosis are culturally based, and reactions to the diagnosis are more emotionally than intellectually determined. Even though the patient understands that tuberculosis is not caused by being "dirty" or "sinful," he may still carry over feelings from his childhood when he was told that tuberculosis only happens to persons who are dirty or sinful.

There is a high incidence of alcoholism among patients with tuberculosis, probably because of the increased possibility of alcoholics coming into contact with tubercle bacilli during drinking bouts and because of their decreased resistance to infection. Some of these patients have been committed to the hospital by legal action after refusal to obtain treatment even though their disease is a threat to the health of their family and community. They present the dual problem of the patient with alcoholism (p. 157) and the patient with tuberculosis who cannot accept his disease.

Increasing attention needs to be given to patients who refuse treatment and thus stand in the way of eradication of tuberculosis. The nurse often is the member of the medical team called on to work with these patients. Patience and understanding as well as flexibility in trying new approaches are essential in working with them. Although the patient needs explanations as to the need for treatment and time to make his own decisions regarding means of obtaining it, delaying tactics should be discouraged by setting limits. Avoidance of questions that permit categorical refusal is wise. It is often helpful to discover the person for whose judgment the patient has the greatest respect and to seek his help in encouraging treatment. This person may be a physician, a clergyman, a family member, or a close friend. Persons who have completed treatment for tuberculosis and are well again often are helpful in answering specific questions the patient may have and may thus relieve many of his anxieties. Every effort should be made to help the patient feel there is sincere concern for his and his family's welfare. In spite of all efforts, some patients will not consent to treatment. Sometimes, if they become suddenly worse, they may then be receptive to treatment, and the opportunity to work with them and help them at this time should not be missed.

Nurses working with patients with tuberculosis must be able to accept the diagnosis if they are to help the patient. Nurses who have a fear of tuberculosis show it in their behavior. Most patients with tuberculosis are extremely sensitive to ways in which various health workers approach them. If personnel are obvious about precautions in giving care, this may make the patient feel rejected. Nurses may be fearful of the disease for various reasons. If the nurse is aware of being fearful, talking it over with an experienced person who is unafraid of tuberculosis may prove helpful. Reassurance that tuberculosis is not highly communicable is usually very helpful to the nurse who has not previously cared for a patient with tuberculosis.

The majority of patients with tuberculosis are able to assume responsibility for their own care. The nurse's major responsibility is to help the patient learn what he should do and why and to give encouragement and supervision in the simple but essential elements of good care. Group teaching often is a very productive method of instructing both patients and family members since they often learn from each other and give each other emotional support.

Activity. Although tuberculosis used to be treated with bed rest, restriction of activity is no longer ordered except as warranted by the patient's general physical condition. If the patient is hospitalized, small day-by-day routine tasks and activities should be planned. The patient should be encouraged to maintain interest in his appearance and grooming. Manicures, shampoos, and hair styling can and should be done. Any patient who has a long-term confining illness may value his smallest possessions in a way quite different from the person who is well and participating actively in life. Personal belongings tend to collect, and the patient needs help in sorting and arranging them.

If an organized occupational therapy department is available, the patient is encouraged to engage in appropriate activities. The interest of others in his projects adds to his own enjoyment. Patients may like to tell the nurse about their projects or even to teach some of the skills involved. When occupational therapy service is not available, the nurse can teach some simple skills to patients or arrange for them to take responsibility for small jobs such as distributing mail and taking orders for papers. Some patients enjoy doing these and similar jobs.

Diet. Adequate nutrition is essential to increase or to maintain natural body resistance and to help in the repair of damaged lung tissue. Some patients may have lost weight, and they may lack appetite. If the patient is hospitalized, members of his family can help by occasionally preparing food and bringing it to him. It may replace the regular hospital meal, or it may be used as a supplement to the meal. The patient's appetite is sometimes improved by serving food requested since, when outlets for their interest are restricted, some patients may be too preoccupied with food and may gain weight. Occasionally persons with tuberculosis are overweight and reasonable dieting may be prescribed.

Surgical treatment

When medical treatment has failed to check and heal the disease process, surgical treatment for tuberculosis may be necessary. Surgical treatment for tuberculosis includes pneumonectomy, lobectomy, segmental lobe resection, and wedge resection. Usually parts of the lungs with active disease are resected, and as much unaffected lung tissue as possible is preserved. The nursing care and descriptions of operative procedures are explained later in this chapter in the section on thoracic surgery (p. 583).

Extrapulmonary tuberculosis

Tuberculosis may affect other parts of the body besides the lungs, such as the larynx, gastrointestinal tract, lymph nodes, skin, skeletal system, nervous system, and urinary (p. 453) and reproductive systems.

Tuberculous meningitis. The onset of symptoms of tuberculous meningitis usually is sudden. The patient has marked constipation, an elevation of temperature, chills, headache, convulsions, and sometimes loss of consciousness. If untreated, this disease causes death, but with the use of antituberculosis drugs it is usually controllable. A 12-month course of chemotherapy is essential, however, and the nurse must help the patient and his family realize that it is absolutely necessary. Streptomycin, isoniazid, and PAS are all given concurrently. Nursing care is the same as that for any other type of meningitis.

Skeletal tuberculosis. Since the advent of antituberculosis drugs, better case finding methods, pasteurization of milk, and tuberculin testing of cattle, skeletal tuberculosis is growing less common. It is most common in children, but adults also are sometimes affected. Although tubercle bacilli may attack any bone or joint in the body, the spine, hips, and knees are most often involved. Deformities occur as a result of bone destruction. Tuberculosis of the spine is now rare in the United States. The "hunchback" deformity it causes can still be seen in some people, particularly in those who have come from countries where standards for pasteurization of milk and tuberculin testing of cattle were not rigid. (For nursing care of patients having tuberculosis of the spine, see specialized texts on orthopedic nursing.)

■ INFECTION WITH ATYPICAL ACID-FAST BACILLI

Pulmonary disease that is indistinguishable from tuberculosis can be produced by a number of species of mycobacteria other than *M. tuberculosis.* These organisms are strongly acid-fast, but differ from *M. tuberculosis* on culture. Four groups have been classified by Runyon: group I, *M. kansasii* (photochromogens); group II, scotochromogens, which are commonly found in soil and water; group III, Battey bacilli (nonchromogens), which are found mainly in Georgia; and group IV, *M. fortuitum* (rapid growers).[33] These atypical organisms are found in various geographic locations. Group I is the most widely distributed and many organisms have been identified in the Midwest. Group III is found more in the southeastern portion of the United States. The pulmonary disease caused by atypical bacilli closely resembles tuberculosis. The disease often causes lung cavities, responds poorly to antituberculosis drugs, and quite often requires surgery. It occurs most commonly in persons in high socioeconomic groups—especially those residing in suburban areas of large cities. As is true with tuberculosis, the disease is three to four times more common in men than in women. Most of those infected are middle-aged or older, and men with emphysema seem to be particularly susceptible. Atypical bacilli are not believed to be airborne; thus isolation is not required. Because of the seriousness of the pulmonary disease caused by these organisms, patients are usually given chemotherapy for at least 2 years and should have careful medical follow-up after discharge from the hospital. It is possible for persons to be infected with both tubercle bacilli and atypical bacilli at the same time.

■ CHRONIC OBSTRUCTIVE PULMONARY DISEASE

Chronic obstructive pulmonary disease (COPD) refers to diseases that produce obstruction of air flow and includes *asthma, chronic bronchitis,* and *pulmonary emphysema.* The disease spectrum associated with this diagnosis ranges from pure obstructive airway disease with the presence of bronchitis but no emphysema, through various combinations, to severe emphysema without significant bronchitis. The pathophysiologic processes that cause these changes are neither static nor are they necessarily progressive. Thus all stages are possible, from reversible abnormalities to relentlessly progressive cardiopulmonary insufficiency. There has been much confusion concerning the clinical usage of the terms "chronic bronchitis," "emphysema," and "asthma"; therefore the term "chronic obstructive pulmonary disease" is now frequently seen rather than a designation of the specific disease. However, as more is being learned regarding the pathophysiology involved in these diseases, the trend is once again to define each specific abnormality more precisely.[104a] These diseases often begin insidiously and progress slowly. Early symptoms may be only a slight morning cough and slight shortness of breath on exertion that the patient does not notice because he gradually reduces his activity to compensate for shortness of breath. By the time medical attention is sought, pathologic changes have occurred and symptoms are often moderately severe.

The incidence of chronic obstructive pulmonary disease has increased spectacularly in recent years. Between 1950 and 1966 the number of deaths from emphysema and chronic bronchitis increased 800%. By 1970 over 30,000 deaths were attributed to these diseases, and in 50,000 other deaths, chronic bronchitis or emphysema was listed as a contributory cause. These diseases are more prevalent among men than women, but the death rates for asthma and emphysema are now showing a higher percentage rate of increase in women than in men.[78]

Chronic bronchitis and emphysema

Chronic bronchitis and emphysema are discussed together for a number of reasons: they are difficult to differentiate clinically; they often co-exist in the same individual; and many of the medical and nursing care measures are similar. In specifying the differences that do exist, however, it is helpful to examine the effect that each disease has on the individual.

Chronic bronchitis is defined as follows:

. . . a clinical disorder characterized by excessive mucous secretion in the bronchial tree. It is manifested by chronic or recurrent cough. . . . Thus, the diagnosis of chronic bronchitis can be made only by excluding other bronchopulmonary or cardiac disorders as the sole cause of the symptoms.[7]

Pulmonary function studies demonstrate reduced expiratory flow rates, reduced vital capacity, and increased residual volume, but the total lung capacity is frequently within normal limits. As the disease progresses, hypoventilation occurs and arterial blood gases usually show a low *resting* pO_2 and, if the obstruction is severe, an elevated pCO_2. During exercise the pCO_2 increases and the pO_2 may also rise, perhaps because of an improvement in ventilation-perfusion relationships. Cor pulmonale (right ventricular hypertrophy, which develops as the result of increased pulmonary vascular resistance in response to hypoxemia and hypercapnia), right-sided heart failure, and respiratory failure are also frequent complications of chronic bronchitis. The patient is short of breath; he uses accessory muscles of respiration and complains of chronic cough and sputum production. His color is dusky to cyanotic and he is often stout to overweight in body build. Such patients are often termed "blue bloaters" because of their color, frequent hypoxia, and right-sided heart failure.[119]

Emphysema is defined in morphologic terms as follows:

. . . an anatomic alteration of the lungs characterized by an abnormal enlargement of the air spaces distal to the terminal non-respiratory bronchioles, accompanied by destructive changes of the alveolar walls.[7]

This destruction of tissue leads to physiologic obstruction by collapse of the airways on expiration. As a result, full exhalation is difficult and air trapping ensues. Pulmonary function studies demonstrate decreased expiratory flow rates, particularly forced expiratory volume and maximal midexpiratory flow, increased total lung capacity, and increased residual volume (p. 549). The vital capacity may be normal or only slightly reduced until late stages of the disease; thus the FEV_1/VC ratio is changed. Arterial blood gas tests of persons with emphysema usually show a normal pCO_2 and a pO_2 that is normal or only slightly low *at rest* but falls during exercise. Late in the course of the disease, the pCO_2 is elevated, and cor pulmonale and respiratory failure may arise as complications.[119]

Clinically, cough and sputum production are not striking symptoms unless there is a superimposed infection. Because of the increased total lung capacity, the diaphragm becomes relatively fixed in a flattened position. Many patients use abdominal muscles as well as other accessory muscles to aid breathing. Pursed-lip breathing is often done naturally by the patient as this aids exhalation. (Pursed-lip breathing on exhalation slows the expiratory flow rates and results in less of an increase in intrathoracic pressure that "pushes in" on the airways.) The patient with emphysema is often not as cyanotic as the patient with bronchitis; he is usually thin and often appears to have a barrel chest. Because *resting* hypoxemia is absent and ventilation is high, maintaining a normal pCO_2 despite abnormal gas exchange function, these patients are frequently termed "pink puffers."[119]

The specific etiology of these two diseases is not known, but their development has been related to inhaled irritants, especially cigarette smoke, and chronic infection. The only exception is the recent discovery of the relationship of familial emphysema to alpha-1 antitrypsin deficiency. Persons who have this deficiency may develop severe, disabling emphysema early in life, usually of the bullous type. (Bullae, large air spaces, are formed by the destruction of many alveoli.) The finding of low levels of alpha-1 antitrypsin in patients with emphysema indicates a need to screen relatives and provide counseling regarding the use of preventive measures.[67,72] The only way to prevent the development of emphysema is to avoid inhalation of irritants, especially cigarette smoke, and to seek prompt treatment of any respiratory infection.

The goals in the treatment of chronic bronchitis and emphysema are to improve ventilation and to overcome hypoxia. There is a variety of means by which these goals can be met and most of them are dependent on skilled nursing care if full benefit is to be derived.

Management. In order to improve ventilation the patient must avoid respiratory irritants. Since the single most important cause of respiratory irritation is cigarette smoke, the patient is urged to give up smoking. If his job involves inhaling dust or fumes, he may have to change occupations. He should also avoid breathing cold air and may benefit from a move to a warm, dry climate. Respiratory allergens to which the patient is sensitive should be avoided (p. 91).

Bronchodilators. Since most patients have a bronchospastic component to their disease, they are treated with bronchodilators. Both direct and indirect bronchodilators are used. *Direct bronchodilators* act on the smooth muscle of the bronchi to relieve spasm. These include aminophylline, isoproterenol (Isuprel), Bronkosol, and ephedrine preparations. Aminophylline is usually given as a rectal suppository or, in the acute situation, intravenously. The usual dose is 250 to 500 mg. ($3^3/_4$ to $7^1/_2$ grains). Isoproterenol is administered as an aerosol. Since it is an adrenergic agent, its side effects include tachycardia, tremor, and vasoconstriction. It should be used in small doses; usually 8 to 10 drops diluted in 4 ml. of saline solution are given. Bronkosol has less effect on cardiostimulating receptors, and therefore the incidence of tachycardia associated with its use is less, although it may still occur. The usual dose is 0.25 to 0.5 ml. in 4 ml. of saline solution. Commercially prepared pressurized cartridges containing these drugs are available. The usual dose is two deep inhalations of the medication three to four times a day. The patient should be instructed to reduce the frequency of administration if side effects occur. He also should be cautioned not to use them too often since high, frequent doses may make him resistant to the bronchodilating effect.

Indirect bronchodilators include the *adrenocortical steroids* and *antibiotics*. Because infections increase mucus production and further limit ventilation, antibiotic therapy is instituted at the first sign of infection. Since organisms causing respiratory infections are usually sensitive to broad-spectrum antibiotics, tetracycline is often initiated before culture and sensitivity studies are available. Some physicians prescribe antibiotics prophylactically either intermittently or continuously, and patients are instructed in the schedule to be followed. Patients with chronic obstructive pulmonary disease should receive flu vaccine (attentuated preparations of the current infecting strains) each fall to protect them from influenza. Because adrenocortical steroids reduce the inflammatory response seen in chronic bronchitis, they may also be prescribed. Prednisone in small doses is frequently used. If the patient has a positive tuberculin test, he will receive isoniazid prophylactically as long as he is receiving steroids. Occasionally a patient with bullous emphysema that is confined to one area of the lung may be treated by surgical resection of the involved area.

Attention is also directed to *liquefying secretions* so that they can be more easily expectorated. The best

liquefying agent is water, and the patient should have a fluid intake of 3 to 4 L./day. In addition, nebulized mist therapy with water, saline solution, or half-normal saline solution is administered using one of several types of equipment. (See discussion on nursing intervention, p. 569.)

Intermittent positive pressure breathing (IPPB). IPPB is often ordered as a means by which to administer aerosolized medications, both the bronchodilators and mucolytic agents. IPPB may also be used to increase alveolar ventilation and to make cough more effective. Positive pressure improves the inspiratory phase of ventilation and enhances the flow of air to the alveoli, since much of the work of breathing is done by the machine rather than the patient. However, this relief from the work of breathing lasts only the length of the treatment—usually 15 to 20 minutes three or four times a day. Also, the use of IPPB has become a controversial issue in recent years. Studies have shown that IPPB as a means for promoting increased alveolar ventila-

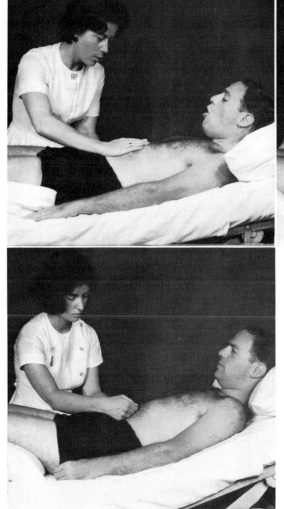

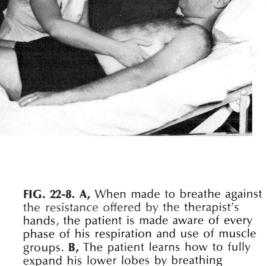

FIG. 22-8. **A,** When made to breathe against the resistance offered by the therapist's hands, the patient is made aware of every phase of his respiration and use of muscle groups. **B,** The patient learns how to fully expand his lower lobes by breathing against counterpressure applied to the side of the chest during inspiration. **C,** The patient is taught diaphragmatic control by breathing against a resistance applied in the costophrenic angle. (From Bendixen, H. H., and others: Respiratory care, St. Louis, 1965, The C. V. Mosby Co.)

tion, delivering aerosols, and removing secretions is no more, and possibly less, effective than other methods in patients who are able to deep breathe effectively by their own effort.[12,25,107] In those who are unable to do this, however, IPPB continues to be a useful method of treatment.[12,25,107] (See p. 594 for further discussion regarding positive pressure ventilators.)

Oxygen therapy. Oxygen may also be used. For patients with carbon dioxide retention, flow rates are adjusted so that the inhaled concentration of oxygen is not greater than approximately 30%. (See section on respiratory failure.) Some patients have to receive supplementary oxygen at home in order to maintain function. They may use oxygen continuously or only with exercise. Others may use it only at night when sleep and a supine position reduce ventilation.[1] Portable units with liquid oxygen are now available so that the patient's activity is not limited by the length of tubing connecting him to the oxygen source.

Pulmonary physiotherapy. Pulmonary physiotherapy, including breathing exercises, teaching the patient to cough effectively, and segmental postural drainage, is an important part of the treatment program. *Breathing exercises* are used to increase the efficiency of the patient's breathing pattern (Fig. 22-8). The patient with chronic obstructive pulmonary disease is taught to use a diaphragmatic pattern. In teaching, exhalation is stressed rather than inspiration. The patient is taught to exhale slowly and fully through *pursed lips,* contracting his abdominal mus-

cles. Manual pressure on the upper abdomen during expiration facilitates this maneuver. On inhalation through the nose, the abdominal muscles are relaxed. This technique will slow the respiratory rate, encourage deep breathing, and facilitate expiration. The patient is taught to use this "controlled" breathing pattern while performing various activities of daily living—from sitting, standing, walking, and climbing stairs to more complex activities. As this pattern becomes natural to the patient, he will be able to use it during periods of increased shortness of breath. Patients who do not know how to use controlled breathing tend to increase their respiratory rate and their work of breathing when they are short of breath. As a result, physiologic obstruction increases, oxygen requirements increase, and effective ventilation decreases. Changing a patient's respiratory pattern requires a great deal of effort by both the patient and those caring for him.

This same method of teaching diaphragmatic breathing can be used to teach the patient to cough. The difference is that expiration is forced down to residual volume. This maneuver often stimulates the cough reflex. If it does not, the patient is taught to actively cough at the end of full expiration. Physiologically, forced expiration simulates the effects of a cough and is therefore more effective than telling the patient to take a deep breath and cough.

Segmental postural drainage with clapping and vibration is a technique used to combine the force of gravity with the natural ciliary activity of the small

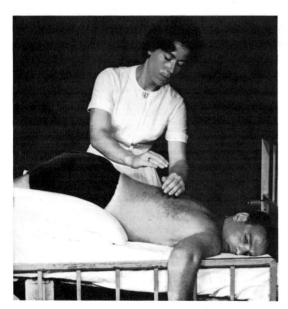

FIG. 22-9. In percussion, cupped hands are used to clap the chest wall with considerable force in order to shake loose sticky, thick secretions. The arm of the patient shown here should have been supported by a pillow. (From Bendixen, H. H., and others: Respiratory care, St. Louis, 1965, The C. V. Mosby Co.)

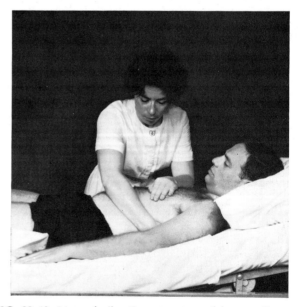

FIG. 22-10. Manual vibration at a rate of four to five per second is applied across the chest during a prolonged expiration, with the aim of shaking loose the secretions. (From Bendixen, H. H., and others: Respiratory care, St. Louis, 1965, The C. V. Mosby Co.)

bronchial airways to move secretions upward toward the main bronchi and the trachea. From this point the patient can cough them up, or they can be suctioned. In the treatment of chronic obstructive pulmonary disease, drainage of all segments is usually done by placing patients in various postural drainage positions (Fig. 22-14). Treatment may also be directed at draining specific areas of the lung. While the patient is in each position, *clapping* with a cupped hand is done over the area being drained. This maneuver helps to loosen secretions and stimulate coughing (Fig. 22-9). After clapping of the area for approximately 1 minute, the patient is instructed to breathe deeply. *Vibrating* (pressure applied with a vibrating movement of the hand on the chest) is done during the expiratory phase of the deep breath (Fig. 22-10). This assists the patient to exhale more fully. The procedure is repeated as necessary. Patients who are acutely ill may need to have some postural drainage positions modified or eliminated. For example, the patient with a tracheostomy often cannot be placed in a prone position. (See p. 575 and Kurihara[64] and Thacker[104] for further details about postural drainage.)

Nursing intervention. Nursing care is of prime importance if treatment programs are to be successful. Alert observation and intelligent, skilled nursing intervention are imperative; the nurse must be a competent teacher. Usually the care program for the patient in the hospital must also be carried out at home since chronic obstructive pulmonary disease cannot be cured. With professional supervision, the patient must continually treat himself if he is to maintain optimal function. Teaching is difficult because the patient is often depressed and anxious. He often has hypoxia, which decreases his mental alertness and acuity and his ability to do physical work.

Although pulmonary physiotherapy activities may be performed by a physical therapist, they are often part of the nurse's responsibility. Regardless of where the primary responsibility lies, nurses must be familiar with the techniques so that they can demonstrate and reinforce them and be sure that the patient is doing them correctly. Also, the need for pulmonary physiotherapy may occur at a time when the physical therapist is not available to the patient.

The nurse must be familiar with techniques of inhalation therapy. When used for intermittent treatments, IPPB is usually ordered at 15 to 20 cm. water pressure for 15 minutes three to four times a day. In acute situations, treatment may be ordered every hour. Many patients are at first unable to tolerate this high level of pressure. Initial treatments, therefore, may be begun at a lower pressure, for example 5 cm. of water, which is then gradually increased to the most effective level as the patient learns to use the machine correctly.

During use of IPPB the patient is taught to main-

tain a slow respiratory rate using a diaphragmatic respiratory pattern. It is important that expiration be prolonged, with the latter part of exhalation being active. Every several breaths the patient should deep breathe and exhale as fully as possible. Correct positioning, with the patient sitting upright unless contraindicated, is necessary to achieve the most beneficial effects. In addition, if clearance of secretions is an objective, he must be taught to cough effectively and should do this several times during the treatment and at the end.

Precautions to be taken when using IPPB equipment include those to protect the patient from cross contamination. Medication or water left in the tubing or nebulizer serves as a medium for bacterial growth, particularly of *Pseudomonas.* Use of individual tubing, nebulizer, and mask or mouthpiece as well as proper cleaning techniques and filters are recommended to prevent such cross contamination.[36,85] Other possible complications of IPPB are dizziness resulting from hyperventilation, which lowers pCO_2 levels; toxic drug reactions; gastric distention; exacerbation of hemoptysis; and ruptured alveoli. IPPB administered sooner than approximately 1 hour following meals may cause nausea and vomiting.

Inhalation therapy also includes *mist therapy.* There are various ways to administer mist. A small particle size is preferred, because large particles of mist are filtered out in the upper airway and never reach the lower airway where secretions collect. If an extremely small particle size is desired (one that can reach the smaller airways and alveoli), ultrasonic mist is used (Fig. 22-11). Nebulizers that are heated can produce a gas flow with a higher water vapor content than can those that are cold. Mist therapy is administered by mask, tent, or IPPB units. Individuals vary in their ability to tolerate mist therapy and in the amount or type of mist necessary to pro-

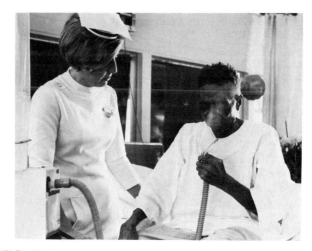

FIG. 22-11. Nurse specialist instructs the patient in the use of ultrasonic mist therapy. (Courtesy University Hospitals of Cleveland, Cleveland, Ohio.)

duce therapeutic effects. The high water content of air often makes patients who are already short of breath and anxious feel that they are suffocating. This is especially common if the patient is using a tight-fitting mask or if he is in a mist tent with an ultrasonic nebulizer. In a heavily misted tent the patient is unable to see out and therefore feels cut off from those caring for him. Claustrophobia is another common complaint. Ultrasonic mist temporarily increases the volume of secretions because of the added volume of water. The patient may therefore complain of increased shortness of breath until the secretions are expectorated. It may also induce bronchospasm; therefore treatment may be preceded by inhalation of a bronchodilating agent and the volume of mist carefully adjusted to avoid this complication. The nurse must closely observe both the physiologic and psychologic response so as to assure optimal therapeutic effects of the treatment without worsening the patient's condition. The patient should be encouraged to cough during and after the treatment. Because mist therapy is so effective in liquefying secretions, it is helpful before postural drainage. Controversy exists as to whether mist should precede or follow IPPB when both treatments are being used. Some feel that IPPB facilitates removal of secretions and therefore should be done after mist therapy has loosened secretions; others believe that IPPB given before mist will help to establish effective breathing patterns so that moisture will better penetrate the respiratory tract and, particularly if bronchodilators are being used, afford a degree of bronchodilation that will increase the effectiveness of the mist therapy and prevent bronchospasm.

Some of the bronchodilators and mucolytic agents are administered in aerosol form via nebulizers. Several types of nebulizers may be used. Some medications come in commercial metered-dose hand nebulizers, or the medication may be diluted with water or saline solution and administered via a hand bulb nebulizer. Another method is to connect a nebulizer by rubber tubing to a source of compressed gas (air or oxygen). Midway in the rubber tubing connection a Y tube is inserted. The air is turned on after the medication is placed in the nebulizer. Usually 4 to 6 L. of gas/minute is sufficient. The nurse should test the amount of spray briefly by placing a finger over the open end of the Y tube. If fine spray cannot be seen, the equipment is not working properly. With all methods the patient needs to be taught how to administer the drugs to himself. First, he should exhale fully (as described previously). Then, with the nebulizer positioned at the mouth but without his lips sealed around it, the patient takes a deep breath through his mouth. At the same time a mist is obtained from the nebulizer by squeezing the bulb or closing the Y tubing. The patient should hold his breath for 3 to 4 seconds at full inspiration and then exhale slowly, pursing his lips. The latter helps to

create increased pressure in the airways and carries the medication further into the bronchioles and alveoli.

Rehabilitation. It is now recognized that patients with chronic obstructive pulmonary disease can maintain a much higher level of functioning for longer periods than was once thought possible. The patient is no longer told, "You have emphysema—there is nothing we do to help you. Go home and don't overexert yourself." Many communities now have programs in pulmonary rehabilitation. Some of these programs are sponsored by the local Christmas Seal agencies, which are affiliates of the American Lung Association (ALA), and others are part of a hospital program.

Pulmonary rehabilitation programs stress the attainment and maintenance of optimal functioning for the individual patient. Emphasis is placed on bronchial hygiene, using all the measures described previously as well as physical retraining. Specific exercise programs vary, but all attempt to rebuild muscle strength so that the patient can undertake activity at a smaller oxygen cost to himself.* The psychosocial

*Details about breathing exercises can be found in Bendixen, H. H., and others: Respiratory care, St. Louis, 1965, The C. V. Mosby Co.; and Hass, A.: Essentials of living with pulmonary emphysema, a guide for patients and their families, Patient Publication no. 4, New York, 1963, The Institute of Physical Medicine and Rehabilitation.

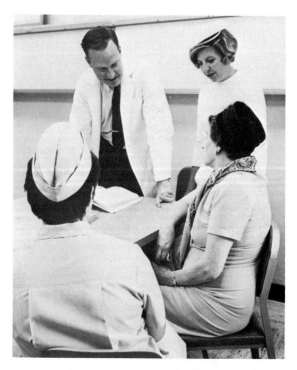

FIG. 22-12. Patient and visiting nurse discuss the patient's progress since discharge with physician and nurse clinician who cared for her during hospitalization. (Courtesy University Hospitals of Cleveland, Cleveland, Ohio.)

aspect of care is also stressed in these programs, which utilize a multidisciplinary approach whenever possible. Therapy is structured according to the individual's medical stability, physiologic need, stamina, personality, and life-style. Studies have shown that while overall lung function may not improve and the course of the disease is not halted, the patient and his family can be helped to cope with the symptoms of his disease and therefore to lead a more satisfying life.

Although it is difficult to measure the physiologic effects of these programs, hospitalization of patients who have participated in them is less frequent and most patients state that they feel better.[4] The patient is seen regularly by the physician, and it is extremely helpful if both the hospital and public health nurses are able to be involved in the long-term care of the patient (Fig. 22-12). In some centers, clinical nurse specialists follow the patients and refer them to the physician when problems requiring medical consultation arise.

Asthma

Asthma is discussed separately from bronchitis and emphysema because it results in intermittent rather than continuous airway obstruction. Its onset is sudden as opposed to the slow insidious progression of symptoms seen in bronchitis and emphysema. In differentiating asthma from other chronic obstructive pulmonary diseases, the American Thoracic Society has described it as follows:

. . . a disease characterized by an increased responsiveness of the trachea and bronchi to various stimuli and manifested by a widespread narrowing of the airways that changes in severity either spontaneously or as a result of therapy.[7]

The specific cause of asthma is as yet unknown. It may be classified as allergic (atopic) or nonallergenic; in some individuals, it may be both. In one third of asthmatics no allergic component can be demonstrated, and in many individuals no obvious cause for an attack can be identified. In individuals with allergic asthma, levels of immunoglobulins (IgE) are higher than normal, although there is no direct correlation between changed serum levels and the severity of an asthmatic attack.[103]

In those whose asthma is caused by allergy, attacks are precipitated by contact with the allergen to which they are sensitized. In nonallergenic asthma, attacks may be precipitated by different factors at different times. Infections, emotional stress, changes in temperature and humidity, irritating fumes and smoke, strong odors, and physical exertion have been known to induce these episodes. Hypoxemia, hypercapnia, and the overuse of bronchodilators may also lead to an acute asthmatic attack.[13,62,84]

Pulmonary function studies done during nonsymptomatic periods may show no significant changes. During periods of airway obstruction, however, FEV_1, FEV, and MVV are decreased, while FRC is increased. Hypoxemia may be present, the degree depending on the severity of the obstruction and the resultant changes in the $\dot{V}/\dot{Q}$ ratio. Pulmonary function studies for asthmatic patients include measurements before and after the use of a bronchodilator to determine therapeutic response.

Persons who have asthmatic attacks usually seek medical care because the attacks are both incapacitating and frightening. The patient must often make an attempt to lessen emotional stress and to control physical exertion since these factors are less amenable to management than are specific allergens. If the underlying cause of an allergy is obscure, if it is resistant to treatment, or if the patient has nonallergenic asthma, the recognition and control of secondary factors may be the main approach to treatment. It is imperative to understand that even though psychologic factors may precipitate an attack, the patient's response to it is physiologic and he requires the same treatment as that prescribed for an attack precipitated by an allergen or any other factor.

Nursing intervention. There is perhaps no disease in which knowing the patient well is more important than in asthma. Since sensitivity tests can be done with only a very small fraction of the substances with which the patient is in contact, the physician usually makes the diagnosis on the basis of a careful history. Knowing how the patient lives, how he spends his leisure time, what he eats, what type of work he does, his social contacts, and many other circumstances may give useful clues as to the cause of his asthma. Although the allergist urges patients to report seemingly trivial and insignificant details, patients often hesitate to do so since they are used to reporting only physical changes within themselves. The alert nurse can be of real help in learning the cause of an allergic reaction. It is often the nurse who may learn that a relative has just visited and was accompanied by a cat or dog. This information would be most important because animal dander is one of the most common allergens for individuals with atopic asthma.

The nurse may make observations regarding emotional stresses that appear to aggravate the patient's condition. Careful observation of his relationships with members of his family may give clues to sources of emotional stress. Some patients remain in the hospital during an acute episode and return home relieved of serious symptoms. However, unless his life circumstances can be altered, family relationships and general socioeconomic conditions that cause stress may send the patient back to the hospital with another attack.

Patients with chronic asthma may gain a sense of security while in the hospital and may be reluctant to return home. Asthmatic attacks can be precipitated by plans for discharge, and the patient's stay may thus be prolonged. Patients with severe emotional problems may find help in psychotherapy.

Signs and symptoms. Asthmatic attacks often occur at night. The person awakens with a feeling of choking. He can neither get enough air into his lungs nor can he breathe air out satisfactorily. The bronchioles react with swelling of the mucosa, muscle spasm (bronchospasm), and increased amount of thick secretions. The patient's breathing has a characteristic wheezing sound as he attempts to draw air through the constricted and obstructed airways. Cyanosis may develop. When an attack starts, the patient should sit upright. He should be given something on which to lean forward, such as an overbed table. During an acute attack the patient uses the accessory muscles of respiration in his effort to get enough air, and leaning forward helps him to use them more effectively. Since his only concern during an acute attack is breathing, he must be protected from falling and from other injury. He should be given medication for relief of the attack as soon as possible, and he should be constantly attended until acute symptoms subside. The attack usually ends with the patient coughing up large quantities of thick, tenacious sputum. He may become completely exhausted from increased physical effort, and he should rest quietly after the attack. He usually perspires profusely, and he may need change of clothing and special protection from chilling. Most attacks subside in $1/2$ to 1 hour, although asthmatic attacks associated with infection may continue for days or weeks.

Patients who are severely affected with asthma and who have attacks that are difficult to control with the usual medications may develop *status asthmaticus*. In this case the symptoms of an acute attack continue despite measures to relieve them. The patient is acutely ill. When he is admitted to the hospital, he needs emergency treatment. A prolonged attack causes exhaustion, and death from heart failure may occur. Oxygen is administered, and positive pressure may be used intermittently. In extreme cases, when the air passages appear seriously obstructed, a mixture of helium and oxygen may be given by endotracheal tube or by mask. Helium has a higher rate of diffusion and a lighter molecular weight than oxygen, so it can be inhaled with less effort. During an acute attack the alveoli progressively distend as in emphysema; actually acute emphysema exists. Unless relaxation of the bronchioles can be accomplished, insufficient oxygen passes through the alveolar membrane into the bloodstream (hypoxemia), and the patient becomes progressively more cyanotic. The patient needs constant observation, and he should have everything done for him. Repeated attacks of status asthmaticus may cause irreversible emphysema, resulting in a permanent decrease in total breathing capacity.

Some patients have *chronic mild asthma*. Symptoms are not noticeable when the patient is at rest. However, after exertion such as laughing, singing, vigorous exercise, or emotional excitement, the patient develops dyspnea and wheezing. These attacks are controlled with medications, and patients usually can continue their usual mode of living with few modifications and no serious lung changes. They are not hospitalized but they sometimes come to outpatient clinics for medical supervision.

Management. The management of asthma is directed toward symptomatic relief of attacks, the control of specific causative factors, and the general care for maintenance of optimum health. The chief aim of various medications is to afford the patient immediate and progressive bronchial relaxation. A drug often given to control mild attacks is *epinephrine* (Adrenalin), which relaxes smooth muscles in the respiratory tract and counteracts the bronchial constriction that occurs during attacks. Epinephrine, 0.2 to 0.5 ml. of a 1:1,000 solution, is given subcutaneously or intramuscularly and may be repeated every 5 to 10 minutes for two or three doses. Sometimes epinephrine in oil, 0.2 to 0.5 ml. of a 1:500 solution, is ordered to be given intramuscularly every 6 to 12 hours. It provides slower systemic absorption and prolongs the effect. Some patients who have frequent mild attacks are taught to give their own injections, or a member of the family may be taught to give the injections.

Patients with chronic bronchial asthma are maintained at home on active drug therapy and return to the physician's office or the clinic for periodic supervision. Many patients take *ephedrine sulfate*, 25 mg. ($3/8$ grain), by mouth every 4 hours during the day. Ephedrine sulfate, like epinephrine, relaxes hypertonic muscles. The stimulating effects of ephedrine sulfate can be lessened by combining ephedrine with a mild sedative such as phenobarbital, 15 mg. ($1/4$ grain), taken by mouth several times a day. *Theophylline ethylenediamine* (aminophylline) may be given during acute attacks. The dosage is 0.25 to 0.5 Gm. ($3^3/4$ to $7^1/2$ grains) intravenously or intramuscularly. Aminophylline suppositories, 0.5 Gm. ($7^1/2$ grains), can also be given rectally every 8 to 12 hours. Tablets are available that combine theophylline, ephedrine, and phenobarbital (Tedral). Many patients are treated with other drugs to dilate the bronchi. These drugs are given by inhalation. The patient who is ambulatory will need instruction in the use of a nebulizer (p. 570). *Isoproterenol hydrochloride,* 0.5 ml. of a 1:200 solution, is often used.

Expectorants such as *potassium iodide* or *ammonium chloride* may be given to help loosen thick bronchial secretions. The dosage of potassium iodide is usually 0.3 Gm. (5 grains) by mouth three times a day after meals. Sedatives help to keep the patient quiet and to provide for better rest. However, they are used with caution to avoid depressing respiratory function and to avoid the danger of addiction. If a narcotic is needed, *meperidine hydrochloride* (Demerol), 50 mg. given intramuscularly every 4 hours, is used in preference to morphine. *Barbiturates* such as phenobarbital, 30 mg. ($^{1}/_{2}$ grain) by mouth every 4 hours during the day, and pentobarbital, 100 mg. ($1^{1}/_{2}$ grains) by mouth at night, help to give the patient steady sedation. *Codeine,* 15 mg. ($^{1}/_{4}$ grain), or *elixir of terpin hydrate with codeine,* 5 ml. (1 dram) every 4 hours, helps to control excessive coughing, thus permitting more rest. In asthma following infection, various antibiotics are used, depending on the organism involved. Adrenocorticosteroids are sometimes used for patients with severe asthma that does not respond favorably to other drug therapy. Their precise method of action is unknown, but it is thought that they may reduce edema of the bronchial airways. *Cromolyn sodium* (Aarane, Intal) is a new drug that inhibits the allergic response following exposure to specific antigens. It is used as a prophylactic measure and is of *no* benefit in the treatment of an acute attack of asthma.

■ MANAGEMENT OF THE PATIENT WITH PULMONARY DISEASE

Difficulty in breathing. The patient with pulmonary disease may have very slight or severe difficulty in breathing. There may be obstruction of the free passage of air through the bronchi and/or damage to lung tissues. The patient may have both of these difficulties. If so, more effort is required for breathing, and the patient is more aware of breathing. This is tiring and unpleasant. With increased difficulty in getting air, most patients become apprehensive and even panicky. A nurse who understands this can be a great comfort to the patient. The presence of another person often helps the patient to control fear and eases his efforts in breathing. The patient with chronic obstructive pulmonary disease has often discovered ways to minimize his breathing difficulties. The nurse should be alert to the patient's wishes about position, exercise, etc. and should utilize these in planning nursing care.

Position. The most comfortable position for more relaxed breathing is a semiupright or upright sitting position. In these positions the lungs and respiratory muscles are not cramped and thus are not working against resistance. A pillow placed lengthwise at the patient's back will support him and will keep the thorax thrust slightly forward, allowing freer use of the diaphragm and therefore deeper breathing. For patients who must be upright, the overbed table with a pillow on top can be used as a support and a resting place for the head and arms (Fig. 22-13). If the patient has marked breathing difficulty and is not sufficiently alert or is very alert and fearful, side rails

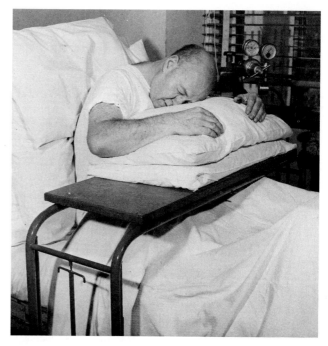

FIG. 22-13. Pillows placed on the overbed table provide a comfortable support for the patient who must sleep in a sitting position.

should be used for additional security. The patient may also use them to pull himself up into a higher sitting position. If the patient is at home, he may prefer to sit up in a large chair that supports him well and to lean toward a smaller chair placed in front of him. This chair should be blocked to prevent it from slipping.

Since the diaphragm becomes flattened and less active, some patients find breathing is helped by wearing an elasticized abdominal support. The support is often made of material similar to that used in elasticized girdles. Men may need to be persuaded to wear this kind of support but, on trial, learn how much the support adds to comfort and accept it quite readily. Pressure from the girdle must be from below the umbilicus upward so that the flattened diaphragm is forced up into the thorax.

Environment

Proper ventilation, humidity, and temperature of the room will help the patient to breathe more easily. Irritants such as smoke should be excluded. Patients may have preferences as to room temperature and amount of fresh air, and the nurse should respect those preferences. In general, most patients breathe more easily if the air is cool. An air-conditioned room may make breathing easier.

For patients with nose, throat, and bronchial irritation, warm, moist air produced by a *humidifier* or *vaporizer* may be beneficial. A vaporizer can be used to humidify the air throughout the room, or it can be put close to the patient so that he can inhale the steam as it is released. The large electrically operated vaporizers used in hospitals serve to moisten the air in the entire room. Water flowing from a gallon-sized jar is heated to form steam that is then directed out through a long, flexible spout. Inhalation of plain steam or of an aromatic medication such as tincture of benzoin or menthol is often ordered.

If the patient is at home, the nurse can help him and his family to improvise equipment for inhalations and for proper humidity. An empty coffee can or a shallow pie tin can be filled with water and placed on an electric plate in the patient's room to increase humidity. If the inhalation is to be directed, an ordinary steam kettle or a kettle with a longer improvised paper spout may be used. The paper should be changed frequently. A few drops of menthol or oil of eucalyptus can be put into the water. Benzoin will cause corrosion in the kettle, which is exceedingly difficult to remove. The kettle and electric plate should be placed a safe distance from the patient's face so that he can breathe the medicated steam, yet not be burned by accidentally tipping the kettle or by touching the hot plate. After the 25- to 30-minute treatment, equipment should be removed from the bedside.

Small electric vaporizers can be purchased at most local drugstores. They usually consist of a pint-sized or larger jar with a heating element extending into the jar. The jar should be filled with ordinary tap water and a pinch of salt added to hasten heating. The top of the jar holds a small, removable perforated cup, to which is attached a small metal spout. Cotton saturated with medication is placed inside the cup, and the small metal spout is fitted over the cup. As the water boils, the medicated steam is directed out through the small spout. Jars for the set are usually replaceable and inexpensive.

If breathing is so difficult that the patient cannot get enough oxygen from the air, it may be necessary to give additional oxygen. Dyspnea and cyanosis are not always present, and increased pulse rate may be the first detectable sign of oxygen shortage. The nurse, therefore, should check the patient's pulse rate carefully as well as his color and the character and the rate of respirations. Oxygen may be administered by nasal catheter, by nasal prongs, or by mask. The method used depends on the patient, his need, and the concentration of oxygen necessary. If oxygen is not readily available, increasing the amount of fresh air may help. The nurse should be familiar with operation of the various devices used to administer oxygen and should check frequently to note whether they are operating properly. (For details of nursing care of patients receiving oxygen, see texts on fundamentals of nursing.)

When the patient is having difficulty in the exchange of inspired and expired air, oxygen or some-times compressed air may be given under *positive pressure*. IPPB machines such as the Bennett respirator are most often used. These are discussed on p. 594. In an emergency, mouth-to-mouth breathing may be necessary (p. 262).

Continued uncorrected difficulty in breathing may cause an excess of carbon dioxide or a deficiency of carbon dioxide in the bloodstream. The former is due to incomplete exhalation and causes acidosis. The latter is due to hyperventilation and causes respiratory alkalosis (p. 118). If the patient's greatest difficulty is exhalation and if inspiration becomes slower and deeper, there is danger of carbon dioxide narcosis, and oxygen should *not* be given, since a low oxygen level in the blood may be the only stimulus for respiration. The nurse must notify the physician at once if this occurs. (See p. 590 for a discussion of respiratory insufficiency and failure.)

Coughing

Two of the most troublesome symptoms of respiratory disease are the increase in mucous secretions secondary to mucous membrane inflammation or allergic response and the stimulation of coughing due to irritation of the respiratory tract. If coughing is productive, the patient should be encouraged to cough in order to keep air passages clear and allow sufficient oxygen to reach the alveoli. Changing the patient's position will help to prevent pooling of secretions in the lungs and will stimulate coughing. The patient should be instructed to breathe as deeply as possible to loosen secretions and to stimulate productive coughing. For an effective cough, the patient should take a deep inspiration, contract the diaphragm and intercostal muscles, and exhale forcefully. Any sputum raised should always be expectorated, not swallowed. If he cannot cough forcefully enough to raise sputum and if his respirations are very shallow or sound very moist, he is given extra fluids or a medication to thin the secretions. The medication may be given as a nebulizer treatment so that it is applied topically to the respiratory passages.

Many patients with obvious, noisy respirations caused by accumulated sputum hesitate to cough because coughing causes pain. To assist such a patient the nurse's hands can be placed on the front and back of the chest to give support as the patient coughs (Fig. 22-16). A towel placed around the chest and held snugly as the patient coughs may also be used.

Although coughing is a physiologic protective reflex, constant nonproductive coughing and hacking can lead to exhaustion. Medications, therefore, are often prescribed for coughing. The type prescribed depends on the nature of the cough and the secretions. The purposes of various cough medications are to increase secretions, to decrease secretions, to thin secretions so that they can be raised and expectorated more easily, or to depress the cough reflex.

Sedative expectorants increase secretions, protect irritated membranes, and lessen the amount of coughing. Increased secretions may result in a productive cough and make paroxysms of coughing less frequent. For this purpose, ammonium chloride in wild cherry or orange syrup is often ordered, and other mixtures such as iodide solutions or ipecac syrup are sometimes used. Aerosolized normal or half-normal saline solution is also effective in thinning secretions. The mucolytic enzymes trypsin (Tryptar) and pancreatic dornase (Dornavac) are useful if the secretions are purulent. Stimulating expectorants such as terpin hydrate diminish secretions and promote repair and healing of the mucous membrane.

When the main objective of treatment is to suppress coughing, drugs depressing the cough center in the medulla are ordered. Codeine is frequently used and may be added to elixir of terpin hydrate, but there is danger of addiction with its prolonged use. Some nonnarcotic drugs with actions similar to codeine have been prescribed widely. Among them are dextromethorphan (Romilar hydrobromide) and noscapine (Nectadon).

When respiratory difficulty is severe, secretions are present, and coughing is unproductive, intratracheal suctioning and occasionally bronchoscopy are necessary. By means of bronchoscopy, mucus plugs may be loosened or removed and intratracheal suctioning made more effective. Equipment for emergency bronchoscopy may be kept in the patient's room. When this procedure is ordered the nurse must see that electrical outlets are adequate and that the necessary equipment is assembled in one place and ready for immediate use. (See p. 551 for care of the patient during bronchoscopy.)

Postural drainage. Segmental postural drainage for the care of patients with chronic obstructive pulmonary disease is described on p. 568. However, patients with other respiratory conditions may also require postural drainage and it is discussed further here (Fig. 22-14). Postural drainage may be used to assist the patient who has difficulty in raising sputum. By means of gravity, secretions flow into the bronchi and trachea and into the back of the throat and can be raised and expectorated more easily. A position providing gravity drainage of the lungs can be achieved in several ways, and the procedure selected usually depends on the age of the patient and his general condition as well as the lobe or lobes of the lungs where secretions have accumulated. The young patient may tolerate greater lowering of the head than an elderly patient, whose vascular system adapts less quickly to change of position. A severely debilitated patient may only be able to tolerate slight changes in position.

Postural drainage achieved merely by putting blocks under the casters at the foot of the bed sometimes produces excellent results. The footboard of the bed may also be supported on the seat of a firm

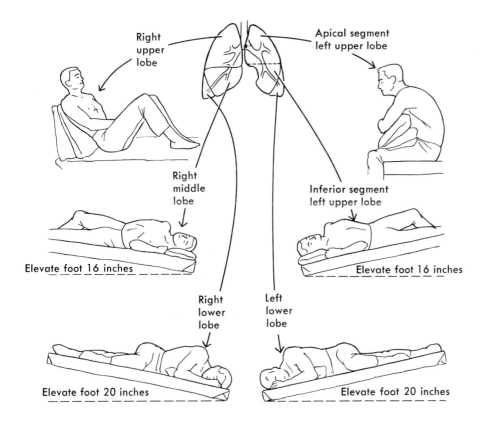

Right upper lobe

Apical segment left upper lobe

Right middle lobe

Inferior segment left upper lobe

Elevate foot 16 inches

Elevate foot 16 inches

Right lower lobe

Left lower lobe

Elevate foot 20 inches

Elevate foot 20 inches

FIG. 22-14. Postural drainage requires that the patient assume various positions to facilitate the flow of secretions from various portions of the lung into the bronchi, trachea, and throat so that they can be raised and expectorated more easily. Drawing shows the correct position to drain various portions of the lung.

chair to provide a position in which the head is lowered. Tilt boards (special tables that can be raised or lowered to any angle) or Stryker frames are sometimes used, but many physicians prefer raising the foot of the bed since this entails much less exertion for the patient.

The nurse should know the part of the lung affected and should help the patient assume a position that is best for draining that portion (Fig. 22-14). For example, if the right middle lobe of the lung is affected, drainage will be accomplished best by way of the right middle bronchus. The patient should lie on his back with his body turned at approximately a 45-degree angle. The angle can be maintained by pillow supports placed under the right side from the shoulders to the hips. The foot of the bed should then be raised about 12 inches. This position can be maintained fairly comfortably by most patients for half an hour at a time. On the other hand, if the lower posterior area of the lung is affected, the foot of the bed

can be raised 18 to 20 inches with the patient assuming a prone position for drainage. A summary of the positions for segmental postural drainage is given in Table 22-1.

Postural drainage and percussion should be planned so as to achieve maximum benefit. The best time is generally in the morning soon after arising and at night prior to retiring. Frequency of treatments will depend on each patient's needs, but care should be taken to avoid exhaustion, which only leads to shallow ventilation and negates the positive effects of the treatment.

Patients having postural drainage of any kind are encouraged to breathe deeply and to cough forcefully to help dislodge thick sputum and exudate that is pooled in distended bronchioles, particularly after inactivity. Humidity, bronchodilators, or liquefying agents often are given 15 to 20 minutes before postural drainage is started, since they facilitate the removal of secretions. The patient may find that he

Table 22-1   Positions for segmental postural drainage, clapping, and vibrating

Area of lung	Position of patient	Area to be clapped and/or vibrated
Upper lobe		
Apical bronchus	Semi-Fowler's position, leaning to right, then left, then forward	Over area of shoulder blades with fingers extending over clavicles
Posterior bronchus	Upright at 45-degree angle, rolled forward against a pillow at 45 degrees on left and then right side	Over shoulder blade on each side
Anterior bronchus	Supine with pillow under knees	Over anterior chest just below clavicles
Middle lobe (lateral and medial bronchus)	Trendelenburg position at 30-degree angle or with foot of bed elevated 14 to 16 inches, turned slightly to left	Anterior and lateral right chest from axillary fold to midanterior chest
Lingual (superior and inferior bronchus)	Trendelenburg position at 30-degree angle or with foot of bed elevated 14 to 16 inches, turned slightly to right	Left axillary fold to midanterior chest
Lower lobes		
Apical bronchus	Prone with pillow under hips	Lower third of posterior rib cage on both sides
Medial bronchus	Trendelenburg position at 45-degree angle or with foot of bed raised 18 to 20 inches, on right side	Lower third of left posterior rib cage
Lateral bronchus	Trendelenburg position at 45-degree angle or with foot of bed raised 18 to 20 inches, on left side	Lower third of right posterior rib cage
Posterior bronchus	Prone Trendelenburg position at 45-degree angle with pillow under hips	Lower third of posterior rib cage on both sides

can raise sputum on resuming an upright position even though no drainage appeared while he was lying with his head and chest lowered.

Since some patients complain of dizziness when assuming positions for postural drainage, the nurse should stay with the patient during the first few times and should report any persistent dizziness or unusual discomfort to the physician. Postural drainage may be contraindicated in some patients because of heart disease, hypertension, increased intracranial pressure, extreme dyspnea, or age. However, most patients can be taught to assume the positions for postural drainage and can proceed without help.

Chest percussion (clapping) is contraindicated in the case of pulmonary emboli, hemorrhage, exacerbation of bronchospasms, and severe pain and over areas of resectable carcinoma. Often patients with a chronic problem need to be taught to do postural drainage independently so that they can continue at home. The position usually is maintained for 10 minutes at first, and the period of time is gradually lengthened to 15 to 20 or even 30 minutes as the patient becomes accustomed to the position. At first, elderly patients usually are able to tolerate these positions only for a few minutes. They need more assistance than most other patients during the procedure and immediately thereafter. They should be assisted to a normal position in bed and requested to lie flat for a few minutes before sitting up or getting out of bed. This helps to prevent dizziness and reduces the danger of accidents.

The patient may feel nauseated because of the odor and taste of sputum. Therefore the procedure should be timed so that it comes at least 1 hour before meals. A short rest period following the treatment often improves the appetite. The patient needs mouth care following postural drainage. Aromatic mouthwashes should be available for frequent use by any patient who is expectorating sputum freely.

Care of sputum. Since the causative organisms may not be known early in the respiratory disease, the nurse should use caution in the disposal of sputum and should instruct the patient how to protect others. The patient who is coughing or clearing his throat forcefully should be instructed to cover his mouth and nose with several thicknesses of disposable tissues to prevent possible spread of infectious organisms. The nurse should be calm and matter-of-fact in doing this so that the patient does not feel that he is dangerous to others or that he has some dread disease. Used tissues should be folded carefully and placed in a paper bag or flushed directly down the toilet. If a bag is used, it should be closed and preferably burned. Used tissues should be collected from the bedfast patient at frequent intervals, and whoever handles the bags should wash his hands thoroughly to avoid transfer of infection to others.

If the patient has a copious amount of sputum, he may be instructed in the use of a sputum cup. Waxed paper cups with lids may be used. In some hospitals the waxed paper cups are placed in metal containers. At least once daily the inner cup should be discarded and a fresh one provided. The metal containers frequently become contaminated with sputum and therefore should be washed and boiled often. Some hospitals have a schedule for boiling them daily.

If the patient cannot care for and dispose of his own sputum, he must have assistance. Tissues may be placed in the patient's hand, and a paper bag may be placed on each side of the bed so that he does not have to turn to dispose of the soiled tissues. The bedfast patient who handles his own sputum should be offered soap and water with which to wash his hands before meals.

Appetite and nutrition

The odor and taste in the mouth caused by frequent raising of sputum may seriously affect appetite and may impair nutrition. Provision should be made for oral hygiene before meals, washing of hands should be encouraged, and sputum cups or other evidence of sputum should be removed before meals are served. Some patients find that a strong, clear, well-seasoned broth helps to make the mouth feel fresher and improves appetite for the rest of the meal. Other patients report that beginning a meal with acid fluids such as grapefruit or tomato juice improves acceptance of other food. The nurse should report food preferences to the dietitian.

Frequently patients with breathing difficulties tolerate regular full meals poorly. Smaller and more frequent meals are taken with greater comfort, and thus nutrition is maintained. Gas-forming foods should be avoided. Taking fluids frequently also helps to keep mucous secretions thin. The patient should try to take fluids every few hours. This measure will also help to counteract constipation and thereby lessen straining and exertion.

Rest

Adequate rest is important in combating respiratory disease. During respiratory illness, however, normal sleep may be interrupted for a number of reasons. The patient may be plagued with frequent coughing, and breathing may be difficult. Airways may become blocked with secretions, and the patient may be awakened by the resultant increased difficulty in breathing.

The nurse should be alert for signs of what irritates the patient, precipitates cough, and therefore prevents rest. For example, excessive talking, smoking, or laughing or sitting in a draft or in a dry, overheated room may predispose to coughing. Cough medications given before the hour of sleep and when rest is disturbed by coughing are often helpful. However, when the patient has noisy breathing and it is obvious that secretions are present in the respiratory tract, he should be encouraged to cough deeply and to expectorate until the airway is free of obstruction before medication is given. A suitable position in bed and changes in position also help the patient to rest more quietly. Room temperature and ventilation should be kept at what the patient feels is best for him.

Prevention of new infection

Patients with any type of respiratory disease should protect themselves against exposure to new infection. They should avoid outdoor exertion in cold weather and extremes of cold or humidity. If they must go out in cold, damp weather, warm clothing should be worn. If the clothing gets wet, it should be changed immediately. Smoking should be discouraged. Undue emotional stress may also lessen the patient's resistance and increase susceptibility to additional infection.

■ OTHER CHRONIC LUNG DISEASES

Bronchiectasis

Bronchiectasis means dilation of the bronchus or bronchi. When infection attacks the bronchial lining, inflammation occurs and an exudate forms. The progressive accumulation of secretions obstructs the bronchioles. The obstructed bronchioles then break down and enlarge, appearing saccular and cylindric in shape (saccular bronchiectasis). Their expulsive force is diminished, and they may remain filled with exudate. Only forceful coughing and postural drainage will empty them. Bronchiectasis may involve any part of the lung parenchyma, but it usually occurs in the dependent portions or lobules. Prior to the widespread use of antibiotics in treating patients with respiratory infections, this disease began in young people, many patients showing symptoms in childhood or by the age of 20. Although the incidence of childhood bronchiectasis is decreasing, it is increasing in individuals with cystic fibrosis, immune-deficiency diseases, or atopic asthma in which repeated respiratory infections have been successfully treated with antibiotics. These patients now survive the acute episodes of bacterial infection that complicate their underlying disease but not infrequently develop bronchiectasis as a sequela. If the disease is widespread, it may resemble other forms of chronic obstructive lung disease, with generalized wheezing and eventual progression to cor pulmonale.[119] A contributing factor in bronchiectasis may be a congenital weakness in the structure of the bronchi that results in impairment of elasticity. Bronchiectasis may occur without previous pulmonary disease, but it usually follows such diseases as bronchopneumonia, lung abscess, tuberculosis, or asthma.

Symptoms of bronchiectasis vary with the severity of the condition. The patient may complain of fatigue, weakness, and loss of weight. Appetite can be affected by the fetid sputum. The condition may develop so gradually that the patient is often unable to tell when symptoms first began. Clubbing of the fingers is common, as it is in other chronic respiratory disease. The patient's chief complaint in bronchiectasis is severe coughing (brought on by changing position) that is productive of large amounts of blood-tinged sputum and causes dyspnea. The patient may have a paroxysm of coughing when he gets up in the morning and again when he lies down.

Treatment of bronchiectasis is not very satisfactory. Surgical removal of a portion of the lung is the only cure (p. 584). Therefore patients who have bronchiectasis that involves both lungs are not candidates for surgery and do not have a good prognosis. The life expectancy usually is considered to be no more than 20 years. Many patients develop cardiac complications resulting from the extra strain on the heart caused by inability of the lungs to oxygenate the blood adequately.

Postural drainage at least twice a day helps to remove secretions and thus helps to prevent coughing (p. 575). During severe episodes of coughing the patient should not be left alone, since a large plug of thick secretion may block a large bronchiole and cause severe dyspnea and cyanosis. Occasionally a bronchoscopy may be done to remove the plug of mucus or to break adhesions that may be interfering with postural drainage by blocking passage to the main bronchi. Antibiotics may be used in the treatment of bronchiectasis. Although they do not cure the condition, they may prevent further infection and are often used prior to surgery. If the involvement of the lung is widespread, oxygen may be used. Nursing care should stress good general hygiene, which may contribute to relief of symptoms. Adequate diet, rest, exercise, and diversional activity are important, and avoiding superimposed infections such as colds should be emphasized. Frequent mouth care is essential, and cleansing the mouth with an aromatic solution before meals often makes food more acceptable.

Pulmonary fibrosis

Pulmonary fibrosis is a diffuse interstitial disease of the lung. It is seen in a wide variety of diseases, but the specific cause and etiology are often unknown. Pulmonary fibrosis may develop as a reaction to noxious gas inhalation, to silicosis, or to radiation; it may develop in collagen disease, extensive tuberculosis, and many other diseases. Hamman-Rich disease is a syndrome of pulmonary fibrosis of unknown cause.

The patient with pulmonary fibrosis is short of breath because of his "small lung" and problems with gas exchange. Blood gas findings demonstrate hypoxemia and often hypercapnia. Clubbing of the fingers is also a common sign. Cardiac complications may follow, since heart action must be increased to make up for respiratory impairment. There is no cure and no specific treatment for pulmonary fibrosis, but adrenocortical steroids are often helpful in reducing pulmonary dysfunction and in relieving symptoms. The patient is cautioned to avoid strenuous exercise that will tax the respiratory and cardiac systems and, above all, to guard against exposure to upper respiratory infection.

Histoplasmosis

Histoplasmosis is a fungus disease that affects the lungs. Its incidence is quite high in the United States, and it is especially common in certain areas of the central and eastern part of the country. Endemic areas have been identified in the St. Lawrence, Ohio, and Mississippi Valley areas. It is not communicable from man to man. Organisms are transmitted to man by inhaling spores that thrive in moist, dark, protected soil. The disease masquerades as either influenza or chronic tuberculosis with cavities. Chest films demonstrate a nodular infiltrate. Special stains are required to see *Histoplasma capsulatum* on sputum smears. Skin tests for histoplasmosis are available, but if active disease is suspected, a serum complement fixation test should be obtained rather than using the skin test. Skin testing with histoplasmin is helpful in screening programs, although it is not as reliable as is tuberculin skin testing.

The signs and symptoms of histoplasmosis show a variable range from those of a slight self-limited infection to fatal disseminated disease. Severe infections are characterized by prolonged fever, chest pain, dyspnea, prostration, weight loss, widespread pulmonary infiltrates, hepatomegaly, and splenomegaly. Some infected persons may have only a benign acute pneumonitis lasting a week or less, while others may be symptom free.

Histoplasmosis responds to treatment with an antibiotic drug, *amphotericin B*. Since it must be given intravenously and causes toxic reactions such as gastrointestinal symptoms, headache, cough, and decreased renal clearances, the patient is hospitalized and observed closely during treatment. The infusion containing the drug is given over a 5- or 6-hour period. It is administered every other day for about 8 weeks. Acetylsalicylic acid and promethazine hydrochloride, an antiemetic antihistamine, are often given a half hour before the infusion is started and repeated as necessary. Hydrocortisone may be given to reduce the side effects. A blood urea nitrogen test or nonprotein nitrogen determination is usually taken every 2 to 3 days during treatment because ampho-

tericin may cause kidney damage. Any symptoms of potassium deficiency (p. 116) or anemia (p. 411) should be reported to the physician at once. The general nursing care is similar to that for the patient with noninfectious tuberculosis.

Nurses working in areas where this disease is prevalent have an important role in helping to locate sources of infection and in teaching the public to prevent inhalation of potentially infected material. Since the disease can be fatal and children appear to be particularly susceptible, the nurse should point out potential danger to rural families when it is known that the soil is contaminated.

■ OTHER CHEST CONDITIONS

Lung abscess

A lung abscess is an area of localized suppuration within the lung. It usually is caused by bacteria that reach the lung through aspiration. The infected material lodges in the small bronchi and produces inflammation. Partial obstruction of the bronchus results in the retention of secretions beyond the obstruction and the eventual necrosis of tissue. Before the advent of antibiotics and specific chemotherapy, lung abscess was a fairly frequent complication following pneumonia. When a lung abscess forms, various organisms are found. Lung abscess may follow bronchial obstruction caused by a tumor, a foreign body, or a stenosis of the bronchus. Children particularly may aspirate foreign material such as a peanut, and a lung abscess results. Metastatic spread of cancer cells to the lung parenchyma may also cause an abscess, and occasionally the infection appears to have been borne by the bloodstream. In recent years the incidence of lung abscess due to infection has decreased, and secondary lung abscess following bronchogenic carcinoma has increased.

Symptoms of lung abscess include cough, elevation of temperature, loss of appetite, malaise, and, if the condition is of long standing, clubbing of the fingers. Unless the abscess is walled off so that there is no access to the bronchi, the patient usually raises sputum. There may be hemoptysis, and often the patient raises dark brown ("chocolate-colored") sputum that contains both blood and pus.

The patient's course in lung abscess is influenced by the cause of the abscess and by the kind of drainage that can be established. If the purulent material drains easily, the patient may respond well to segmental postural drainage, antibiotic therapy, and good general supportive care. When obstruction interferes with drainage into the bronchi, bronchoscopic procedures should be employed not only to improve drainage but to rule out obstructing foreign bodies or neoplasms.[66] Today, surgical treatment to establish drainage has become increasingly less necessary, but if after several weeks of medical treatment a cavity persists, a segmentectomy or lobectomy may be performed.

Medical treatment cannot cause a walled-off abscess to disappear, and surgery may be necessary. If surgery is done, the portion of lung containing the abscess is removed. If the abscess is due to carcinoma, the surgery may be much more extensive.

Empyema

Empyema means pus within a body cavity. It usually applies to the pleural cavity. Empyema occurs as a result of, or in association with, other respiratory disease such as pneumonia, lung abscess, tuberculosis, and fungous infections of the lung and also following thoracic surgery or chest trauma. It is now occurring fairly often as a complication of staphylococcal pneumonia. The patient with any kind of lung infection or chest injury should be observed closely for signs of empyema, which include cough, dyspnea, unilateral chest pain, elevation of temperature, malaise, poor appetite, and unequal chest expansion. The condition may develop several weeks after an apparently minor respiratory infection. The diagnosis can usually be made from the signs and symptoms and the medical history, but it is confirmed by a chest radiograph that demonstrates the presence of a pleural exudate. A thoracentesis is done to obtain a sample of the pus for culture and sensitivity studies and to relieve the patient's respiratory symptoms.

The aim in the treatment of empyema is to drain the empyema cavity completely and thus obliterate the pleural space. This can be accomplished in several ways. Initially the cavity may be aspirated daily and antibiotics instilled in it in an attempt to sterilize this space. If the cavity cannot be evacuated within a few days or if the lung fails to reexpand so as to obliterate the space, surgical treatment is necessary. Depending on the situation, either closed or open chest drainage may be employed. In closed chest drainage a trocar is inserted between the ribs at the base of the empyema cavity. A chest catheter is then threaded through the trocar, the trocar is removed, and the tube is connected to water-seal drainage (p. 586). This allows the pus to drain from the cavity into the water-seal bottle. It will only be effective, however, if the pus is thin and easily removed and if the visceral pleura is capable of moving out to the parietal pleura to eliminate the space. When empyema is chronic and the lung is adherent to the chest wall, rib resection with open drainage is often employed. In this procedure a portion of one or two ribs is removed. A large tube is inserted into the cavity and allowed to drain into a chest dressing. The tube is changed weekly. If this method of treatment is successful, the empyema cavity will gradually be eliminated. In some instances of chronic empyema a fibrinous peel forms on the visceral pleura, keeping the lung from reexpanding and filling the space left after the empyema cavity was drained. In this situation a *decortication* is performed. In decortication the fibrinous peel is removed from the lung by blunt dissection, freeing the lung so that it can expand and fill the pleural space. In order to assure that expansion will occur, chest tubes are inserted into the pleural space and connected to water-seal drainage and suction. When there is evidence that the lung has reexpanded the tubes are removed. (See p. 587 for further discussion of chest drainage.) If none of these methods are successful in closing the pleural space, a thoracoplasty (removal of ribs) may be necessary.

Carcinoma

During the last 40 years there has been a startling increase in the incidence of carcinoma of the lung. There were nearly 72,000 deaths from carcinoma of the lung in 1973.[6] It is the leading cause of cancer deaths in males, the rate being 14 times greater than 40 years ago. The death rate in females, although lower than in males, is increasing at a much faster rate. It was estimated that in 1974 the male death rate would increase 3% over 1973 and the female rate 10%.[6] Most people who develop the disease are over 50 years of age. Some of the factors believed to be involved in this increase in incidence of carcinoma of the lung include more accurate diagnosis and a tendency to name the lung as the primary site.

The cause of carcinoma of the lung is closely related to cigarette smoking. The death rate is 10 times as high among regular cigarette smokers as among nonsmokers. The rate is 20 times as high for those who smoke two packs or more daily.[6] Prevention is the best protection against carcinoma of the lung because early detection of the disease is difficult, and at the present time only about 1 patient in 20 (5%) is "cured" (living at the end of 5 years). From available research data it seems evident that curtailing smoking is a primary preventive measure. The nurse should be active in teaching the dangers in smoking and should set a good example for others in this regard. It is especially important that teenagers be given specific facts concerning the dangers involved in cigarette smoking because they are not likely to be habitual smokers at that age. Recent studies indicate that the incidence of smoking among teenagers is on the increase. People who are already habitual smokers should also be urged to stop smoking, even though it may be very difficult for them to do so. Various types of programs to assist persons stop smoking are described by Hunt and Bespalec.[55] Since air pollution affects the lungs and may predispose to the development of carcinoma, the nurse should encourage and actively support community programs to decrease the amount of air pollution. Industrial exposure, particularly to asbestos, is also associated with an increased risk of carcinoma.

Carcinoma of the lungs may be either metastatic

or primary. Metastatic tumors may follow malignancy anywhere in the body. Metastasis from the colon and kidney is common. Metastasis to the lung may be discovered before the primary lesion is known, and sometimes the location of the primary lesion is not determined during the patient's life.

Since most new growths in the lungs arise from the bronchi the term *"bronchogenic"* carcinoma is widely used. The symptoms that a patient has will depend on whether the neoplasm is located peripherally or centrally. Peripheral lesions may not cause any symptoms and be discovered only on routine chest radiographs. If peripheral lesions perforate into the pleural space, there will be *pleural effusion* (fluid in the pleural space) and direct invasion of ribs and vertebral bodies may follow. If this occurs, the pain may be severe.

Centrally located lesions arise from one of the larger branches of the bronchial tree. They cause obstruction and ulceration of the bronchus with subsequent distal suppuration. Symptoms include cough, hemoptysis, dyspnea, chills, and fever. Unilateral wheezing may be heard on auscultation.

In the later stage of the disease, weight loss and debility usually indicate metastases, especially to the liver. Carcinoma of the lung may metastasize to nearby structures such as the prescalene lymph nodes, the walls of the esophagus, the pericardium, or the heart or to distant areas such as the brain, liver, or skeleton.

Time is very important in the treatment of lung cancer. If carcinoma is detected while it is still confined to a local area, immediate surgery, with removal of all or part of a lung (pneumonectomy or lobectomy), may be successful. The nursing care of the patient following surgery of the lung is discussed later in this chapter. *Unfortunately about one third of the lesions are inoperable at the time the patient seeks medical attention and an additional one-third are found to be inoperable on surgical exploration. Of the one-third who are operable, the mortality rate is about 10% for pneumonectomy and between 2% to 3% for lobectomy.*

Palliative treatment (irradiation, chemotherapy, or both) may be used for those patients who cannot be treated surgically, particularly when there is obstruction of an airway, obstruction of major vessels, severe pain, or recurrent pleural effusion. Irradiation prior to surgery is no longer widely used as studies have indicated no improvement in survival rates. Chemotherapy is used as additional therapy for some patients. (See p. 301 for a discussion of chemotherapy of cancer.)

Efforts to detect malignant lesions of the lung early while curative treatment may be possible must be continued. The nurse should urge all persons, particularly men over 40 years of age, to have an x-ray examination of the chest periodically in addition to a yearly physical examination. As a result of various public education media, many people have become more conscious of early signs of pulmonary cancer, but there is still a great need for them to learn about diagnostic tests that are available, including x-ray examinations, bronchoscopic examinations, and cytologic studies of sputum. The nurse should know of available cancer detection clinics in the community and should assist patients to secure proper medical supervision (Chapter 15).

Pulmonary embolism and pulmonary infarction

Pulmonary embolism is the lodgment of a clot or other foreign matter in a pulmonary arterial vessel, and pulmonary infarction is the hemorrhagic necrosis of a part of the lung parenchyma caused by interruption of its blood supply, usually as a result of embolism.[15]

The source of the embolism may be thrombi originating in the iliac, femoral, or pelvic veins; the prostatic venous plexus; the vena cava; and the right atrium. They are common in older patients who are confined to bed. Postoperative embolism usually comes from a thrombosed vein in the pelvis or the lower extremities. It may cause symptoms before any signs of venous thrombosis appear at its place of origin.

The size of the pulmonary artery in which the clot lodges and the number of emboli determine the severity of symptoms and the prognosis. If the embolus blocks the pulmonary artery or one of its main branches, immediate death may occur and it is often mistaken for a coronary occlusion. A recent study indicates that pulmonary emboli were found on autopsy in 30% to 50% of patients who died after surgery.[75a] If the embolus blocks a smaller vessel, the patient may complain of sudden sharp upper abdominal or thoracic pain, become dyspneic, cough violently, and have hemoptysis; shock may develop rapidly. If the area of infarction is small, the symptoms are much milder. The patient may have cough, pain in the chest, slight hemoptysis, and elevation of temperature with an increase of leukocyte count in the blood. An area of dullness can be detected by the physician on listening to the patient's chest sounds.

The diagnosis of pulmonary embolism is made by the clinical history, by changes in blood chemistries, and by chest films. Lung scans and pulmonary angiography are also done; pulmonary angiography is a definitive diagnostic tool if a sharp cut-off is seen. As recannulization often takes place rapidly, the procedure must be done in the acute phase, or else it may be negative. The diagnosis of pulmonary embolism is often, of necessity, based on clinical criteria alone. If the patient survives a severe pulmonary infarction, he needs immediate medical attention. While awaiting the physician he should be kept in bed and as quiet as possible. A high Fowler's position usually helps breathing. The subsequent medical and nursing care are similar to that needed by the patient who has an acute myocardial infarction (p. 343). If the infarction is a mild one, the treatment is more conservative and resembles that provided for the patient with pneumonia. In either case an immediate attempt is made to locate the original source of the embolus and to treat the thrombosis. (See articles by Le Quense[68] and Sasahari[93] for a detailed discussion of current therapy.)

The development of techniques to provide extracorporeal circulation (p. 365) has made it possible to remove emboli from the pulmonary arteries—a major step forward, since pulmonary emboli cause many deaths. At present this surgery is done quite rarely. The nursing care following pulmonary artery surgery combines that needed after any operation on major blood vessels (p. 390) and the postoperative care of patients having thoracic surgery as well as the care of the patient being treated medically for pulmonary embolism.

The best treatment for pulmonary embolism is prevention. Prevention of thrombophlebitis in patients undergoing surgery is discussed on p. 221. The same nursing measures should be used to prevent emboli in medical patients especially when the patient is elderly and has chronic vascular or cardiac disease.

Pneumothorax

Pneumothorax is a condition in which there is air in the pleural space between the lung and the chest wall (Fig. 22-15). It usually results from the rupture of an emphysematous bleb on the surface of the lung, but it may also follow severe bouts of coughing in persons who suffer from a chronic chest disease such as asthma. It also occurs when wounds have penetrated the chest wall and perforated the pleura. Rather frequently it occurs as a single or recurrent episode in otherwise healthy young people. As atmospheric pressure builds up in the pleural space, the lung on the affected side collapses and the heart and mediastinum shift toward the unaffected lung. If untreated, the patient may die.

A *spontaneous pneumothorax* occurs without warning. The patient has a sudden sharp pain in the chest, accompanied by dyspnea, anxiety, increased diaphoresis, weak and rapid pulse, fall in blood pressure, and cessation of normal chest movement on the affected side. When a spontaneous pneumothorax is suspected, a physician should be summoned immediately. The patient should not be left alone. He should be reassured and urged to be quiet and not to exert himself. Oxygen and equipment for a thoracentesis should be assembled at once. Air is immediately aspirated from the affected pleural space, and the intrapleural pressure is brought to normal if possible. If air continues to flow into the pleural space, contin-

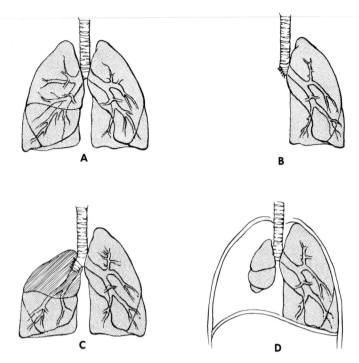

FIG. 22-15. A, Normal expanded lungs. **B,** Surgical absence of the right lung following a pneumonectomy. **C,** Surgical absence of the right upper lobe following a lobectomy. **D,** Complete collapse of the right lung due to air in the pleural cavity (pneumothorax).

uous drainage of air with closed chest drainage equipment is necessary. If the cause of the condition is trauma, the immediate treatment is to seal the chest wound and then to aspirate air from the pleural space.

The patient who has had a spontaneous pneumothorax is usually most comfortable in a sitting position. Physical activity is kept at a minimum for at least 24 hours. The patient is asked to remain as quiet as possible and to avoid stretching, reaching, or moving suddenly. He should breathe normally and not hold his breath. His pulse rate and respirations must be checked frequently. Radiographs are always ordered to determine the amount of air in the pleural space and the amount of collapse of the lung as well as the degree of mediastinal shift. When radiographs are taken, the patient needs help to prevent overexertion.

When air no longer is expelled from the pleural space through the underwater drainage system and a radiograph reveals that the lung has completely reexpanded, the chest tube is removed and the patient is allowed out of bed. He may be advised to avoid strenuous exertion, which increases rate and depth of respirations for a time, but usually he may return to relatively normal activity rather quickly. If there are frequent recurring episodes, some physicians instill silver nitrate into the pleural space to cause adhesions between the visceral and parietal pleurae.

If this procedure is unsuccessful, the portion containing the defect may be resected from the lung and the parietal pleura abraded to produce an adhesion to the faulty lung area.

■ THORACIC SURGERY

Many of the conditions and diseases described in the previous sections of this chapter are either entirely or partially corrected by a surgical procedure. Intelligent nursing care of patients undergoing thoracic surgery depends on knowledge of the anatomy and physiology of the chest, of the surgery performed, and of procedures and practices that assist the patient to recover from the operation. When endotracheal anesthesia became possible, surgery of the chest was given a great impetus. Before that time it had not been possible, except in the rarest of circumstances, to operate on the lung without causing collapse of the good lung and death. By means of endotracheal anesthesia, it is possible to keep the good lung expanded and functioning even when it is subjected to atmospheric pressure. Endotracheal anesthesia is used for surgery involving the lungs and for most chest surgery in which the pleural space is entered.

Principles of resectional surgery

In order to understand resectional surgery and the purpose of chest tubes and water-seal drainage, it is important to review a few points about the anatomy of the lung. The pleura, which lines the chest wall and covers the lung, is one continuous serous membrane. The portion that covers the lung is the *visceral pleura,* and that covering the inside of the chest wall is the *parietal pleura.* Together they form a *potential space,* which normally contains a few milliliters of serous fluid that lubricates the surfaces and prevents friction rub during respiration. The pressure in the pleural space is subatmospheric (less than 760 mm. Hg) and is referred to as being negative. This pressure is usually 756 mm. Hg and goes down to about 751 mm. Hg prior to inspiration. It is this change in pressure that allows air (atmospheric pressure) to enter and expand the lungs. The pressure within the lung itself *(intrapulmonic)* always remains near 760 (758 to 762) mm. Hg.

When the pleura is entered surgically or by trauma to the chest, atmospheric pressure (positive pressure) enters the pleural space and the lung collapses. Thus after resection of the lung (except pneumonectomy) two drainage tubes are inserted into the pleural space and each tube is connected to a water-seal drainage bottle. As long as the tip of the tube in the chest bottle is 1 to 2 cm. under water and all connections between it and the patient's chest tube are secure, the system is "sealed" (Fig. 22-17); that is, air and fluid can escape from the pleural space into the drainage bottles and no air (positive pressure) or fluid can reenter.

In all resectional surgery (except pneumonectomy) the remaining portions of the operated lung must overexpand and fill the space that is left by the removal of the resected portion. *Thus the primary purpose of chest tubes and water-seal drainage is to (1) aid in the expansion of the remaining portions of the lung and (2) reestablish negative pressure in the pleural space.* This is accomplished as air and fluid are removed from the pleural space. Nursing actions necessary to maintain the integrity of this system will be discussed under postoperative care.

Operative procedures

Exploratory thoracotomy. An exploratory thoracotomy is an operation done to confirm a suspected diagnosis of lung or chest disease. The usual approach is by a posterolateral parascapular incision through the fourth, fifth, sixth, or seventh intercostal space. Occasionally an anterior approach is used. The ribs are spread to give the best possible exposure of the lung and hemithorax. The pleura is entered and the lung examined, a biopsy usually is taken, and the chest closed. This procedure may also be used to detect bleeding in the chest or other injury following trauma to the chest. Since the pleural space was entered, a chest tube and water-seal drainage are necessary.

Pneumonectomy. A pneumonectomy, the removal of an entire lung, is most commonly done to treat bronchogenic carcinoma (Fig. 22-15). It may also be used to treat tuberculosis, bronchiectasis, or lung abscess. However, a pneumonectomy is only done in those instances when a lobectomy or segmental resection will not remove all the diseased tissue. A thoracotomy incision is made in either the posterior or anterior chest using the method described under exploratory thoracotomy. Before the lung can be removed, the pulmonary artery and vein are ligated and then cut. The main stem bronchus leading to the lung is clamped, divided, and sutured, usually with black silk. To assure an airtight closure of the bronchus a pleural flap is placed over it and sutured into place. The phrenic nerve on the operative side is crushed, causing the diaphragm on that side to rise and reduce the size of the remaining space. Because there is no lung left to reexpand, drainage tubes are not used. Ideally the pressure in the closed chest is slightly negative. This pressure is taken postoperatively using a pneumothorax machine and air can be removed or added to attain the desired pressure. The fluid left in the space will consolidate in time preventing the remaining lung and heart from shifting toward the operative side (mediastinal shift).

Lobectomy. In a lobectomy one lobe of the lung is removed (Fig. 22-15). It is used to treat bronchiectasis, bronchogenic carcinoma, emphysematous blebs or bullae, lung abscess, benign tumors, fungal infections, and tuberculosis. For a lobectomy to be successful the disease must be confined to one lobe and the remaining portion of the lung must be capable of expanding to fill up the space. Two chest tubes are usually used for postoperative drainage.

Segmental resection (segmentectomy). In a segmental resection one or more segments of the lung are removed. This operation is used in an attempt to preserve as much functioning lung tissue as possible. It is a very taxing operation for the surgeon since the dissection between segments must be done very carefully and slowly, and the identification of the segmental pulmonary artery and vein and bronchus is more difficult than when a lobe is involved. Since there are 10 segments in each lung only a portion of a lobe may need to be removed. The most common indication for segmentectomy is bronchiectasis. It is also used to treat tuberculosis. Chest tubes and water-seal drainage are necessary postoperatively. Because of air leaks from the segmental surface, the remaining lung may take longer to reexpand.

Wedge resection. In a wedge resection a well-circumscribed diseased portion is removed without regard to the segmental planes. The area to be removed is clamped, dissected, and sutured. Chest tubes are used postoperatively.

Decortication. In a decortication a fibrinous peel is removed from the visceral pleura, allowing the encased lung to reexpand and obliterate the pleural space. This procedure is discussed further under the treatment of empyema (p. 580). Chest tubes and chest suction are used to facilitate the reexpansion of the lung. If the lung has been encased for a long time, it may be incapable of reexpanding following decortication. In this situation thoracoplasty may be necessary.

Thoracoplasty. A thoracoplasty is an extrapleural procedure involving the removal of ribs. By removing ribs it is possible to reduce the size of the chest cavity. Prior to the widespread use of resectional surgery, thoracoplasty was the basic surgical treatment for tuberculosis. Today thoracoplasty is used primarily to prevent or treat the complications of resectional surgery. When it is felt that a patient's lung may not be able to expand sufficiently after a resection to fill the space, a thoracoplasty is done 2 or 3 weeks prior to the resection. It also may be done prior to pneumonectomy since this will reduce the chance of mediastinal shift after surgery. This type of thoracoplasty is often called a *preresection* or *tailoring* thoracoplasty; that is, the chest wall is tailored to reduce its size.

If the remaining portions of the lung fail to reexpand sufficiently postresection or if another complication such as empyema occurs, a thoracoplasty is done. In general it is employed when there is a space in the chest that cannot be obliterated by other means. Usually no more than three ribs are removed, and therefore paradoxical motion following thoraco-

plasty is seldom seen anymore. Paradoxical motion is discussed under chest injuries (p. 589).

Management of the patient requiring chest surgery

Preoperative evaluation. In addition to the screening tests that are run on all preoperative patients, special tests are usually required for patients having chest surgery. These are chest radiography, including laminography (p. 547), pulmonary function tests, electrocardiography, blood gas studies, bronchospirometry, bronchoscopy, and in some instances bronchography. If the patient is scheduled for a pneumonectomy the evaluation will be even more precise and often includes a cardiac catheterization. Since the tests may be done on an outpatient basis, the office nurse or clinic nurse must be sure that the patient understands what he is to do and why. Close family members should also be kept informed.

Preoperative care. The operation is discussed with both the patient and his family. The preoperative nursing care is similar to that discussed on p. 193. The patient should understand that he will receive oxygen postoperatively either by mask, nasal prongs, catheter, or tent because this practice is routine for patients undergoing chest surgery. He should know that he will be turned and asked to cough at least every 1 to 2 hours postoperatively in order to maintain a clear airway and to aid in the reexpansion of the remaining portions of the lung.

The nurse should teach the patient how to cough. Patients who practice coughing preoperatively usually will cough more effectively postoperatively. Exercises to preserve symmetric body alignment, full range of motion of the shoulder, and maximum pulmonary function are usually started during the preoperative period and continued postoperatively. In some hospitals the physical therapist instructs the patient. The nurse, however, must provide follow-up instructions and is responsible for seeing that the patient carries out the instructions properly. Many times the nurse must take the responsibility for teaching the exercises. If so, the nurse should find out which exercises the surgeon feels should be used and, if possible, should obtain assistance from a physical therapist in how best to provide each specific exercise.

If a catheter is to be used for drainage of the chest, the patient can be told that it will be used to drain fluid and air that normally accumulates after a chest operation. He should also be told to expect to have pain for some time postoperatively because intercostal nerves are severed, but he should be told that medication can be given for this pain and that he must not let the pain prevent him from coughing. If he has pain on breathing deeply, he should not hesitate to ask whether medication can be given. The patient should also know that the physician may start an infusion in a vein in the leg before he goes to the operating room. The skin is often incised and a polyethylene tube (Intercath) inserted into the vein to obviate the danger of infiltration of the fluid and of collapse of the vein in the event of shock.

Postoperative care. Usually the patient is kept flat in bed until his vital signs are stabilized. After that time he should be turned frequently, and care is taken to be sure he is not lying on his chest tubes. Oxygen is usually administered by nasal catheter at 6 to 8 L./minute. It is continued until the patient has fully reacted from anesthesia.

Vital signs are taken every 15 minutes for 2 hours and then every hour for several hours. It is not unusual for blood pressure to fluctuate during the first 24 to 36 hours, and close monitoring of the patient is essential. *Drainage on chest dressings is unusual and should it occur it should be reported at once.*

When the patient has fully reacted he can usually breathe best in a semi-Fowler's position. He is also most comfortable if a pillow is placed under his head and neck but not under his shoulders and back. The patient should be assisted to cough as soon as he is conscious. If his blood pressure is stable, he is assisted to a sitting position and his incision is supported anteriorly and posteriorly by the nurse's hands. Firm, even pressure over the incision with the open palm of the hands is a most effective method. The nurse's head should be behind the patient when he coughs (Fig. 22-16). The patient is encouraged to breathe deeply and then cough. Sips of fluids, especially

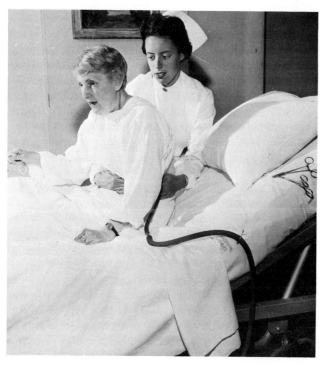

FIG. 22-16. The nurse is splinting the chest by applying pressure; this lessens muscle pull and pain as the patient coughs.

warm ones such as tea or coffee, often facilitate coughing. Coughing keeps the *airway patent, prevents atelectasis,* and *facilitates reexpansion of the lung.* The patient should cough every hour for the first 24 hours and then every 2 to 4 hours. The patient should cough until his chest sounds clear. He will be helped to cough by the nurse's encouragement. Since coughing is essential to the patient's recovery, he must be awakened if asleep. Otherwise secretions will accumulate in the tracheobronchial tree. If the patient is unable to cough effectively, tracheal suctioning may be necessary. The patient can cough most effectively 20 to 30 minutes after he receives his pain medication, and this should be capitalized on by the nursing staff. Mist therapy or IPPB treatment with drugs such as isoproterenol also may be used postoperatively to loosen secretions and to make coughing more effective.

When assisting the patient to and from a sitting position the nurse should use the arm on the patient's unoperated side. The back of his neck should also be supported. When the patient lies back down, the head and neck are supported until they are on the pillow. A pull rope or draw sheet tied firmly to the foot of the bed may be used to help the patient raise and lower himself.

Abdominal breathing exercises such as those described on p. 569 are a valuable adjunct to the care of the patient with chest surgery because they improve ventilation without increasing pain and assist him to cough more effectively. The exercises should be taught preoperatively so that the patient has time to practice them before surgery.

Morphine or meperidine hydrochloride is usually ordered for pain. Medication for pain should be given as needed and may be required as often as every 3 to 4 hours during the first few postoperative days. The patient is extremely uncomfortable and will not be able to cough or turn unless he has relief from pain. In some instances the dosage of the narcotic is decreased so that it may be given oftener and yet not depress respirations. The tubes in the chest cause pain, and the patient may attempt rapid, shallow breathing to splint the lower chest and avoid motion of the catheters. This impairs ventilation, makes coughing ineffective, and causes secretions to be retained. Thus it is a nursing responsibility to do all that is possible to make the patient comfortable as this facilitates deep breathing and coughing. If, despite all efforts, the patient's discomfort is interfering with adequate chest excursion, an intercostal nerve block may be performed.

The patient is encouraged to take fluids postoperatively, and he can progress to a general diet as soon as it is tolerated. Forcing fluids helps to liquefy secretions and makes them easier to expectorate. Usually fluids by mouth and mist therapy are all that is needed to thin and loosen secretions.

Passive arm exercises are usually started the evening of surgery. The purpose in putting the patient's arm through range of motion is to prevent restriction of function. Most patients are reluctant to move the arm on the operative side, but with proper preoperative instruction and postoperative follow-through they do so readily. It is important for both the patient and nurse to understand that the longer the arm is unexercised, the stiffer it will become. The patient should put his arms through active range of motion two or three times a day within a few days. The recommended exercises are similar to those done following mastectomy (p. 810). The exercises are best done when the patient is upright or when he is lying on his abdomen. Exercise such as elevating the scapula and clavicle, "hunching the shoulders," bringing the scapulae as close together as possible, and hyperextending the arm can only be done in these positions. Since lying on the abdomen may not be possible at first, these exercises are done when the patient is sitting on the edge of the bed or standing.

Care of chest tubes and water-seal drainage. Before the patient leaves the operating room the chest catheters are attached to sterile water-seal drainage bottles, the tubes are clamped, and the bottles are placed on the bed. On receiving the patient in the recovery room or surgical unit, the bottles should be placed on the floor and unclamped. The tubing is then fastened to the bed so that there are no dependent loops between the bottles and the bed (Fig. 22-17). The tip of the tube should be kept from 1 to 2 cm. under water so that if the bottle accidentally tips over, the tube will remain under water. The water level in the bottle is marked by placing an adhesive strip at the water line. The date and hour are written on the tape, which gives a ready indication as to the amount of drainage. If considerable drainage accumulates in the bottle, this will increase the amount of subatmospheric (negative) pressure in the system, and it will be more difficult for the patient to expel air and fluid through it. In this instance the glass rod may be pulled up so less of it is under water or the surgeon may order that the drainage bottle be changed. In this case, a sterile setup is prepared. When the bottle with sterile water and tubing are ready, the chest tube is clamped as close to the chest as possible. The chest tube is then disconnected from the drainage tubing, the new setup is connected, and the chest tube is unclamped. The drainage should be measured and may be sent to the laboratory for examination.

As explained under basic principles, most surgeons insert two catheters into the pleural space. One is inserted through the anterior chest wall above the resected area. This is referred to as the *anterior* or *upper tube.* It is used to remove air from the pleural space. The second tube is inserted through the posterior chest and is referred to as the *posterior* or *lower*

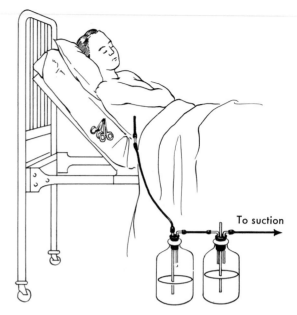

FIG. 22-17. Chest catheter in place. The chest catheter is attached to a closed drainage system. Note that the glass tube in the drainage bottle connected to the tubing of the chest catheter is below the level of the water. The bottle to the right of the drainage bottle is a "breaker bottle" and regulates the amount of suction transmitted to the drainage bottle, the chest catheter, and the pleural cavity. The two hemostats attached to the bed are available should the bottle break or water-seal system be otherwise interrupted.

tube. It is primarily for the drainage of *serosanguineous* fluid that accumulates as the result of the operative procedure. The lower tube may be of a larger diameter than the upper tube to prevent it from becoming plugged with clots. Fig. 22-18 shows the placement of tubes within the pleural space.

As the patient breathes in and out, there will be movement of fluid in the glass tube that is under water. This is known as fluctuation or oscillation, and the column will move up as the patient fills his lungs on inspiration or when he coughs, and it will fall when the patient is exhaling. The tubes should be checked for fluctuation frequently and they should be "milked" or "stripped" every hour to prevent formation of clots that could plug the tubes. If the column of water is not fluctuating, the nurse should be sure that the patient is not lying on the tubes or that they are not blocked by a clot. Changing the patient's position or having him cough often restores visible fluctuation. If fluctuation still does not occur, this should be reported.

Two hemostats should be kept at the bedside at all times (Fig. 22-17). These are to be used to clamp the tube if the water-seal bottle is accidentally broken. For this reason, the patient and all personnel should know what to do if a bottle is broken. When a bottle is broken, the chest catheter should be

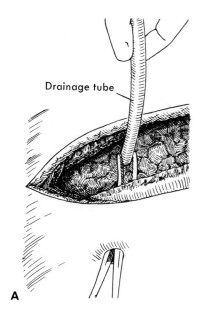
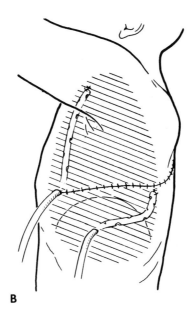

Drainage tube

FIG. 22-18. A, Drainage tube being inserted into the pleural space. **B,** Note that the upper and lower tubes are placed well into the pleural space. (From Johnson, J., and Kirby, C. K.: Surgery of the chest, ed. 3, Chicago, 1964, Year Book Medical Publishers, Inc.)

A

B

clamped and then reconnected to a sterile setup as soon as possible. Sterile water should be used in the bottle. As soon as the system is reconnected with the tip of tube under water, the clamp should be removed. Except in case of emergency such as a broken bottle, most surgeons prefer that tubes not be clamped and a specific order is written if clamping is desired. The reason for this is that when the tubes are clamped, air (positive pressure) leaking from the resected pleural surface further collapses the lung. Air leaks are common the first few hours after surgery and will usually seal off without further attention. Therefore, if the patient is being transported from one place to another such as to the x-ray department, tubes should not be clamped unless it is for a very few minutes. In general, water-seal bottles are changed only when broken or on specific order of the surgeon. If the nurse is expected to change the bottles routinely, the procedure outlined at the beginning of this section should be employed using strict asepsis.

Water-seal bottles should never be lifted above the level of the patient's chest, since this would allow the water in the bottle to be pulled into the pleural space. Although some surgeons insist the bottles be taped to the floor, this should not be necessary if all personnel understand the precautions to be observed in the care of the water-seal bottles. The bottles should be placed on the floor so that they will not be broken by a lowered side rail. When a Hi-Lo bed is being used, care must be taken not to lower the bed onto the bottles.

SUCTION DRAINAGE. If air is leaking from the pleural surface faster than it can be removed by the negative pressure of the water-seal system, additional suction may be necessary to reexpand the lung. Surgeons vary in their use of suction. Some prefer

not to add it until 24 hours after surgery since they believe using it earlier will only make existing pleural air leaks larger, especially if the patient has had a segmental resection. Following decortication, suction is added immediately after the patient returns from surgery.

There are several suction devices that can be used; however, many of them require the use of a suction control or "breaker" bottle between the suction source and the patient's water-seal bottle (Fig. 22-17). The use of a breaker bottle provides for control of the amount of suction that is applied to the water-seal bottle and thus to the patient's pleural space. The stopper in the control bottle has three openings. One is connected to the water-seal bottle, one is connected to the suction source, and the third contains a glass rod that is under water and open to the outside (Fig. 22-17). The amount of suction produced will be determined by the distance between the surface of the water and the tip of this tube. When the suction source is turned on, the level of water in the open tube will sink in proportion to the amount of negative pressure in the system.[66] Thus, if there is 15 cm. of water between the surface of the water and the tip of the tube, the amount of negative pressure in the system will be 15 cm. of water pressure. Since the water will be at the bottom of the tube when this amount of pressure is reached, any increase in negative pressure will cause air to be drawn in from the outside, *breaking* the suction at this level. Therefore it can be expected that the water in the breaker bottle will bubble almost continuously. If it fails to bubble at all, the desired level of suction is not being attained. When the water in the breaker bottle is not bubbling, the tubing should be checked for air leaks. If there are no leaks and bubbling still does not occur, the surgeon should be notified at once since the air leak in the pleura may be so great that the amount of negative pressure is not sufficient to overcome it. In this instance water will be added to the bottle to increase the distance between the surface of the water and the tip of the tube, thereby increasing the amount of negative pressure being exerted on the pleural space.

The distance the tube is placed under water in the breaker bottle is determined by the surgeon. A breaker bottle and suction may be attached to one or both tubes. Most commonly it is attached to the upper tube since this is where air is most likely to be leaking from the pleural surface. A small empty trap bottle is usually attached by tubing between the breaker bottle and the suction source. The purpose of this bottle is to protect the suction motor from becoming wet should the breaker bottle overflow. (Further information about other kinds of chest suction devices in common use can be found in other sources.[26,29a,39,59])

REMOVAL OF CHEST TUBES. Usually the remaining portions of the patient's lung will reexpand within 48 to 72 hours. When the water column is no longer fluctuating and chest radiographs reveal that the lung completely fills the pleural space, tubes are removed. Although both tubes may be removed at the same time, the upper tube is often left in place after the lower tube has been removed since there still may be some residual air left in the apex of the pleural space. This will depend on whether an upper or lower lobe was removed, how distensible the remaining lung tissue is, and how fast pleural air leaks seal. In general, tubes are not left in longer than 5 to 7 days because of the danger of an infection developing along the tube tract.

The patient should be given medication for pain about $1/2$ hour before the tube is to be removed. In preparation for removal of the tube, the nurse should prepare three 2-inch strips of adhesive about 6 inches long. A sterile field with a suture set and a pile of 4 by 4 inch gauze squares should be prepared. The patient is turned onto his unoperated side or he may sit on the side of the bed with his feet in a chair. After the sutures securing the tube are cut, the patient is told to exhale or strain as the tube is removed. The surgeon will remove the tube with one hand while holding the gauze squares in the other. As soon as the tube is out, the gauze squares are placed snugly over the opening. The nurse then applies the adhesive tape to assure an airtight dressing.

AMBULATION. Some surgeons do not allow the patient out of bed until the chest tubes are removed.[66] However, they will allow the male patient to stand beside the bed to void as necessary. Other surgeons want the patient to ambulate as soon as his vital signs are stable, often the evening of surgery. The patient can be safely gotten up with chest tubes connected to water-seal bottles as long as the nursing staff is well versed in the care of these patients. Since the chest bottles do restrict the patient's movement, he can limber his legs at the bedside and then move to a nearby chair. In this case, two persons are necessary—one to assist the patient and the second to move the bottles. Bottles can be lifted from the floor as long as they are not raised above the level of the patient's chest. Some hospitals have bottle holders on wheels that can be used in ambulation of the patient. If the patient is unable to be out of bed, range of motion exercises should be emphasized (Fig. 1-2).

Complications of resectional surgery. The most common complications of resectional surgery include a persistent air space that is not filled by the remaining lung, bronchopleural fistula, and empyema. A thoracoplasty may be necessary eventually to correct any of these complications.

Special care following pneumonectomy. Generally the patient is permitted to be only on his back or his operated side, since some surgeons fear that the sutured bronchus may not stay closed. If it should open while the patient is lying with his operative side uppermost, fluid in the operative side would drain into the good lung and drown the patient. Although the chances of this occurring are small, this precaution is usually observed. Another reason for not allowing the patient to lie on his unoperated side is that this compresses his remaining lung and restricts lung excursion and ventilation. The patient is watched immediately postoperatively for cardiac overload and CVP monitoring (p. 326) is common. The patient should also be watched closely for mediastinal shift. If pressure builds up within the operated side, it can cause the mediastinum to shift toward the unoperated side. Conversely, the unoperated lung may shift toward the empty space left after a pneumonectomy. For this reason, the surgeon will palpate the patient's trachea at least daily to be sure that it is in midline. If a shift occurs toward the good lung, it is treated by removing air (positive pressure) from the empty space. If the shift is toward the empty space, air may be instilled into the space to increase the pressure and cause the mediastinum to shift back. If the mediastinum persists in shifting toward the empty side, a thoracoplasty may be necessary. This will reduce the size of the space and keep the mediastinum in midline. A patient with mediastinal shift resembles the patient in congestive heart failure. His neck veins are distended, his trachea is displaced to one side, his pulse and respirations are increased, and he is dyspneic.

Patients who have had a lung removed may have a lowered vital capacity, and exercise and activity should be limited to that which can be done without dyspnea. Since the body must be given time to adjust to getting along with only one lung, the patient's return to work may be delayed. If the diagnosis is cancer, radiation therapy is usually given, and it may be started before the patient leaves the hospital. (See p. 292 for further discussion of nursing care for patients receiving radiation therapy.) The patient who has had a pneumonectomy for cancer is urged to report to his physician at once if he has hoarseness, dyspnea, pain on swallowing, or localized chest pain, since these difficulties may be signs of metastasis.

Special care following thoracoplasty. Since thoracoplasty is an extrapleural procedure, chest tubes are not necessary unless the pleura is inadvertently entered during surgery. Because portions of several ribs (usually 3 or 4) have been removed, the patient may have considerable pain. Drainage on the dressings may also occur. Although paradoxical motion is rarely seen unless more than three ribs are removed, the patient's breathing pattern should be watched closely. (See p. 589 for description of paradoxical motion.)

Since thoracoplasty is done either prior to or after resectional surgery, the patient is faced with more than one surgical procedure. Therefore the patient may require additional emotional support in accepting the need for two operations.

■ CHEST TRAUMA

Trauma to the chest is a major problem most often seen first in the emergency department. The injuries to the chest range from a few fractured ribs to major trauma to the chest wall, sternum, lungs, heart, and major blood vessels. Injuries to the chest are broadly classified into two groups—blunt and penetrating. *Blunt* or nonpenetrating injuries include fractures of the ribs in which there is no damage to the pleura and lung. These injuries occur most commonly as the result of automobile accidents, falls, or blast injuries. Automobile accidents in the United States kill approximately 55,000 persons each year. Of this number, 40% have a major thoracic injury.[80] The injury is most often sustained when striking the steering wheel or being hurled from the car.

Fractures of the ribs

The fourth, fifth, sixth, seventh, and eighth ribs are most commonly fractured. Fractures of the ribs are caused by blows, crushing injuries, or strain caused by severe coughing or sneezing spells. If the rib is splintered or the fracture displaced, sharp fragments may penetrate the pleura and the lung. Patients with possible rib fractures should have an x-ray examination of the chest and should be observed carefully for signs of pneumothorax or hemothorax.

The patient with a rib fracture complains of pain at the site of the injury that increases on inspiration. The area is very tender to the touch, and the patient splints his chest and takes shallow breaths. Unless the lung has been penetrated, the usual treatment for rib fracture is conservative and includes strapping the chest with adhesive tape from the affected side to the unaffected side or applying a circular strapping, using an Ace bandage. A chest binder also may be used. If adhesive tape is used, the skin may be shaved and painted with tincture of benzoin to prevent blistering and other irritation. When the pain is severe and is not relieved by strapping and analgesic medications, the physician may do a regional nerve block. This procedure consists of infiltrating the intercostal spaces above and below the fractured rib with procaine, 1%. If the lung has been penetrated, the patient may raise bright red sputum.

Paradoxical breathing. When multiple ribs are fractured, the chest wall on that side becomes unstable and the result is a *flail chest.* Thus the chest wall no longer provides the rigid bony support that is necessary to maintain the bellows function required for normal ventilation. This causes paradoxical breathing. In *paradoxical breathing* the portion of the lung underlying the unstable chest wall moves opposite to the remainder of the lung. On inspiration that portion of the lung sucks in while the remaining lung expands. On expiration it balloons out as the remaining lung contracts. This results in a vicious cycle of events leading to *hypoxia.* The treatment of paradoxical motion is to *stabilize the chest wall,* and a variety of methods are used depending on the extent of the injury and the patient's condition. Presently there is considerable controversy about the treatment of flail chest. The treatment may either be by internal or external stabilization of the chest wall.

Internal stabilization is best obtained by use of a *volume-controlled* ventilator attached to a cuffed tracheostomy tube (p. 592). The ventilator is set to automatically control the patient's respirations. If the patient is breathing against the ventilator, he will need to be sedated. Narcotics, sedatives, and even muscle relaxants may have to be given. When the patient also has a head injury, narcotics are contraindicated and muscle relaxants will be used until ventilatory control is achieved. Once the patient is quieted down and is no longer resisting the ventilator, hyperventilation can be used to depress the respiratory center so that ventilatory control is maintained.[80] The patient will require meticulous tracheostomy care in order to maintain a clear airway and to prevent infection. The patient may have to be on the ventilator for as long as 8 to 14 days. During this time he will require the attention of experienced respiratory therapists, frequent blood gas studies, and constant care by skilled nursing personnel. Culture and sensitivity studies of tracheal aspirations should be repeated at least every 4 to 5 days. These can be obtained by collecting the tracheal aspiration in a Luken tube.

External stabilization is achieved by the use of skeletal traction. Under local anesthesia a small incision is made, and stainless steel wire is attached to the ribs or sternum to pull the chest wall outward. The wire is connected to a rope and pulley with about 5 pounds of weight. Usually in 14 to 21 days the chest wall is rigid enough to permit removal of the traction. Towel clips and special clamps may also be used to apply traction.[59] The patient may not be able to cough effectively, and therefore frequent intratracheal aspirations or tracheostomy may be necessary to maintain a patent airway.

In some patients, especially large-chested individuals, a combination of both ventilatory support (internal stabilization) and external traction may be required.

Penetrating wounds of the chest

When a knife, bullet, or other flying missile enters the chest, a penetrating wound occurs. The major problem in penetrating injury is not injury to the chest wall but injury to the structures within the chest cavity. Penetration of the lung can cause leakage of air from the lung into the pleural cavity (pneumothorax) (Fig. 22-15). Blood may also leak into the pleural cavity (hemothorax). As the air or fluid accumulates in the pleural cavity, it builds up positive pressure, which causes the lung to collapse and may even cause a mediastinal shift, thus compressing the opposite lung and interfering with cardiac action. The patient then has serious difficulty in breathing and may go into shock. His pulse may become weak and rapid and his skin cold and clammy, and his blood pressure falls rapidly.

Emergency treatment is directed toward sustaining oxygen exchange and correcting circulatory failure. Often the patient is intubated with an endotracheal tube and then he is checked for air or blood in the pleural cavity. An emergency thoracentesis is done, and air and fluid are removed by syringe. Usually a catheter is inserted into the pleural space and connected to water-seal drainage (p. 586). If the lung fails to reexpand with this treatment or there is evidence of internal bleeding, surgical exploration may be necessary and will be done after shock and other complications are under control.

In order to monitor the patient for hypovolemia, a central venous pressure (CVP) line is inserted (p. 326). This line can also be used to administer intravenous fluids and blood as necessary. If it is suspected that cardiac injury and tamponade may be present, a *pericardicentesis* will be done. The CVP is a very effective way to monitor for tamponade. A pressure above 15 cm. of water or a rising CVP in a patient in shock with penetrating trauma in the region of the heart often indicates cardiac tamponade.[80]

If an open sucking wound of the chest has been sustained, it should be covered immediately to prevent air from entering the pleural cavity and causing a pneumothorax. Several thicknesses of material may be used, and these are anchored with wide adhesive tape, or the wound edges may be taped tightly together. If an object such as a knife is still in the wound, it must never be removed until a physician arrives. Its presence may prevent the entry of air into the pleural cavity, and its removal may cause further damage. The patient who has sustained a penetrating wound of the chest should be placed in an upright position and taken to the nearest emergency room or physician's office.

The treatment of sucking chest wounds centers around relieving pneumothorax (or hemothorax) and preventing further air from entering the chest. A chest tube is inserted and connected to water-seal drainage and the wound is repaired surgically. The patient may be in shock, and blood transfusion and oxygen are commonly administered.

■ RESPIRATORY INSUFFICIENCY AND RESPIRATORY FAILURE

Respiratory insufficiency occurs when the exchange of oxygen and carbon dioxide is not sufficient to meet the needs of the body *during normal activities.* Thus patients with chronic obstructive pulmonary disease may develop respiratory insufficiency. Other clinical conditions in which respiratory insufficiency can occur are muscular dystrophy, Guillain-Barré syndrome, poliomyelitis, myasthenia gravis, and overwhelming pulmonary infection. When the patient is unable to maintain ventilation and gaseous exchange *at rest,* he is in *respiratory failure.* With inadequate ventilation, the arterial pCO_2 rises above 50 mm. Hg and the arterial pO_2 and pH fall. Some patients are able to compensate for the high pCO_2 level and maintain a normal pH; they are considered to have chronic respiratory insufficiency. However, with added stress such as infection, the patient develops acute respiratory failure and his pH falls further as the pCO_2 rises. Patients with a decreased pO_2 (less than 50 mm. Hg) also are considered to have respiratory failure. They may not have an elevated pCO_2; in many instances the pCO_2 is actually below normal. These patients may easily develop carbon dioxide retention if they become tired or if there is further extension of infection or other stress. The diagnosis of respiratory failure is made by arterial blood gas analysis.

Management

The initial medical treatment can often be conservative if the diagnosis is made early enough. Most patients who have an elevated pCO_2 have lost the usual respiratory drive, carbon dioxide stimulation. They no longer respond to increased carbon dioxide levels by increasing their rate and depth of respiration; rather, the elevated pCO_2 depresses the respiratory center. Their respiratory drive is now derived from their low pO_2 level. Therefore, even though these patients lack oxygen, it is extremely dangerous to raise their pO_2 to normal levels. If the patient's arterial pO_2 is normal and he is retaining carbon dioxide *(hypercapnia),* he will have no respiratory drive. Hypoventilation becomes more severe and pCO_2 continues to rise. This situation results in "carbon dioxide narcosis," a markedly elevated carbon dioxide level that causes coma or semicoma (p. 118). Patients are therefore treated with "low-flow" or "controlled-flow" oxygen; that is, inspired oxygen concentrations of 24% to 30%. These concentrations can easily be obtained by using a Venti-mask or a two-pronged nasal cannula with a 1 to 2 L. oxygen flow. This amount of oxygen can significantly increase the amount of oxygen carried by hemoglobin without a significant increase in arterial pO_2. Therefore the patient's blood carries much more oxygen even though he is still hypoxemic. He continues to have respiratory drive and his pCO_2 does not rise. These patients also receive frequent (every 1 to 2 hours) IPPB therapy to aid ventilation and reduce CO_2 levels. Because the IPPB machines deliver 60% to 80% oxygen (not 40%) when set on oxygen with air dilution, the equipment must be modified to administer low-flow oxygen. Low concentrations of oxygen are obtained by using compressed air for the driving force and adding 1 L./minute of oxygen through the nebulizer.

By the use of low-flow oxygen the amount of oxygen carried in the patient's blood can often be increased enough to maintain basic body function without further reduction of ventilation. Patients with a normal pCO_2 and hypoxemia are usually able to tolerate high flows of oxygen (5 to 10 L./minute) without an increase in pCO_2. Throughout treatment, blood gas studies should be done frequently to determine the patient's ventilatory status. When oxygenation is at a safe level, attention can be directed toward reducing the amount of secretions present and correcting factors that precipitated the acute respiratory insufficiency.

Aggressive, constant nursing care is essential for these patients. The nurse must be continually alert to clinical changes that represent changes in the patient's ventilation. Increasing confusion and behavioral changes often indicate an elevated pCO_2. The behavioral changes may range from pugnacious, combative behavior to lethargy. Other clinical signs of *hypercapnia* are flushed skin color (due to reflex vasodilation), muscle twitching, and headache. Signs commonly seen in *hypoxia* include tachycardia, increased pulse rate, cyanosis, changes in blood pressure, and changes in behavior. In *early* stages of hypoxia, the blood pressure is elevated as a result of vasoconstriction and increased peripheral resistance. In *later* stages the blood pressure falls to hypotensive levels and circulatory arrest can occur.

It is important to point out that cyanosis is not an early sign of hypoxia, since it does not occur until arterial oxygen saturation is less than 85%. Thus the nurse needs to be alert to earlier signs of hypoxia.

Because a patent airway is necessary for gaseous exchange, these patients need to be stimulated and encouraged to deep breathe and cough effectively. Mist therapy, liquefying agents, and postural drainage with clapping and vibrating are indicated. If the patient is unable to maintain a clear airway, tracheobronchial suctioning may be necessary. Tracheobronchial suctioning is difficult to do and is very uncomfortable for the patient who is already short of breath. Usually this procedure is carried out by the physician, but nurses who have been specially taught are prepared to do it. When assisting with the procedure, the backrest is raised so that the patient is sitting upright in bed. The nurse pulls the patient's tongue forward as the physician inserts the catheter through the nose. As with other types of suctioning, a Y tube connector should be used. When the catheter is in the trachea, suction is applied. This usually stimulates the patient to cough violently and often he becomes cyanotic. The patient is suctioned for 10 to 15 seconds at a time and oxygen is administered prior to and between aspirations. A small amount (3 to 5 ml.) of saline solution often is introduced through the catheter to assist in removing secretions. Suction is always applied intermittently as the catheter is withdrawn to avoid tracheal injury due to invagination of the mucosa and resultant tearing.

Although patients with respiratory insufficiency are often anxious and frightened, sedation is contraindicated because it depresses respiration. Therefore it is especially important that the nurse be supportive of the patient and be skillful in helping him breathe more effectively. The patient can be extremely demanding and the nurse must understand the fear and anxiety that is often the basis for the patient's behavior. The nurse should also help other personnel to understand the patient's behavior. In this way a therapeutic nurse-patient relationship is established and maintained.

If the patient is unable to maintain ventilation as indicated by a rising arterial pCO_2, mechanical ventilation is necessary. To mechanically ventilate the lung, an artificial airway is needed. Tracheal intubation with an oral or nasal cuffed endotracheal tube is done initially. (The cuffed tube ensures a closed system so that adequate ventilation is possible.) If mechanical ventilation is necessary for more than a few days, a tracheostomy is performed (see p. 612 for discussion of tracheostomy care). Most physicians prefer that the tracheostomy be performed with an endotracheal tube in place. This ensures an adequate airway while the tracheostomy is performed in an operating room under ideal conditions. When an endotracheal tube is removed, the patient's normal airway is restored and he is able to cough effectively. However, when a tracheostomy tube is removed, the patient has an air leak at the incision site. This air leak prevents him from creating high intrathoracic pressures and thereby decreases the effectiveness of his cough and his ability to maintain a patent airway until the incision is healed.

The endotracheal tube may be made of either plastic or rubber with an inflatable cuff so that a closed system with the ventilator may be maintained (Fig. 22-19). The tube is inserted via the mouth or nose through the larynx into the trachea. If an oral endotracheal tube is used, a rubber airway or bite block is often necessary to prevent the patient from biting the tube and obstructing his airway.

The tracheostomy tube is usually made of plastic or metal. It may be either a single-lumen or double-lumen (Jackson) type (Fig. 22-20). Both types of tubes may be cuffed, and the newer plastic tubes come with high-volume, low-pressure cuffs that are less likely to cause damage to the trachea (Figs. 22-19 and 22-21). Single-lumen tubes must be changed every 48 to 72 hours since they are more difficult to clean and more likely to become plugged than are double-lumen tubes (p. 614).

Immediately after insertion of the endotracheal tube and periodically thereafter the chest should be auscultated to ensure that there are breath sounds on both sides. If a cuffed tube is inserted too far, it will slip into one of the main stem bronchi (usually the right) and occlude the opposite bronchus and lung, resulting in atelectasis on the obstructed side. Even if the tube is still in the trachea, airway obstruction will result if the end of the tube is located on the carina (area at lower end of trachea at point of bifurcation of main stem bronchi). This will result

in dry secretions that obstruct both bronchi. Although these complications are more common with the use of an endotracheal tube, they can occur in the patient with a tracheostomy, especially in a small person with a short neck. In either case, the tube is pulled back until it is positioned below the larynx and above the carina. The tube is then fastened securely in place. A replacement tube of the same size should always be kept at the bedside in the event that it is needed.

Nursing care of a patient with a cuffed tube

The use of a cuffed tube (endotracheal or tracheostomy) (Figs. 22-19 and 22-21) requires special nursing care measures. The inflated cuff can restrict the blood supply to that area of the trachea, resulting in erosion and necrosis. It is therefore imperative that the cuff be deflated at least every hour for 5 minutes, or as long as possible if the patient is unable to tolerate the full 5 minutes. The procedure to follow when deflating the cuff is as follows:

1. *Suction the oral and nasal pharynx.* Although the cuff normally prevents aspiration of oral secretions, aspiration can occur with deflation. Suctioning of the upper airway will remove those secretions that might be aspirated.

2. *Deflate the cuff.*

3. *Using a sterile catheter, suction the lower airway through the endotracheal or tracheostomy tube.* See p. 614 for details of tracheostomy suctioning. Because some secretions—especially those pooled directly above the cuff—may not have been previously removed, suctioning after deflation will remove those that have accumulated around the tube. Deflation of the cuff also may cause movement of the tube, which stimulates the cough reflex. The

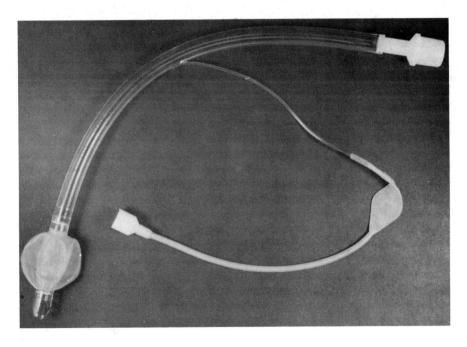

FIG. 22-19. Forregar high-volume, low-pressure cuffed endotracheal tube. The cuff shown here is not inflated. A low-pressure cuff is preferred because it is less likely to cause tracheal damage.

cough will raise other secretions to a level in the tracheobronchial tree where they can be aspirated.

4. *Ensure adequate ventilation while cuff is deflated.* Many patients are able to maintain their own ventilation for short periods off the ventilator. While off the ventilator, the patient should receive heated mist in whatever gas mixture is ordered.

Some patients require mechanical ventilation at all times. These patients should be breathed manually using a self-inflating or anesthesia bag. Usually adequate ventilation can be maintained in this manner for short periods even with the cuff deflated. Occasionally a patient has such high airway resistance that ventilation cannot be maintained without a closed system. In such instances the cuff must be deflated frequently for very brief periods (30 to 60 seconds).

5. *Inflate the cuff.* It is important to remember that the cuff need only be inflated for positive pressure ventilation. If the patient does not require mechanical ventilation, the cuff should not be inflated. When the cuff is inflated, it should be inflated during the positive pressure phase (inspiration) while the patient is on the ventilator. Two different methods may be used to inflate the cuff depending on the patient's condition and the preference of those responsible for care. In the first method, air is injected into the cuff until a full seal is attained. At this point a pressure-cycled respirator will turn off and no air will escape around the tube or through the nose

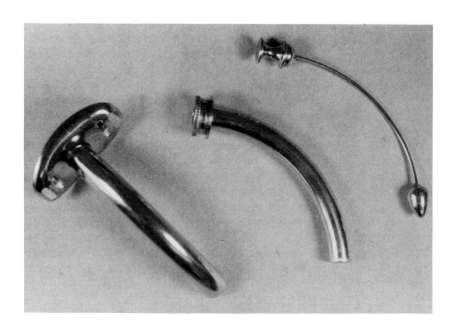

FIG. 22-20. Metal tracheostomy tube showing, from right to left, outer cannula, inner cannula, and obturator.

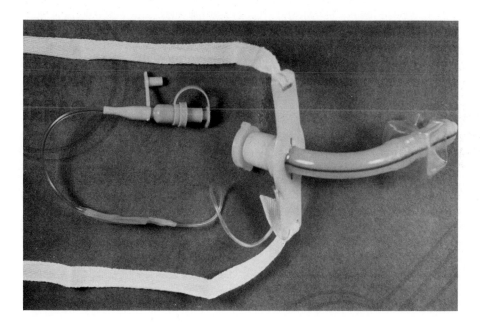

FIG. 22-21. Portex high-volume, low-pressure cuffed tracheostomy tube.

and mouth. The tubing leading to the cuff is then clamped. In the other method, air is injected until a full seal is attained and then 0.5 ml. of air is withdrawn and the tubing clamped. This latter method creates a partial leak for which the respirator can be set to compensate. The nurse should note the amount of air needed to inflate the cuff and use the smallest amount required to attain a seal. Overinflation of the cuff is extremely dangerous because it can lead to the development of tracheomalacia, tracheal stenosis, tracheoesophageal fistula, or erosion through a major blood vessel.

It is important to remember that the patient cannot speak with a cuffed tube in place because air does not pass directly through the larynx. The patient should be told why he cannot speak and that he will be able to speak normally when the tube is removed. Patients who are not informed of the change in function may believe that they have permanently lost their ability to speak.

When the patient has a tracheostomy tube in place, he can often speak when the cuff is not fully inflated. Speech is still difficult as air must be forced around the tube and up through the larynx. For patients who can tolerate it, it is often helpful to obstruct the opening of the tracheostomy tube while the cuff is deflated. This allows the patient to breathe through the upper airway. See p. 613 for discussion of means of communication provided for the patient while he cannot speak.

Suctioning the patient. All of these patients require suctioning and should be suctioned as often as necessary. The frequency of suctioning is a nursing judgment. Many patients in respiratory failure have an infection and accumulation of secretions before intubation or tracheostomy is performed. Once the patient is intubated, the tube produces a natural route for introduction of bacteria into the lower airway and the patient also loses much of his ability to produce an effective cough, as he can no longer build up the pressure needed to create an expulsive cough. Because the patient has difficulty moving secretions up his tracheobronchial tree, it is important to suction as deeply as possible. The depth to which a catheter can be inserted through an endotracheal tube on an adult is approximately 18 to 22 inches. Postural drainage with percussion and vibration (p. 575) is extremely helpful in moving secretions up to a point where they can be aspirated.

If the catheter cannot be inserted as far as usual, a mucus plug may be obstructing passage of the catheter. Saline irrigation (approximately 5 to 10 ml.) will often liquefy the obstructing secretions so they can be aspirated. When plastic catheters and plastic tubes are used, it is not uncommon for the surface of the catheter and tube to stick to each other, inhibiting passage of the catheter. Instilling 1 to 2 ml. of sterile saline solution during insertion of the catheter

will often allow the catheter to be inserted without difficulty. Details of tracheostomy suctioning and care can be found on p. 614.

Because the insertion of the endotracheal or tracheostomy tube creates a bypass of the upper airway, the patient loses his ability to humidify and warm inspired air. Therefore, whether he is on or off the respirator, the inspired air should be heated and humidified to prevent mucosal irritation and drying of secretions. *Large-bore* tubing is needed to provide this mist, as water particles will condense in *small-bore* tubing. A noticeable difference in the viscosity of secretions is evident in patients who do not receive mist for even as short a period as 30 minutes. Other important nursing care measures and observations vary with the route of intubation—via the larynx or from below the larynx. The patient who has an endotracheal tube in place usually has an increased volume of oropharyngeal secretions because of irritation from the tube. The patient also has great difficulty in swallowing (especially if an oral tube is used), necessitating frequent oropharyngeal suctioning. The patient with an endotracheal tube is allowed nothing by mouth. Nourishment will be given intravenously or by nasogastric tube feedings. The patient with a tracheostomy tube in place is usually able to swallow and have a normal oral intake. Some experts prefer that the cuff on the tracheostomy tube be inflated while the patient is eating to prevent aspiration. Others believe that the inflated cuff bulges into the esophagus and makes swallowing more difficult, and they therefore prefer the cuff to be deflated. Nursing assessment will determine which technique to use. In determining if the patient aspirates food it is often helpful to feed the patient red gelatin. The consistency of gelatin makes it easier to swallow than water and the red color makes it easy to detect if aspirated into the lower airway.

Both a tracheostomy tube and endotracheal tube have a direct effect on the airway, but the potential damage of an endotracheal tube is more extensive than that of the tracheostomy tube. Movement with rubbing of the endotracheal tube may produce laryngeal erosion and damage to the vocal cords. There is also the danger of laryngeal edema when the tube is removed. The nurse must be alert to signs of laryngeal stridor and upper airway obstruction. The patient is usually given mist by mask or tent as soon as he is extubated to prevent this complication. If upper airway obstruction occurs, reintubation or tracheostomy is necessary. With both the endotracheal and tracheostomy tubes tracheal stenosis may result from irritation and scarring at the cuff site. Good nursing care can often prevent this complication.

Positive pressure ventilators

The tube is attached to either a pressure-cycled or volume-cycled ventilator. The Bird and Bennett

(PR series) are pressure-limited ventilators while the Möerch, Emerson, Engstrom, Air Shields, Bennett MA-1, and Ohio 560 are volume-limited machines. Both types of machines can be used intermittently or continuously to assist or to control respiration.

When a pressure-cycled ventilator is used, the machine is set to deliver a predetermined amount of pressure (usually 15 to 25 cm. of water). When this pressure is reached, the machine turns off and the patient exhales normally. The volume of gas delivered to the patient is not necessarily constant, because it depends on the resistance of the entire system, including the patient's lungs. For this reason, the expired tidal volume must be monitored frequently and adjustments made in the respirator controls as needed.

With a volume-controlled machine a constant volume of air is delivered to the patient with each breath. The volume is preset and is delivered to the patient at whatever pressure is necessary to attain that volume. A volume-cycled machine should have a pressure cutoff valve. Such a mechanism allows a pressure limit to be set. If the pressure required to deliver the set volume exceeds the pressure limit, the machine will turn off before the entire volume is delivered. The pressure limit on a volume-cycled machine usually has an audible alarm. The nurse can set the limit slightly above (approximately 5 cm. of water) the pressure required to ventilate the patient. The alarm will then go off if the patient coughs, accumulates secretion, or starts to resist the machine.

Regardless of which type ventilator is used, mechanisms for various regulations are necessary if the machine is to be adjusted to each patient. It is preferable to have a respirator that can be used to assist or control the patient's breathing. "Assist" means that the patient trips (turns on) the machine with his own inspiratory effort. Most respirators have a sensitivity control knob that can be adjusted to respond to weak inspiratory efforts. "Control" implies the use of automatic cycling. The patient may be apneic and the machine set at the desired rate; the patient's own respiratory rate may be too slow and the automatic cycling can be used to force him to breathe faster; or the patient's own respiratory efforts can be ignored and an automatic rate used to ventilate the patient. (Some machines with automatic cycling do not allow for the latter adjustment.) It is also helpful to be able to regulate the flow rates at which the gas is delivered to the patient. For example, patients breathing at a rapid rate and high volumes need faster flow rates than those breathing slowly and at moderate volumes. A final necessity is the ability to regulate the inspired concentration of oxygen from 20% (room air) to 100%.

All respirators used for mechanical ventilation must

1. Provide for the heating and humidification of inspired air
2. Provide a means for measurement of expired volumes
3. Be dependable for long periods of use
4. Be easily cleaned

Any patient on continuous mechanical ventilation should be "sighed" (given a deep breath) several times an hour. Some respirators automatically "sigh" the patient, while with others the patient is "sighed" manually using a self-inflating (Ambu) or anesthesia bag. The periodic deep breathing is necessary to prevent alveolar collapse and resultant atelectasis.

A negative-pressure respirator such as the tank respirator (iron lung) may also be available (Fig. 32-1). This respirator is usually used for patients with neuromuscular problems without intrinsic lung disease. The tank respirator creates subatmospheric pressure around the chest. Since there is atmospheric pressure at the mouth and nose, air enters the patient's lung. This type of ventilator does not require tracheal intubation and is usually not used in patients with increased airway resistance.

Weaning from the ventilator. The nurse plays an important role in weaning the patient from the ventilator. Both physiologic studies (blood gases, tidal volume) and clinical status determine the patient's readiness to breathe without mechanical assistance. Prior to weaning, the patient should have been taught breathing exercises. When he is taken off the respirator, a nurse in whom he has confidence should remain with him. It is also helpful if the environment around the patient is calm. Much of the success of weaning is dependent on the interrelationship between the patient's physiologic and psychologic responses. If he becomes very anxious and takes rapid, shallow breaths, he often will not tolerate being off the respirator. If a pattern of controlled breathing can be maintained, success is much more likely. Weaning is usually begun with short periods off the respirator. The amount of time off the respirator is increased according to the patient's tolerance. The nurse must carefully assess the adequacy of the patient's ventilation while he is off the respirator. If, in the nurse's judgment, he cannot tolerate breathing on his own because of inadequate tidal volume, cyanosis, tachycardia, diaphoresis, or restlessness, mechanical assistance should be reinstituted.

Throughout the treatment of the patient in respiratory failure, ventilation should be carefully monitored by blood gas studies and simple spirometry (tidal volume, vital capacity). Alert nursing observation of the patient can determine the adequacy of ventilation. Meticulous attention is given to maintaining a patent airway, which is the prime nursing responsibility. (See specialized material for further detail.[77,85,113])

REFERENCES AND SELECTED READINGS*

1 A report of the Committee on Emphysema, American College of Chest Physicians: Recommendations for continuous oxygen therapy in chronic obstructive lung disease, Chest **64:**505-507, Oct. 1973.

2 A statement by the Committee on Therapy of the American Thoracic Society ALA (1968): Physical adjuncts in the treatment of pulmonary diseases, Am. Rev. Respir. Dis. **97:**725-729, April 1968.

3 A statement of the American Thoracic Society: Guidelines for work for patients with tuberculosis, Am. Rev. Respir. Dis. **108:**160, July 1973.

4 Agle, D. P., and others: Multidiscipline treatment of chronic pulmonary insufficiency. I. Psychologic aspects of rehabilitation, Psychosom. Med. **35:**41-49, 1973.

5 American Academy of Pediatrics: Report of the Committee on Infectious Diseases, ed. 17, Evanston, Ill., 1974, American Academy of Pediatrics, Inc.

6 American Cancer Society, Inc.: 1974 cancer facts and figures, New York, 1974, American Cancer Society, Inc.

7 American Lung Association: Chronic obstructive pulmonary disease, a manual for physicians, New York, 1972, The Association.

8 *American Lung Association: Introduction to lung diseases, New York, 1973, The Association.

9 *Avery, M. E., and others: The lung of the newborn infant, Sci. Am. **228:**75-85, April 1973.

10 Baerel, F. R., and Vance, J. W.: A simplified method for presenting acid-base situations, Chest **57:**480-484, May 1970.

11 Barstow, R. E.: Coping with emphysema, Nurs. Clin. North Am. **9:**137-145, March 1974.

12 Bartlett, R. H., and others: Respiratory maneuvers to prevent postoperative pulmonary complications, a critical review, J.A.M.A. **224:**1017-1021, May 1973.

12a Bates, B.: A guide to physical examination, Philadelphia, 1974, J. B. Lippincott Co.

13 Bates, D., Macklem, P. T., and Christie, R. V.: Respiratory function in disease, ed. 2, Philadelphia, 1971, W. B. Saunders Co.

14 Baum, G. L., editor: Textbook of pulmonary diseases, ed. 2, Boston, 1973, Little, Brown & Co.

15 Beeson, P. B., and McDermott, W., editors: Cecil-Loeb textbook of medicine, ed. 13, Philadelphia, 1973, W. B. Saunders Co.

16 Bendixen, H. H., and others: Respiratory care, St. Louis, 1965, The C. V. Mosby Co.

17 Bergersen, B. S.: Pharmacology in nursing, ed. 12, St. Louis, 1973, The C. V. Mosby Co.

18 *Bloomfield, D. A.: The recognition and management of massive pulmonary embolism, Heart & Lung **3:**241-246, March-April 1974.

19 Boyd, D. R.: Monitoring patients with post-traumatic pulmonary insufficiency, Surg. Clin. North Am. **52:**31-46, Feb. 1972.

20 Brannin, P.: Oxygen therapy and measures of bronchial hygiene, Nurs. Clin. North Am. **9:**111-121, March 1974.

21 *Brooks, W.: Replacing ritual with reason in tuberculosis isolation, Am. J. Nurs. **69:**2410-2411, Nov. 1969.

22 *Broughton, J.: Chest physical diagnosis for nurses and respiratory therapists, Heart & Lung **2:**200-206, March-April 1972.

23 Chapman, J. S.: The atypical mycobacteria: their significance in human disease, Am. J. Nurs. **67:**1031-1033, May 1967.

24 Cherniak, R. M., Cherniak, L., and Naimark, A.: Respiration in health and disease, ed. 2, Philadelphia, 1972, W. B. Saunders Co.

25 Chester, E., and others: Bronchodilator therapy: comparison of acute response to three methods of administration, Chest **62:**394-399, Oct. 1972.

26 Closed drainage of the chest, a programmed course for nurses, Public Health Service Publication no. 1337, Washington, D. C., 1965, U. S. Department of Health, Education and Welfare.

27 Collart, M. E., and Brenneman, J. K.: Prevention of postoperative atelectasis, Am. J. Nurs. **71:**1982-1987, Oct. 1971.

28 Comroe, J. H.: Physiology of respiration, Chicago, 1965, Year Book Medical Publishers, Inc.

29 Crosby, L., and Parsons, L. C.: Measurements of lateral wall pressures exerted by tracheostomy and endotracheal tube cuffs, Heart & Lung **3:**797-803, Sept.-Oct. 1974.

29a Daly, B. J., Gorenshek, N., and Mendelsohn, H.: Chest surgery. In Meltzer, L., and others, editors: Intensive care for nurse specialists, ed. 2, Philadelphia, 1975, Charles Press, Publishers.

30 Davenport, F. M.: Prospects for the control of influenza, Am. J. Nurs. **69:**1908-1911, Sept. 1969.

31 Demers, R. R., and Saklad, M.: Fundamentals of blood gas interpretation, Respir. Care **18:**153-159, March-April 1973.

32 DeWalt, E. M., and Haines, Sister Ann Kathleen: The effects of specified stressors on healthy oral mucosa, Nurs. Res. **18:**22-27, Jan.-Feb. 1969.

33 *Diagnostic standards and classification of tuberculosis, ed. 13, New York, 1974, American Lung Association.

34 Downs, J. B., and others: Intermittent mandatory ventilation: a new approach to weaning patients from mechanical ventilators, Chest **64:**331-335, Sept. 1973.

35 Dunn, C. R., and others: Determinants of tracheal injury, Chest **65:**128-135, Feb. 1974.

36 *Dyer, E., and Peterson, D.: Safe care of IPPB machines, Am. J. Nurs. **71:**2163-2166, Nov. 1971.

37 Edwards, P. Q., and Ogasawara, F. R.: Phasing out the child-centered TB program, ALA Bull. pp. 12-13, Nov. 1971.

38 Egan, D. F.: Fundamentals of respiratory therapy, ed. 2, St. Louis, 1973, The C. V. Mosby Co.

39 Enerson, D. M., and McIntyre, J.: A comparative study of the physiology and physics of pleural drainage systems, J. Thorac. Cardiovasc. Surg. **52:**40-46, July 1966.

40 Farer, L. S.: Infectiousness of tuberculosis patients, Am. Rev. Respir. Dis. **108:**152, July 1973.

41 Farer, L. S.: Preventive treatment of tuberculosis. In American Thoracic Society: Basics of RD, New York, 1973, The Society.

42 Fayerhaugh, S. Y.: Getting around with emphysema, Am. J. Nurs. **73:**94-99, Jan. 1973.

43 Finch, C., and Lenfant, C.: Oxygen transport in man, N. Engl. J. Med. **286:**407-415, Feb. 1972.

44 *Fitzmaurice, J. B., and Sasakara, A. A.: Current concepts of pulmonary embolism: implications for nursing practice, Heart & Lung **3:**209-218, March-April 1974.

45 *Flatter, P. A.: Hazards of oxygen therapy, Am. J. Nurs. **68:**80-84, Jan. 1968.

46 *Foley, M. F.: Pulmonary function testing, Am. J. Nurs. **71:**1134-1139, June 1971.

47 *Furcolow, M. L., and Rakich, J. H.: Histoplasmosis and nursing aspects of histoplasmosis, Am. J. Nurs. **59:**79-83, Jan. 1959.

48 *Grimes, O. F.: Neuromuscular syndromes in patients with lung cancer, Am. J. Nurs. **71:**752-755, April 1971.

49 *Haas, A.: Essentials of living with pulmonary emphysema, a guide for patients and their families, Patient Publication no. 4, New York, 1963, The Institute of Physical Medicine and Rehabilitation.

50 Haberman, P. B., and others: Determinants of successful selective tracheobronchial suctioning, N. Engl. J. Med. **289:**1060-1062, Nov. 1973.

*References preceded by an asterisk are particularly well suited for student reading.

51 Hargreaves, A. G.: Emotional problems of patients with respiratory disease, Nurs. Clin. North Am. **3**:479-487, Sept. 1968.

52 *Helming, M. G., editor: Symposium on nursing in respiratory diseases, Nurs. Clin. North Am. **3**:381-487, Sept. 1968.

53 Hinshaw, H. C.: Diseases of the chest, ed. 3, Boston, 1969, Little, Brown & Co.

54 Hohle, B. M.: The atypical mycobacteria: patient care at home, Am. J. Nurs. **67**:1033-1036, May 1967.

55 Hunt, W. J., and Bespalec, D. A.: An evaluation of current methods of modifying smoking behavior, J. Clin. Psychol. **30**:431-438, Oct. 1974.

56 *Jacquette, G.: To reduce hazards of tracheal suctioning, Am. J. Nurs. **71**:2362-2364, Dec. 1971.

57 *James, G.: A "stop-smoking" program, Am. J. Nurs. **64**:122-125, June 1964.

58 Jenkins, D. E.: Current status of the atypical mycobacteria, Clin. Notes Respir. Dis. **4**:3-12, Fall 1965.

59 Johnson, J., and others: Surgery of the chest, ed. 4, Chicago, 1970, Year Book Medical Publishers, Inc.

60 Johnston, R. F., and Hopewell, P. C.: Chemotherapy of pulmonary tuberculosis, Ann. Intern. Med. **70**:359-367, Feb. 1969.

61 Kinney, M.: Rehabilitation of patients with C O L D, Am. J. Nurs. **67**:2528-2535, Dec. 1967.

61a Klause, M. L.: Mediastinoscopy, A.O.R.N.J. **15**:55-59, March 1972.

62 Kopetzky, M.: Normal and asthmatic lungs: how they work. In Essays in medicine, Asthma, New York, 1972, Medcom Books, Inc.

63 Kudia, M. S.: The care of the patient with respiratory insufficiency, Nurs. Clin. North Am. **8**:183-190, March 1973.

64 *Kurihara, M.: Postural drainage, clapping and vibrating, Am. J. Nurs. **65**:76-79, Nov. 1965.

65 Lagerson, J.: Nursing care of patients with chronic pulmonary insufficiency, Nurs. Clin. North Am. **9**:165-179, March 1974.

66 Langston, H. T., and Barker, W. S.: The adult thoracic surgical patient. In Neville, W. E., editor: Care of the surgical cardiopulmonary patient, Chicago, 1971, Year Book Medical Publishers, Inc.

67 Larson, R. K., and others: Genetics and environmental determinants of chronic obstructive pulmonary disease, Ann. Intern. Med. **72**:627-632, May 1970.

68 Le Quense, D. M.: Relation between deep vein thrombosis and pulmonary embolism in surgical patients, N. Engl. J. Med. **291**:1202-1204, Dec. 1974.

69 *Lewis, E., and Browning, M., editors: Nursing in respiratory disease, New York, 1972, The American Journal of Nursing Co.

70 MacDonald, F. M.: Respiratory acidosis, Arch. Intern. Med. **116**:689-698, Nov. 1965.

71 McCormick, K. A., and Birnbaum, M. L.: Acute ventilatory failure following thoracic trauma, Nurs. Clin. North Am. **9**:181-194, March 1974.

72 Mittman, C.: Chronic obstructive lung disease: the result of the interaction of genetic and environmental factors, Heart & Lung **2**:222-226, March-April 1973.

73 Monto, A. S., and Ullman, B. M.: Acute respiratory illness in an American community, J.A.M.A. **227**:164-169, Jan. 1974.

74 *Moody, L.: Asthma, physiology and patient care, Am. J. Nurs. **73**:1212-1217, July 1973.

75 Moody, L. F.: Nursing care of patients with asthma, Nurs. Clin. North Am. **9**:195-207, March 1974.

75a Morell, M. T., and Dunnill, M. S.: The postmortem incidence of pulmonary embolism in a hospital population, Br. J. Surg. **55**:347-352, May 1968.

76 National League for Nursing: Patient care in tuberculosis, ed. 2, New York, 1973, The League.

77 Nett, L.: The use of mechanical ventilators, Nurs. Clin. North Am. **9**:123-136, March 1974.

78 *Nett, L. M., and Petty, T. L.: Acute respiratory failure: principles of care, Am. J. Nurs. **67**:1847-1853, Sept. 1967.

79 Nett, L., and Petty, T. I.: Oxygen toxicity, Am. J. Nurs. **73**:1556-1558, Sept. 1973.

80 *Neville, W. E.: Care of the surgical cardiopulmonary patient, Chicago, 1971, Year Book Medical Publishers, Inc.

80a Niewoehner, D., and others: Pathologic changes in peripheral airways of young cigarette smokers, N. Engl. J. Med. **291**:755-758, Oct. 1974.

80b Obley, F. A., and Preiser, F. M.: Comprehensive outpatient respiratory care: a program conducted in a suburban private practice, J. Am. Geriatr. Soc. **22**:521-524, Nov. 1974.

81 Perry, P. A.: A perspective on chronic obstructive pulmonary disease. In Andersen, E. H., and others, editors: Current concepts in clinical nursing, vol. 4, St. Louis, 1973, The C. V. Mosby Co.

82 Petty, T. L.: Intensive and rehabilitative respiratory care, ed. 2, Philadelphia, 1974, Lea & Febiger.

83 *Petty, T. L.: Respiratory failure and the heart, Heart & Lung **1**:84, Jan.-Feb. 1972.

84 *Petty, T.: A chest physician's perspective on asthma, Heart & Lung **1**:611-620, Sept.-Oct. 1972.

85 *Phipps, W. J., Barker, W. L., and Daly, B. J.: Respiratory insufficiency and failure. In Meltzer, L. E., Abdellah, F. G., and Kitchell, J. R.: Concepts and practices of intensive care for nurse specialists, ed. 2, Philadelphia, 1975, The Charles Press, Publishers.

86 Pontoppiden, H., Geffin, F., and Lowenstein, E.: Acute respiratory failure in the adult, N. Engl. J. Med. **27**:690-698, 743-752, 799-806, Oct. 1972.

87 *Programmed instruction, an educational design program: Respiratory tract aspiration, Am. J. Nurs. **66**:2483-2510, Nov. 1966.

88 *Rassmussen, D. L.: Black lung in southern Appalachia, Am. J. Nurs. **70**:509-511, March 1970.

89 Rie, M. W.: Physical therapy in the nursing care of respiratory disease patients, Nurs. Clin. North Am. **3**:463-478, 1968.

90 *Riley, R. L.: Air-borne infections, Am. J. Nurs. **60**:1246-1248, Sept. 1960.

91 Riley, R. L.: Protective measures; reasonable or ritualistic? Nurs. Outlook **7**:38-39, Jan. 1959.

92 *Rodman, T.: Management of tracheobronchial secretions, Am. J. Nurs. **66**:2474-2477, Nov. 1966.

93 Sasahara, A. A.: Therapy for pulmonary embolism, J.A.M.A. **329**:1795-1798, Sept. 1974.

94 *Scott, B. H.: Tensions linked with emphysema, Am. J. Nurs. **69**:538-540, March 1969.

95 Sedlock, S. A.: Detection of chronic pulmonary disease, Am. J. Nurs. **72**:1407-1411, Aug. 1972.

96 *Selecky, P. A.: Tracheostomy: a review of present day indications, complications, and care, Heart & Lung **3**:272-283, March-April 1974.

97 Simmons, D. H.: Evaluation of acid-base status. In American Thoracic Society: Basics of RD, New York, 1974, The Society.

98 Sitzman, J.: Nursing management of the acutely ill respiratory patient, Heart & Lung **1**:207-215, March-April 1972.

99 *Sladin, A.: Pathogenesis of the shock lung, R.N. **34**:1-12, Dec. 1971.

100 Slonim, N. B., and Hamilton, L. H.: Respiratory physiology, ed. 2, St. Louis, 1971, The C. V. Mosby Co.

101 *Sorensen, K. M., and Amis, D. B.: Understanding the world of the chronically ill, Am. J. Nurs. **67**:811-817, April 1967.

102 *Sovie, M. D., and Israel, J. S.: Acute respiratory failure: use of the cuffed tracheostomy tube, Am. J. Nurs. **67**:1854-1856, Sept. 1967.

103 Stechschulte, D. J.: Asthma and immunology. In Essays in medicine, New York, 1972, Medcom Press.

104 *Thacker, E. W.: Postural drainage and respiratory control, ed. 2, London, 1965, Lloyd-Luke (Medical Books), Ltd.

104a Thurlbeck, W. M.: Chronic bronchitis and emphysema—the pathophysiology of chronic lung disease. In American Thoracic Society: Basics of R.D., New York, 1974, The Society.

105 *Traver, G.: Assessment of thorax and lungs, Am. J. Nurs. **73:**466-471, March 1973.

106 Traver, G.: The nurses' role in clinical testing of lung function, Nurs. Clin. North Am. **9:**101-110, March 1974.

107 *Traver, G. A.: Effect of intermittent positive pressure breathing and use of rebreathing tube upon tidal volume and cough, Nurs. Res. **17:**100-103, March-April 1968.

108 Tuberculosis facts in the United States: New York, 1968, Epidemiology and Statistics Division of the National Tuberculosis and Respiratory Disease Association.

109 U. S. Department of Health, Education and Welfare, Public Health Service: Tuberculosis programs 1972, Atlanta, 1974, Center for Disease Control.

110 U. S. Department of Health, Education and Welfare: Current trends. Isoniazid-associated hepatitis: summary of the report of the tuberculosis advisory committee and special consultants to the director, Center for Disease Control, Morbidity and Mortality **23:**97-98, March 1974.

111 U. S. Department of Health, Education and Welfare: Current trends, recommendations for health department supervision of tuberculosis patients, Morbidity and Mortality **23:**75-76, Feb. 1974.

112 Vaughan, V. C., III: The place of drug therapy in childhood asthma, Am. J. Nurs. **66:**1049-1052, May 1966.

113 Wade, J. F.: Respiratory nursing care: physiology and technique, St. Louis, 1973, The C. V. Mosby Co.

114 *Wagner, M. M.: Assessment of patients with multiple injuries, Am. J. Nurs. **72:**1822-1827, Oct. 1972.

115 *Weg, J. G.: Tuberculosis and the generation gap, Am. J. Nurs. **71:**495-500, March 1971.

116 West, J. B.: Causes of carbon dioxide retention in lung disease, New Engl. J. Med. **284:**1232-1236, June 1971.

116a White, H.: Tracheostomy care with a cuffed tube, Am. J. Nurs. **72:**75-77, Jan. 1972.

117 Wilson, R. F., and others: Physiologic shunting in the lung of the critically ill or injured patient, J. Surg. Res. **10:**571-578, Dec. 1970.

118 *Winter, P. M., and Lowenstein, E.: Acute respiratory failure, Sci. Am. **221:**23-29, Nov. 1969.

119 Wintrobe, M. M., and others, editors: Harrison's principles of internal medicine, ed. 7, New York, 1974, McGraw-Hill Book Co.

120 Ziskind, M. M.: The acute bacterial pneumonias in the adult. In American Thoracic Society: Basics of R.D., New York, 1974, The Society.

23 Ear, nose, and throat diseases

■ The purpose of this chapter is to give nurses an understanding of the causes of ear, nose, and throat diseases and the sequence of complications so that they are able to teach health and prevention of disease. The close link between minor infections of the ears, nose, and throat and serious disease makes prompt care of these conditions important; therefore every nurse should be concerned with prevention of these common infections.

Diagnostic procedures, treatments, and nursing care of patients with specific diseases of the ear, nose, and throat are discussed only briefly. For detailed information on specialized care, refer to references preceded by an asterisk at the end of this chapter and to other periodicals and special publications.

■ COMMON DIAGNOSTIC PROCEDURES

Visual examinations

The mucous membrane lining the vestibule of the nares is examined easily by using a nasal speculum, a head mirror, and a standing or wall lamp with a spotlight head attached. The light should be bright and should be placed about 9 inches to the right of, and slightly behind, the patient's head. The room can be darkened. The speculum stretches the nasal vestibule so that the light reflected from the head mirror can shine into all parts of the nose. A cotton-tipped applicator may be needed to remove secretions or to take a culture. A vasoconstrictor such as phenylepinephrine (Neo-Synephrine) may be applied to shrink the mucous membrane and give a better exposure. The throat often is examined superficially with a tongue depressor and flashlight. For a more extensive examination of the posterior nares and the throat, a nasopharyngeal mirror, a head mirror, a tongue depressor, and a light are used. The nasopharyngeal mirror is warmed with hot water or in a flame from an alcohol lamp to prevent fogginess and failure to reflect. Because this examination may make the patient gag, he should be instructed to breathe through his mouth while the mirror is being directed toward his pharynx.

The larynx may be examined by an indirect or direct method. For an *indirect laryngoscopy,* the patient sits in a chair with his head tilted back and is asked to stick out his tongue. The physician then grasps it with a gauze sponge and pulls it forward and downward. A warmed laryngeal mirror is introduced into the back of the throat until the larynx is visualized. It is examined at rest and during attempts to speak (phonation). If the gag reflex is very sensitive, the pharyngeal wall may be sprayed with a light, topical anesthetic such as 2% cocaine or 2% pontocaine. Pontocaine is preferred by some physicians because it is less toxic than cocaine. A *direct laryngoscopy* is performed on children, on adults who are unable to cooperate for an indirect examination, and on all patients with suspicious lesions of the larynx. A sedative such as secobarbital, meperidine, or another narcotic and atropine sulfate are given 1 hour before the examination, which is usually performed under local anesthesia for which a drug such as 10% cocaine is used. When general anesthesia is used, the same preanesthetic medications are used. Atropine is essential prior to both local and general anesthesia because it reduces the volume of secretions. For direct laryngoscopy, the patient is placed in a reclining position, with his head in a head holder. If no head holder is available, the pa-

■ STUDY QUESTIONS

1 Review the anatomy and physiology of the ear, nose, sinuses, and throat. What are some specific dangers from disease of these parts?

2 What emotional reactions would probably follow the sudden inability to hear? To speak? What means of communication are available for those who are deaf? Who cannot speak?

3 Review the procedures for throat irrigation, ear irrigation, administration of nose drops, and administration of eardrops.

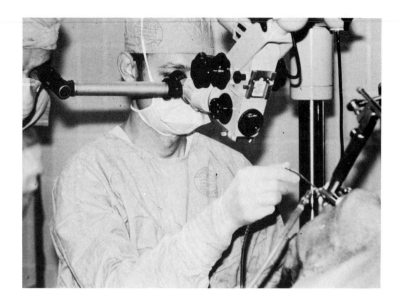

FIG. 23-1. Laryngoscopy using the operating microscope to provide both illumination and magnification. The laryngoscope is self-retaining. (From DeWeese, D. D., and Saunders, W. H.: Textbook of otolaryngology, ed. 4, St. Louis, 1973, The C. V. Mosby Co.)

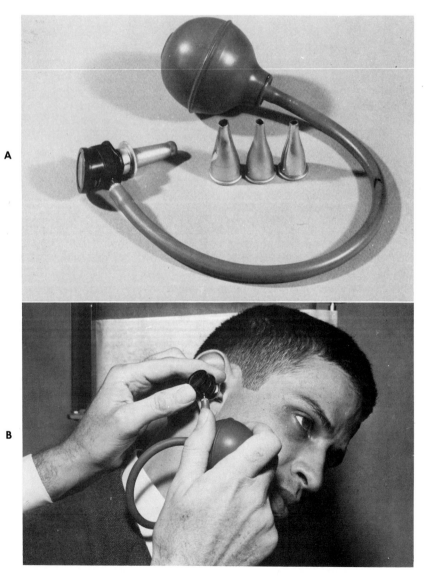

A

B

FIG. 23-2. A, Siegle pneumatic otoscope. The speculum that fits this otoscope is attached. Magnifying lens also may be used with the usual type of speculum if magnification only is desired. **B,** Pneumatic otoscope in use. (From DeWeese, D. D., and Saunders, W. H.: Textbook of otolaryngology, ed. 4, St. Louis, 1973, The C. V. Mosby Co.)

tient's head is extended over the edge of the table and manually supported by a physician or nurse.

The laryngoscope, a hollow, metal tube with a handle at the proximal end and a light at the distal end, is introduced by a doctor through the mouth into the hypopharynx, elevating the epiglottis, and making the interior of the larynx easily visible. Minor surgical procedures such as a biopsy or the removal of a small benign tumor may be performed through this instrument.

After a laryngoscopy under local anesthesia, the patient should not eat or drink anything until the gag reflex returns, usually within 2 hours. The gag reflex can be tested by "tickling" the throat with a tongue blade or applicator. After the gag reflex returns, the patient should try first to drink water since, if it is accidentally aspirated into the trachea or lungs, it is the fluid least likely to cause reaction.

Microlaryngoscopy using an operating microscope is becoming more widely used (Fig. 23-1). This method provides magnification and binocular vision.

The normal frontal and maxillary sinuses can be visualized by illuminating them in a dark room with a specially shaped, lighted bulb or a lighted transillumination tip. This examination is referred to as *transillumination*. If disease is present, the light will not penetrate the sinuses, or it will reveal fluid levels indicative of obstruction to drainage of the sinuses. Radiographs of the sinuses may be ordered to help establish the diagnosis of sinusitis. No physical preparation is necessary and usually no contrast medium is used since the normal sinus is filled with air, which itself casts a shadow in contrast to surrounding structures.

The ears may be examined with an aural speculum and with reflected light supplied by a head mirror. The ear canal often has to be cleansed of cerumen, desquamated epithelium, and other accumulations with a cotton-tipped applicator, a cerumen spoon, or a "loop" before the eardrum can be seen. An array of otologic suction devices and adequate suction are helpful. *Pneumatic* otoscopy may be performed (Fig. 23-2). In this examination, air is compressed into the ear canal, exerting pressure against the drumhead. It is particularly useful in detecting pinhole perforations that otherwise might not be found as middle ear secretions are drawn through them by the suction. The ear may require examination under the microscope, which provides depth perception as well as increased magnification (Fig. 23-3). During this examination the nurse should be prepared to hand the otologic specula, suction, or other instruments to the physician so that his eyes may be kept on the microscope. An *otoscope* with its magnifying lens commonly is used to supplement the examination with the speculum, particularly for the examination of small children. Young children who have difficulty remaining still may have to be restrained for examination of the ears, nose, or throat.

Audiometric testing

The ability to hear pure tones (simple sound waves) and to discriminate speech can be tested with a clinical audiometer. The graph of the hearing levels is called an *audiogram* (Fig. 23-4). Only the weakest intensities (pressures exerted by sound) that can be heard by the patient at each frequency are recorded on the audiogram. Intensity of sound is measured in decibels (dB) (considered the unit of hearing). Threshold is defined as the lowest intensity of sound at which pure tone can be heard. Speech that is comfortably loud to a person with normal hearing ranges in intensity from approximately 40 to 65 dB. The term "frequency" refers to the number of sound waves emanating from a source per second and is expressed in Hertz (Hz). The greater the number of Hertz, the higher its pitch.

A child or young adult with normal hearing can often hear frequencies ranging from 20 to 20,000 Hz. Hearing is most sensitive for frequencies 500 to 4,000 Hz. In audiometric testing the frequencies 125, 250, 500, 1,000, 2,000, 4,000, and 8,000 Hz are commonly employed to assess the hearing sensitivity of an individual. The decibel is the unit of measurement used in defining the degree of hearing loss. (See Fig. 23-4.) If a person's hearing ranges from 0 to 20 dB loss for a tested frequency, it is considered

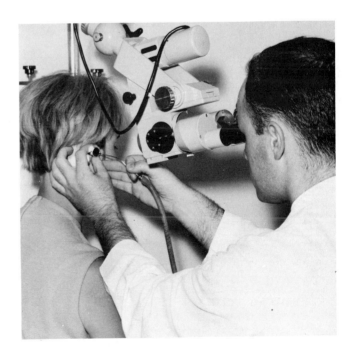

FIG. 23-3. Operating microscope used as diagnostic instrument. Small aural suction tip aspirates serum or pus from ear canal or middle ear. (From DeWeese, D. D., and Saunders, W. H.: Textbook of otolaryngology, ed. 4, St. Louis, 1973, The C. V. Mosby Co.)

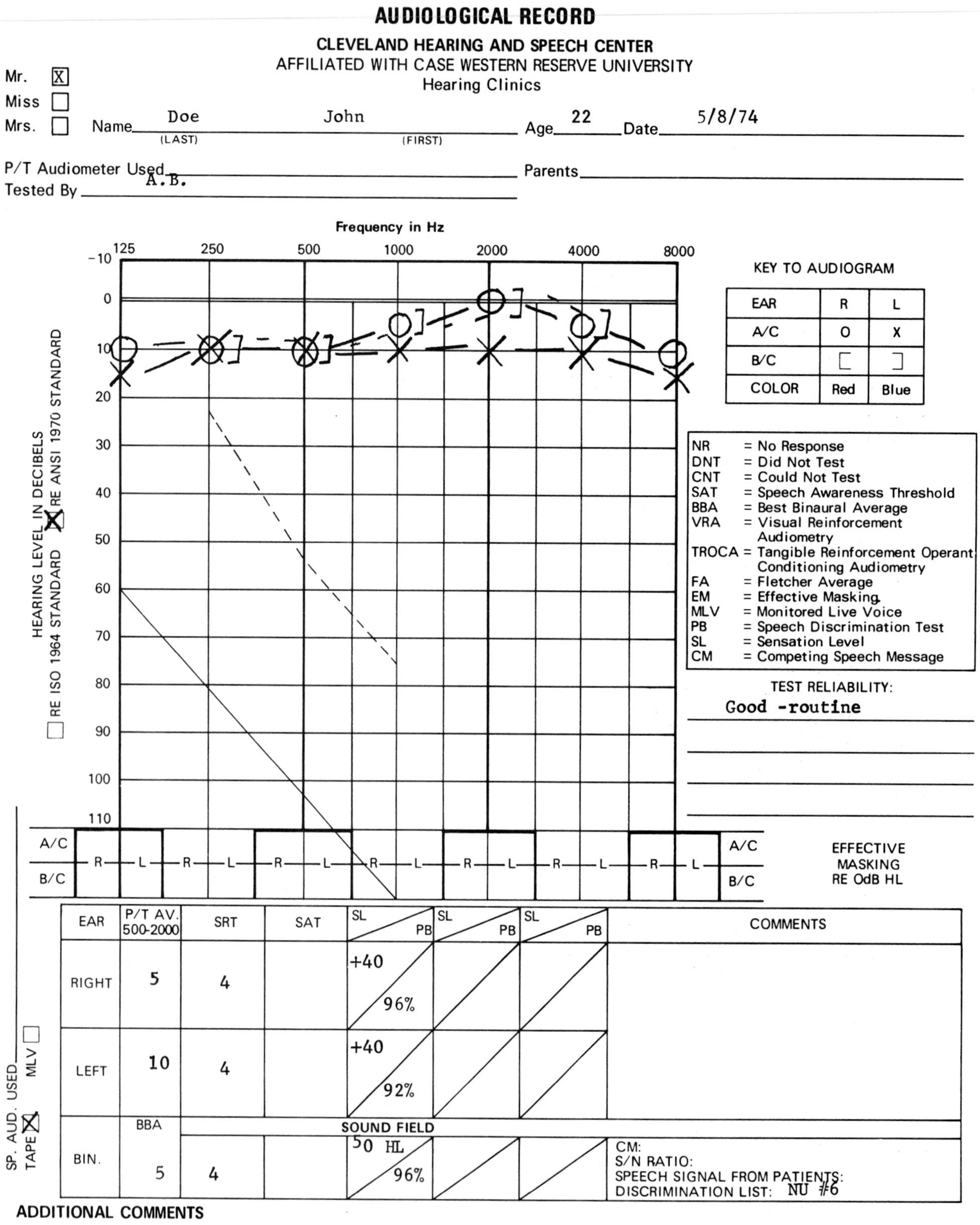

AUDIOLOGICAL RECORD

CLEVELAND HEARING AND SPEECH CENTER
AFFILIATED WITH CASE WESTERN RESERVE UNIVERSITY
Hearing Clinics

Mr. [X]
Miss [ ]
Mrs. [ ]   Name___Doe_____John_____   Age__22__ Date___5/8/74_____
                    (LAST)   (FIRST)

P/T Audiometer Used___A.B._____   Parents_____
Tested By _____

FIG. 23-4. Normal audiogram. (Courtesy Cleveland Hearing and Speech Center, Cleveland, Ohio.)

to be within the normal range. If the hearing loss is greater than 20 dB but less than 50 dB, it is considered a mild hearing loss. A moderate hearing loss ranges from 50 to 69 dB, a severe loss from 70 to 89 dB, and a greater than 89 dB loss is considered a profound hearing loss.

The most important sounds in our environment are those of speech. Generally, normal speech ranges in intensity from about 40 to 65 dB and 500 to 2,000 Hz in frequency. Thus one could generalize by saying a person with a hearing loss of 65 dB or greater in the 500 to 2,000 Hz range cannot hear normal conversation.

In recent years, audiologists (specialists in hearing) have developed some very useful tests to not only determine whether or not a hearing loss is present but also the frequency of the loss, how well the patient can understand speech, and whether the problem site is in the middle ear (that is, conductive loss), inner ear, or auditory nerve system (that is, sensorineural loss).

For best results, audiometry must be performed in a specially constructed soundproof booth. Group screening examinations such as are done in schools are helpful only in discovering children who need individual examination. To test the intensity of sound of air conduction, the patient wears earphones and is instructed to signal with his finger when he hears the tone and when he no longer hears it. The middle frequencies are tested first, and the operator alternately increases and decreases the intensity of sound until he finds the dial setting at which the person being tested can just perceive sound. The point at which the sound can just barely be heard is termed threshold. When testing by *air conduction,* as in most environmental situations, the sound travels through the external and middle ear before reaching the inner ear. Once the air conduction testing is completed, a *bone oscillator* is placed on the mastoid bone behind the ear. This oscillator produces mechanical vibrations that are conducted by the bones of the skull to the inner ear. This enables the audiologist to assess the acuity of the inner ear by bypassing the outer and middle ear. If a person can hear better by bone conduction than air conduction, there is often an implication of some external or middle ear problem.

Speech audiometry is used to determine how well the patient can hear and understand speech. There are two primary tests included in speech audiometry. One is the *speech reception threshold (SRT)* test and the other is a speech discrimination test. The SRT is simply the lowest intensity level in decibels at which the patient can correctly repeat specially selected bisyllabic words 50% of the time. Usually the SRT closely corresponds to the air conduction thresholds. *Speech discrimination tests* require the patient to repeat 50 monosyllabic words common to the English language. These words are usually presented at an intensity level easily heard by the patient (25 to 40 dB above his threshold). The number of correctly repeated words is converted to a percentage score. Individuals with normal hearing generally score 90% to 100% on this test.

Assessment of children. A child's acquisition of speech is critically dependent on proper hearing. Therefore it is imperative that if a hearing loss is suspected by the parents or medical personnel, the child be referred to an audiologist for proper testing and to an otologist for a medical examination and treatment.

Until a child is 4 to 5 years of age, he may be difficult to test by conventional methods. Special testing procedures utilizing rewards for correct responses aid in conditioning the child to behave in an expected manner if he hears the sound. Although child audiology is presently at a very sophisticated level and yields much information as to the child's hearing status, definitive statements often cannot be made. All statements referring to hearing capabilities of very young children should be guarded and interpreted with care. It should be remembered, however, that given the proper testing facilities and setting, it is possible for the audiologist to grossly assess the hearing of a child or infant of any age. Although results may be questionable with a young child, proper management and counseling can only be initiated once the loss is suspected and the child is properly evaluated.

Insufflation

Insufflation of the eustachian tubes may be performed either to test their patency or to force them open mechanically. A simple insufflation procedure is to have the patient compress his nose with his thumb and forefinger and swallow (*Valsalva* procedure). If he can feel the passage of air up the eustachian tube to the middle ear or if the physician, looking through the otoscope, can see the eardrum move outward as the patient swallows, the tube is patent. Another method is to force air into the nostril as the patient swallows water. A Politzer bag (a specially constructed rubber bag equipped with a nasal tip) is inserted into one nostril while the other nostril is compressed by the physician's fingers. As the patient swallows a sip of water, pressure is applied on the bag, forcing air into the nasopharynx and the eustachian tubes. The physician, listening through a rubber tube connecting his ear with the patient's ear, can hear if air passes into the middle ear.

Air may also be forced into the eustachian tubes by means of a catheter inserted through the nose into the nasopharyngeal opening of the tubes. Finding the opening may be a tedious and uncomfortable procedure for the patient. To make the procedure easier, a weak solution of cocaine (1%) may be applied to the mucous membrane to desensitize it as the catheter is maneuvered into place. When the catheter passes into the orifice, the Politzer bag is attached to the catheter and air is instilled as the physician listens to its passage through tubing attached to his ear and the patient's. If passage of air into the tube cannot be heard, it may be due to stenosis or to anatomic irregularities of the eustachian tubes. This procedure is not done when there is an acute infection because of the danger of trauma to the eustachian tube and introduction of infection into the middle ear.

■ INFECTIONS OF THE NOSE AND SINUSES

Infections of the nose, throat, and sinuses are among the most frequent complications of the common cold. The nurse, therefore, should be aware of the signs of these infections and of their complications.

Rhinitis

Acute rhinitis. Simple, acute rhinitis (*coryza,* common cold) is an inflammatory condition of the mucous membranes of the nose and accessory sinuses caused by a filtrable virus. It affects almost everyone at some time in his life and occurs most often in the cold, winter months. It is generally believed that the infecting agent is present in the nose and sinuses at all times and that fatigue and chilling are among many factors influencing susceptibility. The patient usually complains of dryness of the nose, eyes, and soft palate, general malaise, chilliness, and headache. These symptoms are followed in 12 to 24 hours by obstruction to nasal breathing due to swelling of the mucous membrane and a profuse, watery nasal discharge. Sneezing, tearing of the eyes, and nasal irritation also occur, and the postnasal discharge may cause pharyngitis, laryngitis, or bronchitis. Infants and young children are particularly susceptible to this infection, which may spread to the middle ear and cause an otitis media. They should be isolated from persons with colds, and if they develop a cold, they should be observed carefully for symptoms suggesting otitis media. If a high temperature occurs or if the infant becomes restless, rolls his head from side to side in bed, or pulls at his ear, medical attention should be sought.

Most people with colds do not go to their physician unless symptoms persist or make them very uncomfortable. Medical treatment, if sought, usually consists of rest, fluids, moist inhalations, and antihistamines and decongestants. The antihistamines are helpful in alleviating symptoms such as sneezing and tearing of the eyes. Since they cause drowsiness in most persons, they should not be used when driving a car or working near moving machinery. Nose drops may be prescribed if there is prolonged nasal obstruction. Most otologists now believe that nose drops and other topical agents should be used infrequently, since their continued use results in addiction of the nasal mucosa to their use (*rhinitis medicamentosa*).[11] When nose drops are ordered, the individual should be taught how to use them correctly.

No more than three drops or three sprays of solution should be instilled into each nostril at one time unless more medication is specifically prescribed. To administer nose drops a person should either sit in a chair and tip his head well backward, lie down with his head extending over the edge of the bed, or lie down and place a large pillow under his shoulders so that his head is tipped backward. He should remain in this position for 5 minutes after the drops are instilled to allow the solution to reach the posterior nares. If, after 10 minutes, he still has marked congestion, another drop or two of the solution may be used. The mucous membrane of the anterior nares by this time should have become constricted so that the solution may reach the posterior nares more easily. Some physicians feel that the instillation of nose drops is too upsetting for children and order oral nasal decongestants such as pseudoephedrine, 30 mg. ($\frac{1}{2}$ grain), every 3 or 4 hours and steam inhalations. A rubber bulb ear syringe may be used to aspirate the mucous discharge from the nose of infants to clear the nose so that they can breathe and be able to take their feedings. If a rubber syringe is not available, a short piece of rubber tubing should be placed on the tip of a glass syringe. To administer a nasal spray or use an inhalator, the person sits upright with his head tilted slightly backward. The atomizer is placed at the entrance of the nostril and, while occluding the opposite nostril with finger pressure, squeezed. The inhalator is placed in the nostril, and after occluding the opposite nostril, the person inhales. Occluding the opposite nostril prevents the entrance of air and thus allows the medication to be forced high up into the nasal cavity.

If the nasal discharge persists for more than about a week or if the patient develops an elevation of temperature, he should be urged to seek medical attention. Persons who have recurrent colds should seek medical attention because nasal deformity such as enlarged turbinated bones or a deviated septum and chronic sinusitis may cause the repeated attacks. Repeated colds eventually may lead to chronic rhinitis. (For further discussion of the common cold, see p. 553.)

Chronic rhinitis. Chronic rhinitis is a chronic inflammation of the mucous membrane of the nose caused by repeated, acute infections, by an allergy, or by vasomotor rhinitis. Nasal obstruction accompanied by a feeling of stuffiness and pressure in the nose is the chief complaint. A nasal discharge is always present and may be serous, mucopurulent, or purulent, depending on the amount of secondary infection present. Polyp formation may occur, and the turbinates may enlarge as a result of the chronic irritation. Complaints of frontal headache, vertigo, and sneezing are common.

Antibiotics may be used to treat the infection. After the offending allergens have been identified, they should be avoided by the patient. Antihistamines are helpful in alleviating symptoms. The polyps or the hyperplastic tissues may require surgical removal (polypectomy, turbinectomy).

Nasal irrigations may be used in the treatment of chronic rhinitis, and the nurse may be asked to assist with them. Details of this procedure are described in texts on fundamentals of nursing or in textbooks on otolaryngology. Care should be taken to assure that both nostrils are open and that the pressure exerted in them is not greater than that produced when an irrigating can is held 30 to 37.5 cm. (12 to 15 inches) above the level of the nose. Greater pressure increases the danger of forcing infected material into the sinuses or the middle ear. The patient should breathe through his mouth during the procedure, and the irrigating tip should be removed from the nostril if he must sneeze or cough. The position of choice for the irrigation is one in which the patient sits upright with the chin bent forward so that the eustachian tubes will be above the stream of solution. The patient should not blow his nose for ½ hour after the procedure in order to avoid forcing residual irrigating fluid through the eustachian tubes into the middle ears. This procedure is dangerous if performed on a child who is crying or struggling to avoid the procedure.

Sinusitis

Acute sinusitis. Acute sinusitis is an inflammation of one or more of the sinuses. The most common cause of acute sinusitis is obstruction of the paranasal sinuses, which blocks the egress of secretions of the sinuses. These secretions become infected, giving rise to acute sinusitis. Sinusitis also follows acute rhinitis or other respiratory diseases such as pneumonia or influenza and is caused by infection extending through the nasal openings into the sinuses. Abscessed teeth or tooth extraction occasionally causes an acute maxillary sinusitis. Streptococci, staphylococci, or the pneumococcus bacilli usually are the infecting organisms. Sinusitis also can be caused by an allergic reaction.

The patient with acute sinusitis often complains of a constant, severe headache and of pain over the infected sinuses. Maxillary sinusitis will cause pain under the eyes, whereas frontal sinusitis often causes pain over the eyebrows. The patient may have the sensation of "pain in the bone" even on slight pressure over the affected sinus. Pain from the ethmoid and sphenoid sinuses usually is referred and is felt at the top of the head. Occasionally there may be noticeable swelling over the maxillary or frontal sinuses or there may be orbital edema. The patient may have nausea, purulent discharge from the nose if the duct is not closed, obstruction to nasal breathing, fever, and general malaise. Fever usually is proportional to the amount of obstruction present and the virulence of the infection. If the sinus is completely obstructed, the temperature may be as high as 40° C. (104° F.). The throat may be sore from irritation caused by postnasal drainage. Complications of severe untreated sinusitis include osteomyelitis in the adjacent bone, an abscess that may involve the brain, venous sinus thrombosis, and septicemia.

Objectives in the care of patients with acute sinusitis are to establish drainage of the sinuses and to control the infection. Broad-spectrum antibiotics such as tetracycline or erythromycin are given for their specific action on the causative organisms. Drugs such as phenylephrine hydrochloride (Neo-Synephrine), 0.25%, and ephedrine sulfate, 0.25% to 3%, which constrict the blood vessels and thus reduce hyperemia and improve drainage, may be given as nose drops or by inhalation. Mucolytic agents or normal saline solution may be given by inhalation. Antibiotics are usually not ordered because of the danger of sensitizing the individual to them.

If medication is given by atomizer or nebulizer, the adapter is placed in one nostril and the other nostril closed. The patient then should be instructed to breathe through his nose with the mouth closed. Medication is then forced by air pressure (created with a hand bulb) through a small opening in the atomizer. Such pressure breaks the large droplets of fluid into a fine mist. If a nebulizer is used, the solution is usually forced through the apparatus by a current of oxygen or compressed air (p. 569).

Because aspirin may be associated with nasal polyposis, it is usually avoided as a pain medication. Acetaminophen (Tylenol) is a good substitute for aspirin, and occasionally codeine or even morphine sulfate or meperidine may be necessary to relieve the pain. Heat over the sinuses also gives some relief from pain. Hot wet dressings or a heat lamp may be ordered. Moist steam in the room may help to facilitate drainage. Humidity of 40% to 50% will add to the patient's comfort, and the room temperature should be kept constant since room temperature changes aggravate sinusitis.

If conservative measures do not cure an acute sinus infection, the physician may irrigate the maxillary and frontal sinuses with normal saline solution by inserting a trocar and cannula through the openings of the sinuses. If it is impossible to insert the trocar and cannula through the normal opening, the nasal mucosa may be anesthetized with cocaine and the antrum (maxillary sinus) perforated with a trocar and cannula. This procedure is known as an *an-*

trum puncture. The nurse should explain it to the patient and urge him to breathe through the mouth during the procedure. The patient's head is supported while the treatment is given, since, although it is not actually painful, it causes a sensation of pressure and may produce dizziness and nausea.

Since early treatment of acute sinusitis is much more successful than treatment after the condition becomes chronic, patients with symptoms of acute sinusitis should be urged to seek medical attention at once. Chronic sinusitis is difficult to cure and may lead to further complications such as ear infections and bronchiectasis. Organisms associated with chronic sinusitis are usually gram positive but may be anaerobes as well as aerobes.

Chronic sinusitis. In chronic sinusitis the mucous membrane lining a sinus becomes thickened from prolonged or repeated irritation and infection. The patient usually has a chronic purulent nasal discharge, a chronic cough caused by a postnasal drip, and a chronic dull sinus headache that is present on awakening and usually subsides during the day because the varied positions and movement of the head help the sinus to drain. As the passage of air through the nose becomes blocked, there also may be loss of ability to smell.

Treatment of chronic sinusitis may be surgical. Removal of nasal deformities such as a deviated nasal septum, hypertrophied turbinated bones, or nasal polyps that are obstructing the sinus openings may give relief. Sinus irrigations may be done to ensure better drainage. If the condition is caused by an allergy, it responds to general treatment of the allergy.

The person with chronic sinusitis should avoid chilling, and cold, damp atmospheres. Change to a warm, dry climate, though helpful to some people, is not necessarily helpful to all patients. The patient is advised not to smoke, because smoking further irritates the damaged mucous membranes. Air-conditioning often causes discomfort, particularly if the outside air is warm and moist. The person with chronic sinusitis often sleeps poorly and lacks pep and vigor in his living and in his work. Persistent postnasal discharge is believed to contribute, as the person grows older, to bronchiectasis, a chronic lung disease.

Surgery on the sinuses. If the patient has recurrent attacks of sinusitis, it may be necessary to provide better drainage by permanently enlarging the sinus openings or by making a new opening and removing the diseased mucous membrane. Surgery usually is performed during the subacute stage of infection. An opening into the maxillary sinus may be made through the nostril (antrotomy) or through the mouth under the upper lip (*Caldwell-Luc* operation). The Caldwell-Luc operation is not performed on children because they may have unerupted teeth near the site of the incision. While the ethmoid, frontal, and sphenoid sinuses can be approached through the nose, operations through an incision made in the upper half of the eyebrow and extending downward along the side of the nose provide better visualization for the surgeon and are considered safer. (See Fig. 23-5 for location of the sinuses.) Surgery through the nostrils may be (and often is) done under general as well as under local anesthesia, depending on the physician's preference.

Nursing intervention following a sinus operation. To prevent swallowing or aspiration of bloody drainage from the nose and throat postoperatively, the patient who has had a general anesthetic is turned well to the side. On recovery from the anesthesia or following local anesthesia, the patient may be in a mid-Fowler's position, which will help decrease edema at the operative site and promote drainage. Ice compresses are usually applied over the nose or an ice bag is placed directly over the maxillary or frontal sinuses. Ice constricts blood vessels, decreasing oozing and edema, and relieves pain. The patient should be watched carefully for hemorrhage. The nasal drip pad may be changed when it becomes soiled. Excessive bleeding should be called to the surgeon's attention. Repeated swallowing by the patient who is recovering from anesthesia may indicate hemorrhage.

Gauze packing is usually inserted into the nares and usually remains there for 48 hours. Consequently, the patient breathes through his mouth. His lips and mouth become dry and need frequent care. Aromatic solutions are refreshing, and petrolatum helps to prevent dryness of the lips. Warm or cool vapor inhalations often are ordered. The patient should be reminded not to blow his nose, since this procedure may cause trauma to the operative site and bleeding.

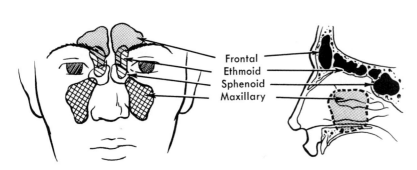

Frontal
Ethmoid
Sphenoid
Maxillary

FIG. 23-5. Location of the sinuses.

If a Caldwell-Luc procedure has been performed, the patient usually is given only liquids for at least 24 hours and a soft diet for 3 or 4 days. Fluids should be given liberally to all patients following surgery of the sinuses. If there is an oral incision, mouth care is given before meals to improve appetite and after eating to decrease the danger of infection.

A gross check of the patient's visual acuity and a check for diplopia are advisable after sinus surgery to be sure that there is no damage to the optic nerve.

Fever or complaints of tenderness or pain over the involved sinus should be reported to the physician, since they may indicate postoperative infection or inadequate drainage. Antibiotics may be given prophylactically. For a week or two postoperatively, there may be swelling of the area or a black eye. Numbness of the upper lip and upper teeth may be present for several months after a Caldwell-Luc operation.

Nasal obstruction

Nasal polyps. Nasal polyps are grapelike growths of mucous membrane and loose connective tissue. They may be caused by irritation to mucous membranes of the nose or sinuses from an allergy or by chronic sinusitis. Since they may obstruct breathing or may bleed, nasal polyps are removed. They are excised through the nose by a snare or biting forceps (a polypectomy).

Deviated septum. The septum, which is normally thin and straight, may be deviated from the midline and protrude more to one side of the nasal passage than to the other. The deviation may cause a nasal obstruction that increases when infection or allergic reaction occurs. If the obstruction is marked, noisy and difficult breathing will result. There may be a postnasal drip, or the mucosa may become dry so that crusts form. This deformity of the septum is common in older children and adults. It may be congenital but usually is the result of an injury. The nurse should encourage persons with trauma to the nose to seek medical attention since, if not treated, a broken nose can lead to chronic sinusitis and chronic rhinitis, even though it may cause no immediate problem.

If the deformity causes nasal obstruction, a *submucous resection* may be performed. After a local anesthetic has been administered, an internal incision is made on one side of the nasal septum from top to bottom. The mucous membrane is elevated away from the bone, the obstructive parts of the cartilage and bone are removed, and the mucous membrane is sutured back into place. Plastic reconstruction may be necessary if a large part of the septum must be removed. Packing is placed in both nostrils to prevent bleeding and to splint the operative area. A newer procedure called a *nasoseptoplasty* is becoming more widely used to treat a deviated septum.

Hypertrophy of the turbinates. If the turbinates hypertrophy and cause nasal obstruction, they can be shrunk by the use of a cautery blade inserted into the inferior or middle turbinate. Sometimes a steroid preparation such as methylprednisolone acetate (Depo-Medrol) is injected into the turbinates to decrease reactivity and make them less responsive to allergens.

Management of the patient requiring nasal surgery. Most nasal surgery on adults is done under local anesthesia. The patient, however, should not be given anything orally for 6 hours preoperatively, since he may become nauseated during the operation. Usually he receives a sedative and a narcotic preoperatively. Children require a general anesthetic and may be given a drug such as atropine to reduce secretions.

The nose is usually packed with 1/2-inch gauze at the conclusion of the operation. The most commonly used packs are petrolatum-impregnated gauze, iodoform gauze with chlortetracycline (Aureomycin), and Cortisporin-impregnated gauze. The latter is particularly effective in reducing the odor of the nasal pack. If the packing should slip back into the throat, the surgeon is notified immediately. The pack is usually removed and replaced as necessary.

Following nasal surgery there is danger of hemorrhage. Blood may be evident on the external dressing that is applied under the nose, or the patient may expectorate or vomit bright red blood. The back of the throat should be examined to see if blood is running down into it. The patient's pulse may be rapid, or he may swallow repeatedly. Some oozing on the dressing is expected, but if it becomes pronounced or if any other symptoms appear, the surgeon should be notified, and material for repacking the nose should be prepared. This material consists of a hemostatic tray containing gauze packing, umbilical tape for posterior packing, a few small gauze sponges, a small rubber catheter (used for inserting a postnasal plug), a packing forceps, tongue blades, and scissors. A head mirror, a good light, epinephrine, 1:1,000, or some other vasoconstrictor, applicators, a nasal speculum, suction, and metal Frazer tip aspirators should be available.

If the dressing under the nose becomes soiled, it may be changed as necessary. This is very important from an esthetic standpoint. Sedation and encouragement are necessary because of general discomfort and apprehension caused by having the nasal passages packed and having to breathe through the mouth. Frequent oral care should be given, and fluids should be given freely. Postnasal drip, the presence of old blood in the mouth, and the loss of the ability to smell lessen the patient's appetite. Antihistamines may be administered to reduce nasal secretions. Because it is difficult to eat while the nose is packed, most patients prefer a liquid diet until the packing is removed, but they can have whatever food is tolerated. In some patients, packing may remain in the nares as long as 1 week, while in others it is removed in 48 hours. Since the packing blocks the passage of air through the nose, a partial vacuum is created when the patient swallows and he may complain of a sucking action when he attempts to drink.

After the nasal packing has been removed, the patient is asked not to blow his nose for 48 hours because blowing may start bleeding. Fever should be reported to the physician because it may be due to infection. Since the patient has swallowed blood, it is normal for the stools to be tarry for a day or two. Because the *Valsalva maneuver* can cause bleeding, the patient should be instructed not to bear down, and milk of magnesia or prune juice is usually ordered p.r.n. The patient is also cautioned about coughing too rigorously.

Following external nasal surgery the patient frequently has discoloration about the eyes and should be told preoperatively that this will occur. To decrease local edema, he is kept in a mid-Fowler's position. Ice compresses usually are used over the nose for 24 hours to lessen discoloration, bleeding, and discomfort. If a bowl of ice and three or four wet 4 by 4 inch gauze sponges are left within easy reach at the bedside, the patient can apply the ice compresses himself.

Similar care is given the patient who has undergone a plastic procedure on the nasal septum. Such a patient should know that the cosmetic result of the operation cannot be evaluated for several weeks. Otherwise he may be disappointed. A protective plaster of Paris splint or a dressing of adhesive tape or a plastic or metal mold usually is placed over the nose after a plastic procedure on the nasal septum and also after a reduction of a fractured nasal septum. When plaster of Paris is used, care must be taken to keep droplets of plaster out of the patient's eyes. If the patient has a fractured nose, however, the surgeon usually removes the protective dressing daily to manually mold the broken parts. Firm healing develops about the tenth day. If a splint is used, the nurse should watch the skin about it to make sure that no pressure areas develop.

Complications of rhinitis and sinusitis

Epistaxis. Epistaxis, or nosebleed, may be caused by local irritation of the mucous membranes due to chronic infections, lack of humidity in the air that is breathed, violent sneezing or nose blowing, or trauma to the nose resulting in damage to or rupture of superficial blood vessels. One of the most common causes of nosebleed is picking of the nose. General or systemic causes may be hypertension and arterial blood vessel changes, blood dyscrasias such as leuke-

mia, or a deficiency of vitamin K or vitamin C. In adulthood, nosebleeds are more common in men than in women. They are most frequent in early childhood and puberty. Patients who have frequent nosebleeds should have a complete medical examination to determine the cause.

Most nosebleeds come from the tiny blood vessels in the anterior part of the nasal septum. This bleeding usually can be controlled at least temporarily by compressing the soft tissues of the nose against the septum with a finger. Firm pressure should be maintained for 5 to 10 minutes, and it may be necessary for as long as $1/2$ hour. Ice compresses may be applied over the nose. If these measures do not control bleeding, the help of a physician should be sought. In order to treat a nosebleed effectively, the physician must first determine the site of the bleeding. This is done best with the patient seated in a chair facing the physician. Both should wear gowns to protect their clothing. An angulated suction tip is used to suck clots from the nose. If suction is not available, the patient is instructed to blow his nose to remove the clot. The physician will then use a bright light (either head mirror or lamp) to inspect the anterior nares. Most anterior nosebleeds come from *Kiesselbach's plexus* (a plexus of veins on the anterior portion of the nasal septum). This bleeding can usually be controlled by inserting a cotton ball soaked in epinephrine, 1:1,000, in the bleeding nostril. Pressure is then exerted against the ala nasi, compressing the cotton ball against the septum for several minutes. The cotton ball is then removed and the bleeding point is cauterized with a silver nitrate stick or an electric cautery.

Bleeding from the posterior part of the nasal septum is more common in the elderly person and is more likely to be severe. If the bleeding point cannot be seen and treated as just described, a postnasal pack may be inserted. Because this procedure is extremely painful and sometimes causes faintness, patients usually are admitted to the hospital. The pack is left in place 2 or 5 days and then removed very gently. If bleeding has been severe, a transfusion may be necessary. To prevent recurrent hemorrhage, the patient should be warned not to blow his nose vigorously.

Nosebleeds can cause real and severe apprehension since bleeding may be profuse, not only dripping from the nose but also flowing into the throat. The patient is usually kept in Fowler's position. The patient should be kept quiet, and stained clothing should be removed. If he remains in an upright position with his head forward, less blood drains into the throat. A basin and tissues are provided for expectorated blood, and the patient is urged not to swallow blood because it may cause nausea and vomiting.

Infections of external tissues about the nose. The skin around the external nose is easily irritated during acute attacks of rhinitis or sinusitis. Furunculosis and cellulitis (inflammation of connective tissue) occasionally develop. (See p. 781 for discussion and treatment of furunculosis.) Infections about the nose are extremely dangerous since the venous supply from this area drains directly into the cerebral venous sinuses. Septicemia, therefore, can occur easily. No pimple or lesion in the area should ever be squeezed or "picked"; hot packs may be used. If any infection in or about the nose persists or shows even the slightest tendency to spread or increase in severity, medical aid should be sought.

■ INFECTIONS OF THE THROAT

Acute pharyngitis

Acute pharyngitis is an inflammation of the pharynx caused by hemolytic streptococci, staphylococci, or other bacteria or filtrable viruses. A severe form of this condition often is referred to as "strep throat" because of the frequency of streptococci as the causative organisms. Dryness of the throat is a common complaint. The throat appears red, and soreness may range from slight scratchiness to severe pain with difficulty in swallowing. A hacking cough may be present. Children often develop a very high fever, while adults may have only a mild elevation of temperature. Symptoms usually precede or occur simultaneously with the onset of acute rhinitis or acute sinusitis. Pharyngitis can occur after the tonsils have been removed, since the remaining mucous membranes can become infected.

Acute pharyngitis usually is relieved by hot saline throat gargles. An ice collar may make the patient feel more comfortable. The physician may prescribe acetylsalicylic acid administered orally, as a gargle, or as Aspergum. Lozenges containing a mild anesthetic may help relieve the local soreness. Moist inhalations may help relieve the dryness of the throat. A liquid diet usually is more easily tolerated, and a generous amount of fluid is encouraged. If the temperature is elevated, the patient should remain in bed, and even if he is ambulatory and has no fever, he should have extra rest. Occasionally sulfonamide drugs or antibiotics are used to treat severe infections, or they are prescribed prophylactically to prevent superimposed infection, particularly in persons who have a history of rheumatic fever or bacterial endocarditis. (See section on rheumatic fever, p. 332.)

Acute follicular tonsillitis

Acute follicular tonsillitis is an acute inflammation of the tonsils and their crypts. It usually is caused by the streptococcus organism. It is more likely to occur when the patient's resistance is low and is very common in children. The onset is almost always sudden, and symptoms include sore throat, pain on swallowing, fever, chills, general muscle aching, and malaise. In children the temperature may rise suddenly to 40.5° C. (105° F.). These symptoms often last for 2 or 3 days. The pharynx and the tonsils appear red, and the peritonsillar tissues are swollen. Sometimes a yellowish exudate drains from crypts in the tonsils. A throat culture usually is taken to identify the offending organism.

The patient with acute tonsillitis should remain in bed and take generous amounts of fluids orally. Warm saline throat irrigations (see fundamental nursing textbooks or specialized texts) are usually ordered, and a sulfonamide preparation or antibiotics are usually given. Acetylsalicylic acid and sometimes codeine sulfate may be ordered for pain and discomfort. An ice collar may be applied to the neck, and if the temperature is over 39° C. (102° F.), an alcohol sponge bath may be given. Until the temperature subsides and the sore throat improves, a bland diet is given. After the temperature returns to normal, the patient should be kept in bed for 48 hours, since heart and kidney damage, chorea, and pneumonia are rather common complications of tonsillitis. Most physicians feel that the patients who have recurrent attacks of tonsillitis should have a tonsillectomy. This procedure is usually done from 4 to 6 weeks after an acute attack has subsided.

Since the patient with acute tonsillitis is usually cared for at home, the nurse should help in teaching the general public the care that is needed. The office nurse, the clinic nurse, the nurse in industry, the school nurse, and the public health nurse have many opportunities to do this teaching.

Peritonsillar abscess

A peritonsillar abscess, or *quinsy,* is an uncommon, local complication of acute follicular tonsillitis in which infection extends from the tonsil to form an abscess in the surrounding tissues. The presence of pus behind the tonsil causes difficulty in swallowing, talking, and opening the mouth. On physical examination the uvula is displaced from midline. In some cases, saliva may drool from the patient's mouth, and he may be unable to swallow at all. Pain is severe and may extend to the ear on the affected side. If antibiotics to which the offending organism is sensitive are administered early, infection subsides. It is felt that some cases of peritonsillar abscess are caused by anaerobic organisms. In these instances, hydrogen peroxide (an oxidizing agent) in the form of a mouthwash may help relieve symptoms. If an abscess forms, incision and drainage are necessary. During the operation, the patient's head usually is lowered and suction applied as soon as the incision is made. This prevents the patient from aspirating the drainage. Warm saline irrigations, an ice collar, or narcotics may help relieve discomfort.

If acute follicular tonsillitis is treated adequately, peritonsillar abscess is unlikely to occur.

Chronic enlargement of the tonsils and adenoids

Tonsils and adenoids are lymphoid structures located in the oropharynx and the nasopharynx. They reach their full size in childhood and begin to atrophy during puberty. When adenoids enlarge, usually as a result of chronic infections but sometimes for no known reason, they cause nasal obstruction. The person breathes through his mouth, may have a dull facial expression, and may have a reduced appetite since the blocked nasopharynx can interfere with swallowing. In children, enlarged adenoids may block openings to the eustachian tubes in the nasopharynx, predisposing to middle ear infections and hearing impairment. Hypertrophy of the tonsil does not usually block the oropharynx but may affect speech and swallowing and cause mouth breathing. Occasionally adenotonsillar hypertrophy in children may so restrict breathing as to precipitate pulmonary hypertension and cor pulmonale. The condition is reversed by surgical removal of the tonsils and adenoids.

Tonsillectomy and adenoidectomy. The tonsils and adenoids are removed when the adenoids become enlarged and cause obstructive symptoms, when they are chronically infected, or when the patient has repeated attacks of tonsillitis. Chronic infections of these structures usually do not respond to antibiotics, and they may become foci of infection, spreading organisms to other parts of the body such as the heart. If a child's tonsils must be removed, the adenoids, even if they are not infected or enlarged, usually are removed too as a prophylactic measure. If possible, the removal of the tonsils is postponed until the child is about 6 years of age, but obstructing adenoids may be removed earlier.

The patient who is to have a tonsillectomy and adenoidectomy usually is admitted to the hospital on the morning of the operation. Some physicians prefer that the child be admitted the evening before surgery so that he can become accustomed to the hospital and have special laboratory tests. These tests would include a thromboplastin time test and for black children a sickle cell preparation test. Children should be carefully prepared for surgery by their parents and the professional staff who care for them (p. 31).

The complete examination is done in the physician's office, but the general physical condition, urine, blood count, and bleeding and clotting times are rechecked before surgery. The surgery will be postponed if there are signs of fever, upper respiratory infection, or other conditions that would complicate the induction of anesthesia or the postoperative course. In children the operation is performed under general anesthesia, while in adults the tonsillectomy may be done under either general or local anesthesia. In the operating room, after the tonsils are removed, pressure is applied to stop superficial bleeding. Occasionally bleeding vessels are tied off with sutures or an electrocoagulation current is used.

Postoperatively the patient who has had a tonsillectomy may have a small amount of dark, bloody drainage from the operative area and may vomit blood that he has swallowed. Until he has reacted fully from the anesthesia, he should be propped on his side or placed on his abdomen with a pillow under his chest (Fig. 23-6). When the patient is awake, he is permitted to sit up in a mid-Fowler's position. Sometimes an ice collar is applied about the throat to make the patient more comfortable and to

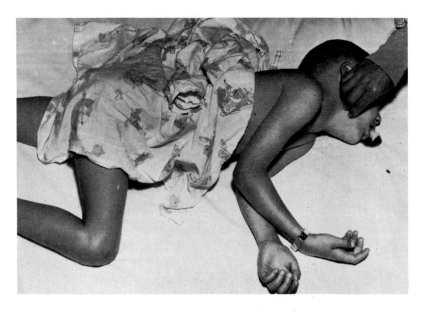

FIG. 23-6. The child is in the recovery room after a tonsillectomy. Note that he is propped on his side. There is an oral airway in place. The nurse is supporting the jaw to assist the airway. (From Havener, W. H., and others: Nursing care in eye, ear, nose, and throat disorders, ed. 3, St. Louis, 1974, The C. V. Mosby Co.)

lessen the chance of hemorrhage. Young children usually resist the application of an ice collar, and therefore it is not used.

Following a tonsillectomy or an adenoidectomy, the patient should be watched carefully for signs of hemorrhage. He is urged repeatedly as he is awakening and thereafter not to cough or attempt to clear his throat, since these actions may initiate bleeding. Efforts should be made to prevent the small child from crying lustily. If he has fully responded from anesthesia, he may be rocked. If the patient swallows frequently, hemorrhage should be suspected, and the throat should be inspected since any signs of hemorrhage must be reported to the physician at once. Vomitus containing bright red blood should be reported at once, and the specimen should be saved for the surgeon's inspection. It is especially important to watch the patient who is asleep for signs of hemorrhage, since he may swallow blood and lose a very large amount of it without any external evidence of bleeding. The pulse rate is taken every 15 minutes for the first hour and every half hour for several hours thereafter.

The physician may be able to control minor postoperative bleeding by applying a sponge soaked in a solution of epinephrine to the site. The patient who is bleeding excessively often is taken to the operating room for surgical treatment to stop the hemorrhage. This may be done by ligating or by cauterizing the bleeding vessel. If sutures must be used, the patient will have more pain and discomfort than he would have following a simple tonsillectomy. He may be unable to take solid food until the sutures have been absorbed.

After a tonsillectomy, the patient usually is kept in bed for 24 hours. When vomiting has ceased, fluids and bland nourishment are offered. While the patient usually will only take small amounts because of pain, he should be urged to take large swallows because they hurt less and because more fluid can thus be taken. Drinking through a straw is not advisable because of the danger of physical trauma and because the suction on the throat may cause bleeding. Ice-cold fluids are most acceptable and are given frequently. Ice cream usually is well tolerated, and ginger ale, cold milk, and cold custard often are offered next, followed by cream soups and bland juices such as pear juice. The morning after surgery the patient is usually offered such food as refined cereal and soft-cooked or poached eggs. When he goes home, he is advised to avoid citrus fruit juices, hot fluids, rough foods such as raw vegetables and crackers, and highly seasoned foods for at least 1 week because they irritate the operative area.

Some otolaryngologists no longer prescribe acetylsalicylic acid for pain since it increases the tendency to bleed. Acetaminophen or another aspirin substitute is usually ordered. Some physicians still suggest that older children and adults gargle gently after the first postoperative day. The gargle solution is prepared by dissolving 0.3 Gm. (5 grains) of acetylsalicylic acid and $\frac{1}{2}$ teaspoon of sodium bicarbonate in half a glass of water. Some of this fluid can be swallowed without harm.

Most patients are discharged from the hospital the day after surgery, but some are permitted to return home the night of the operation. If so, the child's parents are instructed to watch for bleeding and to report it to the physician at once. The child is usually kept in bed for 2 or 3 days and indoors for a week. Adult patients may be up and about as soon as they return home but may be advised to remain indoors for 3 days. Usually the patient is told to avoid exposure to the sun, vigorous exercise, coughing, sneezing, clearing of the throat, and vigorous blowing of the nose since these actions can cause bleeding. If bleeding occurs at any time, the patient should contact the physician immediately. The tough, yellow fibrous membrane that forms over the operative site begins to break away between the fourth and eighth postoperative days, and hemorrhage may occur. The separation of the membrane accounts for the throat's being more painful at this time. Pink granulation tissue soon becomes apparent, and by the end of the third postoperative week the area is covered with mucous membrane of normal appearance.

The adult patient or the parents of a young patient should be given specific instructions for home care. Most hospitals and most laryngologists have these instructions written out. Acceptable foods and fluids should be outlined. The diet can be increased as tolerated. The patient should continue to drink plenty of fluids (2,000 to 3,000 ml. daily) to help relieve the objectionable mouth odor common after any oral surgery. If the patient does not have a bowel movement after a day or two, a mild laxative is usually ordered. Parents should be told that the stool may be dark or black for a day or two because blood has been swallowed during surgery. A temperature of 37.7° to 38.5° C. (99° to 101° F.) may be expected for the first 2 or 3 days, and discomfort in the ears is also expected. Persistence of temperature elevation or discomfort in the ears, however, should be reported to the physician. The patient usually returns to the hospital clinic or to the physician's office for a follow-up examination about 1 week after the operation.

The nurse may need to help some mothers plan ways to amuse a sick child. He should be allowed to play in his bed but should take a short rest in the midmorning and midafternoon. Most children like to be read to, to color, to do puzzles, and to watch selected television programs. A sick child's interest span is short, however, and one must be prepared to have various pastimes ready. Visits from other children should be restricted for the first week since they may expose the patient to upper respiratory infection.

Laryngitis

Simple acute laryngitis. Simple acute laryngitis is an inflammation of the mucous membrane lining the larynx accompanied by edema of the vocal cords. It may be caused by a cold, by sudden changes in temperature, or by irritating fumes. Symptoms vary from a slight huskiness to a complete loss of voice. The patient's throat may be sore and scratchy, and he often has a cough. Laryngitis usually requires only symptomatic treatment. The patient is advised to stay indoors in an even temperature and to avoid talking for several days or weeks, depending on the severity of the inflammation. Steam inhalations with aromatic vapors such as tincture of benzoin, oil of pine, and menthol may be soothing. Cough syrups or home remedies for coughs such as those suggested on p. 554 may be tried. Smoking or being where others are smoking should be avoided.

Acute laryngitis may cause acute respiratory distress and prostration in children under 5 years of age. Because the larynx of the infant and young child is relatively small and is susceptible to spasm when irritated or infected, it easily becomes partially or totally obstructed. After exposure to cold air or as a result of an upper respiratory infection, the child may develop a hoarse, barking cough and an inspiratory stridor (a form of *croup*). He may become restless, the muscles about the clavicle may be visibly retracted as they attempt to help the patient get more air, and his nostrils may flare. The child may sit up and grasp his throat as he tries to breathe. He may be completely well before and after the attack, which may last $1/2$ to 3 hours. The usual treatment is the administration of copious amounts of vaporized cool mist. Some children's hospitals have "croup rooms" where a continuous "fog" of cool mist is generated into the room. If cool mist is not available, warm steam inhalations may be used to provide humidity and liquefy secretions. Occasionally 2 ml. of syrup of ipecac is prescribed to induce vomiting (thereby removing secretions) and to relieve laryngeal spasm.

The child with croup will be less frightened if he is held or if someone stays with him during the attack. Ordinarily sedatives will not be ordered since they tend to depress the patient's limited respiratory effort. However, if the child is very apprehensive and frightened, mild sedation may be used with caution and careful observation following administration. For a severe attack not relieved by this treatment, corticosteroids are usually administered parenterally. If the patient's condition becomes worse despite treatment, a tracheostomy may be necessary.

Chronic laryngitis. Some people who use their voices excessively, who smoke a great deal, or who work continuously where there are irritating fumes develop a chronic laryngitis. Hoarseness usually is worse in the early morning and in the evening. There may be a dry, harsh cough and a persistent need to clear the throat. Treatment may consist of removal of irritants, voice rest, correction of faulty voice habits, steam inhalations, and cough medications. The doctor may order spraying of the throat with an astringent antiseptic solution such as hexylresorcinol (S.T. 37). To do this procedure properly, the patient must use a spray tip that turns down at the end so that the medication reaches vocal cords and is not dissipated in the posterior pharynx. He should place the spray tip in the back of the throat with the bent portion behind the tongue. He should then take one or two deep breaths and on inhalation spray the medication. This procedure may cause temporary coughing and gagging. Many medications used as throat sprays are now sold in plastic squeeze bottles with tube and spray tip attached.

■ ENDOTRACHEAL INTUBATION AND TRACHEOSTOMY

In endotracheal intubation a tube is passed through either the nose or mouth into the trachea. A tracheostomy is an artificial opening made in the trachea into which a tube is inserted. These procedures are used (1) to establish and maintain a patent airway; (2) to prevent aspiration by sealing off the trachea from the digestive tract in the unconscious or paralyzed patient; (3) to permit removal of tracheobronchial secretions in the patient who cannot cough adequately; and (4) to treat the patient who requires positive pressure ventilation that cannot be given effectively by mask.[42] Whether an intubation or a tracheostomy is performed initially depends on the facilities available and the wishes of the physician. Most physicians now consider it safer to do an emergency endotracheal intubation and then perform a tracheostomy as a nonemergency procedure in the operating room if prolonged support of the airway is needed. In this instance the endotracheal tube is not removed until after the tracheostomy opening is made.

A tracheostomy is necessary when an endotracheal tube cannot be inserted or when it is contraindicated as in severe burns or laryngeal obstruction due to tumor, infection, or vocal cord paralysis.[42] Tracheostomy may also be required when a patient is conscious and cannot tolerate an endotracheal tube. Once the patient's airway is secured either by intubation or by tracheostomy, secretions are aspirated and well-humidified oxygen is usually given. If the patient is unable to sustain respiration, a mechanical ventilator (such as a Bennett or a Bird ventilator) is attached to either the endotracheal tube or the tracheostomy tube (p. 594). When mechanical ventilation is required, a cuffed tube is used. Usually an endotracheal tube is not left in place longer than 36 to 48 hours. If the patient is unable to maintain a free airway after this period of time, a tracheostomy is performed.

Depending on the patient's condition, a tracheostomy can be either temporary or permanent; the person who has a laryngectomy will have a permanent tracheostomy. Any patient who has had a tracheostomy is apprehensive and is often fearful of choking. Thus when feasible, the procedure is thoroughly explained to the patient before surgery. Both patient and family need to understand that the patient will be unable to speak but that he will be attended constantly until he has learned to care for himself safely. The nurse should plan with the patient for some means of communication after the surgery. Hand signals such as the OK sign or a raised finger might be used as a means of expressing, for example, the need to void. The patient may want to write on a pad or a Magic Slate. If he cannot write, a word or picture chart can be used.[20] The patient's ideas about how he would like to communicate should be considered. The signal light should be placed within the patient's reach and the nurse should assure him that someone will answer it immediately. He may feel more secure if also given a tap bell to signal for attention.

After the opening is made into the trachea (Fig. 23-7), a silver, nylon, or plastic tube is inserted to keep the tracheostomy open (Fig. 23-8). Twill tapes attached to either side of the tube are tied securely behind the neck to prevent the tube from becoming dislodged when the patient coughs or moves about. Should the tube be coughed out, the opening may close and the patient will be unable to breathe. Therefore a tracheal dilator or curved hemostat is always kept at the bedside so that the opening can be held open if the tube is dislodged. Silver tubes are commonly available in sizes no. 00 to no. 8. (no. 00 is used for the premature or newborn infant, while a no. 6 or 7 is used for most adults). The silver tracheostomy tube consists of two parts, an inner and an outer cannula. The outer cannula is removed only by the physician, while the inner cannula is removed regularly by the nurse for cleaning. The silver tracheostomy tube has a lock that must be turned in order to remove the inner cannula. The lock should be secured when the inner cannula is reinserted after cleaning. Synthetic single cannula tubes are now widely used. They are available in a variety of shapes and sizes, and all have attached cuffs, which can be inflated as necessary.

The operative wound may be sealed with a plastic spray, or a small dressing may be placed around the tracheostomy tube. Although drainage should be minimal, the wound is inspected frequently for

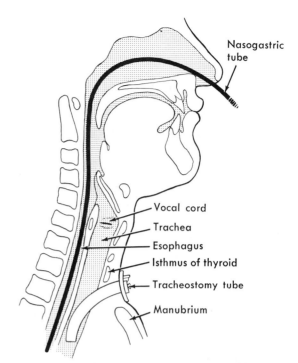

FIG. 23-7. Position of a tracheostomy tube and a nasogastric tube if used.

bleeding during the immediate postoperative period. The dressings are changed as they become soiled with drainage of mucus. Occasionally young children require elbow restraints to prevent them from removing the tube or putting objects into it.

Maintaining a patent airway

One of the nurse's main responsibilities is to see that a tracheostomy remains patent so that the patient has a free exchange of air. The patient is placed in a mid-Fowler's position for comfort and to make breathing easier. He should be attended constantly for 24 to 48 hours because of the possibility of respiratory embarrassment from blockage of the tube by secretions and because he is fearful of not being able to breathe and becomes restless when left alone. Since he needs constant attention, the patient is often placed in an intensive care unit or recovery room.

Oxygen may be administered, and *humidification of oxygen or room air is essential* because the patient has lost his natural humidifying mechanism in the nasopharynx. The most effective form of humidification is a heated (98° F. or slightly above) aerosol. Ultrasonic mist units, ultrasonic room humidifiers, or nebulizers that attach to the tracheostomy tube are efficient systems for providing the patient with adequate moist air (Fig. 22-11). Liquefying agents such as Mucomyst are often employed to make secretions easier to cough up or to remove by suction.

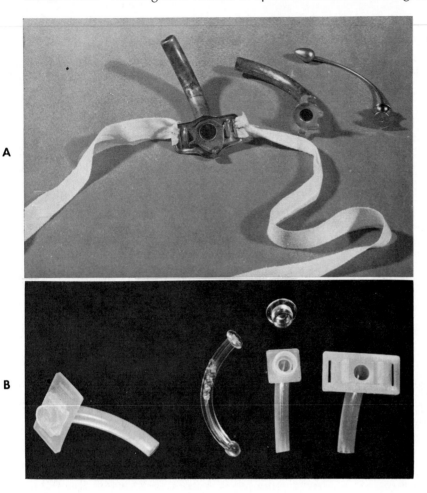

A

B

FIG. 23-8. A, Parts of a silver tracheostomy tube: outer tube with ties attached, inner tube, and pilot. **B,** Plastic tracheostomy tubes. Left to right: Assembled tube, pilot to help introduce tube, inner tube, outer tube, and cork to plug tube to test airway. (From DeWeese, D. D., and Saunders, W. H.: Textbook of otolaryngology, ed. 4, St. Louis, 1973, The C. V. Mosby Co.)

Analgestics and sedatives are given judiciously so as not to depress the respiratory center. The patient is suctioned as often as necessary, possibly every 5 minutes during the first few postoperative hours. The need for suctioning can be determined by the sound of the air coming from the tracheostomy tube, especially after the patient takes a deep breath. If the patient needs to be suctioned, his respirations are noisy and his pulse and respiratory rates are increased. The patient who is conscious can usually indicate when he needs to be suctioned. If he is having any respiratory distress, the tube should be suctioned. If mucus is blocking the inner cannula of a silver tube and cannot be removed by suction, the inner cannula is removed to open the airway. When the mucus is thick, the inner cannula should be cleaned and replaced at once because the outer tube may also become blocked. If, despite these measures, the patient becomes cyanotic, the physician should be summoned at once. A patient who is able to cough up secretions probably will require suctioning less frequently. The amount of mucus subsides gradually and the patient eventually may go for several hours without being suctioned. However, even when secretions are minimal, the patient is apprehensive and needs constant attendance.

Suctioning technique needs to be carefully performed in order to prevent damage to the tracheobronchial mucosa. Some of the problems associated with suctioning are discussed in more detail in various sources.* The purpose of the following section is to provide detailed guidelines about how to suction the tracheostomy tube efficiently and safely.

Suctioning the tracheostomy tube

The aim in suctioning is to remove all secretions that have accumulated in the tracheobronchial tree since the last suctioning. In general, suctioning techniques are the same no matter what type of tracheostomy tube is in use. However, silver tubes have both an inner and an outer cannula, while plastic tubes have only one cannula. Physicians vary in their preference as to the type of tube used. Some otolaryngologists prefer that only metal tubes with an inner cannula be used since they believe that they are safer. When a double-lumen tube is used, the inner cannula can readily be removed for suctioning and cleaning, whereas tubes without an inner cannula may have to be completely removed and replaced should they become plugged with secretions.

*See references 19, 22a, 42, 50a, and 52.

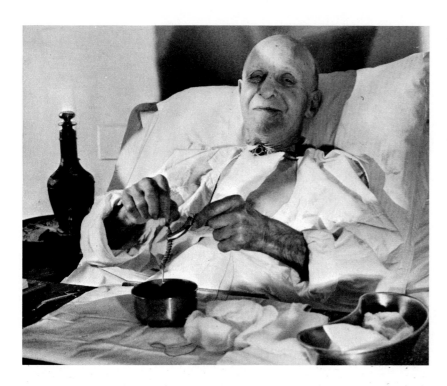

FIG. 23-9. This 82-year-old man cares for his own tracheostomy tube. He is about to clean the inner tube with a small tube brush. (From Anderson, H. C.: Newton's geriatric nursing, ed. 5, St. Louis, 1971, The C. V. Mosby Co.)

This can usually be prevented, however, by adequate humidification and frequent suctioning. The following guidelines apply to the suctioning of any type of tracheostomy tube.

1. Sterile technique is recommended; sterile gloves or forceps and a sterile catheter are used for suctioning. In some hospitals, clean rather than sterile technique is believed to be sufficient when suctioning patients with a permanent tracheostomy who will be caring for their own tube after they go home (Fig. 23-9). In the clean technique the hands are washed well with soap or pHisoHex before suctioning.

2. The catheter must be of a small enough size that it does not occlude the cannula (one-half to two-thirds the diameter of the tube).[44] Commonly, when a silver tube is suctioned, a no. 8 or 10 catheter is used for children, and a no. 14 or 16 for adults.

3. A sterile catheter is used each time the tube is suctioned.

4. Before suctioning, the patient is usually given a few breaths of oxygen to assure that he will not become unduly hypoxic during suctioning. Unless contraindicated, 100% oxygen is used.

5. A fenestrated catheter with a whistle tip is attached to the suction machine. If a nonfenestrated catheter is used, it is connected to the suction machine with a Y tube. The catheter is always inserted without suction. Once the catheter is in place, suction is applied by placing the thumb over the fenestration in the catheter or over the open end of the Y tube (Fig. 23-10).

6. The suction catheter is lubricated with normal saline solution and inserted deep enough into the bronchus to stimulate coughing. Unless otherwise ordered, the recommended depth through the tracheostomy tube is 8 to 12 inches as this permits removal of secretions lying beyond the tip of the cannula (Fig. 23-11). If the patient coughs, the catheter is removed because its presence obstructs the trachea and the patient must exert extra pressure to cough around it. As coughing occurs, the nurse or the patient should have tissues ready to receive mucus, which may be ejected with force. When the patient coughs, the tracheostomy tube is held in place, since it could come out with vigorous coughing.

7. If mucus is tenacious and difficult to remove, the physician may order sterile saline solution instilled into the tube just prior to suctioning. From 5 to 15 ml. is commonly ordered.

8. To aspirate the right bronchus, the patient's head is turned to the left and his chest is tilted to the right. This procedure is reversed to suction the left bronchus (Fig. 23-11). The catheter is always rotated 360 degrees as it is withdrawn, with suction on.

9. To prevent hypoxia, the patient must *not* be suctioned longer than 10 to 15 seconds at a time. He should rest 3 minutes between aspirations, and 100% oxygen should be administered. If secretions are interfering with breathing, suctioning may have to be more frequent.

10. The inner cannula of a silver tube is removed for cleaning every 2 to 8 hours depending on the amount and consistency of secretions. If mucus collects and partially obstructs the lumen, it may be necessary to clean the inner cannula even more

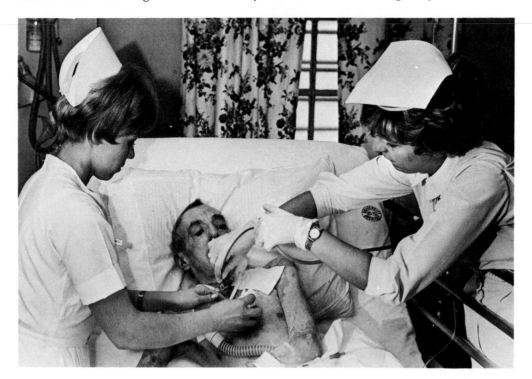

FIG. 23-10. The nurse is wearing sterile gloves and using a Y tube attachment to suction the patient's tracheostomy tube. (Courtesy Medical-World News.)

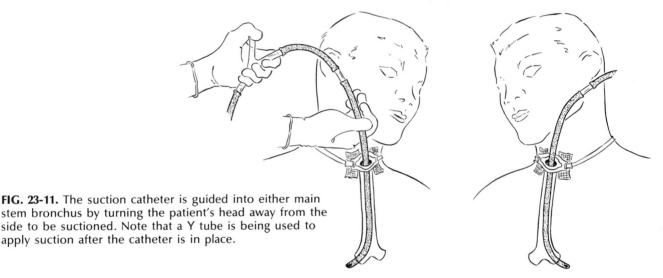

FIG. 23-11. The suction catheter is guided into either main stem bronchus by turning the patient's head away from the side to be suctioned. Note that a Y tube is being used to apply suction after the catheter is in place.

often than every 2 hours. Sterile water, detergent solution, pipe cleaners, and a small test tube brush are used for cleaning. Hot water is not used because it coagulates mucus. The tube may be soaked in a solution of half-strength hydrogen peroxide to soften congealed secretions. The tube is inspected to see that all mucus has been removed. Gauze can be threaded through it to extract excess secretions and solution. After being cleaned, the tube is boiled for 5 minutes and then cooled. Before reinserting the inner tube, the outer tube is suctioned.

Cuffed tubes

Cuffed endotracheal and tracheostomy tubes are now in wide use. Precautions to be observed with a cuffed tube are discussed on p. 592.

616

Management of the patient with a tracheostomy

If a patient is to be discharged with the tube in place, he is taught to care for and change it himself (Fig. 23-9). He will need a mirror so that he can see to do this procedure. He may begin to do this within a few days after surgery and often is happier being able to care for himself. The physician may change the outer tube every few days. Tapes holding the tracheostomy tube can be replaced as necessary, but a second nurse should always be present when this is done. One nurse places one gloved hand firmly behind the patient's neck and, with the other, holds the tube in place by supporting the T portion of the tube with gloved fingers. The second nurse then adjusts the knot or changes the ties.

If the tracheostomy tube comes out for any reason, the passageway for air is immediately obstructed. A tracheal dilator or a curved hemostat and a pair of scissors with which to cut the tape if the tube is only partially out should be conveniently placed in the patient's room. The nurse should use the dilator to maintain an open airway while signaling for assistance. An extra tube that is sterile and of the correct size for the patient should always be kept in the room. Many hospitals require that an emergency tracheostomy set be on the unit at all times. Likelihood of serious interference with breathing if the tracheostomy tube comes out decreases as the wound heals. However, most ambulatory patients are advised to carry a small pair of scissors and a hemostat with them and are told how to use these instruments in an emergency.

The patient who has had a simple tracheostomy may have fluids a few hours after the operation. He needs encouragement in his first efforts to swallow, since he is fearful that food and fluids will be aspirated. This is not a serious danger, although the patient may cough when he first attempts to drink fluids. The suction machine must be available and ready for immediate use at all times. Fluids are usually given parenterally during the first 24 hours. By the second postoperative day, the patient can drink readily and can eat most foods. Occasionally food and water may appear in the tracheostomy tube after swallowing. This occurs because the trachea is fixed in place by the tracheostomy tube and cannot be elevated as easily as in the normal state; therefore some leak exists between the esophagus and the trachea. In persons who have had both a tracheostomy tube and a nasogastric tube for some time the leak may indicate that a tracheoesophageal fistula has developed. The fistula is caused by the tracheostomy tube rubbing against the nasogastric tube and injuring the walls between.

Mouth care is especially important. The patient often has halitosis following this operation and may be sensitive about it. He should be encouraged to drink large amounts of water because this contributes to good mouth hygiene and helps to thin mucous secretions.

The patient usually is advised to avoid talking until the tracheostomy opening is occluded for increasing periods prior to removing the tube completely. Therefore a pad and pencil or Magic Slate should be readily available to him. With the physician's permission, patients who must have the tube left open for extended periods can be taught to cover it momentarily with a finger while they speak.

Use of the tube is discontinued gradually. When a large-size tracheostomy tube is in place, a smaller one is usually inserted. The opening is then partially closed with a rubber or plastic cork, and if the patient can breathe adequately, the tube may then be completely corked for a day before it is removed. When the tube is removed, the skin edges are pulled

together with strips of adhesive tape. After a few days, the wound is healed and air no longer escapes through it. Metal tubes are cleaned and sterilized for future use. Synthetic tubes are discarded after use.

Patients who go home with the tracheostomy tube still in place must be provided with necessary supplies or with instructions as to where to secure them and with knowledge of how to care for themselves. They should have suction equipment. Suction machines can be rented for home use or obtained in many communities through the local chapter of the American Cancer Society. Suction can be provided by attaching a suction hose to a water faucet. Many hardware stores carry the necessary equipment. The amount of suction is controlled by the stream of water.

Persons who have a permanent tracheostomy must take some special precautions. They must not go swimming and must be careful while bathing or taking a shower that water is not aspirated through the opening into the lungs. They are advised to wear a scarf or a shirt with a closed collar that covers the opening, yet is of porous material. This material substitutes for some functions normally assumed by nasal passages, such as the warming of air and the screening out of dust and other irritating substances.

■ CANCER OF THE LARYNX

If treated early, cancer of the larynx is one of the most curable of all malignancies. It is estimated that in the United States there will be 10,000 new cases in 1975. Cancer of the larynx limited to the vocal cords grows slowly because of the limited blood supply. It metastasizes slowly because of the scarcity of lymph vessels in the area. Elsewhere in the larynx, such as the epiglottis, lymph vessels are abundant, and cancer of these tissues often spreads rapidly and metastasizes early to the deep lymph nodes of the neck. Hoarseness is an early symptom of cancer of the vocal cords. If treatment is given when hoarseness (caused by the tumor's preventing complete approximation of the vocal cords) appears, a cure usually is possible. Signs of metastases of cancer in other parts of the larynx include a sensation of a lump in the throat, pain in the Adam's apple that radiates to the ear, dyspnea, dysphagia, enlarged cervical nodes, and cough.

Cancer of the larynx is eight times more common in men than in women, and it occurs most often in persons past 60 years of age. There seems to be some relationship between cancer of the larynx and heavy smoking, chronic laryngitis, vocal abuse, and family predisposition to cancer. Because of the increase in the number of women who are heavy smokers, some specialists believe that the incidence of carcinoma of the larynx among this group will increase. Any person who becomes progressively hoarse or is hoarse for longer than 2 weeks should be urged to seek medical attention at once. The diagnosis of cancer of the larynx is made from the history, from visual examination of the larynx with a laryngoscope, and from a biopsy and microscopic study of the lesion.

Laryngectomy

Partial laryngectomy. If the tumor has not involved the muscles and if the motility of the cord is normal, a partial laryngectomy may effect a cure in early carcinoma of the vocal cords. The most common technique is to make an opening into the larynx through the thyroid cartilage *(laryngofissure)* and remove the involved cord and tumor. As healing takes place, scar tissue fills the defect where the diseased cord was removed and becomes a vibrating surface within the larynx. This tissue permits husky but acceptable speech. A tracheostomy tube is inserted at the time of operation but is removed when edema in the surrounding tissues subsides. For 48 hours postoperatively nutrients may be supplied intravenously or by a nasogastric tube. Fluids and soft foods may then be taken orally. Soft foods may be easier for the pharyngeal musculature to handle than fluids. Foods usually well tolerated are scrambled eggs, cottage cheese, and baked potato. Other care is similar to that given the patient having a tracheostomy for other reasons.

The patient who has had a partial laryngectomy usually is not on absolute voice rest but is not permitted to use his voice until the surgeon gives specific approval (usually 3 days postoperatively). He should then only whisper until healing is complete, after which time he usually adjusts quite readily to his relatively minor limitation of speech.

Total laryngectomy. When cancer of the larynx is advanced, a total laryngectomy may be performed. This includes removal of the epiglottis, thyroid cartilage, hyoid bone, cricoid cartilage, and two or three rings of the trachea. The pharyngeal opening to the trachea is closed, the anterior wall of the esophagus is reinforced, and the remaining trachea is brought out to the neck wound and sutured to the skin. It forms an opening (permanent *tracheostomy*) through which the patient breathes. Because he no longer breathes through his nose, he will have no sense of smell (Fig. 23-12). A radical neck dissection also may be done to remove metastases to surrounding tissues and lymph nodes. In certain selected cases, radiation therapy may be used instead of surgery.

The patient who is to have a laryngectomy is told by the physician that he will breathe through a special opening made in his neck and that he no longer will have normal speech. He is often depressed by this news, which threatens his economic, social, and emotional status as well as his life. In some instances it is helpful for him to be visited by another patient who has made a good recovery from laryn-

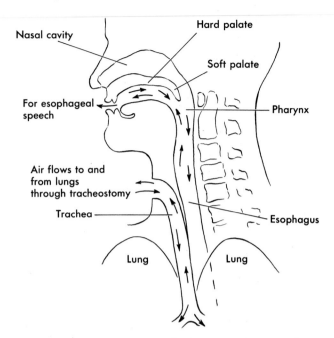

FIG. 23-12. Drawing shows permanent opening in the trachea following total laryngectomy. Note that the nose is not used for breathing and that all air enters through the tracheostomy opening. Air swallowed through the mouth is used to produce laryngeal speech. (Redrawn from Havener, W. H., and others: Nursing care in eye, ear, nose, and throat disorders, ed. 3, St. Louis, 1974, The C. V. Mosby Co.)

gectomy and who has undergone rehabilitation successfully. In other instances this may depress the patient further. Careful assessment must be made of each patient to determine if he will benefit from such a visit and whether the visit should be preoperatively, immediately after surgery, or later in the recovery period. Often no one else can give a patient the reassurance that he can regain speech as well as a fellow patient. Many large cities have a "Lost Chord Club" or a "New Voice Club," and the members are willing to visit hospitalized patients. Information regarding these clubs may be obtained by writing to the International Association of Laryngectomees.* Local speech rehabilitation centers may supply instructive films and other resources. The local chapter of the American Cancer Society and the local health department also have information available. If possible, the family, too, should learn about the method of esophageal speech that the patient will learn to use.

Preoperative and postoperative care of the patient is essentially the same as that described for tracheostomy except that these patients will have a laryngectomy tube in place. Some patients may not have a tube in the tracheostomy after the operation because the sutures keep the stoma open and be-

---

*219 East 42nd St., New York, N. Y. 10017.

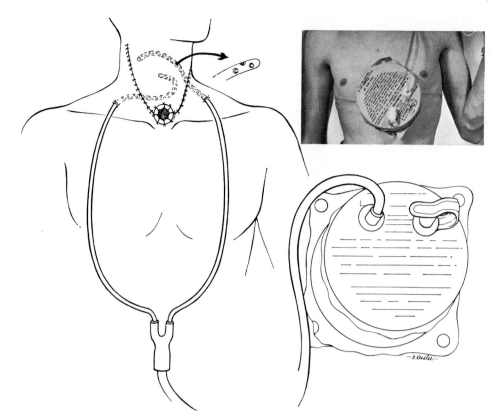

FIG. 23-13. Hemovac apparatus for constant closed suction. In this system of wound drainage, suction is maintained by a plastic container with a spring inside that tries to force apart the lids and thereby produces suction that is transmitted through the plastic tubing. The neck skin is pulled down tight, and no external dressing is required. The container serves as both suction source and receptacle for blood. It is emptied as required, and the drainage tubes are left in the neck for 3 days. (From DeWeese, D. D., and Saunders, W. H.: Textbook of otolaryngology, ed. 4, St. Louis, 1973, The C. V. Mosby Co.)

cause their surgeons believe that there is less tissue reaction and a better stoma if no tube is used. Most otolaryngologists believe that a laryngectomy tube is better than a tracheostomy tube because it is shorter and there is less danger that it will obstruct the right main stem bronchus. The tube will remain there until the wound is healed and a permanent fistula has formed, usually in 2 or 3 weeks. Frequent suctioning is necessary in the early postoperative period to keep the trachea free of secretions.

If a radical neck dissection has also been performed, the patient may have a pressure dressing applied that may interfere with respirations. The patient is more comfortable and can breathe better when placed in a mid-Fowler's position. If drains have been inserted in the wound, drainage may be noted on the dressing soon after the operation. If a catheter has been inserted into the wound and attached to suction, a dressing may be absent and drainage minimal (Fig. 23-13).

A nasogastric tube may be inserted during the surgical procedure for the instillation of food and fluids at regular intervals postoperatively (Fig. 23-7). The use of the tube to give food is thought to minimize contamination of the pharyngeal and esophageal suture lines and to prevent fluid from leaking through these wounds into the trachea before healing occurs. Some surgeons feel that, with modern suturing and drainage techniques, tube feedings are not necessary, and they permit the patient to take food and fluid orally after the second postoperative

day. If the nasogastric tube is used, it is removed as soon as the patient can swallow safely. The patient then needs careful attention in his first attempts to swallow. He may feel that he is choking and may have severe coughing that is frightening and painful. It is extremely important that the nurse be present when the patient first attempts to swallow. Should aspiration occur, the trachea and bronchi must be suctioned at once. Only water should be given until the patient has become accustomed to swallowing.

Speech rehabilitation may be started as soon as the esophageal suture line is healed. In addition to the International Association of Laryngectomees and the local chapter of the American Cancer Society (p. 618), information on alaryngeal speech can be obtained from the American Speech and Hearing Association.* Most persons learn *esophageal speech* best at a special speech clinic. Although some persons may need to go to a nearby city for this instruction, they usually must remain away from home for only 1 or 2 weeks. Motivation and persistent effort are essential in learning this kind of speech; encouragement and support from the professional staff and the patient's family are important to the patient's morale. About 75% of all persons who have their larynx removed master some sort of speech, and the average person can return to work 1 or 2 months after leaving the hospital.

---

*9030 Old Georgetown Rd., Washington, D. C. 20014.

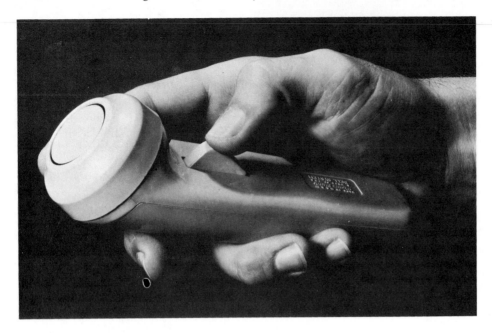

FIG. 23-14. Battery-powered electronic artificial larynx for patient who has a total laryngectomy and cannot learn esophageal speech. (Courtesy Illinois Bell Telephone Co.)

To learn esophageal speech, the patient must first practice burping. This provides the moving column of air needed for sound, while folds of tissue at the opening of the esophagus act as the vibrating surface. The patient must learn to coordinate his articulation with esophageal vocalization made possible by aspirating air into the esophagus. His new voice sounds are natural although somewhat hoarse. The qualities of speech provided by the use of the nasopharynx are still present, however. The patient may have digestive difficulty during the time he is learning to speak, which is due to swallowing air as he practices, to unusual strain on abdominal muscles, and to nervous tension. The patient should be told that digestive difficulty may occur but that it is not cause for alarm. It abates with proficiency in speaking.

If a patient is unable to learn esophageal speech in 60 to 90 days after surgery, a speech aid such as a vibrator or an electronic artificial larynx (Fig. 23-14) may be prescribed for him. An individual who has a hiatal hernia may not be able to accomplish esophageal speech and will have to use another method for speech. Various mechanical devices are available and the new ones permit a natural type of speech, providing pitch inflections and volume control. The local chapter of the American Cancer Society or the local telephone company can provide information about the purchase of these devices.

Several other surgical and prosthetic techniques are being tested. Most have not been widely used because of technical complications and for most patients esophageal speech is still the best method of communication. A summary of some of these procedures can be found in the current literature.[24]

■ DISEASES AND DISORDERS OF THE EAR
Nursing intervention

A few simple rules should be borne in mind when caring for the patient with ear disease. It is important to avoid further infection. Thus hands are washed thoroughly before doing any treatment and all equipment and material used are sterile. Trauma must be avoided. Hard articles such as a glass medicine dropper, a hairpin, or a toothpick or match should never be inserted into the ear lest the eardrum be perforated accidentally. The auditory canal must never be obstructed by a medicine dropper, irrigating tip, wick, or anything else, since obstruction may produce pressure beyond the obstructing object and damage the eardrum. The nurse should never insert any object beyond a point where it can be seen easily, and the patient should be instructed to be careful about placing anything in the ear canal.

A good practice in treating the ear canal is to use an adjustable light such as a standing gooseneck light that does not need to be held. For best visualization of the ear canal, the outer ear is held down and out in an infant or small child and up and back in an adult.

Ears that are draining are often treated by using dry wipes. Sterile applicators may be used, and often they are prepared on the unit, since commercial ones often are hard and ineffectual. *Wicks* (single pieces of gauze picked up at the center, twisted, and then sterilized) may be inserted gently into the ear canal by the physician or the nurse to serve as drains to encourage passage of exudate. The loose end extends outside the ear canal. A wick saturated with a medicated solution may be used both as a drain and for local compress effect. A wick also may be inserted after eardrops have been given to distribute and help retain the medication in the ear canal. It must be changed often and never allowed to become hardened with exudate because this may interfere with the flow of drainage. A wick is never inserted farther than the nurse can see.

Irrigations may be ordered in disease of the auditory canal, and they often are used when wax (cerumen) has become impacted in the auditory canal. However, they are seldom used if the eardrum is ruptured for fear of introducing further infection into the middle ear. When an irrigation is ordered, the irrigation solution should be no warmer than 38° C. (100° F.). The ear is easily stimulated by temperatures that are above or below body temperature, and they may cause vertigo. The patient should sit with the head tilted slightly forward and toward the affected side, holding the emesis basin directly below the ear. The irrigation also may be done with the patient lying down while the nurse sits in a chair. Air should be expelled from the bulb syringe prior to instilling solution, and the tip of the syringe should be directed either toward the roof or toward the floor of the canal but not straight inward. The canal should not be completely obstructed by the syringe since this would keep solution from flowing back and would cause pressure against the eardrum. To assure complete drainage of the irrigation fluid, the nurse should have the patient lie on the affected side for several minutes. The external ear should then be dried thoroughly to prevent excoriation of the skin.

If the patient is to irrigate his ear at home, the nurse should teach him how to do it correctly. By sitting at a wash basin, the patient may be able to manage alone, but it may be better to have the treatment done by a responsible and informed family member. The public health nurse may give this instruction in the patient's home.

Eardrops should be at body temperature because vertigo may result from stimulation of the ear by high or low temperatures. If the bottle of solution is at less than body temperature, it may be warmed by holding it in the hand for a minute or two. The patient should lie on his side with the affected ear uppermost. Lifting the auricles gently upward and backward in the adult and backward in the infant will straighten the ear canal. The external ear should be cleansed with a sponge and the canal straightened with one hand while three or four drops of the prescribed medication are instilled into the ear with a medicine dropper. The drops are instilled so that they run slowly along the wall of the canal and do not entrap air. After the drops are inserted, the patient should remain on the unaffected side for about 5 minutes so that the medication will have a chance to reach all of the ear canal. A piece of cotton moistened with the eardrop solution and gently inserted into the external auditory canal will keep the drops from running out of the ear. The external ear is then dried thoroughly to prevent skin irritation.

The external ear

External otitis. The external ear may be affected by acute and chronic forms of such conditions as eczematous dermatitis, diffuse dermatitis, and fungus and bacterial infections. These conditions may be associated with systemic diseases, with diseases of the skin of the adjacent face, neck, and scalp, or with diseases of the middle ear. They may be caused by trauma or be the result of a primary invasion of organisms. Any symptoms of redness, scaling, itching, swelling, watery discharge, or crusting should be referred to the otologist since, if these diseases are not treated, chronic changes may result, causing thickening of the skin and stenosis of the external canal.

Local treatment may include application of medicated ointments or powders, compresses to provide heat, soften crusts, or supply medication, and cool applications to lessen inflammation and relieve discomfort. Burow's solution (aluminum acetate solution) often is used for its astringent action, which has a cooling and soothing effect. Antibiotic preparations such as those containing bacitracin, neomycin, and polymyxin and the corticosteroids may be prescribed to be applied locally.

When compresses are used, the pillow should be protected, and a loose gauze plug should be placed in the outer ear canal. This plug can either be moistened with solution if the outer ear canal is also involved or be used dry to prevent spread of the infection to the inner part of the canal. Compresses of single-thickness gauze fit the contours of the outer ear best. They should be quite moist yet not dripping. Ice caps are too heavy to use on the sensitive external ear. To apply cold, a light application can be made by placing about two cupfuls of crushed ice in a small sealed plastic bag.

Furunculosis of the external auditory canal. Furuncles, or boils, usually are confined to the external auditory meatus and most often are caused by *Staphylococcus aureus* or *albus*. They cause severe pain because there is little expansile tissue in the area, and as they enlarge, the skin becomes taut and is under great pressure. The swelling may occlude the auditory canal, causing temporary deafness. The administration of antibiotics systemically may resolve the condition, an incision and drainage may be necessary, or wicks treated with antibiotics or drugs such as Burow's solution may be inserted. Acetaminophen, codeine, or hot compresses may be administered to relieve discomfort. When drainage occurs, pain usually subsides.

Impacted cerumen. A certain amount of cerumen in the ear canal is normal, and persons who have no wax have itching and scaling in the ear canal. Occasionally, when the cerumen becomes impacted and causes pain or temporary deafness, it must be removed by the physician. He may ask the patient to instill several drops of warm sweet oil, glycerin, or hydrogen peroxide into the auditory canal for several days to soften the wax. It can then usually be removed by irrigation with a metal Pomeroy syringe or with a cerumen spoon. Since there is danger of perforating the eardrum, this treatment is done by the physician or by a nurse who has received specialized instruction in the procedure.

Foreign bodies in the ear. Children and mentally disturbed adults occasionally insert foreign bodies such as beans, peas, paper, erasers, crayons, chalk, or buttons into their ears. These articles should be removed by a physician because there is danger of traumatizing the canal wall, eardrum, or middle ear while probing for them. Insects may also get into the ear. Their movements cause pain and noise. A few drops of mineral oil, alcohol, or ether instilled into the the ear will either kill or anesthetize the insect. It may then be removed with a forceps or washed out.

The middle ear

Serous otitis media. Serous *(catarrhal)* otitis media is a condition in which sterile serum is present in the middle ear and interferes with hearing. Normally the nasopharyngeal end of the eustachian tubes opens periodically to permit the passage of air up into the middle ear as swallowing or yawning occurs. This air helps to maintain the pressure within the middle ear equal to that of the external ear. When the opening of the eustachian tube is blocked by nasopharyngeal infections or enlarged adenoids or when its lumen is swollen by allergic reactions, air cannot enter. The remaining air eventually is absorbed by the mucous membrane lining, and a negative pressure is created that draws fluid from the surrounding tissues into the middle ear. A sudden change in atmospheric pressure such as that which occurs in flying can also produce this condition. Ascending from a high atmospheric pressure to a low atmospheric pressure moves air from the middle ear out through the eustachian tube, but as a person descends, air may be unable to pass through the eustachian tube back into the middle ear. Chewing gum or swallowing helps to open the tube, thus permitting air to enter the middle ear.

Serous otitis media may be acute or chronic. It may last for a few days or persist for years. The patient may complain of a sense of fullness or blockage in the ear, hearing loss, a low-pitched tinnitus, and an earache. The eardrum usually appears retracted on examination. The condition resolves as the cause of the eustachian obstruction is removed. Gentle inflation of the eustachian tube may bring relief. Aspiration of the fluid with a needle or through a myringotomy incision may be necessary in some instances.

A polyethylene or Teflon tube sometimes is inserted through an opening in the eardrum to equalize pressure and to speed the absorption of the fluid.

Early and adequate treatment of nasopharyngeal infections and allergic conditions can usually prevent chronic serous otitis media from developing. Since this disease is a cause of conduction deafness in children, the nurse should urge mothers of children who complain of persistent earache to seek medical advice. Any person who complains of tinnitus or who seems to have loss of hearing should be advised to seek medical attention promptly.

Acute purulent otitis media. Acute purulent otitis media is an acute inflammatory process in the middle ear. It is common in infants because their eustachian tubes are short and straight, and thus almost any infection in the nasopharynx has direct access to the middle ear. This disease most often follows the common cold or tonsillitis but may complicate measles or scarlet fever. It may also be caused by the forcing of contaminated water into the middle ear through the eustachian tube while swimming or by blowing the nose improperly. People should be urged to avoid swimming in uninspected pools and in stagnant water, and they should be taught to blow the nose gently, lest infected material be forced into the middle ear. The offending organism usually is *Streptococcus* or *Staphylococcus,* which reaches the middle ear by way of the eustachian tube. In children under 6 years of age, however, the most common offending organisms are the *Pneumococcus* and the *Haemophilus influenzae.*

The infection usually begins with local engorgement of the blood vessels, which causes swelling of the mucous membrane lining of the eustachian tubes, middle ear, and mastoid cells. As the inflammatory condition progresses, a serous exudate develops in the middle ear and becomes serosanguineous and, later, mucopurulent. The pressure of the exudate may cause the eardrum to rupture. The fluid may drain into the external auditory canal or it may be forced back into the mastoid cells.

In the early stages the patient complains of a sensation of fullness in the ear. As infection progresses, the eardrum bulges and pain becomes severe and throbbing. The pain may cause the child to tug on his ear, or the infant may roll his head from side to side, cry constantly, and refuse to eat. There may be decreased hearing in the affected ear, tinnitus, and fever, which in a child may range as high as 40° to 41.1° C. (104° to 106° F.).

Since antibiotics have been used to treat acute tonsillitis, pharyngitis, rhinitis, and sinusitis, otitis media is no longer a common complication of these conditions. When otitis media does develop, antibiotics are given at once, and the infection usually subsides before acute, painful symptoms occur. Treatment also may include bed rest, administration of acetylsalicylic acid or codeine for pain, instillation of warm eardrops such as Auralgan (antipyrine and benzocaine in glycerin) to relieve discomfort, administration of nasal vasoconstrictors to open blocked eustachian tubes, application of dry heat such as a hot-water bottle, and forcing of fluids. Usually otitis media is treated on an ambulatory basis, and parents of the infant or young child need careful instruction in his care. In order to prevent otitis media, all parents should be taught to seek medical attention for a child with an earache. The importance of taking prescribed antibiotics for the number of days ordered, even though symptoms have subsided, should also be stressed.

A *myringotomy* (incision into the eardrum) may be performed to permit fluid that has collected in the middle ear to drain. The procedure usually is performed in the physician's office or in the clinic. If necessary, a short-acting anesthetic such as nitrous oxide or a topical anesthetic such as ethyl chloride is used. A single incision is made in the eardrum, and the fluid may be aspirated and cultures taken. It is extremely important that free drainage continue so that it does not cause pressure against the mastoid cells. Cotton may be placed loosely in the outer ear to collect drainage. It should be replaced when it becomes moist in order to lessen the danger of secondary infection. Dry wipes may be used to remove excess drainage. Petrolatum may be placed around the outer ear to prevent it from becoming excoriated from the drainage. Parents and patients should know that the discharge may be infectious and that the hands should be washed after changing cotton plugs or cleaning the ear. Elbow restraints may be necessary to keep the young child from touching his ear and the drainage. Antibiotics usually are continued for several days after the discharge has stopped. If the patient has a rise in temperature, complains of headache, or becomes drowsy, irritable, or disoriented, the physician must be notified at once. These signs may indicate that the eardrum needs to be reopened, that mastoid cells are involved, or that a brain abscess or meningitis is developing. A myringotomy incision usually heals completely and does not affect hearing.

Acute mastoiditis. An acute infection of the middle ear usually is accompanied by some inflammatory reaction in the mucosa of the adjacent mastoid process. If the middle ear infection is not treated early or adequately or if the infection is particularly virulent, acute mastoiditis may occur. *Streptococcus, Pneumococcus, Staphylococcus,* or *Haemophilus influenzae* bacillus may be the causative organism. The inflammatory reaction proceeds from edema of the tissues to the formation of exudate and pus that fill the mastoid cells. Pressure on the blood supply causes necrosis to develop and an abscess to form. There may be pain in the ear, mastoid ten-

derness, fever, headache, and a profuse discharge from the affected ear.

Treatment consists of the use of antibiotics, bed rest, medication for pain, and forcing of fluids. If an abscess forms or if the symptoms persist or become worse and cause an elevation of temperature, vertigo, or facial paralysis, surgery is performed. Because of the availability of more effective treatment, surgery is now rarely necessary except in the underdeveloped countries, where it is common. In a *simple mastoidectomy* an incision is made in front of or behind the ear, the necrotic mastoid cells are removed, a small rubber drain is inserted, and the wound is closed. The middle ear is left intact, and hearing is not affected.

Preoperative preparation for a simple mastoidectomy is similar to the routine preoperative care given any patient. If the earache is severe, an ice bag may be used, and acetaminophen or codeine sulfate may be ordered.

Postoperatively a tight, bulky dressing is applied to provide some hemostasis and to absorb drainage (Fig. 23-15). The dressing may be reinforced as necessary, but it is not changed by the nurse. The surgeon usually changes it every other day. There may be a small amount of serosanguineous drainage apparent on the dressing, but signs of bright blood on outer dressings should be reported at once. If the tissues around the dressing become edematous, the surgeon should be notified because the dressing may need to be loosened. Any signs of facial paralysis

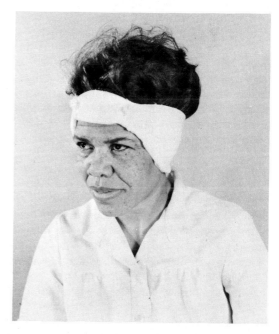

FIG. 23-15. Cling type of 3-inch roller bandage and forehead ties ensure a secure and comfortable head dressing. (Courtesy Eye and Ear Infirmary, University of Illinois Hospitals, Chicago, Ill.)

such as inability to smile or to wrinkle the forehead should be reported. Headache, vomiting, stiff neck, dizziness, irritability, or disorientation may forewarn of a septic thrombosis of the lateral sinus in the brain, meningitis, or brain abscess. A chronic purulent otitis media also occasionally follows this operation, necessitating more radical mastoid surgery.

The patient usually is allowed out of bed within 24 to 48 hours. Fluids are forced throughout the postoperative course.

Chronic purulent otitis media. Chronic purulent otitis media is characterized by chronic purulent discharge from the middle ear. It is a sequela of acute otitis media and involves both the middle ear and the mastoid cells. The mastoid bone cells become thickened, and polyps may develop from the mucous membrane of the middle ear. The patient's main complaint may be deafness, occasional pain, or dizziness. If chronic purulent otitis media is permitted to progress unchecked, meningitis, brain abscess, or facial paralysis may eventually occur because the infection gradually erodes the surrounding bone.

Another complication of chronic purulent otitis media is *cholesteatoma.* It occurs when the eardrum has been ruptured and the ear has drained for some time. Skin cells from the ear canal grow into the middle ear, where their normal excrescences combine with mucus and purulent exudate to form a mass that becomes firm and erodes the tissue surrounding it. This mass must be removed surgically.

The best treatment for chronic purulent otitis media is prevention by early treatment of the acute disease. If the chronic condition does occur, it should be treated as soon as it is recognized. Because the infection is walled off, systemic antibiotics alone are not effective in treating chronic otitis media. They may be effective, however, following meticulous local debridement with suctioning and application of topical antibiotics. Cortisporin eardrops may also be prescribed. When this treatment is not indicated or is not effective, a *radical mastoidectomy* or *modified radical mastoidectomy* is performed. A modified radical mastoidectomy is the more commonly used procedure because it preserves as much of the middle ear structure as possible. In a radical mastoidectomy an incision is made either behind the ear or directly in front of it, and the mastoid cells are completely removed, converting the middle ear and the mastoid space into one cavity. The remnants of the eardrum, malleus, and incus are also removed, but the stapes and facial nerve are preserved. The radical mastoid cavity may be left to gradually reline with epithelium, or a graft of skin or muscle may be applied (musculoplasty). Sterile packing is placed into the wound to keep the graft in position, to hold the external meatus open, and to provide hemostasis. The packing is removed gradually through the external ear. The ungrafted radical mastoid cavity usually is healed 2 to 3 months after the operation. It is very important that sterile technique be observed at all times and that the external ear be kept scrupulously clean. Hearing may be permanently lost in the ear, although many people, even after a radical mastoidectomy, have enough hearing left to manage without a hearing aid.

As already mentioned, mastoidectomy is required much less often now that antibiotic drugs are used to treat acute infections. With continued attacks of acute infection, however, some organisms may become resistant to certain antibiotics, and treatment may become a problem. Nursing care for the patient with a radical mastoidectomy is similar to that given the patient having a simple mastoidectomy.

Surgery of the middle ear

Myringoplasty and tympanoplasty. When chronic perforations of the eardrum cause conductive hearing loss, a *myringoplasty* may be performed. The opening in the eardrum is surgically enlarged, and a piece of skin, vein, or fascia, large enough to fit the opening, is sutured over it. Gelfoam or clotted blood may be used to fill the middle ear space to support the graft, and sterile packing is placed outside, in the external ear, to help keep the graft in position. If the graft takes, a large degree of tympanic function will return.

Other parts of the middle ear also require reconstructive surgery, and the procedures are known collectively as *tympanoplasty.* They may include removal of any scar tissue that interferes with the function of the ossicles, replacement of diseased ossicles with plastic or metal prostheses, and reconstruction of the eardrum. These procedures usually are not performed on children because they are highly susceptible to infections that reach the middle ear by way of the eustachian tubes, and therefore the graft is likely to become infected. The patient should avoid sneezing and blowing his nose postoperatively so as not to disturb the graft. If the patient has to sneeze, he should open his mouth and not cover his nose to prevent pressure building up in a closed space.

The inner ear

Labyrinthitis. Labyrinthitis is an infection of the inner ear (the labyrinth) and usually is a complication of chronic middle ear infection. The inner ear helps maintain equilibrium, and infections there, in addition to producing loss of hearing, disturb the function of the semicircular canals, causing severe vertigo, nausea, vomiting, and nystagmus (involuntary, cyclic movements of the eyeball).

The patient who has labyrinthitis is kept in bed and given massive doses of antibiotics. If vomiting persists, fluids must be given parenterally. However, fluids given orally usually are retained if they are taken in small amounts and if the patient lies with his head perfectly still. Since the patient is quite dizzy, side rails should be placed on the bed to prevent him from falling. An operation such as a radical mastoidectomy is sometimes done to remove the source of the infection. His other nursing care is similar to that for the patient with Ménière's disease.

Ménière's disease. The cause of Ménière's disease is unknown. There is hypertension of the endolymphatic fluid circulation in the cochlea due to increased production or to decreased absorption of endolymph. Atrophy of the hearing mechanism eventually occurs. The patient is incapacitated by severe attacks of vertigo, sometimes to the extent that he is unable to cross a room without falling. He describes a sensation of dizziness, severe tinnitus (ringing in the ears), and a feeling that the room is spinning about him. During an attack, any sudden motion of the head or eyes tends to precipitate nausea and vomiting. The patient may appear withdrawn and irritable as well as acutely ill. Attacks may occur at intervals of weeks or months. They may disappear without treatment or they may continue until the patient is completely deaf in the affected ear. When the eighth nerve (acoustic) dies, symptoms cease.

Diagnosis is made chiefly from the patient's history. Audiometry may be helpful in the diagnosis, and the *caloric test* should still be performed although it is now considered to be of limited value in establishing the diagnosis. Usually a *bithermal caloric test* is performed. In this test, warm as well as cold water is dropped into the ear. The water used is 7° C. above and below body temperature (30° to 44° C.). This procedure usually causes dizziness in a normal patient. If the patient has an *acoustic neurinoma* instead of Ménière's disease, there will be no reaction to the test.

A newer test that is becoming more widely used is *electronystagmography (ENG)*. In this examination, electrodes are applied to each side of the face to measure the movement of the eyes while they are closed (Fig. 23-16). This is possible because the cornea of the eye carries a positive electric charge, while the retina carries a negative charge. Thus when the eyeball moves, charges picked up by the electrodes are amplified and recorded on graph paper as there is a change in the electrical field. Electronystagmography is valuable in diagnosing vestibular disease.

Ménière's disease is characterized by episodic attacks. If the symptoms persist or if the patient has syncope or significant pain, a neurologic consultation is usually obtained to rule out neurologic disease.

There are many types of treatment and all may be prescribed during the course of this disease. In order to reduce hypertension, fluid intake may be limited and diuretic drugs such as chlorothiazide

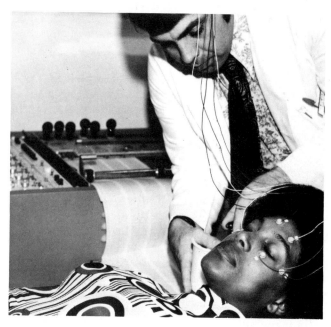

FIG. 23-16. Electronystagmography. Patient undergoing caloric stimulations as nystagmus is recorded on graph. (From DeWeese, D. D., and Saunders, W. H.: Textbook of otolaryngology, ed. 4, St. Louis, 1973, The C. V. Mosby Co.)

(Diuril) may be ordered. If the sodium ion is thought to be a factor in the production of endolymphatic fluid, a salt-free or low-salt diet may be prescribed. Vasodilating drugs such as nicotinic acid often are used. Dimenhydrinate (Dramamine) may be given to control nausea, vomiting, and dizziness. If medical therapy does not control the disease and the patient is incapacitated by vertigo, surgical removal of the membranous labyrinth can be performed, resulting in disappearance of vertigo and loss of hearing in that ear.

Because sudden movement or jarring aggravates vertigo, the patient usually prefers to move at his own rate and to take care of himself. If one stands directly in front of him when talking, so that he does not have to turn his head or his eyes, he will experience less dizziness. Although movement increases the symptoms, the patient should be encouraged to move about in bed occasionally and to permit gentle back care to preserve good skin tone. Lying quietly on the unaffected side with eyes turned toward the direction of the affected ear sometimes is recommended to relieve an acute attack. The patient should not try to read, and bright glaring lights should be avoided. Side rails should be on the bed at all times, and the patient should not attempt to get up and walk without assistance lest he injure himself. Because it is usually very difficult to get the patient with Ménière's disease to take food or fluids, efforts should be made to obtain something that he will eat or drink.

Otosclerosis. Otosclerosis is a progressive condition in which the normal bone of the inner ear is replaced by abnormal osseous tissue. The new growth of bone forms about the oval window and then about the stapes and blocks its movement so that it is unable to vibrate effectively in response to sound pressure. The cause of otosclerosis is not known, but it tends to run in families, and it is more common in women than in men. In some women, pregnancy may be a precipitating factor. According to one source, a focus of otosclerotic bone can be found in one out of eight middle-aged adult white females and one out of fifteen adult white males examined. Hearing loss is gradual and usually becomes noticeable some time between puberty and age 30. Usually both ears are affected—one more than the other—and tinnitus is a troublesome symptom. The treatment for hearing loss due to otosclerosis is a stapedectomy.

Stapedectomy. After a local anesthetic has been administered, an incision is made deep in the ear canal close to the eardrum so that the drum can be turned back and the middle ear exposed. Working through an electric microscope, the surgeon frees and removes the stapes and the attached footplate, leaving an opening in the oval window. The patient can usually hear as soon as this step is completed. The opening in the oval window is closed with a plug of fat or Gelfoam, which the body eventually replaces with mucous membrane cells. A steel wire or a Teflon piston is inserted to replace the stapes and is attached at one end to the incus and at the other to the graft or plug to transmit sound to the inner ear. (See Fig. 23-17.)

Postoperative routines differ in various centers. Some physicians prefer that the patient lie with the operative ear uppermost to prevent displacement of the graft, while others want the patient to lie on the operative ear to facilitate drainage. Some physicians

permit the patient to lie on whichever side is most comfortable for him and does not cause vertigo. If postoperative pain occurs, it is usually relieved by codeine sulfate, 60 mg., or meperidine hydrochloride, 100 mg. Postoperative trauma and edema may cause vertigo for a few days. Dramamine, 50 mg., is given every 6 hours to relieve it. The patient should be cautioned against rapid turning since it may cause vertigo. To prevent falls, side rails should be on the bed and the patient should have supervision and assistance when getting out of bed and walking. Antibiotics may be given to help prevent postoperative infection, and the patient is instructed not to blow his nose for a week to prevent air and organisms from being forced up the eustachian tube. Sneezing should also be avoided, but if a sneeze appears imminent, the patient is advised to open his mouth wide and to sneeze as lightly as possible. He should not lift heavy objects or bend over until such activity is approved by the surgeon. He usually is advised not to wash his hair for 2 weeks and not to get water into his ear for 6 weeks. The patient may be discouraged because hearing may be less than he had experienced in the operating room or be less than he had expected. However, the packing in the ear and postoperative edema may cause some of this loss, and the full effects of the operation cannot be evaluated in the immediate postoperative period. The usual hospital stay is 4 or 5 days. The packing usually is removed in the surgeon's office or in the clinic about the sixth day, and most patients are allowed to return to work in 2 weeks. During the first week the patient may be advised to wear cotton in the ear when outdoors. He should avoid exposure to persons with colds, which might be acquired and lead to middle ear infections. Flying should be avoided for 6 months after the operation.

Hearing impairment

It is estimated that more than 12 million adults and 3 million children in the United States have some kind of hearing defect. Four million of these persons are seriously handicapped, and about 760,000 are totally deaf.[20] For psychologic reasons, hearing loss, hearing defect, or impairment of hearing are the terms used to describe the patient's handicap.

Hearing difficulties may begin in childhood. However, with adequate treatment of upper respiratory infections, treatment of aching and draining ears, and care to avoid foreign objects in the ears, hearing loss often can be prevented. The nurse should be alert to every opportunity for health teaching concerning the conservation of hearing. Screening programs in the communities for detecting children with possible hearing losses are helpful in limiting the handicap by getting the child under medical care. The nurse in industry can help prevent

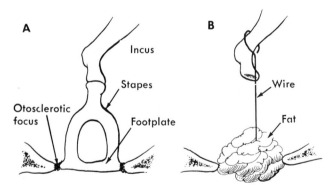

FIG. 23-17. One method of performing a stapedectomy. **A,** Stapes immobilized by otosclerosis. **B,** Replacement of stapes with a fine wire and sealing of the opening in the oval window with a ball of fat removed from the earlobe. The wire and fat apparently cause no reaction.

deafness due to noise of high intensity by teaching the employees why they should wear their earplugs. Concern with noise pollution as well as with other occupational hazards prompted the passage of the *Williams-Steiger Occupational Safety and Health Act* in 1970. The provisions regarding noise protection are too complex to include in detail, but in general, exposure to noise levels in excess of 90 dB (on the A scale) over an 8-hour day are considered excessive and should be avoided (Table 23-1). There are three intensity patterns on which sound is measured; these are called the A, B, and C scales. A copy of the Occupational Safety and Health Act may be obtained from local offices of the Occupational Safety and Health Agency, which are part of the U. S. Department of Labor.

The person who seems to be inattentive or who has a strained facial expression, particularly when conversing or listening to others, may be hard of hearing. Persons with faulty articulation in speech may be deaf. Their faulty articulation may result from not being able to hear themselves speak. The person who habitually fails to respond when spoken to or who makes mistakes in carrying out directions should be encouraged to have his hearing tested. The repetition of "What did you say?" or "uh huh" with a quizzical expression is often a symptom of hearing loss. Persons with marked hearing loss frequently tend to withdraw from others in an attempt to conceal their difficulty.

Hearing is one of man's primary means of communication and helps keep him in touch with reality and his environment. Every effort should be made to develop, protect, and preserve it. As hearing diminishes, the impact of not understanding others and of not being understood may make the person withdraw from social situations, and he may become anxious and insecure. His fear of inadequacy and inferiority

may make him suspicious and depressed. When hearing is completely gone, the individual may find his silent world almost intolerable. Loneliness and isolation eventually may lead to disorientation or the lack of desire to live. The nurse can help find and direct the person with a hearing loss and his family to the appropriate agencies for assistance. There may be ways of improving his hearing through medical or surgical therapy. If the loss is irreversible, aural rehabilitation may make it possible for him to understand and communicate with others again so that he can lead a useful, meaningful life. Unfortunately many persons who have a hearing loss are in the older age group and usually also have some loss of vision, making rehabilitation more difficult.

Types of hearing loss. Hearing loss is classified in several ways. Any interference with the conduction of sound impulses through the external auditory canal, the eardrum, or the middle ear produces a conductive type of hearing loss. The inner ear is not involved, and sound directed to it will be heard clearly. Conductive hearing loss may be due to impacted cerumen or a foreign body in the external auditory canal, a thickening, retracting, scarring, or perforation of the eardrum, pathologic changes in the middle ear that prevent movement of one or more of the ossicles, or a fixing of the stapes due to otosclerosis. At the present time it is only the conductive type of hearing loss that can be treated effectively.

Sensorineural hearing loss results from disease in the inner ear or its neural pathways. Some of the causes include arteriosclerosis; infectious diseases such as mumps, measles, and meningitis; toxicity to drugs such as quinine, dihydrostreptomycin, or neomycin; neurinoma of the eighth cranial nerve; blows to the head or the ears; and degeneration of the organ of Corti due to exposure to noise of high intensity. Treatment usually is not effective for sensorineural loss because the damage has been done by the time the patient goes to the doctor and the process is irreversible. In many cases, sensorineural hearing loss can be prevented by such measures as avoiding toxic drugs, controlling noise in industry and wearing ear protection when exposed to loud noises, and early and adequate treatment of middle ear infections such as otitis media and of systemic diseases such as measles so that the disease does not involve the inner ear. Many persons have hearing losses caused by a combination of the two main types of difficulty.

Rehabilitation. The purpose of rehabilitation of persons with a hearing loss is to reestablish and maintain oral communication by means of hearing aids, maximum application of any remaining hearing ability, and increased use of the other senses. The patient may be fitted with and taught to use a hearing aid. He is taught how to use his remaining hearing ability more effectively by developing his listen-

Table 23-1 Permissible noise exposures

Duration/day (hours)	Sound level (dB [A], slow)
8	90
6	92
4	95
3	97
2	100
1½	102
1	105
½	110
¼	115

From U. S. Department of Labor, Occupational Safety and Health Administration: Noise: the environmental problem, a guide to OSHA standards, Washington, D. C., 1973, U. S. Government Printing Office.

ing skills to improve the hearing he has left and to compensate for what he has lost. Speech reading is taught to supplement the hearing function and includes lipreading and the study of facial expressions, gestures, and body movements used in speech. Speech training is given to develop, conserve, or correct speech. The patient's acceptance of the fact that he has a hearing loss, his desire to seek help, his use of the facilities available, together with high motivation, perseverance, and patience, contribute to the success of rehabilitation.

Recent research has indicated that deaf children's learning abilities can be greatly enhanced by employing the language of signs. In these cases it appears that the "total communication" approach that includes speech reading, auditory training, and sign language is most advantageous.

Services for persons with a hearing loss are offered by audiology clinics sponsored by universities, hospitals, community programs, local or state departments of health and education, or the Veterans Administration. National organizations are available to give information and counseling.*

---

*American Federation of the Physically Handicapped, Inc., 1370 National Press Building, Washington, D. C. 20004; National Association of Hearing and Speech Agencies, 919 18th St. N.W., Washington, D. C. 20006; American Speech and Hearing Association, 9030 Old Georgetown Rd., Washington, D. C. 20014; The John Tracy Clinic, 806 West Adams Blvd., Los Angeles, Calif. 90007.

In working with the person who has difficulty hearing, the nurse should be aware of certain considerations and should teach them to others who are in contact with people who have hearing loss. Speak in a normal voice, and tell the patient when he speaks too loudly that it is not necessary to do so. This will help him to regain his normal modulation. Always talk directly to a deaf patient, making sure that the light is on your face. This helps him lipread. Speak clearly, but do not accentuate words. If the patient does not seem to understand what is said, express it differently. Some words are difficult to "see" in speech reading. Do not smoke or cover the mouth while talking to a person with limited hearing. If he wears a hearing aid, wait until he adjusts it before speaking. Do not avoid conversation with a person who has a hearing loss. It has been said that to live in a silent world is much more devastating than to live in darkness, and persons with hearing loss appear, by and large, to have more emotional difficulties than those who are blind.

Habilitation, rather than rehabilitation, is necessary for one who is born deaf or becomes deaf in early childhood, for this person does not develop language and speech normally. Not only is it medically important to detect deafness or hearing impairment in the young child, but from an educational standpoint, it is imperative that remedial measures be taken during early years when language and speech skills are most easily acquired (between ages 2 and

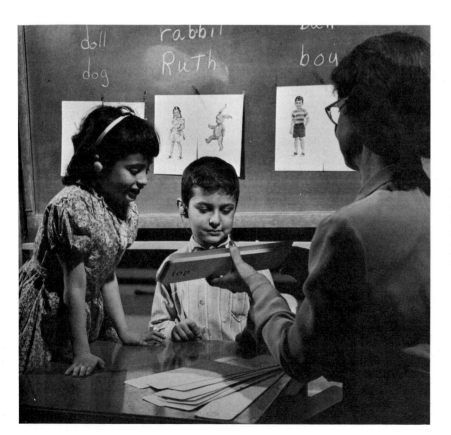

FIG. 23-18. Children with hearing difficulties practice reading preparatory to joining classes for children with normal hearing. Note the hearing aids. (Courtesy New York League for the Hard of Hearing, New York, N. Y.)

5).[20] The child who has never heard speech is unable to imitate it. He is educable, but his education requires more time than that of the normal child. Since a period of about 3 years is required for a child to learn sufficient language to begin the first grade (Fig. 23-18), he should start attending a special nursery school at age 3 or 4. He may then attend classes with children who have normal hearing or go to a public or private school for the deaf. The John Tracy Clinic offers a free correspondence course that helps parents who have preschool children with severe hearing impairment or deafness.[20] Deaf persons often withdraw from others because of their inability to communicate. Therefore there is a great need for programs that focus on finding these individuals and providing service to help them learn the necessary skills for developing a sense of self-worth.

For the person whose vision and hearing both are severely impaired, the catalog distributed by the American Foundation for the Blind* includes a vibrator attachment for the deaf-blind, which is used with a timer or clock. The vibrator is placed under the bed mattress and its vibrations act as an alarm to wake the occupant. A speaking tube or modernized ear trumpet is another aid that is listed. (See p. 844 for further information about this catalog and its braille edition.)

Hearing aids. If a patient's hearing problem indicates a need for a hearing aid, he should be seen both by an otologist and an audiologist. The audiologist can perform various tests and help determine if a hearing aid will benefit the patient and what specific type of hearing aid will be best for him. It is imperative that proper audiologic testing be done be-

_____

*15 West 16th St., New York, N. Y. 10011.

fore a hearing aid is purchased. The otologist can determine the medical nature of the problem and decide whether there is any medical reason why a hearing aid cannot be worn. Hearing aids are instruments used to increase the intensity of the sound reaching the ear of the person with a hearing loss. They do not improve the ability to hear, but they make the sound louder. Hearing aids (Fig. 23-19) usually are recommended when the patient has difficulty in understanding speech in his occupation or in everyday conversations. Patients with a conductive hearing loss benefit most from wearing a hearing aid because their ability to understand speech is usually not impaired if the speech is loud enough. They will not hear as well as they did with normal hearing, but they will be able to hear speech in the frequencies at which most ordinary conversations occur. Because patients with sensorineural loss usually have a hearing loss in the higher frequencies, an intolerance for loud speech and noise, and difficulty in understanding what is being said, they may find the amplification by the hearing aid annoying and impractical for them. Elderly people often have difficulty adjusting to the use of the hearing aid, partially because their hearing loss usually is of sensorineural origin. Their problems also may be due to a lack of patience, concentration, or the mental energy needed to learn to use a hearing aid. Small children with a hearing loss may be fitted with a hearing aid before they begin to crawl and will learn to use it at all times.

The hearing aid usually consists of a microphone used to receive spoken speech and environmental sounds and to convert them into electric signals, an amplifier to strengthen electric signals, a receiver to convert electric signals back to sound, and a battery

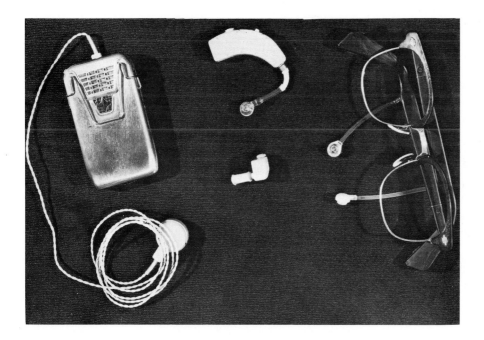

FIG. 23-19. Hearing aids, body and headborne types. A body-type aid is on the left. Its button receiver is coupled to the ear with an insert, and its component housing is either clipped to one's clothing or worn on the body in a harnessed cloth pouch. Remaining are different types of headborne hearing aids. Top center is a behind-the-ear aid, at the right is an eyeglass aid, and in the center is an in-the-ear aid. (From Havener, W. H., and others: Nursing care in eye, ear, nose, and throat disorders, ed. 3, St. Louis, 1974, The C. V. Mosby Co.)

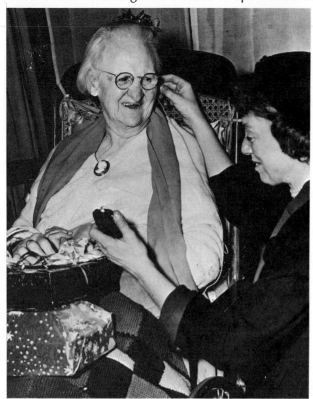

FIG. 23-20. A nurse from New York League for the Hard of Hearing assists an elderly patient to adjust her hearing aid. (Courtesy New York League for the Hard of Hearing, New York, N. Y.)

to supply the electric power. A variety of hearing aids are available. They may be worn on the body (Fig. 23-20), built into the temple bow of eyeglasses, or worn as individual units behind the ear or in the ear canal. The body-worn aids are the most powerful and are generally fitted to people with moderate to severe hearing losses. The eyeglass and behind-the-ear aids are generally equivalent in amplifying power.

The Federal Trade Commission estimated that in 1970 over 500,000 hearing aids were sold to the public. The hearing aid consumer (more than half of whom are over 65 years of age) paid an average retail price of $350 per aid, even though the average cost to the dealer was about $100.

The patient should also be instructed in the care of his hearing aid. The ear mold or plug may be washed daily in mild soap and water, with a pipe cleaner used to cleanse the cannula. It should be thoroughly dried before being reconnected to the receiver. The transmitter of a hearing aid worn on the body should be worn so that the microphone faces the speaker, and it should not be covered by heavy clothing. Men often wear it in their shirt or upper pocket. Women may fit it into a special pocket sewed on the outside of their underclothing. Children often wear it in a fabric harness placed over their undergarments. The person who uses a hearing aid should carry an extra battery and cord at all times.

REFERENCES AND SELECTED READINGS*

1 American Cancer Society, Inc.: 1975 cancer facts and figures, New York, 1974, American Cancer Society, Inc.

2 Bailey, B. J.: Management of sinus infections, Am. Fam. Physician 8:100-107, Dec. 1973.

2a Bates, B.: A guide to physical examination, Philadelphia, 1974, J. B. Lippincott Co.

3 Beeson, P. B., and McDermott, W., editors: Cecil-Loeb textbook of medicine, ed. 13, Philadelphia, 1971, W. B. Saunders Co.

4 *Carty, R.: Patients who cannot hear, Nurs. Forum 11:290-299, 1972.

5 Chadwick, D. L.: Advances in the treatment of diseases of the ear, nose and throat, Practitioner 209:460-473, Oct. 1972.

6 Chiang, T. M., Sukis, A. E., and Ross, D. E.: Tonsillectomy performed on an outpatient basis, Arch. Otolaryngol. 88:307-310, Sept. 1968.

7 Conover, M., and Cober, J.: Understanding and caring for the hearing-impaired, Nurs. Clin. North Am. 5:497-506, Sept. 1970.

8 *Cullin, I. C.: Techniques for teaching patients with sensory defects, Nurs. Clin. North Am. 5:527-538, Sept. 1970.

9 Davison, F. W.: Hyperplastic rhinosinusitis. A twenty year review, Ann. Otol. Rhinol. Laryngol. 82:703-708, Sept.-Oct. 1973.

10 *DeLaney, R. E.: Stapedectomy, Am. J. Nurs. 69:2406-2409, Nov. 1969.

11 DeWeese, D. D., and Saunders, W. H.: Textbook of otolaryngology, ed. 4, St. Louis, 1973, The C. V. Mosby Co.

12 Dison, N.: Tonsillectomy: mother's view, Am. J. Nurs. 69:1024-1027, May 1969.

13 Downs, M. P., and Sterritt, G. M.: A guide to newborn and infant hearing screening programs, Arch. Otolaryngol. 85:15-22, Jan. 1967.

14 Flowers, A. M.: Electronic mechanical aids for the laryngectomized patient, Nurs. Clin. North Am. 3:529-532, Sept. 1968.

15 Frederick, J., and others: Anaerobic infections of the paranasal sinuses, N. Engl. J. Med. 290:135-137, Jan. 1974.

16 Fuerst, E. V., and Wolff, L.: Fundamentals of nursing, ed. 5, Philadelphia, 1974, J. B. Lippincott Co.

17 *Gardner, W. H.: Adjustment problems of laryngectomized women, Arch. Otolaryngol. 83:31-42, Jan. 1966.

18 Gellis, S. S., and Kagan, B. M.: Current pediatric therapy, ed. 4, Philadelphia, 1970, W. B. Saunders Co.

19 Hardy, K. L.: Tracheostomy: indications, technics, and tubes. A reappraisal, Am. J. Surg. 126:300-310, Aug. 1973.

20 Havener, N. H., and others: Nursing care in eye, ear, nose and throat disorders, ed. 3, St. Louis, 1974, The C. V. Mosby Co.

21 Hughes, R. L.: Special devices for the hearing-handicapped patient, Arch. Otolaryngol. 86:522-527, Nov. 1967.

22 Jaffe, B. F.: Sudden deafness, an otologic emergency, Arch. Otolaryngol. 86:55-60, July 1967.

22a *Jacquette, G.: To reduce the hazards of tracheal suctioning, Am. J. Nurs. 71:2362-2364, Dec. 1971.

*References preceded by an asterisk are particularly well suited for student reading.

23 Journal of American Speech and Hearing Association **1:**29, Jan. 1973.

24 Komorn, R. M.: Laryngectomy and surgical vocal rehabilitation, A.O.R.N.J. **17:**73-79, June 1973.

25 Kurland, L. T., and others: Epidemiology of neurologic and sense organ disorders, Cambridge, Mass., 1973, Harvard University Press.

26 Lederer, F. J., and others: Medical problems related to diseases of the larynx, Otolaryngol. Clin. North Am. **3:**599-608, Oct. 1970.

27 *Linnell, C., and Long, Sr. V.: The hearing-impaired infant: diagnosis and rehabilitation, Nurs. Clin. North Am. **5:**507-515, Sept. 1970.

28 Lucente, F. E.: The dying patient in otolaryngology, Laryngoscope **83:**292-298, Feb. 1973.

29 Lucente, F. E.: Psychological problems in otolaryngology, Laryngoscope **83:**1684-1689, Oct. 1973.

29a Maloney, W. H.: Otolaryngology, Hagerstown, Md., 1974, Harper & Row, Publishers.

30 Marlow, D. R.: Textbook of pediatric nursing, ed. 4, Philadelphia, 1973, W. B. Saunders Co.

31 Meadow, K. P.: Self-image, family climate, and deafness, Social Forces **47:**428-433, June 1969.

32 Merenstein, J. H., and Rogers, K. D.: Streptococcal pharyngitis; early treatment and management by nurse practitioners, J.A.M.A. **227:**1278-1282, March 1974.

33 Montgomery, W. W., and Toohill, R. J.: Voice rehabilitation after laryngectomy, Arch. Otolaryngol. **88:**499-506, Nov. 1968.

34 Moore, M. V.: Diagnosis: deafness, Am. J. Nurs. **69:**297-300, Feb. 1969.

35 Nelson, W. E.: Textbook of pediatrics, ed. 10, Philadelphia, 1974, W. B. Saunders Co.

36 Nilo, E. R.: Needs of the hearing impaired, Am. J. Nurs. **69:**114-116, Jan. 1969.

37 Occupational Safety and Health Administration, U. S. Department of Labor: Williams-Steiger Occupational Safety and Health Act of 1970, Federal Register **36:**105, May 1971.

38 O'Dell, A. J.: Emergency care in establishing an effective airway, Nurs. Clin. North Am. **8:**413-424, Sept. 1973.

39 O'Neill, J. J.: The hard of hearing, Englewood Cliffs, N. J., 1965, Prentice-Hall, Inc.

40 Paparella, M. M., and Shumrick, D. A., editors: Otolaryngology, Philadelphia, 1973, W. B. Saunders Co.

41 *Parvulescu, N. F.: Care of the surgically speechless patient, Nurs. Clin. North Am. **5:**517-525, Sept. 1970.

42 Phipps, W. J., Barker, W. L., and Daly, B. J.: Respiratory insufficiency and failure. In Meltzer, L. E., Abdellah, F. G., and Kitchell, J. R., editors: Concepts and practices of intensive care for nurse specialists, ed. 2, Philadelphia, 1975, The Charles Press, Publishers.

43 *Pilgrim, N. C., and others: Reconstructive nasal surgery, Am. J. Nurs. **73:**451-456, March 1973.

44 *Programmed instruction: Respiratory tract aspiration, Am. J. Nurs. **66:**2483-2510, Nov. 1966.

45 *Quimby, M. A.: Care of patients with labyrinthine dysfunction, Am. J. Nurs. **60:**1780-1781, Dec. 1960.

46 *Reeves, K. R.: Acute epiglottis-pediatric emergency, Am. J. Nurs. **71:**1539-1541, Aug. 1971.

47 *Riley, E. C.: Preventing deafness from industrial noise, Am. J. Nurs. **63:**80-84, May 1963.

48 Robinson, M.: A four-year study of the stainless steel stapes, Arch. Otolaryngol. **82:**217-235, Sept. 1965.

49 *Ronnei, E. C.: Hearing aids, Am. J. Nurs. **63:**90-93, May 1963.

50 Sabiston, D. C., editor: Davis-Christopher's textbook of surgery, ed. 10, Philadelphia, 1972, W. B. Saunders Co.

50a *Sackner, M. A., and others: Pathogenesis and prevention of tracheobronchial damage with suction procedures, Chest **64:**284-290, Sept. 1973.

51 *Searcy, L.: Nursing care of the laryngectomy patient, R.N. **35:**35-41, Oct. 1972.

52 *Selecky, P. A.: Tracheostomy: a review of present day indications, complications, and care, Heart & Lung **3:**272-283, March-April 1974.

53 Shaw, E. B.: Endotracheal intubation and tracheostomy—clinical concepts, Disease-a-Month, March issue, 1974.

54 Sheehy, J. L.: Ossicular problems in tympanoplasty, Arch. Otolaryngol. **81:**115-122, Feb. 1965.

55 Spar, H. J.: The deaf-blind. In Garrett, J. F., and Levine, E. S., editors: Rehabilitation practices with the physically disabled, ed. 2, New York, 1973, Columbia University Press.

56 *Stanley, L. M.: Meeting the psychologic needs of the laryngectomy patient, Nurs. Clin. North Am. **3:**519-527, Sept. 1968.

57 Sykes, E. M.: No time for silence, Am. J. Nurs. **66:**1040-1041, May 1966.

58 Vernon, M.: Early profound deafness. In Garrett, J. F., and Levine, E. S., editors: Rehabilitation practices with the physically disabled, ed. 2, New York, 1973, Columbia University Press.

59 Williams, S. R.: Nutrition and diet therapy, ed. 2, St. Louis, 1973, The C. V. Mosby Co.

60 Yates, J. T.: Rehabilitation of hearing impaired adults, J. Rehabil. **39:**20-22, Jan.-Feb. 1973.

61 Yonkers, A. J.: Diagnosing and treating common disorders of the larynx, Geriatrics **28:**150-155, April 1973.

24 Dental and oral conditions

Diseases of the teeth and related structures
Diseases of the mouth and related structures
Trauma

■ This chapter will consider prevention of and nursing care in diseases of the teeth and infections, tumors, and trauma involving the mouth and related structures. In all these conditions, prevention should be stressed before the disease becomes established and treatment is necessary.

The mouth has special emotional significance for every individual, perhaps because it is associated in infancy with food, sucking, warmth, love, and security. It continues to be associated throughout life with survival through the intake of food and with pleasurable sensations related to love and companionship, acceptance and belonging. Therefore severe emotional reactions frequently occur when treatment involving the mouth is necessary. The patient may refuse to visit his dentist, may go into complete panic when the jaws must be wired and normal eating is impossible, and may refuse to accept the fact that a lesion of the mouth is any threat to his health. An understanding of what may be some of the patient's unspoken and often unrealized fears will enable the nurse to give him better care. Patience in explaining tests and treatments often helps. Sometimes merely taking time to explain to the patient how he may be fed following oral surgery may make the difference between his acceptance or rejection of the procedure. Sometimes the patient needs time to accept the need for referral to an oral surgeon and to accept the suggested treatment.

■ DISEASES OF THE TEETH AND RELATED STRUCTURES

Prevention. Teaching the prevention of disease of the teeth and related structures is an important health education responsibility of nurses. Responsibilities vary according to the needs of patients or groups of patients. They include providing public information about overall preventive health measures such as the fluoride treatment of water, proper daily care of teeth and gums to preserve their health, care related to satisfactory use of artificial dentures, diet, general oral hygiene including regular visits to the dentist, and alertness to the possible significance of lesions anywhere in the mouth.

An organized teaching plan may be necessary, and a specific unit of time should be set aside for dental health education. Almost every patient needs to learn about care of the teeth and mouth, whether he is admitted to the hospital with an acute illness or confined to his home because of a heart condition, an infection of his foot, or any other cause.

Nurses will probably be asked about some common misconceptions, and they should know the answers.[18] For example, there is no evidence that any general systemic disease is caused by decayed teeth. There is no evidence that calcium is removed from the mother's teeth during pregnancy and lactation regardless of how deficient in calcium her diet may be. There is, however, abundant evidence that a diet adequate in calcium, phosphorus, and other essential elements during pregnancy contributes to good tooth formation in the growing fetus and that a diet rich in these substances is essential during the years of life when the permanent teeth are being formed.

■ STUDY QUESTIONS

1 Review the anatomy of the teeth, jaws, and mouth. How are the teeth formed? To what is the tongue attached?
2 What main purpose is achieved by chewing food? What enzyme is present in saliva and what is its function?
3 Review the location and function of the thoracic duct.
4 From your notes on fundamentals of nursing, review the measures that can be used to provide optimal oral hygiene of the teeth, gums, tongue, and mucous membranes of the oral cavity.
5 Review the measures that can be used to control unpleasant odors in the mouth.

Calcium is deposited in the buds of the permanent teeth almost immediately after birth. A high-calcium diet after teeth have erupted probably has no effect whatever on their preservation, but local action of other foods such as carbohydrates is of tremendous importance.[19]

Care of the teeth

Removal of plaque. The nurse must realize that the pathogenic site of both dental caries and inflammatory periodontal disease is bacterial plaque. Bacterial plaque is a soft, white mucoid material derived from the breakdown of saliva. Toxin-producing bacteria thrive in its matrix. Their enzymes and other products accumulate within the sulcus (crevice between the gingiva and the crown), causing inflammation and bleeding. Plaque that remains on the teeth for longer than 24 hours begins to mineralize or calcify, forming a hard, tenacious deposit known as calculus (tartar). Calculus has a consistency similar to sandpaper and causes abrasions and ulceration of the internal sulcus. It also has toxin-producing action.[22]

Although plaque can be removed from the teeth by a procedure known as scaling, the most effective means of controlling its formation is by brushing the teeth. The nurse is frequently asked about the kind of toothbrush to use and about general care of the teeth. The points to be emphasized are the use of a proper toothbrush and the correct method and time of brushing.

There is general agreement among dental authorities that toothbrushes should be small enough to reach all tooth surfaces. Usually two or three rows of bristles are recommended, depending on how much space exists between the cheek and the outer tooth surface. Bristles should be soft and cut straight across the brushing surface. Soft bristles conform to the tooth surface by bending or flexing and cleanse more effectively. A dentifrice together with the soft, multitufted bristled brush forms a "matte effect," thereby increasing the amount of friction and the cleansing effect.[21] While nylon bristles are durable, natural bristles are preferred because they are less abrasive. Toothbrushes should dry thoroughly between use to help keep the bristles firm and to prevent bacterial growth. Two brushes may be necessary (particularly if bristles are natural) and should be used alternately. The electric-powered toothbrush is easy to use and safe to operate. Its use may encourage children to brush their teeth more often and may help incapacitated persons to clean their teeth more thoroughly.[31] The individual, detachable brushes make it convenient for use in a family or hospital unit.

Dentifrices containing stannous fluoride help to prevent caries and their value has been officially recognized by the American Dental Association. Other dentifrices simply make brushing the teeth more pleasant. It is estimated that the American public pays approximately $80 million each year for mouthwashes and cleansing agents for their teeth, whereas sodium bicarbonate and salt flavored with peppermint would cost only a fraction of that amount. Ammoniated dentifrices and those containing chlorophyll have been subject to much inquiry, but their benefits have not been proved.

Brushing the teeth should remove debris from between the teeth, stimulate the gums, and yet not traumatize the delicate gingival papillae between the teeth. Many people brush their teeth by passing the bristles quickly across the lateral surfaces of the teeth. This method damages the enamel, does not clean between the teeth, and may injure the gums. The brush should be placed along the gum line with the bristles toward the roots of the teeth. The bristles should then be brought down over the gum and teeth with a gentle sweep, using a downward and upward motion (Fig. 24-1). Although using a longer stroke is easier for the patient, it has a higher potential for traumatizing the gingiva or abrading tooth structure. Also, long strokes will generally pass over irregularly aligned teeth without cleansing adequately. Short strokes, on the other hand, may be more difficult for some patients to perform since they require fine movements and coordination. They are more efficient in the cleansing process because the bristles bend or flex into malaligned or depressed areas. Crosswise motion should be reserved for the top grinding surfaces of the back teeth.

Some dentists recommend a slight vibrating motion over the gums with the brush for further stimu-

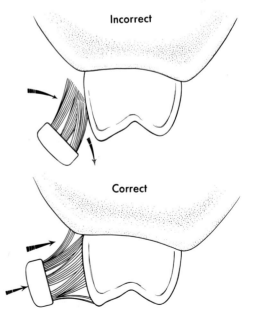

FIG. 24-1. Brushing the teeth. Application of brush so that bristle ends slide gently under the margin of the gingiva.

lation before each downward and upward sweep of the brush, whereas others recommend massage of the gums following brushing. Massage is accomplished by gentle rubbing of the gums with a finger, using very gentle pressure toward the biting surfaces of the teeth. Gum surfaces may be massaged for a few minutes two or three times a day.

A toothbrush will cleanse most surfaces of the teeth adequately except the proximal surface (near the gum line). For cleaning this area, dentists suggest the use of rubber tips, floss, and water irrigation. The rubber tip not only removes plaque from the proximal surface of the teeth but it also massages as it cleans. It should be used in every interdental space where there is room for it and inserted as far into the space as it will go without force. As the tip rests on the interdental tissue, the tip should be activated in a gentle rotary motion so it rubs against the gingiva and proximal surfaces of the teeth.

Dental floss is a useful adjunct for cleaning plaque from interdental spaces. No matter how well instructed, when patients first use floss, they tend to injure the gingiva as they pass the floss through tight contact areas. The tooth surface is cleansed by gently forcing the floss between the teeth with pressure exerted toward the side of the tooth and by moving the floss up and down the tooth surface for several seconds (Fig. 24-2). Water irrigation by means of

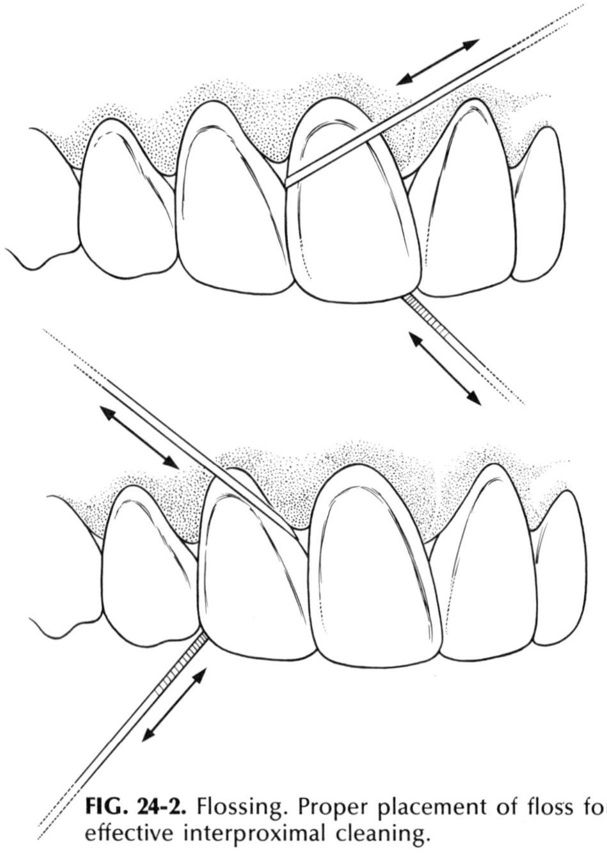

FIG. 24-2. Flossing. Proper placement of floss for effective interproximal cleaning.

the Water Pik is a useful and recommended aid. It acts by flushing away the plaque, food, and debris that has been loosened by the brush, rubber tip, or floss.

Disclosants (vegetable dyes) are important for effective plaque removal as teaching aids in the dentist's office and for the patient at home. They can be used before brushing to alert the patient to the hard-to-clean areas. After brushing, they act as a test of the effectiveness of the technique used. It is suggested that petroleum jelly be applied to the lips and gingiva prior to application of the disclosant to avoid staining of these areas.[23]

Mouthwashes do not significantly inhibit bacterial growth in the mouth. They should not be used by the patient in and effort to treat an oral infection because they may be irritating to an infected mouth, and if used excessively, they may be harmful to natural bacterial flora in the mouth. For the most part, however, they are harmless and are acceptable additions to oral hygiene if desired by the patient and if he can afford them. Most dentists suggest warm water and salt to rinse the mouth if occasional bleeding of the gums occurs. Sodium perborate may be irritating to gum tissues and should not be used without special medical or dental instruction.

When a child has erupted teeth, it is important for the mother to begin brushing the child's teeth, using a small, soft brush. This practice not only provides for effective oral hygiene of the primary teeth, but also begins teaching the child good oral hygiene practices. The child should be taken to the dentist at the age of 3 years, or perhaps earlier, and every 6 months thereafter.

The essentials of good nutrition should be emphasized in the diet of all persons. One of the most effective means of altering plaque formation and the development of dental caries is the restriction in frequency and amount of sucrose intake.

Since limitations have been placed on the consumption of saccharin, other substitutions are being considered by the processed food industry. There is currently considerable interest in modifying the cariogenicity of sucrose by adding various forms of phosphate to such foods as sweetened breakfast cereals. The combination of good oral hygiene and sucrose restriction should effect a reduction in both caries and periodontal disease.[23]

Dental caries. Dental caries (decay of the teeth) is probably the most common, yet the most neglected, chronic ailment of modern man. The American Dental Association reports that tooth decay is occurring in the United States five times faster than it can be repaired.[14] Dental caries is a progressive disease of the teeth related to the consumption of refined carbohydrates such as candy. Within 30 minutes after eating, organisms in the mouth act on the refined sugars left on the teeth and may produce acids that eventually dissolve the enamel surface of the tooth. Decay, cavity formation, inflammation, infection, and loss of teeth follow. Malocclusion gradually develops as teeth are lost. Over 20% of children at the age of 2 years, over 50% at the age of 3 years, and over 75% at the age of 5 years have dental decay. By the age of 14 years, over 95% of children have experienced some dental caries.[12] The average tooth decay rate is about one tooth per person per year.[14] Methods that would control and prevent dental caries include good oral hygiene, dental examinations every 6 months, proper foods, including the avoidance of refined sugars, and the use of fluorides.

The addition of *fluoride* to drinking water in the proportion of one part of fluoride to a million parts of water has been shown conclusively to increase the resistance of tooth enamel to bacterial action during the formative period of young children's teeth and to reduce dental caries by between 48% to 70%.[31] The protection received is permanent and will last a lifetime. Repeated studies have proved that there are no harmful effects to persons who use fluoride in this concentration or even in double this concentration. There is even evidence to indicate that the small amount of fluoride retained and stored in the bones helps to decrease the incidence of fractures and osteoporosis in older people.[14] Mottling of the teeth may occur in parts of the country where the natural water supply contains two or more parts of fluoride per million parts of water, but harmful effects have not been demonstrated.

If the community water is not fluoridated, daily fluoride supplements may be given to children up to 12 years of age. The optimum daily dose for the child up to 1 year of age is 0.25 mg., for the child from 1 to 6 years is 0.5 mg., and for the child from 6 to 12 years is 1 mg.[12] Because the drug must be taken every day from infancy to 12 years of age, some children and their parents find the regimen difficult to follow. The prescription of fluoride supplements to pregnant women for prevention of decay in the teeth of the developing child is not recommended at this time as the data regarding their effectiveness are contradictory. Vitamin-fluoride preparations are available, but there is no evidence that they help control dental caries. The use of these preparations is expensive, and the dosage of fluoride cannot be controlled.[16]

Although less effective and much more expensive than fluoridation of water, local application of fluoride to the teeth of children has been found helpful. Topical application of fluoride cannot prevent cavities from progressing, but it can reduce the development of new cavities by about 40%. It is recommended that children who are not protected by fluoridation of water supplies be given this preventive treatment. Some dentists recommend the local application of fluoride to the teeth in addition to the systemic ingestion of fluoride as an extra protection against the development of caries.[12,16] The treatment consists of one application of stannous fluoride or acid phosphate fluoride to cleaned, dry teeth. It is recommended that the treatment be done when the child is 3 years of age and again at the age of 7 years to protect both the deciduous and the permanent teeth. The treatment is usually repeated at 10 and 13 years of age to protect teeth that appear after 7 years of age. Newly erupted enamel is able to absorb the fluoride ion and form a thin layer of acid-resistant fluorapatite on the enamel surface. Old enamel does not as readily absorb the fluoride ion.[26]

The addition of stannous fluoride to dentifrices helps to prevent tooth decay if used regularly. Acid phosphate fluoride and monofluoride phosphate give evidence that they may equal or surpass the results obtained with stannous fluoride dentifrices.[16] Stannous fluoride recently has been added to prophylaxis pastes used by dentists and dental hygienists to clean and polish teeth. If this method proves effective in reducing caries, cleaning and polishing the teeth and the application of the fluoride may be accomplished in one treatment.[16]

The elimination or drastic curtailment of refined carbohydrate foods would reduce the prevalence of dental caries. In 1823 the average American consumed 8 pounds of sugar a year, whereas now he uses over 100 pounds a year. The consumption of lollipops, ice cream, hard candies, and soft drinks, which are so much a part of American culture, should be curtailed or, preferably, eliminated. The custom of concluding a meal with a sweet dessert and/or candies contributes to tooth decay. The European custom of ending the meal with fresh fruit is an excellent one, since fresh fruit sugars and unrefined starches contain properties that inhibit bacterial enzyme action in the mouth. In fact, eating a raw apple before retiring is an excellent way to clean one's teeth.

Brushing the teeth or even rinsing the mouth with plain water immediately after ingestion of refined carbohydrate foods helps prevent decay. The times when most people brush their teeth are entirely wrong from the standpoint of prevention of dental caries. It is during the first half hour after eating refined carbohydrate that the most harm is done. Immediate rinsing of the mouth with plain water is more helpful than is thorough brushing of the teeth hours afterward when the bacterial damage has been done.

Periapical abscess. A periapical abscess develops around the root of a tooth. It usually is an extension of an infection arising in the pulp caused by dental caries. The abscess may perforate along the gum margin, or it may travel medially to form an abscess over the palate or spread directly to the soft tissues, causing cellulitis and a severely swollen face.

Periapical abscess can cause severe local pain and systemic reactions, including malaise, nausea, and elevation of temperature. The treatment consists of drilling an opening into the pulp chamber of the tooth to establish drainage and to relieve pain. Penicillin may be administered, and warm, saline mouthwashes usually are ordered several times a day. After the acute phase, the tooth may be extracted, or root canal therapy may be started if a sound, permanent tooth is involved. An *apicoectomy* (amputation of the end of the root) may be necessary.[12]

Periodontal disease. Periodontal disease is a disease of the tissues that support the teeth (the periodontium) and affects the gingivae, bone, cementum, and periodontal membrane (Fig. 24-3). Symptoms include infection, bleeding, recession of the gums, and loosening of the teeth. Deterioration of bone structure occurs, and teeth may eventually fall out or have to be extracted. After the age of 40 years, more people lose their teeth from this cause than from dental caries. Periodontal disease is receiving much more attention than formerly, partly because of the recognition of the whole field of dental health as a major public health problem. The Public Health Service is cooperating in studies, and most states now have preventive dental health programs that include attention to other dental diseases besides caries.

Many factors contribute to the development of periodontal disease, among them malocclusion, accumulation of tartar, poor nutrition, including eating too much soft food instead of solid food that requires mastication, poor mouth hygiene, and improper brushing of the teeth. Certain systemic conditions may contribute to the development of periodontal disease. These include alcoholism, diabetes, thyroid imbalance, hormonal imbalance (menstruation and pregnancy), response to chemotherapy, and blood dyscrasias.[22] *Malocclusion* may result in a poor bite with unequal pressure on teeth. It leads to deterioration of bony supportive structures. Removal of teeth without proper replacements permits the teeth to drift backward and alters the bite, again producing unequal pressure on working surfaces of the teeth. Premature loss of deciduous teeth in children should be referred to a dentist. Nonmineralized plaque can form on the calculus surface and destroy the tiny tendrils holding the tooth in the socket. This situation eventually leads to unhealthy receding gums with lessened tooth support (Fig. 24-3). Poor nutrition, improper brushing of the teeth, and local infection may augment the destruction of gums and supportive gum structures to such a degree that they recede. The leverage of daily use then becomes too great on the teeth, and they loosen and finally have to be removed.

Treatment of periodontal disease includes maintenance of oral hygiene and nutrition, control of local irritations and infections by regular visits to the dentist, removal of accumulations of tartar on the teeth, replacement of lost teeth, and correction of malocclusion. Even if treatment has been delayed until there is already a good deal of damage, care by an *orthodontist* (one who specializes in straightening teeth) may be surprisingly helpful. Sometimes bridgework and other forms of splinting can be used so that further erosion of bone and supportive tissue can be halted even if teeth cannot be straightened and the actual bite improved.

Nutrition is so important for patients with periodontal disease that some periodontists have their pa-

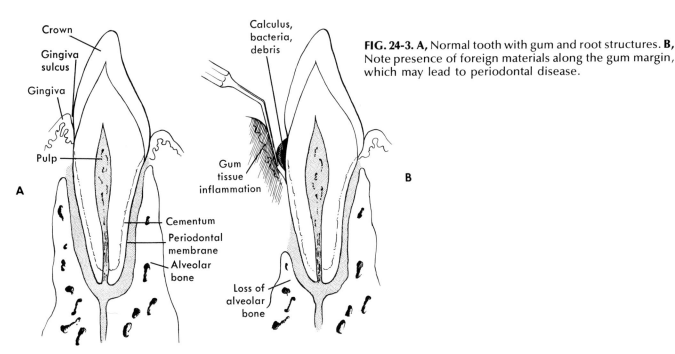

FIG. 24-3. A, Normal tooth with gum and root structures. **B,** Note presence of foreign materials along the gum margin, which may lead to periodontal disease.

Crown

Gingiva sulcus

Gingiva

Pulp

A

Cementum

Periodontal membrane

Alveolar bone

Calculus, bacteria, debris

Gum tissue inflammation

Loss of alveolar bone

B

tients keep weekly food-intake charts to determine what essentials of diet may be lacking. Intake should be evaluated carefully for inclusion of fresh citrus fruits and fresh vegetables, and protein consumption should be noted, since it is so important in gum healing and in gum health.

The nurse must be alert for opportunities to direct patients to the dentist so that periodontal disease may be treated early and the unfortunate results of neglect may be prevented. Many people do not know that malocclusion and space between teeth are of any significance beyond cosmetic effect and lessened efficiency in chewing. The patient may ask the nurse about what seems to him an expensive and possibly unnecessary yet recommended dental procedure. It has been found that people in their forties and beyond can benefit from improvement in equalizing their bite, eliminating space between teeth, better practice in brushing teeth, care of their gums, and regular dental inspection with prophylactic care.

Artificial dentures. Artificial dentures and other dental prostheses are resisted by most people. Serious emotional reactions are manifested when the patient must give up all of his own teeth, no matter how unsatisfactory they may be. In conversation with the patient the nurse should stress the fact that dental prostheses need not be conspicuous, that a proper fit can be obtained in almost all instances, and that there is often cosmetic improvement. The patient should be urged to have patience in learning to use the new teeth. Many elderly people become discouraged easily and are inclined to lay artificial teeth aside and then, because they are embarrassed by their appearance without teeth, avoid people.

Artificial dentures should be cleaned at least twice daily and preferably after each meal. Salt and sodium bicarbonate, a mild tasteless soap such as Ivory, or any good dentifrice can be used. Odor should not be a problem since plastic materials have largely replaced vulcanite materials, which sometimes retained odors. A few drops of ammonium hydroxide or a drop of chlorine household bleach, which is a good deodorant, added to the water used to wash the dentures may make the teeth feel and taste fresher. When artificial teeth are removed for cleansing, the patient should massage his gums thoroughly for a few minutes. Teeth that fit snugly naturally interfere with circulation to some extent. Some dentists encourage their patients to wear their teeth both during waking and sleeping hours since facial contours may be preserved better by this means. Other dentists recommend that the dentures be removed at night to prevent irritation to underlying tissues. Dentures that fit properly should not cause discomfort as soon as the general slight discomfort associated with their newness is overcome. The patient should be advised to report any persistent pressure or irritation to his dentist, since adjust-

ment can usually be made. Any lesion in the mouth associated with the use of dental prostheses should be reported at once since it may be an early malignancy.

Very occasionally there has been so much recession and atrophy of bone structures that it is extremely difficult to fit prostheses properly. A magnetic device has been perfected that can be embedded in the palate and that, by attraction to a magnetized dental plate, helps to hold the dentures in good position.

■ DISEASES OF THE MOUTH AND RELATED STRUCTURES

The mouth, like the eyes and the skin, is an excellent barometer of general health, reflecting general disease and debility as well as good health. In assessment of the mouth, the nurse should note the color of the mucous membrane and of the gum margins, the presence of broken or jagged teeth, deposits on the teeth, and any thickened, irregular areas on the tongue, the gums, or the mucous membrane of the mouth. Pernicious anemia, leukemia, and vitamin deficiencies affect the mouth. Some communicable diseases, including measles and syphilis, produce lesions on the buccal mucosa, tongue, and lips. Specific disease of the mouth most often occurs when general nutrition and oral hygiene are poor, when people neglect their teeth, when smoking is excessive, and when broken teeth irritate the tissues.

Infections of the mouth

Stomatitis. Stomatitis is an inflammation of the mouth that may be caused by drugs such as the barbiturates, pathogenic organisms, mechanical trauma, irritants, or nutritional disorders. Symptoms may include swelling of the mucous membranes, increased salivation, pain, fetid odor of the breath, and occasionally elevation of temperature.

Catarrhal stomatitis is any mild inflammation of nonspecific origin affecting the mouth. It occurs most often in debilitated persons, and the treatment consists of improving the patient's general resistance and using mild alkaline mouthwashes. *Aphthous stomatitis* is the correct name for what are usually called canker sores. These small, painful ulcers may appear singly or in crops. They may follow biting of the cheek or lip, or they may occur spontaneously. Some persons seem to be particularly susceptible to canker sores. Although there is no specific treatment, mild alkaline mouthwashes, better oral hygiene, and more attention to improved nutrition with increased fluid intake and cessation of smoking are beneficial. Local anesthetics may reduce the pain. Topical corticosteroid therapy relieves the pain and improves the gingival response to local treatment, but the results are not predictable.

The virus causing *herpes simplex* often infects the mouths of children between the ages of 2 and 6 years. The gums are swollen and red, and they bleed easily. Vesicles, which are scattered over the tongue and oral mucosa, rupture and result in painful ulcers that interfere with eating. Treatment is supportive since the disease is self-limited to about 14 days. If pain is severe, the physician may advise the patient to rinse his mouth with an aqueous solution of dyclonine hydrochloride (Dyclone), a topical anesthetic. He then may be able to eat a soft diet in greater comfort. The use of antibiotics has not proved beneficial.

Vincent's angina. *Ulceromembranous stomatitis* is commonly known as Vincent's angina. During World War I it was so common that the name "trench mouth" was acquired. It is thought to be caused by a combination of the *Bacillus fusiformis,* which resembles the spirochete of syphilis and *Borrelia vincentii.* There is some question about the communicability of this infection, since causative organisms are found in many mouths although symptoms are absent. The infection causes fever, pain, swelling, fetid breath, and a bad taste in the mouth. Occasionally bleeding of the gums occurs and a gray membrane forms. The patient may have general lassitude and generalized pain about the jaws. If the condition is severe, antibiotics may be given. Since the anaerobic spirochete does not thrive well in the presence of high oxygen concentrations, sodium perborate mouthwashes may be ordered, or half-strength hydrogen peroxide may be applied to the gums. The patient may have to subsist on a liquid or soft diet for a few days. Strongly acid foods, highly seasoned foods, alcohol, and smoking should be avoided.

Ludwig's angina. Ludwig's angina is a rare, deep infection of the tissues of the floor of the mouth caused by the *Streptococcus.* Symptoms include elevation of temperature, toxicity, and local edema that may quickly lead to obstruction of the throat. Once established in the soft tissues, the infection can pass rapidly between the cervical fascial sheaths and reach the mediastinum, where it can cause death. Pressure from infection and edema in the throat as the disease progresses downward can be fatal in a short time.

Treatment for Ludwig's angina requires the immediate administration of large doses of antibiotic drugs. The physician may order hot saline solution mouthwashes hourly during waking hours and hot packs applied externally. Fluids are usually given intravenously. The patient must be watched closely until acute danger is over. A rise in temperature, increased pain, and swelling usually indicate extension of infection. Increased pain on swallowing and on movement of the neck, voice changes, and any difficulty in respiration or evidence of cyanosis must be reported immediately. Surgical incision of the

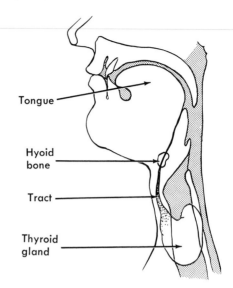

FIG. 24-4. Thyroglossal cyst showing fistulous tract between thyroid gland and base of tongue.

abscess often is done to relieve pressure and to prevent extension of the infection to the mediastinum. Occasionally a tracheostomy is necessary.

Thyroglossal cyst. Thyroglossal cyst is a somewhat rare congenital anomaly that results when certain cells at the base of the tongue do not descend completely to form the middle lobe of the thyroid gland during embryonic life (Fig. 24-4). The cells that are left along the way may form a cyst or a fistula that may empty near the base of the tongue or may form an external fistula anywhere along the tract. The tract is lined with mucous membrane and saliva, and organisms may enter the tract from the base of the tongue. The cyst usually appears as a painless, progressively enlarging mass in the midline of the neck just below the hyoid bone sometime between 2 and 6 years of age. It may become infected acutely or chronically. The treatment is surgical excision of the cyst and of the entire tract, including the center of the hyoid bone. The incision is made between the hyoid bone and the thyroid cartilage, and a drain usually is inserted in the wound postoperatively.

Diseases of the salivary glands

Acute infection can occur in any of the salivary glands, although the parotid gland is the one most often affected. *Parotitis* must be distinguished from *acute communicable parotitis* (epidemic mumps). Parotitis occurs in debilitated patients whose oral hygiene is poor, whose mouths have been permitted to become dry, and who have not chewed solid food regularly. Elderly patients are more susceptible than younger ones. Usually the *Staphylococcus* organism is present. The signs are pain, swelling, absence of salivation, and sometimes purulent exudate from the duct of the gland. Antibiotics often are given. Mouthwashes are used, and either warm or cold compresses applied externally may make the patient more comfortable.

Parotitis usually can be prevented postoperatively by careful attention to oral hygiene, general nutrition, and fluids. Dental prophylactic treatment preoperatively is thought to aid prevention. Having the patient chew gum at times when solid food is not permitted may prevent congestion or obstruction in the ducts of the salivary glands.

Stones may form in the ducts of the salivary glands and within the glands themselves. The submaxillary glands are most often affected. Mucus plugs or tumors may also obstruct normal salivary flow. A radiopaque substance can be injected into the duct *(sialogram)*, thereby visualizing the duct and sometimes the obstruction. Patients who have an obstruction of the salivary glands should be advised to take larger amounts of fluid than usual and to pay particular attention to good oral hygiene. Sometimes probing with a fine probe or gentle massage dislodges the obstruction, but often surgical removal of the stone is necessary. If the entire gland must be removed because of a tumor, paralysis due to trauma of the facial nerve may occur. This paralysis usually disappears within about a month.

Tumors of the mouth

The lips, the oral cavity, and the tongue are prone to develop malignant lesions. The largest number of these tumors are squamous cell epitheliomas that grow rapidly and metastasize to adjacent structures more quickly than do most malignant tumors of the skin. In the United States, oral cancer accounts for 5% of the cancers in males and 3% in females.[1] Recent investigation has revealed a higher incidence of cancers of the mouth and throat among persons who are heavy drinkers and smokers. The combination of high alcohol consumption and smoking causes an apparent breakdown in the body's defense mechanism, as evidenced by an increase in the levels of immunoglobulin A (IgA) in saliva.[24] A good prognosis in treatment of malignant lesions of the mouth depends on early diagnosis and treatment. Every nurse has a real responsibility in interpreting the possible seriousness of any mouth lesion that fails to heal within 2 or 3 weeks and in urging immediate medical care. Pain cannot be relied on as a signal indicating need for medical attention because many advanced malignant lesions in the mouth are painless.

Cancer of the lips usually occurs on the lower lip as a fissure or a painless, indurated ulcer with raised edges. The cause is unknown, but predisposing factors may be prolonged exposure to the sun and wind, constant irritation from the warm stem of a pipe, or chronic leukoplakia. Because metastasis to regional lymph nodes has occurred in only 10% of the patients when diagnosed, the rate of cure is high. In some instances a lesion may spread rapidly and involve the mandible and the floor of the mouth by direct extension. Occasionally the tumor may be a basal cell lesion that starts in the skin and spreads to the lip. Primary lesions of the lip may be treated by cryotherapy, surgical excision, or radiotherapy, depending on the extent and size of the tumor. If extension to the jaw and mandible has occurred, excision and reconstructive surgery are necessary. A complete neck dissection usually is done if the lymph nodes are involved.

Cancer of the anterior tongue and floor of the mouth may seem to occur together because their spread to adjacent tissues is so rapid. They occur as hard plaquelike or ulcerated areas that do not heal. These cancers frequently are found on the under surfaces or lateral portions of the tongue. Irritants such as tobacco, betel leaf, jagged teeth, and poor dental hygiene may contribute to their development. Metastasis to the neck has already occurred in over 60% of the patients when the diagnosis is made. The mortality rate is high. Lesions about the base of the tongue may go unnoticed by the patient and may be far advanced when treatment is started. The prognosis is poor in the patient with this malignant lesion. Treatment depends on the location of the lesion, its stage of development, and the judgment of the surgeon. Intra-arterial infusion of methotrexate, a folic acid inhibitor, into the site of the lesion is sometimes instituted prior to surgical removal of the lesion. Partial or total surgical excision of the tongue *(hemiglossectomy, glossectomy)* sometimes is done. Surgery may be followed by radiation treatment (often interstitial radiation is used, p. 298) and/or by a radical neck dissection in which lymph nodes and adjacent tissues are removed (p. 642). Radiation treatment often is used instead of surgery, and this treatment may or may not be accompanied or followed by a neck dissection.

Leukoplakia is not a cancerous lesion, but if it is allowed to remain untreated, it so often becomes malignant that it is considered here. Leukoplakia begins as chalky, white, thickened patches on the tongue or buccal mucosa of heavy smokers. These patches are not readily removed. Conservative treatment includes good general oral hygiene with use of mild alkaline mouthwashes, dental treatment if needed, and cessation of smoking. The lesions are watched carefully, and if they do not respond to this treatment within a few weeks, they are removed by surgical excision or by cautery. Lesions that seem thickened or papillary are removed at once since they are most likely to undergo malignant degeneration.

Preparation for therapy. The patient who is to have surgical treatment for malignancy of the mouth needs expert and empathetic nursing care. The public is so conscious of cancer that the possibility of spread through metastasis is well known. Dealing with the entirely normal but very real sense of fear that the patient has is an essential part of nursing care.

The treatment for cancer of the mouth, whether by chemotherapy, surgery, or radiation, interferes with normal functions of the mouth. The patient and his family should be told about the changes that will occur and about the methods that will be used to help him communicate and take nourishment. For example, local excisions of the lip or tongue may affect speech to some degree, and the patient may have difficulty making himself understood. Patients having a hemiglossectomy or an intraoral mold inserted will be unable to speak. The provision of a pad of paper with a pencil, a tiny blackboard with chalk, or a Magic Slate will permit the patient to communicate with others. If a hemiglossectomy is done, taking food orally is impossible for a time, and the patient should know that he will be fed by other means. Because it may be difficult for patients with radon seeds in the tongue or for those who have local excisions of the mouth to eat, parenteral fluids, fluids through a catheter or nasogastric tube, or the administration of food through a feeding cup may be necessary. The patient who is to have a hemiglossectomy should be told that suction may be used to remove saliva.

If a radical neck dissection and tracheostomy are to be done at the same time as the treatment of the primary tumor, an explanation of the patient's care after these procedures should be made (pp. 642 and 612). The patient and his family should be assured that he will be attended constantly until he is conscious and able to care for himself. The nurse should get to know the patient in order to judge how much he should be told about his treatment. For example, some patients who are to lose teeth and part of the jaw are relieved to know something about prosthetic devices that are available. Impressions sometimes are taken preoperatively to guide in making suitable prostheses following surgery. Other patients are so overwhelmed by the prospect of the operation itself that they are far from ready to think beyond the most immediate future.

Surgery of the mouth. The preoperative and postoperative care is similar to that discussed on p. 194. Preoperatively, oral prophylactic treatment usually is given, and antibiotics may be administered to decrease the number of bacteria present in the mouth at the time of surgery. The surgery may be done under local or general anesthesia, depending on whether or not a radical neck dissection also is being performed. While recovering from general anesthesia, the patient may be placed in a prone position or on his side to facilitate drainage from the mouth. When he has reacted, he usually is more comfortable in Fowler's position. Bleeding and drainage from the suture line on the lip or tongue should be minimal.

Because of the vascularity of the tongue, patients who have had a wide resection of the tongue should be watched carefully for hemorrhage. If a hemiglossectomy has been performed, the patient will have difficulty in swallowing saliva or expectorating secretions, and the mouth may need to be suctioned frequently. Occasionally a suction device such as is used by dentists is employed to carry away saliva as it accumulates. A gauze wick may be used to direct saliva into an emesis basin. The patient should be provided with mouth wipes and a bag for disposing of them. If he is unable to swallow, the nurse should attend the patient constantly until such time as he is accustomed to the situation and can help to care for himself.

The mouth may be irrigated with sterile water, a mild alkaline mouthwash, hydrogen peroxide, normal saline solution, or a solution of sodium bicarbonate, depending on the physician's preference. Usually sterile equipment is used even though the mouth cannot be kept sterile. A catheter may be inserted along the side of the mouth between the cheek and the teeth and solution injected with gentle pressure, or a spray may be used. Remaining fluid and mucus drains into an emesis basin or is removed with the suction apparatus. Dressings may be protected during this treatment by fitting a plastic sheet snugly over them. As soon as the patient is able to do so, he is encouraged to assist with this part of his care.

The method used to feed the patient will depend entirely on the extent and nature of his surgery. Most patients can suction and feed themselves a few days following mouth surgery and are happier doing so. An Asepto syringe with a catheter attached may be used, and from this apparatus the patient may progress to a feeding cup with a piece of rubber tubing attached. Through practice the patient will develop confidence in caring for himself, and he is often more adept than the nurse in placing the catheter or tube in a position where fluids can be received into the mouth and swallowed without difficulty. A mirror often helps. He needs privacy when he is experimenting with the method that is best for him. He should not be hurried and should be observed very carefully to determine how much assistance he needs. As he begins to take liquids and then soft, pureed foods, he is taught to follow all meals with clear water to cleanse the mouth and foster good oral hygiene.

If the patient has had a hemiglossectomy, he may be fed through a nasogastric tube or through a soft catheter that is passed into the throat and beyond the operative site. Liquid food, 200 to 400 ml., may be given every 3 or 4 hours. The food may be a special formula or regular food that has been blended with liquids in a blender (p. 663). The patient must be watched carefully after the liquid diet is given since nausea and vomiting must be avoided. The sudden arrival in the stomach of fluid through a tube sometimes produces results different from those which occur when food and fluid are taken into the mouth and retained for a few moments during chewing. In addition, the act of swallowing causes some relaxation of the stomach. It is best to give a very small amount of fluid at first, to be certain that it is approximately body temperature, and to wait a few minutes before continuing with the procedure. Diarrhea sometimes occurs when patients must live on liquid foods. The patient should be prepared for it, and the physician should be notified if the condition persists. Sometimes adjustments in the constituents of the liquid feedings help with this problem, and the dietitian may be called on for assistance. At other times a medication such as bismuth is added to the liquid food. If the patient goes home before feeding by these means is discontinued, he or a member of his family should be taught how to prepare the liquid diet, pass the tube, and give the feeding.

While the patient does experience some pain in the area of the incision, most of his difficulty arises from his inability to swallow and speak normally. Medications such as meperidine hydrochloride (Demerol) may be given to relieve the pain, and mouth irrigations and frequent mouth care will make him feel more comfortable. The hospital staff, other patients, and visitors should be alerted to his problem with oral communication. Conversation can be carried out so that the patient's responses can be limited to affirmative and negative gestures or to minimal written replies. The patient usually is permitted out of bed the day after surgery. There usually is no dressing applied to a mouth or lip wound.

The patient may remain in the hospital only 2 or 3 weeks, or he may be hospitalized much longer while further stages of surgery are done or while radiation treatment is given. At this time he needs constant encouragement and careful nursing care. He must be encouraged to mingle with other persons and is often happier in a room with others, provided that there are facilities for privacy when it is needed. The patient should be encouraged to take an interest in his personal appearance. Men should shave as soon as shaving is permitted by the physician. Members of the patient's family should be encouraged to visit, and they, too, should learn how the patient may take food, how he may care for himself, what prosthetic devices are available, and how speech retraining can be accomplished if extensive resection of the tongue or palate or removal of the larynx has been necessary. (Speech training is discussed on p. 619.) Prosthetic devices cannot be fitted until healing has taken place, but pictures of persons who are wearing such devices with resultant marked improvement in their appearance are often encour-

aging to the patient. Prostheses are individually designed to replace portions of the palate and jaw that have been resected and to make the use of dentures possible. Plastic surgery may be done to partially replace lost tissue. Meeting and talking to other patients who have had similar operations with good results and good adjustment are very helpful to the patient.

Radiation. Tumors of the mouth may be treated by radiation in various forms. Needles or molds containing radium, radioactive cobalt, or other radioactive substances may be inserted and left in place for a prescribed time. Seeds containing emanations from radium or radioactive cobalt may be used and left in place indefinitely or else removed. (See Fig. 15-5.) External radiation treatment using x-rays or other radioactive substances may be prescribed.

Whatever method of treatment is chosen should be explained fully to the patient. If needles containing radioactive elements are used, he must know that the needles are fastened to string that must not be pulled lest the dosage or direction of radiation be altered or the needle lost. He must understand that talking with the needles in place will be difficult or impossible. Radioactive needles must be checked several times each day. The nurse should know and should stress to the patient the importance of reporting immediately if one of the needles becomes dislodged. Auxiliary personnel and all other persons in attendance should understand the need to watch all equipment carefully for needles that have been removed or dislodged (for example, when emptying an emesis basin), lest radioactive materials be unwittingly discarded. If radiation is delivered by means of an intraoral mold, the patient must know that he will be unable to talk. He should know that any slipping or change in position of the mold will influence the dosage, so that he must report discomfort and must not attempt adjustment himself. A sling to support the chin helps to alleviate strain and discomfort in the mouth and jaw. Sometimes lying down for short periods is helpful, and occasionally sedatives may be necessary. Attention to mouth hygiene and giving food and fluids are similar to that necessary following surgery of the mouth. Suction equipment should always be ready for immediate use in the event of hemorrhage or choking. If either of these conditions should occur, the patient must be attended constantly since he may become panicky, particularly if a mold is in his mouth.

X-ray therapy usually irritates the gums and mucous membranes of the mouth and inhibits the secretions of the mucous membranes so that saliva may not be produced for months. Sloughing of the tissues may occur and cause a fetid odor in the mouth. Remaining teeth usually are extracted before x-ray therapy is begun. Dentures are not tolerated for some time thereafter because of the sensitivity of the tissues. The physician may order the mouth irrigated once an hour with a solution of $1/2$ teaspoon of sodium chloride and $1/2$ teaspoon of sodium bicarbonate to a quart of water. Some physicians order a solution of 0.3 Gm. (5 grains) acetylsalicylic acid in 2 ounces of water as a gargle that may be swallowed. Gargling may be repeated as often as every 4 to 6 hours. Hydrogen peroxide or Dobell's solutions are ordered sometimes if there is sloughing, and Chloresium (drug preparation containing chlorophyll) may be useful for some patients. Potassium permanganate, 1:10,000, occasionally is used, although its taste is objectionable to some patients. A solution of fifteen drops of common chlorine household bleach in a glass of water helps to control mouth odors and is acceptable to many patients. Inhalation of tincture of benzoin sometimes makes the mouth and throat feel pleasanter and less dry. Mineral oil may be used to relieve dryness of the lips and mouth. If infection occurs in the mouth, antibiotics may be given systemically.

Because smoke is irritating to the mucous membranes, the patient should not smoke. Hot and cold foods or fluids should be avoided because the injured mucous membranes are extremely sensitive to changes in temperature. Some patients complain of a metallic taste, which may be alleviated by sour substances such as lemon candies and citrus fruit juices. Solutions of local anesthetics such as butacaine (Butyn) may be applied to the mucous membranes, or lozenges such as dibucaine hydrochloride (Nuporals) may be prescribed if the discomfort in the mouth caused by the local irritation seriously interferes with eating. (See p. 292 for further discussion of the care of a patient having radiation therapy.)

Radical neck dissection. A radical neck dissection is used in the treatment of malignant tumors of the oropharynx and neck in an attempt to remove metastases and/or prevent the spread of cancer cells to the cervical lymph nodes. The operation usually includes wide removal of the involved tissue and lymph nodes on the affected side. The operation usually is performed in conjunction with the treatment of the primary tumor by surgery or radiation. A tracheostomy may be performed if the surgery has been so extensive that edema is likely to obstruct breathing or to permit suctioning or if a glossectomy has been performed and there is danger of aspiration during normal breathing.

The preoperative and postoperative care is similar to that discussed on pp. 199 and 612. If a tracheostomy has not been performed, an endotracheal tube will probably be in place when the patient returns from the operating room. This tube usually is removed by the surgeon or the anesthetist when the patient is able to breathe safely by himself. When the patient has recovered from the effects of anesthesia, he usually is more comfortable and breathes with

less difficulty in Fowler's position. The patient should be observed closely after removal of the endotracheal tube for signs of respiratory embarrassment caused by irritation of the tube or by tracheal edema. Internal bleeding and pressure from dressings also may obstruct the intake of air. Dyspnea, cyanosis, or changes in the temperature, pulse, respirations, or blood pressure should be reported at once. If the superior laryngeal nerve is cut during the operation, partial anesthesia of the glottis will occur, and the patient may aspirate secretions from the mouth as well as food and fluids. Suction will need to be used frequently, and the patient must be observed carefully for difficulty in breathing.

A few hours after awakening from the anesthesia the patient is urged to sit up and cough. Coughing may be stimulated by placing the tip of the catheter used for suctioning either in the throat or, if a tracheostomy has been done, in the trachea. Coughing must often be followed immediately by suctioning of the mouth and upper throat to remove blood and secretions. If a tracheostomy has been performed, the secretions raised by coughing are suctioned through the tracheostomy tube. Two sterile catheters will be needed since different catheters must be used to remove fluid accumulations from the mouth and to suction the trachea. (See p. 612 for management of the patient who has had a tracheostomy.) Nurses can help patients feel more secure and comfortable by placing their hands firmly in a position to support the neck as the patient coughs. The patient may be instructed to place his locked hands behind his neck and thus support his head and neck when he moves about. (See Fig. 27-4).

Some surgeons place perforated catheters in the wound and attach them to a portable suction unit (Hemovac) to remove secretions and to draw the skin flaps down tightly (Fig. 23-13). From 70 to 120 ml. of serosanguineous fluid may be removed on the first postoperative day. By the third postoperative day, the amount of drainage usually has decreased to 30 ml. or less. No dressings are applied to this wound, and a plastic spray dressing such as Aeroplast may be used. Other surgeons insert one or more drains in the wound and apply massive pressure dressings to obliterate dead spaces, help prevent edema, and splint the part. The dressings are checked for signs of bleeding and for signs of constriction, which may cause edema and hamper respiration. Dressings are usually changed by the surgeon 5 to 7 days following the operation, although the drain may be removed earlier. Some or all of the packing and some of the sutures are removed at this time, and the massive pressure dressings are replaced by a simpler dressing that permits more freedom of movement.

The patient who has had neck surgery usually receives antibiotics in addition to medication for pain. Morphine and other narcotics that depress respiration are used with caution, and an effort is made to limit their use by administering them only before painful procedures such as changes of dressings. Careful support of the neck and of the dressings when the patient sits up, a firm mattress, and gentleness in suctioning and in doing all other necessary procedures make medication for pain less necessary. Atropine sulfate is given with extreme caution because it makes secretions more tenacious and therefore more difficult to remove.

The administration of food and fluids will depend on the site and treatment of the original tumor. If there are no contraindications to the intake of food orally, it may be taken as tolerated. The patient usually is permitted to be out of bed the day after surgery has been performed.

Palliative care. Tissue necrosis and severe pain occur in advanced cancer of the mouth, either from failure in treatment or from death of tissue due to radiation. The patient is harassed by difficulty in swallowing, fear of choking, and the constant accumulation of foul-smelling secretions. The danger of severe, and even fatal, hemorrhage must always be considered. Nursing care of these patients includes the most careful and thoughtful attention to certain details; for example, secretions left in emesis basins or in suction bottles can be most upsetting to the patient. It is exceedingly difficult to induce patients with advanced carcinoma of the mouth to take sufficient nourishing fluids, and the nurse can often help by finding out specifically what fluids or foods the patient likes and believes are easiest for him to take. Relatives may be permitted to prepare and bring special dishes to the hospital if the patient so desires. Sometimes a gastrostomy is done to permit direct introduction of food into the stomach (p. 662). Most physicians prescribe analgesic drugs freely for patients whose disease has progressed beyond medical

control. The patient should be observed for signs of suicidal intent.

Since many terminally ill cancer patients are happier when cared for at home by their loved ones, an important nursing responsibility is teaching a member of the family to feed, suction, and otherwise care for the patient. Relatives may learn how to care for the patient while he is in the hospital and then are often assisted in their homes by a nurse from a community nursing agency. A carefully worded referral including the nursing care plan from the nurse in the hospital to the nurse in the community helps a great deal to make the patient's adjustment from hospital to home care an easier one.

■ TRAUMA

Fracture of the jaw. Fracture of the jaw occurs quite frequently as a result of vehicular accidents and of men's physical encounters with each other. Treatment consists of bringing the separated fragments together and immobilizing them. This is accomplished with wires that are attached to the upper and lower rows of teeth and twisted together or with arch bars fastened by rubber bands or tie wires (Fig. 24-5). Rubber bands are used most often since they can be removed readily and the degree of fixation can be adjusted easily. If an open operation is necessary, interosseous wiring or plating may be done. Because of the excellent blood supply to the jaw, fractures usually heal rapidly (5 to 8 weeks). Tetanus prophylaxis and antibiotic therapy are usually started on admission.

Preoperatively the patient is told that he will be able to breathe normally, to talk, and to swallow liquids but that he will not be able to eat solid food. He should be assured, however, that he will be able to take sufficient food for health. Many times the pa-

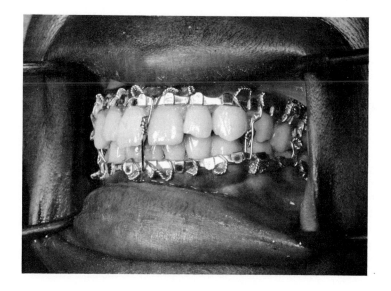

FIG. 24-5. One method of wiring the jaw. (Courtesy Marsh Robinson, D.D.S., M.D.)

tient with a fracture of the jaw can resume quite an active life during convalescence. Most patients are in the hospital a very short time or are treated on an ambulatory basis unless they have sustained other injuries.

Immediately following "wiring of the teeth," the patient is watched for nausea and vomiting, which may be caused by emotional trauma, blood or other swallowed material, or anesthesia. Care must be taken to prevent aspiration of vomitus. Vomitus and secretions must be removed by suction since the patient cannot expectorate them through the mouth. Usually a catheter can be inserted through the nasopharynx or into the mouth through a gap created by missing teeth or in the space behind the third molar. Scissors or a wire cutter should be at the bedside so that the wires can be cut or the elastic bands released if necessary. The nursing care for the patient must have specific orders that state, among other things, the circumstances under which wires or rubber bands should be released.

Patients who have fixation by wiring need much the same care as is needed following surgery of the mouth. They must often subsist on liquids and must learn to take a high-caloric liquid diet through a catheter, an Asepto syringe, a feeding cup, or a straw. They need instruction about mouth hygiene, and they must be instructed to report any sudden swelling, pain, or other symptoms that may occur after dismissal from the hospital. Osteomyelitis is much less common now that antibiotics are available, but it can occur and is more likely to do so in the unusual cases of compound fracture in which bone fragments have penetrated either the outer skin or the inside of the mouth.

Injury to soft tissue. Injuries to soft tissues within the mouth usually are caused by pressure against teeth, direct trauma from a foreign object, or protrusion of bone through the buccal mucosa following fracture of the jaw. Breaks in the skin about the mouth often accompany these injuries. Treatment consists of thorough cleansing of the wounds. Usually an antibacterial solution is used and is followed by irrigation with sterile normal saline solution. Skin wounds are gently debrided and sutured with an extremely fine, nonabsorbable suture for best cosmetic results. Because of the vascularity of the scalp and face, infection is rare following traumatic injury to these areas.

Lacerations within the mouth are cleansed and sutured if their extent and location make these measures necessary. Hemorrhage must be watched for, especially if total injuries necessitate extensive dressing, which may hinder normal expectoration of blood and cause it to be swallowed. Edema may be pronounced following trauma to the mouth and may interfere with respirations. Usually the head of the bed is elevated in a semi-Fowler's position to aid in venous drainage from the area and thereby lessen edema. Tight dressings about the face must be checked carefully since they may contribute to development of edema and may cause headache.

Patients who have sustained penetrating wounds of the mouth are usually given antibiotics and tetanus serum prophylactically. The nurse should question the patient about a history of sensitivity to serum before treatment for prevention of tetanus is given. Mouth care and feeding of patients with these injuries present problems similar to those encountered following surgery or a fracture and have already been discussed in this chapter.

REFERENCES AND SELECTED READINGS*

1 American Cancer Society, Inc.: 1975 cancer facts and figures, New York, 1974, The Society.

2 Barbarosa, J. F., and Bertelli, A.: Surgical treatment of cancer of the base of the tongue, Arch. Otolaryngol. **86:**666-672, Dec. 1967.

3 Beeson, P. B., and McDermott, W., editors: Cecil-Loeb textbook of medicine, ed. 13, Philadelphia, 1971, W. B. Saunders Co.

4 Brown, M., and Alexander, F.: Improved intermaxillary wiring, Arch. Otolaryngol. **88:**193-195, Aug. 1968.

5 Casey, D. E.: Treatment of fractures of the maxilla and mandible, Surg. Clin. North Am. **48:**191-200, Feb. 1968.

6 Collella, R. F. A.: Dental care, Pediatr. Clin. North Am. **15:**325-336, May 1968.

7 *Farr, H. W., and Hislop, R.: Cancer of the tongue and nursing care of patients with mouth or throat cancer, Am. J. Nurs. **57:**1314-1319, Oct. 1957.

8 Ferber, J. R.: Detection of periodontal disease in the aged, J. Am. Geriatr. Soc. **2:**1053-1062, Nov. 1963.

9 *Franks, A. S.: The mouth in old age, Nurs. Times **69:**1292-1293, Oct. 1973.

10 Frazell, E. L., Strong, E. W., and Newcombe, B.: Tumors of the parotid, Am. J. Nurs. **66:**2702-2708, Dec. 1966.

11 Gage, A. A., and others: Cryotherapy for cancer of the lip and oral cavity, Cancer **18:**1646-1651, Dec. 1965.

12 Gellis, S. S., and Kagan, B. M.: Current pediatric therapy, ed. 5, Philadelphia, 1973, W. B. Saunders Co.

13 Glickman, I.: Clinical periodontology, ed. 4, Philadelphia, 1972, W. B. Saunders Co.

14 *Hass, R. L.: The case for fluoridation, Am. J. Nurs. **66:**328-331, Feb. 1966.

15 *Havener, W. H., and others: Nursing care in eye, ear, nose, and throat disorders, ed. 3, St. Louis, 1974, The C. V. Mosby Co.

16 *Horowitz, H. S., and Heifetz, S. B.: Individual fluoridation and fluorides for the individual, Clin. Pediatr. **5:**103-108, Feb. 1966.

*References preceded by an asterisk are particularly well suited for student reading.

17 Jaffe, P. E.: Dental cleansing tape, N. Y. J. Dent. **43:**245-247, Oct. 1973.

18 *Kesel, R. G., and Sreebny, L. M.: Periodontal diseases, Am. J. Nurs. **55:**174-175, Feb. 1955.

19 *Kesel, R. G., and Screebny, L. M.: Toothbrushing, Am. J. Nurs. **57:**186-188, Feb. 1957.

20 Lawton, D. M., and others: Determinants of dental care, Can. J. Public Health **64:**343-350, July-Aug. 1973.

21 *Less, W.: Mechanics of teaching plaque control, Dent. Clin. North Am. **16:**647-659, Oct. 1972.

22 *Levine, P., and others: Safeguarding your patients against periodontal disease, R. N. **36:**38-41, July 1973.

23 *Mandel, I. D.: New approaches to plaque prevention, Dent. Clin. North Am. **16:**661-670, Oct. 1972.

24 Mandel, M. A., and others: Salivary immunoglobulins in patients and bronchopulmonary carcinoma, Cancer J. **31:**1408-1413, June 1973.

25 McDonald, R. E., editor: Dentistry for the child and adolescent, St. Louis, ed. 2, 1974, The C. V. Mosby Co.

26 Nelson, W. E.: Textbook of pediatrics, ed. 9, Philadelphia, 1969, W. B. Saunders Co.

27 Paparella, M. M., and Shumrich, D. A., editors: Otolaryngology, ed. 3, Philadelphia, 1973, W. B. Saunders Co.

28 Redman, B. K., and Redman, R. S.: Oral care of the critically ill patient. In Bergersen, B. S., and others, editors: Current concepts in clinical nursing, vol. 1, St. Louis, 1967, The C. V. Mosby Co.

29 *Reitz, M., and others: Mouth care, Am. J. Nurs. **73:**1728-1730, Oct. 1973.

30 Sabiston, D. C., editor: Christopher's textbook of surgery, ed. 10, Philadelphia, 1972, W. B. Saunders Co.

31 Schlesinger, E. R.: Dietary fluorides and caries prevention, Am. J. Public Health **55:**1123-1129, Aug. 1965.

32 Schultz, R. C.: The nature of facial injury emergencies, Surg. Clin. North Am. **52:**99-106, Feb. 1972.

33 Scopp, I. W.: Oral medicine: a clinical approach with basic science correlation, ed. 2, St. Louis, 1973, The C. V. Mosby Co.

34 Shklar, G., and Schwartz, S. M.: An approach to the diagnosis of diseases of mouth and jaws, Dent. Clin. North Am. **18:**55-75, Jan. 1974.

35 Spouge, J. D.: Oral pathology, St. Louis, 1973, The C. V. Mosby Co.

36 *Stanley, M. K., and Bader, P.: Adult teeth can be straightened, Am. J. Nurs. **62:**94-97, Feb. 1962.

37 Stookey, G. K., and Katz, S.: Chairside procedures for using fluorides for preventing dental caries, Dent. Clin. North Am. **16:**681-692, Oct. 1972.

38 *Weiss, L., and Weiss, E.: Facial injuries and nursing care, Am. J. Nurs. **65:**96-100, Feb. 1965.

39 Williams, S. R.: Nutrition and diet therapy, ed. 2, St. Louis, 1973, The C. V. Mosby Co.

40 Wintrobe, M. M., and others, editors: Harrison's principles of internal medicine, ed. 7, New York, 1974, McGraw-Hill Book Co.

41 Work, W. P.: Therapy of salivary gland tumors, Arch. Otolaryngol. **83:**89-91, Feb. 1966.

25 Diseases of the gastrointestinal system

Physical assessment of the abdomen
Diagnostic examinations and procedures
Gastric and intestinal decompression

Diseases of the upper gastrointestinal system
Esophageal disorders
Hiatus hernia (esophageal or diaphragmatic hernia)
Gastric disorders
Cancer
Pyloric stenosis

Diseases of the lower gastrointestinal system
Appendicitis
Meckel's diverticulum
Mesenteric vascular occlusion
Regional enteritis
Ulcerative colitis
Amebiasis
Salmonellosis
Trichinosis
Diverticulosis and diverticulitis
Cancer of the colon
Hernia
Peritonitis
Intestinal obstruction

Diseases of the rectum and anal canal
Cancer of the rectum
Disease conditions of the anus

■ The term "gastroenterology" is used to identify the study of the gastrointestinal tract in health and disease. Health and comfort are the primary functions of the gastrointestinal system, which provides the body tissues with adequate and continuous amounts of water, electrolytes, and nutrients from the food we eat. Through the process of digestion, secretion, absorption, and excretion, the gastrointestinal tract maintains the body's daily requirements and excretes the waste products of digestion. Food must proceed through the gastrointestinal tract without hindrance and at the proper rate necessary for the aforementioned processes to take place.

The bolus of food must pass from the esophagus into the stomach with ease and without reflux of gastric acid. It remains in the stomach for the time required to reduce the contents to semiliquid consistency through gastric contractions and the activity of the gastric enzymes. As the stomach contents pass through the duodenum and small intestine, there needs to be a sufficient time lapse to ensure adequate absorption. The same principle applies to the large colon and the time necessary for the absorption of water and some electrolytes.

Disorders of gastrointestinal functions, whether caused by psychologic or physiologic factors, interfere in some manner and to some degree with the normal maintenance of gastrointestinal function and the vital process necessary for the maintenance of health. Interruptions of gastrointestinal functions can create acute as well as chronic health problems. Complaints of gastrointestinal disturbances are common and numerous, the major ones include *dysphagia* (difficulty in swallowing), *dyspepsia* (heartburn), abdominal pain, hemorrhage, nausea and vomiting, diarrhea, and constipation. Most people have experienced the stomach upset and diarrhea that often accompany disorders such as influenza, dietary indis-

■ **STUDY QUESTIONS**

1 Review the anatomy and physiology of the gastrointestinal system. What are some factors that stimulate gastric motility?
2 Review the regions of the outer abdomen and locate the left and right epigastric, the hypogastric, and the inguinal regions. What muscles lie under each of these regions?
3 What enzymes are present in the small bowel, and what is their action on normal skin?
4 How can electrolyte balance be affected by excessive vomiting and persistent diarrhea?
5 In your hospital what distinction is made between a liquid, a soft, and a general diet? What foods would you exclude in a low-residue diet?
6 Review the medications that are used to control motility of the gastrointestinal tract.

cretions, or emotional upsets. These experiences are frequently uncomfortable and contribute to temporary abnormalities of gastrointestinal motility and absorption. Too often conditions of the gastrointestinal tract are viewed as short term and functional in nature, and medical opinion is not sought until it may be too late to reverse the damage to the gastrointestinal tract. Unfortunately some diseases of the gastrointestinal system do not produce symptoms until the disease has progressed so far that medical treatment cannot cure it. As an example, cancer of the gastrointestinal tract may not produce symptoms until the condition is far advanced.

There are many laboratory tests and examinations available to help establish the presence or absence of disease in the gastrointestinal system. Some tests are performed only to help establish a diagnosis when definite symptoms of disease occur, whereas others are advocated as part of a yearly physical ex-

amination for persons over 40 years of age in an attempt to detect early signs of disease such as cancer.

The common diagnostic tests and examinations used to help diagnose disease of the gastrointestinal system will be considered in this discussion. Since removal of gastric and intestinal contents may be required in the treatment of patients with many kinds of gastrointestinal disorders, these procedures also will be discussed before nursing care for specific diseases is considered.

The physician writes an order for each test and examination. The nurse is usually responsible for working with the x-ray department and the laboratory in scheduling the tests as well as for the instruction and physical preparation of the patient. It is the responsibility of the nurse to inform the patient about the tests he is to have. He should know what to expect, the purpose of the test, and how he may participate so that informative results can best be

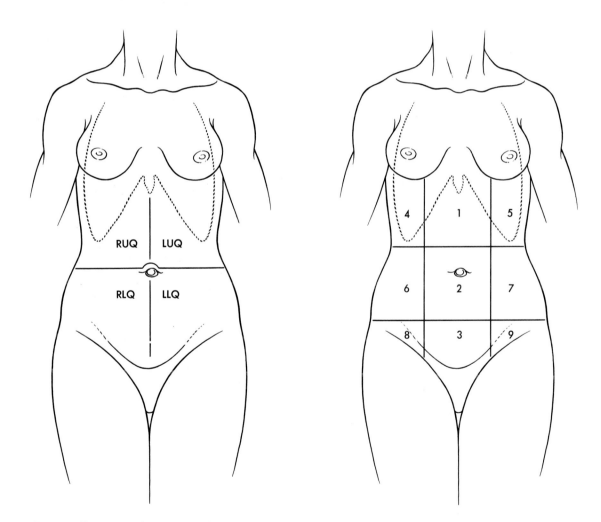

FIG. 25-1. Illustrating the topographic divisions of the abdomen commonly used to localize signs and symptoms and the anatomic location of viscera within the abdomen. *1,* Epigastrium; *2,* umbilical; *3,* suprapubic (bladder and uterus); *4* and *5,* right and left hypochondrium; *6* and *7,* right and left lumbar or flank; *8* and *9,* right and left iliac or inguinal.

obtained. If some time must elapse before the results are known or if tests are to be repeated, he should be so informed. This knowledge lessens anxiety and helps the patient feel that he is participating in his treatment.

When several x-ray examinations are ordered for a patient, they should be scheduled in the following order so that the best results can be obtained with a minimum of delay: intravenous pyelogram, gallbladder series, barium enema, and gastrointestinal series. Since the tests are expensive, time-consuming, and often exhausting, it is important that the patient be properly instructed and prepared so that the examinations will not have to be repeated.

▨ PHYSICAL ASSESSMENT OF THE ABDOMEN

Physical examination of the abdomen requires knowledge of the terms used to designate the divisions of the abdomen (Fig. 25-1) and the anatomic structures located therein.* The structures located in each quadrant of the abdomen are the following:

Right upper quadrant (RUQ)
Liver
Gallbladder
Duodenum
Right kidney
Heptatic flexure of colon

Left upper quadrant (LUQ)
Stomach
Spleen
Left kidney
Pancreas
Splenic flexure of colon

Right lower quadrant (RLQ)
Cecum
Appendix
Right ovary and tube

Left lower quadrant (LLQ)
Sigmoid colon
Left ovary and tube

The examiner must know the appropriate methods for examination and the patient's history and complaints of visceral discomfort before beginning the examination. In patients with a rigid and painful abdomen, for example, the examiner would avoid palpation or manipulation.

The methods for physical examination are performed in the following order: (1) inspection, (2) auscultation, (3) percussion, and (4) palpation. The examination should take place in a warm room, and the patient should have adequate covering to prevent shivering and tensing of the abdominal wall. The patient should void to empty the bladder before the examination and should be placed in the supine position with his head elevated with one pillow and his arms at the sides or across the thorax. A small pillow under the knees may give the patient greater comfort and aid in relaxation of the abdominal musculature. A right-handed examiner should stand to the right side of the patient. The height of the bed should be such that the examination can be carried out by the examiner with ease. If necessary, the patient can be moved to the side of the bed closest to the exam-

---

*Additional information on physical assessment of the abdomen can be found in references 6a and 47a.

iner. The patient should be draped so that the pubis is covered, and the female patient's breasts should be covered with a folded towel. The patient should be informed of each step of the examination.

Inspection

Arrange the illumination to shine across the abdomen and toward the examiner or have the light source lengthwise over the patient. Inspect the skin color and texture and observe for scars, engorged veins, visible peristalsis, masses, or abnormal contour.

	Interpretation
Scars or striae	May be result of pregnancy, obesity, ascites, tumors, edema, surgical procedures, or healed burned areas
Engorged veins	May be due to obstruction of vena cava or portal vein and circulation from abdomen
Skin	Observe for dehydration and evidence of jaundice
Visible peristalsis	May be due to pyloric or intestinal obstruction; normally peristalsis not visible except for slow waves in thin persons.
Visible pulsations	Normally slight pulsation of aorta visible in epigastric region
Visible masses and altered contour	Observe for hernias, distention of ascites, and obesity; instructing patient to cough may bring out hernia "bulge" or elicit pain or discomfort in the abdomen

Auscultation

Auscultation is used primarily to determine the presence or absence of peristalsis and should be done before percussion and palpation to avoid an increase or decrease of peristalsis (or disturbing viscera, causing abnormal activity). Other sounds such as friction rubs or murmurs may be heard (Fig. 25-2). Using the bell, the stethoscope should be placed lightly over the abdominal wall. Most intestinal sounds occur at a rate of five or more per minute and are high pitched and gurgling in quality. A normal peristaltic wave produces audible sounds of air and fluid movement through the intestine. The stethoscope bell is placed to the right and below the umbilicus.

	Interpretation
Absence of sounds	Peritonitis and paralytic ileus
Increased peristalsis	Repeated, high pitched, and occurring at frequent intervals; heard in early pyloric obstruction and early intestinal obstruction

NOTE: Place the stethoscope over the upper middle quadrant of the abdomen above the umbilicus and move to the left and right upper quadrants of the abdomen.

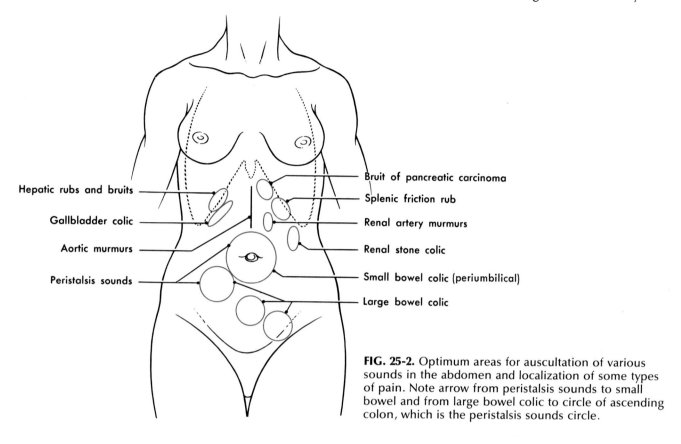

Hepatic rubs and bruits

Gallbladder colic

Aortic murmurs

Peristalsis sounds

Bruit of pancreatic carcinoma

Splenic friction rub

Renal artery murmurs

Renal stone colic

Small bowel colic (periumbilical)

Large bowel colic

FIG. 25-2. Optimum areas for auscultation of various sounds in the abdomen and localization of some types of pain. Note arrow from peristalsis sounds to small bowel and from large bowel colic to circle of ascending colon, which is the peristalsis sounds circle.

Bruit	Presence of abnormal sounds (turbulence of blood flow through partially occluded or diseased artery of the aorta or renal artery)
Hum and friction rub	Heard over liver and splenic areas

Percussion

Percussion is primarily used to confirm the size of various organs and to determine the presence of excessive amounts of fluid or air. Normally, percussion over the abdomen is tympanic due to the presence of a small amount of swallowed air within the gastrointestinal tract. A dull or flat percussion note will be found over a solid structure such as a distended bladder or enlarged uterus and over the liver in the seventh interspace. Tympanic sounds should be heard beginning at the ninth interspace in the left upper quadrant of the abdomen. Dullness or flatness of tone in this area may be due to some enlargement of the spleen or the left kidney.

Percussion is performed by placing the left middle finger firmly against the abdominal wall and striking the distal interphalangeal joint of that finger with the tip of the right middle finger. The fingers of the right hand should be flexed and the wrist relaxed as the procedure is performed. The four quadrants should be percussed beginning with the thorax area and moving downward systematically. The degree of soft to pronounced tympany determines gaseous bowel distention.

Fluid wave. In performing a fluid wave test, the left hand of the examiner is placed on the patient's right flank and the ulnar edge of the hand of the patient or assistant is placed over the upper middle abdomen as the examiner's right hand sharply strikes the left flank of the patient. A sharp wave will be felt by the left hand in the presence of a significantly large amount of fluid (ascites).

Palpation

Palpation is an important procedure that aids in confirming the findings of inspection and history data. Palpation is of value in determining the outlines of the liver, spleen, kidneys, uterus, and bladder when these organs are enlarged and in determining the presence and characteristics of abdominal masses and the degree of tenderness or muscle rigidity. This procedure will elicit subjective as well as objective findings.

A mass found in the abdomen should be described as to its size, location, contour, mobility, and tenderness, since without additional diagnostic studies it is impossible to state the point of origin as to stomach, pancreas, or colon, for example. Asking the patient to tense the abdominal muscles, to cough, or to strain aids in determining the presence of an abdominal hernia that may be classified as ventral, inguinal, femoral, or umbilical.

The examiner should begin with light palpation and proceed to deep palpation only if necessary. The hands should be warm to avoid tension of the abdominal muscles and to ensure adequate relaxation and comfort of the patient. Areas of tenderness or discomfort should be approached gradually. Place the entire palm and extended fingers on the abdomen and press the fingertips gently into the abdomen about 1 cm. Begin at the pubis and work upward to the costal margins with a smooth, gliding motion of the hand about 1 or 2 inches at a time. With deep palpation, the finger pads should move so that the abdominal wall will glide over the underlying structures backward and forward in a range of 4 or 5 cm. Rigidity of the abdominal muscles is produced by irritative lesions involving the peritoneum. This type of muscle spasm cannot be relaxed voluntarily. Two types of pain may be elicited by palpation.

Visceral	Arising from an organic lesion or functional disturbance within an abdominal viscus (for example, intestinal obstruction)
Somatic	Sharp and well localized, involving peritoneum or abdominal wall itself (for example, the localized right lower quadrant sharp pain of appendicitis)
Structures not normally palpable	Spleen, liver, gallbladder, and kidneys

Various techniques for detecting enlargement of specific organs and structures will be described.

Spleen. Stand at the patient's right side, placing the left hand over the patient's left costovertebral angle; work the right hand gently under the left posterior costal margin and press to move the spleen anteriorly as the patient is instructed to take a "deep breath and hold it." If the spleen is enlarged, it will be palpated as a firm mass against the fingers of the left hand. Normally the spleen is not palpable.

Liver. Gently work the fingertips of the right hand deep into the right upper quadrant. The patient is instructed to "take a deep breath and hold it" (Fig. 25-3). The normal liver may not be palpable. When felt as a firm edge against the fingers for more than 1 cm. below the costal margin, it is considered abnormal.

Kidneys. In a thin person the lower edge of the kidneys may be felt high in the flank by deep palpation.

Sigmoid colon. Deep palpation in the left lower

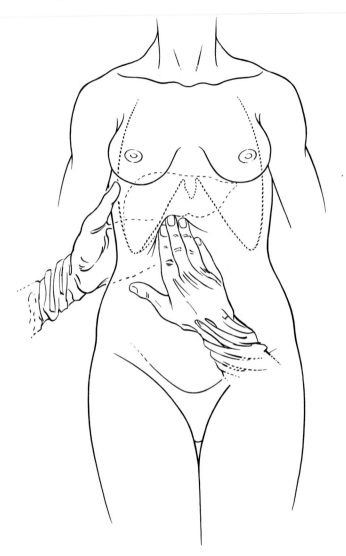

FIG. 25-3. Correct placement of hands for palpating the liver.

quadrant will reveal the sigmoid colon as a mass that is freely movable and frequently tender.

Aorta. The aorta is felt as a soft, pulsatile structure in the midepigastrium that extends toward the pelvis. Aneurysms are felt as pulsatile masses in the midportion of the abdomen.

Gallbladder. The gallbladder normally cannot be palpated. In a jaundiced patient the right upper quadrant will reveal a soft, cystic mass approximately 6 to 8 cm. in diameter on palpation.

■ DIAGNOSTIC EXAMINATIONS AND PROCEDURES

Barium enema. A series of radiographs taken after a barium enema has been given is used to demonstrate the presence of polyps, tumors, and other lesions of the large intestine and to reveal any abnormal anatomy or malfunction of the bowel. As the barium is instilled through a rectal tube, the radiologist, using a fluoroscope and television monitoring screen, observes its passage into the large intestine. The patient is asked to retain the barium while radiographs of the intestines are taken. He is then asked to expel the barium, and another film is taken to see if any pockets of barium are retained. This procedure is commonly referred to as a lower G.I. (gastrointestinal) series.

The preparation for a barium enema includes an explanation to the patient of the x-ray procedure, of the importance of retaining the barium during the examination, and of the need for the preparatory regimen. For the barium to clearly outline the lumen of the bowel, the bowel must be empty. This is best accomplished by giving enemas, laxatives, or rectal suppositories as ordered. Food and fluids are restricted for these x-ray examinations.

Barium that is retained in the bowel becomes hard and difficult to expel. To ensure complete evacuation of the barium from the intestinal tract after this procedure, the physician may order an oil retention enema or a laxative such as magnesium citrate. Since the patient is usually exhausted after a barium enema and the subsequent cleansing regimen, he should have rest. Petroleum jelly or, if ordered, a local analgesic ointment such as dibucaine (Nupercaine) may be applied to the anus to alleviate discomfort. If the patient is not too tired, a warm bath may also be soothing.

Gastrointestinal series. A gastrointestinal series consists of several radiographs of the stomach and intestinal tract and is used to detect tumors, ulcerations, or inflammation of the stomach and duodenum and to reveal any abnormal anatomy or malposition of these organs. As the patient swallows barium (a radiopaque substance), the radiologist makes a fluoroscopic examination, and then he takes radiographs of the stomach and the duodenum. Since the barium tastes like chalk, it is often flavored to make it more palatable. After the patient has drunk the barium, he is asked to assume various positions on the x-ray table, and the table may be tilted so that the barium will outline the stomach wall and flow by gravity into the intestinal loops as the radiologist, using the fluoroscope, watches the television monitor and takes the radiographs. Successive films are taken as the barium moves into the areas to be observed or into the large bowel, thus completing the visualization of the upper gastrointestinal tract, the ileum, or the small intestine. If the patient has a spastic duodenal bulb or increased peristalsis in the duodenal area, atropine may be administered prior to the radiograph to slow down the action of the small intestine, permitting better visualization of the area. This procedure is called hypotonic duodenography.

In preparation for a gastrointestinal series the nurse should explain the procedure to the patient and tell him that he must not take food or fluids for 6 to 8 hours before the examination. The presence of food in the stomach prevents the barium from outlining all of the stomach wall, and the radiographs will be inconclusive and misleading. If the patient eats, the radiographic examination should be postponed until the next day. The patient can be assured that the test will not cause discomfort and that he may eat as soon as the nurse is notified by the radiology department that the series is completed. However, breakfast will probably be omitted, and lunch may be delayed. After a gastrointestinal series, a cathartic may be ordered to speed the elimination of barium from the intestines. Retained barium may become hard and cause obstruction in the intestine or an impaction in the rectum.

Endoscopy

Esophagoscopy and gastroscopy. Esophagoscopy and gastroscopy are procedures performed to visualize the esophageal and gastric mucosa. By these means, a disease process may be located and inspected, and a specimen of tissue may be obtained for microscopic study.

The conventional gastroscope is a hollow, cylindric metal tube that permits visualization of the inner surface of the stomach mucosa except the fundus, the greater curvature, and the pylorus. The *fiberscope,* a type of gastroscope, has a shaft made of rubber or plastic that allows for greater flexibility and permits visualization of the greater curvature, the antrum, the pylorus, and the duodenal bulb. Glass fibers that are incorporated into the shaft of the instrument transmit light to the mucosa and the image back to the examiner. Cameras may be attached to either instrument for the purpose of taking pictures of abnormalities of the gastric mucosa during the examination. (See Fig. 25-4.)

Radiographs of the stomach and esophagus are taken prior to these examinations, since an obstruction of the esophagus might make passing an instrument dangerous. The physician will often use the radiographs to guide him in passing the gastroscope.

Although these procedures are not actually painful, patients find them extremely exhausting and uncomfortable. The nurse should explain the examination to the patient in simple terms, emphasizing that if he carefully follows the physician's instructions and remains quiet during the passing of the instrument, he can help make the procedure a short and successful one. Food and fluids are withheld for 6 to 8 hours before the examination so that the patient does not regurgitate as the tubular instrument is passed through the mouth into the esophagus and so that the lining of the stomach is visible. Occasionally an esophagoscopy or a gastroscopy must be performed as an emergency measure to remove a

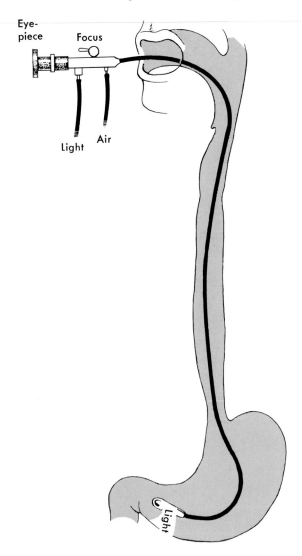

Eye-
piece　Focus

Light　Air

Light

FIG. 25-4. By means of a fiberscope the interior of the stomach may be visualized.

foreign object such as a bone or a pin. In such an emergency the stomach cannot be emptied, but suction should be available for use to prevent aspiration of regurgitated food or fluid. Eyeglasses and dentures should be removed to prevent their being broken. The patient should void before the examination to prevent discomfort or embarrassment. Pajama bottoms should be worn to prevent inadvertent exposure during the procedure. The patient's written permission is obtained before this examination is performed.

The patient is given sedatives ½ to 1 hour before the examination or at the time of the examination to lessen apprehension and to make him less aware of the passage of the instrument. The premedication also decreases the possibility of toxic effects from the local anesthetic. A narcotic such as meperidine hydrochloride (Demerol) and a barbiturate such as soluble phenobarbital are ordinarily used for seda-

tion. To decrease secretions, atropine sulfate may be administered. The patient should be observed carefully for possible reactions to these drugs, and he should be protected from injury while under their influence. Before the examination begins, the physician explains the procedure to the patient and tries to gain his full understanding and cooperation. During the procedure, both the physician and the nurse should reassure the patient and tell him what is happening. The patient is unable to speak and may be very frustrated by his inability to communicate. The patient's posterior pharynx is then sprayed with cocaine or tetracaine (Pontocaine) to inactivate the gag reflex and to lessen local reaction to the instrument. In order to prevent the aspiration of medication, the patient is asked to hold his breath while the posterior pharynx is sprayed and not to swallow saliva but to expectorate it into an emesis basin that is provided. The nurse should watch the patient for any toxic reactions to the anesthetic. An emergency tray containing intravenous barbiturates should be readily available. (See p. 207 for the toxic reactions to cocaine and tetracaine.) When the gag reflex has disappeared (usually within 5 to 10 minutes), the patient assumes a dorsal recumbent position on the treatment table for passage of the conventional gastroscope. For an esophageal examination his head and shoulders extend over the edge of the table, and for the passage of a gastroscope he lies on his side. The nurse supports the patient's head, and he is told again how important it is to remain perfectly still while the instrument is passed. Sudden movement at this time might cause the instrument to perforate the esophagus. Children and patients whose behavior is unpredictable should be firmly restrained if this procedure is attempted without the use of a general anesthetic. For passage of the fiberscope the patient sits or lies on the side of the bed or table facing the physician. If tissue is removed for pathologic examination, it should be placed immediately into a specimen bottle and correctly labeled.

When the examination is finished, the patient is instructed not to eat or drink until the gag reflex returns, lest fluid be aspirated into the lungs. The gag reflex usually returns in about 4 hours. In the hospital the physician or the nurse tests for the return of the gag reflex by gently tickling the back of the throat with a cotton swab or a tongue depressor. If the patient goes home, he should check by touching his throat with a swab or his finger before he attempts to eat or drink.

Following an esophagoscopy or a gastroscopy, the patient may be hoarse and complain of a sore throat. These symptoms should disappear within a few days. The patient should be so informed because he will not notice discomfort until the anesthesia wears off. Warm saline solution gargles may give some relief. These procedures are exhausting to the patient, and provision should be made for him to rest when they are completed.

Anoscopy, proctoscopy, and sigmoidoscopy. Anoscopy, proctoscopy, and sigmoidoscopy are procedures performed to visualize the mucosa of the anus, rectum, and sigmoid. Tumors, polyps, or ulcerations may be discovered, examined, and biopsied. An anoscopy is an examination of the anus; a proctoscopy is an examination of the anus and rectum; and a sigmoidoscopy is an examination of the anus, rectum, and sigmoid. Most often, a sigmoidoscopy is done, and this examination is routinely performed before rectal surgery and as part of the physical examination of patients who complain of chronic constipation or hemorrhoids or have any other symptoms of lower intestinal disease such as bleeding. Many physicians recommend that a sigmoidoscopy be included in the annual physical examination of men over 40 because of the relatively high incidence of cancer of the rectum and sigmoid in this age group.

The preparation for endoscopic examination of the bowel varies in different hospitals and clinics, but the patient should always receive an explanation of the procedure and of the preparation to be carried out. Usually he is instructed to eat a light evening meal prior to the examination. On the morning of the examination, enemas may be given until the return is clear, or a small hypertonic salt solution enema may be ordered. If the patient is suspected of having ulcerative colitis, the physician will probably not order a hypertonic enema, since it would cause inflammation of the mucosa and confuse the findings of the examination. Cathartic rectal suppositories such as bisacodyl (Dulcolax) are also used. If enemas are to be taken at home by the patient, the nurse should be certain that he knows how to carry out this procedure correctly and that he has suitable equipment. Visualization of the bowel mucosa is impossible unless all the fecal material is evacuated. Enema fluid should also be completely expelled before the examination is performed since it, too, will obstruct visualization. Cathartics are seldom used in preparation for this examination because they may cause downward flow of material from the upper bowel when the test is being performed. A light breakfast is usually permitted on the day of the scheduled test.

The nurse collects the necessary equipment for a sigmoidoscopy. Since the examination is upsetting to most patients, all possible preparations should be made before the patient is brought to the examining room to ensure a smooth-running and rapid procedure. The instrument must be checked to see that all the parts are functioning. The electric light bulb should be tested by attaching the instrument cord to the battery or to the electrical outlet. Besides the instrument, a draping sheet, gloves, lubricant, cotton swabs (12 inches in length), an emesis basin, toilet tissue, biopsy forceps, a suction machine with suction tip, and a paper bag for waste are required.

Before the examination begins, the physician again explains the procedure to the patient. It is preferable for the patient to assume a knee-chest position, and he is draped so that only the rectum is exposed. Because it may be difficult for an elderly or a very ill patient to assume or maintain a knee-chest position, a side-lying (Sims) position occasionally may be used. (For a complete description of these two positions, see p. 498.) The nurse should assist the patient in maintaining the correct position. He should be encouraged to remain still, to relax as much as possible, and to take deep breaths. He should also be watched carefully, lest he become faint. Since the lights are turned off during the examination, it is sometimes difficult to note the patient's color. If any doubt exists about his condition, his pulse rate should be taken.

The physician usually first examines the rectum with his gloved finger. He then inserts the lubricated instrument. After the instrument has been passed into the rectum, the solid, round-tipped inner portion (obturator) is removed. The intensity of light is then adjusted with the rheostat so that adequate light is reflected on the mucosa. If the sigmoidoscope is being used, the instrument is advanced slowly through the bowel for about 25 cm. (10 inches). The patient feels the instrument entering the rectum and sigmoid. This process may cause discomfort but should not cause real pain. Most patients are surprised that so little discomfort is associated with the procedure. Air is sometimes pumped into the bowel through the sigmoidoscope to distend the lumen of the bowel, thus permitting better visualization. The air may cause severe "gas pains." If small amounts of fluid or stool are still present in the bowel, they are removed with the cotton swabs and by suctioning. A proctoscopic procedure and maintenance of a knee-chest position usually tires the patient. As soon as the instrument has been removed and the excess lubricant removed from about the anus, he should be assisted to his bed and permitted to rest. The patient who is examined in the clinic is advised to rest for half an hour and should have some food or fluid before he leaves. This is particularly important for the elderly patient.

Other diagnostic tests

Gastric analysis (with histamine). Examination of the fasting contents of the stomach is helpful in establishing a diagnosis of gastric disease. For example, an unusual amount of gastric secretions containing food ingested the night before suggests pyloric obstruction. An absence of free hydrochloric acid in the stomach contents may indicate the presence of gastric malignancy or pernicious anemia, whereas an increased amount of free hydrochloric acid suggests a duodenal ulcer. In a gastric ulcer the amount of acid may be either decreased or normal in amount.

To obtain fasting stomach secretions, a nasogastric tube must be passed. The procedure must be explained to the patient, and food and fluids are withheld for 6 to 8 hours before the test is to be done. Anticholinergic drugs are omitted for 24 hours before the test. The nurse assembles the equipment needed for the procedure and at this time gives the patient any additional information about the test that he needs.

If the patient sits up with his head hyperextended, the tube is inserted more easily. This position can be accomplished by raising the head of the bed and arranging pillows under the shoulders, allowing the head to rest on the mattress. The head is then slightly flexed to a more normal position as the patient swallows the tube. The procedure may also be performed with the patient seated in a chair. The nurse should make sure that the chair supports the patient so that he does not become unsteady if he leans backward. As the physician reviews the procedure with the patient, the nurse may draw screens about his bed and cover his gown with a protective plastic sheet or disposable pad. He should be provided with an emesis basin and paper tissues. A nasogastric tube (Levin, no. 12, 14, or 16) is used. The tip of the tube may be lubricated with a water-soluble lubricant, and the physician inserts it through either nostril or through the mouth. Then he gently passes it into the posterior pharynx. The patient is asked to swallow hard and repeatedly, and he may be given sips of water as the physician quickly advances the tube into the stomach. A syringe is then fitted onto the end of the tube, and all the stomach contents are aspirated and placed into a specimen bottle. The physician may want to test the reactions of the aspirated secretions by using litmus paper. Blue litmus turns pink in the presence of acid. The tube is then secured to the nose and to the forehead with adhesive tape. Care should be taken that the tube does not pull or press against the nostril or cross in front of the eye. The end of the tube is closed with a clamp or with an elastic band to prevent leaking. Most patients are inclined to hold themselves very rigid while the tube is in the stomach, and they may be afraid to move. They are encouraged to assume any position that is most comfortable and instructed to expectorate saliva because it may act as a buffer and invalidate the examination.

After a fasting specimen has been collected, histamine phosphate, 0.25 to 0.5 mg. of a 1:1,000 solution, or betazole hydrochloride (Histalog) is given subcutaneously. Any patient receiving histamine should have his pulse and blood pressure taken immediately after administration. Normally the pulse is increased and the blood pressure is lowered slightly.[9] Betazole hydrochloride is usually preferred since it does not cause the side effects associated with histamine. When histamine is administered to a patient who has a peptic ulcer, there is a definite increase in the total output of gastric secretions and an increase in the amount of free hydrochloric acid in the stomach. If histamine is used, the patient should be told that he will look and feel flushed and warm and that he may develop a pounding headache. These symptoms are caused by the vasodilating effects of histamine and will subside fairly rapidly. If vasogenic shock occurs, the patient should be placed flat in bed and a vasoconstrictor drug such as 1:1,000 epinephrine (Adrenalin), 0.5 to 1 ml. subcutaneously, is usually administered. Vasogenic shock may also occur if the patient is given an accidental overdose of histamine. After the histamine injection has been given, the stomach contents are aspirated every 10 to 20 minutes until three or more specimens of gastric secretions have been obtained. The peak in hydrochloric acid secretion usually occurs about $\frac{1}{2}$ hour after the administration of histamine.

When the test is completed, the tube is clamped and quickly withdrawn. The nurse may be asked to perform this procedure. The patient should be given paper tissues because he usually has secretions in his eyes, nose, and throat. Mouth care should then be given, and if the hospitalized patient is not nauseated, breakfast may be served.

If the patient is not hospitalized, this test often is performed in the physician's office or in the clinic, and the nurse may do the entire procedure. The nurse must have an order to administer epinephrine should the patient have a reaction to histamine.

Tubeless gastric analysis. This procedure is thought to be useful as a screening technique for detection of gastric achlorhydria. The test will indicate the presence or absence of free hydrochloric acid but cannot be used to determine the *amount* of free hydrochloric acid if it is present. Quantitative determinations must be done through aspiration of stomach contents.

For a tubeless gastric analysis, a gastric stimulant such as caffeine or histamine phosphate is given to the patient. One hour later he is given 2 Gm. (30 grains) of a cation exchange resin containing 90 mg. (1½ grains) of azure A (Azuresin, Diagnex Blue) with 240 ml. of water orally on an empty stomach. If there is free hydrochloric acid in the stomach, on the introduction of this resin a substance will be released in the stomach that will be absorbed from the small intestine and excreted by the kidneys within 2 hours. Absence of detectable amounts of dye in the urine indicates that free hydrochloric acid probably was not secreted.

Insulin tolerance test. An insulin tolerance test is another test used to evaluate the secreting action of the gastric mucosa. The test is carried out in the same way as a gastric analysis, except that instead of histamine a specified amount of regular insulin is administered intravenously. The drop in blood sugar produced by the insulin stimulates the vagus nerve, and the flow of gastric secretions may be increased. A normal stomach responds only slightly to stimulation of the vagus nerve, and there will be no significant increase in the gastric secretions. In the patient with a peptic ulcer, however, there will be a marked increase in the total gastric output and in the amount of free hydrochloric acid. The insulin tolerance test may be used to determine the success of a resection of the vagus nerve in decreasing the hyperactivity of the stomach. It is therefore often performed before and after a vagotomy. In the event that symptoms of insulin reaction appear, orange or other fruit juice should be available as well as 50% glucose for intravenous injection.

Exfoliative cytology. Exfoliative cytology is the study of the individual cell or clumps of cells to identify or to exclude the presence of malignancy. Because malignant cells tend to exfoliate (separate from the tumor), methods of accelerating exfoliation are used by passing a Levin tube and lavaging the stomach vigorously with quantities of saline solution or by passing stomach tubes to which gastric brushes or abrasive balloons are attached to collect fragments of mucosa. Chymotrypsin may be administered to digest the overlying protective coat of mucus and thereby expose the mucosa to the irrigating solution or abrasive collecting agent. All the aspirated irrigating solution, cells, and bits of tissue obtained are sent to the laboratory for study.

Peroral small bowel biopsy. Biopsy of the mucosa and of lesions of the small intestines is possible through the passage of a biopsy capsule. The capsule consists of inner and outer shells that are attached to the distal end of a Miller-Abbott tube or to special tubes constructed for this purpose. The inner shell encloses a cylindric cavity that contains a blade. The biopsy opening is located in the distal end of the capsule (Fig. 25-5). The tube with the capsule is passed as previously described, and by swallowing and peristaltic activity it reaches the biopsy site as established by fluoroscopy. At this point the biopsy port is opened and the blade is operated by hydrostatic pressure and vacuum created by syringes attached to the double lumen openings at the other end of the tube. The specimen is guillotined off and collected in the capsule. After the tube is removed, the tissue is sent to the laboratory for study.

Stool examination. Gross, microscopic, chemical, and bacterial examinations of the stool supply information that is helpful in establishing a diagnosis of gastrointestinal disease. Stools that are abnormal in color, odor, amount, consistency, and number are significant. Abnormal stools should be accurately described and a specimen saved for examination by the physician. The physician may order further laboratory studies to be performed. Stool examinations are required for the complete evaluation of all patients with gastrointestinal complaints.

The nurse is responsible for seeing that specimens are collected. If the patient is ambulatory, he may be given a specimen box and spatula and instructed in obtaining a specimen. Otherwise the specimen should be collected by the nursing personnel. The nurse should be familiar with and also inform auxiliary staff of any special techniques that are required to preserve stools for special examinations. For example a specimen to be examined for amebae must be kept warm and taken immediately to the laboratory for examination. It can be kept warm by placing the specimen box in a pan of warm water or on a hot-water bottle. If an enema must be given to collect a stool specimen, it is important that plain tap water or normal saline solution be used, since soaps or hypertonic solutions may change the consistency of the stool and alter any abnormal contents. If the stool is to be examined for occult (hid-

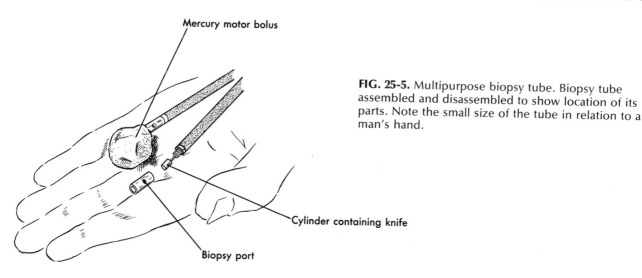

FIG. 25-5. Multipurpose biopsy tube. Biopsy tube assembled and disassembled to show location of its parts. Note the small size of the tube in relation to a man's hand.

Mercury motor bolus

Cylinder containing knife

Biopsy port

den) blood, red meat is eliminated from the diet for 24 hours before the specimen is collected. The reason for this should be explained to the patient.

■ GASTRIC AND INTESTINAL DECOMPRESSION

Decompression of the stomach. Decompression, or removal of flatus, fluids, and other contents, from the stomach, usually is accomplished by attaching a suction apparatus to a nasogastric tube. It may be used to prevent and to treat postoperative vomiting and distention caused by the lessening of peristalsis following anesthesia, by manipulation of the viscera during surgery, or by obstruction from edema at the site of operation. In pyloric obstruction it is used to relieve dilation of the stomach, and in gastric hemorrhage it may be used so that the blood loss can be accurately measured and replaced. When a nasogastric tube is to be used to keep the stomach deflated postoperatively, it usually is inserted before surgery, since it is easier to pass at that time. (Passage of the nasogastric tube is described on p. 654.)

The length of time that the tube remains in the stomach depends on the reason for its use and the physician's opinion of the physiologic effects of intubation on electrolyte balance and the psychologic effects on the patient. It may be left until normal peristalsis returns postoperatively (from 48 to 72 hours). It may be removed soon after surgery and reinserted only if distention or vomiting occurs, or it may be removed and reinserted once or twice a day to aspirate stomach contents. When the nasogastric tube is used in the treatment of pyloric or intestinal obstruction, it usually is left in place until the obstruction is relieved. The tube used in conjunction with gastric or esophageal surgery is carefully placed by the surgeon during the operation so that it does not intrude on the suture line. The nurse should never manipulate this tube, lest injury be caused. If there is some question about the tube's position or function, the surgeon should be consulted. If the tube is inadvertently removed or pulled out by the patient, the physician may decide not to reinsert it because of the danger of perforating or otherwise injuring the anastomosis.

The need for continuous intubation should be explained to both the patient and his family. If the purpose of the tube is not fully understood, its use may cause apprehension and fear. Acceptance by the patient usually facilitates passage of the tube, and there is less possibility that he will pull it out. The presence of the tube in the nasopharynx soon causes local discomfort, and the patient may complain of a lump in his throat, difficulty in swallowing, a sore throat, hoarseness, earache, or irritation of the nostril. He may also expectorate and wish to blow his nose often because the irritation of the tube causes an increase in mucous secretions. Many patients report that discomfort from the tube far exceeds that from the incision. To lessen this discomfort, the tube should be secured so that there is no pressure against the nostril. Excess secretions from around the nares should be removed, and a water-soluble lubricant such as K-Y jelly should be applied to the tube and to the nostril to prevent crusting of secretions. When the tube is in the nostril, the patient tends to breathe through his mouth, and his lips and tongue may become dry and cracked. Frequent mouth rinses and the application of petroleum jelly or cold cream to the lips help prevent dryness. Fluids usually are restricted, but the patient may be permitted to chew gum to increase salivation or to suck small pieces of ice. Warm saline solution gargles may relieve dryness and soreness of the throat, and the physician may order throat lozenges. He also may spray the throat with a local anesthetic such as tetracaine. Phenylephrine (Neo-Synephrine), 0.25%, nose drops are sometimes helpful in relieving nasal stuffiness. Frequent changing of the patient's position helps to relieve pressure from the tube on any one area in the throat. The patient often is inclined to be tense and fearful. The nurse should assist him with turning and physical care, showing him how much activity is possible without displacing the tube. If the patient finds the presence of the tube particularly uncomfortable, the nurse should consult the physician about ordering a sedative or tranquilizer. Unless contraindicated, all patients who have a nasogastric tube should have the head of their bed elevated 30 degrees to prevent esophageal reflux and subsequent esophagitis.

Nasogastric tubes usually are attached to suction to ensure drainage, since the stomach contents must flow against gravity. The nurse should understand how the suction apparatus functions. Before the tube is attached, the nurse checks the suction apparatus to be sure that it is working properly. Various types of apparatus may be used. Regardless of the type, if, after it has been assembled and turned on, it will draw up water from a container, it can be assumed that it is working properly. The tubing from the suction apparatus is then attached by a connecting tube to the nasogastric tube, permitting observation of the fluid being removed from the stomach. A clamp, pin, or adhesive sling should be used to support the weight of the additional drainage tubing so that tension is not placed on the nasogastric tube. Sufficient tubing should be attached so that the patient can turn freely, and the device used to secure the tubing to the bed should be placed so as not to obstruct the drainage or inhibit the patient's movement.

Mechanical failure of the suction apparatus or blockage of the drainage tubing or of the nasogastric tube itself may stop the suction, impeding drainage and causing distention, discomfort, and sometimes vomiting. The apparatus should be checked frequently to minimize this possibility. The physician may wish the tube irrigated with small amounts (30 ml.) of normal saline solution at specified intervals to keep the lumen of the tube open and free from plugs of mucus or clots of blood. After the fluid is inserted into the tube, it should be aspirated, if possible. The amount of fluid inserted and withdrawn from the tube should be recorded accurately. Fluid that is instilled but not immediately withdrawn will be removed by suction, and if the irrigating fluid is not taken into consideration, the measurement of the total gastric drainage will be inaccurate. If the fluid does not flow easily into the tube or if it does not return at irrigation, the physician should be consulted.

When continuous gastric suction is used, the gastric secretions collected in the drainage bottle should be measured every 24 hours, since the total amount of fluid and the electrolytes lost through drainage must be replaced by parenteral routes. It is the responsibility of the nurse to see that the drainage is collected and measured and that there is a record of all fluid intake and output.

Decompression of the stomach may also be accomplished by attaching a *gastrostomy tube* that is in place in the stomach to suction. Decompression by this method is used when gastric or intestinal distention is anticipated following extensive operations such as radical resection and obstructing carcinoma of the colon and total colectomy for ulcerative colitis. Some surgeons use a gastrostomy tube after limited gastric resection combined with vagotomy. The tube is inserted through the abdominal incision into the stomach at the time of surgery, and suction is maintained postoperatively until the hazard of paralytic ileus is over. The patient is much more comfortable than with nasogastric suction, especially if the need

for suction is prolonged, and there also is less danger of respiratory complications. Irrigation of the tube, care of the suction apparatus, and measuring and recording of the drainage are carried out as described previously.

Decompression of the intestinal tract. Decompression, or deflation, of the intestinal tract is accomplished by attaching a tube passed by way of the nose or mouth into the intestine to the suction apparatus. This procedure is used to drain fluids and gas that accumulate above the mechanical intestinal obstruction, to deflate the intestines during paralytic ileus, and to deflate the bowel before or after intestinal surgery.

The tubes most often used for intestinal decompression are the Miller-Abbot tube and the Cantor tube. The length of these tubes permits their passage through the entire intestinal tract. There is a small balloon on the tip of each, which, when inflated with air or injected with water or mercury, acts like a bolus of food. This balloon stimulates peristalsis, which advances it along the intestinal tract. If peristalsis is absent, the weight of the mercury in the balloon will usually carry it forward. When a Miller-Abbott tube is used, the mercury is inserted into the balloon of the tube after the tube is passed.

The choice of tube depends on the physician's preference. The Miller-Abbott tube is a double-lumen tube. One lumen leads to the balloon and the other to the "eyes" along its course, permitting drainage of intestinal contents and irrigation. The external end of the tube contains a metal adapter with two openings—one for drainage of secretions and the other for inflating the balloon. (See Fig. 25-6.) In irrigating this tube, the nurse must be careful that the correct opening is used—the one marked "suction." The other opening is for inflating or deflating the bal-

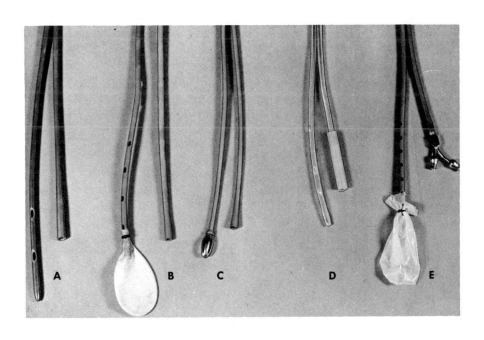

FIG. 25-6. The tips and the ends to be attached to suction for the various types of tubes used for gastrointestinal intubation. **A,** Rubber nasogastric tube. **B,** Cantor tube. **C,** Rehfuss tube for duodenal drainage. **D,** Plastic nasogastric tube. **E,** Miller-Abbott tube.

loon. It should be clamped off and labeled "do not touch."

The Cantor tube is a single tube with only one opening, which is used for drainage. Before the tube is inserted, the balloon is injected with mercury with a needle and syringe. The needle opening is so small that the globules of mercury cannot escape through it. The mercury can be pushed about so that the balloon is elongated for easy insertion.

Another intestinal tube, the Harris tube, is a single tube also and similar to the Cantor tube except that there is a metal tip on the end of the tube, which is followed by the small bag containing the mercury. Other modifications of intestinal tubes may be used (p. 227).

Intestinal tubes are passed in the manner described under gastric analysis. The addition of the balloon on the tip of the tube makes its insertion through the nose doubly difficult for the patient. The tube can be mechanically inserted only into the stomach. Its passage along the remainder of the gastrointestinal tract is dependent on gravity and peristalsis. The weight of the mercury in the balloon helps propel the tube through the intestines. After the tube reaches the stomach, its passage through the pylorus and into the duodenum can be facilitated in many ways. Position and activity aid in its passage. After passage of the tube, the patient is usually encouraged to lie on his right side for 2 hours, on his back in a Fowler's position for 2 hours, and then on his left side for 2 hours. Passage of the tube through the pylorus is usually ascertained by radiographic or fluoroscopic examination. After the tube has passed the pylorus, the patient may be encouraged to walk about to increase peristalsis and to speed the advancement of the tube through the intestines with the help of gravity. During this time the physician or the nurse advances the tube 7 to 10 cm. (3 to 4 inches) through the nose or mouth at specified intervals. The intestinal tube should not be secured to the face until it has reached the desired point in the intestines, since taping the tube will prevent it from advancing with peristalsis. The pull of the mercury on the end of the tube may move the bowel along with the tube and cause telescoping of the bowel. This results in intussusception, which is a serious complication. The tube should be monitored carefully by radiographic examination at least once daily to assure that coiling of the tube or telescoping of the bowel has not occurred. Extra tubing should be coiled on the bed or, if the patient is up, pinned to his clothing.

Decompression is accomplished by attaching a suction apparatus to the tube either as the tube advances or after it has reached the obstructed portion of the bowel. Drainage should be measured every 24 hours, and the fluid and electrolytes lost are replaced by the parenteral routes. If the tip of the tube is far down in the intestine and if the patient is not nauseated or vomiting, he may be permitted light foods such as clear or cream soups, custards, gelatins, milk, or fruit juice, all of which can be absorbed in the upper part of the small intestine. The physician may wish the tube irrigated at intervals with normal saline solution or tap water to check its patency. Because the fluid has a longer distance to travel than in a nasogastric tube, it is difficult to aspirate the solution used. The nurse should record the amount instilled into the tube. If no return flow can be obtained, only a small amount of solution should be used. If she is able to aspirate the fluid, this also should be recorded.

The intestinal tube is usually left in the intestine longer than the nasogastric tube remains in the stomach. It is often left in for from 4 to 6 days after intestinal surgery, depending on the amount of edema around the anastomosis and the return of peristalsis. In most cases of intestinal obstruction, the tube must be left in for 7 to 10 days, but the amount of time in which the tube remains depends on the disease and the patient's response to treatment. Nasal and pharyngeal discomfort usually is pronounced, and the nursing measures described under gastric intubation should be employed. Signs of the return of peristalsis and of the reduction of edema at the operative site, such as the passage of gas rectally or a spontaneous bowel movement, should be reported to the physician since they usually indicate that the tube is no longer needed.

The intestinal tube is always removed gradually, several centimeters at a time. Some resistance may be felt as it is withdrawn because of the pull against peristalsis. The patient may feel a tugging sensation and become nauseated. When the tip of the tube reaches the posterior nasopharynx, it may be brought out through the mouth so that the balloon and mercury can be removed. The tube is then pulled through the nose. Since the tube usually has a fecal odor and may cause nausea, the tubing should be removed from sight at once and the patient should be given oral care as soon as it is removed. For several days after removal of an intestinal tube, the patient's throat may be sore and he may be hoarse. Gargles and lozenges can be continued until these symptoms subside.

Occasionally the balloon of an intestinal tube may extrude from the anus. If this occurs, the upper end of the tube is usually cut off and the tube is disconnected from suction and removed through the rectum. Removal is usually done slowly and with the help of peristaltic action.

Diseases of the upper gastrointestinal system

The following discussion considers the more common diseases of the upper gastrointestinal system as well as specific treatment and related management.

■ ESOPHAGEAL DISORDERS

Achalasia (cardiospasm, aperistalsis)

Achalasia is a condition in which there is an absence of peristalsis in the esophagus, and the esophageal sphincter fails to relax following deglutition (swallowing). The cause is unknown, but the disorder is a direct result of disruption of the normal neuromuscular mechanism of the esophagus. Anxiety and tension seem to aggravate the symptoms and bring on exacerbations. The disease is most common in middle life, and is the most common cause of dysphagia in women. Because the condition is found in older persons, cancer of the lower end of the esophagus must be ruled out by esophagoscopy.

In the early phases of achalasia there is no gross lesion, but as the disease persists, the portion of the esophagus about the constriction dilates, and the muscular walls become hypertrophied. The dilated area becomes atonic, and esophageal peristalsis may be absent so that little or no food can enter the stomach. While varying degrees of the condition exist, in extreme cases the esophagus above the constriction may hold a liter or more of fluid.

The patient may first complain of substernal fullness following the hasty ingestion of bulky or cold foods. He may have to make a determined, conscious effort to pass food beyond the constricted area. He may even have difficulty swallowing liquids. In time there is frank dysphagia with or without malnutrition. The patient loses weight and may suffer from avitaminosis. He may also complain of chest pain similar to that of angina pectoris. As the condition progresses, there is regurgitation rather than vomiting of esophageal contents onto the pillow or into the larynx when the patient is asleep. The diagnosis is confirmed by radiographs taken as the patient swallows barium and by esophagoscopy.

If the constriction is not severe, the patient usually is advised to eat a bland diet, avoiding bulky foods. Meals should be eaten slowly, and drinking fluids with meals helps the food to pass through the narrowed opening. Frequent changes of position during eating may also help. The patient should sleep with his head elevated to avoid the possibility of aspiration of esophageal residue.

If the patient cannot pass food beyond the constriction, forceful dilation of the narrowed opening with the specific purpose of tearing some of the muscle fibers in the area may be done. This procedure is accomplished by passing graduated mercury-tipped bougies, passing tubes with bags attached that can be inflated under pressure, or passing a mechanical (Starck) dilator. The generally accepted surgical procedure is a cardiomyotomy. The muscular layer is incised longitudinally down to, but not through, the mucosa. The incision is so done that two thirds of its length is in the esophagus and the remaining one-third is in the stomach. This permits the mucosa to expand so that food can pass more easily into the stomach.

Postoperatively the nursing care is the same as the routine care given any patient who has had chest surgery. A rare complication is accidental perforation of the esophageal mucosa so that leakage may contaminate the mediastinum. Regurgitation occasionally occurs after surgery but can usually be controlled by the administration of antacid medications. Since overflow may still occur at night, the patient is advised to refrain from food or fluid for several hours before retiring.

Esophageal diverticulum

An esophageal diverticulum is the bulging of the esophageal mucosa and submucosa through a weakened portion of the muscular layer of the esophagus. It is most often located at the pharyngoesophageal junction, in the lower end of the thoracic esophagus, or just above the diaphragm (epiphrenic diverticulum). As food is ingested, some of it may pass into the diverticulum. After a sufficient amount has accumulated in the pocket, it overflows into the esophagus and is regurgitated. There is always danger that some of the regurgitated material may be aspirated into the trachea and lungs during sleep or that the diverticulum may enlarge and cause esophageal obstruction.

The patient may complain of pain on swallowing, of gurgling noises in the area, and of a cough due to tracheal irritation. His breath usually has a foul odor caused by decomposition of food in the diverticulum. The odor can be alleviated somewhat by frequent brushing of the teeth and the use of aromatic mouthwashes.

If the symptoms become severe, surgery is performed. The herniated sac is excised, and the resultant esophageal opening is closed. These procedures are well tolerated, and the administration of antibiotics makes postoperative infections rare. If a supraclavicular approach has been used, fluids are usually permitted as soon as nausea subsides, and a bland diet is prescribed soon afterward. If a transthoracic approach is utilized, chest drainage may be used, and the patient usually is allowed nothing by mouth for several days.

Stricture of the esophagus

The deliberate or accidental swallowing of caustic materials such as lye may cause serious strictures in the esophagus as the mucosa heals. Unfortunately many of the patients are small children, and they may suffer from the effects of such an accident for the remainder of their lives. Although the patient may be able to swallow fluid for a while after the accident, strictures develop as healing occurs, and sometimes no food can pass into the stomach. Careful attempts are made to dilate the stricture by passing bougies. Usually this is done under the fluoroscope so that danger of causing damage that would result in further stricture formation is lessened. If the destruction of the esophageal mucosa is extensive, a *gastrostomy* (permanent opening into the stomach) may be performed. Care of the patient with a gastrostomy is discussed later in this chapter. Braided silk thread is then inserted through the mouth and esophagus into the stomach and brought out through the gastrostomy opening. The two ends of the thread are tied together to form a complete loop, and the thread is used for pulling bougies or beads tied to it through the esophagus to dilate it and to prevent complete closure of the lumen. Such treatment may be necessary for months or years after the ingesting of a caustic substance. If a satisfactory esophageal lumen cannot be maintained, surgery may be performed. The stricture may be resected or bypassed with a segment of jejunum or colon.

Tumors

Carcinoma is the most common condition causing obstruction of the esophagus and accounts for about 2% of all cancer deaths in the United States and in the United Kingdom.[8] The tumor may develop in any portion of the esophagus, but it is most common in the middle and lower thirds.

The only possible hope for successful treatment lies in very early diagnosis and surgical treatment. The nurse should urge any patient who has difficulty in swallowing, no matter how trivial it may seem, to seek medical advice at once. This applies particularly to persons over 40 years of age since cancer of the esophagus occurs more often in middle and later life than at younger ages.

The patient who has cancer of the esophagus initially complains only of mild and intermittent dysphagia. Gradually he finds it extremely difficult to swallow solid food, and by the time he seeks medical attention he often has resorted to strained foods and liquids. He may regurgitate after eating and has gradual weight loss. Pain in the back may indicate that the growth has extended into surrounding structures. Unfortunately, even if the patient reports to a physician when the first symptoms appear, the disease is often already well established, has metastasized, and is incurable. Diagnosis is made by radio-graphs of the esophagus taken as the patient swallows barium (Fig. 25-7) or by examination of tumor cells obtained during esophagoscopy.

Treatment for cancer of the esophagus is surgical. If obvious metastasis is present or if the patient's physical condition is poor, only palliative surgery may be attempted. If major surgery is performed, the type of surgery depends on the site of the lesion. Upper thoracic lesions are resected through a right thoracotomy or thoracic abdominal incision. An *esophagogastrostomy* may be performed or a segment of colon may be anastomosed to the resected areas of the esophagus and stomach. Lower esophageal lesions are removed through a left thoracotomy or thoracic abdominal incision. The operation includes an *esophagogastrectomy,* splenectomy, and wide resection of lymph nodes. A major portion of the acid-secreting portion of the stomach is removed to reduce the occurrence of reflux esophagitis.

If the patient cannot tolerate major surgery, or if the lesion is inoperable, a *gastrostomy* may be performed. This procedure is usually done under local anesthesia. An opening is made into the stomach through a small upper left abdominal incision. The

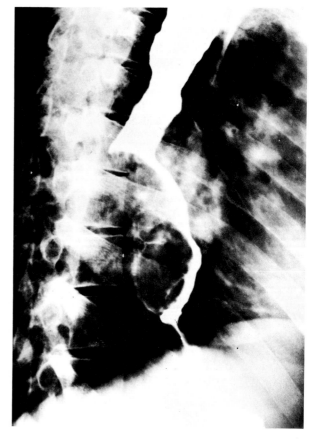

FIG. 25-7. This radiograph, taken after the patient had swallowed barium, shows the location of a lesion in the esophagus as it approaches the stomach.

anterior wall of the stomach is exposed, drawn forward, and sutured to the anterior abdominal wall about the incision, thus preventing the stomach contents from entering the abdominal cavity. A small incision is then made into the stomach, and a catheter, tube, or special prosthesis is inserted into it (Fig. 25-8). A Foley or mushroom catheter is often used. The opening is sutured tightly around the catheter so that leakage of stomach contents cannot occur. Food can then be introduced directly into the stomach. Instead of a catheter, a special prosthesis (Barnes-Redo) may be used. Radiation therapy is sometimes used to inhibit growth of tumor cells.

Management of the patient requiring an esophagectomy or an esophagogastrostomy

Preoperative care. Because the nutritional status of most patients with esophageal cancer is poor, an attempt is made preoperatively to improve nutrition and to reestablish fluid and electrolyte balance. Glucose, amino acids, electrolytes, and vitamins usually are prescribed to be administered intravenously. An accurate record of the intake and output should be kept since this information is important in ordering fluids to be administered parenterally. If food and fluids can be taken orally, they should be high in protein and in total calories. Occasionally a temporary gastrostomy may be performed to supply food preoperatively. It is closed a few weeks after the esophageal resection if this operation has been successful in reestablishing a communication between the esophagus and the stomach.

The patient with esophageal cancer requires special skin care to prevent decubiti. Protection of bony prominences, frequent massage of dependent parts of the body, and frequent changes of position are necessary. Because of weakness, malaise, and depression, the patient may forget to change position as often as necessary unless he is reminded to do so.

Since the breath may be foul, special oral care should be given. The patient may raise a mixture of pus, blood, and decomposed food. He must be assured privacy when he is attempting to clear his throat and particularly when he is attempting to get food and fluids past the obstruction. The emesis basins should be changed often, and a cover should be provided. Mouthwashes are useful in making the mouth feel fresher and should be offered to the patient before he attempts to take food. They should be varied from time to time unless the patient has one he prefers, because sometimes the flavor of the solution becomes identified with the unpleasant throat secretions and becomes almost as distasteful as the secretions.

Preoperative teaching should include instructions for the patient about chest drainage, coughing and turning after the operation, postoperative exercises, restriction of oral fluids, oxygen, frequent observation of pulse and blood pressure, intravenous injections, and the nasogastric tube. This teaching is described in detail in the chapters concerned with preoperative care of the general surgical patient and the patient undergoing chest surgery (pp. 196 and 585). The nasogastric tube is usually inserted immediately preoperatively if the esophagus is not completely obstructed.

Postoperative care. The immediate postoperative care for the patient who has had esophageal surgery centers about the maintenance of an airway, obser-

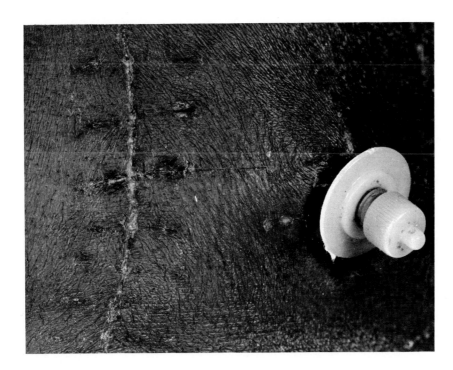

FIG. 25-8. The Barnes-Redo prosthesis is sutured into the gastrostomy opening. The cap can be unscrewed easily for tube feedings. (Courtesy Dr. William Barnes and Dr. Frank Redo, The New York Hospital–Cornell Medical Center, New York, N. Y.)

vation for circulatory or respiratory difficulties, protection from injury, care of the chest drainage system, and care of the nasogastric tube (as described earlier in this chapter).

Small amounts of bright red blood may drain from the nasogastric tube for a short time (6 to 12 hours). The color of the drainage should then become greenish yellow. Because esophageal tissue is very friable and because the anastomosis may be under tension, the tube is usually left in until complete healing of the esophageal anastomosis has occurred. If the tube is removed, oral fluids are not permitted for several days. Fluids are given parenterally to meet fluid, electrolyte, and caloric needs. When fluids are permitted orally, a small amount of water (30 to 60 ml.) is given hourly, and the patient is observed for such signs of leakage of fluid into the mediastinum as pain, a rise in temperature, and difficulty in breathing. If no untoward symptoms occur, foods are introduced and gradually increased until the patient is receiving several small meals of bland food daily. If the stomach has been brought up into the chest cavity (esophagogastrostomy), the patient may complain of a feeling of fullness in the chest or difficulty in breathing after eating. Serving smaller meals more frequently may help to relieve these problems.

When the cardia of the stomach has been removed, some patients complain of nausea and vomiting. This difficulty is usually caused by irritation of the esophageal mucosa by the gastric juices. After an esophagogastrectomy (resection of the lower esophagus and the cardia of stomach), the gastric secretions can readily flow into the esophagus when the patient lies flat. He should be advised to rest his head and shoulders on pillows when he lies down.

Resumption of activity must be gradual. Because surgery for cancer of the esophagus is extensive, the patient may require several months of convalescence. In addition, since the malignant lesion is seldom completely removed, only a small percentage of patients live more than 5 years after the operation, and many are chronic invalids during that time. The physician usually informs the family of the patient's prognosis, and sometimes the patient is also told. Both the patient and his family should be told of the need for close medical supervision. Upper respiratory infections should be carefully avoided, and medical help should be sought at once if signs of even minor indisposition occur.

Many patients with cancer of the esophagus receive terminal care at home and are cared for by a public health nurse and by members of the family under the nurse's supervision. The patient and his family should always be asked if they would like to have a nurse visit the patient in his home. Occasionally the nurse also helps the family to prepare for the patient's return home. The nurse who goes into the home can often give helpful suggestions regarding the preparation of suitable food, care of the mouth, rest, and prevention of accidents. (See p. 304 for care of the terminally ill cancer patient and p. 255 for description of home care programs.)

Some patients with cancer of the esophagus are not found to be suitable candidates for esophageal surgery. Their skin care, mouth care, and nutrition are similar to that described for the patient being prepared for esophageal surgery; sometimes a gastrostomy is done as a palliative procedure.

Management of the patient requiring a gastrostomy

It is usually very difficult for the patient to accept the need for gastrostomy—probably partly because of the deep psychologic significance of food and eating. After a long period of vomiting, discomfort, and inability to eat, however, the patient may become so debilitated that both he and his family are willing for the surgery to be performed.

After a gastrostomy the catheter is secured to the abdominal wall by a suture or adhesive tape to prevent its slipping out. A clamp is applied to the end of the catheter to prevent leakage of gastric secretions onto the skin. A small dressing covers the incision, and there should be very little bloody drainage postoperatively.

The skin around the gastrostomy should be inspected frequently, because if there is leakage of gastric secretions around the tube, the skin will become irritated and excoriated from the action of the digestive enzymes. The skin should be kept clean with frequent use of soap and water and should be kept dry; a protective ointment such as zinc oxide and a dressing of oiled silk and gauze may be applied around the tube (Fig. 20-18). After about 10 days to 2 weeks the tube may be removed and reinserted only when food is given. The patient is taught to perform this procedure himself. The tube is kept clean by washing it with soap and water after each meal. It is inserted 10 to 15 cm. (4 to 6 inches). A catheter plug or rubber-tipped hemostat may be used to close the catheter and prevent leakage from the gastrostomy tube between meals. There is less likelihood of leakage if the patient relaxes for a short time after the meal and if the meals are not too large.

When the Barnes-Redo prosthesis is used, the problems of feeding and skin care are somewhat simpler. The prosthesis consists of a cap that unscrews, an external and internal flange, and a nylon shaft that is 4 to 6 cm. (1.6 to 2.5 inches) long. When foods are to be introduced, the cap is unscrewed and an 18 Fr. whistle-tip catheter is inserted into the shaft of the prosthesis as far as it will go. After the feeding is completed, the cap is replaced. Drainage is minimal, and skin care consists of keeping the area between the skin and the flange clean and dry. The prosthesis protrudes somewhat from the abdomen, but is not noticeable under loose clothing (Fig. 25-8).

Soon after the operation, fluid nourishment may be given through the catheter. The initial meal, consisting of a small amount of tap water or glucose in water, is usually given by the surgeon. Fluids are given every 4 hours at first. If there is no leakage of fluid around the tube and if the patient appears to tolerate the clear fluids, foods blended into a mixture may be added until a full diet is eventually given through the tube. The meal should be warmed to room or body temperature before it is given, and it should be diluted if it is too thick. It should be given with screens drawn about the patient for privacy if he does not occupy a single room. A funnel or glass syringe is used to introduce the liquid into the catheter. Before the meal is given, a small amount of water should be introduced through the tube to make sure it is patent. In order to prevent air from entering the stomach, the catheter should not be unplugged until the nurse is ready to give the feeding. The fluid should flow in by gravity. Sometimes a small amount of pressure from the bulb of the Asepto syringe on the barrel of the glass syringe is necessary to pass thicker fluids through the tube. The usual amount of each meal is 200 to 500 ml. and should take 10 to 15 minutes to flow through the tube. If the patient feels "full" or nauseated, meals may be decreased in amount and their frequency increased. A small amount of water is instilled to cleanse the tube at the end of the meal. In order to aid digestion the head of the bed should be elevated for at least $\frac{1}{2}$ hour following a feeding.

The meals may be a special formula or regular food blended so that it will pass through the tube. The use of regular foods helps maintain the patient's nutritional state, prevents diarrhea that often accompanies the use of specially prepared tube feedings that are high in fat, and makes it easier for the patient and his family to prepare his food at home. Food that is normally cooked should be cooked until it is soft, and the juices from cooking should be included since they contain essential vitamins and minerals. Solid and liquid foods are blended into a mixture with a food blender, fork, potato masher, or egg beater and are strained. Water should be given through the tube between feedings so that approximately 2,500 to 3,500 ml. of fluids are received daily. If diarrhea occurs, camphorated tincture of opium (paregoric) may be ordered and given with the meal.

The patient should see, smell, taste, and chew small amounts of food before taking his feeding, in order to stimulate the flow of gastric secretions and give him some of the satisfaction of normal eating. It is sometimes recommended that the patient chew his food normally and then deposit it into a funnel attached to the gastrostomy tube. If he can accept this sensible although somewhat unesthetic procedure, it is unquestionably beneficial because saliva

is mixed with the food. The teeth and mouth also maintain better health. Privacy must, of course, be assured the patient who takes his meals in this way.

If the patient is not upset by sitting down to meals with his family when he cannot eat, he should be encouraged to do so since this socializing usually helps his digestion and is good for his morale.

The psychologic trauma of not being able to eat normally is usually severe. The patient may become depressed, and he needs a great deal of encouragement. Most patients, however, as they become proficient in feeding themselves, gradually accept this method of obtaining nourishment as inevitable and adjust remarkably well.

Both the patient and his family should learn how to care for the skin and the tube and how to prepare the liquid meals as well as how to insert the tube and instill the nourishment through it. They should be told of the need for close medical supervision, and they should be encouraged to consult the physician, the nurse, or the dietitian when problems arise. It may be desirable for a public health nurse to visit the patient at home to supervise the initial preparation of food and giving of the feeding and to answer any other questions in regard to the patient's care.

■ HIATUS HERNIA (ESOPHAGEAL OR DIAPHRAGMATIC HERNIA)

There are three variations of hiatus hernia, but the *sliding hiatus hernia* is by far the most common and is now known to be one of the most common patho-

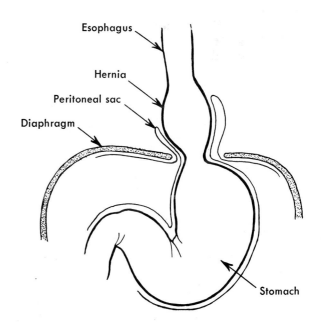

FIG. 25-9. Displacement of a portion of the cardia of the stomach through the normal hiatus into the thoracic cavity (sliding hiatus hernia). (From Anderson, H. C.: Newton's geriatric nursing, ed. 5, St. Louis, 1971, The C. V. Mosby Co.)

logic conditions of the upper gastrointestinal tract[19] (Fig. 25-9). In this condition, part of the stomach "slides" or follows the normal path of the esophagus through an enlarged hiatal opening in the diaphragm into the thorax. The cause of this abnormal enlargement may be trauma, congenital weakness, relaxation of ligaments or skeletal muscles, or increased abdominal pressure. Hiatus herniation can occur at any age but is more often found in persons who are middle-aged or elderly. The condition is often misdiagnosed, or diagnosis is delayed. Sometimes the hernia is not apparent when swallowing barium unless the patient is placed in a Trendelenburg position.

When a hiatus hernia develops, the function of the cardioesophageal sphincter is lost, permitting a reflux of unneutralized gastric juices into the esophagus, which in turn produces inflammation of the lower esophagus. If this condition persists over weeks and months, ulceration occurs, accompanied by hemorrhage and formation of fibrous tissue. An occasional complication is incarceration of a portion of the stomach in the chest with constriction of the blood supply and possibly necrosis, causing peritonitis and mediastinitis. Another problem may be caused by regurgitation of gastric contents during sleep and subsequent aspiration into the lungs. The elderly patient may visit his physician with signs of pneumonitis, since, because his reflexes are less acute, he aspirates fluid into the lungs more easily than the younger person.

Symptoms of hiatus hernia vary greatly. Some small hernias may cause no symptoms, whereas others cause the patient serious difficulty. Often the patient will complain of heartburn after meals and during the night. Heartburn and pain beneath the sternum may occur after meals, on physical exertion, particularly when bending forward is entailed, or on any sudden change of posture. Food may be regurgitated several hours after meals, and the patient may complain of the sensation of food "sticking" as he swallows (dysphagia).

If the hiatus hernia causes no symptoms, treatment is usually not necessary. The treatment for hiatus hernia with symptoms may be either medical or surgical, depending on how well the hernia responds to medical treatment. Medical treatment of hiatus hernia includes a regular schedule of meals, avoiding highly seasoned foods, coffee, and fruit juices. The patient is instructed to eat slowly, to reduce weight if obese, and to avoid heavy weight lifting. He is advised to eat small meals, to avoid carbonated beverages, and to sit in an upright position during meals and for sometime thereafter. When the patient is in the hospital for other causes and there is no reason why he cannot sit upright, the head of the bed should be raised to an upright position for meals and left in this position for $1/_2$ hour following meals. Antacids such as aluminum hydroxide gel may be prescribed to be taken $1/_2$ hour after meals and at bedtime.

The problem of regurgitation of food during sleep can be minimized by elevating the head of the bed on 4- or 6-inch blocks. The patient is often advised to avoid wearing tight, constricting clothing about the waist. He should be taught to go about usual activities, but give attention to changes in posture, particularly if they involve sharp forward bending. For example, in picking up an object from the floor, he should use proper body mechanics and stoop rather than bend from the waist. Kneeling rather than bending or even stooping may be better for some activities.

Hiatus hernia can be corrected surgically by a repair that may involve entering the abdominal and/ or the thoracic cavity to return the stomach to the abdominal cavity and to repair the diaphragm. Surgery is used only for persons with unrelieved and persistent symptoms.

■ GASTRIC DISORDERS

Gastritis

Gastritis is an inflammation of the gastric mucosa and is the most common pathologic condition of the stomach. It may be acute or chronic.

Acute gastritis. Acute gastritis follows the ingestion of large amounts of alcohol and injudicious eating. Occasionally it may be caused by certain drugs such as aspirin, indomethacin, and prednisone. The gastric mucosa becomes red, congested, inflamed, and edematous and may be covered with thin gray or green patches that may exude a white, purulent material. The main symptom of acute gastritis is severe and sometimes prolonged vomiting. (Symptoms and care of persons suffering from gastritis and diarrhea secondary to food poisoning with organisms such as the *Staphylococcus aureus* is described on p. 270.) The treatment is to withhold everything by mouth until vomiting ceases. Some patients develop severe dehydration and electrolyte imbalance. This is treated with intravenous fluids and appropriate electrolytes. When food can be tolerated, tea, milk, gelatin, toast, and simple bland foods are given until a normal diet can be resumed. Drugs to relax smooth muscles, such as the atropine derivatives and propantheline bromide (Pro-Banthine) may be ordered.

Acute episodes of gastritis may become chronic, with pathologic changes occurring. At first the gastric glands show obstruction with disappearance of the acid secretion, followed by disappearance of pepsin and the intrinsic factor. About one third of persons having gastritis develop gradual degeneration of the gastric mucosa, leading to eventual loss of gastric secretion. In time, perhaps within a few years, and after utilizing the vitamin B₁₂ stored by the liver, the patient will develop pernicious anemia and require vitamin B₁₂ injections for the remainder of his life.

Chronic gastritis. Chronic gastritis is diagnosed only after tests and examinations have eliminated the possibility of other gastric diseases. Gastroscopy aids in the diagnosis. The patient usually gives a history of prolonged dietary indiscretions such as eating large amounts of very hot, spicy foods or drinking alcoholic beverages excessively. Symptoms may range from chronic gastric distress to massive gastric hemorrhage. The patient is placed on a bland diet, given antacids such as aluminum hydroxide gel, and instructed to avoid foods and situations that have brought on symptoms in the past. Abstention from alcohol, coffee, and tobacco may aid in controlling gastric hypersecretion.

Peptic ulcer

A peptic ulcer is an ulceration involving the mucosa and deeper structures and is due in part to action of the acid gastric juices. The acid induces a chemical inflammation that lowers the pain threshold of the nerve endings in the margins and in the base of the ulcer. Vascular engorgement with or without acute inflammation further decreases the threshold for pain. The site of the peptic ulcer may be the distal esophagus, the stomach, the upper duodenum, or the jejunum, as, for example, a marginal ulcer following a gastroenterostomy (Fig. 25-10) or as seen in the Zollinger-Ellison syndrome, p. 672. It is believed that 10% of the male population suffer from this condition some time during their lifetime.[51] Peptic ulcer occurs four times as commonly in men as in women, but the incidence in women seems to be increasing. At the present time, peptic ulcer of the stomach and duodenum afflicts more than 10 million citizens of the United States and is most common in persons between 20 and 60 years of age. The incidence of peptic ulcer as well as the number of people who die of the disease is steadily increasing.

The cause of peptic ulcer is not known, but it is believed that there are three factors that greatly influence its development: a source of irritation such as an increase of hydrochloric acid with a decrease of alkaline mucus secreted by the surface cells; a breakdown of the local tissue resistance and defense mechanisms; and the influences of heredity, hormones, and personality. The hormones appear to have some effect on ulcer formation since ulcers are more prevalent in men than in women. In the Zollinger-Ellison syndrome a gastrinlike hormone released by the noninsulin-producing islet cell tumor of the pancreas is known to produce extreme gastric hypersecretion and hyperacidity and severe recurrent peptic ulceration.[24]

Certain so-called ulcerogenic drugs such as corticotropin and the adrenocorticosteroids, the salicylates, and phenylbutazone (Butazolidin) are known to contribute to the development of peptic ulcers in some patients. The mechanism of these ulcerogenic drugs is varied. With the anti-inflammatory steroids, it involves mucosal injury secondary to increased gastric acid secretion and reduced gastric mucus secretion. The latter is due to the steroid antiprotein synthetic action. With aspirin, there is an increased exfoliation of mucous cells and a decrease in mucus production.[40]

The tendency for ulcers to occur runs in families. It has been demonstrated that emotional factors influence the function of the stomach and cause changes in the gastric mucosa. Persons who are under continuous pressure and who are nervous, tense, perfectionists, and unhappy may develop symptoms of peptic ulcers. It has not been proved, however, whether these symptoms truly follow or precede the development of the ulcer.

Acute ulcers usually are superficial, involving only the mucosal layer. In most cases they heal within a relatively short time, but they may bleed, perforate, or become chronic.

A chronic peptic ulcer is a deep crater with sharp edges and a "clean" base. It involves both the mucosa and the submucosa. If the ulcer penetrates the stomach wall and becomes adherent to an adjacent organ such as the pancreas, the organ may become the base of the ulcer.

Peptic ulcers are described as gastric or duodenal, depending on their location. An ulcer (usually of the jejunum) occurring near the site of anastomosis is termed a *marginal ulcer.* Most gastric ulcers occur on the lesser curvature of the stomach. Such ulcers tend to be larger and deeper than duodenal ulcers, and they have a tendency to undergo malignant changes. Duodenal ulcers are not as well defined as

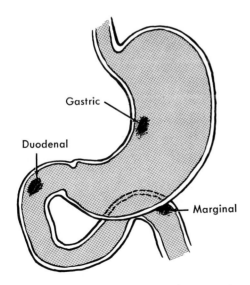

FIG. 25-10. Most common locations of peptic ulcers.

gastric ulcers, but the pathology is the same. Most of them occur on the first part of the duodenum. They are more common than gastric ulcers.

The patient who has a peptic ulcer usually complains of pain that is characteristic in its nature, intensity, radiation, location, and periodicity. Initial attacks of pain often occur in the spring and the fall, last for a few weeks, and then disappear. Each succeeding attack is more severe and more prolonged than the preceding one. The pain is described as gnawing, aching, or burning. It is usually located in the upper abdomen, near the midline, and it is confined to a small area. However, it may radiate around the costal border or to the back. Pain from a duodenal ulcer is usually located in the right epigastric area, whereas that from a gastric ulcer is usually located in the left epigastric area. Pain usually starts 1 or 2 hours after eating, when the stomach begins to empty, and it may disappear spontaneously, after the ingestion of food, or after the ingestion of an antacid medication such as aluminum hydroxide gel. If the ulcer is severe, it may cause pain at night. It is not unusual for the patient to awaken with pain at 2 or 3 A.M. when gastric secretion is at its peak.[58]

Although pain is felt at the site of the existing lesion, it is known that normal stomach mucosa does not have pain sensation. It is thought, therefore, that the inflamed mucosa around the ulcer must be sensitive to the gastric secretions because inflammation lowers the pain threshold.[8] Eructation is common in peptic ulcer but differs from that occurring in gallbladder disease in that it occurs more often when the stomach is empty and does not follow the ingestion of fatty foods. If edema around the lesion obstructs the pylorus, gastric retention with dilation of the stomach may occur, causing nausea and vomiting. This occurrence, however, is not common in peptic ulcer.

The diagnosis of peptic ulcer is made from the patient's history, a gastrointestinal series, a gastric analysis, and stool examinations for occult (hidden) blood. Gastroscopy can also be done, but the diagnosis may be established without it. The most common reason for gastroscopy is to differentiate between a gastric ulcer and gastric carcinoma.

Treatment is directed toward relief of symptoms, healing of the ulcer, and prevention of recurrence. The majority of peptic ulcers heal under medical treatment. Surgery is used most often in the treatment of complications.

Management. Ulcer management consists of rest and sedation, a bland diet, restriction of irritating substances such as coffee, tea, alcohol, and tobacco, and the use of antacids and anticholinergic medications, and an attempt to relieve undesirable emotional stimuli by medical counseling or psychotherapy. *Radiation* of the stomach is used in some centers for

selected patients in an attempt to decrease or eliminate the secretion of hydrochloric acid so that the ulcer may heal. Gastric hypothermia as described on p. 108 may be used to suppress gastric secretions. When the ulcer is covered with normal mucosa, it is considered healed. Healing may occur in a few weeks, or it may require months.

Rest. Both physical and mental rest are necessary for the healing of a peptic ulcer. If the patient has domestic problems, a change in environment may be indicated, possibly hospitalization for a week or two. If he has severe pain or complications that do not respond to treatment at home, hospitalization will be necessary. It may take the combined efforts of the physician, the nurse, the family, and the social worker to help the patient understand the need for complete rest and to secure his cooperation in achieving it. The patient should be on bed rest and removed from activity and disturbing noise. Usually he is permitted visitors and is allowed to participate in activities that keep him interested and occupied but that do not involve physical or mental effort (such as playing games with other patients or watching television). The nurse can gain the confidence of the patient by giving thoughtful, intelligent nursing care, by explaining procedures, and by promptly attending to his needs. Although the patient may appear outwardly calm, his emotional makeup may make him react strongly to the slightest unfavorable stimulus. Foresight on the part of the nurse will prevent the occurrence of incidents that aggravate the patient. Nursing care that provides a regular, smooth routine is best for the patient. Meals, medications, and treatments should be given at correctly spaced intervals and on time. Noise, rush, confusion, and impatience on the part of members of the staff should be avoided. The nurse should plan to spend time listening to the patient in an attempt to obtain clues to problems that should be relayed to the physician.

When symptoms of peptic ulcer are severe and acute, large doses of sedatives such as phenobarbital and tranquilizers may be prescribed to help the patient rest. These drugs may make him so drowsy that close supervision will be necessary to prevent circulatory and respiratory complications. He should be turned from side to side at frequent intervals and encouraged to move his legs and arms and to take several deep breaths every 1 or 2 hours. Side rails should be placed on the bed of a heavily sedated patient to prevent falling and injury. The patient's skin should be inspected frequently for rashes that might indicate a toxic reaction to barbiturates or other drugs.

Diet. There are several approaches to dietary treatment of patients with peptic ulcers. Some physicians feel that rigid dietary restrictions result in no more rapid healing of the ulcer than does a liberal diet. Food is both an antacid and a stimulus for acid secretions, and the neutralizing action of food (especially protein) is soon overcome by an increased rate of acid secretion that irritates the ulcer and produces pain. For these reasons, some physicians prescribe a liberal, bland diet, restricting only those foods that cause the patient distress and dividing the total food intake into five or more meals. As the diet is liberalized, the patient is taught to eat frequently or between meals and to avoid feelings of hunger because hunger permits unbuffered acid to act on the mucosa and thus undo the healing that has occurred.

Other physicians prescribe a modified Sippy diet based on the fact that the acid-combining power of food proteins neutralizes the free hydrochloric acid secreted by the stomach. Theoretically the ulcer will then heal since it is no longer constantly irritated by the gastric juices. Constant dilution of stomach contents and neutralization of acid are achieved by giving whole milk, skim milk, or half milk–half cream punctually every hour. Vitamins and minerals are usually ordered to help make up for the nutritional deficiencies of this diet. Gradually small meals of cereal, soft-cooked eggs, white toast, creamed soups, and other bland foods are added until three meals are substituted for some of the liquid nourishment. The liquid nourishment of milk or milk and cream is still taken between meals.

Patients on either regimen should avoid chemically irritating foods that stimulate the flow of gastric juices and that may cause pain. These foods include meat extracts, meat soups, gravies, certain spices, and beverages containing alcohol and caffeine such as coffee, tea, and cola products.

When hourly feedings are an essential part of the patient's treatment, the nurse must see that they are taken as prescribed. If the patient objects to the taste of milk or tires of the sameness of his diet, small amounts of strawberry, malt, maple, or other flavoring may be added to the mixture. If the patient is acutely ill or has received much sedation, the responsibility for the hourly feedings must be assumed entirely by the nursing staff. If the patient is reliable and capable, a pitcher of milk or milk and cream may be left at his bedside in a container of ice so that he can take his own nourishment. When this is done, it is important that the nurse not forget about the patient. The patient with a peptic ulcer needs attention as much as he needs food, and he benefits from a kindly inquiry from the nurse as to whether or not he has taken the feeding, whether there is enough milk in the pitcher, and whether or not it is sufficiently cool. Many patients find that the feedings give them relief from discomfort and therefore anticipate a quick cure with such treatment. They are very upset if meals are delayed. Since much of the patient's time is spent thinking about himself and his treatment and about the implications of his illness for his family, it is understandable that he becomes irritable when the schedule is not carefully adhered to.

It may be necessary to administer the milk and the antacids by a continuous drip tube feeding so that the gastric secretions will be continuously neutralized. This is particularly important during night hours. The nasogastric tube is passed in the manner described earlier in this chapter. A Kelly flask or an infusion bottle containing the milk and the antacids is connected by plastic tubing to the nasogastric tube. A screw clamp regulates the flow of solution through the tube. A prescribed amount of fluid is usually allowed to run into the stomach over a 24-hour period. It should include enough water to supply the patient's daily needs. To prevent the milk from becoming sour, the nurse should keep only a small amount of mixture in the bottle at any one time. The flask should be changed frequently and should be washed and boiled before reuse. Special pump machines such as a Barron food pump are now available.

Drugs. Drugs that are given to lower the acidity of the gastric secretions include nonsystemic antacids such as aluminum hydroxide gel (Amphojel), magnesium trisilicate and aluminum hydroxide gel (Gelusil), magnesium aluminum hydroxide gel (Maalox), magnesium aluminum hydroxide gel and simethicone (Mylanta), calcium carbonate, and magnesium oxide. Monalium hydrate (Riopan) is often prescribed for patients on restricted sodium intake. These drugs reduce gastric acidity by physical absorption or by chemical neutralization. They are poorly absorbed from the stomach and therefore do not alter the pH of the blood or interfere with normal acid-base balance. When they are prescribed in the initial stages of treatment for an ulcer, they are given hourly. Because milk may be given hourly, a schedule is usually set up in which the milk is given every hour on the hour and the antacids every hour on the half hour. In order to maintain this schedule, it is important that the patient be well instructed so that he can assume some responsibility for this regimen under nursing supervision.

Since sodium bicarbonate is readily absorbed from the intestine into the bloodstream, patients should be advised against taking it when gastric pain occurs. If a large quantity is taken, the acid-base balance of the blood will be upset. Also, the reaction of sodium bicarbonate and hydrochloric acid forms carbon dioxide, which may increase distress by causing distention.

Drugs used to decrease gastric motility are anticholinergic agents of the belladonna group. Most of the drugs presently used as antispasmodics are synthetic substitutes for atropine. Some of the more commonly used ones are methscopolamine bromide (Pamine bromide), methantheline bromide (Banthine bromide), propantheline bromide (Pro-Banthine bromide), pipenzolate bromide (Piptal), and Donnatal (containing atropine sulfate, phenobarbital, and hyoscyamine hydrobromide). Because these drugs are cholinergic blocking agents, certain side effects may occur. These include dryness of mouth, blurred vision, headache, constipation, urinary retention, palpitation, and flushing and dryness of the skin. Because of the high incidence of side effects, the physician may have to change the antispasmodic ordered for the patient until the one with the fewest untoward effects for the patient is determined.

Patients who are on milk diets or who are receiving drugs such as aluminum hydroxide gel and anticholinergic drugs often become constipated. The physician may order a mild cathartic, but no cathartic should be taken without a physician's order, since it may increase gastrointestinal motility when it is undesirable.

Preventive health teaching. To prevent exacerbations of an ulcer, the patient must learn to avoid the foods and situations that tend to reactivate the ulcer. The physician usually evaluates the problems or pressures in the patient's home life or at work that may bring about attacks of ulcer pain. If the patient cannot be removed from his environmental influence, he may be given help in accepting stressful situations. He should be encouraged to allow time for periods of rest and relaxation in his daily schedule. Occasionally the physician may advise the patient to have psychotherapy so that he may understand his problems better and thus be more able to cope with them.

The patient should practice moderation in diet, work, and play. He should be aware that he has had an ulcer and that excesses may cause the ulcer to become reactivated.

The planning, preparation, and serving of food should be thoroughly discussed with the patient and his family, and cultural and religious preferences should be considered. Highly seasoned foods, very hot or cold foods, fried foods, raw fruits and vegetables, coffee, and alcohol should be avoided. The patient should learn to eat slowly in a quiet environment, and he should try to avoid situations that cause emotional disturbance before and during meals. It is usually necessary for him to remain on a bland diet for at least a year. It is common for him to want to resume his former eating pattern as soon as pain disappears, but he should know that doing so may cause an immediate return of symptoms. Some patients do not have pain as a symptom and in these patients dietary management assumes even greater importance. The patient's work sometimes makes the selection of suitable meals difficult. If the selection of food is limited, the patient can take milk with him in a vacuum bottle to supplement the limit-

ed selection. If the patient becomes emotionally upset by situations at work or at home, he should learn to eat a bland diet and to drink milk between meals. These measures may prevent a serious exacerbation of the ulcer.

There seems to be a relationship between smoking and irritation of a peptic ulcer. Therefore most physicians believe that the patient who has a peptic ulcer should give up smoking permanently. To do so is often very difficult for the patient, since often his life and work situations as well as his personality makeup are such that a change of this sort is a major one. The patient needs constant encouragement and understanding when he is endeavoring to give up smoking if the habit is well established.

Because alcohol tends to increase the secretion of acid and is irritating to the gastric mucosa, it should not be taken on an empty stomach. However, some physicians allow their patients to take small amounts of alcohol with their meals.

Ulcerogenic drugs such as salicylates, corticosteroids, and phenylbutazone are generally not prescribed for patients with a history of peptic ulcer. The treatment of headache in these patients is often a problem. However, newer medications such as acetaminophen (Tylenol) and Ascriptin (aspirin and magnesium aluminum hydroxide) can often be used safely.

For the successful treatment of an ulcer and the prevention of future exacerbations, the physician must have the complete confidence of the patient. The nurse can often help to augment the patient's confidence in his physician and in the prescribed treatment. The nurse can also learn about doubts and worries of the patient and report them to the physician so that reassurance or explanation may be given as needed. If every consideration is given to adjusting the prescribed regimen to fit the patient's physical, economic, and social pattern, he will be better able to follow the treatment. When plans are being made by the health team for the patient's discharge from the hospital, the patient and his family should be included. In this way, existing problems can be discussed realistically in relation to future care.

The patient who has had a peptic ulcer must remain under medical supervision for about a year. He may have periodic x-ray examinations of the stomach to determine the extent to which the ulcer has healed. After that time, if healing is complete, he should be advised to report to his physician at once if symptoms reappear since peptic ulcers can recur after the patient has enjoyed several years of good health.

Complications requiring surgery. Emergency surgery is necessary when a peptic ulcer perforates and causes peritonitis or erodes a blood vessel, causing severe hemorrhage. Elective surgery may be performed if an ulcer does not respond to the medical regimen and continues to produce symptoms, if it causes pyloric obstruction, or if a chronic recurring gastric ulcer is thought to be precancerous.

Perforation. Acute perforation of a peptic ulcer is a surgical emergency and is the most frequent cause of death in patients with peptic ulcer. Between 1% and 2% of all ulcers will perforate. After the perforation occurs, gastric contents pour into the peritoneal cavity, causing peritonitis. Both gastric and duodenal ulcers may perforate.

The patient who has a perforated ulcer has symptoms similar to those occurring when any abdominal organ or other part of the gastrointestinal tract perforates. The extremely irritating qualities of the gastric contents released into the abdominal cavity, however, may be quite overwhelming and lead to prostration and severe shock in a short time. There is a sudden sharp pain that spreads quickly over the abdomen. Characteristically, the patient bends over with pain and draws up his knees to prevent pull on the abdominal wall. He is reluctant to move, holds himself tense, and protests against having his abdomen touched. On palpation, the abdomen is found to be boardlike and very tender. The patient usually perspires profusely, and his facial expression is one of agony and apprehension. Since his breathing is rapid and shallow to prevent pull on abdominal muscles, he may be cyanotic. The patient's temperature is usually normal or subnormal, and his pulse is usually rapid and weak. A positive diagnosis is made by taking a radiograph of the abdomen with the patient standing. If the ulcer has perforated, air under the diaphragm is visible on the film. It is important for the nurse to remember that patients on corticosteroids may develop a peptic ulcer and perforation without exhibiting any of the usual symptoms.

Some perforations are minor and close within a short time or wall themselves off. However, most perforations require surgery and should be closed surgically as soon as possible. The longer the perforation exists, allowing the irritating (and infected) gastrointestinal secretions to pour into the abdominal cavity, the higher the mortality rate becomes.

Immediate therapy consists of passing a nasogastric tube and connecting it to continuous suction to drain gastric contents. Nothing is given orally. Parenteral fluids are given to combat fluid and electrolyte imbalance, and antibiotics are administered. The patient is kept in a low Fowler's position so that the gastric contents that have escaped will collect in the pelvic cavity and will be more accessible surgically. The patient is very frightened and apprehensive and the nurse should stay with him to explain what is being done, what will be done in surgery, and to offer reassurance.

The operation used to close a perforation consists of suturing the opening and reinforcing the area with an omental graft; it is known as a *plicating* operation. The gastric contents that have escaped into the peritoneal cavity are aspirated by suction during the operation. A solution containing antibiotics may be placed in the abdominal cavity before the abdomen is closed. In selected patients, *gastric resection, vagotomy* and *antrectomy,* or *vagotomy* and *pyloroplasty* may be performed. Some physicians believe that early perforations seal rapidly if the stomach is kept empty by continuous gastric aspiration and if the patient is maintained on intravenous fluids and antibiotics.

Routine postoperative care is carried out as described on p. 213. As soon as the patient recovers from anesthesia, however, he is returned to a low Fowler's position. Large doses of antibiotics are administered, and the nasogastric tube is left in place until peristalsis returns. Fluids are given parenterally, and nothing is given by mouth. Drainage from the nasogastric tube is greenish yellow, and there is usually no blood present. Nursing care of patients with nasogastric tubes in use was discussed on p. 654.

Postoperatively the patient should be watched carefully for signs of continuing peritonitis and for abscess formation. Elevation of temperature, respiratory distress, continued abdominal pain, and signs of paralytic ileus such as distention and the inability to pass flatus or stool should be reported to the physician. The physician may also perform periodic rectal examinations to determine the presence of pelvic masses caused by abscess formation. Such an abscess may need to be incised and drained. The nurse should explain to the patient why the rectal examinations are necessary. (A full discussion of the complications of peritonitis is given on p. 687.)

When the nasogastric tube is removed, the patient is given small amounts (30 to 60 ml.) of clear fluid by mouth each hour. If this amount of fluid is well tolerated, he usually is given 90 ml. of milk every hour and, after 2 or 3 days, a bland diet with milk between meals. Most patients are discharged from the hospital on a medical regimen for ulcers. The nurse should review this regimen carefully with the patient who has never had this treatment and also with the patient who has been on this regimen previously.

Chronic peptic ulcers. Patients who have chronic peptic ulcers often require surgery. Even under medical treatment some ulcers persist or keep recurring. Others do not respond to medical treatment and cause the patient so much pain that he is unable to work, sleep, or eat. These intractable chronic ulcers usually occur in the middle-aged or older patient. Surgery is also indicated in gastric ulcers that do not respond to medical treatment quite rapidly, since many of them become cancerous if allowed to persist, and many times it is impossible to diagnose the condition with certainty even with the many diagnostic measures available.

Several different operations may be used in the treatment of chronic peptic ulcers (Fig. 25-11). The *Billroth II* operation or variations thereof (such as Polya and Hofmeister) consist of the removal of one half to two thirds of the stomach *(subtotal gastrectomy).* In this type of gastric resection the ulcer and a large amount of acid-secreting mucosa are removed. The duodenal stump is closed, and the remaining segment of the stomach is anastomosed to a loop of jejunum *(gastrojejunostomy, gastroenterostomy).* Gastric contents now will pass directly from the stomach to the jejunum. Since the distal end of the duodenum still connects with the jejunum, bile now flows from it to the jejunum to mix with the food.

The *Billroth I* operation (or variations thereof) consists of the removal of the lower half to two thirds of the stomach. The remaining portion of the stomach is anastomosed to the duodenum *(gastroduodenostomy).*

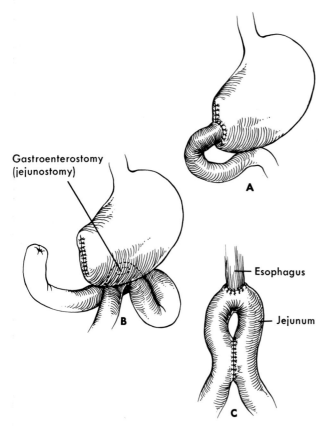

Gastroenterostomy
(jejunostomy)

A

B

Esophagus

Jejunum

C

FIG. 25-11. Types of gastric resections and anastomoses. **A,** Gastric resection with anastomosis of the remaining segment of the stomach with the duodenum (Billroth I type). **B,** Gastric resection with closure of the duodenum and anastomosis of the remaining segment of the stomach to the jejunum (Billroth II type). **C,** Total gastrectomy with anastomosis of the esophagus to the jejunum. The duodenum has been closed.

An *antrectomy* consists of the removal of the entire antrum (area between the fundus and the pylorus) of the stomach and the anastomosing of the remaining stomach to the duodenum *(gastroduodenostomy).* A *vagotomy* is performed by resecting the vagus nerve branch to the stomach 6 to 7 cm. above the junction of the esophagus and the stomach. An antrectomy with a vagotomy may be performed. Theoretically, resecting the entire antrum of the stomach removes the source of the hormone gastrin, and the gastric hormonal phase of gastric hypersecretion is eliminated. (See Fig. 25-12.) In addition, by eliminating the cerebral stimuli to the stomach by a vagotomy, the motility of the stomach muscle and the volume of gastric secretions are lessened. A *pyloroplasty* is a procedure performed to facilitate gastric emptying by enlarging the pyloric opening and eliminating its sphincteric action.[51] A *vagotomy* (via the parasympathetic system) causes considerable reduction in gastric secretion and greatly suppresses gastric motility. More than half of the persons who have a vagotomy alone will later require some procedure to enhance emptying of the stomach. The poor emptying of the stomach results in antral stasis and distention, causing release of the hormone gastrin from the gastric mucosa. The secretion of acid and pepsin is thus enhanced further through the response to gastrin.

A *gastrojejunostomy* (gastroenterostomy) or a vagotomy combined with a gastrojejunostomy may be the treatment of choice for elderly patients who cannot tolerate extensive surgery, for very young patients whose nutritional state suffers irreparably from removal of large amounts of stomach, or for patients with penetrating ulcers of the duodenum or with a deformed duodenum where a Billroth I type of anastomosis would be technically difficult to perform. In a gastrojejunostomy (gastroenterostomy), the jejunum is pulled up and anastomosed with the

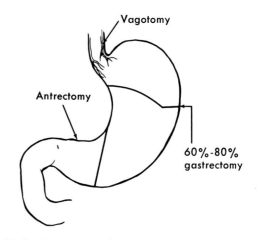

Vagotomy

Antrectomy

60%-80%
gastrectomy

FIG. 25-12. Some surgical approaches used in treatment of peptic ulcer.

stomach. A new opening for the food to pass from the stomach is then made between the stomach and the jejunum without removal of any portion of the stomach.

After a gastric resection the *"dumping syndrome"* sometimes occurs. It may also occur in patients who had a vagotomy, antrectomy, or gastroenterostomy. Mild symptoms occur in approximately 50% of all patients and usually disappear in a few months to a year. They remain troublesome in approximately 5% to 15% of all patients who undergo gastric resection.[8] The onset may occur during the meal or from 5 to 30 minutes after the meal. The duration of the attack may last 20 to 60 minutes.[24] The patient complains of weakness, faintness, palpitations of the heart, and diaphoresis. A feeling of fullness, discomfort, and nausea often occurs, and diarrhea may also develop. These symptoms are thought to be due to the entrance of food directly into the jejunum without undergoing usual changes and dilution in the stomach. The food mixture, more hypertonic than the jejunal secretions, causes fluid to be drawn from the bloodstream to the jejunum. The reaction appears to be greater after the ingestion of highly concentrated and refined carbohydrate foods. The symptoms just described are also attributed to the sudden rise in blood sugar (hyperglycemia), with the entrance of glucose into the bloodstream, and the subsequent fall in the blood sugar level. Blood glucose falls to subnormal levels, producing the symptoms of hypoglycemia. The rapid gastric emptying and the propulsion of chyme into the small intestine is felt to initiate an intensive gastrocolic reflex and cause diarrhea and a feeling of fullness and discomfort.

Fear of symptoms makes the patient reluctant to eat, and he may lose weight. He should be advised to avoid concentrated carbohydrates such as heavily sweetened cereals and sweet desserts that are rapidly dissolved into a concentrated solution. A diet high in protein and high enough in fat to compensate for the carbohydrate restriction should be encouraged. The patient should lie down after eating, should eat frequent, small, dry meals, and should avoid drinking fluid for 2 or 3 hours after meals. The dumping syndrome may be a serious postoperative complication that severely hampers the patient in his work and in many other experiences of normal living. The nurse should observe all patients for early signs of this condition following gastric surgery and report her observations to the surgeon. This may help him to treat the patient early and prevent the discomfort, malnutrition, and psychic reactions to the entire experience, which compound the difficulty of treating this condition satisfactorily.

Pyloric obstruction. Pyloric obstruction may be caused by edema of tissues around an ulcer or by scar tissue from a healed ulcer located near the py-

lorus. It may be only partial and cause dilation of the stomach, or it may be complete. Patients with this complication may have severe projectile vomiting that may or may not be preceded by nausea. A positive diagnosis is made by gastrointestinal x-ray examination and gastric analysis. Obstruction caused by edema and spasm generally responds to medical management. A nasogastric tube is usually passed and connected to gastric suction or the tube may be clamped and aspirated twice daily. Sometimes continuous drip feedings of milk and cream are given to neutralize the stomach secretion and permit the inflammation to subside. After the feeding has been running for several hours (commonly 8), the tube will be clamped for 15 to 30 minutes, and then the stomach contents will be aspirated to see how much of the feeding has passed through the pylorus. If the patient does not vomit during the continuous feeding period, it can be assumed that the feeding is passing through the pylorus and that the obstruction will respond to medical treatment. If the patient does vomit, the nasogastric tube will be attached to continuous suction and fluids and electrolytes will be given intravenously.

When the obstruction is relieved and the patient's condition permits, surgery may be performed. The operation performed is usually a gastric resection, involving the pylorus or the antrum section of the stomach with a part of the duodenum. Either a Billroth I or II procedure or a gastroenterostomy and vagotomy may be performed.

Hemorrhage. Peptic ulcers cause bleeding in at least 25% of all persons who have the disease.[8] If the ulcer has perforated a major blood vessel, the patient may have a severe hemorrhage, vomiting large amounts of blood and passing tarry stools. Vomiting of blood usually occurs with a gastric ulcer, whereas tarry stools are more common with a bleeding duodenal ulcer. Both symptoms may be present in either condition. The patient may also complain of feeling faint, dizzy, and thirsty. He may become dyspneic, apprehensive, and restless as the blood volume is reduced, the blood pressure drops, the pulse rate increases, and signs of shock become apparent. The systemic signs of hemorrhage may appear before (or without) hematemesis and before passage of blood or tarry stools.

The patient with a bleeding ulcer is placed on bed rest and is usually given a sedative such as phenobarbital sodium to alleviate restlessness and apprehension. Morphine sulfate may be used since it aids rest and also helps to slow down intestinal peristalsis. The physician usually orders the blood pressure, pulse rate, and respirations to be checked and recorded frequently (as often as every 15 minutes when acute bleeding is suspected). Blood transfusions are often given to raise the blood volume. They are given slowly to avoid increasing the blood pressure and thereby increasing the bleeding. Vital signs are monitored frequently to determine the body's response to fluid replacement and possible continuation of the hemorrhage.

If the patient is not vomiting and only a small amount of blood is being passed rectally, he usually is given milk every hour, and antacids are prescribed. A full bland diet may be ordered because it maintains nutrition, neutralizes gastric acidity, reduces absorption of the formed clot, and slows peristalsis. If the patient is vomiting blood, however, he is given nothing orally. All bloody vomitus should be measured and described. The physician may wish it saved for his inspection. A nasogastric tube may be passed and attached to suction to collect the blood so that it can be more accurately measured and replaced by transfusion. The fluid and electrolyte balance are maintained by infusions. Sometimes there is an order to irrigate the tube with iced physiologic saline solution or iced water. If so, the irrigating fluid usually must be suctioned back, as the iced fluid causes blood to clot not only in the stomach but also within the tube. The patient who is vomiting blood will need special mouth care. A weak solution of hydrogen peroxide may be used to more easily remove blood from the tongue, teeth, and gums.

The number of tarry (or currant jelly-like) stools should also be measured and recorded, and they may be saved for laboratory examination. Since the patient may be alarmed at the sight of blood, all evidence of bleeding should be quickly removed from the bedside, and the linen should be changed as needed without disturbing the patient any more than necessary. The patient should be told that he is receiving blood transfusions to replace the blood he has lost and that rest and quiet will help stop the bleeding. The sedative or narcotic should be given regularly to allay anxiety and apprehension. If large doses of sedative and narcotic drugs are given, attention must be taken to turning the patient hourly and to encouraging him to breathe deeply to prevent the possibility of respiratory congestion.

Most ulcer hemorrhages respond to medical management. The operations performed for continued and/or massive hemorrhage include partial gastric resection; excision of the ulcer, if possible, and ligation of the bleeding vessel; and vagotomy and pyloroplasty for bleeding duodenal ulcers in patients who are poor risks.[8]

The general principles of nursing a patient after gastric surgery that are discussed on p. 673 are applicable. The drainage from the nasogastric tube is usually dark red for 6 to 12 hours after surgery. It should turn greenish yellow within 24 hours. The patient may continue to pass tarry stools for several days postoperatively, but this is usually because the blood from the hemorrhage before surgery has not yet passed completely through the gastrointestinal tract.

Gastric hypothermia. Although used less frequently than in the past, some physicians use local cooling in the treatment of massive gastric hemorrhage. The goal of the procedure is to stop the bleeding permanently or until the patient is able to tolerate surgery.[12a,52] These physicians believe that hypothermia is effective in the treatment of some patients with peptic ulcers because the cooling suppresses gastric secretions and digestion, relieves symptoms, and permits the ulcer to heal by decreasing gastroduodenal blood flow and by permitting contraction of the muscular gastric wall. This makes it possible for granulation tissue and collagen fibers to develop. A triple-lumen tube with a large balloon is passed through the mouth into the stomach. The coolant, a mixture of alcohol and water, is gradually instilled into the balloon until it contains approximately 600 to 850 ml. of solution and touches all of the gastric mucosa. Pumps circulate the solution at a temperature of $-17°$ to $-20°$ C. ($2°$ to $-4°$ F.). The tube can remain in place for as long as 72 hours or until the bleeding has stopped. Cold normal saline gastric lavage at a temperature of $0°$ C. ($32°$ F.) in volumes of 10 L. may be used to lavage the stomach intermittently over a 30- to 60-minute period to produce local hypothermia. Ice water may be substituted for saline solution in patients with cardiac decompensation in order to avoid sodium overload.[12a]

Gastric irradiation. Radiation therapy to the stomach to reduce activity of the acid-producing glands may be used for selected elderly patients who cannot be operated on and who do not respond favorably to any other form of medical treatment.

Zollinger-Ellison syndrome. The Zollinger-Ellison syndrome, first described in 1955, refers to the peptic ulceration associated with a noninsulin-producing islet cell tumor of the pancreas.[57] The syndrome is characterized by one or more peptic ulcerations occurring in the lower end of the esophagus, stomach, duodenum, and jejunum and by enormous gastric hypersecretion and acidity and the presence of nonbeta islet cell adenomas of the pancreas. Frequently the syndrome is accompanied by diarrhea and steatorrhea. The latter is thought due to lack of pancreatic lipase needed for fat digestion, whereas the diarrhea may result from large quantities of acid passing into the duodenum. Diarrhea of long duration can cause serious loss of electrolytes (potassium and sodium in particular) and may prove to be fatal.

These tumors of the pancreas have been found to produce enormous quantities of gastrin or a gastrin-like substance that is responsible for the excessive stimulation of gastric acid and the subsequent ulcerations. Because of the repeated reappearance of the peptic ulcers and the multiple and aberrant locations, it is usually impossible to resect all areas involved. Total gastrectomy is often performed, and in many cases it is the only method that proves lifesaving. Even a small amount of gastric tissue not resected has led to recurrent ulcerations.[24]

Management of the patient requiring gastric surgery

Except in emergencies, all patients who are to have gastric surgery undergo extensive diagnostic studies before surgery is performed. If the patient is to have surgery for an ulcer, he is maintained on a medical regimen during the preoperative period. The nursing responsibilities related to caring for patients undergoing diagnostic procedures have already been described. Specific nursing responsibilities related to caring for patients with intestinal obstruction and with gastrointestinal hemorrhage are discussed in the appropriate sections. The general preoperative instructions and preparation are those given any patient preceding major surgery (p. 196). Special instructions for the nursing care of patients in whom a chest approach is used are discussed on p. 585.

Routine postoperative nursing care is given as described on p. 217. Because the incision is made in the upper abdomen, the patient is inclined to breathe shallowly to limit pain in the incision. The prescribed medications for pain should be given as necessary, and special attention should be given to encouraging the patient to breathe deeply and to cough productively. The patient with a high abdominal midline incision is usually more comfortable in a modified Fowler's position. Drainage from the nasogastric tube after gastric surgery usually contains some blood for the first 12 hours, but bright red blood, large amounts of blood, or excessive bloody drainage should be watched for and its occurrence reported to the surgeon at once. While the nasogastric tube is used, and until peristalsis resumes, fluids by mouth are restricted. Mouth care is therefore needed frequently to keep the mucous membranes of the throat and mouth moist and clean. Until the tube is removed and until the patient is able to drink enough nutritious fluids, fluids are given parenterally. The average patient is given about 3,500 ml. of fluids intravenously each day (2,500 ml. for his normal body needs plus enough to replace fluids lost through the gastric drainage and vomitus). It is important that gastric drainage and urinary output be accurately measured and recorded.

The patient is encouraged to change his position every 2 hours to prevent distention of the stomach that can occur with adherence of the nasogastric tube to the mucosa. Vitamins are usually prescribed until the patient is eating a full, well-balanced diet. Fluids by mouth are usually restricted for about 12 to 24 hours after the nasogastric tube is removed. Small amounts of fluid are then given frequently. If water is well tolerated, small amounts of bland food may be added until the patient is able to eat six small meals a day and to drink 120 ml. of fluid every hour between meals. This dietary regimen, however, usually must be adapted to the individual patient since some patients tolerate increasing amounts of food and fluids better than others. Regurgitation after meals may be caused by eating too fast, by eating too much, or by postoperative edema about the suture line that prevents the food from passing into the intestines. If regurgitation occurs, the patient should be encouraged to eat more slowly, and the size of the meals should be decreased temporarily. If the gastric retention continues, it is probably caused by edema about the suture line, and food and fluids by mouth usually are discontinued for a time. A nasogastric tube may be passed and attached to a suction apparatus, and fluids may be administered parenterally until the edema subsides.

After most gastric surgery, drainage on the dressings is minimal. If a total gastrectomy is performed, however, drains are usually inserted from the site of the anastomosis, and there may be serosanguineous drainage. The patient usually gets out of bed the day after surgery, and his activity is increased progressively thereafter.

The patient is usually discharged from the hospital 2 to 3 weeks after surgery. Before discharge, a gastrointestinal series is often done to observe the functioning of the gastroenterostomy. Barium studies may be repeated 6 weeks after surgery to establish a baseline for comparison should symptoms recur. The patient still may be eating six small meals a day, or he may tolerate three larger meals of bland food. He should be advised to eat slowly and to decrease the size of the meals if he is uncomfortable after eating. The remaining stomach gradually is able to accept larger amounts of food and fluids. Within 6 months to a year, the patient is usually able to eat three regular meals. He requires about 3 months to convalesce before he regains his strength completely and is able to resume full activity. After discharge, he needs medical supervision and should be advised to keep appointments either in his physician's office or in the hospital clinic. During these visits the nurse can help to determine the patient's understanding of his condition. He may need to discuss problems about his diet with the dietitian.

■ CANCER

Cancer of the stomach is responsible for approximately 16,000 deaths each year in the United States, or a little less than 10% of all deaths from cancer.[2] The incidence has decreased in the United States over recent years, although the reason for this is unknown. It is found more often after the age of 45 years and is more common in men than in women. There is no known cause for this disease, but it is believed that heredity is a factor in its development and that chronic gastritis and chronic gastric ulcer may be precursors of cancer of the stomach.

Cancer may develop in any part of the stomach but is found most often in the distal third. It may spread directly through the stomach wall into adjacent tissues, to the lymphatics, to the regional lymph nodes of the stomach, to the esophagus, spleen, pancreas, and liver, or through the bloodstream to the bones. Involvement of regional lymph nodes occurs early and is found in about 60% to 75% of all patients who would seem to be curable at the time of surgery.

Unfortunately the patient with cancer of the stomach usually has no symptoms until the growth spreads to adjacent organs. Symptoms may occur only after the disease has become incurable. Vague and persistent symptoms of gastric distress, flatulence, loss of appetite, nausea, gradual weight loss, and loss of strength may be the only complaints of the patient. These vague symptoms should never be ignored. If the nurse knows of anyone with them, they should be encouraged to seek immediate medical advice. However, since such symptoms are not necessarily symptoms of cancer, the patient should not be unduly frightened. Pain does not appear usually until late in the disease, and the absence of this symptom is often the reason for the patient's delay in seeking medical help. If the disease progresses untreated, marked cachexia develops, and eventually a palpable mass can often be felt in the region of the stomach. Often no early gastric symptoms appear, and fatigue and persistent anemia may be the only signs. Cancer of the stomach occurs three times more frequently in persons who have pernicious anemia than in others. This is primarily due to achlorhydria associated with chronic gastritis and gastric atrophy.

A positive diagnosis of gastric carcinoma is usually made by means of a gastrointestinal series. The tumor may not be evident in its early stages, and the x-ray examinations may have to be repeated at intervals. An absence of free hydrochloric acid in stomach secretions obtained by gastric aspiration is suggestive of a gastric neoplasm. When other examinations are negative, cytologic studies may demonstrate the presence of malignant cells in the stomach. Occult blood is frequently found in the stools.

The operative treatment for cancer of the stomach is either a subtotal gastrectomy or a total gastrectomy. Whichever procedure is used, the omentum and the spleen usually are also removed because of the common occurrence of metastasis to these areas. A subtotal gastrectomy has already been described. When the cancer is spread diffusely throughout the stomach, when it extends high in the lesser curvature, or when it arises in the cardia, a *total gastrectomy* is performed. The entire stomach is removed, and then continuity of the gastrointestinal tract is reestablished by anastomosis of a loop of the jejunum to the esophagus (Fig. 25-11). The two portions of the jejunum meeting the esophagus are then sometimes joined to form a reservoir for food.[51] A total gastrectomy is never done when signs of metastasis to other abdominal organs such as the liver are evident. A palliative resection of the stomach is usually done for patients who have cancer of the stomach with metastases.

The nursing care of a patient who has had a total gastrectomy differs in some ways from that of patients undergoing other types of gastric surgery. Since the chest cavity must be entered, the patient will have a catheter for chest drainage, and the nursing care will be that of the patient who has had chest surgery (p. 585). There is little or no drainage from the nasogastric tube because there is no longer any reservoir in which secretions may collect, and there is no stomach mucosa left to secrete. When normal peristalsis returns, the nasogastric tube is removed. The patient is given clear fluids hourly, and if after 2 or 3 days there is no evidence of leakage through the anastomosis, the diet is increased to several small meals (usually six) of bland foods a day. An elevation of temperature or dyspnea should make one suspect leakage from the anastomosis, and all oral intake should be stopped until the physician has been consulted.

Following a total gastrectomy, the maintenance of good nutrition is difficult because the patient can no longer eat regular meals and because the food that is taken is poorly digested and therefore poorly absorbed from the intestines. Since the patient also becomes anemic, ferrous sulfate is often prescribed. Patients who have had a total gastrectomy rarely regain normal strength. Most of them are semi-invalids as long as they live. Survival rate for gastric cancer is unusual beyond 5 years because of early and extensive metastasis. X-ray therapy is sometimes used, but for cancer in this location it is of limited use.

■ PYLORIC STENOSIS

Pyloric stenosis in the adult is usually the result of previous duodenal ulceration or carcinoma. Persistent copious vomiting requires urgent attention because fluid and salt loss follow rapidly. Pyloric stenosis is one of the most common conditions requiring surgery in infancy. It occurs most often in tense infants of tense, apprehensive parents and is seen most often in firstborn children. Pyloric stenosis causes vomiting that usually is forceful and occurs soon after the formula is taken. Vomiting is followed immediately by eagerness to take food. As the condition persists and loss of weight occurs, peristaltic waves can be seen passing across the abdomen from right to left and reversing immediately prior to vomiting. Symptoms usually appear in the second or third week of life and seldom develop after 3 or 4 months of age. The cause of this condition is hypertrophy of the sphincter muscle of the pylorus, which often may be felt as a tumor mass in the right upper quadrant of the infant's abdomen.

Pyloric stenosis is treated medically before surgery is considered. If it is treated early before hypertrophy is pronounced and malnutrition is severe, surgery may be avoided. Medical treatment consists of administering small amounts of sedative drugs such as phenobarbital or the alkaloids of belladonna such as atropine in regular doses several times a day, usually preceding meals, and modifying the diet. Smaller feedings may be given at more frequent intervals, and cereals may be substituted for some of the milk, since solid foods are less easily vomited. The infant needs a quiet, relaxed environment. In the hospital the nurse should see that all his needs such as a change of diapers or extra warmth are met at once so that he does not become upset. Very gentle rocking prior to and immediately following meals sometimes helps. If the infant is at home, the public health nurse can often help the family to ensure a more relaxed environment for the infant. Sometimes, for example, it appears that a mother's fears about whether or not she is properly caring for her baby contribute to the infant's difficulties.

Surgical treatment for pyloric stenosis is used when the condition does not respond to medical treatment alone. It consists of incision into the sphincter muscle of the pylorus (pylorotomy, Ramstedt operation), and the response to this treatment is almost uniformly good. All the measures described in Chapter 11 relating to surgery in infancy and childhood should be considered. Usually a nasogastric tube is passed and stomach contents are aspirated just prior to surgery. Since only the muscle layers are cut and the stomach is not entered during the surgery, many surgeons permit the infant to have water and sometimes formula almost as soon as he has reacted completely from the anesthesia.

Diseases of the lower gastrointestinal system

Many disease conditions affect the lower gastrointestinal system. Only some of the more common ones and the related nursing care will be discussed here.

■ APPENDICITIS

In the United States there are still some deaths each year from appendicitis. If symptoms had not been neglected or if the patient had not been given a cathartic, some of these deaths might have been prevented. It is important, therefore, that the nurse continue to help teach the public that symptoms of right lower quadrant or periumbilical pain accompanied by loss of appetite, elevation of temperature, and possibly nausea, vomiting, and diarrhea should be reported to a physician. Patients with these symptoms should not be treated at home by local heat, enemas, or cathartics.

Appendicitis is an inflammatory lesion of the vermiform appendix. It is more common among men, and it occurs most frequently between the ages of 10 and 30 years. It may occur at any age, however. Although there is no certain cause of the disease, occlusion of the lumen of the appendix by hardened feces (fecaliths), by foreign objects, or by kinking of the appendix may impair the circulation and lower resistance to organisms within the body such as the colon bacillus or the *Streptococcus.* A small part of the appendix may be edematous, inflamed, or necrotic, or the entire appendix may be so involved. An abscess may develop in the appendiceal wall or in the surrounding tissue. The serious danger is that the appendix will rupture and cause a generalized peritonitis.

The typical symptoms of acute appendicitis are pain about the umbilicus and throughout the abdomen (which may soon become localized at a point known as *McBurney's point,* exactly halfway between the umbilicus and the crest of the right ilium), nausea, anorexia, and often vomiting. Acute appendicitis is remarkable for the suddenness of its onset. The patient may have felt quite well an hour or two before the onset of severe pain. Approximately 90% of these patients will have a white cell count above 10,000/mm.[3], and approximately three fourths of the patients will have a neutrophil count above 75%. The temperature usually is irregularly elevated about 2 to 4 degrees above normal and is accompanied by an increase in pulse. These symptoms are present in about 60% of all patients with acute appendicitis.[51] Other patients have less well-defined local symptoms because of the location of the appendix. It may be retrocecal, or it may lie adjacent to the ureter. If the patient has questionable symptoms, a urinalysis and an intravenous pyelogram may be made to rule out an acute pyelitis or a ureteral stone. There are many other diseases that produce symptoms similar to appendicitis, and they sometimes need to be ruled out before a positive diagnosis can be made. Some of these are acute salpingitis, regional ileitis, mesenteric lymphadenitis, and biliary colic. The older patient with acute appendicitis may experience only dull pain. Children who develop appendicitis may have only slight abdominal pain, although usually they vomit. Because the abdominal omentum is not well developed in children, if the appendix perforates, peritonitis can easily develop because the infection cannot be walled off so quickly. It is recommended, therefore, that the ill child who refuses food and who vomits be taken to a physician for diagnosis and treatment. He should *never* be given a cathartic for these complaints.

Management

When appendicitis is suspected, the patient usually is hospitalized at once and placed on bed rest for observation and the necessary diagnostic procedures that must be performed. Since an operation may be performed shortly after admission, the patient is not given anything by mouth while reports of the blood count are awaited. Sometimes a nasogastric tube is passed and attached to suction. Parenteral fluids may be given during this time. Narcotics are not given until the cause of the pain has been determined since they would mask signs or symptoms. Sometimes an ice bag to the abdomen is ordered to help relieve pain. A rectal examination is done to help establish the diagnosis, and the patient should be given an explanation as to why the procedure is necessary.

An appendectomy is usually scheduled as an emergency operation. The patient is given a general or regional anesthetic, and the appendix is removed through a small incision over McBurney's point or through a right paramedial incision. The incision usually heals with no drainage. Drains are used when an abscess is discovered, when the appendix has ruptured and peritonitis has developed, and sometimes when the appendix appears edematous and ready to rupture and is surrounded by clear fluid.

Bowel function is usually normal soon after surgery. Nausea and vomiting disappear with surgical treatment, and the patient is permitted food as tolerated. Convalescence is usually short. The patient gets out of bed the day after surgery and may resume normal activity within 2 to 4 weeks.

■ MECKEL'S DIVERTICULUM

Meckel's diverticulum is a fibrous tube or cord located usually about 50 cm. (20 inches) above the ileocecal valve. It is the remnant of a duct used in fetal life and is found in about 2% of the population.[67]

The diverticulum can become inflamed, causing symptoms similar to those of appendicitis or hemorrhage from the bowel. Differential diagnosis is particularly difficult in children. The diagnosis is usually made at surgery. At this time the diseased diverticulum and the involved intestine are resected.

■ MESENTERIC VASCULAR OCCLUSION

Mesenteric vascular occlusion is common, occurring frequently in patients with extensive arteriosclerosis or serious heart disease resulting in emboli to the intestines. Often the patient is elderly. It also may occur in patients who are recovering from recent abdominal surgery. Thrombosis of the mesenteric vein may occur as a complication of cirrhosis of the liver, following splenectomy, or as a result of an extension of a thrombophlebitic process in the ileocolic veins. The superior mesenteric arteries usually are occluded. Causes other than atherosclerosis or intravascular thromboses of the mesenteric vessels include polycythemia, sickle cell disease, other blood dyscrasias, and pancreatic disorders.

The blood supply to the lower part of the jejunum and ileum is usually interrupted by a mesenteric vascular occlusion. The walls of the intestine become thickened and edematous, then reddened, and finally black and gangrenous. Infarction of the small bowel may develop over a period of several weeks or may appear suddenly. In partial blockage of the superior mesenteric artery by an atherosclerotic plaque, pain is crampy and colicky in nature and may last for several hours after a meal. The pain is associated with the demand for oxygen needed for the increased intestinal muscular activity. In the event of sudden occlusion the patient complains of an acute onset of sharp abdominal pain, nausea, and vomiting. He has disturbed bowel function and may pass blood from the rectum or may have no bowel action. The white blood cell count is elevated. The patient may be in shock when first seen, even when the condition is reported at the onset of symptoms. The patient is hospitalized at once. Nothing is given orally, and a nasogastric tube is inserted and attached to suction. Parenteral fluids may be started. Treatment depends on the suddenness and cause of the occlusion. If a clot can be found and removed after opening the superior mesenteric artery, the blood flow will be restored. If necessary, damaged bowel tissue is removed. Chronic occlusion may be corrected by endarterectomy or a bypass procedure.

The preoperative and postoperative care of patients having a bowel resection is described later in this chapter. The patient who has surgery for vascular occlusion usually is given heparin and bishydroxycoumarin (Dicumarol) to prevent further clot formation. This treatment not only requires close medical supervision but also careful nursing care, as discussed on p. 380. The patient may also be given antispasmodic drugs such as papaverine hydrochloride. He may be very ill both preoperatively and postoperatively and may need constant nursing care. The mortality rate from mesenteric vascular occlusion is high, particularly among elderly patients.

■ REGIONAL ENTERITIS

Regional enteritis is a nonspecific inflammation of the small bowel, predominantly the terminal ileum.

It is characterized by cobblestone-like ulcerations along the mucosa, a thickening of the intestinal wall, and the formation of scar tissue. The disease usually occurs between the ages of 20 and 30 years. Its cause is unknown. The inflammation begins at the ileocecal valve and extends upward, sometimes skipping whole areas of intestinal mucosa. The ulcers are likely to perforate and form fistulas that connect with the abdominal wall or with any hollow viscus such as the colon, sigmoid, bladder, or vagina. Scar tissue may form as the ulcers heal, preventing the normal absorption of food, and strictures may form and cause intestinal obstruction.

The patient with an acute regional enteritis usually has severe abdominal pain or cramps localized in the right lower quadrant, moderate fever, and mild diarrhea. The white blood cell count is elevated. Often the disease is diagnosed as acute appendicitis, but when the patient is operated on, he is found to have a normal appendix but an inflamed ileum.

Chronic regional enteritis is characterized by a long history of diarrhea, abdominal pain, loss of weight, anemia, fistula formation, and, finally, intestinal obstruction. Weight loss and anemia result from chronic, persistent inflammation of the bowel, decreased food intake, and malabsorption. The diarrhea may consist of three or four semisolid stools daily containing mucus, pus, and sometimes undigested food. The abdominal colicky pain is relieved with a bowel movement. A mass sometimes can be felt in the area of the appendix or cecum.

The treatment for both acute and chronic enteritis is essentially medical. The patient is given a high-calorie, high-protein bland diet together with vitamins to help maintain good nutrition. Patients with regional enteritis utilize fats poorly and do not tolerate high-fat diets well. Iron compounds may be necessary to treat anemia. Anticholinergic drugs such as propantheline bromide (Pro-Banthine) may be administered. Intestinal antibiotics such as phthalylsulfathiazole (Sulfathalidine) and salicylazosulfapyridine (Azulfidine) may be administered orally, and antibiotics may be administered systemically for control of secondary infections. Steroid therapy may be used in acute states of the disease.

If intestinal obstruction occurs or if there are fistulas, surgery is necessary. Occasionally an ileostomy is done above the involved bowel. The diseased bowel may be resected and the remaining segments anastomosed, or it may be left and a "short-circuiting" operation performed. This operation consists of dividing the ileum, closing the distal portion with sutures or removing it, and anastomosing the proximal portion to the transverse colon *(ileotransverse colostomy).* If the diseased bowel is adherent to the surrounding organs and tissues, an ileotransverse colostomy may be performed. The inflammation is treated with antibiotics.

■ ULCERATIVE COLITIS

Ulcerative colitis is an inflammatory disease of the colon. Although its cause is unknown, it is thought to be the result of either an infectious process or a psychogenic disturbance. Vascular factors have been suggested as a possible cause of ulcerative colitis as have food allergies. The latter relates especially to a hereditary deficiency of lactase, thus supporting the autoimmune theory of the bowel becoming inflamed in the presence of an osmotic-acid load imposed by the lactose in milk. None of the possible causes, however, has been proved. Many patients with this disease have personality disorders, and they often are perfectionistic, sensitive, frustrated, and dependent people.

Ulcerative colitis may occur at any age in either sex, but it is found most often in adolescents and young adults. In 75% of those with ulcerative colitis the onset has been between the ages of 15 and 49 years. When seen in the elderly patient, the condition is attributed to ischemic disease of the bowel. The disease varies in severity, and the patient may be symptom free between periods of acute distress. A severe attack may be brought on by an acute infection, an emotional upset, or unknown factors.

In the early stages of ulcerative colitis, only the rectum or rectosigmoid is affected, with the rectal mucosa containing many superficial bleeding points. As the disease progresses, advancing up the colon, the bowel mucosa becomes edematous and thickened. The superficial bleeding points gradually enlarge and become ulcerated. The ulcers may bleed or perforate, causing abscess formation or peritonitis. The edematous mucosa may undergo changes and form pseudopolyps, which may become cancerous. The continuous healing process, with formation of scar tissue between the frequent relapses, may cause the colon to lose its normal elasticity and its absorptive capability. Normal mucosa is replaced by scar tissue, and the colon becomes thickened, rigid, and pipelike. The diagnosis is based on the patient's history and symptoms, on results obtained from barium enemas, from proctoscopic and sigmoidoscopic examinations, and on failure to find any causative organisms in the stools.

The main symptom of an acute attack of ulcerative colitis is diarrhea. The patient may pass as many as 15 to 20 or more liquid stools a day. They contain blood, mucus, and pus. Abdominal cramps may or may not occur before the bowel movement. The patient may have loss of appetite, low-grade fever, and occasionally nausea and vomiting. With the persistence of these symptoms, as well as the marked depression of colonic absorption, the patient becomes weak, dehydrated, debilitated, and cachectic.

Ulcerative colitis is a serious disease with a fairly high mortality rate. The personality makeup of many patients with this disease seems to be such that they accept the disease stoically but are unable always to conform to the regimen that is prescribed; for example, it may be impossible for the patient to eat the foods that he knows are necessary.

Medical treatment for ulcerative colitis is directed toward restoring nutrition, combating infection, reducing the motility of the inflamed bowel, and treating the psychogenic factors that may be involved. Blood transfusions may be necessary if anemia is severe. If the patient is vomiting and is severely undernourished and dehydrated, parenteral fluids may be given. A high-protein, high-calorie, high-vitamin, low-residue diet is usually urged to help the patient regain nutritional losses and to foster healing. Because there is no conclusive evidence that the diet affects the condition, the patient may be permitted to eat what he chooses. Sedatives or tranquilizers are often prescribed to alleviate nervous tension, and antispasmodic drugs such as belladonna preparations are given to slow down peristalsis. Drugs such as kaolin and bismuth preparations (bismuth subcarbonate) are used to help coat and protect the irritated intestinal mucosa and give better consistency to the stools, and opium preparations such as paregoric may be used to lessen the frequency of stools. Antibiotics may be ordered to prevent or to treat secondary infection.

Salicylazosulfapyridine (Azulfidine) is now widely used in the treatment of ulcerative colitis, and many physicians consider it the drug of choice. Like all sulfa drugs, salicylazosulfapyridine can cause serious side effects; therefore, the nurse may wish to review these when administering this drug. The side effects of oliguria and crystalluria are particularly apt to be a problem in patients with ulcerative colitis unless they maintain a liberal fluid intake.

ACTH and the adrenal steroids such as prednisone may be prescribed in the treatment of ulcerative colitis. They often produce dramatic results in severe cases of the disease by decreasing the toxemia and fever, diminishing diarrhea, bleeding, and rectal urgency, and promoting a sense of well-being in the patient. It should be understood, however, that while corticotropin and the corticosteroids suppress the inflammation associated with ulcerative colitis, they do not cure the disease. A relapse rate as high as 80% has been reported when patients were withdrawn from steroid therapy.[8] Nevertheless, many patients' lives have been saved since these drugs became available. (For nursing care of patients receiving steroid therapy, see p. 82.) Since some experts believe that ulcerative colitis may be caused by an autoimmune reaction, azathioprine (Imuran) may be prescribed in addition to steroids.

About 20% of patients with ulcerative colitis require surgery because of complications such as hemorrhage or perforation.[8] An ileostomy and a subtotal colectomy may be performed in an attempt to cure the condition when the disease is so incapacitating that it makes an invalid of the patient or when no improvement has been obtained from medical treatment over a period of time. Choice of surgery depends on the individual patient and on the physician. It is recognized that surgery does not remove the basic condition that led to development of the disease. Many patients, however, seem to recover almost completely following a total colectomy and are able to lead normal, useful lives.

Nursing intervention

The patient with ulcerative colitis may be admitted to the hospital for immediate supportive treatment during an acute exacerbation of the disease or for preparation for surgery during a remission. In either instance, if the disease is of long duration, the patient is usually thin, nervous, and apprehensive and is inclined to be preoccupied with his physical condition. These qualities, which are caused by the illness, are superimposed on the basic personality pattern of many patients with this disease—sensitivity, insecurity, and dependence are common characteristics. This makes it hard for the nurse to get to know the patient and sometimes hard for her to understand him. The nurse should not hesitate to seek guidance from the physician in her approach to the patient. Sometimes specialized medical and nursing consultation is available. All members of the nursing staff should use the same approach to the patient. Although the patient may accept treatment and nursing care, he may remain restrained and withdrawn; often he is depressed even though he appears resigned to his problems. Hostility may also be a form of behavior exhibited by the patient. The nurse needs to see this as the patient's way of testing his environment and the professional staff and in effect is a way of asking, "Do you really care for me and want to help me?" Acceptance of his behavior, together with gentle, intelligent nursing care, will help the nurse gradually gain the patient's confidence and will increase his ability to accept certain essentials of his treatment, such as the diet regimen.

All procedures and treatments should be carefully explained to the patient. Telling him, for example, that medication is available to him for controlling bowel movements sometimes seems to reduce his apprehension. The nurse should listen carefully to the patient's own report of things that seem to stimulate peristalsis and cause frequency of bowel movements. If he has found that certain foods or combinations of foods cause diarrhea, this fact should be noted on the nursing care plan and reported to the dietitian. Other information such as the best time for bathing, whether soon after a meal (to permit a long rest period afterward) or later (when food is partially digested), should be on the nursing care plan.

The acutely ill patient may have bed rest prescribed. If he is very thin, care must be taken that bony prominences are protected. An alternating air-pressure mattress is often helpful. If it is not available, a large piece of sponge rubber should be placed under the buttocks. Sponge rubber mattresses are also useful in the prevention of pressure sores. Areas of friction against linen should be watched for. If the patient braces himself on the bedpan by leaning on his elbows, thereby causing pressure areas, these areas should be massaged frequently with a lubricant. If the patient spends most of his time on the bedpan, it should be padded with sponge rubber, or a fracture pan can be used. If he uses the commode, it can also be protected with a piece of sponge rubber or with a rubber ring.

A record must be kept of the number, amount, and character of the stools, and specimens of stool should be sent to the laboratory as requested. Although each bowel movement may be very small, the commode or bedpan should be emptied as often as it is used. The patient wants the bedpan accessible at all times. He may even insist on keeping it in bed with him, and usually he is permitted to do so. Air-Wick or electric deodorizers are sometimes used to dispel unpleasant odors in the room. Linen should be kept fresh, and the patient's perineum, buttocks, and anal region should be washed thoroughly several times a day. Dibucaine (Nupercaine) or other prescribed ointment may be applied to the anus to relieve discomfort. Sitz baths are beneficial to the skin and circulation and are often permitted two or three times a day provided that the patient is carefully protected from chilling.

The patient should be kept warm, and drafts and chilling must be avoided. Extra covers should be provided so that the patient may use them as he wishes. Heat in the room and covers should provide enough warmth and protection to permit regular airing of the room to help remove odors and to supply fresh air.

Seeing that the patient eats the prescribed foods in adequate amounts and takes supplementary nourishment are essential parts of nursing care. Protein foods are very important. The ingenuity of the nurse will often be taxed in getting the patient to eat enough, since sometimes a real distaste for food is a symptom of this disease. Any concession or consideration that promises to increase food intake should be made. The family may be permitted to prepare favorite foods at home and to bring them to the patient provided that the foods are bland and otherwise conform to the prescribed diet.

If infusions and transfusions are necessary, these procedures must be carefully explained to the patient since they often cause apprehension. Because the patient's blood pressure is often low and his veins poor, and because he tolerates the annoyance

of these procedures poorly, care is taken to anchor the needle securely and to use an arm board so that the needle does not become dislodged.

During the patient's convalescence the nurse should be alert for any suggested problems. Because the physical causes of this condition are unknown, and the condition itself is not cured but only alleviated by the variety of treatments available, effort is made to learn of and control the emotional components of the disease. The social worker may be asked to talk to the patient and attempt to learn of social, economic, or other problems that are bothering him. The public health nurse may make a home visit before the patient leaves the hospital to determine whether or not he can be cared for properly at home and to report any other pertinent information. The family should be guided in ways to help the patient when he is at home, such as preparing food and thus helping to maintain nutrition, and understanding and accepting the disease and the patient's behavior. The patient needs careful follow-up on an outpatient basis.

Surgical management

An ileostomy usually is an operation that the patient accepts so that he may again be an active member of society without the constant annoyance of the symptoms of ulcerative colitis. An *ileostomy* is an opening into the small intestine (ileum) through the abdominal wall to the outside. Fecal material no longer passes through the large bowel to the rectum but is discharged through the opening in the abdominal wall. Special bags have been developed to collect this drainage, since the contents of the ileum are semiliquid. Preoperative visits and talks with patients who have made successful adjustments to ileostomies are helpful and tend to make the patient less fearful of the operation and its consequences. Persons who have had this operation sometimes gladly offer their services, and filmstrips about ileostomy care are available.

A few days before the operation, the patient is placed on a low-residue diet, and for 24 hours before surgery he receives only fluids. This decreases intestinal residue. Intestinal antibiotics such as phthalyl-sulfathiazole or neomycin are administered to lower the bacterial count of the intestine, which helps to prevent postoperative infection of the suture line. Immediately before surgery a nasogastric or intestinal tube is passed to keep the bowel empty.

One of three surgical procedures may be chosen in the treatment of a particular patient: an *ileostomy* and a *partial colectomy* may be performed, leaving a rectal stump, which may be anastomosed to the ileum at a later date; a *total proctocolectomy* through an abdominal perineal incision may be done, leaving the patient with a permanent ileostomy; or the large bowel may be resected and the ileum anastomosed to the remaining segment of colon at the time of the surgery.

A more recent surgical procedure is one that includes an ileal pouch with the ileostomy that eliminates the necessity of wearing an applied appliance and the problem of skin irritation.[7] An intra-abdominal reservoir with a potential capacity of 500 ml. is fashioned in 6 months so that the patient can intubate and evacuate the ileal contents several times daily. In 90% of the cases this procedure has successfully eliminated the need for wearing an external ileostomy bag.

After a partial colectomy, the patient returns from the operating room with two openings, sometimes called buds or stomas, on the abdominal wall. The proximal opening, which is usually on the right side, is the ileostomy from which liquid stool will flow. The distal opening, usually on the left side, leads to the remnant of lower bowel that has not yet been removed. If a total colectomy was performed, the patient will have only an ileostomy since the large bowel and rectum are removed.

The operation and nursing care of the patient undergoing an abdominal perineal resection are described later in this chapter. The patient having a colectomy and ileorectal anastomoses will have no opening in his abdomen. His nursing care is similar to that described on p. 690.

Ileostomy bag. After the resection, the proximal ileum is brought out onto the abdomen and sutured so that it is flush with the skin. Many surgeons prefer having the ileum project above the skin surface about $1/2$ to $3/4$ of an inch, since they have found that the appliance can then be worn with greater comfort.[47] A hole is cut in the back plate of a tempo-rary ileostomy bag so that it is large enough for fecal contents to drain into it but small enough so that drainage does not escape onto the skin. The purpose of the temporary ileostomy bag is to keep fecal drainage from running onto the abdomen and the incision while the wound is healing. The first few days after surgery the amount of drainage from the stoma may be very small. However, as soon as peristalsis returns and the patient begins to eat, fecal drainage begins. Enzymes in the contents of the small intestine can digest skin. The bag prevents these enteric enzymes from draining onto the skin and causing ulcerations that are difficult to heal and that make later use of a permanent collection appliance less successful. If the wound is healed, and swelling from the stoma has receded, the permanent bag may be applied before the patient leaves the hospital.

The temporary ileostomy bag usually is a disposable type (Fig. 25-13). It is held to the skin with skin adhesive. If the skin is intact and the bag properly applied, it will remain in place until lifted off or removed with ether or benzene. It usually needs to be changed every 3 or 4 days. Because the skin must be clean and dry for the application of the skin adhesive and the bag, the bag should be applied before the patient eats or several hours after eating, when there is likely to be little or no drainage from the ileostomy. The bag should be applied with the opening to the side so that the contents can be drained and the bag rinsed. Tincture of benzoin may be used to protect the skin. However, if the skin becomes irritated despite all efforts, an antacid such as Maalox can be applied to the area and allowed to dry until powdery. Tincture of benzoin is then applied over this. While the skin is still sticky, karaya powder is

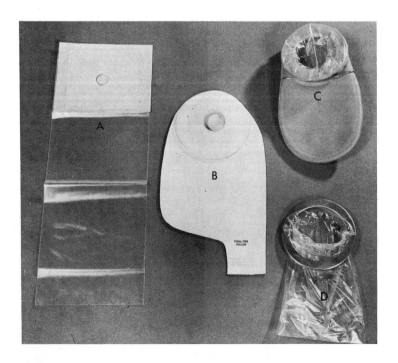

FIG. 25-13. Various types of drainage bags are available for patients with an ileostomy or a colostomy. **A,** Temporary disposable drainage bag; the opening may be enlarged to fit any orifice. **B,** Permanent ileostomy bag. **C,** Permanent colostomy bag. **D,** Colostomy bag with metal frame and disposable bag.

applied; then another coating of tincture of benzoin is added before the bag is affixed to the skin. Another method of skin protection is the use of a karaya gum doughnut around the stoma that is then used as a means of attaching the ileostomy bag. The karaya gum is water soluble and easily removed from the skin.

A permanent ileostomy bag is usually made of plastic material and lasts for 1 to 2 years. Bags are now available that can be discarded after each use. Since these bags are expensive for long-term use, the patient is encouraged to begin using a permanent bag before his discharge from the hospital. The patient should be taught how to change the bag and how to care for the skin and bag. Many patients leave the bag in place for several days. When this is done, some patients have found it helpful to make a cotton or felt covering for the bag. This prevents the bag from irritating the skin. They usually wear a belt to hold it securely. It can be emptied without being removed from the body. The elastic band at the bottom of the bag is removed and the contents allowed to flow into the toilet bowl. Then, with the use of a small glass syringe or an Asepto syringe, the inside of the bag may be washed with lukewarm water and soap and rinsed. When the bag is changed, the skin under it should be washed well. Most patients keep at least two bags so that the one most recently worn can be washed and soaked in a weak solution of vinegar (1 teaspoon to 1 quart of water) and then aired thoroughly. This care will prevent odors and increase the life of the bag.

Many patients are concerned lest the bag show under their clothing. If loose, full clothing is worn, the bag is not noticeable at all. In fact, many women patients wear pantyhose or a girdle over the bag and are able to wear fitted clothes. As the patient gains weight and his strength returns, he may engage in any activity he wishes. Many engage in active sports, and even swimming is possible. If a woman wears a bathing suit with a full skirt and a man wears loose trunks, no one will notice the bag. Some women have become pregnant and had normal antenatal courses and normal deliveries after having an ileostomy.

Preparation for discharge. Some patients have difficulty in adjusting to the care of the ileostomy and need a great deal of encouragement and instruction. The patient should be able to care for his ileostomy before he leaves the hospital. However, if he seems reluctant to learn self-care, it may be advisable to teach a member of his family. Later, when the patient feels better physically, he usually takes over his own care. Groups of patients who have ileostomies have banded together to form "ileostomy clubs" in various parts of the country (Q.T. clubs). They hold regular meetings to discuss mutual problems. Nurses are welcome to attend ileostomy club meet-ings as observers or as speakers. The journal *United Ostomy Quarterly* and other manuals are available on request by subscription to the United Ostomy Association.* The patient who is too far away to attend club meetings may want to arrange for the magazine to be sent to him. It will keep him aware of new developments in the care of ileostomies. He should be urged, however, to discuss any changes he contemplates making with his physician. Although most patients learn to accept their ileostomy and to care for it during a small part of their day, an occasional patient, unfortunately, will center most of his time and attention on it.

Diet. There are few dietary restrictions for persons who have an ileostomy. However, the patient needs to know that some foods such as corn will come through the ileostomy undigested and that foods such as cabbage will cause flatus. He also needs to know that beets may make the irrigating fluid red and lead the patient to believe that he is bleeding. Certain foods such as fresh fruits usually make the stool more liquid and profuse and therefore should be taken in small amounts or avoided. Each patient learns what foods cause him difficulty and avoids them. Any food that has caused diarrhea or flatus before the operation probably should be avoided. Before the patient leaves the hospital his food intake should be reviewed carefully with him. He should know how to plan his meals so that the essential foods are included. Much good illustrative material is available and can be secured from local health departments and voluntary agencies such as the National Dairy Council.

Complications. Gastrointestinal upsets are much more serious for patients with an ileostomy than for other people. Fluid and electrolyte balance is easily upset, and the patient may develop acidosis or alkalosis (p. 118). If nausea, vomiting, and diarrhea continue, medical attention should be sought.

Follow-up care. The patient who has an ileostomy must remain under medical supervision for some time. If he had a partial colectomy, he may be readmitted to the hospital later to have the ileum anastomosed to the rectum or to have the rectum removed. Before he leaves the hospital, he should be advised to have a public health nurse visit him in his home. The patient often does better if he knows that there is someone in the community to whom he may turn for advice and help in the simple details of daily care. He may have trouble with skin irritation, in obtaining new equipment, and in deciding on use of a new paste for the skin. He may have questions related to marriage, work, or recreation. The nurse can help him decide which of his questions and problems require medical advice. It must be remembered that the basic personality of the patient is not changed

---

*United Ostomy Association, 1111 Wilshire Blvd., Los Angeles, Calif. 90017.

by the operation, although the activities that the operation may make possible often produce remarkable changes in his attitudes and reactions toward himself and toward his problems.

■ AMEBIASIS

Amebiasis is caused by the protozoan parasite *Entamoeba histolytica,* which primarily invades the large intestine and secondarily invades the liver. The active, motile form of the protozoa, the trophozoite, is not infectious and, if ingested, is easily destroyed by digestive enzymes. The inactive form, or cyst, however, is highly resistant to extremes in temperature, most chemicals, and the digestive juices. When the cyst is swallowed in food or water, it easily passes into the intestines, where the active trophozoite is released and enters the intestinal wall. Here, it feeds on the mucosal cells, causing ulceration of the intestinal mucosa. Although the disease varies in severity, the onset is usually acute, with symptoms developing within 2 to 4 days of exposure. Weakness, prostration, nausea, vomiting, and a gripping pain in the right lower quadrant of the abdomen and tenesmus usually occur. Each day the patient has numerous semifluid, foul-smelling stools containing mucus and pus.

Prevention

It is estimated that at least 10% of the population of the United States have amebiasis in the acute, chronic, or asymptomatic stages.[8] Although the disease exists chiefly in the tropical countries, it also prevails wherever sanitation is poor. The cyst, which is the infectious agent, can survive for long periods outside the body, and it is transmitted by direct contact from man to man, by insects, and by contaminated water, milk, and other foods. For this reason, people traveling in tropical countries should drink only boiled water and eat only cooked foods. The most infectious agent is the "carrier," who, although having a few or no symptoms of the disease, passes the cysts in his stools. If his hygienic habits are poor and if he is a food handler, he can easily transmit the cysts to the food he prepares for consumption by others.

Management

If either the trophozoite or the cyst can be found in the stool, a positive diagnosis of amebiasis can be made and definitive treatment started. It is easier to find the parasite in the stool during the acute stage of the disease than later. Immediately after defecation, a warm stool should be sent to the laboratory for examination. Several stool specimens from successive bowel movements may be requested. If the laboratory is at a distance, the specimen container should be transported on a hot-water bottle or in a pan of warm water. When special laboratory facilities are required, a fresh stool can be placed in a preservative and sent to the Center for Disease Control, Atlanta, Georgia, for diagnosis.

The patient with a mild or asymptomatic form of amebiasis is treated on an outpatient basis; 90% of all patients usually respond to a course of amebicidal therapy.[8] The nurse should be familiar with drugs that are prescribed for this disease and should know their effects on the patient. If the halogenated hydroquinolines such as diiodohydroxyquin (Diodoquin) are given, the patient may have some diarrhea caused by them. Neurotoxicity to this agent has been reported recently.[1] The drug is administered in a dose of 650 mg. three times a day for 20 days. Tetracycline may be prescribed alone or in combination with diiodohydroxyquin. The maximum daily dose of tetracycline is 2 Gm. daily for 7 days.

Emetine hydrochloride may be used in the treatment of the disease, especially when liver abscess is suspected. The patient receiving emetine hydrochloride is placed on strict bed rest, and pulse rate and blood pressure are watched carefully since the drug is very toxic. Some of the many signs of toxicity to this drug include nausea, vomiting, diarrhea, generalized weakness, cardiac irregularity, fall in blood pressure, neuritis, desquamation of the skin, loss of the sense of taste, and mental depression. Emetine hydrochloride usually is given for 7 to 10 days. Recently, metronidazole has been used to treat symptomatic disease. It is administered two or three times per day with the maximum daily dose being 800 mg. for 7 days.

Amebiasis is a disease with remissions and exacerbations, and it may persist for years. During acute exacerbations the patient may become dehydrated, exhausted, or anemic and require hospitalization. During these times the nurse gives general care and assists with special treatments such as infusions and blood transfusions. The patient's diet should be reviewed with him. He should eat a bland, low-residue diet, and may be advised to avoid alcohol and tobacco.

A careful record of the patient's intake and output should be kept, and he should be encouraged to take generous amounts of fluid orally. The number and character of the stools should be described, and the bedpan should be sterilized after each use. In handling the bedpan, precautions should be taken since some cysts are usually passed. Cleanliness should be stressed, and the patient should know why it is so important to wash his hands after bowel movements. Particular emphasis should be placed on careful washing of hands before meals to avoid reinfection.

Persons known to be exposed to amebiasis should have stool examinations weekly for 3 weeks. If infected, they will be treated as described for the asymptomatic form of the disease.[1]

SALMONELLOSIS

The salmonella infections are a group of acute infections caused by variations of the motile gram-negative *Salmonella* bacillus. There are more than 1,200 strains of the bacillus, many of which are capable of producing disease in both animals and man. The *Salmonella* organisms cause gastroenteritis and food poisoning; septicemia and localized infections such as endocarditis, pneumonia, osteomyelitis, meningitis, and pyelonephritis; paratyphoid fever; and typhoid fever.[1] In recent years the incidence of typhoid fever in the United States has stayed at about 500 cases per year.[8]

Infection with *Salmonella* organisms is acquired through the oral route. The source of infection may be through milk, water, ingestion of infected animal tissues, or ingestion of other foods contaminated by persons who have the organisms on their hands. Eggs have been found to carry the organisms and cracked eggshells allow the organism to enter and contaminate the egg. One large metropolitan hospital had several cases of salmonellosis develop among their hospitalized patients, and this outbreak was traced to contaminated eggs. Persons with subclinical disease and carriers can pass the infection to others who are more susceptible. Bone meal fertilizer and domestic animal and pet foods have been known to harbor the organism.

Gastroenteritis usually appears within 8 to 48 hours of ingesting the organisms in large numbers. It is more common in children than in adults. Diarrhea may vary in amount from 1 to 10 L./day and result in moderate to critical fluid and electrolyte losses. Enteric fever and bacteremia usually appear within 1 to 10 days of exposure and last from 1 to 3 weeks. In both of these conditions the patient's temperature may be elevated markedly, and he may have nausea, vomiting, and other signs of a severe systemic infection. In bacteremia, blood cultures will be positive for the organism, and in both enteric disease and in bacteremia caused by *Salmonella* organisms, the stools are usually positive 1 or 2 weeks after acute symptoms appear.

The treatment of *Salmonella* infections depends on the disease present and the patient's symptoms. Fluids are usually forced, and a diet that is bland and largely liquid is ordered. If the patient is unable to take sufficient fluids and calories orally, fluids are given parenterally.

In *Salmonella* food poisoning, usually no chemotherapy is given since it does not seem to alter the course of the disease or shorten the period of time the individual will be a carrier of the organism. For patients with paratyphoid fever and typhoid fever, ampicillin is the drug of choice; chloramphenicol (Chloromycetin) is administered when the organisms are resistant to ampicillin.[1] Ampicillin may also be administered for 3 to 6 weeks to typhoid carriers in an attempt to rid them of the organism. It is not effective, however, in treating carriers of paratyphoid. Removal of the diseased gallbladder may eradicate the carrier state.

Nursing care of the patient with salmonellosis depends on the severity of the infection and the symptoms present. Excreta may need to be disinfected. Precautions should be taken in handling all body discharges. Other aspects of nursing care depend on the symptoms and may include general nursing measures for headache, excessive diaphoresis, restlessness, and poor mouth hygiene as well as depression and discouragement.

The nurse has a responsibility in teaching the prevention of *Salmonella* infections. Prevention can be accomplished best by adequate washing of the hands before eating and by all who handle food, adequate refrigeration of uncooked and prepared foods, and thorough cooking of meats, eggs, and egg products. Because of the increased incidence of these infections, the use of uncooked eggs is no longer recommended. At the present time no immunization is being given for any of the *Salmonella* group except *Salmonella typhosa,* which causes typhoid fever. Immunization against typhoid fever is indicated only in the following situations: (1) exposure to a carrier in a household, (2) outbreaks of typhoid fever in a community, and (3) travel to areas where typhoid fever is endemic.[1]

■ TRICHINOSIS

Autopsy reports show that at least 5% of the population of the United States is affected with trichinosis. No immunization is possible and no specific treatment is available, yet the disease could be eradicated with the knowledge that we now possess.[8] The disease is caused by the larvae of a species of roundworm, *Trichinella spiralis,* which become encysted in the striated muscles of man, hogs, and other animals, particularly those (such as rodents) that consume infected pork in garbage. Trichinosis is transmitted through inadequately cooked food. Pork is the most common source of infection. When infected food is eaten, live encysted larvae develop within the intestine of the host, mate, and produce eggs that hatch in the uterus of the female worm. The larvae are discharged in huge numbers (approximately 1,500/worm) into the lymphatics and lacteals of the host's small intestine at the rate of about two an hour for about 6 weeks. They pass to the muscles of the host, where they become encysted by the reaction of the host's body and may remain for 10 years or longer.

Signs and symptoms of trichinosis are varied. Although the reason is unknown, edema appears as puffiness about the eyes, particularly involving the upper lids. If a very large number of larvae have been ingested, nausea, vomiting, and diarrhea due to intestinal irritation usually occur about 4 days after the infected food has been eaten. On about the seventh day, when the larvae migrate throughout the body to the muscles, there are usually muscle stiffness, weakness, and remittent fever. The extent of these symptoms depends on the number of larvae present and the resistance of the host. There may be pain in the back, the muscles of the eyeballs, the muscles of chewing, and elsewhere in the body. Muscles of the diaphragm are often affected, causing pain on breathing. An increase in the eosinophil count is a characteristic finding in trichinosis and persists for several weeks after the onset of acute symptoms. Trichinosis can cause death, which usually occurs from pneumonia or cachexia from 4 to 6 weeks following the onset of symptoms. Death may also occur from paralysis of the respiratory muscles.

The incidence and prevalence of trichinosis are higher in the United States than in any other country in the world. It occurs much more often in hogs that have been fed garbage than in those fed on grain. The larvae do not form cysts in pork. Therefore they are not visible to the naked eye and cannot be seen by food inspectors.

Basic scientific facts necessary for the complete prevention of the disease in human beings have been known for years. Trichinae can be killed by cooking and by freezing at a temperature of $-18°$ C. ($0°$ F.) for 24 hours. They are not killed by smoking, pickling, or other methods of processing. Sausage and other infected pork products carelessly prepared are a common source of infection in man. Other meats ground in the same machine without thorough cleaning or cut on the same meat block may also cause infection. There is a need for thorough cooking of all pork products consumed at home regardless of how sanitary the local meat market may appear to be. A safe rule to follow is to never eat pork products in a restaurant—only at home, where adequate cooking can be assured—and never eat any ground meat without thoroughly cooking it.

■ DIVERTICULOSIS AND DIVERTICULITIS

A diverticulum of the colon is an outpouching of mucosa (through a weak point in the muscular layer of the bowel wall) resulting from persistent and abnormally high intracolonic pressure. The presence of many diverticula in the sigmoid and the descending colon is called "diverticulosis." If diverticula become inflamed, the term "diverticulitis" is used. The cause of diverticula is unknown. Recent studies postulate that the removal of indigestible fiber from the diet may contribute to the development of the disease.[12b] At least 10% of the total population has this condition, which is much more common in middle-aged and elderly persons than in the young. Some experts have described it as the most common disease of the colon.[12b] In itself, a diverticulum is a benign condition usually causing no symptoms. It may, however, become impacted with feces and become irritated, inflamed, and infected. Diverticulitis may sometimes be prevented by care in selection of food and avoidance of constipation. A fairly bland, low-residue diet is usually recommended, and a stool softener may be prescribed.

The patient with diverticulitis complains of general discomfort or pain in the left lower quadrant. There may be local tenderness, leukocytosis, and fever. Hemorrhage occurs in about 10% to 20% of all patients and may be chronic and mild or severe. The patient is usually treated conservatively with a low-roughage diet, daily doses of a softening agent or a demulcent such as Metamucil, antispasmodics, and sedation. More recently, smooth but bulky foods have been prescribed with good results.[50a] Antibiotics are given when there are signs of infection.

A possible complication of diverticulitis is perforation, with resultant abscess formation or generalized peritonitis. The inflammatory process may also cause bowel obstruction. The patient may require surgery for treatment of these conditions, and occasionally surgery is also done to remove a portion of the seriously involved bowel. A colostomy is sometimes necessary.

■ CANCER OF THE COLON

Malignant tumors of the large bowel and rectum are the most common forms of cancer. Approximately one fourth of all gastrointestinal cancers arise in the colon. In 1975, it is expected that 69,000 Americans will be affected, and there will be 39,000 deaths. The number of cases are thought to be increasing in frequency because of the increase in the life span. Although the cause of cancer of the colon is unknown, various possible contributory factors called carcinogens have been suggested such as food additives, bacteria, and stool bulk (roughage) as well as bowel transit time (bowel stasis). In addition, isolated polyps are known to undergo malignant changes.[14] *Familial polyposis,* therefore, may predispose to the development of cancer of the lower bowel. Because, in the early stages, symptoms of cancer of the colon are vague and may be absent, it is now recommended that the yearly physical examination of persons over 40 years of age includes examination for the presence of this disease. Since carcinoma of the lower bowel is more common in men than in women, it has also been recommended that all men over 40 years of age have this examination. In some cancer detection clinics, proctoscopic examinations are made routinely on all men past 35 years of age.

Anyone in whom constipation, diarrhea, or alternating constipation and diarrhea develops should seek medical attention at once. Changes in the shape of the stool, the passing of blood rectally, and any change in bowel habits also should be reported. Weakness and fatigue are sometimes the first signs of cancer of the colon since constant loss of blood in the stool may go unnoticed, and a severe anemia may develop.

Early discovery of the growth and its immediate removal offer a fairly good chance for cure. In the beginning stage of the cancer growth the tumor is confined to the intestinal mucosa, gradually extending around the bowel to form a stricture and causing early symptoms of bowel obstruction. Eventually the cancer penetrates the wall of the colon and spreads either directly into the peritoneum or into abdominal organs or indirectly through the lymphatics into the surrounding lymph nodes and through the blood vessels to the liver and other structures.

Symptoms of cancer of the colon vary with the location of the growth. Carcinoma of the colon on the right side (ascending colon) usually is a large cauliflower-like growth. It causes severe anemia, nausea, vomiting, and alternating constipation and diarrhea. A mass is usually palpable on the right side of the abdomen. There are no symptoms of obstruction as a rule because the fecal contents in this portion of the colon are still liquid and able to flow past the growth.

Carcinoma of the colon on the left side (descending colon) often produces symptoms of partial obstruction because the stool is harder on that side. Although tumors in this area are usually smaller than those found in the colon on the right side, they proliferate fibrous tissue which, as it contracts, causes narrowing of the lumen of the bowel. Because the stool in the bowel on the left side is formed, it has difficulty passing by the tumor and through the stenosed area. The patient becomes progressively constipated, the stool may be small or flattened, "pencil-shaped," or "ribbon-shaped." Blood, mucus, and pus may be passed with the bowel movement. The abdomen may become distended, and rumbling of flatus and fluid may be heard. Seventy-five percent of the cancers of the lower bowel occur in the rectum and sigmoid part of the colon.[51]

Diagnosis of cancer of the colon is made by physical examination, sigmoidoscopy, and barium enema examination. The treatment is always surgical, and the tumor, surrounding colon, and lymph nodes are resected. If possible, the remaining portions of the bowel are anastomosed. If cancer of the ascending colon is found, the colon on the right side is entirely removed (right colectomy), and the ileum is anastomosed to the transverse colon (ileotransverse colostomy). Growths of the descending colon or upper sigmoid are removed by a left colectomy, and the remaining sigmoid is anastomosed to the transverse colon. If the cancerous growth is such that it is not resectable, or if the growth has caused an obstruc-

tion with accompanying inflammation, an opening may be made into the cecum (cecostomy) or into the transverse colon (transverse colostomy) as a palliative measure to permit the escape of fecal contents. When the edema and the inflammation around the tumor subside, the growth is resected, the bowel sections are anastomosed, and the cecostomy or colostomy usually is closed. The preoperative and postoperative nursing care of patients who have resection of the bowel, a cecostomy, or a colostomy is discussed later in this chapter.

Carcinoma of the colon may cause a complete obstruction, and the acute symptoms of obstruction may be the first indication that anything is wrong. Occasionally the tumor perforates into the peritoneal cavity and peritonitis occurs before any other signs of illness have been noticed by the patient.

■ HERNIA

A hernia is a protrusion of an organ or structure from its normal cavity through a congenital or acquired defect. Depending on its location, the hernia may contain peritoneal fat, a loop of bowel, a section of bladder, or a portion of the stomach. If the protruding structure of the organ can be returned by manipulation to its own cavity, it is called a *reducible* hernia. If it cannot, it is called an *irreducible* or an *incarcerated* hernia. The size of the defect through

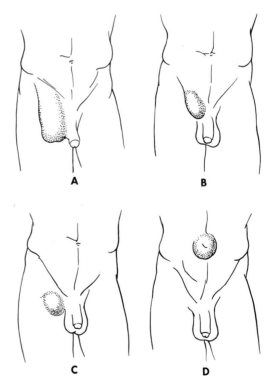

FIG. 25-14. Types of hernias. **A,** Large indirect inguinal hernia. **B,** Direct inguinal hernia. **C,** Femoral hernia. **D,** Umbilical hernia.

which the structure or organ passes (the neck of the hernia) determines largely whether or not the hernia can be reduced. When the blood supply to the structure within the hernia becomes occluded, the hernia is said to be *strangulated.*

The patient with a hernia complains of a lump in the groin, around the umbilicus, or protruding from an old surgical incision (Fig. 25-14). The swelling may have always been present, or it may have suddenly appeared after coughing, straining, lifting, or other vigorous exertion.

A hernia may cause no symptoms except swelling that disappears when the patient lies down and reappears when he stands up or coughs. If pain is present, it may be due to local irritation of the parietal peritoneum or to traction on the omentum. An incarcerated hernia may become strangulated, causing severe pain and symptoms of intestinal obstruction such as nausea, vomiting, and distention. These complications require emergency surgery, and a portion of bowel may have to be resected if it has become gangrenous from impairment of its circulation.

Unless there are contraindications due to age or physical condition, most hernias can be treated successfully by surgery. When the patient is in good physical condition and when the hernia is causing little or no discomfort, elective surgery may be done. Surgery obviates the serious complications of untreated hernias such as strangulation and incarceration. Patients who have unusual abdominal protrusions or enlargements, therefore, should be advised to seek medical advice. If a hernia is found during a preemployment physical examination, employment may be deferred until the hernia is repaired. This is particularly likely when the work involves physical labor. Since the hernias that occur as a result of employment are compensable, the time and money involved in their treatment are of economic concern to the employer. Unfortunately the patient too often seeks medical attention only if the protrusion becomes troublesome, if he fears it is malignant, or if he must have it repaired before he can be accepted for employment.

An *indirect inguinal hernia* is one in which a loop of intestine passes through the abdominal ring and follows the course of the spermatic cord into the inguinal canal. The descent of the hernia may end in the inguinal canal, or it may proceed into the scrotum (and occasionally into the labia). It is caused by the intestines being forced by increased intra-abdominal pressure into a congenital defect resulting from failure of the processus vaginalis to close after the descent of the testes in the male and after fixation of the ovaries in the female. Indirect hernias are much more common in men than in women. This higher incidence in men may be explained in part by their participation in more vigorous exercise and by the size of the testes, which must pass through the inguinal ring during fetal life.

A *direct inguinal hernia* is one that passes through the posterior inguinal wall. It is caused by increased intra-abdominal pressure against a congenitally weak posterior inguinal wall. These hernias are more common in men. They are the most difficult to repair and are likely to recur after surgery.

A *femoral hernia* is one in which a loop of intestine passes through the femoral ring and down the femoral canal. It appears as a round bulge below the inguinal ligament and is thought to be due to a congenital weakness in the femoral ring. Increased intra-abdominal pressure due to pregnancy or obesity probably causes the herniation through weakened muscle. Femoral hernias are more common in women than in men. This is thought to be because of the inclination of the female pelvis.

An *umbilical hernia* is one in which a loop of intestine passes through the umbilical ring. It is caused either by the failure of the umbilicus to close at birth or by a congenital defect in the umbilical scar, which opens in adult life under conditions causing increased intra-abdominal pressure such as pregnancy, intestinal obstruction, or a chronic cough. Infantile umbilical hernias occur frequently in nonwhite babies. Umbilical hernias that occur in adults are seen most often in elderly, obese women.

An *incisional hernia* is one that occurs through an old surgical incision. It is caused by the failure of the resected and approximated muscles and fascial tissues to heal properly because of wound infections, drains, or poor physical condition. As a result of increased intra-abdominal pressure, a portion of the intestine or other organs and tissues may protrude through the weakened scar.

Management

The patient can very often reduce the hernia (return it to its normal position) by lying down with his feet elevated or by lying in a tub of warm water and pushing the mass gently back toward the abdominal cavity. If his physical condition does not permit surgery, the physician sometimes advocates the use of a *truss* to keep the hernia reduced. However, this device is not a cure, and its use is somewhat rare. A truss is a pad made of firm material that is placed over the opening through which the hernia protrudes and is held in place with a belt. The truss should be applied before the patient gets out of bed and after the hernia has been reduced. If the hernia cannot be reduced, the truss should not be applied and the patient should seek medical treatment. The truss should be applied next to the body, since underclothing worn under it causes it to slide and decreases its effectiveness. Irritation of the skin under the truss can be overcome by daily bathing and the use of talcum powder. Unless the patient has a chronic cough, the truss should be removed when he is in bed.

The only cure for a hernia is surgical treatment. The herniating tissues are returned to the abdominal cavity, and the defect in the fascia or muscle is closed with sutures *(herniorrhaphy).* To prevent recurrence of the hernia and to facilitate closure of the defect, a *hernioplasty* may be performed using fascia, filigree wire, tantalum mesh, stainless steel mesh, or a variety of plastic materials to strengthen the muscle wall.

The preoperative preparation for a hernia repair includes examination to detect any diseases of the respiratory system that might cause increased intra-abdominal pressure postoperatively. A chronic cough due to excessive smoking or other causes or excessive sneezing due to an allergy might cause weakening of the repair before the incision has completely healed. The operation is postponed until the patient recovers from any respiratory disorder that is discovered. The nurse should report to the surgeon any signs of incipient upper respiratory infection since such an infection may occur after he has examined the patient.

In addition to good general postoperative care, the nurse, in caring for the patient who has had an operation for a hernia, should prevent tension on the newly repaired tissues. Postoperatively the nurse should be alert for signs of respiratory infection. If a cough occurs, medications are usually prescribed to depress the cough reflex. They should be given as ordered to prevent paroxysms of coughing and subsequent strain on the repair. The patient should be instructed to hold his hand firmly over the operative area when coughing or sneezing.

Since urinary retention may occur after a herniorrhaphy, appropriate nursing measures should be taken to prevent the bladder from becoming overdistended. Catheterization is sometimes necessary. The patient is usually permitted to get out of bed to void on the operative day, and after the first day he has full ambulatory privileges.

The patient who has elective surgery for a hernia usually is permitted a full diet as soon as it is tolerated. If a spinal anesthetic is used and the abdominal cavity is not entered, there is usually no loss of peristalsis, and the patient is able to eat normally at once. If a general anesthetic is used, fluid and food are restricted until peristalsis returns. When an umbilical or a large incisional hernia has been repaired, a nasogastric tube attached to suction may be used to prevent postoperative vomiting and distention with subsequent strain on the suture line. Fluids are given parenterally, and food and fluids by mouth are restricted. Abdominal distention following a hernia repair should be reported at once. The physician may pass a nasogastric tube, or he may order a rectal tube inserted. Mild cathartics may be prescribed since straining during defecation increases intra-abdominal pressure and should be avoided.

Because of postoperative inflammation, edema, and hemorrhage, swelling of the scrotum often occurs after repair of an indirect inguinal hernia.

This complication is extremely painful, and any movement of the patient causes discomfort. It is difficult to turn, to get into or out of bed, and to walk. Ice bags help to relieve pain. The scrotum is usually supported with a suspensory or is elevated on a rolled towel. Narcotics may sometimes be necessary for pain, and antibiotics may be administered to prevent the development of epididymitis. When a patient has a swollen scrotum, the nurse must check his voiding carefully. He may delay voiding because moving about increases pain and discomfort.

Wound infection occurs occasionally. It interferes with healing, and if it is not recognized early and treated adequately, the repair may weaken. Infections are treated with antibiotics systemically and with dressings or packs locally (p. 88).

The patient who has had elective surgery for a hernia is usually hospitalized for 5 to 7 days, but he is restricted from strenuous activity for at least 3 weeks. He should be advised to consult the surgeon about when he may return to work. If his work entails lifting, he should be certain that the physician knows this, and he should be instructed in good body mechanics.

■ PERITONITIS

Peritonitis is an inflammatory involvement of the peritoneum caused by trauma or by rupture of an organ containing bacteria, which are then introduced into the abdominal cavity. Some of the organisms found are *Escherichia coli,* streptococci (both aerobic and anaerobic) staphylococci, pneumococci, and gonococci. Peritonitis also can be caused by chemical response to irritating substances such as might occur following rupture of the fallopian tube in an ectopic pregnancy, perforation of a gastric ulcer, or traumatic rupture of the spleen or liver. Inflammation due to chemical causes, however, is so closely followed by invasion of blood-borne bacteria that it is only a few hours before organisms may be isolated from most fluids that accumulate in peritonitis.

Local reactions of the peritoneum include redness, inflammation, edema, and the production of large amounts of fluid containing electrolytes and proteins. Hypovolemia, electrolyte imbalance, dehydration, and finally shock develop due to the loss of fluid, electrolytes, and proteins into the peritoneal cavity. The fluid usually becomes purulent as the condition progresses and as bacteria become more numerous. Peristalsis is halted by the severe peritoneal infection, and all the symptoms of acute intestinal obstruction may occur. They include nausea, vomiting, pain in the abdomen, severe distention, rigidity of the abdominal wall, and failure to pass anything rectally. The patient's white blood cell count is usually high. Peritonitis also causes serious systemic symptoms, including high temperature, tachycardia, weakness, diaphoresis, pallor, and all other signs of severe systemic reaction and of shock. Peritonitis is a very serious disease that had an extremely high mortality rate before antimicrobial and bacteriostatic drugs and other modern treatment became available.

Management

Management usually consists of emergency measures to combat infection, restore intestinal motility, and supply lost electrolytes and fluids. Massive doses of antibiotics are administered parenterally. Intestinal or gastric intubation is usually ordered at once, the tubes are attached to suction, and a rectal tube is inserted. Fluids and electrolytes are given intravenously. The patient is not given anything orally, and narcotics and sedatives are given for severe pain and apprehension as soon as the diagnosis is confirmed and there is no danger of masking symptoms.

Nursing care of the patient having gastric and intestinal intubation was discussed earlier in this chapter. The patient who has acute peritonitis needs constant nursing care since he is extremely apprehensive. Pain and discomfort may also be so severe that he cannot be expected to use good judgment in leaving the nasogastric tube in place and in keeping his arm still on a board when an infusion is being given. The patient should be given mouth care, and protection is needed to prevent drying and cracking of the lips since dehydration is usually marked.

Usually the patient is placed in a semi-Fowler's position so that gravity may help localize pus in the lower abdomen or the pelvis. Also, in this position the patient can take deeper breaths with less pain, which helps to prevent respiratory complications. Heat may occasionally be applied to the abdomen, but some doctors feel that heat is not advisable.

Natural barriers are used in the body's attempt to control the inflammation. Adhesions quickly form in an attempt to wall off the infection, and the omentum helps to enclose areas of inflammation. These processes may result in involvement of only part of the abdominal cavity and may finally narrow the infected area to a small, enclosed one (abscess). As healing occurs, fibrous adhesions may shrink and disappear entirely so that no trace of infection can be found on exploration of the abdomen at a much later date, or else they may persist as constrictions that may permanently bind the involved structures together. Sometimes they cause an intestinal obstruction by occluding the lumen of the bowel. If abscesses form, they are usually in the lower abdomen. They may, however, be walled off elsewhere. For example, abscess formation following a ruptured appendix may develop under the diaphragm (Fig. 4-1) and may even perforate that structure and cause an empyema.

If the peritonitis is caused by a perforation which is releasing irritating or infected material into the abdominal cavity, surgery is performed as soon as the patient's condition permits. However, if the patient is in shock, it may be several hours before shock can be relieved and before surgery can be safely performed. The operation usually consists of closure of the abnormal opening into the abdominal cavity and removal of the fluid that has accumulated. (See discussion of perforated peptic ulcer for further details of nursing care, p. 669.) If peritonitis is due to the rupture of a fallopian tube, as in an ectopic pregnancy, the tube must be removed (p. 518).

■ INTESTINAL OBSTRUCTION

Intestinal obstruction develops when intestinal contents cannot pass through the lumen of the bowel. It may be due to mechanical causes, neurogenic causes (paralytic ileus), or vascular abnormalities (Fig. 25-15). *Mechanical obstruction* is most often caused by strangulated hernias and adhesions, although cancer of the large bowel accounts for the majority of cases of mechanical obstruction in the colon.[51] Other mechanical causes are *volvulus* (a twisting of the bowel) and *intussusception* (telescoping of a segment of the bowel within itself, most common in emaciated infants and small children). Volvulus occurs most often in elderly persons, and the sigmoid loop of the large bowel is usually affected. Bands, strictures, and adhesions that cause obstruction of the bowel lumen may be congenital but usually result from previous abdominal surgery or peritonitis.

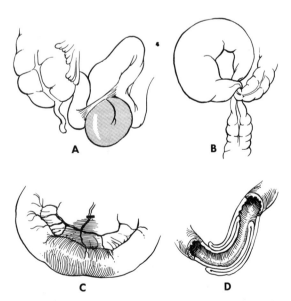

FIG. 25-15. Some causes of intestinal obstruction. **A,** Constriction by adhesions. **B,** Volvulus. **C,** Mesenteric thrombosis. **D,** Intussusception.

In *neurogenic obstruction* there is interference with the innervation of the bowel, which causes peristalsis to cease or to be markedly retarded. Paralytic ileus may be a complication of peritonitis, acute medical illness such as pneumonia, a reaction to severe pain, or changes in circulatory supply to the bowel. Other causes of paralytic ileus include handling of the bowel during surgery, spinal cord lesions, electrolyte imbalance, or toxic conditions such as uremia.

Obstruction due to vascular disease is relatively rare and usually occurs in persons who have evidence of other vascular disease. Occlusion usually occurs in the superior mesenteric vessels, cutting off the blood supply to a large segment of the bowel. When the affected portion of the bowel is unable to perform its muscular function, peristalsis ceases, and the bowel becomes distended with fluid, gas, and food residue and rapidly becomes gangrenous.

The symptoms of intestinal obstruction vary according to the degree and site of obstruction. In general, sudden acute mechanical occlusions located high in the intestinal tract produce more intense and earlier symptoms than those occurring lower in the system. When the lumen of the bowel first becomes obstructed, there is an increase in peristalsis above the occlusion in an attempt to move intestinal contents past the obstruction. As the peristaltic waves become more forceful, they cause sharp intermittent or cramping abdominal pain. The increased peristaltic activity also injures the intestinal wall, causing edema around the obstructed area, and the intestine proximal to the obstruction becomes distended. Normally most of the fluid in the intestinal tract is absorbed through the intestinal wall, helping to maintain fluid and electrolyte balance. When the intestine is obstructed, however, the normal absorptive power of the intestinal mucosa is lacking because of irritation from hyperactivity and/or impairment of circulation. Most of the gas consists of swallowed air that contains about 79% nitrogen and is slowly absorbed from the intestinal tract. The combined presence of fluid and this gas in the bowel causes increased tension and may occlude the blood supply, causing gangrene to develop. The bowel distal to the obstruction remains empty and constricted so that there is no passage of gas or stool rectally.

Vomiting that occurs with intestinal obstruction may be frequent, abrupt in onset, copious, often spontaneous, and foul in odor (often fecal). Such vomiting is caused by reverse peristalsis, as the intestinal contents are regurgitated into the stomach, from which they are ejected. In general, the higher the obstruction, the earlier and more severe is the vomiting. If the obstruction is in the large bowel, vomiting may not occur as the ileocecal valve permits fluid to enter the colon but prevents its passage back into the ileum.

Intestinal obstruction is an extremely serious condition which, if not treated promptly, can cause death within a few hours. Failure of the normal absorptive powers of the intestinal wall to continue and the loss of fluid through vomiting cause severe fluid and electrolyte imbalance. Bacteria and toxins escaping through the affected bowel may cause toxemia and peritonitis. The patient develops all the signs of shock and requires immediate treatment.

General principles of management

The treatment for intestinal obstruction is intestinal intubation, the administration of fluids and electrolytes by infusion, and the relief of mechanical and vascular obstruction by surgery. Paralytic ileus is not treated surgically unless gangrene of a portion of the bowel has occurred. The operative procedure varies with the cause and the location of the obstruction and the general condition of the patient. If constricting bands or adhesions are found, they are cut, and it may be necessary to resect the occluded bowel and to anastomose the remaining segments. It may be necessary to do a temporary cecostomy or colostomy and, later, when the patient is in better physical condition, a resection and anastomosis of the bowel may be performed.

Nursing intervention includes caring for the intestinal tube, maintaining intestinal decompression, and keeping an accurate record of all intake and output. Intravenous fluids are ordered to maintain fluid and electrolyte balance. The nurse should report any increase in temperature because it may indicate more obstruction or peritonitis. Good supportive care must be given. Pain and vomiting often leave the patient physically and emotionally exhausted. He may need assistance in simple activities such as turning in bed, and he needs encouragement and assurance that the intubation and other treatment usually result in lessening of symptoms within a short time. Skin and mouth care are essential. Any vomitus should be immediately removed from the bedside since its foul odor may increase nausea. Pulmonary ventilation should have the nurse's careful attention. Since intestinal distention may cause respiratory distress, the patient usually is more comfortable in a Fowler's position. He should be encouraged to breathe through the nose and not to swallow air because it increases the distention and discomfort. A rectal tube may be used to provide relief from lower abdominal distention. Enemas or colonic irrigations may be ordered, and the nurse must carefully observe and record the results of these treatments. The nurse should be alert for signs that peristalsis has returned and should report the passage of flatus and any abnormal substances such as blood or mucus. Urinary retention due to pressure on the bladder may occur, and the patient should be observed for this and the amount at each voiding recorded. A total

24-hour urinary output below 500 ml. should be reported to the physician.

Management of the patient requiring resection and anastomosis of the bowel

Preoperative care. Preoperative preparation of the patient who is to have surgery of the bowel varies in some aspects from that of preparation for other abdominal surgery. During the preoperative period the patient is usually given a low-residue diet so that the bowel will contain little or no stool at the time of surgery. Bowel cleansing methods plus the inability of the bowel to absorb vitamins necessitate the administration of supplemental vitamins such as vitamins K and C. Parenteral fluids and electrolytes are given to replace losses from the bowel preparation, the restricted food and oral intake, and the bowel absorptive failure. Intravenous hyperalimentation may be used to administer fluid (p. 112), electrolytes, and proteins in the debilitated patient in preparation for surgery. Twenty-four hours prior to surgery a clear liquid diet may be given if tolerated. The reasons for diet restriction as well as for the intravenous fluids should be explained to the patient and his family.

Antibiotics specific for organisms found in the bowel may be administered 3 to 5 days before surgery in an attempt to decrease the bacterial count of bowel contents, which helps to decrease the incidence of postoperative wound infection. Oral antibiotics used to "sterilize" the bowel include succinylsulfathiazole (Sulfasuxidine), phthalylsulfathiazole (Sulfathalidine), and neomycin. These drugs are poorly absorbed from the gastrointestinal tract and thus their concentration in the bloodstream is low. A cathartic such as magnesium sulfate may be given before they are administered, and then the drugs are given in large doses every 4 hours until the operation is performed. The patient may also receive a daily cathartic or enemas followed by instillation of phthalylsulfathiazole into the bowel. Some surgeons do not use oral antibiotics because they do not believe the bowel can be sterilized and because use of antibiotics may cause pseudomembranous enterocolitis, an infrequent but serious disease of the colon.

Still others believe intestinal antibiotics are of little value without significant reduction of stool mass. Rigorous purging and diet reduction may be poorly tolerated by the elderly or the acutely ill patient. Therefore the general physical state of the patient is carefully assessed as well as the degree of bowel obstruction in order to modify preoperative preparation. Many patients require a high-calorie intake in order to survive, and 5% dextrose alone is not sufficient to meet their needs. Intravenous hyperalimentation is often used to provide adequate nutrients and prevent negative nitrogen balance.[27]

A nasogastric or intestinal tube is inserted before the operation. Since the passage of a tube into the intestines may take as long as 24 hours, intestinal intubation is usually started the day before surgery. As the tube passes through the small intestine, the bowel becomes "threaded" on it and thus is compactly held together and shortened while the operation is performed. Before and after surgery, the intestinal tube is usually attached to a suction apparatus for the aspiration of intestinal contents. This prevents the accumulation of gas and intestinal fluid around the suture line. If a nasogastric tube is used, it is inserted the morning the operation is scheduled.

Postoperative care. Until peristalsis returns and the anastomosis is partially healed, the nasogastric or intestinal tube is used, and special attention must be given to keeping the tube draining and to maintenance of fluid and electrolyte balance. The surgeon carefully checks the amount of solutions needed and reviews the daily output from voiding and from aspiration through the tube. The nurse must be very certain that recording of these fluids is accurate and that all fluids given as infusions or by other means the previous day are also carefully included in the patient's record. The patient should have mouth care frequently, and an antibiotic solution may be ordered for this care, since colon bacteria may reach the mouth via a "wick action," especially when an intestinal tube is used.

Because the patient may have some difficulty voiding after bowel surgery, all available nursing measures should be instituted to prevent urine retention. If these fail, a Foley catheter may be used (p. 455). Pain in the incision may be severe and may interfere with full respiratory excursion. The patient should be given narcotics as necessary for pain and must then be encouraged to cough and to breathe deeply. He must also be encouraged to change his position every hour or two and often needs encouragement and assistance in doing so during the first day or two postoperatively.

A rectal tube can be inserted to facilitate the passage of flatus. Drugs to stimulate expulsion of flatus such as dexpanthenol (Ilopan) or neostigmine (Prostigmin) may be administered. Since ambulation is of great assistance in starting peristalsis, the patient is assisted out of bed a day or two after surgery, even while the nasogastric or intestinal tube is still in use. The passage of gas or stool rectally should be reported to the surgeon at once, since it usually indicates the return of peristalsis and means that the patient may begin to take something orally and that the intestinal tube can be removed.

Until the intestinal tube is removed, the patient is not given anything by mouth, and total food and fluid needs are met by the parenteral route. After the tube is removed, the patient gradually is given additional foods until he has a full diet, although occasionally bland foods may be given for some time after surgery. It is not unusual for patients who have had a resection of the bowel to have some diarrhea after peristalsis returns. Usually it is temporary and soon disappears. When the stool becomes normal, the patient is advised to avoid becoming constipated because a hard stool and straining to expel it could possibly injure the anastomosis, depending on its location. If he has a tendency to develop constipation postoperatively, he should try drinking fruit juice and water before breakfast or taking a glass of prune juice daily. He should not take laxatives without medical approval. Stool softeners or a mild bulk cathartic such as psyllium (Metamucil) is prescribed frequently.

Management of the patient requiring a cecostomy

Although the treatment of choice for growths in the ascending colon is a resection and anastomosis or a transverse colostomy, a temporary cecostomy is occasionally performed to relieve obstruction if the patient cannot tolerate major surgery. With the use of local anesthesia to control pain, an opening is made into the cecum through a small incision in the right lower quadrant of the abdomen, and a catheter is inserted into the bowel. The catheter is sutured to the skin and provides an outlet for feces, which is still fluid in the ascending colon. Tubing is attached to the catheter, which is attached to a bottle that is capped to control odors but that is provided with an air vent so that drainage can occur. The tubing should be long enough so that the patient can move about freely. In order to keep the tube open, it is usually irrigated every 4 hours with a physiologic solution of sodium chloride. The fluid is allowed to run in by gravity and flows out by inverting the syringe or funnel or by aspiration.

The dressings around the tube should be changed as frequently as necessary, and the skin should be kept clean and dry. After the tube is removed, skin care and changes of dressing should be continued until all drainage ceases (Fig. 20-18). Occasionally an ileostomy bag is used to keep drainage off the skin (Fig. 25-10). A water-soluble chlorophyll derivative (Chloresium) may be applied for its soothing, antipruritic, and deodorizing effects.

Management of the patient requiring a colostomy

A colostomy is an operation in which an artificial opening is made into the colon. It is performed to permit escape of feces when there is an obstruction of the large bowel or a known lesion such as cancer that will eventually cause an obstruction. It also may be done to permit healing of the bowel distal to it after an infection, perforation, or traumatic injury since it diverts the fecal stream from the affected area. It is sometimes done as a palliative measure in the treatment of an obstruction caused by an inoperable growth of the colon, or if the rectum must be removed to treat cancer, a colostomy may be performed to provide a permanent means of bowel evacuation.

When the physician first tells the patient of the probable need for a colostomy, the patient's immediate response is likely to be one of shock and disbelief. Whether the colostomy is to be temporary or permanent, he finds it very difficult to accept. Knowledge that it is a lifesaving measure, confidence in the surgeon, and sometimes explanation and acceptance of the proposed operation by members of his family may convince him to consent to the operation. It is not unusual for the patient to be sad, withdrawn, and depressed, especially as he is threatened by the change or altered body image as the result of a colostomy.[30]

Occasionally a patient commits suicide in the hospital or abruptly signs himself out of the hospital when he knows that a colostomy is necessary. The nurse should anticipate and prepare for possible events and should help auxiliary nursing personnel to understand the emotional turmoil the patient is experiencing. The patient's reaction to a proposed colostomy will be based on the way he sees it affecting his life, his physical stature, his place in his family, his economic welfare and that of his loved ones, his social life, and many other situations that have meaning for him. His response will depend on his social and cultural background and on his emotional makeup as well as on a number of other circumstances.

The nurse should be prepared to supplement any information given to the patient by the physician and to assess how much information to give him preoperatively on care of the colostomy. Some patients definitely benefit from discussing the care, reading materials, seeing equipment, and talking to persons who are living normal lives following a colostomy. Others find this approach upsetting. The patient should, however, have a simple explanation of the anatomy of the colon, how surgery will alter the normal bowel function, and how the colostomy can be managed as a routine part of his daily activities.[37] The nurse needs to assess the patient's readiness for this kind of learning and plan accordingly.

Some hospitals have prepared printed materials for patients who have had a colostomy. Booklets on colostomy care also may be packaged with colostomy bags and equipment sold commercially. If printed material is used, it should be carefully discussed with the patient before it is left with him. After he has perused it, the nurse should plan to spend additional time answering any questions he may have. One of the advantages of this type of material is that the patient has a reference available after his discharge from the hospital. It adds to his security in caring for himself.

Members of the patient's family should be encouraged to visit him often since it is essential that the patient who has had a colostomy feel loved and accepted. During the preoperative period, effort should also be made to augment the patient's confidence in the members of the medical and nursing staff, since the patient who has complete confidence in the persons who will treat and care for him is more likely to accept his situation postoperatively and be more willing to start to learn self-care. The patient watches every facial expression or gesture of the nurses and is extremely sensitive to evidence of distaste. If other persons accept the colostomy as not unusual, it helps the patient to feel that it is not a calamity that has happened to him alone.

Occasionally a patient may reject the colostomy completely postoperatively and will make no attempt to learn to care for it. With help however, most patients will learn to care for themselves. As soon as the patient indicates that he is ready, the nurse should take every opportunity to have him look at the colostomy and to assist in small ways in his care. In this way, fear and distaste for the task can usually be gradually overcome. Every effort should be made to keep the patient as clean and dry as possible. He may become emotionally upset and depressed at the sight of fecal drainage and particularly when the drainage is liquid and soils the bed and his gown in addition to dressings. Soiled dressings and linen should be disposed of neatly and quickly. They make the patient depressed, interfere with his activity and his desire to eat, and delay his acceptance of the colostomy. Soiling of the bedclothes and the patient's clothing should be prevented if at all possible, but the patient should understand that, until defecation through the colostomy has been regulated, occasional soiling of bedclothes may occur. He should be reassured that it is not of major importance and that he should not let fear of continuous drainage keep him from moving about freely in bed. This is very seldom a problem in colostomy care. If it is, however, a disposable colostomy bag should be tried.

Although it is useless and even detrimental to urge the patient to participate in his own care before he is able to accept self-care, the nurse should quietly, calmly, but persistently encourage increasing participation. Usually, a major psychologic hurdle for the patient is seeing the colostomy for the first time and observing while it is cared for. The nurse should observe the patient's physical and emotional status and determine how much participation is appropriate for him. The nurse may need to assist the patient in accepting his altered self-image prior to teaching self-care. Allowing the patient to ventilate his feelings may prove to be the most important goal of the rehabilitative process.[30] It is sometimes necessary to work with a member of the family and to teach him to care for the patient. If this is not possible or if there are no relatives, plans may need to be made for care in a nursing home or for a public health nurse to visit the home to give part of the regular care.

Transverse colostomy

A transverse colostomy eliminates function of all the bowel distal to it and is performed to relieve an obstruction, to divert the fecal stream and thus permit healing of a portion of the bowel, or as a palliative measure to prevent obstruction in inoperable lesions of the lower bowel. Two types of procedures may be performed. The transverse colon may be divided and the ends brought out at the margins of the skin incision. This type is called a *double-barreled colostomy.* The proximal opening, or stoma, in the right margin of the incision is the outlet for the stool, and the distal left opening (stoma) leads to the now nonfunctioning lower bowel. This type of colostomy may begin to drain feces as soon as peristalsis returns after surgery.

In another method a loop of the transverse colon is brought out into the abdominal wall, and the skin and underlying tissues are sutured *(loop colostomy)* (Fig. 25-16). A glass rod, the ends of which are connected to a piece of rubber tubing, usually is placed between the loop of the bowel and the skin to prevent the bowel from slipping back into the abdominal cavity. The rod is left in place until the wound is well healed and the loop of bowel has become adherent to the abdominal wall. This takes about 10 days. The bowel usually is not opened to permit the escape of intestinal contents for 3 to 5 days after the operation, which allows the skin incision to heal and prevents contamination of the abdominal cavity. A nasogastric tube is used until the loop of bowel is opened, and the passage of gas and stool indicates the return of peristalsis. The bowel is usually opened by an incision made with a scalpel. The lumen is exposed but is not divided completely. It may also be opened by electric cautery to minimize bleeding. The colostomy is usually opened in the treatment room since it does not cause pain and no anesthetic is necessary. Because the bowel has no sensory nerve endings, the patient may be assured that he will have no pain, If cauterization is done, however, the odor of burning flesh may disturb the patient and may cause nausea. The opened bowel now has a proximal opening leading to the functioning gastrointestinal tract from which stool and flatus will flow and a distal opening leading to the colon and rectum similar to the double-barreled colostomy. Since it may be difficult to establish which is the distal opening, the nurse who assists the surgeon in opening the bowel or with the first irrigation should obtain this information and make a drawing on the nursing care plan, indicating the proximal and distal openings. However, if such information has not been recorded, inspection will reveal the opening from which fecal material is coming; this is the proximal opening.

Care of the colostomy. Because semiliquid drainage from the opening may be fairly constant, the skin should be washed with soap and water, and the

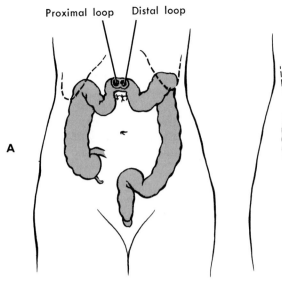

Proximal loop   Distal loop

A

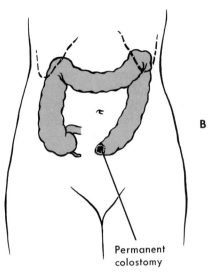

B

Permanent
colostomy

FIG. 25-16. A, Transverse colostomy that may or may not be permanent. **B,** Permanent colostomy following an abdominoperineal resection.

dressings should be changed as often as necessary to prevent skin irritation. A piece of plastic film or other waterproof material, cut large enough to envelop the dressings and with an opening in the center cut to fit snugly around the colostomy bud yet not compress it, may be used to prevent fecal contents from getting onto the skin and staining the patient's gown or bed linen. This dressing is similar to that used for patients who have had ureteral surgery (p. 439 and Fig. 20-18). Montgomery straps may be used to hold the dressing in place and obviate the need for frequent removal and application of adhesive tape. Petroleum jelly gauze or a protective ointment is sometimes placed around the opening to keep the skin from becoming irritated. However, the ointment must be removed at frequent intervals to ascertain that the skin under the protective coating remains in good condition. The use of ointments may make the appearance of the colostomy more objectionable to the patient.

The patient's bedside unit should be equipped with supplies needed for changing the dressings. It is best to keep the equipment on a tray that is easily available to both the patient and the nurse. The tray should be stocked with paper bags or newspapers for disposal of waste, gauze for dressings, cotton for cleansing the skin, abdominal pads for extra protection over the dressings, petroleum jelly gauze or protective ointments and tongue blades for their application, tincture of benzoin, and extra Montgomery straps.

As soon as the patient is physically able, he should be encouraged to assist in changing the dressings. Since this procedure is not a sterile one, washed, used gauze or unsterile pieces of gauze may be used. The gauze should be rolled and placed about the opening in doughnut fashion, thus preventing drainage from easily seeping out the bottom and sides of the dressing. If the gauze is opened and fluffed, it will be more absorbent than a flat piece.

A colostomy irrigation may be done regularly through the proximal opening. However, elimination through the opening rarely can be completely regulated so that there is no drainage between irrigations. The irrigation procedure is described in the discussion on care of the patient who has had a permanent colostomy. A colostomy bag usually is necessary for the patient who has a transverse colostomy. Without it, he may have difficulty in engaging in daily activities. Often it is when the bag is to be worn that the patient first takes an interest in his own care. The bag tends to give him a feeling of security. If disposable bags are not used, the colostomy bag must be cleansed daily and immediately following its removal. It should be washed thoroughly with soap and water, dried, powdered to prevent the two surfaces from sticking together, and allowed to air for at least 12 hours. If this procedure does not remove odors, the patient may be advised to soak the bag for $1/2$ hour in a weak solution of chlorine household bleach or vinegar.

Materials needed for the colostomy should be obtained early so that they will be available for use before the patient leaves the hospital. He should not be discharged from the hospital until he or a member of his family is competent in caring for the colostomy or until other arrangements for his care have been made. This is extremely important since it may color the patient's ultimate adjustment to his situation. It is advisable to ask a public health nurse to visit the patient in his home to evaluate the adjustment he has made and to give him and his family additional help if necessary. The public health nurse should report her findings to the physician or the nurse in the hospital or clinic. Most patients welcome the suggestion that a nurse may be available to visit them at home. The patient should remain under medical care and should feel that there is a nurse in the physician's office, the hospital clinic, or the public health agency to whom he can turn for help in overcoming problems related to normal living following the colostomy.

Closure of the colostomy. If the colostomy was performed to relieve obstruction or to divert the fecal stream to permit healing of a portion of the bowel, the patient will be readmitted to the hospital at a later date for a further examination and for possible resection of the diseased portion of the bowel. The opening may subsequently be closed.

In preparation for a resection of the bowel and closure of the colostomy the physician may order irrigations of the distal loop. Fluid, usually normal saline solution, is instilled into the distal loop through a catheter attached to a funnel or Asepto syringe. For this irrigation the patient should sit on the bedpan or on the toilet since, unless there is complete obstruction, the solution may be expelled rectally. Mucus and shreds of necrotic tissue may be passed. The returns should be inspected before they are discarded. A nonabsorbable sulfonamide derivative such as phthalylsulfathiazole dissolved in a small amount of water may be slowly instilled into the distal loop and rectum after the irrigation. The patient should be asked to retain this solution as long as possible since the antibiotic lowers the bacterial count of the bowel contents and lessens the risks of postoperative infection.

Permanent colostomy

A permanent colostomy is usually performed in conjunction with an abdominal perineal resection for cancer of the rectum. After the sigmoid colon is resected, the proximal end is brought out through the abdominal wall and sutured to it to become the permanent opening for the elimination of feces. Although there is no sphincter control, bowel movements from a sigmoid colostomy can be regulated or controlled by regular habits of eating and by giving an enema at a specific time each day. The time interval for the enema may be altered later as an evacuation pattern is established.

At the time of the operation the proximal end of the resected sigmoid is brought out through the incision and sutured to the skin so that the opening, called a stoma or bud, is flush or level with the abdominal wall. The patient returns from the operating room with a dressing over the colostomy. There is usually no drainage from the opening until peristalsis returns, approximately 24 to 48 hours after the operation.

As soon as peristalsis returns, as evidenced by the passage of gas or stool, the nasogastric tube is removed. The patient may then progress from a liquid to a regular diet as tolerated. The dressing should be changed as frequently as necessary, and the skin should be kept clean and dry, as described in the discussion of care of a transverse colostomy. The incision may be protected with collodion or a water-soluble tape.

Colostomy irrigation. About the fifth to the seventh postoperative day the surgeon usually does the first irrigation through the artificial opening. If the returns are satisfactory and the opening is unobstructed, the nurse then assumes responsibility for subsequent irrigations. It is a nursing function to teach the patient how to establish regularity of evacuation through the colostomy and how to irrigate it. Some patients need to irrigate the colostomy every day, whereas others may need to do so only every 2 to 3 days. The latter is likely to be true if the patient normally has not had a bowel movement every day. Some patients find that a very small amount of water stimulates normal evacuation. An occasional patient may not have to irrigate at all. He may find that at the regular time for evacuation the colostomy empties spontaneously.

Equipment needed for the irrigations should be assembled on a tray, and the patient should be encouraged to keep it in a convenient place when he returns home. While commercial irrigation sets are used by most patients, it is possible to improvise equipment; for example, a soft plastic container from the grocery store may be used as an irrigating cup. Some clinics are using a bulb syringe technique.[56] Various types of commercial irrigation sets are available, but the principles of all are the same. The cup that fits over the opening has a small hole in the center through which to insert the catheter. The cup is usually plastic so that returns can be easily seen, and it is held snugly in place against the abdominal wall with elasticized straps. Outlet tubing attached to the cup allows drainage of the fecal material into the toilet or into a bucket if the patient does the irrigation in bed. The irrigator prevents uncontrolled drainage of the fluid and feces. The nurse should know that special cups are available for the patient who has an unusually large or high opening, although in modern practice the opening is made to be flush with the skin so that no protrusion should exist. Representatives of the various manufacturers are glad to give advice and assistance in such matters. In addition to the irrigator, the patient needs a 2-quart enema can or bag, tubing 2 feet long, a glass connecting tip, a 16 or 18 Fr. catheter (usually a whistle-tip catheter is employed), a tubing clamp, a pitcher for extra water, toilet tissue, petroleum jelly to lubricate the catheter, a paper bag or newspaper, dressings, and an irrigating pole or a hook on which to hang the bag. The patient may install a hook in his bathroom at home or he may use a clotheshorse. The hook should be so placed that there are no more than 18 to 24 inches between the irrigating fluid and the colostomy opening. A small table or shelf on which to place equipment within easy reach should also be provided.

As soon as the patient is ambulatory, the irrigation should be done on a commode or on the toilet. Bathrooms that have poor ventilation and that do not afford privacy should be avoided since the procedure is a long one, taking at least 1 hour and often longer at first, and the patient is extremely self-conscious. At first it may be necessary to pad the toilet seat with sponge rubber and to provide some support for the patient's back. Several bath blankets in a pillowcase can be used. When the equipment has been assembled, water obtained for the irrigation, privacy assured, and the patient comfortably settled on the toilet, the dressing is removed, and the area around the colostomy is cleansed with reclaimed gauze or with disposable tissues that can be discarded in the toilet. Warm tap water, about 40.5° C. (105° F.), is used, although cool water has been used because it is believed to stimulate peristalsis and thereby lessen the time necessary for the procedure.[61] After the air has been expelled from the tubing, the lubricated catheter is inserted through the opening in the cup and through the colostomy opening into the bowel. The cup is fastened snugly against the skin, and the outlet tubing is allowed to hang between the patient's legs into the toilet bowl. When the catheter is inserted 10 to 20 cm. (4 to 6 inches), the clamp on the tubing is released and the solution is allowed to flow into the bowel. After about one third or one half of the solution has run into the bowel, the inlet tubing should be clamped until the fluid and fecal contents drain out. If, during the insertion of the fluid, the patient has abdominal cramps, the inflow should be clamped for several minutes. Excessive cramping usually means that the irrigating can is too high and the fluid is running in too rapidly. This should be avoided in order to lessen discomfort and because markedly increased peristalsis may hamper passage of material through the intestine. The procedure is continued until a normal amount of fecal material is expelled. For some patients, this may require only 500 ml. of fluid, whereas others may need more fluid.

The patient usually benefits psychologically from sitting on the toilet during the irrigation. Discarding tissues into the toilet and draining the bag directly makes him feel that his situation is not so far from normal as he had feared. If possible, the same nurse should assist the patient with this procedure for several successive days (Fig. 25-17). This saves the patient embarrassment and enables the nurse to give appropriate encouragement, reassurance, and assistance without the patient's having to repeat his particular difficulties and problems.

When the irrigation is completed, the patient should be encouraged to massage the abdomen, to bend forward and from side to side, and to stand up once or twice before the cup is removed. Considerable variation in the time necessary for an irrigation

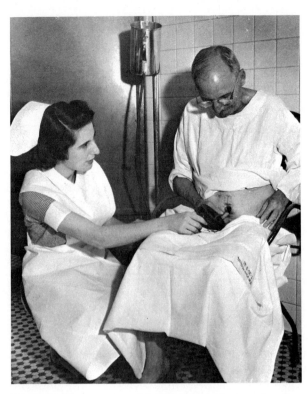

FIG. 25-17. The nurse assists the patient in learning to irrigate his colostomy. (From Anderson, H. C.: Newton's geriatric nursing, ed. 5, St. Louis, 1971, The C. V. Mosby Co.)

exists among patients. Since it may take 20 minutes or longer for the bowel to completely empty, some patients read during that time. Most patients leave the cup on and clamp off the bottom of its outlet while they take a shower, do household chores, or shave since there may be a small amount of drainage after they start to move about. If elimination has been regulated, only a small dressing such as a piece of cleansing tissue needs to be worn over the colostomy. This dressing prevents the clothing from being stained with the small amount of mucus that may drain from the opening. When elimination is well regulated, it is preferable that the patient not wear a colostomy bag, thus obviating any possibility of odors. Some patients, however, worry lest they have drainage and can become regulated only when a bag is worn. Because emotional upsets and worry hinder regulation, it is not always advisable to insist that the patient with a permanent colostomy go without a bag.

As the nurse helps the patient with the irrigations, he is given step-by-step directions. Gradually the patient should take over one step of the procedure after another until, before discharge from the hospital, he is assembling his own equipment, doing the irrigation, and cleaning the equipment. The nurse should continue to do some part of the procedure occasionally so that the patient will feel that she is interested in his welfare.

Regularity of evacuation through the colostomy depends on setting up and maintaining a regular routine in its care. Before irrigations are started in the hospital, the nurse and the patient should try to determine the time of day it will be most convenient for him to do the irrigations when he returns home. He should remember that the procedure will probably prevent use of the bathroom by others for some time, and he must plan for his family's needs as well as his own. If possible, the irrigations should be done in the hospital at the time that will be best to do them at home, so that a pattern of regularity will not have to be reestablished when the patient goes home. Because the amount of solution needed to completely empty the bowel and to prevent any leakage until the next irrigation varies among individuals, it must be tested for each patient. After the irrigation, the nurse should note any incontinence. If incontinence has occurred, the amount of fluid should be increased.

A permanent colostomy may need to be dilated because of narrowing of the opening due to shrinkage during and after healing. The procedure is usually initiated by the surgeon after the intestines become adherent to the abdominal wall, usually within 10 days postoperatively. If the patient has difficulty inserting the irrigation tube, he should report this to the physician immediately. In an effort to avoid stoma stricture the physician may advise the patient to insert his finger into the colostomy opening about once a week.

The patient may eat the food that he enjoys and that he was accustomed to before his operation. However, he should avoid foods that have caused diarrhea in the past. Fruits and vegetables may be increased in the diet when constipation is a problem. Most patients who have had a colostomy avoid gas-forming foods such as beans and cabbage, since the flatus is not retained by the artificial opening, which has no real sphincter.

When the skin incision is healed and the patient is physically able, he may bathe, swim, work, and engage in any physical or social activities he chooses. The convalescent period usually lasts from 2 to 4 months. However, the care of the colostomy should be mastered and regularity should be established within 2 to 4 weeks. The patient should be encouraged to have a public health nurse visit him in his home since he often finds that some unanticipated adjustments need to be made after he is home.

The family is not always able to accept the patient who has a colostomy. There may be strong feelings of disgust or revulsion at the colostomy and its function, fear of cancer, or less well-defined rejection of body mutilation. If difficulties of this kind seem apparent for any patient, the nurse should discuss them with the physician. Sometimes the social worker can help to work out a solution for the patient in the hospital, and often a public health nurse can help in the transition from hospital to home.

Surgical bypass procedure for massive obesity

In recent decades it has been clearly recognized that obese individuals have a shortened life span.[12] Statistics of insurance companies have shown a substantial increase in mortality from arteriosclerotic cardiovascular disease and cirrhosis of the liver in those who are considered morbidly obese. It is generally agreed that massively obese persons have an increased predisposition for diabetes, hypertension, bronchitis, osteoarthritis, and other serious ailments.

Since medical treatment in the form of dietary restriction, medications for appetite control, as well as hypnosis and psychiatric therapy often is unsuccessful, surgical procedures have been tried in an attempt to alleviate the problem of obesity. Various surgical procedures have evolved in the past 20 years in an effort to "shunt" or bypass a portion of the small intestine and limit the area available for absorption of fats and carbohydrates. The most recent procedure is the jejunoileal bypass in which approximately 14 inches of the jejunum and 4 inches of the ileum are preserved for the bypass anastomosis.[50] The 14 inches of the proximal jejunum is anastomosed to the side of the ileum 4 inches from the ileocecal valve. The retention of the ileocecal area is an important factor in retarding the intestinal transit time and thus permitting longer contact of the chyme to the intestinal mucosa. The long length of bypassed jejunoileum is anastomosed with the ileal end to the transverse colon or sigmoid colon.

Patients selected for surgery are carefully evaluated physically and mentally. Studies are carried out with special attention being given to the cardiopulmonary and endocrine status as well as the gastrointestinal assessment of the stomach, small bowel, and colon function. Preoperative measurements of serum calcium, potassium, magnesium, and other electrolytes plus assessment of vitamins A, B_{12}, and C and folic acid are made. Psychologic evaluation is considered essential by most physicians in determining the patient's response to weight loss and change in body image and his acceptance of the close surveillance of metabolic changes that may occur postoperatively.[50]

The majority of the patients have an uneventful recovery. In some, hypokalemia and hypocalcemia may occur and supplementation may be necessary. Malabsorption of the fat-soluble vitamins A, D, E, and K and particularly vitamin B_{12} may cause a deficiency and require replacement therapy. Some patients may have diarrhea as a result of diminished fat digestion and absorption. These patients are taught to avoid excessive liquid intake and excessive fat intake as a means of controlling bowel function.

Occasionally medication may be necessary to control persistent diarrhea.[54]

Weekly follow-up is essential in the immediate postoperative period, and periodic clinical evaluation in the subsequent years must be impressed on the patient. After discharge, the patient's rehabilitation and desired loss of weight is achieved by his physician's long-range metabolic and nutritional follow-up.[12,13a,50]

Diseases of the rectum and anal canal

Patients having surgery involving the rectum and anal canal may present special nursing problems. After these operations, the tissues around the anus may be very sensitive to pain. Careful attention to this area is needed to provide maximum comfort for the patient while healing takes place.

■ CANCER OF THE RECTUM

Cancer of the rectum and lower sigmoid is quite common. It occurs most frequently in men between 50 and 60 years of age. Cancer of the rectum metastasizes slowly, since the tumor extends by direct extension through the rectal wall to surrounding tissues before metastasis through the lymphatic and venous systems occurs.

The most common symptoms of cancer of the rectum and sigmoid are the passage of small amounts of bright red blood in the stool and alteration in bowel habits. Either constipation or diarrhea may occur, or these two conditions may alternate. Early diagnosis and treatment are possible only if the patient reports early symptoms to a physician. The importance of reporting these seemingly unimportant but most significant symptoms cannot be overemphasized to the public, since pain does not occur until the disease is far advanced. Cancer of the rectum can be accurately diagnosed by pathologic examination of a biopsy of the lesion taken during a proctoscopic examination.

Usually growths in the middle and lower third of the rectum require removal of the entire rectum, leaving the patient with a permanent colostomy. For growths in the upper third of the rectum, it may be possible to resect that portion containing the tumor and then anastomose the remaining segments so that the anal sphincter is maintained and normal bowel evacuation is possible. The nursing care of patients having a resection of the rectum would be similar to that described on p. 690.

Abdominoperineal resection of the bowel

Most malignant growths in the rectum are removed by an operation known as an abdominoperineal resection of the bowel. The operation is performed through two incisions: a low midline incision of the abdomen and a wide circular incision about the anus. Through the abdominal incision, the sigmoid colon is divided and the lower portion is freed from its attachments and temporarily left beneath the peritoneum of the pelvic floor. The proximal end of the sigmoid is then brought out through a small stab wound on the abdominal wall and becomes the permanent colostomy. Through the perineal incision the anus and rectum are freed from the perineal muscles, and the anus, the rectum containing the growth, and the distal portion of sigmoid are removed. The perineal wound may be closed around Penrose drains, or it may be left wide open and packed with gauze and a rubber dam to cause it to heal slowly from the inside outward.

Preoperative care. Preoperative nursing care of the patient who is to have an abdominoperineal resection of the bowel is similar to that given the patient having other intestinal surgery. Such care is described earlier in this chapter. Some surgeons pass ureteral catheters preoperatively so that the ureters are not inadvertently tied off during surgery. A Foley catheter is inserted into the bladder and attached to a straight drainage system to keep the bladder empty during surgery and thus prevent operative injury.

Postoperative care. Postoperatively the patient has a permanent sigmoid colostomy. The care of this colostomy was discussed earlier in this chapter. Because a large amount of tissue is removed at this operation, the patient is frequently in shock immediately postoperatively. Vital signs should be noted frequently, and urinary output may be checked hourly. A urinary output below 30 ml./hour may indicate impending renal failure, which may necessitate fluids and other means to elevate the blood pressure and thus increase perfusion through the kidneys. Rectal dressings should be watched carefully for signs of excessive bleeding. The usual drainage is serosanguineous and profuse. The mattress, therefore, should be adequately protected, and pads that can be changed without unduly disturbing the patient should be used. The dressing may need to be reinforced during the first few hours postoperatively. After the surgeon has changed the first dressing (usually 24 hours postoperatively), the nurse may be requested to change the dressings as necessary. Since the dressing requires frequent changing, a T binder gives the best support without causing skin irritation.

Bed rest may be prescribed for several days because of the effect of the extensive surgery on the patient. The surgeon may also wish to avoid having the patient get up too soon so that the pelvic floor can heal partially and the danger of a perineal hernia can be avoided.

Since the patient usually has severe pain while lying on his back, and because he finds it very difficult to turn, he usually prefers to lie on one side and remain there. He must, however, be encouraged to change his position frequently, to breathe deeply, and to cough productively. IPPB treatments may be ordered to improve ventilation. During the first few days the nurse should assist him in turning as necessary and should help him to do exercises in bed. For example, he must be encouraged to straighten out his knees, to dorsiflex the feet, and to tense the muscles of the legs. In an effort to make the patient comfortable the nurse must see that positions such as flexion of the knees that may predispose to development of postoperative thrombophlebitis are avoided. Pillows should be used to add to the patient's comfort, but the nurse *must* assist him in changing positions at regular and frequent intervals. Some patients are comfortable in a flat position lying on a rubber air ring. Others find that this position causes a pull on the incision. The patient is most comfortable on a firm bed with pieces of sponge rubber placed to relieve pressure on weight-bearing areas and to support the perineal dressing when he is lying on his back.

The patient usually needs a narcotic for pain at regular intervals for the first 2 or 3 days postoperatively. If he is in the older age group, however, the narcotic should be given judiciously so that respirations and physical activity are not decreased too much. Smaller doses may be sufficient for older patients. If the nurse finds that the dose appears to depress the patient too much, this should be discussed with the surgeon.

The Foley catheter usually is left in the bladder postoperatively to prevent the bladder from becoming distended and from pressing against the repaired pelvic floor until it heals. Its use also eliminates the need for women patients to use the bedpan to void (a very painful procedure after this operation) and prevents contamination of the wound and dressings with urine. The catheter, however, fairly frequently causes irritation and infection of the bladder. After it is removed, the patient may be unable to void or may void inadequately. It may then have to be reinserted for several more days, or the patient may be catheterized at specified intervals as necessary until he is able to void normally. Occasionally, following this operation, the male patient requires a prostatectomy for benign prostatic hypertrophy. Antibiotics

and large amounts of fluid are given when an indwelling catheter is used. Special care should be taken that the catheter drains constantly so that residual urine does not remain in the bladder. (See p. 455 for discussion of care of patients needing catheters.)

If the perineal wound has been packed, the packing is removed gradually. If a drainage tube or drain has been sutured in the perineal wound, it usually is removed by the second or third postoperative day. After it is removed, the wound is usually irrigated once or twice a day to remove secretions and tissue debris, to prevent abscesses from forming in the dead space that may be left, and to help ensure healing of the wound from the inside outward. If a catheter is to be inserted into the wound for the irrigation, the nurse should ascertain from the surgeon how deep it can be inserted and in what direction to insert it. Precise directions as to how to do the irrigation should be recorded on the nursing care plan.

Normal saline solution or diluted hydrogen peroxide is frequently used as the irrigating solution. When the patient is permitted out of bed, sitz baths may be substituted for the irrigations, and as drainage from the wound decreases, a perineal pad may be substituted for the dressing. A rubber ring should be used when the patient takes a sitz bath so that water can flow freely around the incision. The response in healing is often quite remarkable when this is done. Since the patient is usually ready to leave the hospital before the perineal wound has completely closed, arrangements must be made for him to continue to take sitz baths at home. If he does not have a bathtub available, a large basin may be used. A public health nurse should always be called on to assist the patient and his family in procedures of this kind to avoid accidents and to give the patient the assurance of professional help as he cares for himself.

Because a longer period of bed rest may be necessary than following many operations, the patient is usually weaker than most patients when ambulation is attempted. He should be very carefully assisted and closely observed until he is strong enough to get about alone with safety. If a plastic-covered pillow, a piece of sponge rubber, or a flotation pad is placed on the chair, the patient is usually more comfortable and is able to sit up for a longer time.

Convalescence after an abdominoperineal operation is prolonged and may require months. During this time the patient should remain under close medical supervision. A well-prepared and detailed interagency referral from the nurse in the hospital to the nurse in the public health agency helps a great deal in assuring continuity of care for the patient. By this means the nurse in the home may contact one of the nurses who gave the patient care in the hospital or the physician to discuss any problems encountered while giving guidance and assistance to the patient and to his family. This helps to prevent minor differences in procedures or in other instructions which may be upsetting to the patient.

■ DISEASE CONDITIONS OF THE ANUS

Although most conditions of the anus usually do not endanger the life of the patient, they are often a source of chronic discomfort and concern. They may cause a great deal of pain because the anus is well supplied with nerves. These diseases may prevent the patient from walking or sitting comfortably, may increase or initiate constipation, and may even cause so much local discomfort that the patient is unable to work. Even after treatment, local discomfort may continue for some time, and although the treatment is minor, the patient may have difficulty in readily resuming normal activity. The nurse should be aware of the problems that patients with disease of the anal area encounter, and she should try to anticipate nursing care that will prevent and relieve discomfort.

Hemorrhoids

Hemorrhoids are one of the most common afflictions of man, and they cause an enormous amount of pain and discomfort. Congestion occurs in the veins of the hemorrhoidal plexus and leads to varicosities within the lower rectum and the anus. The cause for the development of this condition is not definitely known, but many factors seem to be involved. Heredity, occupations requiring long periods of standing or sitting, the erect posture assumed by man, structural absence of valves in the hemorrhoidal veins, increase of intra-abdominal pressure caused by constipation, straining at defecation, and pregnancy all are factors predisposing to development of hemorrhoids.

Internal hemorrhoids appear above the internal sphincter and are not apparent to the patient unless they become so large that they protrude through the anus, where they may become constricted and painful. Internal hemorrhoids often bleed on defecation, and although the amount of blood lost may be small, continuous oozing over a long period of time may cause an iron deficiency anemia. *External hemorrhoids* are those which appear outside the anal sphincter. They bleed relatively rarely and seldom cause pain unless a hemorrhoidal vein ruptures and a so-called thrombosis occurs. If this occurs, the hemorrhoid becomes inflamed and extremely painful.

Many patients have both internal and external hemorrhoids. Constipation often predisposes to the development of hemorrhoids and usually becomes worse after they occur because the patient tries to restrain bowel movements that produce pain or bleeding. Other people resort to laxatives without competent medical supervision. Although hemorrhoids rarely undergo malignant degeneration, constipation and bleeding are symptoms of cancer of the rectum. For this reason all patients with these symptoms should have a medical examination to rule out cancer. The nurse is often in a position to advise persons who have what they assume to be painless bleeding hemorrhoids of long duration to visit their physician.

Management. The treatment of hemorrhoids consists of local treatment, sclerosing by injection, ligation, and surgery. The local application of ice, warm compresses, or analgesic ointments such as dibucaine (Nupercaine) gives temporary relief from pain and reduces the edema around external hemorrhoids or prolapsed internal ones. Sitz baths are also extremely helpful in relieving pain. The physician may prescribe agents to soften the stool. Thrombosed external hemorrhoids usually respond to this treatment with lessening of pain and absorption of the confined blood. Finally, only a painless skin tag remains, and it is not removed surgically unless it causes strictures or its presence interferes with cleanliness enough to aggravate the patient seriously. If a thrombosed external hemorrhoid does not respond to medical treatment, it may be incised to release the encased blood. This procedure usually is done in a physician's office and results in immediate relief of pain.

Injection is used in the treatment of moderate-sized internal hemorrhoids that cause bleeding or are protruding. A sclerosing solution such as 5% phenol in oil is injected carefully into the submucous areolar tissue in which the hemorrhoidal veins lie to produce an inflammatory reaction. Fibrous induration, which surrounds and constricts the veins, occurs at the site of the injection in 2 or 3 weeks. Bleeding from the hemorrhoids usually stops within 24 to 48 hours. There is some local pain at the time of the injection but there usually is no limitation of activity following this treatment.

Internal hemorrhoids may be treated by ligating them with rubber bands. The hemorrhoid is grasped with a forceps and pulled down into a special instrument which, when the trigger handle is pressed, slips an elastic band over it. The rubber band constricts the circulation and causes necrosis. The destroyed tissue usually sloughs off within a week. An enema is given prior to the treatment to prevent a bowel movement for 24 hours so that there is no straining which would cause the rubber band to break or slip off. No anesthesia is required and the procedure usually is performed in the physician's office. Local discomfort is minimal and usually is relieved by aspirin or Darvon.

Surgical excision with ligation *(hemorrhoidectomy)* is the treatment used most often for all external hemorrhoids and for internal ones that do not respond well to sclerosing or ligation. There are several methods by which a hemorrhoidectomy may be performed. However, the classic procedure involves excising each hemorrhoid and tying the pedicle with a ligature. The raw areas in the anus then heal by secondary intention.

Preoperatively the patient may be given a laxative, and he is encouraged to eat a full, normal diet until a few hours before the anesthetic is given. Stool softeners are often given to soften the stool and facilitate its passage through the rectum postoperatively, and a bulk laxative such as Metamucil may be given to increase the bulk of the stool.

To prevent pressure on the anal area following a hemorrhoidectomy, the patient may be placed on his abdomen, although many patients prefer to lie on the back, with a support such as a flotation pad under the buttocks. Since the patient may have severe pain postoperatively, ice packs, warm wet compresses, analgesic ointments, and narcotics may be given. Because the operation is usually considered minor and dressings may not be used, the tendency may be to minimize this operative procedure. In reality it can cause the patient more discomfort than some more serious operations.

Complications can occur and the most serious one is hemorrhage, which may happen within 24 hours after surgery if a ligature on one of the pedicles slips off. It can also occur between the seventh and tenth postoperative day when the suture may slough off and separate from the pedicle.[51] Hemorrhage can go undetected in these patients since the blood will gather in the anal canal and not be expelled immediately. Therefore the patient's vital signs should be checked frequently for the first 24 hours to rule out internal bleeding. If hemorrhage does occur, a Foley catheter may be inserted into the rectum and the balloon inflated to put pressure on the bleeding areas.[49]

The patient may be permitted out of bed the evening of surgery or the day after, and sitz baths usually are ordered to be taken twice a day. They often give relief from pain and discomfort. They should be supervised by nursing personnel until the patient can manage safely alone.

The patient often has difficulty voiding after a hemorrhoidectomy. This difficulty can usually be overcome by getting the patient out of bed to urinate. Sitz baths are also very helpful in stimulating voiding.

If the patient is not nauseated, a full diet is permitted immediately after surgery. Stool softeners are continued as preoperatively, and the patient is encouraged to have a bowel movement as soon as the inclination occurs. Passing a stool of normal consistency as soon as possible after surgery prevents the formation of strictures and preserves the normal lumen of the anus. The incidence of wound infection is slight after rectal surgery due to local tissue resistance to the bacteria normally present in the rectum. It is most likely to occur if bowel action has been delayed and healing tissues have become adherent. If the patient complains of much pain about the area and is fearful of having a bowel movement, the surgeon often orders medication such as dextropropoxyphene hydrochloride (Darvon) or Darvon Compound (32 to 65 mg.) to be taken a short time before a bowel movement is attempted. The patient needs careful nursing attention when he attempts the first bowel movement since it may cause dizziness and even fainting.

If a spontaneous bowel movement does not occur within 2 or 3 days postoperatively, laxatives are increased and an oil retention enema followed by a cleansing enema may be given through a small rectal tube. The patient is advised to take a sitz bath after each bowel movement to keep the operative area clean and to relieve local irritation. This practice should be continued until he returns to the physician (usually within 1 or 2 weeks).

Following a hemorrhoidectomy, the patient is advised to avoid constipation by eating a diet containing adequate fruit and roughage, exercising moderately, drinking plenty of fluids, and establishing a regular time for daily bowel movements. The physician may prescribe stool softeners or a mild laxative to be taken daily or every other day for a time.

Anal fissure

An anal fissure is a slitlike ulcer resembling a crack in the lining of the anal canal at or below the anorectal line. Usually it is the result of trauma caused by passage of hard-formed stool that overstretches the anal lining. The ulcer does not heal readily. Defecation initiates spasm of the anal sphincter, and the patient has severe pain that lasts for some time. Slight bleeding may occur, and constipation is usually caused by the patient's restraining his bowel movements to avoid pain.

Anal examination causes muscle spasm of the sphincter. Since spasm results in pain, the fissure must be examined under anesthesia. Treatment usually consists of digital dilation of the sphincter under anesthesia, or the anal ulcer may be surgically excised.

Local pain and spasm sometimes can be relieved by warm compresses, sitz baths, and use of analgesic ointments. Colace is usually ordered to lubricate the canal and to soften the stool. Postoperatively the care is similar to that given the patient who has had a hemorrhoidectomy.

Anal abscess

An anal abscess is located in tissues around the anus. It is caused by infection from the anal canal and may follow an anal fissure. If the abscess involves the anal, para-anal, or perineal tissues, there is throbbing local pain caused by pressure on the somatic sensory nerves in the perineum and local signs of inflammation. The patient finds it difficult to sit or lie on the area. In fact, any position is uncomfortable since he suffers from reflected pain.

If the abscess is located deep in the ischiorectal tissues, however, the patient is aware only of vague discomfort until the disease spreads into an area where there áre nerve fibers. The patient with an *ischiorectal abscess* is usually very ill. He has fever, chills, and malaise. The abscess must be incised and drained.

Postoperative care. Postoperatively the patient usually prefers to lie on his side or abdomen. Because most patients have some difficulty voiding, nursing measures should be initiated to prevent bladder distention. To void, the female patient needs to lie on her abdomen. This position prevents pain and contamination of the wound. A small child's bedpan or an emesis basin is more comfortable for the patient to use in this position.

There is usually a large amount of seropurulent drainage from the wound, and the physician may order that the dressings be changed as necessary. The wound is usually packed with gauze, and the nurse may be asked to wet the pack with warm normal saline solution or to repack the wound with warm normal saline dressings at specified intervals. The packs should be inserted into the bottom of the wound since it is important that it heal from the inside outward. The skin around the wound should be protected with petroleum jelly to prevent irritation from drainage. The wet dressing should be covered with oiled silk or plastic material to prevent wick contamination and to prevent wetting the bed. The dressing can be held in place by Montgomery straps or a T binder.

As healing progresses, sitz baths are usually ordered. If the wound is located near the anus, the patient is advised to cleanse the area carefully after defecation and to take a sitz bath after each defecation. Until healing is complete and all drainage disappears, a small dressing should be worn over the wound. A stool softener may be given to prevent or to treat constipation. Antibiotics usually are administered.

The patient is often discharged from the hospital before the wound has completely healed. He should continue to take sitz baths at home. If any difficulties are encountered he should report them to the physician.

Anal fistula

An anal fistula is an inflammatory sinus or tract with a primary opening in an anal crypt and with a secondary opening on the anal, para-anal, or perineal skin or in the rectal mucous membrane. It results from the rupture or drainage of an anal abscess. The patient has a periodic drainage that stains his clothing. An anal fistula is usually a chronic condition, and unfortunately many patients attempt to treat themselves with patent remedies before they seek competent medical care. The patient should be encouraged to have a gastrointestinal examination to rule out regional enteritis or other colon diseases.

The treatment of an anal fistula is a *fistulectomy* or a *fistulotomy*. A fistulectomy consists of an excision of the entire fistulous tract. The overhanging edges, if any, are trimmed away to leave an open, saucer-shaped wound. This procedure is usually performed when the fistula is quite straight and somewhat superficial. When a fistulotomy is performed, the entire tract is laid open, and the overlying skin margins are excised to leave a wide, saucer-shaped wound. The membranous lining of the remaining half of the fistulous tract quickly acquires a covering of granulation tissue. This procedure is usually used when a deep fistulous tract exists.

Postoperatively, patients with both procedures usually have warm, wet dressings applied. They generally are permitted to get up to void. A stool softener or mild laxatives may be given orally daily until the first bowel movement occurs, and sitz baths are prescribed to keep the area clean and to relieve discomfort. The patient who has had an operation for a fistula is more comfortable sitting on a protected pillow or a piece of very thick sponge rubber rather than on a rubber ring.

Pilonidal disease

Pilonidal cysts occur in the sacrococcygeal area and are thought to be congenital in origin. The cyst is lined with epithelium and hair. Pilonidal means "nest of hair." The cavity of the cyst communicates with the overlying skin by means of one or more short channels, each opening onto the skin in the

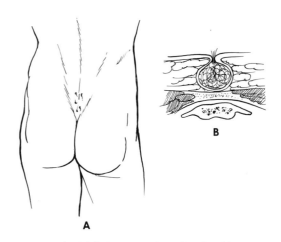

FIG. 25-18. Pilonidal sinus. **A,** Opening in skin over sacrococcygeal area. **B,** Cross section through cyst and pilonidal opening.

midline (Fig. 25-18). The lining of the channel or sinus is the same as the cyst, and tufts of hair are often seen protruding from the opening on the skin. These cysts or sinuses cause no symptoms unless they become infected. The patient then complains of pain and swelling at the base of the spine. An abscess forms, and it may rupture spontaneously or may require surgical incision and drainage. If the infection becomes chronic and the sinuses continue to drain, surgery becomes necessary.

Several types of operations may be done. The cyst may be excised and the wound closed. The patient remains in bed for several days after this procedure. To prevent contaminating the wound, the woman patient should void while lying on her abdomen. It is best if she practices this procedure before the operation. The patient should be observed for complications of bed rest such as urinary retention and should be encouraged to cough, breathe deeply, and move his arms and legs often. Ambulation is gradual. The patient should not take large steps, and he should not sit for long periods since these activities cause tension on the incision. A low-residue diet is usually given, and foods such as orange juice or prune juice that may stimulate peristalsis are avoided for the first few days. Defecation usually is delayed several days if possible, and a small oil retention enema is sometimes ordered before the first defecation takes place. When the patient does have his first bowel movement, the surgeon usually wishes to be notified so that the dressing can be changed. Antibiotics are usually given prophylactically, and narcotics may be needed for pain.

The cyst may be excised and the wound left open to heal by secondary intention. The wound is packed, and the patient remains in bed until the packing is removed 24 to 48 hours later. The patient is then permitted out of bed, and the wound is dressed daily. Sitz baths may be prescribed to be taken three or four times daily and after each bowel movement.

If an exteriorization operation or marsupialization is performed, the cyst cavity and all the channels are opened. The overhanging margins of skin are excised down to the base of the wound, providing a flat, saucer-shaped wound, the floor of which is formed by the deep half of the lining of the cyst or channel. The area to be covered by granulation tissues is thus decreased, and healing will occur within 6 weeks. A pressure dressing is applied and the patient usually remains in bed until the dressing is removed 24 to 48 hours later. Baths or showers are permitted and dry heat is usually applied to keep the area dry. Fluffed gauze squares may be placed in the wound to help keep its edges separated. Hair adjacent to the wound is removed as it appears. The patient usually is discharged from the hospital in 5 to 7 days and returns to work in 2 to 3 weeks.

REFERENCES AND SELECTED READINGS*

1 American Academy of Pediatrics: Report of the Committee on Infectious Diseases, ed. 17, Evanston, Ill., 1974, The Academy.

2 American Cancer Society, Inc.: 1975 cancer facts and figures, New York, 1974, The Society.

3 *Amshel, A. L.: Hemorrhoidal problems—medical and surgical treatment; Sheridan, B. A.: After hemorrhoidectomy—postoperative nursing care, Am. J. Nurs. 63:87-91, Dec. 1963.

4 Ayulo, J. A.: Hiatus hernia: a review, Am. J. Gastroenterol. 58:579-593, Dec. 1972.

5 Barnes, C. M.: Support of a mother in the care of a child with esophageal lye burns, Nurs. Clin. North Am. 4:53-57, March 1969.

6 Barton, K. M., and Kirsner, J. B.: Gastric ulcer—individualization in diagnosis and therapy, Med. Clin. North Am. 48:103-115, Jan. 1964.

6a Bates, B.: A guide to physical examination, Philadelphia, 1974, J. B. Lippincott Co.

7 Beahrs, O. H., and Adson, M. A.: Ileal pouch with ileostomy rather than ileostomy alone, Am. J. Surg. 125:154-158, Feb. 1973.

8 Beeson, P. B., and McDermott, W., editors: Cecil-Loeb textbook of medicine, ed. 13, Philadelphia, 1971, W. B. Saunders Co.

9 Bergersen, B. S.: Pharmacology in nursing, ed. 12, St. Louis, 1973, The C. V. Mosby Co.

10 Bockus, H. L.: Gastroenterology, ed. 3, vol. 1, Philadelphia, 1974, W. B. Saunders Co.

11 Boros, E.: Hiatus hernia, Am. J. Gastroenterol. 37:438-441, April 1962.

12 Braasch, J. W.: The surgical treatment of obesity, Surg. Clin. North Am. 51:667-672, June 1971.

12a Bryant, L., and others: Comparison of ice water and ice saline solution for gastric lavage in gastroduodenal hemorrhage, Am. J. Surg. 124:570-572, Nov. 1972.

12b Burkitt, D. P., Walker, A. R. P., and Painter, N. S.: Dietary fiber and diseases, J.A.M.A. 229:1068-1073, Aug. 1974.

13 Byrne, J. J., and Hennessy, V. L.: Diverticulitis of the colon, Surg. Clin. North Am. 52:991-999, Aug. 1972.

13a *Chandler, J. G.: Surgical treatment of massive obesity, Postgrad. Med. 56:124-132, Aug. 1974.

14 Cole, J. W.: Carcinogens and carcinogenesis in the colon, Hosp. Practice 8:123-130, Sept. 1973.

15 *Cole, W. H.: Cancer of the colon and rectum, Surg. Clin. North Am. 52:871-881, Aug. 1972.

16 Cole, W. H., and Zollinger, R. M.: Textbook of surgery, ed. 9, New York, 1970, Appleton-Century-Crofts.

17 Colley, R., and Phillips, K.: Helping with hyperalimentation, Nursing '73 3:6-17, July 1973.

18 Culp, C. E.: Pilonidal disease and its treatment, Surg. Clin. North Am. 47:1007-1014, Aug. 1967.

19 Dagradi, A. E., and Stempien, S. J.: Symptomatic esophageal hiatus sliding hernia, Am. J. Dig. Dis. 7:613-633, July 1962.

20 Davidsohn, I., and Henry, J. B.: Todd-Sanford clinical diagnosis by laboratory methods, ed. 15, Philadelphia, 1974, W. B. Saunders Co.

*References preceded by an asterisk are particularly well suited for student reading.

21 Deitel, M.: Intravenous hyperalimentation, Can. Nurse **69**:38-43, Jan. 1973.

22 Drummond, E. E., and Anderson, M. L.: Gastrointestinal suction, Am. J. Nurs. **63**:109-113, Dec. 1963.

23 Earlam, R. J., and Ellis, F. H.: The surgical repair of hiatal hernia: current controversy, Surg. Clin. North Am. **47**:813-826, Aug. 1967.

24 Egdahl, R. H., and Mannick, J. A.: Modern surgery, New York, 1970, Grune & Stratton, Inc.

25 Ellis, F. H., Jr.: Esophageal hiatal hernia, N. Engl. J. Med. **287**:646-649, Sept. 1972.

26 Ferguson, J. H.: Acute intestinal obstruction, Practitioner **209**:164-169, Aug. 1972.

27 Fischer, J. E., and others: Hyperalimentation as primary therapy for inflammatory bowel disease, Am. J. Surg. **125**:165-175, Feb. 1973.

28 Friedrich, H. N.: Oral feeding by food pump, Am. J. Nurs. **62**:62-64, Feb. 1962.

29 Fuerst, E. V., and Wolff, L. V.: Fundamentals of nursing, ed. 5, Philadelphia, 1974, J. B. Lippincott Co.

30 Gallagher, A. M.: Body image changes in the patient with a colostomy, Nurs. Clin. North Am. **7**:669-676, Dec. 1972.

31 Giannella, R. A., and others: Salmonella enteritis. I. Role of reduced gastric secretion in pathogenesis. II. Fulminant diarrhea in and effects on the small intestine, Am. J. Dig. Dis. **16**:1000-1013, Nov. 1971.

32 Gibbs, G. E., and White, M.: Stomal care, Am. J. Nurs. **72**:268-271, Feb. 1972.

33 *Given, B., and Simmons, S.: Nursing care of the patient with gastrointestinal disorders, St. Louis, 1971, The C. V. Mosby Co.

34 Goldstein, F.: Newer approaches to the management of peptic ulcer, Med. Clin. North Am. **49**:1253-1270, Sept. 1965.

35 Grafe, W. R., Loehr, W., and Thorbjarnarson, B.: Gastroenterostomy and vagotomy in the treatment of duodenal ulcer disease, Ann. Surg. **168**:966-970, Dec. 1968.

36 *Grant, J. N.: Patient care in parenteral hyperalimentation, Nurs. Clin. North Am. **8**:165-181, March 1973.

37 Gutowski, F: Ostomy procedure: nursing care before and after, Am. J. Nurs. **72**:262-267, Feb. 1972.

38 Harrower, H. W.: Management of colostomy, ileostomy and ileal conduit, Surg. Clin. North Am. **48**:941-953, Aug. 1968.

39 *Herter, F. P.: Preparation of the bowel for surgery, Surg. Clin. North Am. **52**:859-869, Aug. 1972.

40 Hunt, T. K.: Injury and repair in acute gastroduodenal ulceration, Am. J. Surg. **125**:12-18, Jan. 1973.

41 Jackman, R. J.: Innovation in anorectal procedures, Surg. Clin. North Am. **47**:999-1005, Aug. 1967.

42 Jones, H. L., and Nielsen, O. F.: Colitis: management based on pathologic mechanisms, Med. Clin. North Am. **49**:1271-1294, Sept. 1965.

43 *Kaplan, M. H., Bernheim, E. J., and Flynn, B. M.: Esophageal varices and components of nursing care, Am. J. Nurs. **64**:104-108, June 1964.

44 Katona, E. A.: Learning colostomy control, Am. J. Nurs. **67**:534-541, March 1967.

45 *Klug, T. J., and others: Gastric resection—and nursing care, Am. J. Nurs. **61**:73-77, Dec. 1961.

46 *Kurihara, M.: The patient with an intestinal prosthesis, Am. J. Nurs. **60**:852-853, June 1960.

47 *Lyons, A. S., and Brockmeier, M. J.: Mechanical management of the ileostomy stoma, Surg. Clin. North Am. **52**:979-990, Aug. 1972.

47a *Mansell, E., Stokes, S., and Adler, J.: Patient assessment: examination of the abdomen, programmed instruction, Am. J. Nurs. **74**:1679-1702, Sept. 1974.

48 *McKittrick, J. B., and Shotkin, J. M.: Ulcerative colitis, Am. J. Nurs. **62**:60-64, Aug. 1962.

49 Nankin, P., and others: Hiatus hernia, Surg. Clin. North Am. **51**:1347-1353, Dec. 1971.

50 Payne, J. H., and others: Surgical treatment of morbid obesity, Arch. Surg. **106**:432-437, April 1973.

50a *Plumley, P. F., and Francis, B.: Dietary management of diverticular disease, J. Am. Diet. Assoc. **63**:527-530, Nov. 1973.

51 Sabiston, D. C., editor: Davis-Christopher textbook of surgery, ed. 10, Philadelphia, 1972, W. B. Saunders Co.

52 Sandlow, L. J., and Spellberg, M. A.: Gastric hyperthermia for control of upper gastrointestinal bleeding, Am. J. Gastroenterol. **59**:307-314, April 1973.

53 Schwartz, S. I., and others: Principles of surgery, ed. 2, New York, 1974, McGraw-Hill Book Co.

54 Scott, H. W., and others: New considerations in use of jejunoileal bypass in patients with morbid obesity, Ann. Surg. **177**:723-735, June 1973.

55 *Secor, S. M.: Colostomy rehabilitation, Am. J. Nurs. **70**:2400-2401, Nov. 1970.

56 *Sill, A. R.: Bulb-syringe technique for colonic stoma irrigation, Am. J. Nurs. **70**:536-537, March 1970.

57 Sleisenger, M. H., and Fordtran, J. S.: Gastrointestinal diseases: pathology—diagnosis—management, Philadelphia, 1973, W. B. Saunders Co.

58 Spiro, H. M.: Clinical gastroenterology, New York, 1970, Macmillan Publishing Co., Inc.

59 Steigmann, F.: Are laxatives necessary? Am. J. Nurs. **62**:90-93, Oct. 1962.

60 Steigmann, F., and Shlaes, W. H.: The treatment of amebiasis, Med. Clin. North Am. **48**:159-175, Jan. 1964.

61 Turrell, R., and others: Symposium on new perspectives in colorectoanal surgery, Surg. Clin. North Am. **45**:1067-1329, Oct. 1965.

62 U. S. Bureau of the Census: Statistical abstracts of the United States, 1972, ed. 93, Washington, D. C., 1972, U. S. Government Printing Office.

63 *Vukovich, V., and Grubb, R. D.: Care of the ostomy patient, St. Louis, 1973, The C. V. Mosby Co.

64 Welch, C. E., editor: Advances in surgery, ed. 4, Chicago, 1970, Year Book Medical Publishers, Inc.

65 *Werrin, M., and Kronick, D.: Salmonella control in hospitals, Am. J. Nurs. **66**:528-531, March 1966.

66 Williams, S. R.: Nutrition and diet therapy, ed. 2, St. Louis, 1973, The C. V. Mosby Co.

67 Wintrobe, M. M., and others: Harrison's principles of internal medicine, ed. 7, New York, 1974, McGraw-Hill Book Co.

68 *Woodward, E. R., and Eisenberg, M. M.: Gastric physiology, with special reference to gastric and duodenal ulcers, Surg. Clin. North Am. **45**:327-343, April 1965.

69 Zimmerman, J. M., and King, T. C.: Use of the Souttar tube in the management of advanced esophageal cancer, Ann. Surg. **169**:867-871, June 1969.

70 Zimmermann, W. J., and Zinter, D. E.: The prevalence of trichiniasis in swine in the United States, 1966-1970, HSMHA Health Rep. **86**:937-945, Oct. 1971.

26 Diseases of the liver and adjacent structures

■ The liver and the biliary system are affected by a variety of diseases. In this chapter, nursing related to diagnostic tests and to general problems commonly seen in patients with hepatic and biliary diseases will be discussed before specific nursing care involved in some of the more common diseases is considered.

Since the public is becoming better informed about diseases such as viral hepatitis, fear is usually present when disease of the liver is suspected. Many people have friends or acquaintances who have died of a hepatic disease or who have been handicapped for long periods of time because of it. However, certain diseases of the liver need not necessarily occur, and the nurse can help in their prevention. For example, the spread of viral hepatitis can be controlled substantially if the public is taught to use good hygienic practices and proper sterilization techniques. Certain degenerative diseases of the liver can be prevented if people are informed about the proper use of substances such as carbon tetrachloride that are harmful to hepatic cells. Serious damage to hepatic tissue may be prevented by referring persons with signs of disease of the liver such as dark urine, light stools, and jaundice to a physician.

■ PHYSICAL ASSESSMENT OF THE LIVER AND GALLBLADDER

Normally the liver and gallbladder cannot be felt by the examiner on palpation of the abdomen. For details of the procedure to follow in further assessment of the abdomen as well as the liver and gallbladder, see p. 648.

■ DIAGNOSTIC EXAMINATIONS AND TESTS

Several tests are used to determine whether or not disease of the liver is present and to distinguish the various causes of symptoms if some derangement of the liver or of the biliary system is evident. They include tests of hepatic function, procedures that demonstrate the amount and distribution of bile pigment, and radiographs that may show biliary malfunction. The patient should be told the purpose of each test, what preparation is necessary, and what to expect during the test or examination.

Liver function tests

Liver function tests are used to determine the presence and the extent of hepatic damage and to check the progress of disease of the liver. They are of great importance in determining whether or not signs and symptoms are due to disease of the hepatic cells themselves (hepatocellular) or to pathologic processes outside the hepatic cells (extracellular). Since the liver has many functions that are closely interrelated, single tests of liver function usually give information about the efficiency of several of

■ STUDY QUESTIONS

1 Review the main functions of the liver.
2 Review the anatomy of the biliary system. What are the important constituents of bile? What is its function in digestion?
3 What are the practices in your hospital regarding use and sterilization of needles and syringes? Are disposable needles and syringes used?
4 List some drugs you have learned about that are toxic to the liver.
5 Review procedures and the nursing care given when a paracentesis is done.
6 Review the blood vessels leading to and from the liver, the spleen, and the kidneys. Review the portal circulation. How does it differ from other venous systems?

the organ's activities. This is particularly true when metabolic functions are considered.

Most liver function tests involve taking samples of the patient's blood, and many require that he fast preceding the test, causing inconvenience and discomfort for the patient. If the nurse makes sure that the tests are scheduled as ordered, laboratory slips filled in correctly, blood samples correctly labeled, urine specimens collected on time, and food withheld as necessary, this will help prevent the need for repetition of the tests. Since the rules of laboratories vary as to whether or not fasting should precede the taking of blood for some tests, the nurse should learn the practice within the hospital. If in doubt, it is usually best to have the patient fast, although the importance of regular meals for persons with disease of the liver must be kept in mind.

Bilirubin metabolism. Tests may reveal the functional capacity of the liver in breaking down, reusing, and excreting bile pigment by measuring the amount of bilirubin present in the blood, stools, and urine. Bilirubin is formed by the heme portion of the hemoglobin molecule from fragile and aged red blood cells. The released bilirubin combines with plasma proteins, mainly albumin, and is transported to the liver where it is conjugated with other substances into a soluble state. Normally it is excreted with bile into the duodenum and is broken down by bacteria in the lower intestines into urobilinogen. Most of the urobilinogen is excreted in the feces, becoming stercobilin, which gives the characteristic brown color to stools. The remainder returns to the liver, where it is reconverted to bilirubin, or it is eliminated in the urine. Only minute amounts of bilirubin are found in the blood and urine of well persons. When the hepatic and biliary ducts become blocked or damaged, conjugated and unconjugated bilirubin is no longer excreted into the bowel but returns to the blood *(jaundice)* and is excreted by the kidneys *(bilirubinuria).* Serum levels of bilirubin are increased and stercobilin (urobilinogen), which gives color to the stool, is not excreted. Therefore the stools become clay colored (acholic). With biliary or hepatic obstruction, urobilinogen will be decreased or absent in the urine. With complete biliary obstruction, urobilinogen is absent from the urine, since the kidneys excrete soluble bilirubin but not protein-bound urobilinogen.

The *quantitative van den Bergh test for serum bilirubin* is one that measures the total serum bilirubin in the blood and can differentiate between protein-bound and soluble (conjugated) bilirubin. The total serum bilirubin content indicates the intensity and progress of jaundice; determination of the amount by the direct or by the indirect method gives some indication as to the cause of the jaundice. For example, the bile pigment in the serum of patients with hemolytic jaundice is determined by the indirect test (unconjugated bilirubin), whereas in obstructive jaundice there is bile in the blood serum, and values can be obtained in the absence of alcohol (direct method, or conjugated bilirubin). Normal values for total serum bilirubin range from 0.1 to 1 mg./ 100 ml. Fasting is not necessary for this test.

The *icterus index* occasionally is used to determine the amount of bile pigment in blood serum. The normal reading is 4 to 6 units, but it may reach 15 units before jaundice is evident. Fasting usually is required for this test. Carrots eaten the day before the test will interfere with results because they contain carotene, which increases the level of bilirubin in the blood serum.

Changes in the color of urine or stools may be early specific signs of hepatic or biliary disease. The nurse who observes a change in the color of either the urine or the stool should examine both and report the findings to the physician.

Urine containing abnormal amounts of bilirubin has a characteristic mahogany color, and if the specimen is shaken, a yellow foam appears (the *foam test).* Urobilinogen in a fresh urine specimen is colorless but turns to brown urobilin on standing. The normal amount of *urinary urobilinogen* ranges from 0 to 4 mg. in 24 hours. This amount is increased in nonobstructive liver disease and will cause the urine to be darker than usual. If the flow of bile into the intestines is obstructed, urobilinogen is not formed and it disappears from the urine. Determination of urine urobilinogen levels is used to distinguish between extrahepatic and intrahepatic obstruction. If the obstruction is extrahepatic, no urobilinogens will be found in the urine. There are several methods used to determine the amount of urobilinogen present in urine. A random sample of urine, a 2-hour afternoon specimen, or a 24-hour specimen may be used.[17] A urine specimen collected in the early afternoon gives maximal values, since bile concentration in the intestine is highest in the midafternoon and early evening.

The normal range for *fecal stercobilinogen* is from 40 to 280 mg. daily. In hemolytic jaundice, as much as 4,000 mg. may be excreted each day.[7] A decrease in or absence of stercobilinogen in the stool (acholia) would suggest an obstruction to the flow of bile that prevents it from reaching the intestines. The stool gradually becomes lighter and may be clay colored or almost white.

Protein metabolism. Some of the most important functions of the liver are concerned with protein metabolism, including the deamination of amino acids and the maintenance of normal levels of albumin, globulin, and fibrinogen in the blood. Determination of the *ratio of serum proteins* (A/G ratio) is a measure of hepatic function. An alteration in the normal ratio may indicate degenerative disease of the liver. The serum albumin tends to drop below 4 Gm./100 ml. of blood, whereas the serum globulin tends to rise above 2.4 Gm./100 ml. of blood in patients with disease of the liver. No fasting is necessary for this test.

The *cephalin-cholesterol flocculation test* is performed to distinguish jaundice due to disease of the liver from obstructive jaundice and to screen for early detection of subclinical disease of the liver. A colloidal suspension of a cephalin-cholesterol mixture shows distinct flocculation and sedimentation when serum from the blood of a patient with liver damage is used. The latter is caused by failure of the diseased liver to make certain changes in the protein constituents of the plasma. A reading of 1+ at the end of 24 hours or 2+ at 48 hours is considered a positive test.

The *thymol turbidity test* depends on the presence in the serum of increased amounts of gamma globulin, beta globulin, and serum lipids. The test is particularly valuable in acute hepatitis in determining the degree of hepatic damage and in following the course of the disease through the late convalescent stages.

Protein electrophoresis involves the use of an electric current to separate protein fractions. The fractions migrate in a characteristic direction in an electric field. After the fractions are separated by electrophoresis, the specimen is stained and a densitometer is used to measure the amounts of the various serum proteins. In the normal test the various amounts of the fractions in relation to total protein (100%) would be as follows: albumin, 53%; alpha globulins, 14%; beta globulins, 12%; and immune serum globulins, 20%.[17] This test is valuable in determining the degree of hepatic damage. In portal cirrhosis the level of serum albumin is decreased.

Since prothrombin (and fibrinogen), necessary for blood clotting, is manufactured by the liver, the *prothrombin level* may be determined when disease of the liver is suspected. Normal plasma clots in 20 seconds or less. A prothrombin-complex activity below 80% is considered abnormal; when below 40%, it may be associated with bleeding.[7] The prothrombin level is often lowered in cirrhosis of the liver, in metastatic carcinoma of the liver, and in acute hepatic necrosis or in chronic liver disease. Failure of a low prothrombin level in a patient with jaundice to respond to bile salts given by mouth and to parenteral administration of synthetic vitamin K indicates that the jaundice may be due to liver damage and not to biliary obstruction. Fasting is not necessary for this test.

Since most of the ammonia resulting from protein catabolism is converted into urea in the normal liver, a high concentration of *ammonia* in the blood is a good indicator of potential or existing hepatic coma. The normal range is less than 75 μg of ammonia nitrogen/100 ml. of blood.

Carbohydrate metabolism. There is a decreased ability to use both glucose and galactose when hepatic cells are damaged. The galactose tolerance test may be used to differentiate between hepatocellular jaundice and obstructive jaundice. The galactose tolerance test is done as follows: The patient is given nothing by mouth on the morning of the test. The first morning specimen of urine is discarded, and the patient drinks 40 mg. of galactose dissolved in 500 ml. of water and flavored with lemon juice. After ingestion of this solution, urine specimens are collected hourly for 5 hours, numbered, and sent to the laboratory. The urine is examined for the total amount of sugar excreted. An excretion exceeding 3 Gm. of sugar is considered indicative of disease of the liver. This test may also be performed by giving the galactose intravenously; 1 ml. of 50% solution of galactose/kg. body weight is given after a sample of blood has been drawn. Another blood sample is taken 75 minutes after injection of the galactose. A test on normal blood should reveal less than 5 mg. of sugar/100 ml. of blood in this blood sample. Patients with hepatic disease have higher levels; however, the blood sugar level is often low in patients who have chronic liver damage. These carbohydrate tests are often inaccurate and they are used less often than in the past.[43]

Serum lipid metabolism. The liver is the main source of *serum cholesterol* and *serum phospholipids* and influences the concentration of other blood lipids.

A *quantitative determination of serum cholesterol* helps to determine hepatic function. It is known that patients with hepatic disease have a decrease in cholesterol esters in relation to total cholesterol. The normal blood serum cholesterol level is between 140 and 220 mg./100 ml., approximately 70% of which is the cholesterol ester. In suspected or known hepatic disease a figure of 40% or lower in cholesterol esters or a steady decrease in cholesterol esters is indicative of progressive disease of the liver with poor prognosis, whereas an increase in the cholesterol esters indicates improvement in the condition. Fasting usually is required for this test.

The concentration of *serum phospholipids* tends to be low in severe hepatocellular disease and increased in diseases associated with obstruction to the flow of bile. An elevation of serum phospholipids reflects corresponding elevation in cholesterol. The normal range of serum phospholipids, expressed as lecithin, is 110 to 250 mg./100 ml.

Detoxification. The detoxifying capacity of the liver may be tested by means of the *hippuric acid test.* Hippuric acid results from the synthesis of benzoic acid and glycine by the liver and is normally excreted at a regular rate in the urine. The test is done as follows: The patient is given a light breakfast of toast and coffee. One hour later, 6 Gm. of sodium benzoate dissolved in 30 ml. of water and flavored with oil of peppermint, cherry syrup, or lemon juice is given by mouth. This may be followed by 100 ml. of water. The patient is then asked to void immediately, and this specimen is discarded. Then he fasts and voids each hour for 4 hours. The specimens are labeled, numbered, and sent to the laboratory. Normal excretion should total 3 Gm. of hippuric acid in the four specimens. In the intravenous hippuric acid test, 1.77 Gm. of sodium benzoate is administered after the patient has voided and taken a glass of water. One urine specimen is collected an hour later and should contain more than 0.7 Gm. of hippuric acid. Abnormal findings may show poor hepatic function such as occurs in hepatitis, cirrhosis, and malignant disease of the liver. In conditions in which jaundice is the result of obstruction in the biliary passages and in which the liver has not yet been damaged, the test is normal.

Dye excretion. Since one of the functions of the liver is excretion, tests that measure the rate with which a dye such as *Bromsulphalein* (BSP) is removed from the bloodstream are useful. Fasting is necessary for this test. The patient is weighed, and the dosage of the dye is calculated on the basis of 5 mg./kg. body weight. The dye is injected slowly into the vein, and a blood sample is taken in 45 minutes from the opposite arm. Normal persons have less than 5% retention at 45 minutes. The nurse participates in the scheduling of tests and should know that phenolsulfonphthalein tests for kidney function should not be scheduled for at least 24 hours after dye for a liver function test has been given. *Rose bengal* or *indocyanine green* also may be used as a dye for a test of liver function.

The BSP test may be used in patients with upper gastrointestinal bleeding in order to differentiate cirrhosis with esophageal varices from other gastrointestinal bleeding.

Serum enzyme determinations. Necrosis of liver cells such as occurs in hepatitis brings about an increase in serum enzymes. Three enzymes frequently studied are *serum glutamic oxaloacetic transaminase* (SGOT), *serum glutamic pyruvic transaminase* (SGPT), and *lactic dehydrogenase* (LDH). While SGPT is specifically elevated in diseases of the liver, SGOT is raised in myocardial infarction, pulmonary embolism, and other diseases as well as in hepatic diseases. LDH determination is primarily used to diagnose myocardial infarction but the levels are also elevated when there is hepatic necrosis (p. 324).

Serum cholinesterase is believed to be synthesized in the liver and involved in protein metabolism. Its activity is depressed in cirrhosis particularly.

The *alkaline phosphatase test* is significant in that the level is only slightly elevated in diseases of the liver such as hepatitis and cirrhosis but is markedly elevated in biliary obstruction. Depending on the method used, normal levels range from 0.5 to 4.0 Bodansky units or 3 to 13 King-Armstrong units. Alkaline phosphatase is also elevated in diseases of the bone.

Radiologic examination

Radiologic examinations are used to diagnose diseases of the liver, the portal system, the gallbladder, and the biliary ducts and to determine the ability of the gallbladder to concentrate bile and to expel it through the common bile duct into the duodenum.

Cholecystography. A normal liver will remove radiopaque drugs such as iodoalphionic acid (Priodax), iopanoic acid (Telepaque), and iodipamide methylglucamine (Cholografin methylglucamine) from the bloodstream and store and concentrate them in the gallbladder. Because the roentgen rays cannot penetrate the dye, the dye-filled gallbladder shows up as a dense shadow on x-ray examination *(cholecystogram, gallbladder series)*. A satisfactory gallbladder shadow would indicate a functioning gallbladder. A total absence of opaque material in the gallbladder would suggest a nonfunctioning gallbladder. After ingestion of a fatty meal, a functioning gallbladder should contract and expel the radiopaque dye along with the bile through the common bile duct into the duodenum. X-ray examination at this point would outline the bile ducts. Stones, which are not radiopaque, show up as dark patches on the film. Visualization of the gallbladder depends on absorption of the dye through the intestinal tract, isolation of it by the liver, and a free passageway from the liver to the gallbladder. Therefore, if the results show a nonfunctioning gallbladder, sometimes the test is repeated to be sure that failure to visualize the gallbladder by x-ray examination was not due to insufficient dye.

On the evening before cholecystography is scheduled, the purpose of and preparation for the test should be explained to the patient. The importance of following instructions regarding food restriction the morning of the test as well as the need for the high-fat meal, which may cause nausea, should be discussed.

The average adult dose of both Priodax and Telepaque is 3 Gm. (45 grains) given orally following a low-fat evening meal, after which no food is given. These drugs may cause nausea, vomiting, and diarrhea in some people. The nurse should check dosages accurately and watch carefully for toxic signs, which should be reported to the physician. If vomiting occurs soon after ingestion of the drug, the physician may ask that the tablets be repeated when nausea subsides, or he may delay the test for several days. If the patient cannot tolerate the drug by mouth, a radiopaque substance such as Cholografin may be given intravenously by the physician in the x-ray department. The radiopaque dyes are organic iodine compounds and may cause allergic reactions when given intravenously. Symptoms may include dyspnea, chills, diaphoresis, faintness, and tachycardia and are identical to symptoms that can occur when radiopaque substances containing iodine are injected intravenously for other tests such as pyelography or arteriography. (See p. 430 for a discussion of precaution and care.)

On the morning of the examination the patient may have only black coffee, tea, or water. One or more enemas may be given to help remove gas from the intestinal tract so that it will not interfere with a clear radiograph. The patient goes to the x-ray department, and two radiographs are taken during the morning. He is then given a high-fat noon meal, after which another radiograph is taken. Ingestion of fat should stimulate flow of bile and emptying of the gallbladder. The dye is finally excreted in the urine, and some patients report slight temporary pain on urination following the test.

Cholangiography. Cholangiography is the x-ray examination of the bile ducts to demonstrate the presence of stones, strictures, or tumors. The radiopaque substance may be administered intravenously or injected directly into the common bile duct with a needle or catheter at the time of surgery. Following operations on the common bile duct, the radiopaque drug, usually Cholografin, may be instilled through a drainage tube such as the T tube to determine the patency of the duct before the tube is removed. This dye also may be injected through the skin and abdominal wall into a bile duct in the main substance of the liver *(percutaneous transhepatic cholangiography)*. This technique is useful in visualizing the

location and extent of a pathologic process such as obstructive jaundice and permits decompression of the liver for improved function. The procedure helps the surgeon identify the location prior to surgery or may indicate that surgery is not necessary. The hazards of the examination occasionally may include bile leakage leading to bile peritonitis or bleeding due to accidental rupture of a blood vessel.[15]

Splenic portography and splenic pulp manometry. The injection of radiopaque solution through the skin into the spleen *(percutaneous splenic portography)* is done to visualize the venous inflow into the liver. It is also possible to measure the actual pressure in the portal vein by use of *splenic pulp manometry.* This test is valuable in determining the degree of portal hypertension.[30]

Hepatic vein catheterization. In hepatic vein catheterization a radiopaque catheter is inserted through the subclavian vein and right atrium into the right or left hepatic vein to occlude the flow of blood coming into the vein. This allows the pressure from the sinusoidal tract to be exerted on the head of the catheter. Hepatic vein catheterization makes possible not only measurement of hepatic vein pressure but also estimation of hepatic blood flow and visualization of the outflow tract of the liver.[30]

Radioisotope scanning. The liver may be outlined by radioisotope scanning techniques. After radioactive isotopes such as colloidal gold (^{198}Au), molybdenum (^{99}Mo), technetium (^{99}Tc) or rose bengal tagged with radioactive iodine (^{131}I), all of which selectively localize in the liver, are administered, the patient assumes a supine position and a scintillation detector is passed over the abdomen in the area of the liver. The radiation coming from the isotopes immediately

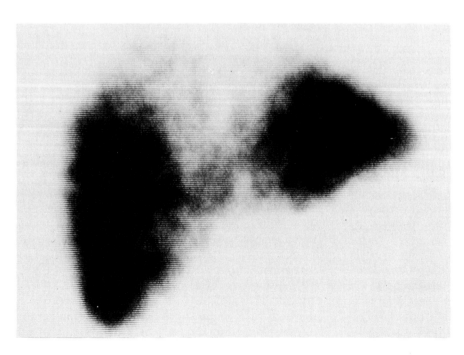

FIG. 26-1. Liver scan showing metastasis to the liver (light area on the right) of carcinoma of the colon. (Courtesy Abbas M. Rejali, M.D., Department of Radiology, Case Western Reserve University, Cleveland, Ohio.)

beneath the probe is detected, amplified, and record- ed by photoscanning. This technique helps differen- tiate nonfunctioning areas from normally active liver tissue and helps identify hepatic tumors, cysts, and abscesses (Fig. 26-1). In cirrhosis there is a gen- eralized decreased uptake. As reactions to the drugs usually do not occur, the procedure is considered safe and does not cause the patient any discomfort. Only small amounts of the radioactive material are given, and precautions are not necessary. Radioiso- tope scanning techniques are used to detect diseases in many areas of the body.

Duodenal drainage

In this test, also known as the biliary drainage test, bile obtained from the duodenum is examined for occult blood, pancreatic enzymes, tumor cells, leukocytes, cholesterol crystals, and pigment gran- ules. It may be done when the patient is ambulatory or while he is hospitalized. The patient should be prepared for a somewhat lengthy procedure, but he should know that once the tube has been passed he will have little or no discomfort. The preparation is similar to that for a gastric analysis (p. 653). The pa- tient is not permitted anything by mouth except small sips of water for 12 hours. A slender tube weighted at its tip with metal and marked with a series of rings to indicate the distance it travels to the cardia, pylorus, and duodenum, respectively, is passed through the patient's mouth (Fig. 25-6). Other modified gastroduodenal tubes are available and may be used for this purpose. After the tube is in the stomach, the patient is placed on his right side with his hips elevated about 6 inches so that gastric motility will be aided by gravity to carry the tube into the duodenum. The physician may have to manipu- late the tube into place with the aid of the fluoro- scope. It may take from 1 to 5 hours for the tube to reach the duodenum. The nurse may aid passage of the tube into the duodenum by talking to the patient about food. Thus by stimulating the flow of digestive juices, peristalsis increases and the tube can progress faster.

When the tube reaches the duodenum, several specimens are taken. The first specimen is usually light in color and consists of bile coming from the common duct. After this specimen is obtained, ap- proximately 50 ml. of magnesium sulfate (25% solu- tion) is introduced through the tube to stimulate the flow of bile, and a second specimen is collected in 10 to 15 minutes. This specimen is usually darker and more viscid, containing bile from the gallbladder that has flowed in response to the cholagogue action of magnesium sulfate. A third specimen, containing bile coming from the hepatic duct and freshly secret- ed by the liver, is sometimes collected.

Olive oil may be instilled through the tube to stim- ulate the gallbladder to contract and expel bile into the duodenum, or cholecystokinin, a synthetic preparation of the substance normally found in the intestinal mucosa, may be administered intrave- nously. An intravenous injection of synthetic secre- tin may be given. It should cause an increase in the flow of bile and pancreatic secretions.

Biopsy of the liver

A biopsy of the liver may be taken in an attempt to establish a diagnosis of hepatic disease. In this procedure a specially designed needle is inserted through the chest or abdominal wall into the liver and a small piece of tissue is removed for study. This procedure is contraindicated if the patient has an in- fection of the right lower lobe of the lung, ascites, a blood dyscrasia, or is unable to cooperate by hold- ing his breath. To avoid hemorrhage, vitamin K may be given parenterally for several days before the biopsy is taken. A biopsy may not be done if the prothrombin time is below 40%. The physician should explain the procedure to the patient; for example, the patient should know that he must hold his breath and remain absolutely still when the needle is intro- duced. Movement of the chest may cause the needle to slip and to tear the liver covering. Most hospitals require that the patient give written permission for the procedure to be done. Food and fluids may be withheld for several hours preceding the test, and a sedative usually is given about $^1/_2$ hour before the biopsy is to be taken.

The method is as follows: With the patient lying on his back, the skin over the area selected (usually the eighth or ninth intercostal space) is cleansed and anesthetized with procaine hydrochloride. A nick is made in the skin with a sharp scalpel blade. Then the patient is instructed to take several deep breaths and to hold his breath while the needle is introduced through the intercostal or subcostal tissues into the liver. The special needle assembly is rotated to sepa- rate a fragment of tissue, and then is withdrawn. The specimen is placed into an appropriate contain- er, which is then labeled and sent to the pathology laboratory. A simple dressing is placed over the wound, and the patient must remain on bed rest for 24 hours to prevent hemorrhage. Some physicians prefer that the patient lie on his right side with his right arm flexed under the hypochondrium after the biopsy.[30]

The dangers of this procedure, which is done rela- tively "blind," are accidental penetration of a small blood vessel, causing hemorrhage, and accidental penetration of a biliary vessel, causing a chemical peritonitis from leakage of bile into the abdominal cavity. Occasionally a laparotomy must be done to treat complications of liver biopsy. The nurse should check the equipment used and the specimen very carefully for any signs of discoloration from bile and should report the findings to the physician. The patient's pulse rate and blood pressure should be taken every half hour for the first few hours and then hourly for at least 24 hours. The physician may order pressure applied to the biopsy site to help stop any bleeding. Pressure may be applied by having the patient lie on his right side with a small pillow or folded bath blanket placed under the costal margin for several hours after the biopsy.

■ MANAGEMENT OF THE PATIENT WITH HEPATIC OR BILIARY DISEASE

Jaundice, difficulty with nutrition because of poor appetite, nausea and poor tolerance of food, and secondary infections are problems confronting many patients with hepatic and biliary disease, regardless of its cause. Therefore these problems and the medical and nursing care essential to alleviating them will be discussed before the management of persons with a specific disease is considered.

Jaundice

Jaundice is a symptom complex caused by a disturbance of the physiology of bile pigment and is present in many diseases of the hepatic and biliary system. There is an excess of bile pigment in the blood, which eventually is distributed to the skin, mucous membranes, and other body fluids and body tissues, giving them a yellow discoloration. Jaundice, caused by faulty hepatic function due to disease of the hepatic cells, is described as *hepatocellular.* When it results from intrahepatic or extrahepat-

ic obstruction that interferes with the flow of bile, it is described as *obstructive. Hemolytic* jaundice presumably is caused by destruction of great numbers of blood cells, which results in the production of excessive amounts of bilirubin and inability of the liver to excrete the bilirubin as rapidly as it is formed. Therefore the plasma concentration rises, the amount of urobilinogen in the intestines is greatly increased, and much of the urobilinogen is absorbed back into the blood and excreted in the urine. The results of these changes are summarized in Table 26-1.

Pruritus. The presence of bile pigment in the skin causes pruritus (itching) in about 20% to 25% of the patients who have jaundice. Bathing or sponging the skin with tepid water, followed by the application of an oil-based lotion, often helps relieve itching. The antihistaminic drugs are sometimes used to control pruritus. Tranquilizing drugs such as chlordiazepoxide (Librium) have been effective in helping to decrease the patient's reaction to pruritus. Relief from itching can be obtained by administering cholestyramine (a resin), which binds bile salts in the intestines and increases their excretion in feces. The usual dose is 4 Gm. three or four times a day and beneficial results may not be obtained before 4 days.[5]

Only soft, old linen should be used for the patient who has pruritus. Profuse diaphoresis sometimes accompanies jaundice, and bile-stained perspiration may color the bed linen. The linen should be changed at once for psychologic reasons as well as for physical comfort. The patient's fingernails should

Table 26-1   Bile pigment metabolism: jaundice

Types of liver cell dysfunction	Serum bilirubin (conjugated)	Serum bilirubin (unconjugated)	Total serum bilirubin (conj. and unconj.)	Urine urobilinogen	Urine bilirubin	Stool	Jaundice (icterus)
Normal		<0.2 mg%	+	±	0	Brown	0
Hemolytic	<0.2 mg%	>0.2 mg%	++	++++	0	Dark brown	Light reddish yellow
Familial	<0.2 mg%	>0.2 mg%	++	±	0	Brown (normal)	Reddish yellow
Hepatitis	+	>0.2 mg%	++	+++	++	Light brown	Deep reddish yellow
Cirrhosis	+	>0.2 mg%	++	+++	++	Light brown	Deep reddish yellow
Incomplete biliary obstruction	++	>0.2 mg%	+++	Variable and fluctuating	+++	Light	Light to deep greenish yellow
Complete biliary obstruction	+++	>0.2 mg%	++++	0	+++	Clay colored	Deep greenish

be cut short and his hands kept clean, since itching may be so severe that the patient may excoriate the skin by scratching and may cause skin lesions, which heal very slowly when jaundice is pronounced.

Emotional factors. The patient with marked jaundice is usually sensitive about his appearance. If he is ambulatory, dark glasses can be worn to conceal the yellow color of the sclerae. The hospital room should be kept softly lighted. White or yellowish light bulbs make jaundice much less obvious than does fluorescent lighting. The patient who is particularly concerned with his appearance may rest better in a room by himself and may wish to have visitors restricted.

Hemorrhage. Because the jaundiced patient has a low blood prothrombin level, the coagulation time of his blood is prolonged and he bleeds easily. Therefore he is a poor risk for surgery and may bleed profusely from minor medical procedures such as a venipuncture or an intramuscular injection. Normal production of prothrombin is dependent on four things: (1) ingestion of foods that can undergo synthesis in the intestine, (2) presence of bile in the intestine, thus enabling the intestine to produce vitamin K from food constituents, (3) absorption through the intestinal wall of the vitamin K produced, and (4) use of the vitamin K by the liver in the formation of prothrombin.

Since vitamin K depends on the presence of bile salts for its manufacture and absorption in the intestine, bile salts are often given by mouth to patients who are jaundiced. Vitamin K may be given both orally and parenterally in the hope that it will enable the liver to form more prothrombin. If vitamin K, which is not water soluble, is given by mouth, bile salts must be given as well. However, menadione sodium bisulfite (Hykinone), a water-soluble preparation of vitamin K, usually is ordered. The usual dose is 0.5 to 2 mg. ($\frac{1}{120}$ to $\frac{1}{30}$ grain) daily, given parenterally. If the jaundice is due to obstruction in the biliary tract and not to hepatic disease, it can be treated satisfactorily. If the liver is severely diseased and unable to make use of the vitamin K provided, the prothrombin level will remain low despite the administration of bile salts and vitamin K. Fresh blood then may have to be given to provide the prothrombin essential for clotting.[5]

Since the jaundiced patient may bleed more than usual from such minor procedures as drawing blood from a vein, plans should be made for samples of blood to be taken at the same time for several tests. If an infusion is ordered, it should be started at the time blood is obtained. When giving intramuscular and hypodermic injections, the nurse should select the smallest needle that can be used safely and should be particularly careful that the needle is sharp and that, following an injection, firm pressure is exerted for longer than is normally necessary. The patient should be instructed to take special care when brushing his teeth. If prothrombin time is very low, the patient should not use a toothbrush but mouthwash or cotton swabs may be used instead to prevent bleeding gums. The patient's urine and stools should be checked for either old or fresh blood, and if bleeding is suspected, specimens should be saved. Steady oozing of blood from hemorrhoids is not unusual in severe jaundice. Incisions heal more slowly when jaundice is present, and the nurse should inspect dressings frequently for bleeding. The patient's activity may be restricted until the wound has healed completely.

Nutrition. Seeing that the patient with hepatic or biliary disease eats enough of the necessary foods is one of the most important nursing responsibilities. The patient usually has difficulties with food. Disturbance of hepatic function and interference with normal flow of bile into the intestine upset the entire digestive system, causing indigestion, poor appetite, flatulence, and constipation. The patient may not tolerate fatty foods well. He may have learned over a period of months or years, or may need to be taught, to avoid high-fat foods, which tend to produce gas in the stomach and intestinal tract. Food often provokes nausea and vomiting, and the patient may be apprehensive about eating.

In recent years a great deal of attention has been given to diet and its relation to chronic degenerative disease of the liver. It is suspected that the liver's ability to excrete toxins and carry on its many other functions is seriously hampered by inadequate intake of protein and of vitamin B. If liver damage has occurred, the organ's ability to store glycogen and vitamins A, B complex, C, and D may also be lessened, and the patient may be in much greater need of regular intake of complete foods than before his illness. In the absence of bile salts, a major component of bile, the digestion and absorption of fats and the absorption of vitamin K are seriously hampered.

A diet high in calories, protein, and vitamins, fairly high in carbohydrates (unless weight reduction is desired), with moderate amounts of fat is often ordered for patients with diseases of the liver. Many physicians believe that the patient who has hepatic damage should have 100 to 300 Gm. of protein/day, but it is exceedingly difficult to have the patient eat this amount. Lean beef (broiled steak if it can be afforded), broiled chicken, and fish are some of the best high-protein foods. Egg white, gelatin, and cottage cheese provide large amounts of protein and can be prepared in a variety of ways. Yeast is particularly high in protein and in vitamin B. Dried skim milk is very useful for fortifying drinks taken between meals and can be added to muffins, sauces, and many other foods.

The nurse should learn what the patient likes to

eat, what particular foods cause him most distress, and what foods he tolerates well. Nurses should learn what meal schedule for the day seems to suit the patient best. For example, does he tolerate and enjoy frequent small meals? Does he like snacks between meals? Does he like the heaviest meal at noon or at the end of the day? The nurse should convey this information to the dietitian so that meals for the hospitalized patient may be similar to those eaten at home.

Often the patient eats best when comment about his appetite is kept to a minimum. Mouthwashes before meals help to relieve the unpleasant sensation and taste in the mouth that interfere with appetite and that are so common in patients with hepatic disease. Meals should be attractively served, with hot foods hot and cold foods cold. Diversion during meals helps to improve appetite. Some patients find that drinking effervescent fluids instead of water during the meal helps to relieve nausea and flatulence after meals. The patient should rest for a half hour immediately after concluding a meal. Almost any exceptions in dietary regulations should be made to get what the patient needs and will eat. If the patient is hospitalized, members of his family may be permitted to bring foods that he likes and will eat, provided that these foods conform to the diet prescribed and that this practice is approved by the physician. The dietitian should be informed if this is done. Alcohol, however, to stimulate appetite or for any other purpose is usually not ordered for patients with hepatic disease since it may be taxing to the diseased liver.

Protection from infections and drugs

The patient with severe hepatic or biliary disease is a ready candidate for *infection* because protein metabolism and utilization of vitamins are decreased. His resistance is so low that infections are easily acquired and shed with difficulty. Also, infections produce toxins that must be dealt with by the liver. The patient should be protected from exposure to infection of any kind. If he is seriously ill, he should be in a single room, and no one who has a cold should be admitted, including medical and nursing staff as well as visitors.

A large number of *drugs* such as morphine sulfate and chlorpromazine are toxic to the injured liver, since the inactivation process is diminished or absent, thus creating accumulation within the liver.[41] Therefore the effect of drugs such as morphine is unusually potent and prolonged. Furthermore, drugs such as the barbiturates are also poorly tolerated and cause an increased cerebral sensitivity to central nervous system depressants of any type. Therefore physical symptoms such as restlessness should be alleviated by nursing care so that medications can be avoided. The usual nursing measures

such as a back rub, attention to ventilation, and a warm drink should be tried before resorting to sedatives for sleep, and an ice cap should be tried before codeine or other drugs are given for a headache. Even if the patient has little or no jaundice, the liver should be protected from possible additional injury by drugs.

■ DISEASES OF THE LIVER AND PANCREAS

Viral hepatitis

Viral hepatitis is by far the most important infection attacking the liver. Although the disease is not new, it assumed serious proportions during World War II when 50,000 men developed jaundice after receiving yellow fever vaccine containing human serum.[4] Since that time it has become a major public health problem in the United States as well as in many other countries and has been studied intensively. There are two types of viral hepatitis: infectious hepatitis (IH) and serum homologous hepatitis (SH).

Incidence. Viral hepatitis is a reportable disease in most states. In 1971 the Center for Disease Control (CDC) reported approximately 69,000 cases of hepatitis in the United States.[21] The report concedes that the figures may be grossly underestimated, since carriers with subclinical manifestations also exist. It is well recognized as a major public health problem in most communities.

Most of the reported cases were of infectious hepatitis. The incidence of serum homologous hepatitis is felt to remain fairly constant, while the incidence of infectious hepatitis has two distinct patterns. First, it is more common in the fall and winter months, peaks in the late winter and early spring months, and falls to low levels in the summer. Second, the annual frequency rates seem to peak at 7-year intervals. The latest peak year was in 1968-1969.[37] Both infectious and serum hepatitis have a high incidence among drug abusers. The increased rates are due to communal living under poor sanitary conditions (infectious hepatitis), and the sharing of unsterilized needles (serum hepatitis) in parenteral drug use.[37]

Homologous serum hepatitis has a somewhat higher mortality rate than infectious hepatitis, but it is thought that its higher rate may be due to the fact that many patients who are given plasma or blood transfusions are already quite ill. It is also believed that lowered host resistance, rather than a higher virulence of the virus, may be the cause of death.

Most persons recover from viral hepatitis within 3 to 4 months. Rarely the disease may run a mild, but prolonged course, with enlargement of the liver and abnormal liver function studies persisting for 1 to 2 years. Approximately 5% of all persons with viral hepatitis have an exacerbation of the disease within 6 months of the onset. In 15% to 45% of patients with postnecrotic cirrhosis, a history of hepatitis or symptomatology resembling viral hepatitis is given. More often the disease seems to be initiated by acute hepatitis that progresses to cirrhosis.[41]

One attack of viral hepatitis confers immunity for that strain of virus infection but does not protect against attack by the other virus. However, the disease can become chronic, with acute exacerbations occurring months after the first acute symptoms have subsided. Hepatic damage following attack by one virus naturally lessens the body's defenses if attack by the second virus should occur.

Viral hepatitis seems to be most prevalent in low-income areas where there is crowding and limited sanitation. Children's homes, schools, and housing projects with a high concentration of children produce optimum settings for contact spread. Susceptibility to the disease is highest between 6 and 25 years of age, but there is a trend toward an increased incidence in adults, particularly in the older age groups.[7] Recent studies show that pregnant women are highly susceptible to viral hepatitis during the second and third trimesters of pregnancy and that the mortality rate is extremely high in the last trimester.

Causative agents—conduct and mode of transmission. Viral hepatitis is believed to be caused by filtrable viruses. Since these viruses are not transmissible from man to experimental animals, study of the disease is difficult. Recently, tests have revealed the presence of circulating antigens (substances that induce formation of antibodies) in persons with acute viral hepatitis. One antigen previously referred to as Australia antigen and currently as hepatitis B antigen (HB-Ag) has been discovered as a lipoprotein in the serum of many patients with serum hepatitis. Chemical analysis of the lipoprotein shows no relationship to human serum constituents. Tests demonstrate that the HB-Ag particles have the appearance of a virus, but to date, researchers can only say it is a lipoprotein resembling an incomplete virus particle that is detectable in the blood of patients with the infection.[21] The viruses of hepatitis appear to be extremely resistant to the usual methods of destruction of pathogenic agents, such as drying, freezing, and exposure to various disinfecting agents. There is no proof that boiling for less than 30 minutes is effective in its destruction. Autoclaving is the best way to destroy the virus.

Viral hepatitis is caused by two distinct but similar viruses that produce almost identical symptoms but that vary in their incubation period and mode of transmission. These viruses are known as the "A" or IH virus (short-incubation virus), which causes infectious hepatitis, and the "B" or SH virus (long-incubating virus), which causes homologous serum hepatitis. The latter is associated exclusively with HB-Ag.

Some investigators prefer the older terminology of type A and type B in referring to infectious hepatitis and serum hepatitis, respectively. The reason given is the possibility that agents not yet discovered (type C, D, etc.) may be responsible for some forms of hepatitis.[21] The incubation period for the IH virus is 10 to 40 days and for the SH virus, probably 2 to 6 months. The source of the virus causing *infectious hepatitis* is human blood and human feces. The infection is spread by the oral intake of food, milk, or water contaminated with the virus or by the parenteral introduction of the hepatitis virus through blood, blood products, or the equipment used for venipuncture or other procedures that require penetrating the skin. Biting insects, urine, and nasopharyngeal secretions also may be sources of the virus, but this possibility is still unproved. The virus is excreted in the feces long before clinical symptoms appear, and they may remain for long periods of time in the feces of persons who have had the disease and in carriers. It is not known whether carriers are natural carriers or whether they have had the disease in a less severe and unrecognized form. It is known that mild, subclinical disease that is not severe enough to cause jaundice can occur.

The source of the virus that causes *homologous serum hepatitis* is the blood of persons who have the infection or who are carriers of the virus. The virus is transmitted parenterally through blood, serum, or plasma or through equipment used for venipuncture or pricking the skin. It has now been confirmed that the virus is also spread if the blood of infected persons comes in contact with the mouth, the mucous membrane of the nose, or an open cut in the skin of persons caring for or associating with a patient.[1] The disease can be transmitted from infected patients to medical, nursing, and other hospital personnel by accidentally pricking the skin with a needle contaminated by a patient's blood. Since HB-Ag has been found in stool, urine, and other body secretions of infected persons, the possibility that the virus can be spread by way of the oral route into the gastrointestinal tract seems more plausible.[21] A summary of the differences between type A and type B hepatitis can be found in Table 26-2.

Prevention. It is in the area of prevention that the nurse can make the greatest contribution to the control of viral hepatitis. Since there is no specific treatment for the disease and no adequate immunization, it is only by making use of what is known about the viruses that control can be accomplished.

Methods of destroying the viruses of hepatitis are limited. There is the possibility that the undiagnosed patient may be most infectious; therefore particular emphasis should be placed on *thorough washing of hands* with soap and running water after possible

Table 26-2   Viral hepatitis: clinical, epidemiologic, and immunologic comparison

	Infectious hepatitis (type A)	Serum hepatitis (type B)
Incubation period	10 to 40 days	60 to 160 days
Route of infection	Oral or parenteral	Parenteral or personal contact
Type of onset and severity	Usually acute and mild	Usually insidious and severe
Presence of HB-Ag (previously referred to as Australia antigen)	Not present	Present during incubation period and acute phase; may persist in "carrier" state
Age group affected	Children and young adults	All age groups
Presence of jaundice	May be absent in mild cases (anicteric); rare in children; more common in adults	Rare in children; more common in adults
Abnormal transaminase (SGOT, SGPT)	Transient variations in first to third week	Prolonged for 1 to 8 months
Thymol turbidity	Usually increased	Usually normal or slightly increased
Immune serum globulin prophylaxis (ISG)	Excellent in depressing severity; questionable in prevention	Poor or questionable

determined, and for this reason many hospitals have converted to autoclave sterilization and the use of sterile, disposable syringes and needles almost entirely. Although the nurse cannot set the policy in such matters for the hospital or the public health agency, careful planning can often ensure that almost all equipment is autoclaved and that boiling is resorted to only in emergencies. When boiling is the only way to sterilize needles and other equipment, the nurse should see that everything placed in the sterilizer is *covered completely and boiled for at least a half hour.*[18] (See fundamentals of nursing texts for the proper method of sterilizing equipment by boiling.)

Both infectious hepatitis and homologous serum hepatitis can be transmitted from one patient to another when multiple doses of a drug are put into one syringe and only the needle is changed between patients. This practice should be deplored! Regardless of the extra expense involved and the extra time and work entailed in preparation of materials for each injection, separate needles and syringes that have been autoclaved or disposable syringes and needles should be used. School immunization programs and practices in large outpatient clinics such as allergy clinics have been affected by recent recommendations in this regard. The nurse often must help explain the need for the extra cost to administrative personnel.

The nurse who is responsible for obtaining blood specimens should ensure that only autoclaved lancets or needles are used to prick the skin and that only autoclaved or sterile, disposable needles and syringes are used in taking blood. All syringes that are to be reused should be autoclaved, since a vacuum may be created when the blood is being taken that can draw contaminants such as viruses from the syringe into the patient's vein. Soaking equipment in alcohol or any of the commonly used antiseptics is useless. In fact, no chemical sterilization is safe against the virus of homologous serum hepatitis.[18]

Since there are carriers of the IH and SH viruses, all needles and other equipment that have penetrated the skin of any patient should be handled with the greatest care. Homologous serum hepatitis occurs quite frequently among hospital personnel. This is not surprising considering how often the nurse, laboratory worker, or other member of the nursing staff may unwittingly prick himself with needles that have been used for a wide variety of parenteral treatments. The safest way to handle any needle that is to be sterilized and reused is to rinse it carefully in plain water after use and to place it in a rack that can be immersed in a solvent or soap solution. This practice is now in use in some institutions and agencies where all needles are cared for by a central sterile supply department or by a special staff. Also, special washers that provide efficient cleansing of both

exposure. The staff must regard all feces, blood, and other body fluids as potentially infectious and not just those of the hepatitis patient or the patient who is jaundiced. The patient should be taught how to wash his hands thoroughly, and should know why this is necessary, particularly after having a bowel movement. Thorough washing of all equipment that might be contaminated lessens the danger to persons who must handle it and may help protect the next patient for whom the equipment is used. Since infectious hepatitis can be transmitted by infected stool and contaminated foods and water, food handlers should be encouraged to pay careful attention to handwashing regulations.

At the present time dry heat and steam heat under pressure (autoclaving) are the only safe ways to sterilize needles and other equipment used to penetrate the skin. The adequate boiling time is still un-

needles and syringes with a minimum of handling are available. Needles from infusion sets should be removed from the tubing immediately when an infusion is discontinued so that persons cleaning the equipment at a later time will not accidentally prick themselves. Special precautions should be used when disposing of disposable syringes and needles both to protect garbage handlers from accidental infection and to keep them out of the hands of drug abusers. The needle should be broken at the hub immediately after using it and then placed in a covered container. Plastic syringes are subjected to hot water sterilization, which melts them and makes them unusable. All nurses must be aware of their responsibility in preventing children and adults from finding and using disposable syringes and needles in unauthorized ways.

It is recommended that patients with infectious hepatitis be placed on enteric and blood precautions. The reasons for the precautions and how the patient can assist with them should be carefully explained to him. The greatest caution should be taken in handling his stool and in performing treatments that involve contamination of the hands. Bedpans should be isolated and should be autoclaved following the patient's discharge from the hospital. Rubber gloves are often advised when enemas are given. In most localities feces need not be treated if proper sewage disposal is available. If there is any doubt, the local health department should be consulted.

To prevent spread of IH viruses by carriers, it is suggested that individual toilet paper packages, rather than rolls, be used in any public bathroom and that toilets be cleaned with 1% aqueous iodine. The use of disposable seat covers and foot pedals for flushing the toilet would help to reduce the chances of spread of the infection.

All patients should have individual thermometers, and the thermometer used for a patient with infectious hepatitis should be discarded on his discharge from the hospital. Since there is no really safe and satisfactory method of sterilizing a thermometer, discarding it is the only way to be certain that the disease will not spread by it. The cost of the thermometer is relatively small. For the protection of the nursing personnel, the patient's temperature should be taken by mouth whenever possible. When small children must have the temperature taken rectally, the greatest care should be given to washing hands thoroughly. Poor technique in carrying out temperature-taking procedures has been suspected as a cause of widespread infection from the IH virus in foundling homes and similar sheltered care facilities for children.

Even though the virus of infectious hepatitis, unlike that of serum hepatitis, has not been found in urine, special precautions should be taken in handling urine because of the possibility that urine may

be contaminated with any of the potential hepatitis viruses as yet undiscovered.[21] Because both of the viruses may be transmitted by the oral route from contaminated hands and food, special care should be taken in handling nose and mouth secretions. The patient should be instructed to use tissues, which are placed in a paper bag and burned. Disposable dishes are best to use. Food waste should be burned and dishes boiled for 30 minutes or (ideally) autoclaved. If feasible, utensils may be washed in the patient's room and autoclaved on his discharge. Rooms should be cleaned well and aired when the patient leaves the hospital. When the patient has homologous serum hepatitis, utmost care must be given to syringes, needles, and other instruments that are contaminated with the patient's serum. They should be autoclaved at 121° C. (15 pounds pressure) for 15 minutes or dry heat sterilized at 170° C. for 2 hours. Use of disposable syringes and needles is recommended. Known or suspected carriers should not be blood donors.[1] Patients should also be placed on stool precautions because of possible transmission via the fecal-oral route. If any doubt exists as to which of the virus diseases a patient has, it is safest to take the precautions necessary in the care of patients with infectious hepatitis.

Anyone who has been exposed to viral hepatitis should be urged to report this fact to the physician. This is especially important for a woman in the second or third trimester of pregnancy. Although the role of transplacentally transmitted viral hepatitis in causing injury to the liver in newborn infants has not been determined, the disease is believed to increase the likelihood of abortion, stillbirth, and congenital abnormalities.[7] Immune serum globulin (ISG, formerly called gamma globulin) offers some protection against infectious hepatitis, but it does not protect against the SH virus of homologous serum hepatitis. However, since often it cannot be determined which of the two diseases is involved, immune serum globulin usually is given in the hope that exposure was to the IH virus. Although immune serum globulin and serum albumin are obtained from the blood, they do not transmit the virus of homologous serum hepatitis. Therefore their administration cannot expose the patient to this disease. It is also recommended that persons planning travel to areas where hepatitis is endemic receive immune serum globulin. The dose for an adult is approximately 2 ml. (0.01 ml./pound of body weight) intramuscularly. Currently, a hyperimmune anti-HB globulin is undergoing clinical testing for effectiveness against serum hepatitis.[21]

A simple test for bilirubinuria, the *Ictotest,* has been developed. Since bilirubin is present in the urine of the person who has viral hepatitis before clinical signs appear, it has been suggested that, as part of a disease detection program, this test be done on anyone exposed to infectious hepatitis, all school-children, hospital patients and employees, blood donors, employees in public institutions and industrial plants, and food handlers. Early recognition of the disease would make control of its spread easier. The test is done by placing five drops of urine on the Ictotest reagent tablet.

Symptoms and pathology. The clinical symptoms of viral hepatitis vary. Patients may be asymptomatic and show minimal laboratory evidence of hepatic disturbance. Some patients may have many symptoms of the disease but no jaundice. A few may have fulminating necrosis of the liver and die. In most instances, however, viral hepatitis is a mild disease, and complete recovery is the rule.[7] Symptoms and pathology in infectious hepatitis and homologous serum jaundice are almost identical, except that acute symptoms may be more severe in infectious hepatitis. Symptoms usually appear from 4 to 7 days before jaundice is apparent and may consist of headache, anorexia, nausea and vomiting, chills, elevation of temperature, aches and pains, malaise, and tenderness over the liver. Often the patient who smokes has a sudden distaste for tobacco. Examination of blood cells reveals a leukopenia. The temperature usually returns to normal when jaundice appears, but the anorexia and nausea persist. Children usually have a milder, nonicteric form of infectious hepatitis with symptoms predominantly those of an intestinal or respiratory illness.

Viral hepatitis causes diffuse degeneration and necrosis of liver cells. Degeneration, regeneration, and inflammation may occur simultaneously and will distort the normal lobular pattern and may create pressure within and about the portal vein areas. These changes may be associated with elevated serum transaminase levels, prolonged prothrombin time, and slightly elevated serum alkaline phosphatase level. Because the pathologic process is usually distributed evenly throughout the liver, biopsy has been particularly useful in studying and diagnosing the disease. In most instances of nonfatal viral hepatitis, regeneration begins almost with the onset of the disease. The damaged cells and their contents eventually are removed by phagocytosis and enzymatic reaction, and the liver returns to normal.[7] The outcome of viral hepatitis may be affected by such factors as the virulence of the virus, the amount of hepatic damage sustained during the patient's life before exposure to the virus, his natural barriers to damage and disease of the liver, and the supportive care he receives when symptoms appear. The disease may take several courses, and different terms describe each of them.

Fulminating viral hepatitis designates a sudden and severe degeneration and atrophy of the liver. This condition may follow acute poisoning, but it most often is associated with an overwhelming infection with the hepatitis virus that progresses rapidly to cause death unless corticosteroids are successful in arresting the process. The liver may shrink in size to as little as 600 grams, in contrast to a weight of 1,500 grams in a normal adult.

Subacute fatal viral hepatitis causes acute massive necrosis, which, even though it is not evenly distributed throughout the organ, finally destroys enough of the liver to cause death. This form of the disease may vary in duration from several weeks to several months, with apparent short remissions followed by exacerbations. In its late stages, subacute fatal viral hepatitis is almost impossible to distinguish from cirrhosis of the liver in clinical manifestations and in liver function tests. However, history of exposure to viral hepatitis and symptoms of acute infection aid in diagnosis.

Chronic forms of the disease are still not well understood. Signs of chronicity may persist in biopsied hepatic tissue when liver function tests show no abnormality and when no clinical signs are evident. However, the opposite may be true. Acute exacerbations of chronic viral hepatitis can progress to acute fatal hepatic necrosis.

Management. There is no specific medical treatment for viral hepatitis. Physical activity is restricted during the acute phase, and the patient is kept in bed. The amount of bed rest required will depend on the individual patient. It will be longer in patients with severe hepatitis and in the elderly. General care, including attention to good oral hygiene, skin care, and elimination, is necessary. Special attention should be paid to protecting the patient from infection. The nurse who cares for the patient in his own home should observe carefully for changes in the color of urine and stool and for jaundice and should report the findings at once to the physician.

During the acute stage of the disease, fluids are encouraged by mouth if nausea is not a problem. The desirable fluid intake usually is considered to be at least 3,000 ml./day. If the patient's temperature is high and nausea and vomiting are severe, infusions containing glucose are given, and occasionally solutions containing other electrolytes and protein hydrolysates are ordered. Fluid intake and output are recorded. Occasionally a record of daily weight is requested to determine whether there is water retention in acute stages of the disease. When chronic disease has developed, the patient is weighed daily if ascites or edema is suspected.

When the appetite has returned to normal, a diet high in calories, proteins, and moderate carbohydrates usually is ordered. Fats may or may not be limited, and vitamins may be given. If necessary, all the nursing measures described on p. 711 should be used to encourage the patient to eat.

During the first few days after the onset of symptoms, the patient feels ill, and keeping him contented in bed is not difficult. However, restlessness becomes a nursing problem if the patient must remain in bed several weeks. When the patient begins to feel well, he becomes anxious to resume normal living and is irritated by the circumstances requiring enforced inactivity. His irritation may be expressed, for example, by tiring of the hospital menu, regardless of the quality of the food. The family should realize that in the home he may also be critical of food for the same reason. Wheeling the patient in his bed to the recreation area, where he may view television or converse with others, often helps him pass the day without boredom. Occupational therapy activities that can be brought to the bedside are useful in keeping the patient relatively content during the tiresome convalescent period.

There is a trend toward earlier ambulation of patients with viral hepatitis. When acute symptoms subside and the jaundice begins to recede, the patient may be permitted to walk about in his room with periods of rest after each meal. Activities are increased gradually, and if there are no adverse effects, the patient may be permitted to convalesce at home under close medical supervision. Recurrence of anorexia, enlargement or tenderness of the liver, or lack of progress as shown by studies of hepatic function indicate a need to return to bed rest. Some patients are cared for at home from the onset of symptoms to complete recovery. With the assistance of a public health nurse, many families are able to care for the patient safely and adequately.

Some patients develop a fulminating type of hepatitis, which may lead to hepatic collapse and death. These patients are treated with corticosteroids. When hepatic coma is imminent, they will receive the same treatment given any patient in hepatic coma. This condition is discussed on p. 724.

Abscess of the liver

The most common cause of an abscess of the liver is infection with *Entamoeba histolytica,* the causative organism in amebic dysentery. Signs of hepatic involvement may appear several months after an attack of amebic dysentery. An abscess of the liver also may be caused by a variety of pyogenic organisms such as *Escherichia coli* or *Staphylococcus aureus,* which are carried by the bloodstream or travel from the biliary ducts. Occasionally an infection in abdominal organs or other structures such as the appendix may lead to an abscess in the liver. A highly specific and sensitive indirect hemagglutination test now provides over 95% accuracy in the diagnosis of amebic liver abscesses. A liver scan may also be useful in making a diagnosis.

Nausea, vomiting, and jaundice are frequent symptoms of abscesses of the liver. Chills and sweats are common and are followed by temperature elevation, malaise, and dull, constant pain in the area of the liver. Most pyogenic abscesses can be prevented by prompt treatment of intra-abdominal infections with surgery and antibiotics. The treatment of a single abscess consists of aspiration or drainage of the abscess and administration of antibiotics. Emetine hydrochloride and chloroquine are used in the treatment of the amebic hepatic abscess, followed by aspiration or drainage as indicated. (See p. 682 for discussion of treatment of amebiasis.)

Carcinoma of the liver

Primary carcinoma of the liver is exceedingly rare. Secondary carcinoma, however, is very common and occurs in about one third of all patients in whom carcinoma has not been controlled by surgery before metastasis occurs. Metastasis to the liver should always be suspected when a patient with a history of carcinoma develops anorexia, weakness, loss of weight, secondary anemia, pain in the right upper quadrant, and general ill health. Jaundice and ascites are signs that the process is quite far advanced. The patient may live only a short time after their onset.

Until recently there was no treatment for carcinoma of the liver beyond symptomatic medical and nursing care. Now, provided that the growth is limited to a single lobe and there is no evidence of metastases elsewhere, a *hepatic lobectomy* may be done to remove metastatic as well as primary carcinoma. The remarkable regenerative capacity of the liver permits resection of 70% to 80% of the organ.[7] Preoperatively the patient is given massive doses of vitamin K, blood volume is ascertained and necessary blood given, and preparation of the bowel is done as for intestinal surgery. Postoperative care may include the care given a patient who has had chest and abdominal surgery plus the general care needed by any patient with dysfunction of the liver. A nasogastric tube usually is inserted and attached to suction. Nothing is given by mouth for several days. Cortisone may be given to enhance liver regeneration. The patient is acutely ill following this surgery and must be attended constantly, with the most careful attention given to changes in vital signs. Hemorrhage is the complication most feared, and myocardial infarction seems to occur readily.

Following surgery of the liver, the patient may be out of bed by the third postoperative day, but he must be attended constantly, and his pulse, blood pressure, and respiratory rate must be checked before, during, and after any exertion, since complications such as hemorrhage may occur.

If the growth has spread throughout the liver, irradiated yttrium or radioactive gold (^{198}Au) may be injected into the metastatic tumor masses through the abdominal wall (percutaneous route). Continuous infusions of antitumor agents such as methotrexate or 5-fluorouracil (5-FU) into the liver through a catheter inserted into the hepatic artery also may cause regression of the tumor and alleviate symptoms. (For further details and for care of the terminally ill cancer patient, see p. 304.)

Current interest in transplantation of many organs has produced two approaches used in liver transplantation. In one a donor liver is implanted in the site of the excised liver, and in the other a donor liver is transplanted in an ectopic site to supplement the residual function of the host's own liver. Hepatic transplantation in humans remains limited and experimental.

Trauma to the liver

Trauma to the liver is fairly commonly associated with automobile accidents or other injuries. There may be rupture of the liver with severe internal hemorrhage and death. Attempts are sometimes made to operate and suture the ruptured organ or to apply local pressure to stop the bleeding.

Trauma to the liver can cause severe contusion, with subsequent degeneration of injured hepatic cells. The prognosis depends on the amount of tissue damaged and other factors, and the final outcome for the patient may not be known for many years after the injury has been sustained.

Degeneration of the liver

Degeneration of the liver can follow injury, infection, and damage by toxic agents such as incompatible blood. It can be caused by obstruction of biliary passages with subsequent pressure and damage to hepatic cells. It can also be due to the ingestion of substances toxic to the liver, to faulty nutrition, and possibly to other factors not yet understood.

Prevention. The nurse can help in the prevention of degenerative liver disease by teaching the danger of injudicious use of materials that are known to be injurious to the liver and by emphasizing the need for a diet that is protective to the liver.

Since cleaning agents, solvents, and related substances sometimes contain products that are harmful to the liver, the public should read instructions on labels and should follow them implicitly. Dry-cleaning fluids may contain carbon tetrachloride, which can cause injury if warnings to avoid inhalation of the fumes and to keep windows open are not heeded. If people must use these agents inside their home, a good practice is to open the windows wide, clean the materials as quickly as possible, and then vacate the room, the apartment, or the house for several hours, leaving the windows open.

The "do-it-yourself" movement has increased the danger of hepatic damage from poisons. Many solvents that are used to remove paint and plastic material and to stain and finish woodwork contain injurious substances and should be used outdoors and not even in the basement, since dangerous fumes may spread throughout the house. Cleaning agents and finishes for cars should be applied with the garage door open or outdoors. Nurses in industry have a responsibility to teach the importance of observing regulations to avoid industrial hazards. Nitrobenzene, tetrachlorethane, carbon disulfide, and dinitrotoluol are examples of injurious compounds used in industry.

Some drugs that are known to cause mild damage to the liver must be used therapeutically. However, the nurse should warn the public regarding the use of preparations that are available without prescription that may be injurious. Many drugs reach the market before dangers of their extensive use have been conclusively ruled out; for example, chlorpromazine, which was being widely used to control "nerves," is known to cause stasis in the canaliculi of the liver, which may lead to serious hepatic damage. A safe rule to follow is to avoid taking any medication except that specifically prescribed by a physician for a specific ailment.

For many years alcohol has been incriminated as the cause of cirrhosis. While this seems to be true in certain susceptible persons, another probable cause of cirrhosis is an inadequate protein intake resulting from the haphazard fashion in which the alcoholic eats. An inadequate diet can result in degenerative changes in the liver and subsequent blockage of the portal blood vessels, causing cirrhosis. Since many people have poor eating habits, teaching the principles of proper nutrition and checking on eating habits is an important nursing function for prevention of hepatic damage.

Toxic hepatitis. Toxic hepatitis may be caused by drugs (chlorpromazine), by poisons taken for suicidal purposes (phosphorus), and by substances used in manufacturing certain products (carbon tetrachloride or methylenedianiline [MDA]). A report of an industrial outbreak of toxic hepatitis secondary to inhalation of MDA can be found in recent literature.[30a] The toxic effects and the subsequent damage to the liver parenchyma depend on the size of the dose and the amount of time that the toxic agent has been present. The more massive the dose, the greater is the injury to the hepatic cells and liver structure.

The treatment for toxic hepatitis is to remove or eliminate the cause if it is known. Lavage and catharsis may be indicated to remove the hepatotoxin from the intestinal tract. Antidotes such as BAL have been used with some degree of success in binding the agent for accessible excretion by the kidneys. Liver function tests such as tests of serum transaminase levels are valuable in evaluating the severity and the progress of the hepatic injury.

Rest in bed and general supportive care are presently all that can be done beyond the general measures used for patients with any hepatic disease. Some patients who have severe toxic hepatitis recover with apparently little, if any, residual hepatic damage. Others have severe permanent damage and may develop all the signs and symptoms of cirrhosis of the liver. The patient who recovers from an attack of toxic hepatitis should be instructed to avoid additional injury to the liver for the rest of his life.

Cirrhosis of the liver

Cirrhosis of the liver is a term applied by pathologists to several diseases that are characterized by diffuse inflammation and fibrosis of the liver resulting in structural changes affecting normal liver function. One type is *portal cirrhosis,* which is also known as Laennec's cirrhosis. Portal cirrhosis has also been called nutritional, fatty, and alcoholic cirrhosis.

Portal cirrhosis continues to be the most common type of chronic hepatic disease. Microscopically, the most important feature is loss of hepatic architecture as hepatic tissue is destroyed and replaced with fibrous tissue; regeneration of the parenchyma occurs in an irregular and disorganized fashion.[41] In European and American studies of persons with cirrhosis, chronic alcoholism was present from 50% to 80% of the time.[41] However, chronic alcoholism is by no means the only cause of portal cirrhosis. Alcoholics often develop fatty degeneration of the liver that may lead to hepatic cirrhosis, but the same histologic changes have been seen to occur in persons who are abstainers. One of the most common causes of cirrhosis is malnutrition. Other causes of cirrhosis are viral or toxic hepatitis, cardiac failure, schistosomiasis, metabolic disorders, and obstruction of the extrahepatic biliary tract.

Incidence. Portal cirrhosis is worldwide in distribution and not related to race, age, sex, or nationality. Studies of the incidence and data on the mortality in China, India, Africa, Western Europe, and South and North America, for example, suggest that environmental factors such as malnutrition may be of greatest significance. In the United States, cirrhosis as a cause of death is outranked only by heart disease, cancer, and cerebral hemorrhage in the 45- to 61-year-old age group.

Pathology. In portal cirrhosis, because of the changes listed previously, the liver is usually enlarged and firm. In cirrhosis resulting from viral or toxic hepatitis, the liver is usually shrunken and irregular, and large regeneration nodules and broad areas of fibrous tissue are present. When cirrhosis develops secondarily to congestive heart failure, the liver is firm, tender, and enlarged, and there is progressive fibrosis and accumulation of fat, without prominent regeneration nodules.

The symptoms of cirrhosis are caused by the progressive destruction of hepatic cells. The resultant regeneration and proliferation of interstitial tissue with fibrosis cause obstruction of the portal vein, which the body attempts to circumvent by establishing collateral circulation. *Ascites,* or fluid in the peritoneal cavity, usually follows obstruction of the portal vein and occasionally is one of the first signs of cirrhosis, although it usually does not occur until the disease is quite far advanced and jaundice has become marked.

Once the disease is established, it usually advances slowly to cause death. Many patients, however, can be helped to live for years if they follow instructions to protect their liver from further damage. The liver has remarkable powers of regeneration. Sometimes sufficient collateral circulation can be established and sufficient repair of hepatic tissue can be accomplished so that symptoms subside for long periods of time. At other times the patient appears to be doing fairly well when he suddenly goes into coma and may die within a few days.

Signs and symptoms. The patient with cirrhosis may have a long history of failing health, with vague complaints of gastrointestinal distress, fatigue, and low resistance to mild infections. There may be weight loss, depression, headache, and slight elevation of temperature. As the disease advances, typical signs of severe anemia, including malaise and memory loss, may occur. Venules on the head and upper body become markedly distended, and spider angiomas (tiny, bright red, pulsating arterioles that disappear on pressure) frequently appear. Veins may be prominent in the lower extremities as the patient loses weight. The skin becomes thin and dry, and edema appears in the lower trunk and lower extremities. Sometimes jaundice, first apparent in the sclerae of the eyes, is the first sign that something is wrong. Increased pressure may develop in the portal system. This pressure, in turn, increases the pressure in the esophageal veins, and varicosities may develop in them. Occasionally gastric hemorrhage following rupture of a varicosed esophageal vein and drainage of blood into the stomach are the first indications that the patient has advanced cirrhosis of the liver. The increased portal pressure may cause hypersplenism, which is characterized by anemia, neutropenia, and thrombocytopenia. Furthermore, increased erythrocyte destruction occurs within the enlarged spleen.[7]

Management. There is no specific treatment for cirrhosis of the liver; the emphasis is on preventing further damage to the liver and on supportive care of the patient. Thus an adequate diet compatible with the ability of the patient's liver to handle protein will be ordered. Rest, moderate exercise, avoidance of exposure to infections, and protection from toxic agents of any kind are emphasized. Alcohol is forbidden. The patient is often disinterested in food and needs constant encouragement to eat the prescribed diet. As the disease progresses, more and more effort must be made to compensate for the failure of the several functions of the liver. Vitamins may be given to compensate for the organ's lost ability to store vitamins A, B complex, D, and K. Bile salts are usually given if the patient is jaundiced because absorption of fat-soluble vitamin A and synthesis of vitamin K are poor due to insufficient bile salts in the intestine.

Because alcohol is thought to interfere with the hepatic conversion of folic acid to its active metabolites, many of these persons have a folic acid deficiency anemia that usually responds well to treatment with oral doses of folic acid.[4]

To achieve a remission of threatened hepatic failure in cirrhosis may take a long time. There may be setbacks and periods when there is no improvement. The patient and his family often become discouraged and require support from the physician and nurse. On discharge from the hospital, visits from the public health nurse may be requested to give whatever care, supervision, and support seem necessary. The patient must be taught to avoid substances potentially toxic to the liver, such as alcohol and chlorpromazine.

Complications of hepatic disease

Ascites, or the accumulation of serous fluid in the peritoneal cavity, is the result of many factors, both local and systemic. These factors include (1) decreased hepatic synthesis of albumin necessary for plasma osmotic pressure, (2) increased portal vein pressure creating transudation from the intestines and mesentery, (3) increased serum aldosterone level due to impaired degradation by the liver, and (4) transudation from the liver due to obstruction of hepatic lymph outflow.[7] The patient with cirrhosis frequently retains abnormal amounts of water and sodium. The sodium retention would seem to be related to the excessive aldosterone activity. It has been postulated that water is retained by excessive secretion of antidiuretic hormone, possibly caused by the liver dysfunction.[7]

Ascites is a fairly common complication of advanced hepatic disease and is treated in several ways. Restriction of sodium aids greatly in limiting the formation of ascitic fluid in disease of the liver. The patient with cirrhosis usually is on a low-sodium diet. The lack of salt in the food makes it less palatable, and the patient may not consume enough protein and total calories. The nurse should report the patient's food intake to the physician and dietitian, as adjustments may need to be made in the salt restriction. Salt substitutes such as potassium gluconate may be permitted.

Many physicians try to control edema and fluid accumulation in the abdomen by giving diuretics. Removal of fluid through the kidneys has the advantage of usually not removing essential body protein, which is contained in fluid removed from the abdom-

inal cavity. Since a single diuretic usually is not successful, a combination is used. Thiazide diuretics such as chlorothiazide (Diuril), which inhibits the reabsorption of sodium in the proximal tubules, and spironolactone A (Aldactone A), which prevents the reabsorption of sodium in the distal tubules, may be given. Occasionally, one of the glucocorticoids such as prednisone may be added. Complications do occur from the administration of these drugs but can be prevented in some instances. For example, the loss of potassium due to the administration of the thiazides can be compensated for by increasing the intake of potassium in foods. Spironolactone A may increase the amount of potassium in the blood, and it may be necessary to decrease the potassium intake. The nurse should list the food and fluids that are high in potassium for the patient and his family so that they can make the necessary adjustments in his diet. (See p. 126 and references 26 and 53.)

When renal function is impaired or when it is felt that diuretic therapy may precipitate hepatic coma, paracentesis may be necessary (Fig. 26-2). However, paracentesis is used with caution in patients with severe and chronic liver disease since it may also precipitate hepatic coma. If the abdomen is tight with fluid and is producing dyspnea and anorexia, paracentesis may be necessary. In general, only enough

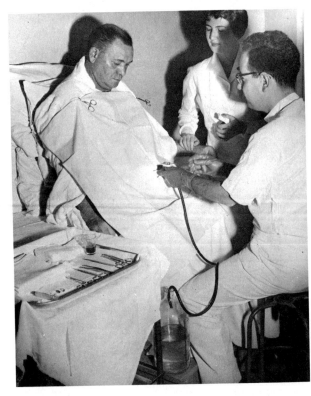

FIG. 26-2. Careful observation is necessary during a paracentesis. Note the pillows supporting the back and arms of the patient. The patient's feet are resting on a stool.

fluid to make the patient comfortable is removed. Other dangers of paracentesis include shock and hypovolemia, which occur as the fluid from the general circulation shifts to the peritoneal cavity as the ascitic fluid is withdrawn. One liter of ascitic fluid contains as much protein as 200 ml. of whole blood. Salt-poor human blood albumin may be administered to counteract the loss of fluid and protein. (For details of paracentesis and the nursing care involved, see texts on fundamentals of nursing.)

Patients with cirrhosis are often *jaundiced* and this will cause severe itching. Keeping the skin clean, dry, and well lubricated will improve the itching. Calamine lotion may also be helpful. Because these patients are often emaciated and have edema, this presents another problem in skin care. The patient should be turned frequently to help prevent pressure areas from developing over the sacrum. Many of these patients also have presacral edema which leads to skin breakdown. The use of alternating pressure mattresses and flotation pads (p. 188) may be helpful. When edema is severe, the skin may "weep" as the accumulation of fluid seeps through the pores in the skin. Frequent change of bed linen will then be necessary.

Esophagogastric varices are varicosities occurring in the cardiac end of both the stomach and the esophagus and are caused by pressure within the portal venous system with subsequent backing up of venous blood. Esophagogastric varices occur in approximately 30% of all patients with cirrhosis of the liver[39]; however, any patient with cirrhosis of the liver is a potential candidate for varices. The varices

may rupture, with flow of blood into the stomach. Severe hematemesis and resultant shock follow, requiring emergency treatment.

Management. Management of bleeding esophagogastric varices consists of restoring blood volume and controlling the bleeding. Measures that may control the hemorrhage include gastric lavage with ice water, local gastric hypothermia using an esophagogastric balloon, or intravenous injection of vasopressin (Pitressin), which reduces portal pressure and blood flow by constricting the splanchnic arterioles. Since vasopressin also decreases the blood supply to the liver, it should be used with caution. Esophagogastric tamponade (with a Blakemore-Sengstaken tube) may be used to control massive hemorrhage. In selected persons, emergency surgical procedures such as direct ligation of the varices, esophagogastric resection, or splenorenal or portacaval anastomosis may be performed.

The esophagogastric tube (Blakemore-Sengstaken) is a three-lumen tube with two balloon attachments. One lumen serves as a nasogastric suction tube, the second is used to inflate the gastric balloon, and the third is used to inflate the esophageal balloon (Fig. 26-3). The tube is passed through the nose into the stomach with the balloons deflated. When the tube is in the stomach, the gastric balloon is inflated with 100 to 300 ml. of air and the lumen is clamped; the tube is then pulled out slowly so that the balloon is held tightly against the cardioesophageal junction. A cube of foam rubber called a nasal cuff is placed between the tube and the nares, and the tube is secured to the face with adhesive tape.

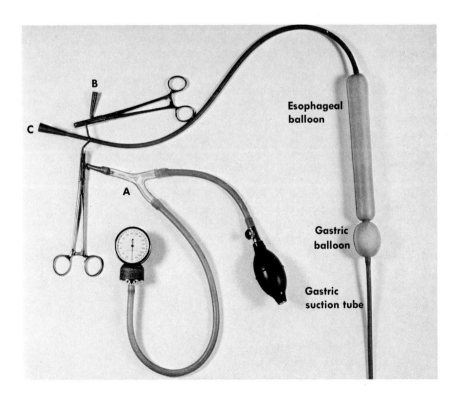

FIG. 26-3. The esophagogastric tube (Blakemore-Sengstaken tube). **A,** Lumen leading to the esophageal balloon. **B,** Lumen leading to the gastric balloon. **C,** Lumen for gastric suction. (See text.)

Esophageal balloon

Gastric balloon

Gastric suction tube

The cube of foam rubber absorbs excess nasal secretions and reduces trauma to the nostril. It also provides traction which maintains the tube in the proper position. If after the gastric balloon is inflated there is further hematemesis or if bloody fluid is returned on aspiration, one can assume that the bleeding is from the esophagus and the esophageal balloon should be inflated (Fig. 26-4). The esophageal lumen is connected by a Y tube to a manometer and the balloon is inflated with 20 to 45 mm. Hg and clamped. In order to stop bleeding, the pressure will have to be greater than the patient's portal venous pressure. If bleeding is from esophageal varices, blood will no longer be aspirated from the stomach. If there is still blood present, the stomach may be lavaged with a small amount of ice water, or a solution of iced alcohol and water may be circulated through the balloon to provide vasoconstriction as well as pressure. The nasogastric lumen is usually connected to intermittent gastric suction, which permits easy appraisal of whether or not bleeding has ceased and also serves to keep the stomach empty. It is important to remove all blood from the stomach because it may precipitate hepatic coma.

The person who is being treated for esophagogastric varices is very ill and may be disoriented. He requires constant attention and if there is any chance he will pull on the tube, his arms should be restrained. The nurse must be constantly alert to the pressure in the balloons. If the gastric balloon should collapse or rupture, the entire tube may move up and obstruct the patient's airway. Should the gastric balloon rupture, the esophageal balloon is deflated at once and the entire tube is removed.

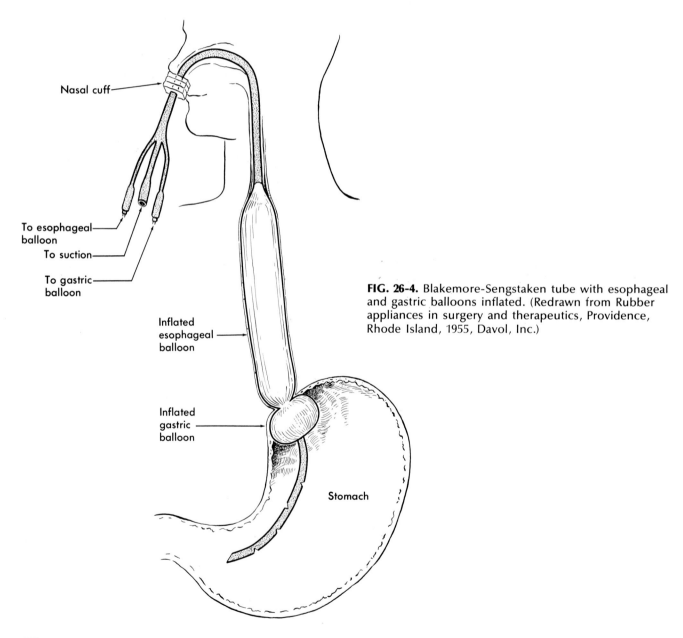

Nasal cuff

To esophageal balloon

To suction

To gastric balloon

Inflated esophageal balloon

Inflated gastric balloon

Stomach

FIG. 26-4. Blakemore-Sengstaken tube with esophageal and gastric balloons inflated. (Redrawn from Rubber appliances in surgery and therapeutics, Providence, Rhode Island, 1955, Davol, Inc.)

The esophageal balloon can be left inflated up to 48 hours without tissue damage or severe discomfort for the patient. The fully inflated gastric balloon with traction exerted on it, however, compresses the stomach wall between the balloon and the diaphragm, causing ulceration of the gastric mucosa, and is severely uncomfortable for the patient. To offset the possibility of necrosis, the physician may release the traction and balloon pressures periodically. A second tube should be in the patient unit ready for immediate use in case of damage to the one being used (the tubes are not reused). Before the tube is inserted, the balloons should be tested. The tubes have the date of manufacture stamped on them, and those over a year old should be discarded because of deterioration of the rubber. Before removal of the tube, the balloons are deflated gradually, and the tube is then gently withdrawn by the physician. The patient then should be observed closely for any indications of renewed bleeding.

As soon as the balloons are in place and bleeding has been controlled, transfusions of *fresh* whole blood are given to combat the hypovolemic shock. Fresh blood is used for several reasons: (1) whole blood develops an increasing concentration of ammonia due to hydrolysis of various unstable compounds, and hepatic coma can be precipitated with blood that is only 3 to 4 days old[26]; (2) the damaged liver may be unable to metabolize citrate from the sodium citrate used to preserve stored blood, and citric intoxication can result; (3) patients with cirrhosis excrete sodium poorly; and (4) refrigerated blood is virtually devoid of prothrombin and coagulation factors essential for clotting.

Oxygen is usually administered to increase the oxygen available to the blood. A saline cathartic such as magnesium sulfate may be given through the nasogastric tube to hasten the expulsion of blood that has passed from the stomach to the intestine, and enemas may also be given. This is in an effort to lessen bacterial action of the blood in the intestinal tract. This action produces ammonia, which passes to the bloodstream and in turn puts a burden on the liver, which must detoxify it to form urea. An antibiotic that destroys intestinal bacteria, such as neomycin, also may be given to lessen their activity in the decomposition of protein in the intestine. Antacids are commonly prescribed to reduce stomach acidity and to prevent a reflux of acid into the esophagus. They are given through the nasogastric lumen of the tube.[30]

Nursing intervention. The patient with bleeding esophagogastric varices is acutely ill and extremely apprehensive. Discomfort from the tamponade tube and the potential onset of encephalopathy must be considered in the patient's behavior. He must be attended constantly, given reassurance, and kept absolutely quiet. All procedures and his part in them should be quietly and calmly explained to him and carried out with the minimum of activity. The family generally is very frightened and should be given as much information as necessary to relieve their concern. Some member of the family should be permitted to see the patient or to stay with him for a short time.

The nurse is responsible for checking the vital signs, which may be observed as often as every 15 minutes until there are signs that hemorrhage is controlled. The blood pressure cuff should be left on the arm deflated, and care should be taken to inflate it only a few degrees above the anticipated level. In this way many patients may sleep through the taking of blood pressure. Care should be taken to see that the transfusion and the infusions are running. The patient in shock may feel cold and must be kept warm but not perspiring. If iced solutions are used in the balloons, chills may occur. They should be reported to the physician, who may order a warming blanket.

When an esophagogastric tube is in use the nurse must also check the manometer attached to the esophagogastric tube. If the pressure rises or falls below the prescribed level, the amount of air or solution in the balloon must be adjusted. Often this adjustment is made by the physician, but it may be made by the nurse if there are orders to that effect.

Because the inflated esophageal balloon occludes the esophagus, the patient cannot take anything by mouth or even swallow his saliva. He should be provided with cleansing tissues and an emesis basin. The patient needs frequent mouth care, and all blood in his mouth should be removed. If he is very weak or if he is not permitted to move at all, gentle suctioning of the mouth and throat may be needed to prevent aspiration of saliva. The nostrils should be kept clean, lubricated, and protected so that tissues do not sustain injury because of pressure from the tube. Care must be taken not to disturb the tube, and the nurse should consult with the physician as to how much movement the patient is permitted. Passive moving of extremities usually is allowed.

Surgical care. Because bleeding from esophagogastric varices usually is caused by portal hypertension due to obstruction of blood flow somewhere in the portal venous system, curative treatment is aimed at locating the site of obstruction by x-ray examination and then reducing the flow of blood through that portion of the portal system. Depending on the location of the obstruction, various elective operative procedures may be employed. If the splenic vein is blocked, a *splenectomy* may be done. If the block is intrahepatic, a *portacaval anastomosis* (portacaval shunt) may be done. The portal vein is anastomosed to the inferior vena cava so that the blood from the portal system bypasses the liver (Fig. 26-5). When the portal vein is blocked, the splenic vein is anasto-

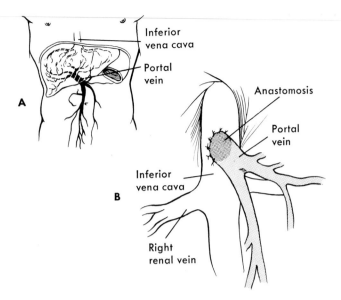

FIG. 26-5. Portacaval shunt. **A,** Normal relationship of the portal vein to the inferior vena cava. **B,** Anastomosis of the portal vein to the inferior vena cava.

mosed to the left renal vein. This procedure is called a *splenorenal shunt* and relieves pressure on the portal vein since approximately 30% of the blood in the portal vein comes from the splenic vein.[39] If there is no portal hypertension, the varicosed vessels may be ligated through a thoracotomy incision.

Careful preoperative preparation is necessary since it must be remembered that the patient with liver damage severe enough to cause bleeding varices is not a good operative risk. Preoperative criteria for a portacaval shunt include at least one hemorrhage from esophageal varices, absence of ascites and hepatic coma, a bilirubin level below 1.5 mg., and an albumin level above 3 Gm./100 ml. It is generally felt that a *prophylactic* shunt is not usually justified. The patient is usually apprehensive about the recommended operation, yet in *selected* cases it is known that the operative risk is much less than the risk from recurring hemorrhage. Vitamin K, antibiotics, and transfusions are usually given preoperatively.

Following surgery the patient needs close observation and often constant nursing attention. Narcotics should be given for severe pain, but sedative drugs usually are avoided because of their toxic effects on the diseased liver. Generally, narcotics are given in guarded amounts and infrequently in the presence of liver disease. When they are given, the patient must be observed carefully for impending hepatic coma. The patient must be encouraged to breathe deeply and to cough hourly. Fluid intake and output must be recorded accurately, and lessening of output must be reported, since renal function sometimes decreases for a time following this operation.

Hemorrhage may occur since prothrombin levels may be lowered. Hepatic coma may also be a postoperative complication. The nurse can recognize impending hepatic coma by beginning signs of mental confusion, slowness in response, and generally inappropriate behavior.

Some surgeons do not pass a nasogastric tube because of danger of injury to the varices. Others pass a nasogastric tube and attach it to suction postoperatively since it is believed that postoperative distention may predispose to thrombosis of the portal vein. In either instance the patient is fed intravenously and given nothing by mouth until signs of active peristalsis are apparent. The patient is observed closely for pain, distention, fever, and nausea, which may be signs of thrombosis at the site of anastomosis. *Regional heparinization* may be employed to prevent thrombus formation at operation. A fine polyethylene catheter is inserted into the right gastroepiploic vein, brought out through the wound, and attached to a continuous drip of heparin and saline solution. The surgeon determines the rate of flow. The catheter may be left for 5 to 7 days, and during this time the nurse must see that it is not obstructed or subjected to tension in any way. During heparinization, the patient remains in bed or sits by the bedside. Particular attention should be paid, therefore, to exercising the lower extremities in an attempt to prevent thrombi from developing.

Some surgeons prefer to keep the patient flat in bed for several days until the anastomosis is healed. Others have their patients get out of bed on the day after the operation. Leg and arm exercises are begun on the day after surgery. The lower extremities must be observed carefully for signs of edema, which may follow the sudden increase of blood flow into the inferior vena cava. Elevation of the lower extremities may be ordered, and the length of time the patient spends standing and walking should be medically prescribed.

After a shunting procedure, none of the venous blood passes through the liver, and protein end products are not completely detoxified. For this reason, the patient is occasionally placed on a low-protein diet. Neomycin or chlortetracycline (Aureomycin), both of which destroy the bacteria in the intestine, may be given so that fewer bacteria remain to break down protein.

Hepatic coma

Hepatic coma (hepatic encephalopathy) is a degenerative disease of the brain associated with liver failure. Dysfunctions of the central nervous system are thought to be precipitated by elevated ammonia concentrations, hypoxia, changes in electrolyte concentrations with disturbances of acid-base balance, infections, and depressant drugs. Many patients with hepatic coma have an increase in their blood ammo-

Table 26-3 Factors commonly precipitating hepatic coma

Factors depressing liver function	Factors increasing level of ammonia
Hypoxia	Gastrointestinal ammonia (old blood in bowel from gastrointestinal hemorrhage)
Secondary to hemorrhage and hypovolemic shock	High-protein intake
Secondary to morphine and other sedatives	Transfusions, especially with stored blood
Intercurrent infection	Thiazide diuretics and acetazolamide (Diamox)
Exercise	Hypokalemia
In patients with chronic liver disease who are in impending coma	Secondary to thiazide diuretics
In patients with acute hepatitis	Secondary to potassium loss from the bowel
Acute hepatitis during pregnancy, especially during last trimester	Shunting of blood into systemic circulation without passing through hepatic sinusoids
Abdominal paracentesis	Natural collateral bypass of liver
Secondary to reduction of plasma volume	Surgical bypass of liver
Patients may also have hyponatremia, especially if natriuretic diuretics were being administered before paracentesis	Alkalosis secondary to hyperventilation and hypokalemia
	Hyperbilirubinemia (serum bilirubin level greater than 35 mg./100 ml.)

nia concentration. Normally, ammonia, which is formed in the intestines from the breakdown of protein by intestinal bacteria, is converted to urea through the Krebs-Henseleit cycle in the liver. When liver failure occurs, ammonia is not converted into urea and ammonia concentration in the circulating blood is increased. The factors that may cause depression of liver function and/or an increase in the level of ammonia in the blood and thus may precipitate hepatic coma are summarized in Table 26-3. The signs and symptoms of hepatic failure include changes in personality and behavior, lethargy, confusion, twitching, and a characteristic flapping tremor of the extremities, dizziness, stupor, and coma. A peculiar sweetish odor can frequently be detected on the breath (fetor hepaticus). The patient's temperature may rise markedly. Symptoms may follow a sudden increase in jaundice or in ascites.

Treatment of hepatic coma centers around (1) finding and treating the precipitating cause, (2) general supportive measures, and (3) avoidance of additional trauma to the liver.[26] This is accomplished by eliminating protein from the diet completely for several days, giving carbohydrates by mouth or nasogastric feedings, and administering antibiotics such as neomycin that destroy bacteria in the intestine and subsequently reduce the amount of ammonia formed. Enemas and cathartics such as magnesium sulfate may be given to empty the bowel and prevent further ammonia formation. Some physicians prefer to rely on cathartics and on the use of cation exchange resins to help remove toxic substances from the bowel rather than to give the antibiotics. Antibiotics destroy bacteria, which are active in the manufacture of vitamin K, and the absence of bacteria causes diar-

rhea and other symptoms. Sodium glutamate and L-arginine are sometimes given intravenously in a solution of glucose in an attempt to stimulate the formation of urea and reduce the amount of ammonia in the blood, but these two substances have not been proved to be of definite benefit.[1] Recently lactulose has been used experimentally in an attempt to decrease the production of ammonia. Lactulose, which is given orally, is a synthetic disaccharide that cannot be utilized in the small intestine. It produces diarrhea, lowers the pH, and alters the bacterial flora of the colon, thereby decreasing the production of nitrogenous substances.

In some patients, large doses of the adrenocortical steroids are effective in reversing hepatic coma, providing that hepatic cell destruction has not been overwhelming.

Many patients in hepatic coma die of renal failure secondary to an inadequate circulating blood volume (hypovolemia). In some patients, renal function progressively deteriorates without any apparent cause. The treatment of hepatic coma requires a careful balancing of fluid administration to maintain adequate perfusion of the kidney without creating an excessive load on the cardiovascular system. Therefore, when intravenous solutions are being administered, the nurse must be cognizant of the desired flow rate and be alert to signs of cardiovascular overload. These would include tachycardia, dyspnea, and sudden chest pain (p. 124). In order to adequately monitor renal function, an indwelling catheter is often inserted, especially if the patient is being maintained on intravenous fluids. Central venous pressure (CVP) monitoring (p. 326) is also commonly used. The nurse must be alert to changes in the CVP readings suggestive of either hypervolemia or hypovolemia.[30] The supportive nursing care required by any patient with hepatic disease as well as by any unconscious patient should be given.

Tracheostomy may be performed as a prophylactic measure. Intermittent positive pressure breathing with oxygen may also be used to improve oxygenation.[30] (See pp. 567 and 617 for details of care of patients with these treatments.) Since most narcotics and sedatives must be detoxified by the liver, they are contraindicated in patients with impaired liver function. If a sedative must be used, drugs such as chlordiazepoxide (Librium), barbital, or phenobarbital, which are excreted by the kidney, are prescribed.[30]

Exchange transfusions have been used to combat hepatic coma on the premise that toxic substances are both diluted and removed from the blood. In selected patients a colon bypass operation may be performed to stop function of the colon and prevent absorption of material from the intestines. Attempts have been made to replace nonfunctioning livers with those of recent cadavers.[8] To date these transplants have not been successful because immunosuppressive therapy is inadequate and the transplanted organs have been rejected by the recipient's body.

The patient in hepatic coma is very ill and is vulnerable to any increase in stress. He should receive the meticulous nursing care necessary for any patient who is unconscious. Particular care should be taken to protect the patient from infection. If the patient survives, long-term care as discussed for the patient with cirrhosis of the liver should be planned. The patient who has had definite or threatened hepatic coma may be kept indefinitely on a diet low in protein. When protein is added to the diet, it will be added gradually and often will not exceed 50 Gm. daily (normal intake is 70 to 80 Gm. daily). Patients with chronic liver disease may go in and out of coma; therefore the patient should be observed for any change in behavior, which would indicate early coma. The patient and his family should also be taught to be alert to subtle changes in his behavior.

Pancreatitis

Pancreatitis is an inflammation of the pancreas. There may be edema of the tissues, suppuration and abscess formation, necrosis, or hemorrhage, depending on the cause and the severity of the disease. The chief cause is the obstruction of the pancreatic duct by stones, tumors, or inflammatory strictures that prevent the free flow of pancreatic secretions into the duodenum. Regurgitation of bile through the pancreatic duct and activation of proteolytic enzymes in the pancreatic juice also cause pancreatitis. It may be caused by infection carried by the bloodstream or traveling from the biliary system or the duodenum. Many of the patients with acute pancreatitis have

associated disease of the biliary tract or are chronic alcoholics.[39]

The most common type of *acute pancreatitis* is known as the edematous type and often is associated with chronic biliary tract disease. The patient has constant pain radiating to the back, which may be so severe that he is unable to lie on his side. The pain may be so excruciating that it causes shock. Nausea and vomiting, elevation of temperature, and elevation of white blood cell count often are present, and jaundice may occur. Elevated serum and urine amylase levels often help the doctor to distinguish acute pancreatitis from other acute conditions of the abdomen or from coronary artery disease. The urinary amylase level remains elevated for a longer period of time than does the serum amylase level.

Meperidine hydrochloride (Demerol), 100 to 200 mg. every 4 to 6 hours, may be necessary to reduce pain. Occasionally the intravenous administration of procaine hydrochloride or a splanchnic nerve block may be necessary to relieve the pain. Nothing is permitted by mouth because of nausea and because it would stimulate pancreatic secretions and aggravate symptoms. Propantheline bromide (Pro-Banthine bromide) or methantheline bromide (Banthine bromide) may be given parenterally to depress vagal stimulation of pancreatic secretions. Recently aprotinin (Trasylol) has been administered. It inhibits trypsin, inactivates kallikrein (an enzyme normally present in an inactive form, which is activated during acute pancreatitis), and relieves pain.[34] Antibiotics may be administered to control infections. Paralytic ileus may occur as a response to the severe abdominal pain. A nasogastric tube usually is inserted and attached to suction. Intravenous fluids and appropriate electrolytes are administered. If shock is present, it may be treated with transfusions of blood, plasma, or dextran. ACTH or corticosteroids may be used to treat patients with severe and fulminating pancreatitis.

An exploratory laparotomy may be performed in acute pancreatitis when a diagnosis cannot be established and the possibility of general peritonitis, perforation of an organ, or a bowel obstruction cannot be excluded. If cholecystitis or cholelithiasis is present, an operation may be performed when the patient can tolerate surgery. An operation also is sometimes done in an attempt to divert or increase bile flow at the sphincter of Oddi (entrance to the duodenum) and thereby reduce regurgitation of bile into the pancreatic duct.

A much less common but more severe form of acute pancreatitis is known as acute hemorrhagic pancreatitis. In this fulminating process, pancreatic enzymes erode major blood vessels, causing hemorrhage into the pancreas, the retroperitoneal tissues, and the colon. The patient may develop ascites, and the exudate obtained on paracentesis is described as "beef broth."[4] The patient goes quickly into shock and must be treated with transfusions of whole blood. An operation may be done to drain blood or other fluid from the abdominal cavity. Despite intensive medical treatment and the best of nursing care, the mortality rate is high.

Pancreatitis can become *chronic* with calcification and fibrous replacement of normal duct tissue. Nausea, persistent pain, loss of weight, and occasionally jaundice occur. The danger of addiction to narcotics becomes a problem with patients who have chronic pancreatitis, particularly alcoholics. If there is extensive damage to the islet cells, diabetes mellitus may complicate the disease.

Tumors of the pancreas

Tumors of the pancreas are usually malignant and occur most often in the head of the pancreas, causing jaundice and obstruction. Men are affected much more often than women. Usually the patient is past middle life, and obvious signs such as severe pain and jaundice may have been preceded by vague anorexia, nausea, and weight loss over a period of months. Surgery is usually done in an attempt to remove the tumor from the head of the pancreas.

If the tumor is operable, a pancreaticoduodenal resection (Whipple procedure), which includes removal of the head of the pancreas, the lower end of the common bile duct, the duodenum, and the distal stomach, may be done. The common bile duct and the remaining portion of the pancreas and stomach are then anastomosed to the jejunum. If the tumor is not resectable, a palliative operation such as a cholecystojejunostomy, a choledochojejunostomy, or a palliative gastrojejunostomy may be done to help restore temporarily a normal flow of bile and some pancreatic enzyme to the intestinal tract. The type of procedure performed depends on the involvement found at operation. Palliation of the symptoms also may be achieved by the administration of chemotherapeutic agents such as 5-fluorouracil.[39]

In addition to routine postoperative care following abdominal surgery, the patient who has had pancreatic surgery must be watched for signs of peritonitis, gastrointestinal obstruction, and jaundice until sufficient time for healing has elapsed and until it is determined that all the anastomoses are secure and patent. Stools should be observed, and frothy, light-colored stools containing conspicuously undigested fat should be reported. If most of the pancreas was removed, the patient may have to take pancreatic enzymes in tablet form by mouth to aid the digestion of fat. The patient should be watched for signs and symptoms of diabetes mellitus following this procedure, although it rarely occurs unless the entire pancreas has been removed. If hypoinsulinism occurs, treatment with insulin will be necessary for the remainder of the patient's life (p. 748). The average

duration of life after the Whipple procedure is about a year.

Occasionally a patient may have an islet cell tumor of the pancreas. It is a benign lesion in the tail of the pancreas and results in overproduction of insulin, causing symptoms of hypoglycemia (p. 756). Surgical removal of the tumor relieves symptoms.

■ DISEASES OF THE BILIARY SYSTEM

There are no specific means to prevent disease of the biliary system. However, since disease of this system occurs much more often in obese persons, it is reasonable to suppose that control of obesity may contribute to its prevention. Women are more often affected than men, and the description "fair, fat, and forty" is a fairly accurate one. Married women who spend most of their time at home may add more calories than they realize by "eating up leftovers." In all health education the nurse should stress the importance of avoiding excess weight. Patients with biliary tract disease are usually advised to keep fat intake to a fairly low level for the remainder of their lives, although no rigid dietary regulations are needed. Patients who tend to form stones in the ducts are usually advised to be particularly careful of their fat intake and to take generous amounts of fluids. The nurse should emphasize the physician's instructions in this regard.

Cholecystitis

Inflammation of the gallbladder is called cholecystitis. This condition may be acute or chronic and usually is associated with gallstones or other obstructions of bile passage.

A large variety of organisms may contribute to acute disease of the gallbladder. Colon bacilli, staphylococci, streptococci, salmonellae, typhoid bacilli, and many other organisms have been found. Infection may reach the gallbladder through the bloodstream, the lymph system, or the bile ducts. Inflammation may be confined to the mucous membrane lining, or the entire wall of the gallbladder may be involved. Sometimes damage to the wall of the gallbladder results from distention caused by obstruction of bile flow and from contractions of the smooth muscle as it attempts to dislodge a stone occluding the lumen of one of the bile ducts. Cholecystitis is more common in women than in men, the ratio being 2.5:1. Sedentary, obese persons are affected most often, and the incidence is highest in the fifth and sixth decades of life. The incidence of cholecystitis and the mortality rate are high in the elderly.[40]

Acute cholecystitis may be abrupt in onset, although the patient often has a history of intolerance to fatty foods and some general indigestion. Nausea and vomiting usually occur, and there is severe pain in the right upper quadrant of the abdomen. The patient's pulse rate and respiratory rate are increased, and temperature and white blood count are elevated. The chronic form of the disease is usually preceded by several acute attacks of moderate severity, and the patient gives a history of having learned to avoid fried foods and certain other foods such as nuts that are high in fat.

The treatment of choice for most patients with cholecystitis is surgery. The decision as to when to operate depends largely on the age and condition of the patient and the way he responds to treatment. Although some surgeons favor conservative treatment until the acute infection has subsided, others believe that the danger of rupture and subsequent peritonitis is so great that immediate surgery to drain the gallbladder is advisable (*cholecystostomy*). All recommend removing the gallbladder (*cholecystectomy*) when the acute condition has subsided. Infection may spread to the hepatic duct and liver, causing inflammation of the ducts (*cholangitis*) with subsequent strictures that may cause obstruction of bile flow and that are exceedingly difficult to correct surgically.

When medical treatment is prescribed, it includes the administration of antibiotics and infusions of glucose and appropriate electrolytes. Food is withheld until acute symptoms subside. If vomiting persists, a nasogastric tube is passed and attached to suction. Meperidine hydrochloride may be given for pain, although it is thought by some authorities to increase spasm of the biliary sphincter. The inhalation of amyl nitrite may diminish intestinal and biliary spasms.

When food is tolerated, a reducing diet and careful avoidance of too much fat usually are recommended by the doctor. Patients who have had acute attacks are more strongly motivated to follow dietary instructions, and the nurse may be of real help to them in planning attractive dishes that are low in fat and total calories.

Cholelithiasis

Cholelithiasis means the presence of stones in the biliary tract. The stones are composed largely of cholesterol, bile pigment, and calcium. Cholelithiasis may occur in either sex at any age, but it is more common in middle-aged women. The incidence increases gradually thereafter, and one out of every three persons who reach the age of 75 years will have gallstones.[39] It is not known why stones form in the gallbladder and in the hepatic duct. They may be present for years and cause no inflammation. Sometimes they appear to be preceded or followed by chronic cholecystitis. Chronic cholelithiasis is aggravated by pregnancy, perhaps because of the increased pressure in the abdomen.

Gallstones vary in size and number. The small stones are more likely to cause attacks of acute biliary colic, since they pass more easily into the ducts.

Stones may lodge anywhere along the biliary tract where they may cause an obstruction which, if unrelieved, leads to jaundice, or they may cause pressure and subsequent necrosis and infection of the walls of the biliary ducts (Fig. 26-6). Occasionally a stone, because of its location, blocks the entrance of pancreatic fluid and bile into the duodenum at the ampulla of Vater. This condition is difficult to differentiate from obstruction caused by malignancy.

There may be no signs of cholelithiasis until a stone becomes lodged in a biliary duct, although the patient often gives a history of indigestion after consuming rich, fatty foods, occasional discomfort in the right upper quadrant of the abdomen, and more trouble than the normal person with gaseous eructations after eating. Gaseous eructations in cholelithiasis characteristically occur almost immediately following meals, in contrast to those associated with gastric ulcer, which occur when the stomach is empty (usually several hours after a meal).

Gallstone colic, or *biliary colic,* can cause what is probably the most severe pain that can be experienced. The pain may come on suddenly and is probably caused by spasm of the ducts as they attempt to dislodge the stone. There is severe pain in the right upper quadrant of the abdomen, and it radiates through to the back under the scapula and to the right shoulder. Pain may be so severe that the patient writhes in agony despite large doses of analgesic

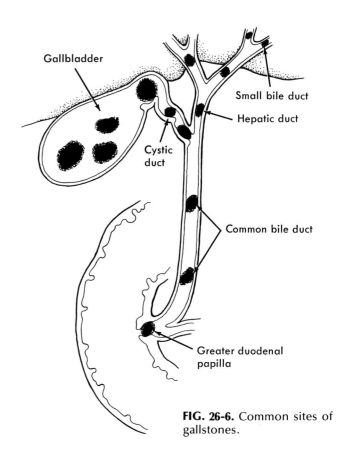

FIG. 26-6. Common sites of gallstones.

drugs. Morphine sulfate and meperidine hydrochloride are avoided if possible because they are thought to increase spasm of the biliary sphincters and increase pressure, which can cause further trauma to the walls of the biliary passages. Nitroglycerin or inhalations of amyl nitrite are sometimes helpful, and papaverine hydrochloride, atropine, and calcium gluconate often are given to help produce relaxation of the biliary ducts. The patient usually has nausea and vomiting, profuse diaphoresis, tachycardia, and occasionally complete prostration. A nasogastric tube attached to suction often helps to relieve distention in the upper gastrointestinal tract and thereby lessens the pain. Occasionally, following an acute attack of biliary colic, the stools are saved to determine whether or not a stone has passed into the intestines. The stools may be sent to the laboratory, or they may be strained for examination on the patient unit.

The treatment for cholelithiasis is surgical removal of the gallbladder and exploration of the common bile duct as soon as the acute attack subsides and the patient can withstand an operation safely.

Carcinoma

Carcinoma can occur anywhere in the biliary system, and unfortunately at present there is no way of diagnosing early carcinoma in the abdominal viscera. Jaundice may be the first sign and indicates that the lesion has developed sufficiently to obstruct bile passage at some point. The treatment for carcinoma of the biliary system is surgical, and an operation is performed as soon as the patient's condition warrants it in the hope that complete surgical removal of the lesion is possible. Patients often benefit from surgery even when cure of the carcinoma is impossible, since various operations that help to restore the flow of bile into the gastrointestinal tract produce remarkable relief of symptoms, and the patient may feel relatively well for a time.

Biliary atresia

Biliary atresia is a condition in which there is a congenital absence or obliteration of the bile ducts. There is no known cause. Jaundice appears about 2 to 3 weeks after birth and progresses until the infant is a greenish bronze color. Tears and saliva may be pigmented, the urine is dark, and the stools are white or clay colored. The child may not be alert and may move slowly, but he usually has a good appetite. The treatment consists of an operation to establish a pathway for bile into the intestines. As surgery is possible for only a small percentage of these children, the prognosis is poor.

Surgical care and management of the patient with biliary disease

Terminology. The terminology used to indicate specific biliary tract surgery sounds somewhat complicated but actually is self-explanatory. *Cholecystectomy* is the removal of the gallbladder, whereas *cholecystostomy* refers to the creation of a new opening into the gallbladder for decompression and drainage. *Choledochotomy* is a surgical incision into the common bile duct, usually for removal of a stone *(choledocholithotomy)*. When carcinoma has been found or when strictures in the ducts make other methods of treatment unsatisfactory, *choledochoduodenostomy* and *choledochojejunostomy,* which refer to anastomoses between the bile duct and the duodenum and between the bile duct and the jejunum, respectively, also may be done. *Cholecystogastrostomy* is the surgical formation of an anastomosis between the gallbladder and the stomach.

Preoperative care. A general medical examination done prior to biliary surgery includes a radiograph of the chest, x-ray study of the gallbladder, and examination of the urine and stools. Usually an electrocardiogram is ordered to detect heart damage. Various tests of hepatic function may be made if disease of the liver is suspected; and if the patient is jaundiced, tests are done to determine the cause. The prothrombin level usually is checked preoperatively.

If there is jaundice, the prothrombin level usually is low, and vitamin K preparations such as phytonadione (vitamin K_1, Mephyton) may be given preoperatively. Occasionally when the prothrombin level is quite low, yet surgery is imperative, transfusions of whole blood may be given immediately preoperatively to provide prothrombin, which is essential for blood clotting. If the patient is taking food by mouth poorly, infusions containing glucose and protein hydrolysates may be given in an effort to protect the liver from potential damage and to ensure wound healing. Signs of upper respiratory disease should be reported at once since upper respiratory infections can lead to serious complications following surgery of the upper abdomen. A nasogastric tube may be inserted before the patient goes to the operating room.

Postoperative care. The patient is usually placed in a low Fowler's position on his recovery from anesthesia. Because the wound is fairly high in the abdomen, breathing is painful, and the patient may hold his breath and take shallow breaths in order to splint the incision and lessen pain. Analgesic medications for pain should be given fairly liberally during the first few days, and the patient should then be urged to cough and to breathe deeply at regular intervals. He must also be helped and encouraged to change his position and to move about in bed frequently. If a nasogastric tube is in use, it is attached to suction. Because essential electrolytes as well as gas are removed by this procedure, it is discontinued as soon as possible—usually within 24 hours. Infusions of 5% glucose in distilled water usually are administered. Sometimes solution containing electrolytes and protein hydrolysates are ordered. When the naso-gastric tube is removed, the patient is given clear fluids by mouth. Sweet, effervescent drinks such as ginger ale usually are tolerated best at first. Within a few days the patient usually is able to eat a soft low-fat diet. Appetite will probably remain poor if bile is not flowing into the duodenum.

The nurse should check the dressings as often as every 15 minutes for the first few hours postoper-atively because, although hemorrhage from the wound is rare, it can occur. Internal hemorrhage also occasionally follows surgery of the gallbladder and bile ducts, particularly when the inflamed gall-bladder was adherent to the liver and was removed with difficulty. Lowering of blood pressure, increase in pulse rate, and other signs of hemorrhage should be reported to the surgeon at once.

The nurse should know exactly what surgical pro-cedure has been done to be able to care for drains and check dressings intelligently. If the gallbladder is removed, the cystic duct is ligated and a drain usually is inserted near its stump and brought out through a stab wound. This tube drains bile and small amounts of blood and other serous fluid or exu-dates onto the dressings. It usually is removed with-in 5 to 6 days when drainage has largely subsided.

If a cholecystostomy has been performed, a self-retaining catheter is inserted through an opening in the gallbladder and is attached to straight drainage. Bile will drain out through this tube until it is re-moved, usually between 6 weeks and 6 months.

If exploration of the common duct has been done, a T tube, with the short ends placed into the common duct, will probably be used (Fig. 26-7). The long end of this soft rubber tube is brought through the wound and sutured to the skin. The section of the T tube emerging from the stab wound may be placed over a roll of gauze anchored to the skin with adhesive tape to prevent it from occluding (Fig. 26-8). The T tube is inserted to preserve patency of the common duct and to ensure drainage of bile out of the body until edema in the common duct has subsided enough for bile to drain into the duodenum normally. If the T tube was clamped while the patient was being transported from the recovery room, it must be released *immediately* on arrival in his room. The nurse should check the operative sheet carefully and make inquiries if directions are not clear. The tube usually is connected to closed gravity drainage simi-lar to that used to drain the urinary bladder. Suffi-cient tubing should be attached so that the patient can move without restriction. The purpose of the tube should be explained to the patient, and he should be told why it must not be kinked, clamped, or pulled. The drainage should be checked for color and amount at least every 2 hours on the operative day. The tube may drain some blood and blood-

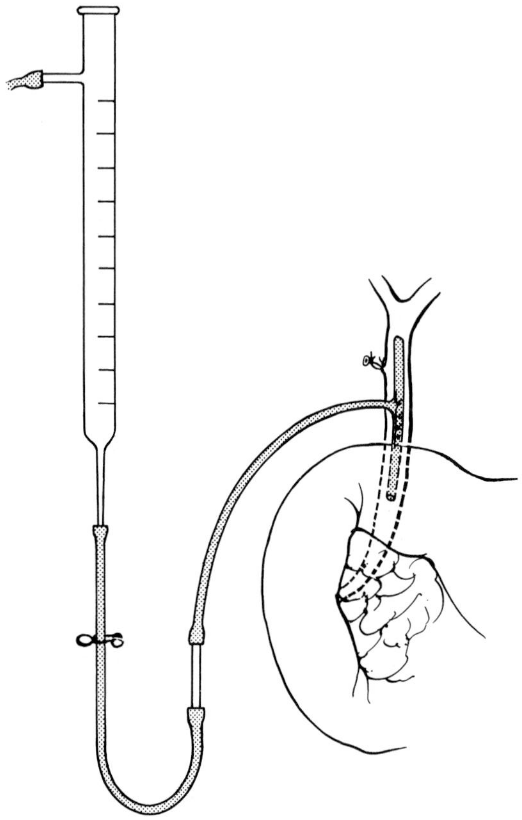

FIG. 26-7. A T tube placed in the common bile duct and attached to a manometer for a burette test. The common bile duct has been brought from its normal position for better visualization of the T tube.

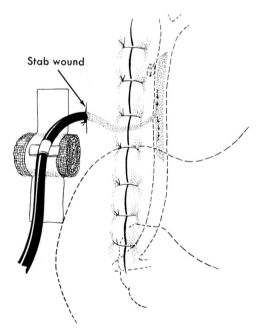

Stab wound

FIG. 26-8. The section of the T tube emerging from the stab wound may be placed over a roll of gauze anchored to the skin with adhesive tape to prevent its lumen from being occluded by pressure.

stained fluid during the first few hours, but drainage of more than a small amount of blood should be reported to the physician. After this, the amount should be measured and recorded each day. At first the entire output of bile (normally 500 to 1,000 ml. daily) may flow through the tube, but within 10 days most of the bile should be flowing into duodenum.

Usually the T tube is removed in 10 days to 2 weeks. Before this is done, a *burette test,* similar to that performed prior to removing a nephrostomy tube (p. 436), is done to determine the patency of the biliary system (Fig. 26-7). If the common bile duct is patent, the pressure readings will fluctuate very little from the initial reading unless the patient is moving, coughing, talking, or laughing just prior to the reading. If the common bile duct is still obstructed, the level of bile will rise in the burette beyond the set point, usually 15 cm. above the level of the common bile duct. If this happens, the physician should be notified. A cholangiogram usually is made following the burette test to confirm the patency of the duct (p. 708). Following the removal of the T tube, the patient may have chills and fever, but they usually subside within 24 hours. They are caused by edema and a local reaction to the bile. Occasionally flow of bile into the abdominal cavity causes peritonitis, and therefore any abdominal pain should be reported at once.

Postoperatively the bile should either drain out through the drainage tubes or flow into the intestine. If it does not do so, it can be assumed that the flow of bile is obstructed and that bile is being forced back into the liver and into the bloodstream. The nurse should observe the patient closely for jaundice, particularly the sclerae. Urine should be examined grossly for the brown color that is indicative of bile pigment. A specimen should be saved for the physician's inspection when bile pigment is observed in the urine. The nurse may observe the patient's progress by noting the stools: a light color is usual if all the bile is flowing out through the drainage tubes (unless bile salts are being given by mouth), but the normal brown color should gradually reappear as drainage diminishes and finally disappears.

The patient should be told about any drainage tubes that have been used. He should know if much bile is expected on the dressings so that he will not become alarmed by soiling of dressings, his gown, or bedclothes. Outer dressings usually should be changed frequently when there is excessive drainage, since the drainage is irritating to the skin and wet dressings interfere with the patient's comfort and rest. Soap and water will remove bile from the skin. Montgomery straps make the changing of dressings much easier.

The patient usually is permitted out of bed the day after the operation. If a T tube or a cholecystostomy tube is present, it may be attached to a small drainage bottle to permit greater freedom of movement. It may be placed in a pocket of the patient's bathrobe or attached to his robe below the level of the common duct. The patient may need help and encouragement because dressings are uncomfortable and he fears "spilling" the drainage when he moves about. He may still be receiving infusions, and transporting the infusion bottle is necessary. He often benefits from a regular schedule of getting up and sitting in a chair or walking with assistance.

Special diets are seldom prescribed by the physician following biliary surgery, but the patient is advised to avoid excessive fats in his meals. The nurse should help to teach the patient the essentials of good nutrition, with emphasis on foods that are low in fat.

Occasionally, if excessive drainage through the T tube or cholecystostomy tube continues for a long time, the bile collected in the drainage bottle is administered to the patient through a nasogastric tube to improve digestion. If this is done, the funnel or Asepto syringe should be covered, and the bile should be in a receptacle so that the patient does not see it. Sometimes the bile may be diluted with grape or other juices to disguise its appearance. The patient generally is not told that he is receiving bile.

Usually from 10 days to 2 weeks of hospitalization are required following biliary surgery when no complications occur. The length of convalescence depends on the individual patient, but usually at least a month is needed before normal activities can be resumed safely. The nurse should emphasize to the patient the importance of keeping medical appointments as requested.

REFERENCES AND SELECTED READINGS*

1 American Academy of Pediatrics: Report of the Committee on Infectious Disease, ed. 17, Evanston, Ill., 1974, The Academy.
2 American Public Health Association: Control of communicable diseases in man, ed. 11, New York, 1970, The Association.

*References preceded by an asterisk are particularly well suited for student reading.

3 Anderson, W. A. D., and Scotti, T. M.: Synopsis of pathology, ed. 8, St. Louis, 1972, The C. V. Mosby Co.
4 Beeson, P. B., and McDermott, W., editors: Cecil-Loeb textbook of medicine, ed. 13, Philadelphia, 1971, W. B. Saunders Co.
5 Bergersen, B. S.: Pharmacology in nursing, ed. 12, St. Louis, 1973, The C. V. Mosby Co.
6 *Bielski, M. T., and Molander, D. W.: Laennec's cirrhosis, Am. J. Nurs. **65:**82-86, Aug. 1965.

7 Bockus, H. L.: Gastroenterology, vol. 3, ed. 2, Philadelphia, 1965, W. B. Saunders Co.

8 Brown, H.: Treatment of hepatic failure and coma, J.A.M.A. **201:**547-548, Aug. 1967.

9 Child, C. G., and Frey, C. F.: Pancreatico-duodenectomy, Surg. Clin. North Am. **46:**1201-1213, Oct. 1966.

10 Cole, W. H., and Roberts, S. S.: Exploration of the common duct, Surg. Clin. North Am. **46:**1113-1128, Oct. 1966.

11 Conn, H. F.: Current therapy, Philadelphia, 1970, W. B. Saunders Co.

12 *Conn, H. O., and Simpson, J. A.: A rational program for the diagnosis and treatment of bleeding esophageal varices, Med. Clin. North Am. **52:**1457-1481, Nov. 1968.

13 *Cunningham, L. M.: The patient with ruptured esophageal varices, Am. J. Nurs. **62:**69-71, Dec. 1962.

14 Davidsohn, I., and Henry, J. B.: Todd-Sanford clinical diagnosis by laboratory methods, ed. 15, Philadelphia, 1974, W. B. Saunders Co.

15 Evans, J. A., and Mujahed, Z.: Percutaneous transhepatic cholangiography, Postgrad. Med. **53:**182-185, Jan. 1973.

16 Foster, J. H., and others: Recent experience with major hepatic resection, Ann. Surg. **167:**651-668, May 1968.

17 French, R. M.: Nurses guide to diagnostic procedures, ed. 3, New York, 1971, McGraw-Hill Book Co.

18 Fuerst, E. V., and Wolff, L. V.: Fundamentals of nursing, ed. 5, Philadelphia, 1974, J. B. Lippincott Co.

19 Garb, S.: Laboratory tests in common use, ed. 5, New York, 1971, Springer Publishing Co., Inc.

20 *Glenn, F.: Surgical treatment of biliary tract disease, Am. J. Nurs. **64:**88-92, May 1964.

21 Gocke, D. J.: New faces of viral hepatitis, Disease-a-Month, pp. 1-32, Jan. 1973.

22 Head, H. B., Kukral, J. C., and Preston, F. W.: Helmet-mounted constant traction spring for maintenance of position of Sengstaken tube, Am. J. Surg. **112:**465-468, Sept. 1966.

23 *Henderson, L. M.: Nursing care in acute cholecystitis, Am. J. Nurs. **64:**93-96, May 1964.

23a Hospitals: Statement on hepatitis B antigen carriers, Hospitals **48:**95-98, Nov. 1974.

24 Host, W. R., Serlin, O., and Rush, B. F.: Hyperalimentation in cirrhotic patients, Am. J. Surg. **123:**57-62, Jan. 1972.

25 Howard, J. M.: Pancreatico-duodenectomy: forty-one consecutive Whipple resections without an operative mortality, Ann. Surg. **168:**629-640, Oct. 1968.

26 Jones, P. N., and Capps, R. B.: The management of hepatic coma, Med. Clin. North Am. **48:**37-51, Jan. 1964.

27 *Kaplan, M. H., Bernheim, E. J., and Flynn, B. M.: Esophageal varices, Am. J. Nurs. **64:**104-108, June 1964.

28 Krugman, S.: Etiology of viral hepatitis, Hosp. Pract. **5:**45-49, March 1970.

29 Linton, R.: The treatment of esophageal varices, Surg. Clin. North Am. **46:**485-498, June 1966.

30 McDermott, W. V., and Supple, A.: Hepatic failure. In Meltzer, L. E., Abdellah, F. G., and Kitchell, J. R., editors: Concepts and practices of intensive care for nurse specialists, Philadelphia, 1969, The Charles Press, Publishers.

30a McGill, D. B., and Motto, J. D.: An industrial outbreak of toxic hepatitis due to methylenedianiline, N. Engl. J. Med. **291:**278-282, Aug. 1974.

31 *Molander, D. W., Brasfield, R. D., and Virgadamo, B. T.: Liver surgery and care of the patient with liver surgery, Am. J. Nurs. **61:**72-76, July 1961.

32 Nadkarni, S. V.: Amebic abscess of the liver, Int. Surg. **58:**112-115, Feb. 1973.

33 Nelson, W. E., Vaughn, V. C., and McKay, R. J.: Textbook of pediatrics, ed. 9, Philadelphia, 1969, W. B. Saunders Co.

34 Nugent, F. W., and Zuberi, S.: Treatment of acute pancreatitis, Surg. Clin. North Am. **48:**595-599, June 1968.

34a Pastorek, N.: Hepatitis, Today's Health **52:**4-49, 67-69, Sept. 1974.

35 Popper, H., and Schaffner, F., editors: Progress in liver diseases, vol. 3, New York, 1970, Grune & Stratton, Inc.

36 Redefer, A. G.: Viral hepatitis: current concepts, Postgrad. Med. **53:**77-81, Jan. 1973.

37 Rosenthal, M. S.: Viral hepatitis. In Current trends in communicable diseases—a monthly report, vol. 3, no. 3, Cleveland, Feb. 1970, Cleveland Dept. of Health, Metropolitan General Hospital, Academy of Medicine of Cleveland and Cuyahoga Health Department.

38 Rutherdale, J. A., and others: Hepatitis in drug users, Am. J. Gastroenterol. **58:**275-287, Sept. 1972.

39 Sabiston, D. C., editor: Davis-Christopher textbook of surgery, ed. 10, Philadelphia, 1972, W. B. Saunders Co.

40 *Schaffner, F., and others: Symposium: liver disease, J.A.M.A. **191:**466-486, Feb. 1965.

41 Schiff, L., editor: Diseases of the liver, ed. 3, Philadelphia, 1969, J. B. Lippincott Co.

41a Schwartz, S. I., and others: Principles of surgery, ed. 2, New York, 1974, McGraw-Hill Book Co.

42 Sherar, L.: Ascites: pathogenesis and treatment, Postgrad. Med. **53:**165-170, Jan. 1973.

43 Sherlock, S.: Diseases of the liver and the biliary system, ed. 4, Philadelphia, 1968, F. A. Davis Co.

44 Small, D. M.: Gallstones diagnosis and treatment, Postgrad. Med. **51:**187-193, Jan. 1972.

45 Stahl, W. M.: Major abdominal surgery in the aged patient, J. Am. Geriatr. Soc. **11:**770-780, Aug. 1963.

46 Starzl, T. E., and others: Orthotopic homotransplantation of the human liver, Ann. Surg. **168:**392-415, Sept. 1968.

47 Stauffer, M. H.: Needle biopsy of the liver, Surg. Clin. North Am. **47:**851-860, Aug. 1967.

48 *Taylor, K., Commons, N., and Jack, M. S.: Liver transplant, Am. J. Nurs. **68:**1895-1899, Sept. 1968.

49 Thorbjarnaroon, B.: The anatomical diagnosis of jaundice by percutaneous cholangiography and its influence on treatment, Surgery **61:**347-354, March 1967.

50 Warren, K. W., Braasch, J. W., and Thum, C. W.: Carcinoma of the pancreas, Surg. Clin. North Am. **48:**601-617, June 1968.

51 Warren, R., and others: Surgery, Philadelphia, 1963, W. B. Saunders Co.

52 Wenzel, R. P., and others: Patterns of illicit drug use in viral hepatitis patients, Milit. Med. J. **138:**345-350, June 1973.

53 Williams, S. R.: Nutrition and diet therapy, ed. 2, St. Louis, 1973, The C. V. Mosby Co.

54 Wintrobe, M. M., and others: Harrison's principles of internal medicine, ed. 7, New York, 1974, McGraw-Hill Book Co.

27 Endocrine diseases

Hormonal replacement therapy
Thyroid dysfunction
Parathyroid dysfunction
Diabetes mellitus
Hypoglycemic states
Diseases of the adrenal glands
Diseases of the pituitary gland

■ The endocrine glands are special glands, or groups of cells, located in various parts of the body. Knowledge as to exactly how they function is still incomplete, but more is being learned about them each year. They are known to secrete and release highly specific chemical compounds (hormones) into the bloodstream. These substances are synthesized in the endocrine glands under genetic control, and they are continually lost from the body either by excretion or by metabolic inactivation. None are secreted at a uniform rate; some seem to have a rhythmic pattern (daily or periodic), while others seem to be secreted in response to the blood level of a specific substance such as sugar, sodium, water, or another hormone.

The hormones, in conjunction with the nervous system, communicate information about conditions in the internal and external environment to all parts of the body and help the body maintain a homeostatic state. It is still unclear exactly how hormone production is stimulated or how the hormones act in the cells. They probably do not initiate any physiologic processes, but by a complex yet unified action they seem to augment and regulate many vital functions such as energy production, metabolism of foodstuffs, water and electrolyte balance, growth and development, and reproductive processes. They also integrate the responses of the body to stress. Authorities now believe that the production of most hormones is directly or indirectly under the control of the nervous system.

The anterior pituitary gland, often called the "master gland" because it seems to be an important regulator of the hormone environment, secretes two

■ STUDY QUESTIONS

1 Where is each of the endocrine glands located? Review the hormones secreted by each.
2 In what way does giving a large amount of a hormone to a patient who already is producing a normal amount affect his own production of the hormone? Why does this reaction take place?
3 What is the difference between secretion and excretion?
4 What vitamin is essential for the body to use calcium efficiently? Why is it necessary?
5 List the signs and symptoms of respiratory obstructions that might be caused by pressure on the trachea.
6 How would you explain to a patient who has a high basal metabolic rate that he needs increased amounts of foods? Name some foods that are high in carbohydrates.
7 Review the procedure for giving a medication by hypodermic injection, and outline a plan for teaching this procedure to a patient.
8 What is the price of a bottle of regular insulin? Of NPH insulin? If the patient is to take a daily dose of 30 units, how long would one bottle of insulin last? What would be the monthly cost?
9 Review the physiologic action of the sympathetic nerves.
10 Where is the hypothalamus located?
11 Review the physiology of stress in Chapter 4.
12 In what ways would the nursing needs of a patient having a hypophysectomy as treatment for cancer of the breast be likely to vary from those of a patient having a hypophysectomy to control the vascular complications of diabetes mellitus?

types of hormones—one type that affects specific tissues directly and another (the tropic hormones) that regulates the output of hormones from other glands (Fig. 27-1). These target glands, the gonads, thyroid, and adrenal cortex, increase their rate of secretion as a result of an increase in the tropic hormones. One of the tropic hormones, adrenocorticotropic hormone (ACTH), stimulates the secretion of glucocorticoids by the adrenal cortex by a negative feedback mechanism. Thyroid-stimulating hormone (TSH), secreted by the anterior pituitary gland, causes the secretion of thyroid hormones. The gonadotropic hormones stimulate secretion of testicular and ovarian hormones. The growth-stimulating hormone (GH) produced by the anterior pituitary gland seems to interact with other hormones such as thyroxin and insulin to regulate the body's growth and development. The posterior pituitary gland secretes antidiuretic hormone (ADH), pituitrin, which stimulates smooth muscles of the blood vessels and intestine to contract, and oxytocin, which stimulates uterine contraction.

The adrenomedullary hormones seem to control the emergency system for quickly mobilizing the body defense system, including the activation of other hormones. Further information as to the action of each hormone and what stimulates its secretion is included with the discussion of diseases of the endocrine gland producing it.

The actions of the endocrine glands are interrelated by a number of control mechanisms: (1) The closed-loop negative feedback system is illustrated in Fig. 27-2. Gland A produces hormone X, which stimulates organ B. In turn, organ B produces substance Y, which then inhibits secretion of gland A. (2) A second negative feedback loop is regulated by the hypothalamus. This complex system controls the adrenal cortex, thyroid gland, and the gonads. Fig. 27-3 outlines this relationship from the hypothalamus to the target tissue and identifies known negative feedback effects. Internal rhythm is another regulating phenomenon. The diurnal variations of ACTH and cortisol production provide examples. While a person is asleep at 2 A.M., production of ACTH and cortisol is at the lowest level, but it rises sharply between 6 and 8 A.M. The human menstrual cycle also illustrates this mechanism. External stimuli such as pain, stress, or infection can each increase the secretion of ACTH and cortisol, while exposure to cold is thought to increase thyrotropic release.

In health, the amount of each hormone in the blood is kept within definite limits. Disturbance in

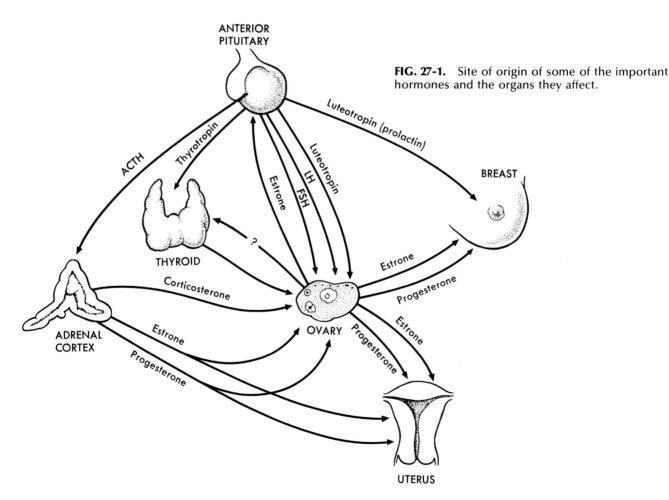

FIG. 27-1. Site of origin of some of the important hormones and the organs they affect.

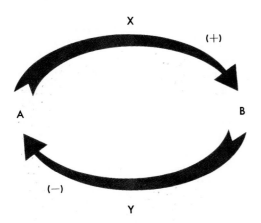

FIG. 27-2. Closed-loop negative feedback system. A principle of control that is applicable to all endocrine glands. (Redrawn from Harvey, A. M., and others: The principles and practice of medicine, ed. 18, Englewood Cliffs, N. J., 1972, Prentice-Hall, Inc.)

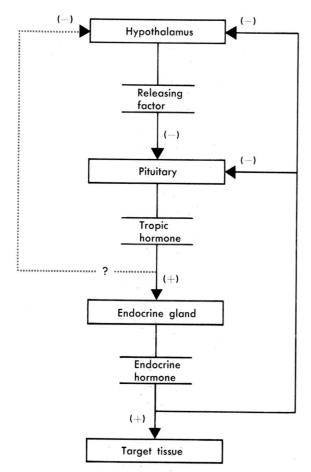

FIG. 27-3. Complex negative feedback loop system. The hypothalamus regulates this complex feedback system. (Redrawn from Harvey, A. M., and others: The principles and practice of medicine, ed. 18, Englewood Cliffs, N. J., 1972, Prentice-Hall, Inc.)

the functioning of an endocrine gland may be caused by malfunction in the regulatory mechanism or by failure of the body processes to respond to regulation. Because the endocrine system is so closely interrelated and because the production of each hormone is dependent not only on other hormones but also on nervous stimulation, genetic controls, enzymatic action, and available energy and nutrients, it is obvious that endocrine dysfunction can arise from diverse causes. Dysfunction of one gland is likely to affect the function of one or more of the others. The structure and thus the function of an endocrine gland may be changed by abnormal embryonic development of the endocrine tissue, deprivation of blood supply to the gland, infection of the gland, tumor (benign or malignant) growths in it, overstimulation of it, or overgrowth of its tissues (hypertrophy and hyperplasia). In *hyperplasia* the size of the gland increases because it is continuously overstimulated, and there is a proliferation of active secreting cells. In *hypertrophy* there is an increase in the size of the gland caused by the increase in functional demands on it. Hypertrophy may or may not be accompanied by hyperplasia. *Hypoplasia* is a decrease in the amount of functioning tissue, and consequently, there is a decrease in the amount of hormone produced. It may be caused by anything that inhibits tissue growth. It is believed that both the production of hormones and the effect of hormones on body cells can be affected by age, race, sex, season, climate, and disease.

Atrophy, or a decrease in the size of a gland, is caused by a decrease in functional demands. This could result from a failure of the gland to perform its function or from an exogenous supply of the hormone that makes the endogenous hormone produced by the gland unnecessary.

Disease of an endocrine gland usually causes a decrease or an increase in the secretion of its hormones, and the symptoms are those of increased or decreased regulation of the processes normally controlled by it. Owing to the diverse physiologic functions under hormonal control, symptoms of endocrine dysfunction may be reflected in many parts of the body, and because many of the functions controlled are vital ones, endocrine disorders may be extremely serious.

The specific treatment of endocrine diseases consists basically of decreasing the output of hormones from hyperactive glands and supplying or compensating for deficient hormones. Occasionally, in hypofunction, treatment may be designed to lessen the need for the hormone or to stimulate its production. Overproduction of a specific hormone often can be controlled by resecting part of the gland secreting the hormone or, if a tumor is stimulating the gland, by removing the tumor. However, the entire endocrine gland sometimes must be removed surgically or destroyed. Occasionally the pituitary gland may be removed or destroyed if it stimulates the secretions of the overactive gland. Sometimes radiation of either the specific endocrine gland or the pituitary gland destroys enough tissue to bring the symptoms under control. If endocrine glands are completely removed or destroyed, essential hormones must be supplied regularly for the remainder of the patient's life. Regular replacement also is necessary to control disease when there is hypofunction of the endocrine gland.

Only a few of the more common diseases of the endocrine system will be discussed in this chapter. Those occurring less often should be reviewed in appropriate specialized texts. Since replacement of hormones is common to most endocrine diseases, replacement therapy will be discussed before some specific diseases are mentioned.

■ HORMONAL REPLACEMENT THERAPY

Long-term replacement. The patient who requires hormonal substitution for the remainder of his life often presents a serious rehabilitative problem. His prognosis may depend largely on his acceptance of the situation and his understanding of his limitations and his treatment. Although hormonal replacement treatment may seem to restrict the patient's life seriously, the person who has been helped to accept his limitations and live within them is able to have a relatively normal life and is far less restricted than he was with the uncontrolled disease. It is important for the patient to have the support of the members of his family and for them to understand and be willing to assume responsibility for his treatment should he be unable to do so himself.

The patient must know that his treatment cannot be discontinued for a single day without specific direction from the physician and that it does not usually provide for the excessive hormonal demands produced by unusually stressful physical or emotional situations. Because of this he should strive to recognize and to avoid stress-producing situations such as tensions on the job, family quarrels, and sudden bouts of unaccustomed exercise. Fasting, extremes of temperature, and fatigue should be avoided also. If any infection, no matter how minor, or any illness occurs, the person should seek medical advice. Pregnancy produces stresses, and therefore the physician should be consulted about family planning; additional hormones may be needed during the period of gestation and delivery. Because sudden, unexpected, stressful situations such as accidents or incapacitating illness may occur, the patient receiving hormones regularly always should carry an identification card on which is noted his name and the name of his physician, with address and telephone numbers and the prescribed hormone being taken as well

as the dosage to be used in event of an emergency.

Even in the absence of stressful situations, the normal person has changing needs for hormones. In replacement therapy, however, a specified amount of hormone must be given. Therefore it is not unusual for the patient to develop symptoms of hypofunction or hyperfunction of the gland for which the hormone is being given. Both the patient and his family should be able to recognize symptoms of dysfunction of the gland and know what to do about them. If there is a means of compensating for too much or too little of the hormone, such as taking sugar for insulin reaction, the method should be taught. If this is not possible and the symptoms are acute, the patient must be taken at once to his physician or the emergency department of a hospital. Many times, if medical advice is sought at the first evidence of even minor symptoms of dysfunction, the dosage of the hormone can be adjusted and further trouble avoided.

Patients receiving hormone replacement always should have at least a 2-month supply of the special drugs and equipment they need, lest an emergency prevent them from obtaining supplies. As new supplies are bought, they should be kept in reserve and the old ones used. Continuous hormonal therapy is expensive. If the patient finds it difficult to pay for the drugs he needs, help should be sought from the social service department in the hospital or from an appropriate social agency in the community.

Temporary replacement. The patient requiring only temporary replacement of hormones may be at home while he is taking them, and if so, he must be taught the importance of taking the prescribed dosage regularly. Usually the dosage is reduced gradually and finally discontinued. While therapy is being tapered off, the patient should be observed for symptoms of hypofunction of the gland that produces the hormones that have been given. The patient and his family should know the signs and symptoms of hormonal deficiency and should understand the need to seek immediate medical attention if these symptoms occur. They also should know that symptoms of hypofunction of the gland may occur even after the therapy has been discontinued. Regular medical follow-up should be continued until the physician determines that it is no longer needed. Glands that have been partially destroyed by radiation or partially removed by surgery eventually increase in size so that their function is normal. The patient may be advised to lead a less stressful life than usual until normal function has returned.

■ THYROID DYSFUNCTION

An oversimplified description of the function of the thyroid gland is that it is the regulator of the rate of metabolic processes in the body. Thyroid hormones stimulate the consumption of oxygen by the tissues, influence the rate of growth, and affect the metabolism of protein, carbohydrates, and lipids. They also stimulate the myocardium and increase the force and rate of contraction.[3] The thyroid gland performs three basic functions: (1) trapping of iodide, (2) synthesis of organic iodine, and (3) storage and secretion of hormones. Iodine is an essential element in the production of thyroid hormones, while the pituitary hormone, TSH, regulates the synthesis and release of the major thyroid hormones, thyroxine (T_4) and triiodothyronine (T_3).

Both of these thyroid hormones influence the metabolic rate. Most circulating T_4 is bound to plasma proteins, primarily thyroxine-binding globulin (TBG) and thyroxine-binding prealbumin (TBPA). Free T_4 denotes the small portion of T_4 that is unbound. It is thought that free T_4 regulates the release of pituitary TSH. T_3 is not bound as tightly to plasma proteins and has a more rapid onset of action than T_4.

Tests of thyroid function

In general, laboratory tests for endocrine disorders are used to demonstrate changes in related physiologic control pathways such as the more complex negative feedback systems as well as to provide isolated analyses of gland function. Indirect measurements such as serum cholesterol levels and Achilles tendon reflex testing, which provide information about the metabolic consequences of thyroid hormone action, are not as precise as today's direct measurements, but they are helpful adjuncts in many cases. Tests are now available at different levels of function: the pituitary, the thyroid, the serum, and peripheral tissues.

Pituitary level tests. A hypothalamic hormone, thyrotropin-releasing hormone, has recently been synthesized and a radioimmunoassay technique has been devised. It provides a direct means of testing pituitary reserve for TSH.

Tests of pituitary-thyroid interrelationship. Radioimmunoassay of serum TSH is becoming a more widely available diagnostic technique. In hypothyroid patients, determination of the TSH level aids in differentiating primary hypothyroid disease (resulting from disease within the thyroid) from secondary hypothyroidism (resulting when a healthy thyroid fails because of the influence of the pituitary). In patients with primary hypothyroidism, TSH levels are elevated. A lack of thyroid hormone decreases feedback inhibition of the pituitary thyrotopin and a rise in TSH results. Low levels of TSH are seen in hyperthyroid patients with Graves' disease and toxic nodular goiters.

Thyroid level tests

Radioactive iodine uptake test. The radioactive iodine uptake test determines the ability of the thyroid gland to accumulate iodine that is ingested.

A tracer dose of radioactive iodine (^{131}I), which is colorless and tasteless, is given by mouth. The drug is absorbed from the gastrointestinal tract and accumulated in the thyroid gland, and the excess is excreted by the kidneys. Approximately 2, 6, or 24 hours following the administration of radioactive iodine, a shielded Geiger counter or a scintillation detector is placed over the neck in the region of the thyroid gland, and the amount of accumulated radioactive iodine is calculated. The normal thyroid usually will accumulate 5% to 35% of the drug within 24 hours. If the patient has thyrotoxicosis, an increase may be shown.

Excess iodine in any form can suppress radioactive iodine uptake. Apprehension at the thought of taking a radioactive substance usually is allayed by explanations. No isolation for radioactivity is necessary.

Thyroid scan test. The thyroid scan is used to determine if there are elevated concentrations of iodine in a particular node or portion of the thyroid gland or in adjacent tissue. The procedure is similar to that for a radioactive iodine uptake test except that the scintillation detector moves back and forth across the neck, recording on a drum a picture of the distribution of radioactivity.

Thyroid suppression test. When hyperthyroidism is suspected but other tests are inconclusive, a thyroid suppression test may be ordered. A radioactive iodine uptake test is done first to establish a baseline. A fast-acting thyroid hormone is given for 8 days, and then the uptake is retested. Failure of the hormone to suppress the uptake indicates hyperthyroidism, since normally the excess thyroid hormone in the blood should depress the patient's thyroid function.

Tests related to serum levels of thyroid hormone

Protein-bound iodine test. The protein-bound iodine (PBI) test indirectly determines the total circulating T_4 concentration. The normal range is from 4 to 8 μg/100 ml. of serum. Results of this test can be falsely elevated by iodides or organic dyes. The patient should receive no medications containing iodine during the week before the test lest the readings be abnormally high. Cough syrups containing iodine as well as specific iodine preparations should be avoided. Tests in which iodine preparations are used, such as x-ray series of the gallbladder or intravenous pyelograms, also interfere with accurate results. Estrogens cause readings to be abnormally high and therefore should be discontinued prior to the test. Mercury causes readings to be abnormally low. Mercurial diuretics should be omitted for 24 to 48 hours before the test. This test is less reliable today because of the increased presence of iodine in the environment.

Thyroxine (T_4) radioassay. T_4 radioassay directly measures thyroid hormone. This test determines the ability of T_4 extracted from serum to displace radioactive T_4 from T_4-binding proteins. This radioassay is not affected by iodides or organic dyes that elevate the protein-bound iodine level and depress the radioactive iodine uptake for varying periods of time. It is now possible to obtain the total circulating T_4 as well as the "free T_4." This small fraction of unbound T_4 denotes the metabolically effective fraction of circulating T_4.

Triiodothyronine (T_3) resin or red cell uptake test. The T_3 resin or red cell uptake test is an indirect measure of T_4-binding proteins. When there is a disproportionate amount of T_4 in the blood relative to the amounts of TBG present, there will be a measurable change in the number of binding sites available to bind radioactive T_3 when it is added to the serum. Radioactive T_3 will attach to the TBG sites, and then the resin added will absorb any unattached T_3. The radioactivity of the resin is then determined. In hypothyroidism there will be many extra available binding sites, more radioactive T_3 will attach to the TBG, and the T_3 resin uptake will be low.

This test does not measure the patient's endogenous T_3 level.

Tests related to peripheral effects of thyroid hormone

Basal metabolism test. The basal metabolism test determines the amount of oxygen used by a person at rest during a given period of time. It is a crude indicator of thyroid function. Results of the test are compared with the mean values obtained from testing a group of normal people of the same age, sex, and size (body surface). The results are expressed in percentage of deviation from the mean values. Thus, if the patient needs 10% more oxygen than the control group, he has a basal metabolic rate (BMR) of plus 10%. Normal basal metabolic rate ranges from minus 15% to plus 15%. Although this test is still used, newer and more accurate diagnostic measures are now available.

Achilles tendon reflex recording. Achilles tendon reflex recording is a simple method of estimating thyroid function. Electrodes attached to a recording drum are applied to the patient's ankle. The physician taps the ankle tendon, and the response time for the reflex is recorded on the drum. A slow ankle jerk correlates with an underactive thyroid, and a rapid one correlates with an overactive thyroid.

Cholesterol test. A blood cholesterol test may be used in diagnosing thyroid diseases, but there is variation of opinion on its reliability. In hyperfunction of the thyroid the blood serum cholesterol level usually tends to be subnormal, whereas in hypofunction it usually is increased.

Simple goiter

Any enlargement of the thyroid gland is spoken of as a goiter. A goiter may be caused by various disorders, such as congenital metabolic defects that prevent synthesis of thyroid hormones or chronic thyroiditis. Simple goiter or hyperplasia results from impaired thyroid function. Inability to secrete sufficient quantities of necessary hormones results in increased secretion of TSH, which stimulates glandular growth. It frequently is seen in girls, appearing at puberty, when the metabolic rate is highest and the body's need for thyroid hormones is greatest. It may diminish or disappear spontaneously after the age of 25 years. In temperate climates the greatest incidence of simple goiter occurs in late winter and in spring. The incidence of simple goiter in the United States is greatest in the Great Lakes Basin, Minnesota, the Dakotas, the Pacific Northwest, and the Upper Mississippi Valley because of the limited amount of iodine in the water and food supply of these regions. Iodine normally is found in seafood, and small amounts of iodine are found in green leafy vegetables that have been grown where iodine is present in the water and soil. Using iodized table salt is an easy and inexpensive way of assuring sufficient iodine intake, since the average adult can obtain more than twice his daily iodine requirement from the amount of salt he normally uses.

A simple goiter may grow unnoticed, or the patient may ignore it unless it becomes nodular or symptomatic. Toxicity or difficulty in breathing, resulting from pressure of the goiter on the trachea, may occur. In the early stages of simple goiter, one drop of saturated solution of potassium iodide a week usually provides enough extra iodine for the thyroid gland to use to produce thyroid hormones, and the hyperplasia will decrease gradually. If the goiter is moderately large, it may be necessary for the patient to take thyroid extract as well as iodine to decrease its size. When the goiter is causing symptoms of pressure, it may have to be removed surgically. Very large goiters also may be removed surgically for cosmetic improvement.

The nurse can help to prevent simple goiter by teaching the importance of eating foods that contain iodine. The patient should be asked about the quantity of leafy vegetables and seafoods he eats and the kind of table salt he uses. Encouraging use of iodized salt is important in parts of the country where there is a known deficiency of iodine in the natural water. The nurse should notice the contour of the neck whenever giving care to any patient. If there seems to be enlargement, the patient should be questioned as to his awareness of it and asked whether he has consulted a physician about it. If not, he should be encouraged to do so.

Cancer of the thyroid gland

Although cancer of the thyroid gland is less prevalent than other forms of cancer, about 1,000 people in the United States die of it each year. It usually is first diagnosed by palpation of a hard nodule on physical examination, but it sometimes is first recognized because it produces symptoms of hyperthyroidism. The cell type determines the rapidity with which the malignancy will advance and therefore influences the type of therapy used and the prognosis. Surgical removal is usually indicated. Radioactive iodine in large doses may also be given in conjunction with surgery. Regular administration of thyroid hormone is started following the operation, and it must be continued throughout the patient's life.

The nurse should urge people to have yearly physical examinations since this may help to detect cancer of the thyroid gland in its early stages. The nursing care of the patient is the same as that for any patient having an operation on the thyroid gland (p. 741). (The care given to the patient who is being treated with radioactive iodine is described on p. 740.)

Hyperthyroidism

The disease characterized by hyperactivity of the thyroid gland commonly is known as hyperthyroidism, but it may be called *thyrotoxicosis, toxic goiter, Graves' disease,* or *Basedow's disease.* In this condition the gland usually enlarges, and it always secretes excessive quantities of thyroid hormones, speeding up all metabolic processes. More oxygen is used, more fuel is burned, and heat output rises markedly. The patient becomes nervous and jittery, tense, overly alert, and irritable. His reactions to situations may be exaggerated, and he may weep or laugh out of proportion to what is expected normally. There is a fine tremor of the hands, and the patient may drop articles easily and may appear awkward or clumsy in his movements. He usually complains of weakness and fatigue, and he often loses weight, although he may eat enormous amounts of food. There is heat intolerance and increase in perspiration. The palms of the hands typically are warm and moist. Palpitations and breathlessness sometimes occur. Gastrointestinal motility is increased, and diarrhea may occur. Today the patient usually seeks treatment fairly early, and his only obvious signs may be nervousness and slight weight loss. Hyperthyroidism is a serious disease which, if not checked, can lead to death from heart failure.

Exophthalmos, or protrusion of the eyeballs, is a characteristic, although not uniformly present, sign of hyperthyroidism. This condition may become so severe that the eyes cannot be closed. In this event the eyes should be protected to prevent irritation and possible corneal ulceration. Soothing eyedrops such as methylcellulose may be helpful. Dark glasses will afford some protection from wind, sun, and dust.

Hyperthyroidism is more common in women than in men. It can occur at any age, but it is most likely to occur at puberty, following pregnancy, or at the menopause. Emotional trauma such as loss of a parent, divorce, or financial crisis sometimes precedes thyroid hyperplasia, but it is not clear whether emotional trauma precipitates the hyperplasia or whether the presence of hyperplasia may cause the severe emotional responses to crises. Toxic thyroid disease often occurs in persons who have other endocrine disturbances such as diabetes mellitus.

Every nurse should be alert to early signs and symptoms of hyperthyroidism. The public health nurse, particularly, may encounter people with beginning signs and symptoms. Physical signs may be obvious, but the patient's expressed complaints about his or her changes in behavior and management of usual activities may give many additional clues. Since the disease gradually becomes more serious and treatment is more effective and less difficult in the initial stages, people suspected of having hyperthyroidism should be urged to seek medical attention early.

Management. Management of the patient with hyperthyroidism is directed toward reducing the output of thyroid hormone. This can be approached in two ways: by using antithyroid medications to block the synthesis of thyroid hormones or by ablation of thyroid tissue surgically or by means of radioactive iodine. Antithyroid medications are usually indicated in treating children, adolescents, young adults, and pregnant women. Radioactive iodine treatment may be used in older patients, patients with drug toxicity, or individuals who demonstrate noncompliance with the medical regimen. Since surgery or radiation can produce permanent effects, hypothyroidism may occur anytime after treatment. Surgery may be used in younger patients when antithyroid treatment has not been successful.

Until the symptoms are controlled, measures to keep the patient emotionally and physically quiet and thus reduce his metabolic needs are necessary. The patient often is given a diet high in calories to provide adequate fuel for the increased energy requirements and to prevent further weight loss as well as to replace weight already lost.

Propylthiouracil and *methimazole* (Tapazole) are the most commonly used *antithyroid drugs.* The action of these drugs is slow, and it usually takes 2 weeks to a month before improvement is noticeable. The patient usually is started on a relatively large dose of an antithyroid drug, and then the dosage is gradually reduced to a maintenance dose. When antithyroid drugs are used as the primary therapy, they usually are continued for 6 to 18 months. It is important to give the drugs at regularly spaced intervals since their effect wears off in about 8 hours. Patients should know this. The patient should be instructed to look for toxic signs of the drug, such as fever, sore throat, and skin eruptions. He should call his physician if they appear. If toxic reaction occurs, blood counts may show leukopenia. Continued use of antithyroid drugs may not be tolerated by some patients.

In addition to the antithyroid drugs, preparations of *iodine,* such as Lugol's solution (strong iodine solution), are still widely used in the treatment of hyperthyroidism. They reduce glandular vascularity and help to prevent postoperative hemorrhage when a partial thyroidectomy is necessary. They also are used when the metabolic rate must be reduced rapidly because their action is more rapid than that of the antithyroid drugs, although less sustained. When Lugol's solution is ordered, it is more palatable given in milk or fruit juice. It should be taken through a straw because it may stain the teeth. A brassy taste in the mouth and sore teeth and gums are signs of toxicity, but this complication rarely occurs.

When antithyroid drugs are not tolerated or do not produce permanent remission of hyperthyroidism, *radioactive iodine* is used for treatment. ^{131}I is the preparation most often used. Usually a single dose of the drug is given. As in the iodide uptake test, the drug is given by mouth (a radioactive "cocktail"). If an unusually large dose of radioactive iodine is given, the patient is hospitalized and isolated for radioactivity for 8 days (the half-life of radioactive iodine). Following administration of large doses of radioactive iodine, the patient must be watched for thyroid storm (p. 742). Patients requiring usual amounts of the drug may go directly home, and no precautions are advised. It takes about 3 weeks for the symptoms of hyperthyroidism to subside and over 2 months for thyroid function to become normal. Occasionally remission is not achieved with one dose, and the treatment is repeated after an interval of several months. Hypothyroidism also may result if too much glandular tissue has been destroyed, and the patient will then need to take thyroid hormones either temporarily or permanently. The patient must be urged to keep appointments with his physician or with the hospital clinic, since it is important that he be followed medically for months to be certain that a normal rate of function remains.

Patients who receive radioactive iodine for hyperthyroidism need to have the treatment explained to them with special care, and they usually need repeated reassurance that the radioactive properties are quickly dissipated. Since they often are more emotional than other patients, they sometimes think they are experiencing reactions to the drug long after this is possible.

Since the advent of the antithyroid drugs and the trend toward early treatment, most patients with hyperthyroidism can be cared for at home. Although patients allowed to stay at home usually are not particularly overactive, they are likely to be very nervous and irritable. It is important for the patient's family and friends to understand that extreme sensitivity and excessive irritability are part of the disease. Otherwise they may become upset with the patient and aggravate the situation. Plans for maintaining a quiet environment should be made with the patient and his family. The patient who must be hospitalized usually is *very* restless, overactive, and jittery, and his behavior must be explained to all nursing personnel as well as to his family and friends. Special adjustments in routine nursing measures may be needed to help the patient rest.

The physical and emotional environment of the patient with hyperthyroidism should be kept as quiet and restful as possible. Whenever possible the patient should have his own room, and it should be kept cool. Patients with this disease often tolerate heat poorly. Often the patient will want no top bedding, and he may want the windows wide open even in cold weather. His wishes should be granted because the patient with hyperthyroidism is generating enough heat to keep from being chilled. If the patient is extremely restless, the base of the bed may need to be made with two full-sized sheets so that it can be tucked in securely at both the head and foot. This measure usually obviates the need for frequent straightening of the bed, which may be embarrassing and upsetting to the patient. The linen may need to be changed frequently because the patient with hyperthyroidism often perspires profusely. Lightweight pajamas are preferable to nightgowns because covers can then be left off or thrown off as necessary.

If the patient is very nervous, he may drop articles or may not be able to handle objects securely. This usually upsets him and may become a source of real frustration. Therefore it may be necessary to do small things for the patient that he may seem physically able to do for himself. For example, he may need water or other beverages poured for him, and some patients may even need help in buttoning their clothes and tying shoelaces. This help should be given as inconspicuously as possible.

Rest. The greatest nursing problem in care of patients with severe hyperthyroidism is providing enough rest. The activities around the patient should be quiet ones, but some limited and guided activity may help the patient more than enforced absolute quiet and rest. Quiet activity such as nonintricate handicrafts or reading keeps the patient occupied and actually may provide rest. The unoccupied patient who is allowed out of bed may use a great deal of energy in wandering about. If he is hospitalized, he may have upsetting contacts with other patients, who may misunderstand him, and he may disturb others. Modifying routines also may be necessary. For example, if the patient on bed rest becomes very upset by having to use the bedpan, he may expend less energy in walking to the bathroom, and orders permitting him to use the bathroom may be needed. Visitors should be restricted if they seem to make the patient more overactive, and the patient should be protected from surprise visits or disturbing news. Persons around the patient, either personnel or family, should try to remain calm, and discussion of controversial subjects should be avoided. When the patient has real difficulty resting, a sedative such as phenobarbital may be ordered to be given regularly. Consistently assigning a staff member who has established good rapport with the patient to care for him also may help to lessen his anxiety and permit him to rest.

Diet. Since appetite usually is increased in hyperthyroidism, the nurse should see that the patient is getting sufficient food. If weight loss has occurred, extra protein may be needed to help rebuild lost tissues, and extra carbohydrate is needed to meet the increased fuel requirements brought on by the disease. Stimulating drinks such as tea and coffee should not be given unless withholding them upsets the patient. Decaffeinated preparations may be substituted for patients who are accustomed to a hot liquid with meals.

The patient should know that persons around him understand his increased need for food, so that self-consciousness does not keep him from eating as much as he really needs. Occasionally the patient's appetite is not good, and yet he needs extra food. Finding out what he likes to eat and trying to obtain it often helps. The patient should be given repeated helpings of foods he likes, and he should be given food between meals.

Operative treatment of diseases of the thyroid

The patient with hyperthyroidism usually undergoes a fairly lengthy program of medical treatment before surgery is scheduled. This treatment may be given at home or in the hospital. The management of the patient has already been discussed. The patient usually is considered ready for surgery when thyroid function has returned to normal (euthyroid) and the patient has a consistent weight gain and a marked diminution of signs of thyrotoxicosis such as tachycardia. An ECG is made before surgery in order to detect evidence of heart damage. Patients with heart damage are preferably treated with radioactive iodine.

Part or all of the thyroid gland may be removed surgically, depending on the purpose for which the operation is done. In the case of a malignancy the gland may be removed completely *(total thyroidectomy),* and the patient must then take thyroid hormones regularly for the remainder of his life. When antithyroid drugs do not correct the hyperthyroidism and treatment with radioactive iodine is contraindicated, hyperthyroidism may be treated surgically by removing approximately five sixths of the gland *(subtotal thyroidectomy).* In most cases this operation permanently alleviates symptoms, while the remaining thyroid tissue provides enough hormones for normal function.

Postoperatively the patient who has had either a total or a subtotal thyroidectomy should be protected from strain on the suture line, helped to raise secretions from the lungs, and observed closely for complications such as hemorrhage, obstruction of breathing, and hypocalcemia, each of which requires immediate medical treatment. He also should be helped to swallow by using measures to relieve the sore throat that usually lasts for several days.

Care of the incision. As soon as the patient has reacted from anesthesia, he usually is placed on his back in a low Fowler's or semi-Fowler's position with the head, neck, and shoulders supported so that the neck is neither flexed nor hyperextended. This position prevents strain on the suture line and avoids the sensation that "the neck is falling off." The patient should be cautioned not to flex or hyperextend his neck, and the nurse should support it while he turns, sits up, or lies down. Support can be given by placing a hand on either side of the neck. As soon as the patient is able (usually by the second postoperative day), he is taught to support his own neck by placing both hands at the back of his head (Fig. 27-4) when he changes position. After the sutures or clips and the tissue drain have been removed from the incision (usually 2 to 4 days postoperatively), and when the surgeon feels that sufficient healing has occurred, the patient should begin gradually to practice full-range neck motion (Fig. 1-2) to prevent permanent limitation of head movements.

General care. A narcotic such as morphine sulfate or meperidine hydrochloride (Demerol) may be given at regular intervals to relieve pain and to ensure rest.

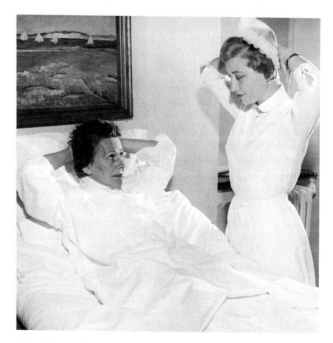

FIG. 27-4. The nurse is teaching the patient who has had a thyroidectomy how to support the weight of her head as she attempts to sit up in bed.

However, it must be given judiciously; respirations should not go below 12/minute. As soon as postoperative nausea subsides, the patient should take high-carbohydrate fluids by mouth and a soft diet if tolerated. Since the throat usually is sore for several days following surgery, the patient may have some difficulty taking nourishment. Analgesic throat lozenges or a narcotic may be ordered. These medications should be given as necessary to relieve the discomfort, which may be severe and prevent the patient from raising secretions, but the time of administration should be planned so that a dose can be given about a half hour before meals to make swallowing easier. Humidification may be used in the room to soothe the mucous membranes of the throat and trachea and thus relieve discomfort.

Postoperative complications. The complications following thyroid operations are extremely serious, and if they are not recognized and treated at once, they can result in death. Complications that the nurse should be alert for are recurrent laryngeal nerve injury, hemorrhage, tetany, and respiratory obstruction. Since the thyroid gland partially surrounds the larynx and trachea, there is danger of respiratory obstruction from a variety of causes, and a tracheostomy set should be kept readily available.

Hemorrhage. The patient's pulse rate, respirations, and blood pressure usually are checked every 15 minutes for several hours postoperatively and then, if they continue within normal limits, at longer intervals. The dressings should be watched for signs of hemorrhage. Since blood may drain back under the patient's neck and shoulders, the nurse's hand should be slipped gently under the neck and shoulders each time the patient is observed to be certain that any bleeding will be detected early. A choking sensation, difficulty in coughing and swallowing, or tightening of the dressing usually means there is bleeding into the surrounding tissues, causing pressure on the trachea and epiglottis. If these symptoms occur, the dressing should be loosened at once and the surgeon notified. If loosening the dressing does not relieve the respiratory difficulty and medical assistance will not be immediately available, the surgeon may instruct the nurse to remove the clips or sutures from the wound to relieve pressure on the trachea. The procedure to follow until the surgeon arrives should be ascertained whenever the nurse is caring for a patient having a thyroidectomy. The surgeon may need to perform an emergency tracheostomy and the patient often must be taken to the operating room for retying of the blood vessels and resuturing of the wound.

Respiratory obstruction. The patient and his family should know that he will be a little hoarse and have some difficulty swallowing after the operation due to irritation caused by the endotracheal tube through which the anesthesia is given. This condition is temporary and will subside after local irritation and edema disappear. Although slight hoarseness is normal, the nurse should observe the patient for any increase in it and for any respiratory difficulty accompanying it, since these conditions may be caused by injury to the recurrent laryngeal nerves, hemorrhage, or excessive edema about the vocal cords and larynx. The most common condition to suspect when the patient has difficulty in speaking or breathing is edema, but if the recurrent laryngeal nerves have been injured during an operation on the thyroid gland, the patient may have vocal cord spasm. If the nerve to one vocal cord only is injured, hoarseness may develop. If the nerves on both sides are injured, the vocal cords will become tight and close off the larynx, causing the patient to show signs of respiratory obstruction. As he attempts to pull air in through tightened vocal cords, a crowing sound is made and the tissues around the neck are retracted (appear sucked in). To recognize early symptoms of recurrent laryngeal nerve injury, the nurse should ask the patient to speak as soon as he has reacted from anesthesia and at intervals of 30 to 60 minutes. The patient with any hoarseness should be observed closely for any other symptoms such as crowing respirations or retraction of the tissues of the neck, and they should be reported to the surgeon at once. A tracheostomy usually is necessary. The injured nerve heals within a few weeks. Respiratory problems disappear and the patient's speaking voice becomes normal. The singing voice, however, often is permanently affected by a recurrent laryngeal nerve injury. A very rare complication of surgery on the thyroid gland is severance of the nerves supplying the vocal cords, which results in permanent loss of speech.

Tetany. A rare but serious complication following thyroid surgery is the accidental removal of one or more of the parathyroid glands. This may cause symptoms of calcium deficiency (tetany), which is fully described on p. 744. This complication may appear from 1 to 7 days postoperatively. If not treated in time, it can cause contraction of the glottis, respiratory obstruction, and death. Calcium gluconate is given intravenously as immediate treatment. Daily oral doses of calcium chloride are then started. If not all of the glands are removed, the remaining ones hypertrophy, so that the hypoparathyroidism is only temporary. If all are removed, the patient must have medical treatment for the deficit for the rest of his life. The nurse should be alert for signs of *thyroid storm,* which can be a complication of surgery.

Thyroid storm. A rare but life-threatening disorder may occur in patients with uncontrolled hyperthyroidism. It may be precipitated by trauma to the thyroid region, intercurrent infection, emotional stress, and thyroid surgery undertaken on hyperthyroid patients who have been inadequately treated with antithyroid drugs prior to surgery. Increased amounts of thyroid hormones are released into the bloodstream and metabolism is markedly increased. The patient's temperature may rise to 41° C. (106° F.) as the body becomes unable to release the heat formed with increased metabolism. The pulse may be very rapid, and there is marked apprehension, restlessness, irritability, and prostration. The patient may become delirious and finally comatose, with death resulting from heart failure. Treatment and nursing care will depend on the severity of the symptoms and the laboratory findings. Treatment includes oxygen and hypothermia blankets to lower the fever, antithyroid drugs, intravenous fluids as necessary, narcotics, sedative drugs, and cardiac drugs such as digitalis preparations or quinidine, as indicated by the heart action. Hydrocortisone, 100 mg., is commonly given intravenously.

Hypothyroidism

The patient with hypothyroidism has signs and symptoms almost directly opposite to those of the patient with a hyperactive thyroid gland. There is a general slowing of the body's activities. This condition may occur at any age and is caused by reduction in the secretion of thyroid hormones due to physiologic atrophy, deprivation of stimulation from pituitary TSH, overtreatment for hyperthyroid states, or total removal of the gland for a neoplasm.

Congenital absence or atrophy of the gland in infancy leads to the condition known as *cretinism,* in which both physical and mental growth is stunted. Early recognition and treatment prevents retarded physical growth, but it does not seem to prevent mental retardation.

The adult with hypothyroidism may notice that he is more sensitive to the cold than in the past, that he perspires little, and that his skin and hair are dry. If the condition has come on slowly, the hair may have become thin. He may have become forgetful and slow to grasp new situations, and he may have noticed that he is slowing up at work, falling asleep in the evening, and perhaps having an increase in minor accidents. Very often family members misjudge the person and feel that he has grown lazy, or a new acquaintance may consider him slow mentally. Speech is slowed, and the patient may have to plan sentences before speaking. All changes may occur so gradually that family members scarcely notice them. Since the gastrointestinal tract becomes sluggish, as do all other body functions, constipation with fecal impactions can occur. Even though appetite may be decreased, the patient tends to gain weight. Menstrual disorders such as anovulation, amenorrhea, functional menorrhagia, and infertility are common in women, and the normal sexual drive is reduced in men.

Most adults have *myxedema* as a complication of hypothyroidism. This general or localized nonpitting edema is caused by accumulations in the tissues of mucopolysaccharides, which are chemical substances that hold water. Periorbital edema and puffy hands and feet are rather common. The tongue often is edematous and may protrude slightly. Edema of the vocal cords may cause the patient to be hoarse. The tissues of the heart also frequently become edematous, and this condition may cause cardiac symptoms.

Treatment of hypothyroidism is the administration of the deficient thyroid hormone. The drugs used to treat hypothyroidism are listed in Table 27-1. It is important that dosages be increased gradually because a sudden increase in metabolic rate can cause death from heart failure. The daily maintenance dose of thyroid hormones required varies widely. The correct dose for each patient is determined by a remission in the symptoms of hypofunction. The nurse should carefully note and report all changes that may indicate either excessive or inadequate dosage. Adults with hypothyroidism respond quickly to the administration of thyroid hormones. Changes in appearance and physical symptoms occur within 2 or 3 days. If hypothyroidism is caused by malfunction of the thyroid gland itself and if treatment is started early, mental and physical characteristics may be restored to normal. Treatment must be continued throughout the patient's life, however, since failure to take the prescribed medication will result in an exacerbation of the disease. When derangement of the adrenocortical and pituitary hormones is also involved, treatment is more complicated and sometimes less successful.

General nursing care for the patient with hypothyroidism is determined by his symptoms. The family should be helped to understand the patient's behavior and to meet his needs. They must give the

Table 27-1 Replacement therapy in hypothyroidism

Preparation	Composition	Daily dosage
Thyroid (thyroid extract)	Combination of T_4 and T_3	15-180 mg.
Thyroglobulin (Proloid)	Combination of T_4 and T_3	60-180 mg.
Levothyroxine sodium (Synthroid sodium, Letter, Levoid)	Synthetic L-Thyroxine	150-400 μg
Liothyronine sodium (Cytomel)	Synthetic tri-iodothyronine	5-100 μg
Liotrix (Euthroid, Thyrolar)	Synthetic combination of T_4 and T_3	Equivalent of 15-180 mg. of thyroid extract

patient time to carry out any activity since he is almost always slow but not necessarily incapable. The patient usually complains of feeling cold and measures should be taken to place him in a room where the temperature can be adjusted to his needs. A minimum of soap should be used for bathing, and creams, bath oils, and lotions should be used to keep the skin in reasonably good condition. If constipation is a problem, the diet should consist largely of foods that are high in roughage. The physician usually orders a diet fairly high in protein and low in total calories. If myxedema is a problem, fluids may be restricted.

Since the early symptoms of hypothyroidism in both children and adults are rather vague, people may not recognize them, or if they do, they may not consider them significant enough to require medical attention. Regular physical examinations by the same physician should be urged, since he may be able to recognize symptoms of hypothyroidism earlier than would otherwise be possible.

Myxedema coma. An emergency situation can arise in hypothyroidism. It may be precipitated by infection or trauma and is characterized by unresponsiveness, hypotension, bradycardia, hypoventilation, and hypothermia. Treatment is directed toward improving pulmonary ventilation and replacement of thyroid hormone. Levothyroxine sodium for parenteral use is available. Thyroid replacement therapy is usually sufficient to correct the hypotension. No attempt should be made to correct the hypothermia by using means to warm the patient. This may result in increased oxygen requirement and further compromise of the patient's circulatory status.

■ **PARATHYROID DYSFUNCTION**

The parathyroid glands are four or more tiny glands located in proximity to the thyroid gland. The secretion, parathyroid hormone, regulates the level of calcium and phosphate ions in the body fluids by increasing the rate of release of calcium from the bones, enhancing its absorption from the intestine, and increasing the renal excretion of phosphorus and the renal absorption of calcium. Its secretion is thought to be stimulated by a fall in the level of blood calcium.

As with other endocrine glands, the parathyroid glands may become hyperactive or hypoactive. Benign neoplasms are the most frequent cause of hyperfunction, but malignant tumors and hyperplasia may occur. Inadvertent removal of all or some of the parathyroid glands during surgery on the thyroid gland or during other surgery in the region and idiopathic atrophy are the commonest causes of hypofunction. Any upset in the function of the parathyroid glands causes symptoms of electrolyte imbalance. (See the discussions of hypocalcemia and hypercalcemia, p. 117.)

Hypoparathyroidism

When there is insufficient hormone production or hypofunction of the parathyroid glands, blood calcium decreases and neuromuscular symptoms appear. (These symptoms are described in the section on hypocalcemia on p. 116.) They appear because a certain level of calcium in the body fluids is essential for the normal transmission of nerve impulses. As the level decreases, the irritability of all the muscles increases, and tetany may develop. Spasm of the laryngeal muscles may cause hoarseness of the voice. Manifestations of prolonged hypocalcemia are prematurely gray hair with alopecia (loss of hair), enamel defects of the teeth, and the development of cataracts in the lenses of the eyes.

The patient with hypoparathyroidism is usually given calcium salts and dihydrotachysterol (Hytakerol) or calciferol by mouth daily until the serum calcium level stabilizes. Dosages are then reduced and a maintenance dose determined. A diet high in vitamin D must also be taken. Vitamin D appears to be the principal regulator of the level of calcium ions in the body fluids and consequently is essential. Because of the danger that hypercalcemia will develop, serum calcium level tests must be done at intervals.

Immediate treatment of tetany is the intravenous administration of calcium gluconate or calcium chloride. Maintenance doses of calcium salts may then be given by mouth, and vitamin D may be given to ensure efficient use of the calcium by the body. Nursing care of patients with tetany includes careful observation of beginning symptoms of neuromuscular disorders so that prompt treatment can be given and severe reactions such as convulsions can be prevented. If the patient does have a convulsive seizure, he should be protected against physical injury, and his tongue should be prevented from slipping backward in his throat, preventing passage of air. (See care of the patient with convulsions, p. 878.)

Hyperparathyroidism

In hyperparathyroidism too much parathyroid hormone is released into the bloodstream, causing the serum calcium to be higher than normal and the serum phosphorus level to be lower than normal. There is increased urinary excretion of both calcium and phosphorus, and renal calculi frequently develop. Other symptoms are anorexia, nausea, vomiting, weakness, fatigue, bone pain, polyuria, polydipsia, and constipation, all of which may be due to electrolyte imbalance. Behavior changes may also occur. If the calcium intake is not increased, calcium is removed from the bones and *osteoporosis* (a demineralization of the bones) results. Osteoporosis causes the bones to become fragile and to fracture easily. Pathologic fractures (fractures resulting from weight bearing or pressure, not from trauma) often occur. Hyperparathyroidism is a chronic illness in which symptoms can be present for years before the problem is recognized.

Treatment for hyperparathyroidism is the surgical removal of part or all of the glands. If the parathyroidism is caused by an adenoma, this tumor is excised. If there is generalized hyperplasia, a subtotal parathyroidectomy is performed. All of the parathyroid tissue may be removed if the patient has a malignancy of the gland, and he then must be treated for hypoparathyroidism for the remainder of his life.

Following surgery the patient must be watched carefully for signs of hypoparathyroidism, especially tetany. Dihydrotachysterol and calcium supplements may be given in decreasing doses for several weeks following surgery, and a high-calcium diet supplemented with vitamin D is continued for many months.

Until treatment is well under way, the patient needs to take generous amounts of fluid so that the calcium is less likely to precipitate out in the urine, causing renal calculi. Until the bones have become recalcified, special care needs to be taken to prevent injury.

■ DIABETES MELLITUS

Diabetes mellitus is a chronic metabolic disease involving a disorder of carbohydrate metabolism and subsequent derangement of protein and fat metabolism. Disturbance in production, action, or metabolic rate of utilization of insulin, a hormone secreted by the islands of Langerhans in the pancreas, is involved in the disease.

Etiology

Normally, insulin speeds the oxidation of glucose in the cells and the conversion of glucose to glycogen and facilitates the conversion of glucose to fat in adipose tissue. It is uncertain how insulin actually acts to accomplish these activities, but the most generally accepted theory is that it facilitates the transport of glucose across cell membranes. The secretion of insulin is stimulated by a rise in the glucose level in the blood and inhibited by a fall in it.

In diabetes mellitus there appears to be insufficient insulin available for use in carbohydrate metabolism. It is now known that this insufficiency may be caused by at least three factors: a failure in production of insulin, blockage of its use, or its destruction by the body. The beta cells in the islands of Langerhans may fail to produce enough insulin. The need for insulin may be greater than the available supply, usually because metabolism is increased excessively for some reason. The use of insulin by the cells may be prohibited by some antagonistic factor such as the growth hormone from the anterior pituitary gland or adrenocortical glucocorticoids. It may be bound to immune serum globulin fractions in the serum (anti-insulin activity) so that it is not available for use. Insulin also may be destroyed by the liver or other tissues. It is felt that anti-insulin activity (a sensitization to the protein in insulin) may be a factor in the adult type of diabetes, and that years of hyperfunction of the insulin-producing cells in the pancreas also may be a cause. Children who develop diabetes are thought to have a primary derangement in the insulin-producing cells or in some other hormonal or enzymatic activity necessary for regulating the secretion or the utilization of insulin.

The predisposition to develop diabetes is known to be hereditary and transmitted as a mendelian recessive characteristic. If both parents have diabetes, all their children, if they live long enough, will eventually develop the disease. If a person with diabetes marries one with no inherited tendency to the disease, none of the children will have diabetes although they will carry the recessive trait and in turn pass it on to their own children.

In 85% of adults with diabetes mellitus, obesity precedes the disease. According to one theory, obesity presents an increased demand for insulin, the special cells within the pancreas that secrete insulin become exhausted, and diabetes develops. Diabetes mellitus is more common in women than in men, and it is thought that this may be due to the higher incidence of obesity among women. It is also more common among married than among single women. This may be linked to the frequent occurrence of obesity in women who have borne children or to hormonal influences related to pregnancy.

Signs and symptoms

The most common and characteristic symptoms of diabetes mellitus are increased appetite (polyphagia), increased thirst (polydipsia), and increased urine volume (polyuria). The signs and symptoms are directly related to faulty oxidation of carbohydrate and the chain of events that follows. Normally, glucose is oxidized by the body to form carbon dioxide and water, with production of energy to meet body needs. Any excess is changed to glycogen in the liver and is stored in the liver and in the muscles, or it is converted to fat and stored. However, insulin is needed for the formation of glycogen. In diabetes, glucose remains in the bloodstream and cannot be converted to glycogen because the insulin is not present or is unusable. The amount of sugar in the blood increases (hyperglycemia) and some of it is eliminated in the urine (glycosuria). The glycosuria promotes polyuria because the increased glucose being filtered by the kidney acts as an osmotic diuretic and increases the volume of urine excreted. This eventually leads to dehydration and polydipsia as a consequence of losing large amounts of water and salt in the urine. Pruritus vulvae, caused by the irritating effect of the urine with its high sugar content, may occur.

Since the patient with untreated diabetes mellitus is unable to utilize carbohydrates satisfactorily, essential carbohydrate starvation results and the body attempts to compensate by an increased appetite (polyphagia). To provide energy for the body unable to utilize carbohydrates, large amounts of fat, including body fat, are oxidized. This utilization of fat depots may lead to weight loss. Fats, upon oxidation, form ketone bodies (fatty acids), which in normal amounts are neutralized with bases such as bicarbonate in the blood plasma to maintain the normal acid-base balance of the body. When excessive amounts of fat are burned, the bases in the blood plasma may become exhausted. Acidosis (ketosis) develops (p. 117) and acetone bodies are then excreted in the urine. Weakness and fatigue are common because of the difficulties in meeting energy requirements.

The onset of symptoms in the young person often is rapid, but in the older, obese patient, the onset usually is insidious. Complications often cause the elderly patient to seek medical care. Diabetes in children frequently is diagnosed when severe acidosis develops during the course of an acute infectious illness.

Incidence

Diabetes mellitus is found most frequently in persons over 40 years of age who are obese and who have a family history of diabetes, although the disease does occur in children and in young adults. The incidence increases steadily until the seventh decade of life. Elderly persons usually have a much less severe form of the disease than younger ones, although complications may be severe. An estimated 2.5 million persons in the United States have diagnosed diabetes, and it has been estimated that there are approximately 1.5 million persons with undiagnosed disease.[10] Although the incidence was once felt to be higher among Jewish than non-Jewish people, a recent study showed that the incidence in Israel is the same as that in the United States.[2]

In general, the increased incidence of diabetes can be attributed to the longer life span (with more people in the older age group), to the lower mortality rate among young people with diabetes mellitus since the discovery of insulin, to the increase in the number of persons with diabetes who now marry and have children, to the public's increased awareness of the disease, and to the availability of detection facilities.

Significance as a public health problem

The fact that diabetes mellitus probably occurs in 1 out of 50 persons presents a sizable public health problem of particular economic and social significance. The establishment of community diabetes programs is being urged in the United States by the Public Health Service. These programs should be directed toward (1) detection of diabetes and follow-up of suspected cases to confirm the diagnosis and to give treatment, (2) prevention or correction of obesity, (3) keeping patients with diabetes under medical supervision and their condition under control, (4) promotion of understanding of diabetes mellitus through education of professional groups, the patient, his family, and the community as a whole, and (5) mobilization of community resources such as medical, nursing, social, and nutrition groups to aid persons who have diabetes.

The American Diabetes Association, Inc., furthers patient education, professional education, diabetes detection, public education, and research. It publishes both a professional journal, *Diabetes,* that helps to keep health professionals informed and a bimonthly magazine, *Forecast,* for persons with diabetes. Each year there is a National Diabetes Week. This week is sponsored by the Association to stimulate early case finding in persons who do not know that they have diabetes and to educate the public about the disease. The Association has 50 local groups that work in their own areas. They sponsor camps for diabetic children and cooperate on nationwide projects.

Local health departments have established multiphasic screening programs to detect diabetes. A test of the blood for sugar level or a test of the urine for sugar is used to detect diabetes, but the blood tests are considered best. Urine testing may give inaccurate results. Because fasting blood sugar tests may be misleading, a 2-hour postprandial test is becoming the procedure of choice in screening for diabetes. To improve screening efficiency, it has been recommended that diabetic detection projects concentrate their efforts on the high-probability groups such as older persons, obese persons with a family history of diabetes, and persons with prior symptoms or an elevated blood sugar level. At the present time, some form of mass screening is being carried out in many states. These programs vary in scope, methods, and goals. Case finding programs can be carried out in health department clinics, hospital outpatient clinics, physicians' offices, industry, or the community (at health fairs or by mobile testing units). Selected groups or whole communities can avail themselves of these services. Follow-up of any positive findings is essential for a successful program. Public health nurses can help by making home visits if diabetes is definitely established, if retesting needs to be done, if individuals have indicated that they have no physician or are under no medical supervision, or if persons being tested request home visits by a nurse at the time of the first testing. Through the nurse's visits, misunderstandings about retesting can be clarified, and family reactions to the possibility of diabetes can be determined.

Prevention

Since the cause of diabetes mellitus is unknown, specific measures for primary prevention are limited. However, much can be done by every nurse who is aware of the hereditary nature of the disease and its probable association with obesity. If diabetes is part of a family history, the nurse can explain to relatives of the patient the significance of periodic testing for detecting the disease early and can encourage all members of the family to maintain normal weight. Women who have had large babies also should be urged to avoid gaining weight and to have periodic tests for diabetes. Statistics show that 17% of mothers with babies weighing over 9 pounds develop diabetes later in life, and 80% to 90% of those with babies weighing over 13 pounds do.

Studies of women with diabetes have shown that there is a high fetal and neonatal death rate, a high proportion of large babies with a high mortality rate, and a great tendency toward other abnormalities in pregnancy. Thus there is now greater emphasis on preventive intensive prenatal care.[9] With improved monitoring devices available to determine placental function and fetal maturity, the pregnant woman with diabetes may be subjected to less risk to herself and the fetus.

It has also been discovered that women who have repeated spontaneous abortions, although giving no signs of carbohydrate intolerance by a regular glucose tolerance test, often show evidence of a decreased insulin reserve when cortisone is given prior to the glucose tolerance test. A significantly large number of relatives of persons with diabetes also respond in this manner. Therefore it is suspected that these people may need close medical supervision during stress situations such as pregnancy, extensive surgery, or serious illness to determine a need for insulin or oral hypoglycemic agents. The nurse should look at the medical history of patients and watch those with family histories of diabetes mellitus closely for symptoms of the disease.

There is much the nurse can do to prevent complications in the person with known diabetes. These measures will be discussed as part of nursing care.

Diagnostic tests

Urine tests. Urine testing is familiar to most of the public. Testing of urine for sugar is part of a complete urinalysis, and the urine of patients with known or suspected diabetes mellitus is tested frequently for sugar and acetone by one of the following methods. Patients with known diabetes mellitus may be asked to do the tests themselves at regular intervals as an indication of adequate control of the blood sugar level.

Clinitest is a copper reduction method of testing the urine for sugar. It comes in a compact kit and is convenient for use because it is small and easy to carry and store. The kit contains a test tube, a medicine dropper, caustic tablets, and a color chart. Two or five drops of urine are placed in the test tube with ten drops of water, and a Clinitest tablet is added. The tablet generates heat and the color of the solution is graded by comparing it with the two-drop or five-drop color chart. Certain drugs can affect the accuracy of this testing product. Large amounts of vitamin C and cephalosporin preparations such as Keflin can give false positive readings.

Tes-Tape, Clinistix, and *Diastix* are strip tests for glucose. Since color charts vary for each product, caution must be exercised in interpreting results. Also, test results must be read at specified time intervals to be accurate. *Acetest* tablets may be used to test for acetone. Urine is dropped on the tablet. If acetone is present, varying shades of lavender will appear and can be compared with a color chart. *Ketostix* is a strip product that can also be used to detect the presence of ketones.

Although single specimens of urine may show the presence of sugar, the physician may wish to find out what time of day the most sugar is excreted and prescribe insulin accordingly. To determine this, *fractional* or *group urines* may be collected. All the urine voided from before breakfast to just before lunch is collected, and a sample is tested for sugar. This is the first specimen; the second is collected from before lunch to just before dinner; the third, from dinner to before bedtime; and the fourth, from bedtime until the next morning.

Twenty-four-hour urine collections also may be obtained to determine the quantity of sugar excreted in a day. In this collection the first specimen of the morning is discarded. All urine excreted for the next 24 hours is collected in a gallon bottle and sent to the laboratory. It is important that the patient knows he must add the first urine voided the next morning to the specimen.

Blood sugar tests. Blood sugar levels are determined when diabetes mellitus is suspected or to check on the effectiveness of the treatment for diabetes. The normal fasting blood sugar ranges from 80 to 120 mg./100 ml. of blood. The blood specimen for sugar usually is taken when the patient is in a fasting state or an hour or two after a heavy meal (a postprandial specimen).

Glucose tolerance test. This test is done to detect abnormalities of carbohydrate metabolism such as may be present in hypoglycemia, diabetes mellitus, and adrenocortical disease. No food is allowed after midnight the night before the test. Samples of blood and urine to test for sugar are obtained at the beginning of the test, and the patient is then asked to drink a mixture containing glucose. Samples of blood and urine are taken at intervals of $1/2$, 1, and 2 hours following the ingestion of the glucose mixture. Interpretation of results differs according to the source of blood samples, the methods of analysis, and critical levels established by various authorities.

In patients with hypofunction of the adrenal cortex, the initial rise in the blood sugar is less than normal, and it returns rapidly to normal levels. The blood sugar of a person with diabetes mellitus or hyperfunction of the adrenal cortex goes up rapidly and will remain high for a longer time than normal. The patient who has hypoglycemia may have a drop in his blood sugar much below normal levels and must be watched during the test for signs of hypoglycemic reaction.

Cortisone-glucose tolerance test. This test is more sensitive than a glucose tolerance test and is used when the results of the glucose tolerance test are inconclusive. It is performed by a method similar to the glucose tolerance test except that cortisone, which is known to cause an abnormal rise in the blood sugar level of people who are predisposed to diabetes, is administered at the start of testing. It is considered positive when the blood sugar is 140 mg./100 ml. or more at the end of 2 hours.

Tolbutamide tolerance test. This test is another useful diagnostic tool. Tolbutamide can be administered by the oral or intravenous route.

Management

Control. Although diabetes cannot be cured, it can be controlled to a large extent by regulating the diet and taking insulin or oral hypoglycemic agents. There are two schools of thought on the control of diabetes. One medical group believes that the patient's urine must be kept sugar free and the blood sugar at a normal level. The other group believes that the disease can be controlled in the presence of an above-normal blood sugar level and of sugar in the urine provided enough insulin is taken and

enough food is eaten to meet metabolic needs. This is demonstrated by disappearance of signs and symptoms such as loss of weight and fatigue.

Emotional factors. The emotional response to a diagnosis of diabetes is often severe and is not easily dealt with. Part of this may result from fear of disability and eventual death. Since diabetes is so widespread, many people know of relatives and friends who have had the disease and who have eventually had amputations or have become blind. Perhaps an even greater cause of emotional reaction is that diabetes affects the patient's life pattern in regard to food. Food and eating have meaning beyond the actual meeting of nutritional needs, and changes in eating habits are extremely hard for patients to accept. Adolescents, perhaps more than any other age group, find restriction in eating almost intolerable and need much understanding in their early adjustment to the disease.

Getting started on a suitable plan of care for diabetes will often make a great difference in how the patient continues with care. It can help him and his family avoid undue stress and concern that may make it difficult to control the diabetes. Since most patients with diabetes are now treated in a physician's office or a hospital clinic, the public health nurse may need to help them with the initial adjustments. Patients whose disease is particularly difficult to control, those with complications such as infection, and those who are unusually apprehensive often are hospitalized for a period of time. The hospital nurse should work closely with these patients to try to help them adjust to their disease. On discharge from the hospital, they, too, often need to be visited by the public health nurse.

The patient's response to the persons who work with him at the time the diagnosis is made and

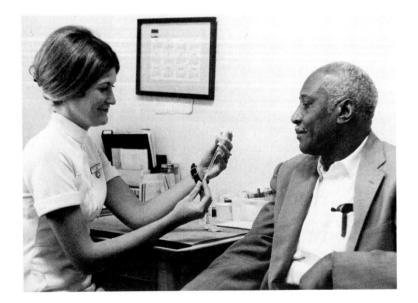

FIG. 27-5. The clinic nurse begins instruction in insulin administration by demonstrating the procedure to the patient.

shortly thereafter is tremendously important in determining his attitude toward his disease and, in turn, his ability to accept the treatment and restrictions that are necessary. Most medical authorities believe that the patient must know the potential seriousness of untreated diabetes. On the other hand, they believe that the more simply and easily the necessary changes can be made, the better for all concerned. If the patient with diabetes mellitus continues with the prescribed dietary regimen, takes the medication ordered, follows other instructions, and has periodic medical checkups, his life can be very much like that of anyone else. Only occasionally do adjustments in the patient's work need to be made. With careful planning, patients can continue to work various shifts. Today the patient who takes insulin regularly finds fewer employment restrictions. By avoiding a job that might create a hazard for him or others in the event of an insulin reaction, the diabetic can enjoy a satisfying career.

Nursing intervention. Whether care and teaching are done in the hospital, in the clinic, or in the patient's home, it is important that the nurse get to know the patient (Fig. 27-5). The patient should be given an opportunity to express what he thinks having diabetes will mean to him, and the nurse should attempt to learn what the patient knows about the disease. In the clinic, provision should be made for every newly diagnosed patient to have a conference with the nurse, preferably in a private conference room. Plans should always be made with him for future teaching conferences.

Since diabetes is a chronic disease and patients often must take daily medication and must adhere to a diet, both children and adults are taught early to take care of these particular needs for themselves unless this is not possible for some reason. Children as young as 6 or 7 years of age can begin to learn to take care of their particular needs. The nurse works out a plan for the patient for self-administration of medication, self-testing of urine, preparation and measurement of food, regular exercise, and recognition of unusual symptoms. The nurse also has the responsibility to review with him the general rules of good hygiene and of healthful living. The patient is taught special care of the feet since circulatory difficulties of the lower extremities often occur, especially in elderly patients. The family members should always be included in the teaching plan even though they may not take an active part in the procedures involved. This helps them to understand what is necessary and to encourage the patient to carry out instructions and enables them to take over if necessary.

The teaching plan should be arranged so that the patient is not rushed and has enough time for sufficient practice in self-care. If a member of the patient's family is to learn to give the care, arrange-

ments may need to be made for this person to come to the hospital or the clinic at other than regular hours. Work or home responsibilities may make attendance at the usual times impossible. A public health nurse may be asked to give this instruction in the home.

Group teaching, combined with individual conferences, is desirable whenever possible. Patients as well as family members often gain reassurance and consolation from contact with others who have similar problems. Emphasis in teaching, in groups or individually, however, should be on the fact that the patient is essentially a *normal* person and quite capable of living a completely *normal* life if he follows a few simple rules of health and adheres closely at all times to the prescription for insulin or other medication and to the diet given to him by his physician. Filmstrips such as *Taking Care of Diabetes** or *Just One in a Crowd*† are useful for group sessions. They should be followed by a discussion period. Booklets are available to supplement teaching, and patients often find them helpful. *Facts About Diabetes,** *ADA Meal Planning Booklet,** and *Forecast,** a bimonthly publication, may be helpful to some patients. Various teaching aids are also available through the Department of Health, Education and Welfare, and several pharmaceutical companies publish material that is helpful in patient teaching. These materials should be reviewed with the patient to be sure that he understands the concepts being presented. One drug company produces pamphlets in several languages that are helpful for those who do not comprehend English well.‡ These are usually available from the local pharmaceutical representative free of charge.

In assisting each patient, the nurse should give him encouragement and note how he appears to be accepting his disease. The necessity of having to take injections and perhaps to limit his diet for the rest of his life is more than some patients can accept. The patient may feel that he is different and must live a life different from that of other people. He may be self-conscious about eating with others because he must avoid certain foods. Each patient will need individual understanding and help to live as normal a life as possible. Satisfactory arrangements can usually be made in his social life. Help in learning diet substitution will aid him in overcoming unnecessary embarrassment when eating meals away from home. Also, he often can be assisted in planning a schedule for injections that will control

---

*American Diabetes Association, Inc., 18 East 48th St., New York, N. Y. 10017.
†Available from the Public Health Service Audiovisual Facility, Center for Disease Control, Atlanta, Ga.
‡E. R. Squibb & Sons, 909 Third Ave., New York, N. Y. 10022.

his diabetes, yet allow him as much freedom as possible. Throughout this adjustment period the patient needs emotional support and interest from his family and from nursing personnel who are familiar with his particular needs.

The nurse assigned to care for a patient with diabetes in the hospital should know whether the diagnosis is recent or whether the patient has had diabetes for some time. Patients who have diabetes often enter the hospital for treatment of another condition. If so, the nurse should find out early the usual diabetic regimen of the patient. If his general condition permits, he usually can continue self-care such as giving his own insulin and making his own food selection. If he is not allowed to continue his routine, he may have difficulty readjusting to it on discharge from the hospital. Self-care, however, is not always desirable. Some patients need to be dependent when a new illness occurs and want others to assume complete responsibility for their care. The nurse should help to determine whether it is best for the patient to be allowed to be dependent in this aspect or whether he should be urged to continue self-care while providing for his dependency needs in other ways. Some patients may be seriously ill and actually physically unable to continue self-care.

Diet. All patients with diabetes mellitus will be placed on some type of a restricted diet. Some obese patients who develop diabetes may be able to control it by diet alone. In these patients the emphasis is on gradual weight reduction to a level that is considered normal or slightly below normal for their height and body build. Those patients who are unsuccessful in weight loss or whose diabetes cannot be controlled by diet alone will receive either oral hypoglycemic agents or insulin in addition to a diet planned to meet their particular needs. Depending on the physician's experience and belief, the patient is placed on a weighed diet, an unweighed diet using a food exchange list, or an unmeasured diet with the elimination of concentrated sweets. The patient on a *weighed diet* actually weighs out specific amounts of food on a small scale. However, if the patient eats away from home, practice in estimating usual weighed amounts will be necessary. Specific amounts of carbohydrates, protein, and fat are prescribed. A usual diet consists of 150 to 200 Gm. of carbohydrate, 75 to 100 Gm. of protein, and fat in an amount that will make up the needed number of calories. An *unweighed diet* is one in which the amounts are calculated according to household measurements or usual-sized portions. Meal plans are based on six lists of foods. If the patient has a *self-chosen, unmeasured diet,* he should eat a well-balanced selection of food in moderate quantity and should avoid overindulgence in sweets. He should eat regularly and at the accustomed time without skipping or delaying meals.

The nurse can do much to help the patient with diabetes to understand food values and to follow his prescribed diet. In each instance the patient's age, weight, activity, medical condition, and general nutritional state should be considered when planning his meals. His social and economic background as well as his eating habits and emotional needs, should be considered. The patient who is accustomed to the foods of a specific culture should have his diet planned around them. Working people may find that they need to increase their caloric intake on return to work since they use more of their food for energy, causing the blood sugar level to drop and leaving an excess of insulin, which may cause signs of insulin reaction. Also, extra food is often necessary after unexpected exercise or emotional stress.

It must be emphasized repeatedly to all patients who have diabetes that insulin or oral hypoglycemic agents, if ordered, *should* be taken, the usual amount of daily exercise *should* be taken, and meals *should* be eaten. Regulation of the blood sugar level depends on maintaining a balance of these three factors. A decrease or an increase in physical activity seems to change the need for glucose and thus the need for insulin or hypoglycemic agents. Normally the body would adjust its secretion of insulin to the changes, but regulation of the insulin level is not possible when standardized doses must be given.

Many patients assume that medications for diabetes and food can be safely omitted if they have a cold or other minor ailment and do not feel like eating. This is not so. Full-liquid or clear-liquid diets can be prepared to provide the essential food for a short time, and the patient and his family should know how to prepare them. Any patient taking medication for diabetes who cannot eat or who is physically incapacitated should consult his physician.

A clinical dietitian, if one is available, may initiate or participate in the diet teaching program. However, the nurse often must give the diet instructions. If the dietitian does the teaching, the nurse and dietician should work closely together to assure adequate follow-up supervision. A good time for teaching the patient is during his meal. Current periodicals contain many useful suggestions for teaching the patient about his diet.

In planning the patient's diet, the six food exchange lists prepared jointly by the American Diabetes Association, The American Dietetic Association, and the Public Health Service are useful and should be available to the nurse. These lists have been published in a booklet* and are available for patients. They are set up according to calories and show how each food listed is equal in nutritional

---

*Department of Health, Education and Welfare: Six food exchange list, Washington, D. C., U. S. Government Printing Office.

value to any other food on the list; they also give suggested menus. The exchange lists allow for substitution of one food for another, depending on the patient's likes or dislikes or the general menus for the day. Exchanges are set up in seven categories: foods not needing measurement, milk, vegetables, fruits, bread, meat, and fats. The patient may take as much as desired of foods not needing measurement such as coffee, tea, bouillon, sour pickles, asparagus, cabbage, celery, cucumber, greens, lettuce, and tomatoes. He must be cautioned not to use sugar, cream, or dressings on these foods, however, without planning for these "extras" in the total intake. Substitutes for sugar are available. Nonnutritive sweeteners that do not contain sodium can be purchased for use with sodium-restricted diets.

If the nurse can help with menu planning on a weekly basis, the patient can learn through demonstration how the diet can be varied and how he can have the food that he likes even though restrictions are necessary. Most patients find it helpful to see food portions, especially such "unmeasurable" things as a small potato, an ounce of meat, or a slice of cheese. When possible, foods are measured using standard household measures such as an 8-ounce measuring cup, a teaspoon, or a tablespoon. All measurements are level, and cooked foods are measured after cooking. The patient with diabetes usually does not need to buy special foods but can select his diet from the same foods purchased for the rest of the family. Fruits may be fresh, dried, cooked, canned, or frozen as long as no sugar is added. Dietetic fruits packed in water or a sugar substitute are also available but are more expensive. Vegetables can be prepared with those for the rest of the family except that the patient's portion should be removed before such things as extra butter, milk, flour, or cheese are added. Meats should be baked, broiled, or boiled. Any fat used must be accounted for in the measurements for the meal. However, patients who drink skim milk can have two additional fat exchanges for each cup of milk prescribed in their diet. Special cookbooks with recipes that can be used for diabetics as well as for other members of the family are now available. They may help patients make meals more varied and appetizing. Special diabetic foods are expensive, and the patient should be reminded that they usually are not calorie free and should be counted in the daily dietary allowance.

Medications used to control diabetes. Either oral (hypoglycemic agents) or parenteral (insulin) medications may be used to treat diabetes mellitus. As a result of a study conducted by the University Group Diabetes Program, the Food and Drug Administration now recommends that oral hypoglycemic agents "be limited to those patients with symptomatic adult onset nonketotic diabetes mellitus which cannot be adequately controlled by diet or weight loss alone and in whom the addition of insulin is impractical or unacceptable."* The oral hypoglycemic agents are most effective in the treatment of elderly patients; they are not used to treat diabetes in the young or in middle-aged or older persons whose blood sugar level fluctuates widely. They are useless in treating diabetic ketoacidosis.

If patients are taking oral hypoglycemic medication instead of insulin, they often feel that they do not need to be as careful about taking the prescribed dosage of the drug, following the prescribed diet, maintaining the usual amount of exercise, testing their urine for sugar, or taking general health precautions. This is particularly true of the elderly patient. However, the dangers of not following the prescribed regimen are the same for these patients as they are for patients taking insulin. Patients on both types of medication may develop hypoglycemic reactions, hyperglycemia, and all the other complications of diabetes. In fact, the patient on oral medications needs to be especially cautious if he develops an infection or is subjected to great stress. Oral medication usually becomes ineffectual then, and he will need to take insulin at least temporarily to control his blood sugar level. The nurse may need to supervise the care of the patient taking oral medication even more closely than that of the one on insulin.

Insulin. Insulin is used in the treatment of 50% to 70% of the patients with diabetes in the United States. There are now eight types of insulin in general use, and each is effective in lowering the blood sugar level by aiding in the metabolism of carbohydrates.

Insulins are classified as to their time of action as rapid, intermediate, and slow acting. Food should be taken within an hour after the injection of rapid-acting insulin to prevent an insulin reaction. *Regular insulin* is a clear liquid that begins to act approximately 45 minutes to an hour after injection. *Crystalline insulin* looks the same as regular insulin but is a more refined product. It remains effective 1 hour longer than regular insulin and is less likely to cause local reaction at the site of injection.

Six types of *modified* insulin are currently used and all of these insulins contain substances that slow their action. *Globin zinc insulin* is modified by the addition of the globin factor of beef and zinc chloride. It has a clear but slightly amber appearance. *Protamine zinc insulin* (PZI) contains insulin plus protamine and a zinc salt. It has a milky appearance. *Neutral protamine Hagedorn insulin* (NPH) is also a cloudy insulin and its action is equivalent to that of one part of regular insulin and two parts of protamine zinc insulin. There are three *lente insulins: lente, semilente,* and *ultralente.*

*FDA current drug information, Department of Health, Education and Welfare, Oct. 1970.

Table 27-2 Action of insulin preparations

Type of insulin	Time of onset	Peak of action	Duration of action
Rapid acting			
Crystalline zinc	Within 1 hour	2 to 4 hours	5 to 8 hours
Regular	Within 1 hour	2 to 4 hours	4 to 6 hours
Semilente	Within 1 hour	6 to 10 hours	12 to 16 hours
Intermediate acting			
Globin zinc	2 to 4 hours	6 to 10 hours	18 to 24 hours
NPH	2 to 4 hours	8 to 12 hours	28 to 32 hours
Lente	2 to 4 hours	8 to 12 hours	28 to 30 hours
Prolonged acting			
Protamine zinc	4 to 6 hours	16 to 24 hours	24 to 36+ hours
Ultralente	Within 8 hours	16 to 24 hours	36+ hours

These insulins consist of insulin precipitated with zinc crystals but suspended in an acetate buffer rather than in a phosphate buffer. By varying the size and form of the particles, the suspensions of this insulin can be adjusted for rapid, intermediate, or prolonged action. These insulins are most valuable for patients who have developed an allergy to protamine or globin. They are also used to treat patients whose diabetes is difficult to control. The time of onset, peak of action, and duration of action depend on whether the insulin is classified as rapid, intermediate, or slow in action (see Table 27-2).

Protamine zinc insulin, NPH insulin, and lente insulins all separate into layers if allowed to stand. To obtain an accurate dose of the active ingredient, the solution should be mixed by rotating the bottle between the palms of the hands and inverting the vial from end to end several times.

Each individual patient has his own particular insulin need, and suitable amounts as well as types are carefully selected by the physician. Patients receiving only rapid-acting insulin need more than one injection a day to enable them to use the carbohydrates eaten. Many patients are given the prolonged-acting insulins since they eliminate the need for several doses during the day. Other patients may need a combination of regular insulin and protamine insulin.

It is important that the nurse understand the type and the time of peak activity of each kind of insulin prescribed. Patients on rapid-acting insulin must have food soon after the insulin is given, while those on intermediate or long-acting insulins will require a supplementary feeding in the midafternoon and/or a bedtime feeding. The between-meal snacks are timed to meet the peak action of the insulin being used.

U-100 INSULIN. This strength of insulin (100 units/ml.) has been introduced to eventually replace the 40 and 80 units/ml. strengths of insulin. Hope-fully, this will eliminate dosage confusion and errors. This strength was recommended since it is compatible with the decimal system. The U-100 insulin is available in all types. All U-100 insulins are prepared in round vials with orange caps and black lettering. The U-100 syringes are available in glass and disposable form. For small insulin doses, a miniature 35-unit glass syringe is available. Other special syringes such as a 2 cc. insulin syringe will soon be available.

To educate and assist patients in converting to U-100 insulin, nurses must have a thorough understanding of insulin concentration. U-100 insulin is a more concentrated insulin in less volume. The U-100 syringe makes the adjustment in volume; there is no need to calculate a conversion of the patient's insulin dose. For example, if the patient's requirements are 24 units of U-80 insulin, then he will take 24 units of U-100 insulin. The patient must understand that U-100 insulin must be used with a U-100 syringe (Fig. 27-6).

TEACHING THE PATIENT TO ADMINISTER INSULIN. Typical trays for the injection of insulin can be set up for use in demonstrations and for patients to use in practice. The materials are gathered in a cardboard box or on a tray. The nurse can discuss boxes or trays that the patient might have at home or suggest suitable purchases, suggest that when the equipment is not in use it be covered, and remind the patient that the set should be stored on a shelf or in a closet out of the reach of children. The time-saving value of having all necessary equipment in one place and accessible is obvious.

Equipment needed for the *injection of insulin* includes an insulin syringe, several hypodermic needles, a small jar for cotton or a box roll of cotton, a bottle of alcohol, and a small saucepan of sufficient depth to boil the syringe and needle. Many public health nursing agencies include a strainer that can be set into the saucepan, making it easier for the

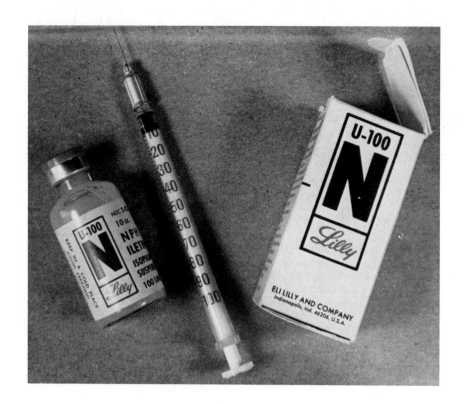

FIG. 27-6. U-100 insulin and disposable U-100 insulin syringe.

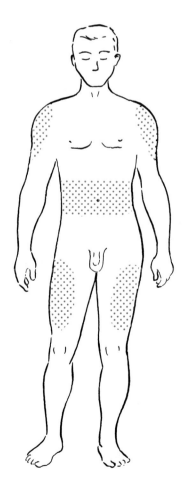
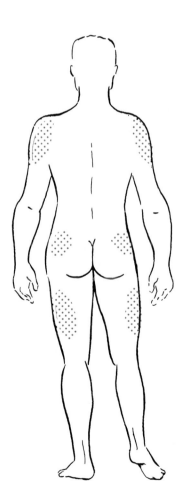

FIG. 27-7. Arms, legs, buttocks, and abdomen can be used for insulin injection. A different site should be used for each injection.

patient to drain and handle the equipment without breakage or contamination. Disposable syringes and needles may be used and facilitate the administration of the medication and teaching of the patient. If the patient cannot afford to use disposable equipment, he should be taught proper techniques of sterilizing and caring for the needle and syringe. The patient can choose between daily sterilization by boiling or soaking the syringe and needle in alcohol with weekly boiling of equipment.

Since repeated injections are necessary, *the site of injection must be rotated* to assure proper absorption of medication (Fig. 27-7). Irritation from repeated injections at the same site can cause induration of the tissue, so that the insulin is absorbed too slowly or not at all. Injections should never be given in any one spot more often than every 2 weeks, and a safe rule to follow is not to use the same site more often than once every 30 days. A diagram of the thighs with the possible sites numbered can be made as a guide. The site of injection is then rotated according to the plan.

It may be necessary for a patient to take two types of insulin. If so, the nurse may teach him to *mix the two insulins* in the same syringe so that they may be given in one injection. A simple way of mixing insulins in the same syringe is to inject the correct amount of air into the second insulin bottle first. Then the correct amount of air is injected into the first insulin bottle and the insulin withdrawn. As a final step, the correct dose is withdrawn from the second insulin bottle. Regular insulin can be mixed with any other type of insulin. The lente insulins can also be mixed together. The syringe should be rotated gently to obtain a well-distributed solution. The injection is then given in the usual manner. The most important point to remember in mixing insulins in the same syringe is that regular (unmodified) insulin is always drawn into the syringe first, since if some of the regular insulin inadvertently enters the vial of modified insulin, it will not significantly change the action of the modified insulin.

At times *modification in methods of administration of insulin* may be necessary because of particular problems; for example, the patient may be elderly, may have unsteady hands, or may have failing vision. In these instances, measurement of insulin as well as proper injection technique will require close attention. Adaptation of equipment may also be necessary (Fig. 27-8). The usual insulin syringe may be too slender to grasp, and numbers may be too small for the patient to read easily. The True-Set syringe has a capacity of 1 cc. and an adjustable metal marker that can be placed in the correct position. This prevents the plunger from drawing farther back. The patient draws up insulin until the plunger of the syringe will not go any farther. Even with very limited vision he can tell by feeling that he has the

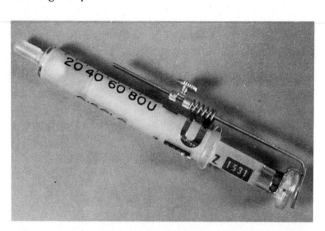

FIG. 27-8. Special syringes are available for the diabetic patient who has visual difficulty. The Tru-Set syringe can often provide independence for a visually handicapped patient.

correct amount. Patients who have failing vision also may use a small magnifying adapter (C-Better Magnifier) that can be clipped to a syringe.

A new insulin syringe with an adjustable positive stop that must be set by a sighted person (Fig. 27-9) and an insulin needle guide (Fig. 27-10) to assist patients with limited vision to insert the needle into the center of the rubber stopper on the insulin vial are available from the American Foundation for the Blind. The Foundation's publication *Aids for the Blind** is a valuable source of information. Special syringes and other equipment may be purchased at surgical supply houses and disposable syringes and needles are available at most drugstores.

Patients with poor vision have the danger of drawing air instead of insulin into the syringe. They must be cautioned to invert the bottle completely and to insert the needle only a short distance. Often they are advised to use only about two thirds of the bottle of insulin and to have on hand another full bottle. Some patients have a public health nurse or a friend withdraw the last doses in a bottle of insulin for them or go to a clinic for the last few injections. The positive stop syringe (Fig. 27-9) also makes it possible for the patient to remove air bubbles from the syringe by filling and emptying the syringe twice, and then slowly refilling it with the preset dose.

A patient may not be able to prepare the insulin dose accurately due to motor and sensory handicaps. He may, however, be capable of giving his own injections. A family member or neighbor could be taught to prepare the correct dose of insulin, or a public health nurse could fill a week's supply of syringes and store them in the refrigerator. The patient would need to rotate the syringe gently before use to mix the insulin. In some instances a member of the

---

*American Foundation for the Blind, Inc., 15 West Sixteenth St., New York, N. Y. 10011.

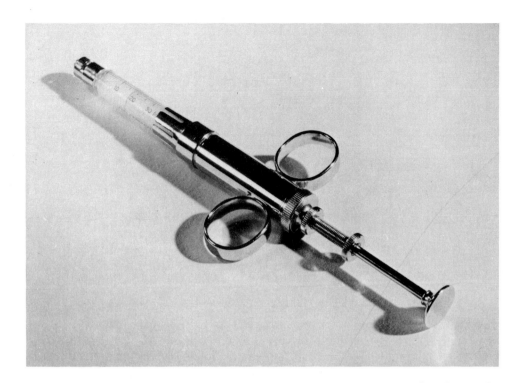

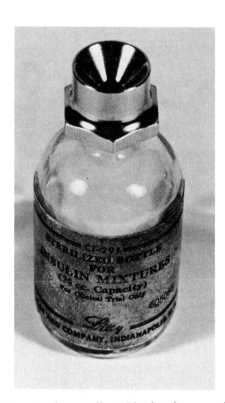

FIG. 27-9. Adjustable positive stop holder fitted over a Cornwall insulin syringe. Adjustment must be set by a sighted person. The syringe can be taken apart for sterilizing without disturbing the setting of the stop. (Courtesy American Foundation for the Blind, Inc., New York, N. Y.)

FIG. 27-10. Insulin needle guide that fits over the top of the insulin vial. Patient cleans the stopper and the guide with alcohol before placing guide on vial. Needle is laid in the V of the guide and vial is pushed toward it. (Courtesy American Foundation for the Blind, Inc., New York, N. Y.)

patient's family may have to give the insulin. A family member should always know how to do this in case impending coma or other illness makes it impossible for the patient to give the insulin to himself.

Oral hypoglycemic agents. Several oral agents are now available for use in controlling blood sugar levels in patients with diabetes mellitus. These agents have proved effective in the treatment of many adults whose diabetes is stable. However, they are not effective in the treatment of juvenile diabetes, severe diabetes, or diabetic ketoacidosis. These drugs are not hormones and it is a misnomer to refer to them as oral insulin. There are two groups of oral agents in use today: the sulfonylureas and the biguanide derivatives. The sulfonylureas are thought to act by increasing the ability of the islet cells of the pancreas to secrete insulin. The mode of action of the biguanide derivatives is not well understood; however, it is felt that they act by supplementing insulin effects in the peripheral utilization of glucose. The biguanide derivatives can be used alone, in combination with other oral agents, or in combination with insulin. They require some insulin, either endogenous or exogenous, to be effective.

The sulfonylurea compounds include acetohexamide (Dymelor), chlorpropamide (Diabinese), tolazamide (Tolinase), and tolbutamide (Orinase). The biguanide derivatives are phenformin hydrochloride tablets (DBI) and phenformin extended release capsules (DBI-TD). The dosages for these agents are presented in Table 27-3. In the University Group Diabetes Program Study (p. 751), tolbutamide was the oral hypoglycemic agent investigated. Death rates from cardiovascular diseases were two and a half

Table 27-3   Oral hypoglycemic agents

Classification	Proprietary name	Usual daily dose	Divided dose per day
Sulfonylureas			
Acetohexamide	Dymelor	250 mg. to 1.5 Gm.	1 to 2
Chlorpropamide	Diabinese	100 to 500 mg.	1
Tolazamide	Tolinase	100 mg. to 1 Gm.	1 to 2
Tolbutamide	Orinase	0.5 to 2 Gm.	2 to 3 after meals
Biguanides			
Phenformin hydrochloride tablets	DBI	50 to 150 mg.	2 to 3
Phenformin extended release capsules	DBI-TD	50 to 150 mg.	1 to 2

times as high in the patients receiving tolbutamide as in those receiving a placebo. The Food and Drug Administration has therefore recommended that oral hypoglycemic drugs be used with caution and that emphasis be placed on diet and weight control for the management of diabetes mellitus of adult onset type.

COMPLICATIONS. Hypoglycemic reactions can occur with the sulfonylurea compounds and are most likely to happen if the patient engages in an unusual amount of exercise or omits some of his diet. Reactions are most common in patients with mild diabetes. Side effects and toxic effects can also occur with the sulfonylureas and these include gastrointestinal upset, weakness, paresthesia, headache, ringing in the ears, and intolerance to alcohol. These drugs are usually not given to patients with liver damage, since they may interfere with certain enzymatic actions. The sulfonylureas also depress radioactive iodine uptake and will give an inaccurate result when radioactive iodine is used to test thyroid function. Phenformin (DBI) side effects include a metallic or bitter taste in the mouth, anorexia, abdominal cramps, nausea and vomiting, and diarrhea. The drug is discontinued if vomiting occurs.

Patients receiving oral hypoglycemic agents should be taught as carefully as those patients receiving insulin. They must understand personal hygiene, foot care, and especially the importance of diet in controlling diabetes.

Hypoglycemic reaction (insulin reaction). All persons with diabetes and their immediate families should know the signs and symptoms and the treatment of hypoglycemia (too much insulin for the available glucose in the blood). Even if the patient follows his usual schedule of medication for diabetes and the prescribed diet, he may have slight reactions at times. Severe reactions, however, are usually caused by too large a dose of insulin or oral antidiabetic drug or too little food. If the patient does not eat all of his food or if he skips between-meal and bedtime supplements of food that have been prescribed, he may have a reaction. Some patients alter the dose of medication to cover excesses in eating, which may cause them to have a reaction. Vomiting, diarrhea, added exercise, or emotional stress may also be the cause of insulin reaction. Every person who has diabetes should carry a card giving his address, the name and address of his physician, the fact that he has diabetes, and his daily insulin or oral hypoglycemic drug dosage. Some diabetics wear Medic-Alert bracelets or necklaces (p. 84).

If for any reason the patient feels shaky, is slightly nervous, perspires, is irritable, or feels dizzy, he should take or be given additional food. These difficulties are the beginning signs of too much insulin. He may also feel weak or hungry and may have headache, palpitation, tremor, blurring of vision, or numbness of the lips or tongue. Many persons with diabetes carry lump sugar or hard candies to be eaten in such emergencies. If the patient is at home, he should drink a glass of orange juice, other fruit juice, ginger ale, or any other readily available source of glucose. Sometimes the reaction comes on suddenly, and the patient may not sense early signs. In such an instance a family member may have to give the orange juice or some other sweet fluid. One of the safest ways to administer sugar to a groggy patient is to place a teaspoonful of corn syrup or honey in his mouth. This will be rapidly absorbed by the mucous membrane of the oral mucosa, and the patient will usually arouse sufficiently to be able to drink a glass of juice or sweetened coffee or tea. If impending hypoglycemia is not treated immediately, the patient becomes stuporous and unconscious. Because hypoglycemia interferes with the oxygen consumption of nervous tissue, there can be irreparable brain damage if sugar is not administered promptly. The symptoms of insulin reaction vary both with the type of insulin used and with the individual patient. The pattern in a given patient is usually the same, however, and the patient can generally tell when he is becoming hypoglycemic. If question exists concerning the validity of a patient's feeling about an impending insulin reaction, blood should be drawn immediately for a blood sugar test and *sugar given at once.* The nurse should understand that when in doubt it is always safer to give sugar to the patient than to risk nervous system damage from hypoglycemia. Usually 20 to 25 Gm. of carbohydrate will be sufficient to overcome hypoglycemia. This can be obtained from 8 ounces of fruit juice or sweetened soft drinks, four teaspoons of sugar, two tablespoons of syrup, or four pieces of hard candy. If the patient is already unconscious, 50% glucose will usually be given intravenously.

Glucagon, a pancreatic hormone that acts primarily by mobilizing hepatic glycogen may be given to treat patients having insulin reactions. The effects of this glycogen conversion lasts about $1\frac{1}{2}$ hours and therefore the patient will also require treatment with sugar to prevent a recurrence of the hypoglycemia. Glucagon is given intramuscularly and some physicians instruct their patients to take it when an insulin reaction occurs. If the patient is unconscious, the family administers the drug and then seeks medical assistance.

Teaching the patient to test urine for sugar. The urine testing equipment used will depend on the stability of the disease, the degree of glycosuria anticipated, the life-style of the patient, his visual acuity, and his physical limitation. Different urine testing products can give 0.5%, 2%, or 5% maximum readings of glycosuria. Some require accurate timing or an ability to measure drops of urine. A patient may be able to distinguish shades of color more accurately on one specific color chart.

What the patient *does* if his test is abnormal depends entirely on the particular patient and the instructions he has received. Instructions should be in writing. The physician may, for example, instruct the patient to do nothing except repeat the test again during the same day and to keep a careful record of urine reactions, or he may instruct him to increase or decrease his insulin or oral drug dosage, increase or decrease his food intake, or get in touch with him at once. Some physicians may want certain patients to show a trace or even 1% sugar in their urine once daily as evidence that the blood sugar is not going too low, whereas for other patients this would not be considered good control. The age of the patient and the stability of his disease affect the physician's decision in advising a course of action. The nurse can assist the patient in interpreting his urine test results and in understanding the rationale for his specific instructions.

Care of the skin and feet. Because patients with diabetes are more susceptible to infection and generally heal more slowly than other persons, special attention must be given to skin care. Ideally, the patient should bathe or shower daily. If this is not desired by the patient, or if it is not possible for him to do so, then emphasis should be placed on daily bathing of areas most likely to become infected. These include the back of the neck, the axillae, and the groin, since it is in these areas where carbuncles are most likely to develop. In obese women, special care should also be given to the areas under the breasts. Any area where two skin surfaces meet is a likely place for infection to develop; therefore these areas should be bathed daily and dried thoroughly. In order to avoid dry skin, a lubricant can be used when bathing or showering, or it can be applied to the skin after a daily bath.

Women with pruritus vulvae may need to sponge the area after each voiding, dry it carefully, and apply cornstarch, which is usually more effective and cheaper than talcum powder. Usually a tub is more soothing than a shower and relieves a great deal of the discomfort. Medicated ointments may also be prescribed.

Because persons with diabetes are prone to develop more severe atherosclerosis and arteriosclerosis, and at an earlier age than nondiabetics, special emphasis should be placed on daily care of the feet in order to prevent infection and diabetic gangrene. All patients with diabetes should be carefully instructed in care of their feet and should see a podiatrist regularly if at all possible (Fig. 27-11). The general rules for foot care in patients with diabetes are the same as those for any patient with diminished peripheral circulation and may be found on pp. 376 and 377. Two pamphlets that are helpful in teaching patients are *Foot Care for the Diabetic Patient** and *Feet First.** Patients over 40 years of age should also be encouraged to inspect their feet carefully as a part of their foot care regime. Their cooperation may be ensured by a frank explanation of the increased incidence of neuropathy for patients with diabetes, which may produce insensitivity to pain. As a result, blisters or cuts can become infected before they are even noticed.

Exercise. All patients with diabetes need regular exercise and this should be discussed with them as

---

*Published by the Department of Health, Education and Welfare, Public Health Service, Division of Chronic Diseases, and available from the Superintendent of Documents, U. S. Government Printing Office, Washington, D. C., 20402.

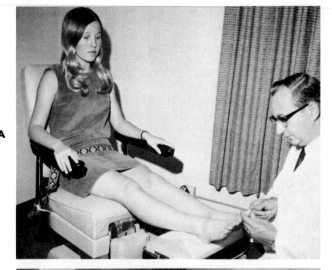

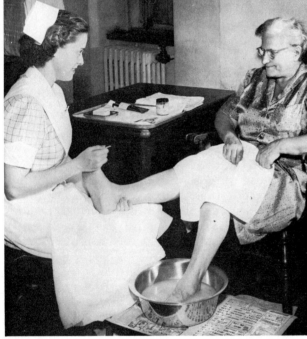

FIG. 27-11. Diabetic patients of all ages need special foot care and may receive it during visits to the clinic. **A,** The podiatrist cuts the nails of a patient. **B,** The nurse teaches a patient how to give herself daily foot care.

part of the overall treatment plan. Patients receiving insulin or oral hypoglycemic agents should understand that the amount of medication prescribed by the physician will be planned around their usual exercise pattern. Because an increase in activity will decrease the need for insulin or the hypoglycemic agents, patients should know that if they are going to exercise more than usual they should plan their dietary intake so that they eat a quick-acting form of glucose just before starting the activity. Also, many physicians will teach patients taking insulin how they may reduce their insulin dose or increase

their food intake when they are planning more exercise than usual.

It may be helpful for young diabetics to know that several well-known athletes with diabetes have been able to perform at championship level in such sports as tennis and professional baseball. In these cases they adjusted their insulin and food consumption to meet their athletic schedule.

Because an increase in exercise does decrease the need for insulin or hypoglycemic agents, an unusual amount of exercise can precipitate a hypoglycemic reaction. This can usually be handled by the patient himself as long as he recognizes the symptoms and he carries some form of rapid-acting glucose such as sugar cubes or hard candy with him at all times.

Diabetic ketoacidosis

Diabetic ketoacidosis (which if allowed to continue will result in diabetic coma and death) occurs when there is not sufficient insulin available to metabolize glucose. When this happens, as explained in the beginning of this section (p. 745), glucose is excreted in the urine, taking with it large amounts of water. Fats must then be burned for energy and ketosis results. This increase in hydrogen ions in the blood calls on the alkali reserve of the body to combat the acidosis. Thus there is a loss of sodium, chloride, potassium, and more water. As the alkali reserve of the body is depleted, the pH of the blood goes down. At the same time the body attempts to rid itself of the increased acids by respiratory and renal means. Carbon dioxide is exhaled through the lungs in increasing amounts as the respirations become more deep and rapid (Kussmaul breathing). The kidneys attempt to excrete more of the acids in the urine and even more water is lost. This results in hemoconcentration and, in time, in generalized hypoxia. In the presence of hypoxia, increased amounts of lactic acid are produced, which further increase the hydrogen ion concentration of the blood. If the process is allowed to continue, the patient will lapse into coma since hypoxia and acidosis interfere with the function of the cerebral hemispheres. The signs and symptoms of diabetic ketoacidosis can be directly linked to the severe dehydration, loss of essential electrolytes, and acidosis. These signs and symptoms include weakness, dull headache, fatigue, general malaise, insatiable thirst, epigastric aching pain, and nausea and vomiting. Accompanying these signs and symptoms are the physical findings of one in severe dehydration and acidosis. The mucous membranes are dehydrated and there is loss of skin turgor, the eyeballs may be soft or sunken, the lips and tongue are red and parched, the face is usually flushed, and hyperpnea (Kussmaul breathing) is present. The temperature will be elevated at first, and then may go down with the resultant hypovolemia. Hypovolemic shock is common and the systolic blood pressure may be as low as 60 to 70 mm. Hg; in time the patient will become anuric, and circulatory collapse can occur. In elderly patients a myocardial infarction may occur as the coronary circulation is curtailed.

Causes. The most common cause of diabetic ketoacidosis is an infection, because infection increases the body's need for insulin. The usual sites of infection are the respiratory or urinary tract or the skin (carbuncles). Other causes of ketoacidosis are failure to take prescribed insulin, inadequate food and fluid intake, and an increased need for insulin such as occurs with surgery, trauma, or excessive food intake. In all these situations the body will be forced to burn fats for energy since glucose either is not available (inadequate intake) or the glucose that is available cannot be metabolized because of an inadequate supply of insulin.

Treatment. Diabetic ketoacidosis is a medical emergency that requires intensive care of the patient both by the physician and nurse. Therapy is directed toward correcting the acidosis, dehydration, and electrolyte disturbances and other factors such as infection that precipitated the ketoacidosis. It can be expected that all of these will be carried on simultaneously.

The severity of the patient's condition is determined by the level of ketones in the blood (ketonemia); therefore the patient's plasma is tested for a 4+ reaction for ketones. Then dilutions of the patient's plasma are made to determine the extent of the ketonemia. The greater the number of dilutions in which ketones remain 4+, the more severe the ketoacidosis.[3] These dilutions are converted to an approximation of the acetone values/100 ml. of blood. Values over 50 mg./100 ml. are considered severe ketosis, while those 80 mg. or over are considered to be evidence of clinical coma.

The amount of insulin ordered for the patient is based on the initial level of ketonemia. The first doses of insulin may be given both intravenously and subcutaneously. The total amount of insulin needed to correct the ketoacidosis will depend on the patient's response to therapy. Some patients require as little as 200 or 300 units of regular insulin to correct ketoacidosis, while others may require 1,000 units or more.

To correct dehydration, normal saline solution or half-strength normal saline solution (0.45%) is given in large amounts—often 4 L. or more is required in the first 24 hours. If normal saline solution is not sufficient to replace the sodium loss, additional sodium is given either as sodium bicarbonate or sodium lactate. Potassium ordinarily is not given early in the treatment because patients with severe dehydration and hemoconcentration usually have hyperkalemia, which is caused by the movement of potassium from the intracellular to the extracellular fluid. As the dehydration is corrected, the potassium moves back into the cells and hypokalemia may occur. Because of the effect of potassium on cardiac muscle, the patient should be carefully monitored via ECG tracings to determine the need for potassium (p. 345).

Nursing intervention. The nursing intervention planned for the patient depends on the severity of the ketoacidosis and the prescribed treatment. In addition to carefully monitoring vital signs and levels of consciousness, the nurse must see that blood and urine specimens are obtained as ordered and that necessary blood and urine tests are carried out. If the patient is in severe ketoacidosis, blood is drawn frequently to test for ketones, sugar, and electrolyte levels. If the patient is unconscious, an indwelling catheter is usually inserted.

As the patient's condition improves, the ketone levels in the blood can be expected to drop and the blood sugar will return to more nearly normal levels. It is at this time that the patient should be watched most closely for signs of insulin reaction. It should be remembered that blood levels of ketone and sugar will return to normal before urinary levels will. When the patient is able to take fluids by mouth, he will usually be given fruit juices, broth, cooked cereal, and milk. Solid foods are added as soon as possible to improve gastric tone and prevent further ileus.

As the patient recovers, the cause of his acidosis should be reviewed with him so that he understands how to avoid a recurrence.

Before the discovery of insulin, diabetic ketoacidosis often caused death. *Immediate* care and treatment are still necessary, but with this care the outcome is usually good. The patient or his family should contact their physician at once if any signs or symptoms of acidosis occur. Carrying a card stating that he has diabetes helps to ensure prompt treatment in the event that coma develops while the patient is away from home. Such a card also helps prevent this condition from being mistaken for head injury, cerebrovascular accident, or drunkenness. A summary of the differences between insulin reaction and diabetic ketoacidosis is presented in Table 27-4.

Hyperosmolar nonketotic coma. Another form of diabetic coma can develop in the diabetic patient who is ketosis resistant. It is more apt to occur in the older patient with mild diabetes, usually noninsulin-dependent, or in patients whose diabetes has been poorly controlled over a number of weeks or months. It is characterized by high concentrations of glucose in the blood with no acetone in the urine. The plasma hyperosmolality that develops creates the osmotic force that pulls water from the cells, particularly the cerebral cells. Coma is the end result.

The most important aspect of treatment is correction of dehydration with half-strength normal saline solution (0.45%) and insulin. The mortality rate from hyperosmolar coma has been high, possibly due to

Table 27-4   Summary of differences between insulin reaction and diabetic ketoacidosis

	Insulin reaction	Ketoacidosis
Onset	Rapid	Slow (days or weeks)
Precipitating factors		
Food	Insufficient	Excessive
Complications	None	Infection
Insulin	Excess	Too little
Exercise	Increased	Too little
Symptoms		
Thirst	Absent	Increased
Vomiting	Absent	Frequent
Hunger	Frequent	Absent
Abdominal pain	Absent	Frequent
Vision	Double	Dim
Signs		
Temperature	Normal or below	Elevated
Respirations	Normal	Hyperpnea (Kussmaul breathing), acetone odor to breath
Blood pressure	Normal or elevated	Lowered, may be in shock
Skin	Moist and pale	Hot, dry, and flushed
Dehydration	None	Loss of skin turgor, sunken eyeballs
Tremors	Frequent	Absent
Laboratory findings		
Urine		
Glycosuria	May be positive, but negative in second specimen	4+
Ketonuria	Negative	4+
Blood		
Sugar	Below normal	Elevated, usually above 200 mg./100 ml.
Ketones	Normal	Elevated, usually 4+
Electrolytes	Normal	Decreased, except serum potassium

the patient's advanced age and concomitant vascular diseases. On recovery, these patients often have the same teaching need as those recovering from ketoacidosis.

Continuity of care

The nurse in the hospital or in the home should always pass information along to other medical personnel as to what care has been given, what teaching has been accomplished, and probable future needs of the patient with diabetes mellitus. This information enables the nurse and patient to continue his care without delays and repetition. Sometimes the patient may not be capable of learning the care he needs to give himself. If the patient lives alone and has no relative or neighbor who can be taught to give daily injections of insulin and to check on other aspects of care, it may be necessary for a nurse to visit the home to carry out these procedures. In teaching the patient with diabetes, the nurse should stress the need for him to have enough medication,

equipment, and foodstuffs on hand so that he can withstand any unexpected situation. He should also know that stress situations may change his need for medication since more glucose will be used, leaving a surplus of insulin in the blood. Therefore it will be imperative for him to test his urine for sugar more frequently so that he may regulate his medication according to his physician's instructions or seek medical advice in regulating the dosage.

Complications of diabetes mellitus

All diabetics have some changes in blood vessels that result in vascular complications. It is well known that diabetics are prone to develop atherosclerosis at an earlier age than nondiabetics. This appears to be related to the high levels of triglycerides found when diabetes is poorly controlled. In addition, diabetics have small vessel (microvascular) changes that are not seen in nondiabetics. These small vessel changes most commonly cause clinical effects in the kidneys, retinas, nervous system, and skin. The cause and rate of progression of these complications is controversial. Factors that may contribute to them include inadequate blood sugar control, diabetes of long standing, or a hereditary defect linked with diabetes that causes vascular difficulties in some diabetics.

Kimmelstiel-Wilson syndrome, a nephrotic syndrome with proteinuria, edema, and hypertension, has an unfavorable prognosis. Treatment is the same as for nephrotic syndrome from other causes. Pyelonephritis is treated with antibiotics.

Retinopathy occurs in time in about 70% of all diabetics.[2] Some patients have some retinal changes at the time of diagnosis; however, it may be years before the patient complains of impairment of vision. Patients with retinopathy may have serious handicaps because failing vision makes it difficult, if not impossible, for them to inject insulin, test urine, prepare their own food, and give themselves general care. Helping them to accommodate to visual changes presents a great challenge to the nurse. (See discussion of diabetic retinopathy on p. 841.)

It is presumed that most diabetics have asymptomatic polyneuropathy. When disabling symptoms do occur, they are most likely to be manifested in the toes and feet and are symmetric. The most common symptoms are numbness, burning paresthesia, and stabbing pains. The patient's limbs are very sensitive to touch and pressure, and the pain may be so severe that the patient cannot walk or wear shoes. Sometimes narcotics are required for pain relief.

Atherosclerosis can result in impaired circulation to the limbs, and diabetic gangrene of the toes and feet can result. Sometimes amputation is required to treat gangrene.

The nurse can help the patient to understand what he can do to help himself (proper foot care) and what the physician will check on the patient's visit to him. It can be reassuring to the patient if he realizes that the physician will be examining his urine for early signs of kidney complications and his eyes for any beginning changes. The nurse can also stress the need to be alert for any underlying problem such as an infection so that it can be promptly treated.

Patients with diabetes mellitus are particularly susceptible to tuberculosis. It is recommended that young diabetics have a chest film at least every 2 years.[2]

■ HYPOGLYCEMIC STATES

Hypoglycemia is a relatively common disorder characterized by blood sugar levels below 50 mg./100 ml. The blood sugar falls more rapidly than normal after eating and may drop to abnormally low levels several hours after a meal or after exercise. The patient usually has a sudden onset of faintness, hunger, weakness, and tremor. Headache and feelings of anxiety sometimes occur. In more severe cases, pallor, diaphoresis, rapid pulse, and even twitching, convulsions, and coma can occur. The symptoms may be intermittent, being relieved by food, or they may last for hours or for days.

Hypoglycemia is often functional, with no known cause demonstrable. It may also be due to a pancreatic adenoma, causing extra insulin to be released, by liver disease, causing inability to store glycogen, or by pituitary or adrenal dysfunction. If possible, the primary cause is treated.

A high-protein, high-fat, low-carbohydrate diet often relieves symptoms. Carbohydrates, especially simple sugars, are used quickly, but protein in excess of the normal body needs is converted gradually to glycogen. This helps to maintain the blood sugar at a more nearly normal and more stable level from meal to meal. The patient should eat meals that are spaced regularly. Many physicians advise their patients to carry lump sugar or candy with them at all times for immediate use if faintness occurs. Candy with nuts is best, since the nuts are a source of protein. The patient must understand that he should not rely on these sugars as a substitute for regularly spaced meals, however, since functional hypoglycemia is provoked by glucose stimulation and more frequent attacks of hypoglycemia may occur.

■ DISEASES OF THE ADRENAL GLANDS

Each kidney is capped by an adrenal gland consisting of two parts, the medulla and the cortex. When stimulated by the sympathetic nervous system, the *adrenal medulla* secretes two hormones, epinephrine and norepinephrine. (Their physiologic action is described on p. 96.) Both are apparently secreted continuously in small amounts, but their output is markedly increased by any stressful situation. When they are secreted in large amounts into the bloodstream, they rapidly stimulate the physiologic functions needed for responding to emergency situations in both the internal and the external environment. However, they are not essential to life because the sympathetic nervous system produces similar though slower and less extensive responses.

The *adrenal cortex* is essential to life. Without its hormones, the corticosteroids, the body's metabolic processes seem to respond inadequately to even minimal physical and emotional stresses such as changes in temperature, exercise, or excitement. Severe stresses such as those caused by serious infections or extreme anxiety may result in shock and death. Although in recent years many steroid compounds have been isolated from the adrenal cortex, only a few appear to affect metabolism significantly. Hydrocortisone, cortisone, corticosterone, and aldosterone seem to be produced in the largest amounts. Small amounts of the sex hormones, especially androgens, also are secreted. The physiologic actions of the corticosteroids are complex and affect a wide variety of vital functions. In fact, it is felt that they may influence the function of all body cells. The corticosteroids are classified according to their major physiologic action as *glucocorticoids* (hydrocortisone and cortisone), *mineralocorticoids* (aldosterone), and sex hormones secreted by the adrenal cortex. All the corticosteroids to some degree cause sodium (and therefore water since it is always held by sodium) to be retained in the body and potassium and chloride to be excreted by the kidneys. However, this seems to be the primary function of the mineralocorticoids.

The glucocorticoids seem to affect numerous metabolic processes, although their exact actions are not known. They apparently enhance protein catabolism and inhibit protein synthesis, and they appear to be insulin antagonists and to increase the synthesis of glucose by the liver. These actions all tend to raise the blood sugar level. They also seem in some way to influence the defense mechanisms of the body. High concentrations of glucocorticoids in the blood suppress inflammation, inhibit the formation of scar tissue, and may prevent allergic responses. Because of this action, they are useful in treating inflammation (p. 81). In man, glucocorticoids seem to be essential in the body's adjustment to stress, and they appear in some way to influence emotional responses. For example, patients with adrenal insufficiency typically are depressed and anxious. Patients receiving large doses of cortisone over a long period of time may become euphoric (unrealistically optimistic and cheerful). Glucocorticoids also apparently play a role in the regulation of melanin metabolism, which determines the pigmentation of the skin and mucous membranes. When there is a deficiency of glucocorticoids, such as in Addison's disease, the skin takes on a bronze coloring.

The action of the adrenal sex hormones apparently is identical to that of the sex hormones that are secreted by the sex glands. Therefore, in treating conditions such as cancer of the breast, in which inhibition of secretion of all sex hormones is considered essential for controlling metastasis, bilateral adrenalectomy may be done.

The secretion of the glucocorticoids and the mineralocorticoids seems to be stimulated by adrenocorticotropic hormone produced by the anterior pituitary gland, and a high blood level of glucocorticoids suppresses the secretion of adrenocorticotropic hormone. Secretion of aldosterone does not seem to be dependent on hormones from the anterior pituitary gland, but rather is regulated by the concentration of sodium and potassium in the body fluids. When the sodium level in the body fluids is low, the secretion of aldosterone is increased, causing the body to retain salt and also water. A high sodium level inhibits its secretion and allows the kidneys to excrete sodium and water and to retain potassium.

Diseases of the adrenal cortex

Diseases of the adrenal cortex usually are related to *hyperfunction* or *hypofunction* of the cortical portion of the adrenal glands. The malfunction may be from a variety of causes both within and without the gland.

Since the adrenal cortex affects so many physiologic functions, tests that are diagnostic for many disorders may be done. Chemical analyses of the blood usually are ordered to ascertain the stability of electrolyte balance. A glucose tolerance test may be done to determine the ability of the patient to use carbohydrates. Tests of renal tubular function may be done to determine the ability of the kidneys to concentrate and dilute urine and thus maintain water balance. X-ray films of the kidney area may be taken to delineate any adrenal tumor. The physician usually orders urine collected so that he may study the *urinary excretion of 17-ketosteroids* (androgenic components) and *17-hydroxycorticoids* (glucocorticoids and related fractions). More accurate diagnosis of adrenal disorders is possible today with improved hormone radioimmunoassay methods as well as more refined stimulation and suppression tests.

Only two of the most common, yet rare, diseases of the adrenal glands will be discussed here. Other related diseases are fully discussed in specialized texts.

Addison's disease. In Addison's disease there is *hypofunction* of the adrenal cortex and an insufficient secretion of both the *mineralocorticoids* and the *glucocorticoids.* Since these hormones are essential for maintaining life, the patient with Addison's disease will die unless he receives adequate exogenous replacement therapy. In the past, it was felt that most cases of Addison's disease were caused by tuberculosis of the adrenal gland. This is no longer believed to be true and now the disease is thought to be due to idiopathic bilateral atrophy of the gland. The disease usually develops insidiously and sometimes it is first manifested when a patient is subjected to the stress of infection, trauma, or surgery. Only then does the latent hypofunction of the adrenal cortex become evident.

The symptoms of Addison's disease include asthenia, fatigue, and gastrointestinal complaints such as anorexia, nausea, vomiting, abdominal pain, and diarrhea. The patient with Addison's disease may also give a history of frequent hypoglycemic reactions with nervousness, headache, trembling, and diaphoresis. He is usually hypotensive, and frequently a chest radiograph will reveal a small heart. In addition, he usually has a severe deficiency of sodium and chloride (*hyponatremia* and *hypochloremia)* and an increase in serum potassium (*hyperkalemia).* These imbalances in electrolytes are related to a deficiency in the *mineralocorticoids,* while a decrease in the *glucocorticoids* is responsible for the hypoglycemic reactions. Most patients with chronic Addison's disease develop a bronzelike pigmentation of the skin and mucous membrane. Thus they always appear to be tanned on those areas of the body that are exposed to the sun. They may also have hyperpigmentation of pressure points such as the knees and elbows and along the belt line.

The diagnosis of Addison's disease may be confirmed by an 8-hour corticotropin test. In primary Addison's disease the urinary level of 17-hydroxycorticosteroids does not rise; in adrenal insufficiency secondary to pituitary dysfunction the level rises slowly. A 30-minute response test may also be of diagnostic value. Plasma cortisol levels are measured before and after an injection of ACTH. If a significant rise does not occur, Addison's disease is suspected.

The treatment of Addison's disease consists of administration of a *glucocorticoid,* either cortisone or hydrocortisone, and a *mineralocorticoid,* usually 9-alpha-fluorohydrocortisone (Fludrocortisone). The usual dose of cortisone is 37.5 mg. daily, with 25 mg. given on awakening and 12.5 mg. given before 4 P.M. Since cortisone is ulcerogenic for some patients, it should always be given after meals or with milk. Antacids may also be prescribed. The dose of Fludrocortisone is 0.1 to 0.2 mg. daily.[2] Other forms of these drugs may be prescribed, but these are the most widely used ones at present.

The patient with Addison's disease should understand the serious nature of his disease and the importance of taking his replacement therapy daily as ordered. He should also know that he should never omit a dose of the drug and that if he has a gastrointestinal disturbance and is unable to retain the drug, his physician should be notified at once. Since the prescribed replacement therapy is planned to meet normal requirements of daily living, the patient will require additional glucocorticoids and mineralocorticoids if he is subjected to increased stress such as that of infection, trauma, surgery, or emotional upset. For this reason the patient with chronic Addison's disease should carry an identification card with him at all times. The card should include his physician's name, address, and telephone number and the name, address, and telephone number of his next of kin. It is also recommended that the card state which of the adrenocortical hormones is to be given in case of illness or injury. In addition, it is recommended that patients with little or no function of the adrenal glands carry an emergency supply of cortisone, hydrocortisone, and desoxycorticosterone at all times.

The patient with Addison's disease who is on adequate replacement therapy can live a normal, productive life as long as he avoids undue stress. The nurse should teach the patient about his disease and about his replacement therapy (Fig. 27-12).

Addisonian crisis. Addisonian, or adrenal, crisis is a severe exacerbation of Addison's disease. It is a very serious condition in which there is severe hypotension, shock, coma, and vasomotor collapse, and it quickly leads to death unless treated promptly. It may occur in any person with an insufficient amount of adrenocortical hormones, regardless of the cause, and may be precipitated by strenuous activity, infection or other stressful situations, or by failure to take prescribed steroids. It often is a complication of surgery or other treatment of the pituitary or adrenal glands. The signs of impending crisis are those of the disease in exaggerated form.

When addisonian crisis occurs, a large dose of hydrocortisone phosphate is given immediately by the intravenous route. A continuous infusion of normal saline solution is started to provide for the maintenance of fluid balance and the administration of drugs. Cortisone may be given intramuscularly also. The patient must do *absolutely nothing* for himself.

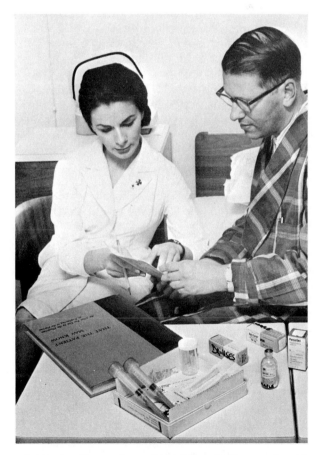

FIG. 27-12. The patient with Addison's disease should be taught about his disease, about the hormones he must take, and how he can live safely with his disease. (Reprinted, with permission, from Shea, K. M., and others: Am. J. Nurs. **65:**80-85, Dec. 1965.)

If he is conscious, the nurse should caution him not to attempt to turn or otherwise help himself. The nurse should not move the patient unless absolutely necessary and should consult the physician before doing so. All forms of stimuli such as loud noises and bright lights should be eliminated. Vital signs usually are taken every 15 minutes and temperature every hour. If hypotension is severe, a vasopressor drug such as phenylephrine (Neo-Synephrine) may be given. Whole blood and concentrated serum albumin are given if hypotension persists, since the protein in these fluids tends to hold fluid in the vascular compartment. The patient often complains of severe headache; an ice bag may be used to relieve it. The patient has an extremely low resistance to infection, and reverse isolation usually is used to protect the patient from exposure to infection. He always must be protected from anyone, including members of his family and from hospital personnel, who has a cold or other infection. If the addisonian crisis was precipitated by an infection, appropriate antimicrobial therapy will be instituted.

Cushing's syndrome. In Cushing's syndrome there is an excessive secretion of the glucocorticoid cortisol. The causes of this increase in secretion include (1) an adrenocortical tumor that secretes cortisol without ACTH stimulation, (2) a nonpituitary neoplasm that secretes ACTH and stimulates the production of cortisol (ectopic ACTH syndrome), and (3) excessive secretion of ACTH by the pituitary gland, stimulating increased levels of cortisol. The latter is referred to as Cushing's disease. This oversecretion results in disruption of normal metabolic processes. Excessive amounts of water and salt may be retained in the body; the potassium level in the body fluids is reduced and other electrolyte balances such as the calcium-phosphorus balance are upset; protein catabolism is increased; the blood sugar level rises and insulin production decreases; the eosinophil count decreases; there is loss of elasticity of vessel walls with increased vascular fragility, predisposing the patient to capillary hemorrhage (petechiae); and there are changes in the secondary sex characteristics.

Signs and symptoms of Cushing's syndrome include muscle wasting with resultant weakness, susceptibility to hemorrhage, and peculiar fat distribution with deposition of fat in the face (moonface), neck, and trunk. Osteoporosis is also common, and fracture of vertebrae may occur. The patient usually has hypertension and is irritable and changeable in mood. Diabetes mellitus that is resistant to insulin may develop. Women patients show signs of masculinization, and the menses often cease. Adolescent or preadolescent boys may have precocious sexual development. Resistance to infection is often lowered and may lead to death.

Treatment of Cushing's syndrome depends on the cause. If a tumor of the adrenal cortex is the cause,

the tumor may be surgically resected. When there is a tumor of one of the adrenal glands, the increase in corticosteroids produced by that gland will cause suppression of ACTH (by negative feedback) and subsequent atrophy of the unaffected gland. In this situation the treatment of choice is the removal of the affected gland with replacement therapy given until the atrophic gland resumes normal functioning.[2] If there is hyperplasia of both glands, then a bilateral total adrenalectomy is usually done. In this case, the patient must be on lifetime replacement therapy.[2] In nonpituitary neoplasms (ectopic ACTH syndrome), surgical removal is the treatment of choice. However, it is often not possible to remove the tumor surgically. When this happens, the patient is treated with metyrapone, which inhibits the final step in cortisol synthesis.

Pituitary tumors can be abated by irradiation, or a hypophysectomy may be performed. The goal in all of these procedures is to reduce the amount of cortisol being produced by the adrenal glands. Sometimes the treatment causes the level of cortisol to be so severely reduced that replacement therapy is required.

The patient with Cushing's syndrome needs skilled nursing care and the utmost consideration. The patient usually is seriously ill and debilitated. Helping him to maintain adequate nutrition, some level of emotional balance, and an acceptance of his situation will challenge the best efforts of all members of the nursing staff. The patient, especially a woman, is greatly upset by the change in appearance. The moonface with acne, the buffalo hump on the back of the neck, the purple striae, and the obvious obesity of the trunk (often with slender arms and legs) makes the patient look very unattractive. He usually is sensitive about his appearance, and he may withdraw from others. The nurse needs to be aware of the patient's feelings and should attempt to protect him from upsetting situations. If the patient is to have surgery on either the adrenal glands or the pituitary gland, he will need careful preparation. Patients who are untreated usually die of infection or from cerebrovascular accidents secondary to severe hypertension.

Primary aldosteronism. Primary aldosteronism is a rare disorder that is usually caused by an aldosterone-secreting tumor of the adrenal cortex. It is reported to be twice as common in females as in males. Hypersecretion of aldosterone increases the renal tubule exchange of sodium for potassium and hydrogen ions; hypernatremia, hypokalemia, and hypertension result. The hypertension is related to the increased sodium reabsorption, whereas severe muscle weakness is the result of potassium depletion.

The most definitive diagnostic tools are elevated urinary and plasma aldosterone levels. Spironolactone, an aldosterone antagonist, has been tried in an attempt to pinpoint the diagnosis. If this drug restores a normal serum potassium level, hyperaldosteronism is suspected.

The treatment goal is surgical removal of tumors or resection of hyperplastic glands. Successful surgery reverses the hypertension in about two thirds of the patients. Early diagnosis and treatment are the goal since patients who are untreated will, in time, develop the sequelae of hypertensive cardiovascular disease and renal insufficiency.

There is considerable controversy about the incidence of primary aldosteronism. Some experts believe that as many as 7% of the patients who appear to have essential hypertension may, in fact, have primary aldosteronism.[2]

Diseases of the adrenal medulla

Pheochromocytoma is a catecholamine-producing tumor (usually benign) of the sympathetic-adrenal system. Although pheochromocytomas account for less than 0.1% of cases of hypertension, it is important that they be diagnosed since they can be cured.[2]

The diagnosis is confirmed by assays of catecholamines and their metabolites in the urine. In pheochromocytoma the levels of these compounds are increased. About 80% of the tumors are located in the adrenal glands and more than 95% are situated in the abdominal and pelvic areas. Only a small percentage of the tumors are malignant. The usual treatment is surgical excision of the pheochromocytoma, which results in complete remission of the symptoms unless there is metastasis to another site. During surgery there may be excessive production of catecholamines as the tumor is manipulated. This causes very high blood pressure levels and cardiac arrhythmias. Administration of phenoxybenzamine (Dibenzyline) daily for 7 to 10 days prior to surgery may be used to control preoperative hypertension and reduce these complications of surgery.

Hypotension may occur postoperatively and is treated with whole blood and volume expanders. If hypotension persists, norepinephrine is given intravenously. Adrenal cortical insufficiency can occur postoperatively if cortical tissue was resected in removing the tumor.

Surgery of the adrenal glands

Both adrenal glands may be removed surgically *(bilateral adrenalectomy)*. In this procedure all the adrenal cortical and medullary tissue is removed. A bilateral adrenalectomy is done most often for patients with cancer of the breast with metastasis, but occasionally it is used for patients with cancer of the prostate with metastasis. Only one adrenal gland or a part of one may be removed *(subtotal adrenalectomy),* or a tumor and the tissue immediately surrounding it may be resected from either the cortex *(adrenocortical tumor resection)* or the medulla *(adrenal medullary tumor resection).*

Management of patients requiring adrenal surgery. When any surgery on the adrenal glands is planned, treatment with steroids usually is discontinued for several weeks preoperatively to prevent the danger of infection after surgery (p. 82). This also allows postoperative control of blood levels of steroids to be more accurately regulated. If antihypertensive drugs have been used, they, too, are discontinued, since the surgery may cause a rather severe drop in the blood pressure. Phenobarbital may be given for sedation during this time.

The operative incision for any type of adrenal surgery is made in the flank close to the diaphragm. Special care should be taken postoperatively to have the patient turned frequently and to encourage him to breathe deeply and to cough. Usually a narcotic is ordered and it should be given about a half hour before coughing is attempted; the incision should be supported. Dyspnea or sudden chest pain should be reported at once because a spontaneous pneumothorax may occur. A nasogastric tube is often passed and attached to suction to relieve the abdominal distention that may accompany this surgery.

Usually the patient remains in bed for 2 or 3 days postoperatively and is kept flat during this time. When he is permitted out of bed, elastic bandages may be applied to the lower extremities because of the instability of the vascular system. The patient's blood pressure must be taken every 15 minutes when ambulation is first attempted. If the blood pressure drops, he should be assisted back to bed, and orders for further attempts at ambulation must be obtained from the physician.

Special care needed by patients requiring adrenocortical surgery. The immediate postoperative care for patients having any type of adrenocortical surgery is quite similar. Adrenocortical function is very labile when part of the adrenocortical tissue is removed and, of course, it is labile when all the tissue is removed since maintenance of the hormonal level then must be controlled completely by replacement therapy. The patient's special needs center around maintaining appropriate amounts of adrenocortical hormones in the blood. The patient undergoing a total adrenalectomy also requires the care needed by a patient with surgery of the adrenal medulla, which is described below.

Immediately after surgery, replacement of corticosteroids is started. Hydrocortisone is given continuously by intravenous drip, and dosage is adjusted at intervals according to the clinical findings. Since hormonal replacement is delicately regulated on the basis of continuous observations of electrolyte balance, blood sugar, and blood pressure determinations, the patient, following any adrenal surgery, needs to be given constant nursing attention until hormonal stability is regained or a maintenance regimen established. Drugs to raise the blood pressure may be given. The rate of infusions containing vasopressor drugs such as metaraminol (Aramine) is regulated in accordance with frequent blood pressure readings (usually every 15 minutes). The nurse is responsible for taking accurate blood pressure readings and adjusting the rate of flow according to the surgeon's orders. When there is no order to decrease or increase the flow, the surgeon must be notified at once about any significant changes in blood pressure. The nurse should also observe the patient carefully for signs of *hypoglycemia*. This condition is most likely to occur if the patient had diabetes mellitus as a symptom, but it can occur in any patient who has adrenal surgery. Intravenous solutions containing glucose are usually ordered. If the patient is able to eat, the nurse should check to see that he has eaten the food served. If not, the surgeon should be notified since the diet is prescribed to meet the patient's particular needs and the surgeon may wish to give nourishment intravenously. Hypoglycemic reactions are most likely to occur in the early morning, and they may follow any unusual physical activity or any emotional upset. The nurse also should be alert for symptoms of *addisonian crisis,* which requires immediate treatment. *Markedly increased* urinary output may indicate the need for vasopressin (Pitressin) to control excessive diuresis.

If the patient had hyperfunction of the gland, his preoperative symptoms will continue for several weeks following surgery. The nursing care started in the preoperative period, therefore, must be continued.

Most patients will require adrenocortical hormones at least temporarily even after being discharged from the hospital. Those who have had a total adrenalectomy must take adrenocortical hormones regularly for the remainder of their lives. All patients usually must take cortisone, and many must take fluorohydrocortisone. Testosterone may be given to the patient who has had surgery for Cushing's syndrome, especially if he continues to have muscle weakness and lethargy. Testosterone is never given to the patient whose surgery has been done for cancer of the breast or prostate because the purpose of the surgery was to remove this hormone.

Special care needed by patients requiring adrenal medullary surgery. Marked hypotension often follows removal of a medullary tumor (pheochromocytoma). It is well to remember that these patients have usually had hypertension, and therefore a blood pressure reading within normal limits may represent hypotension for them. Changes in the blood pressure are more significant when several readings are considered. Infusions containing vasopressor drugs such as metaraminol always are given until the blood pressure stabilizes, and very accurate and frequent regulation of the infusion, similar to that described under adrenocortical surgery, is required. Cerebro-vascular accidents and circulatory collapse may complicate the postoperative course. The nurse caring for these patients should review the care of the patient with hypertension, heart failure, cerebrovascular accident, and shock.

■ DISEASES OF THE PITUITARY GLAND

The pituitary gland, located deep in the cranial cavity at the bifurcation of the optic chiasm, is made up of two parts, the anterior pituitary lobe and the posterior pituitary lobe. The functions of some of the better known hormones secreted by this very important gland are described in a simplified way earlier in this chapter. Actually the action of each hormone is complex and incompletely understood, and it is felt that not all the hormones have even been isolated. New information about the pituitary gland is being learned each year, and each new fact seems to reemphasize the complexity of this gland. What initiates the secretion of pituitary hormones is not clearly understood. It is known that the tropic hormones are secreted in response to lowering of the blood level of the hormones whose secretions are stimulated by them (negative feedback mechanism). It also is known that the antidiuretic hormone is secreted in response to a decrease in the blood volume. How this information reaches the posterior pituitary lobe, however, is still not known, but it is generally believed that the hypothalamus of the brain may be involved.

Because of the influence of the anterior pituitary hormones on other endocrine glands, dysfunction of the anterior pituitary gland may cause symptoms of malfunction in the glands whose secretions are dependent on its tropic hormones. By irradiating or surgically removing the pituitary gland, the secretion of hormones from other glands can be reduced. Sometimes this is done rather than performing a total adrenalectomy, as in treatment for metastatic cancer of the breast or prostate gland.[20] The pituitary gland may also be irradiated or surgically removed in an attempt to slow retinal deterioration associated with diabetic retinopathy. Because of its location near the optic chiasm, tumors of the pituitary gland may press on the optic nerves and cause visual field defects such as bitemporal hemianopsia and loss of visual acuity.

Anterior lobe hypofunction

Hypofunction of the anterior lobe of the pituitary gland may result from compression of the gland by a tumor within the gland itself or tumors associated with contiguous structures. Metastatic carcinoma or inflammatory disease such as meningitis also can damage it, or it may be congenitally malfunctioning.

If a tumor is present, the patient may have visual disturbance caused by pressure on the optic nerve, severe headache due to increased intracranial pressure, and symptoms associated with disturbance of the gland itself. These symptoms may vary according to which hormone insufficiency is manifested. One result of hypofunction is the effect on body growth. In the adolescent, sexual growth and development may be arrested. If TSH is decreased, symptoms of hypothyroidism may occur. If ACTH secretion is impaired, the patient may have symptoms of Addison's disease. A combination of many endocrine deficiency diseases may be present. *Dwarfism* results from congenital deficiency of the growth hormone.

Treatment of anterior pituitary gland disorders depends on their cause. Pituitary extract has been used successfully in some patients with dwarfism, but at present this hormone is extremely hard to obtain and very costly. Tumors causing pressure on the gland are removed surgically if possible. Some tumors of the gland itself, such as a chromophobe adenoma, are amenable to radiation therapy. Sometimes a hypophysectomy (removal of the entire gland) must be done.

Anterior lobe hyperfunction

Congenital hypersecretion of the growth hormone from the anterior pituitary gland causes excessive growth *(gigantism)*. Hyperfunction of the anterior lobe of the pituitary gland in the adult results in *acromegaly* and usually is caused by a tumor in the eosinophil cells. The main symptoms or signs of both acromegaly and gigantism are those of excessive body growth. In gigantism, symptoms become apparent soon after birth, and since the child is in the growth period, the bones enlarge both in length and in width. In acromegaly, since epiphyseal lines have fused with completion of growth, bones enlarge transversely. The features become coarse and heavy, with the lower jaw becoming particularly large. Frontal sinuses are pronounced. Hands and feet become conspicuously wider, necessitating larger-sized gloves and shoes. Lips are heavier, and the tongue is enlarged. Striking changes in the patient's appearance may be noticed in comparing his appearance with pictures of him taken before the onset of symptoms. Patients may be asked to bring pictures of themselves to the hospital to help in diagnosis.

During diagnosis and treatment the patient and his family need understanding care. Changes in appearance often produce emotional reactions. Since physical changes are irreversible even if the disease is arrested, they may be doubly difficult to accept.

Posterior lobe hypofunction

Diabetes insipidus is a disease caused by failure of the posterior lobe of the pituitary gland to secrete antidiuretic hormone. Primary diabetes insipidus is a rare disease, but its symptoms are seen fairly frequently since they may occur when a tumor develops in the gland and because they follow hypophysectomy or irradiation of the pituitary gland.

The antidiuretic hormone increases reabsorption of water from the renal tubules, and in its absence a very large amount of urine is excreted; as much as 15 L. may be excreted daily. This causes fluid and electrolyte imbalance. Patients with diabetes insipidus also have insatiable thirst (polydipsia), anorexia, weight loss, and weakness.

Specific treatment for diabetes insipidus usually consists of giving extracts of the posterior pituitary lobe. Vasopressin tannate (Pitressin tannate) in oil, 5 units given intramuscularly, will give relief for up to 72 hours and is usually used for immediate treatment. It is important to warm the vial and shake thoroughly since the active ingredient tends to precipitate out. This hormone also is available as a powder that the patient sniffs to deposit it on the nasal mucosa, where it is absorbed. It should not be inhaled. A synthetic lysine-vasopressin solution can be used as a nasal spray or drops instead of the powder. It may eliminate the local allergic reaction to foreign protein found in posterior pituitary preparations of animal origin. The patient is taught to use the medication whenever he notices polyuria or polydipsia.

Hypophysectomy

A hypophysectomy is the complete removal of the hypophyseal gland. Following this procedure, the patient's hormonal levels must be evaluated carefully and replacement therapy instituted as necessary.

Following a hypophysectomy, the patient must be attended constantly for several days. In addition to giving care needed by any patient having a craniotomy (p. 925), the most alert attention must be paid to detect early signs of thyroid crisis, addisonian crisis, or sudden electrolyte imbalance, all of which require immediate treatment. Cortisone is given throughout the postoperative period and, of course, must be continued throughout the patient's life. Pitressin may be needed for several weeks but is usually not needed thereafter since the hypothalamus maintains the secretion and excretion of the antidiuretic hormone. Thyroid extract usually is not restarted until several weeks after surgery, since the action of thyroxine continues for about 3 weeks. The operation causes gonadal function to cease and thus causes sterility. Testosterone is ordered frequently for the impotence that occurs in men. Since women rarely have severe menopausal symptoms as a result of this surgery, they usually are not given sex hormones. If the hypophysectomy has been done to treat metastatic cancer of the breast or prostate gland, sex hormones are never given.

Any patient who is hospitalized for this type of surgery has been given explicit information as to its results by the neurosurgeon. The nurse should listen attentively to the patient as he expresses feeling about it both preoperatively and postoperatively. Any misunderstandings should be corrected. Most patients appear to accept their limitations surprisingly well, especially if the symptoms of metastasis or of other disease are ameliorated. They always should be observed closely for the need of emotional support, however, and appropriate help for them should be obtained. The patient and his family must, of course, be taught the precautions he must observe in taking the hormones.

Removal or destruction of the pituitary gland

Various approaches are being used to destroy or remove the pituitary gland: implantation of yttrium 90, external radiation coagulation with radiofrequency, transphenoidal microsurgical hypophysectomy, and total or partial removal by craniotomy. One of these procedures may be used as treatment for advanced breast carcinoma, diabetic retinopathy, or pituitary tumors.

The care of the patient who has yttrium 90 implanted is not very different from that following a hypophysectomy, except that the symptoms of hormonal deficiencies develop slowly, and therefore the patient must be carefully observed so that replacement of hormones can be started or increased as necessary. The precautions used for any radiation therapy also must be observed. The patient has not had cranial surgery, but meningeal infection may be a complication. The patient also needs attention similar to that given a patient who has intranasal surgery of the sinuses. The patient having this treatment usually is hospitalized for a much shorter time than is the one having a hypophysectomy. Therefore special care must be taken to ensure that he is adequately instructed in self-care either in the hospital or by a nurse visiting him at home.

After transphenoidal hypophysectomy, the patient should be observed carefully for signs of hemorrhage. Also, a clear nasal drip or constant swallowing by the patient may indicate a cerebral spinal fluid leak.

Both anterior and posterior pituitary function may be temporarily or permanently impaired by external radiation of the pituitary gland. Therefore replacement of cortisone and vasopressin may be essential. However, these hormones are given only if symptoms develop. The nurse should very carefully note and report changes in the vital signs, the patient's general appearance, weight, emotional state, and mental alertness. The urinary output should be measured carefully and recorded every 2 hours for several days, and an output of 300 ml. or more in any 2-hour period should be reported to the physician at once. Vasopressin must be started before serious fluid and electrolyte imbalance develop. Prolonged replacement therapy with various hormones may be necessary after external radiation of the pituitary gland, especially if most of the glandular tissue has been destroyed.

Osteoporosis

Osteoporosis is an exceedingly common yet poorly understood disease in which there is a defect in the bone matrix formation, with resultant decrease in bone substance and in the ability of the bones to withstand normal stresses. A variety of hormonal derangements are known to cause osteoporosis, including hyperthyroidism, acromegaly, diabetes, hyperparathyroidism, and Cushing's syndrome, as already mentioned in this chapter. By far the larger number of patients with osteoporosis, however, have the condition either associated with disuse of the bones or occurring after the climacteric in the absence of other obvious endocrine dysfunction. It is known that lack of the anabolic steroids permits a negative nitrogen balance to occur and that osteoporosis is a disease primarily of protein metabolism and not of use of calcium. Although unproved, it is believed that hormones (notably estrogen) in some way affect bone metabolism and that their lack permits the resorption of bone at an increased rate.

Osteoporosis is much more common in women than men and occurs frequently in women in their sixties. It is so common that it has almost been considered "physiologic" when it occurs in women after the menopause, and little attention has been paid to it.[2] So frequent is the condition in elderly women that it has been listed as the most commonly seen abnormality of the vertebral column on radiographic examination and exceeds even arthritis in incidence. It is now believed likely that almost all elderly women have some osteoporosis, since approximately 40% demineralization of the bones occurs before radiographs show pronounced disease.

Osteoporosis (other than that caused by bone disuse) develops most often in the vertebrae and in the pelvis. By far the most common symptom is low back pain. Many times, however, the patient has no knowledge that anything is wrong until a fracture occurs or until severe symptoms follow collapse of a vertebra. Pain occurs when bone changes have altered alignment so much that pressure occurs or strain is placed on nerves and supportive structures. Sometimes compression of the vertebral bodies occurs, and this may decrease the height of the trunk and increase the curve of the thoracic spine. A feeling of lack of stability, noted most when walking on uneven surfaces, and difficulty in maintaining balance may also be described by the patient. The nurse should advise any elderly person with any of these signs and symptoms to visit his physician so that treatment, if needed, can be started before a fracture occurs or other serious limitations develop.

Treatment of osteoporosis usually consists of measures to prevent further damage if possible. Daily exercise is felt to be imperative, and many physicians insist that the patient do some walking each day. If severe pain occurs from further collapse or from injury, it usually is treated with the judicious use of muscle relaxants and analgesics, and with rest on a firm bed. If a fracture is sustained, it may be treated by applying a cast and having the patient mobilized. Estrogen and androgen therapy has been effective for many patients and is widely used at this time. Even when administration of estrogens seems to produce no marked regeneration of bone as seen by radiograph, it often lessens pain and enables the patient to be more active. Usually an estrogen preparation such as Premarin is given for one week out of four. A diet high in protein, calcium, and vitamin D may be ordered, although some physicians believe that the person taking a normal, adequate diet receives enough of these essentials, provided he is helped to use them by the administration of hormones.

Most physicians prescribe a firm corset or brace. Whether it is worn continuously or only during periods of special activity depends on the individual patient and the physician. Usually the corset or brace enables the patient to be more active than would otherwise be safe or comfortable for him. A firm bed for sleeping hours and rest periods is always pre-scribed, and a careful balance between rest and activity to avoid overfatigue is usually advised.

The patient with osteoporosis must guard against accidents. Walking on uneven surfaces and when lighting is poor should be avoided, and often the use of a cane is recommended. The patient should be taught the correct method of stooping to pick up an object from the floor and to avoid direct bending, which places pressure on lumbar vertebral bodies. The patient should not lift any heavy object and should distribute any small weight he carries between his two arms to lessen strain on one side of the body. Since his future well-being depends on his being up and about, the patient with osteoporosis should be taught to give special attention to care of his feet and selection of his shoes. Any difficulties should be discussed with his physician.

The nurse who cares for any aged patient should bear in mind that the patient may have undiagnosed osteoporosis. Since the condition can be made worse by confinement in bed, all elderly patients who have been in bed for some time, regardless of the cause, should be treated with the greatest care when mobilization is permitted. They also should be observed closely for indications of pathologic fracture.

REFERENCES AND SELECTED READINGS*

1 *American Diabetes Association: Learning about diabetes: a programmed course of instruction, New York, 1969, The Association.

2 Beeson, P. B., and McDermott, W., editors: Cecil-Loeb textbook of medicine, ed. 13, Philadelphia, 1971, W. B. Saunders Co.

3 Beland, I. L., Rice, V. H., and Power, L.: Metabolic crises. In Meltzer, L. E., Abdellah, F. G., and Kitchell, J. R.: Concepts and practices of intensive care for nurse specialists, Philadelphia, 1969, The Charles Press, Publishers.

4 Bergersen, B. S.: Pharmacology in nursing, ed. 12, St. Louis, 1973, The C. V. Mosby Co.

5 Bondy, P. K., and Rosenberg, L. E.: Duncan's diseases of metabolism, Philadelphia, 1974, W. B. Saunders Co.

6 Brodie, B., and Von Haam, J.: Children born with adrenogenital syndrome, Am. J. Nurs. 67:1018-1021, May 1967.

7 Brown, J. H. U., and Barker, S. B.: Basic endocrinology, Philadelphia, 1966, F. A. Davis Co.

8 *Burke, E. L.: Insulin injection: the site and the technique, Am. J. Nurs. 72:2194-2196, Dec. 1972.

9 *Cranley, M. S., and Frazier, S. A.: Preventive intensive care of the diabetic mother and fetus, Nurs. Clin. North Am. 8:489-499, Sept. 1973.

10 Diabetes source book, U. S. Department of Health, Education and Welfare, Washington, D. C., 1969, U. S. Government Printing Office.

11 Dillon, R. S.: Handbook of endocrinology, Philadelphia, 1973, Lea & Febiger.

12 Dolger, H., and Seeman, B.: How to live with diabetes, New York, 1965, W. W. Norton & Co., Inc.

13 Duncan, G. G.: A modern pilgrim's progress—with further revelations—for diabetics, ed. 2, Philadelphia, 1967, W. B. Saunders Co.

13a *Elliott, D. D.: A self-instruction unit: adrenocortical insufficiency, Am. J. Nurs. 74:1115-1130, June 1974.

14 *Fulton, M., and others: Helping diabetics adapt to failing vision, Am. J. Nurs. 74:54-57, Jan. 1974.

15 Gorman, C. A.: Some problems in thyroid diagnosis, Med. Clin. North Am. 56:841-847, July 1972.

16 *Gribbons, C. A., and Aliapoulios, M. A.: Treatment for advanced breast carcinoma, Am. J. Nurs. 72:678-682, April 1972.

17 *Grim, R. A.: Mr. Edward's triumph, Am. J. Nurs. 72:480-481, March 1972.

18 *Guthrie, D. W., and Guthrie, R. A.: Coping with diabetic ketoacidosis, Nursing '73 3:17-23, Nov. 1973.

18a *Guthrie, D. W., and Guthrie, R. A.: The infant of the diabetic mother, Am. J. Nurs. 74:2008-2009, Nov. 1974.

19 Harvey, A. M., and others: The principles and practice of medicine, ed. 18, Englewood Cliffs, N. J., 1972, Prentice-Hall, Inc.

20 *Hawken, P.: Hypophysectomy with yttrium 90, Am. J. Nurs. 65:122-125, Oct. 1965.

21 *Huang, S. H.: Nursing assessment in planning care for a diabetic patient, Nurs. Clin. North Am. 6:135-143, March 1971.

22 Krupp, M. A., and Chatton, M. J.: Current diagnosis and treatment, Los Altos, Calif., 1973, Lange Medical Publications.

23 *Krysan, G. S.: How do we teach four million diabetics? Am. J. Nurs. 65:105-107, Nov. 1965.

24 *Lawrence, P. A.: U-100 insulin: let's make the transition trouble free, Am. J. Nurs. 13:1539, Sept. 1973.

*References preceded by an asterisk are particularly well suited for student reading.

25 *Leiner, M. S., and Rahmer, A. E.: The juvenile diabetic and the visiting nurse, Am. J. Nurs. **68:**106-108, Jan. 1968.

26 Martin, M. M.: Insulin reaction, Am. J. Nurs. **67:**328-331, Feb. 1967.

27 Moore, M. L.: Diabetes in children, Am. J. Nurs. **67:**104-107, Jan. 1967.

28 Mountcastle, V. B., editor: Medical physiology, ed. 13, St. Louis, 1974, The C. V. Mosby Co.

29 *Nickerson, D.: Teaching the hospitalized diabetic, Am. J. Nurs. **72:**935-938, May 1972.

30 *Porter, A. L., and others: Giving diabetics control of their own lives, Nursing '73 **3:**44-49, Sept. 1973.

31 Rodman, M. J.: The pituitary hormones, RN **31:**55-67, June 1968.

32 Rodman, M. J.: The thyroid and antithyroid drugs, RN **31:**52-59, Feb. 1968.

33 Rosenthal, H., and Rosenthal, J.: Diabetic care in pictures, ed. 4, Philadelphia, 1968, J. B. Lippincott Co.

34 Scheie, H. G., and Albert, D. M., editors: Adler's textbook of ophthalmology, ed. 8, Philadelphia, 1969, W. B. Saunders Co.

35 Schneeberg, N. G.: Essentials of clinical endrocrinology, St. Louis, 1970, The C. V. Mosby Co.

35a *Schumann, D.: Coping with the complex, dangerous, elusive problems of those insulin-induced hypoglycemic reactions, Nursing '74 **4:**56-60, April 1974.

36 Selenkow, H. A.: The normal and abnormal thyroid: an approach to diagnosis and therapy, New York, 1973, Medcom Books, Inc.

37 *Shea, K. M., and others: Teaching a patient to live with adrenal insufficiency, Am. J. Nurs. **65:**80-85, Dec. 1965.

38 *Soika, C. V.: Combatting osteoporosis, Am. J. Nurs. **73:**1193-1197, July 1973.

39 *Stowe, S. M.: Hypophysectomy for diabetic retinopathy, Am. J. Nurs. **73:**632-637, April 1973.

40 Strachan, C. B.: The diabetic's cookbook, Houston, 1969, Medical Arts Publishing Foundation.

41 U. S. National Institutes of Health: Nursing care of patients with pheochromocytoma, Washington, D. C., 1968, U. S. Government Printing Office.

42 *Watkins, J. D., and Moss, F. T.: Confusion in the management of diabetes, Am. J. Nurs. **69:**521-524, March 1969.

43 *Williams, S. M.: Diabetic urine testing by hospital nursing personnel, Nurs. Res. **20:**444-447, Sept.-Oct. 1971.

44 Williams, S. R.: Nutrition and diet therapy, ed. 2, St. Louis, 1973, The C. V. Mosby Co.

45 Winter, C. C., and Barker, M. R.: Sawyer's nursing care of patients with urologic diseases, ed. 3, St. Louis, 1972, The C. V. Mosby Co.

46 Wintrobe, M. M., and others, editors: Harrison's principles of internal medicine, ed. 7, New York, 1974, McGraw-Hill Book Co.

28 Dermatologic conditions

General skin care and prevention of disease
General management of patients with skin conditions
Diseases of the skin

■ People vary in their resistance to dermatologic or skin disease. Some are born with skins that can resist irritation and infection quite well, whereas others have delicate skins that have little resistance to trauma, irritation, and infection. Usually the person with blond coloring has a more delicate skin than the person with a dark complexion.

General condition of the skin, color, and texture provide an excellent barometer of the state of a person's general health. Many conditions existing within and outside the body affect the skin. Nutritional and vitamin deficiencies predispose to skin disease and slow the rate of healing. Hormonal influences are believed to have a part in the progress of some skin diseases. A very nervous person may develop skin lesions. For example, nervousness may lead to itching and to subsequent scratching; infection may then be introduced. Occupational exposure to irritating substances and the removal of natural skin secretions also predispose to skin diseases. A person who handles fabrics or who washes dishes steadily may develop chapped hands and susceptibility to infection unless natural skin oils are replaced by creams and lotions. He may also develop a sensitivity to substances such as dyes and soaps.

The skin is affected by age. The skin of a baby is very delicate, thin, and vascular. It may become irritated easily. In the elderly person the skin undergoes atrophy of underlying tissues and hardening of superficial arterioles that nourished the skin during youth. Sebaceous glands are less active, and the skin is thin, dry, and easily traumatized. Infections occur easily and often heal slowly.

■ GENERAL SKIN CARE AND PREVENTION OF DISEASE

The nurse can contribute to the prevention of skin disease by teaching good care of normal skin and by encouraging people to seek medical attention for abnormal skin conditions. This can be done as the nurse encounters people at work, in their homes, in school, in the hospital, and elsewhere in the community.

Cleansing

The old saying that cleanliness is next to godliness is probably not entirely true. People from cultures who do not have high standards of cleanliness do not necessarily have more skin disease than others. The outer layer of skin cells and the perspiration are acid in reaction, and their presence inhibits the life and growth of bacteria. Strong soaps that are alkaline in reaction may neutralize this protective acid condition of the skin. They may also remove the oily secretion of the sebaceous glands, which lubricate the outer skin layers and contribute to their health. However, mechanical removal of dead skin and excess oil appears justified because they can coat bacteria and prevent the antibacterial action of perspiration. Also, since these substances have an unpleasant odor after undergoing bacterial decomposition, bathing is necessary for esthetic reasons.

The skin should be washed often enough to remove skin excretions and prevent odors but not often enough to cause drying and irritation. Detergent cleansers that are neutral in reaction probably are better than soaps for cleansing the skin. Both soaps and detergents may cause skin reaction in some people, however. There is a great deal of individual variation in the bathing necessary to ensure cleanliness without causing skin irritation. The person who has an oily skin and who perspires freely may need to

■ STUDY QUESTIONS

1 Review the anatomy and physiology of the skin. What are its main functions?
2 What have you learned in fundamentals of nursing about skin care for the elderly patient, the malnourished patient, the dehydrated patient, the emaciated patient, the obese patient, and the patient with neurologic deficits?
3 Review techniques for bandaging various parts of the body.
4 What drugs may fairly often cause skin eruptions?
5 Review the various forms in which external medications can be applied. What are some good features and some limitations of each?

bathe twice daily in warm weather and wash his face several times, whereas the person who has a dry skin may have to use creams and lotions to protect the skin even when he bathes but once a day.

Skin secretions are decreased during cold weather, and most people need to use protective creams and lotions to prevent skin irritation at this time. There are many bath oils on the market today. They leave a residue film of oil over the entire body and may relieve itching from dryness. However, many dermatologists discourage their use because the oily film may prevent normal excretion from the pores. Hard, thickened skin areas should be rubbed daily with a substance such as cold cream, lanolin, or vanishing cream that contains less than 1% to 2% of salicylic acid and helps to soften dry, thickened skin. Elderly people need to take special precautions in the care of their skin (p. 38).

Observation of abnormalities

Care of normal skin should include regular observation of pigmented skin areas, moles, or other apparently minor skin lesions. Any change in size, color, or general appearance should be reported to a physician at once. Pigmentation (lentigo) occurs on the face, neck, and backs of hands and arms of elderly people (Fig. 28-1). These freckles, which are a source of annoyance to many elderly women, are harmless. They can be removed by abrasion, but so-called freckle creams are useless.

Dangers of self-treatment

People should be urged to seek competent medical help when skin conditions develop. Although skin diseases rarely cause death, they do account for much human discomfort and for serious interruption of work and other activities. Many persons are inclined to rely on the advice of friends or of the local druggist or on medications they may have on hand. Each individual's skin reacts differently to treatment, and the skin that is already irritated or diseased may respond violently to inexpert treatment. Since the skin changes, medications prescribed even for a similar skin ailment in the same patient some time previously may not produce a favorable response. Also, drugs may deteriorate, and for this reason old medications are not safe. The patient may be spared much discomfort and expense if he turns to a specialist when symptoms first develop and before a mild skin condition becomes really troublesome. He should be advised to present himself to the physician without changing dressings or otherwise "cleaning up" the lesion.

■ GENERAL MANAGEMENT OF PATIENTS WITH SKIN CONDITIONS

Certain general principles of management apply to most skin conditions and will be discussed before a few of the more common diseases are mentioned. Most nursing care is directed toward making the patient as comfortable as possible, controlling pain and itching, preventing infection, and encouraging healing of the lesions.

Relief of pruritus

Pruritus, or itching, was defined centuries ago as a disagreeable sensation that stimulates the urge to scratch. Actually, very little is known about the physiologic mechanism that causes pruritus. It is believed to be closely associated with the nerve mechanism that causes pain. The sensation arises in the nerve endings in the skin; it is unknown in lesions in which skin layers have been destroyed. Pruritus is known to be aggravated by dilation of capillaries, tissue anoxia such as occurs in venous stasis, and the presence of abnormal constituents such as bile pigment in the skin. Some skin diseases such as tumors and tuberculous and syphilitic lesions are not accompanied by pruritus.

Pruritus can be exhausting and demoralizing to the patient. It is useless, however, to tell him not to scratch, for he may be unable to comply with this advice. Admonishing the patient may only increase

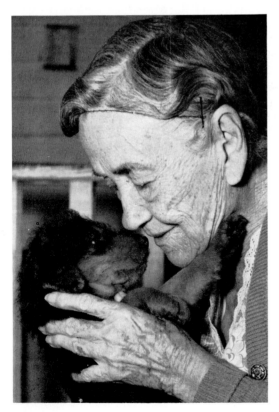

FIG. 28-1. Elderly patients have skin changes. Note discolored spots on skin and tiny raised area on this woman's eyelid. (VanDerMeid from Monkmeyer Press Photo Service.)

his frustration and may make the pruritus worse. It is safe to assume that the normal person who has pruritus will stop scratching when the condition has been sufficiently controlled. Antihistaminic drugs often are prescribed for treatment of pruritus, and the adrenocorticosteroids are used widely. External medications with antipruritic action and colloidal baths also may be ordered and are discussed later in this chapter.

Trauma from scratching can be partially prevented by cutting the fingernails short and by urging the patient to try such measures as pressing the itching lesion with the finger or with the back of the fingernail instead of using the ends of the nails. Hands should be kept scrupulously clean so that danger of introducing infectious organisms is reduced. Infants and young children may need protective mittens or elbow restraints.

Diversions may take the person's mind off the urge to scratch. Sedatives may be given since they help to make the person less irritable. Irritability increases the urge to scratch and decreases willpower. By counting to 100 before scratching, some patients are able to control the urge until the strongest impulse is dissipated.

Cool, light clothing or bedclothes may help to allay itching. It is well known that wool is particularly likely to cause itching even in persons who have no skin disease but who have somewhat dry skin. Any clothing that constricts, rubs, or retains body moisture and heat in local areas should be avoided.

Soft, old sheets should be used on the bed, and sometimes *"neutral" linen* is necessary. It is prepared by rinsing the linen in a mild acid solution, which counteracts the excess alkaline of ordinary laundry soap or detergent. A tablespoon of vinegar to a quart of water may be used in the home.

Pruritus usually increases when the body temperature goes up. Therefore the patient with pruritus should be kept quiet. Activities of all kinds, both physical and mental, increase metabolism and body heat. Activities causing perspiration should be avoided also, because perspiration moistens the skin and increases pruritus, particularly under dressings and on parts of the body where skin surfaces touch each other. Excessive drying of the skin caused by high room temperature and low humidity can also increase pruritus. It occurs easily in the elderly patient who already has a dry skin. Usually a room temperature of 20° to 21° C. (68° to 70° F.) and a humidity of 30% to 40% are best for the patient with pruritus.

Gentleness in handling

Gentleness in treatment and handling of all skin lesions is important. Skin lesions should be patted, never rubbed, and irritation of the area surrounding the lesion should be avoided because it stimulates circulation and leads to increased warmth and pruritus. Touching, rubbing, scratching, removing dressings, and inspecting the lesion are activities that interfere with healing and yet are a temptation to the patient both in the hospital and at home.

Skin lesions may be overtreated easily. The conscientious, ambitious nurse and the patient and his family should know that too much cleansing and treating can do more harm than good. The nurse must understand exactly how much treatment the physician wishes. Usually the more acute the skin disease, the gentler the treatment should be.

Warmth in special situations

The patient who has a generalized flush, or erythema, and the one who has an extensive exfoliative dermatitis may be losing body heat at an abnormally increased rate and may need a room temperature of 32.2° C. (90° F.) or more to maintain normal body temperature. Care must be taken to avoid chilling, particularly after baths and when compresses are used or when parts of the body are exposed. It is surprising how much body heat can be lost when cool, moist compresses are applied to even a relatively small portion of the total body surface. For example, the patient who has cool compresses on a hand and arm or who has an uncovered weeping skin condition of one limb may suffer from generalized chilling if adequate covers are not provided for the rest of his body and if the room is not kept sufficiently warm.

Rest

All dermatologic patients need sleep and rest, yet skin conditions often interfere with these requirements. Skin ailments and accompanying pruritus tend to become worse at night when surroundings are quiet and there are fewer distractions. The patient needs the benefit of nursing measures to induce sleep, such as a warm drink, a back massage, elimination of light and noise, and attention to ventilation. Every effort should be made to help him get enough sleep without the aid of medications since they may cause further pruritus or may even cause increased restlessness, which is harmful. A sedative such as chloral hydrate, which seldom causes skin reaction, or a tranquilizing drug sometimes is given.

If the patient awakens, he should be urged to call the nurse or to turn on the light and read or otherwise occupy himself while resisting the temptation to scratch the skin lesions. It may be necessary for the patient to have a private room in the hospital, but he should be taken to the sun porch or recreation room during part of the day so that he will have contact with others. This not only helps to keep him happier, but it may divert his attention from the itching. If he sleeps during the day, however, he should not be disturbed.

Emotional support

Because many skin lesions are unsightly and slow in healing, the patient often becomes discouraged and upset. He may fear that he is not accepted, wanted, or liked by others, particularly if there are unsightly lesions on exposed parts of the body. This response may be due in part to the idea that unsightly complexions often are linked with unwholesome living and communicable disease. Such a response also may be due to the fact that no one likes to be conspicuous. Members of the patient's family may need interpretation of the patient's reactions.

The nursing staff should try to make the patient feel that he is socially acceptable to persons about him. Care must be taken not to show any distaste or rejection no matter how difficult care of the skin lesions may be. When the lesion is not communicable, the use of gowns and rubber gloves should be kept to a minimum.

The nurse must know each patient and plan individual care accordingly. For example, one patient may be happier if he is permitted to change his own compresses and otherwise care for himself, whereas another patient, because he needs the attention and reassurance of having things done for him, may feel discriminated against if self-care is suggested. However, in almost all instances the nurse should give some care to the skin lesion, even though the patient may attend to his other needs. It affords the nurse an opportunity to observe the lesion carefully, and it helps the patient to feel accepted.

Occupational and diversional therapy is helpful in the care of most dermatologic patients. Any activity that keeps the patient busy and thus distracts his attention from the skin ailment or its feared consequences is justified. A program including occupational therapy during the day will often help the patient sleep during the night. Occupational therapy should be carefully prescribed, however, because in some instances the patient's skin may be sensitive to materials used in the activities.

Bathing and cleansing

The patient with skin disease should not be bathed until he has been examined by a physician. Clothing, dressings, and the lesions themselves with crusts or exudates should be left undisturbed unless a definite order has been given for their care.

After the initial inspection by the physician, oil may be ordered for cleansing the skin. Mineral or cottonseed oil may be used. It should be warmed slightly and applied with a soft cotton ball, with care taken not to rub or irritate the lesions or the surrounding skin. Gauze should not be used because of the danger of trauma. Hard crusts or thickened exudates often are soaked with physiologic solution of sodium chloride, peroxide, pHisoHex in water, or a mild solution of tincture of green soap in warm water. Whether or not a sterile technique is used depends on the lesions, but in any event clean techniques should be used. Care should be taken to avoid reinfection from soiled outer dressings or other sources.

Regular bathing is seldom permitted for dermatologic patients. Cool sponge baths without the use of soap are often ordered, and the genital area usually can be cleansed as often as necessary. The water may be softened with a handful of bran or oatmeal or a tablespoon of uncooked laundry starch to a basin of water. Borax and sodium bicarbonate are sometimes used to soften water and allay itching, but they are drying and therefore are seldom ordered if the patient is elderly or has dry skin.

Many patients simply do not feel clean and are greatly distressed when not permitted a shower or tub bath for several days. Although perfumed cleansing preparations also are usually prohibited, some of the detergents, pharmaceutically approved rose ointment, and cold cream may be permitted by the dermatologist. The use of these products may make the patient feel more comfortable and acceptable to himself and to others.

Colloidal baths are often ordered. Some colloid substances make the enamel surface of the tub slippery. Therefore a rubber mat should be placed in the tub before the patient steps into it. Usually the patient should stay in the bath only for 20 to 30 minutes. Occasionally, when itching is particularly severe, he may remain for over an hour. In this event, small amounts of hot water should be added to the bath at intervals to prevent its becoming too cool. The patient must be watched closely for signs of fatigue and should not be left unattended.

After the bath, the skin should be patted dry with a soft towel. Skin medication should be conveniently placed so that it may be applied immediately, since pruritus may otherwise recur with intensity. Following a bath, the patient should remain in bed for at least $\frac{1}{2}$ hour to avoid chilling.

An *oatmeal, soybean,* or *bran bath* may be prepared as follows: (1) add 2 cups of cereal to 2 quarts of boiling water and stir while boiling for 5 minutes; (2) fill tub to three-fourths its capacity with tepid water, 35° C. (95° F.); (3) pour the cooked cereal into a mesh or gauze bag and stir the bag about in the bath for a few minutes until the water becomes opalescent. The bag may also be used as a mop to gently pat the skin and remove crusts and debris.

A boiled-starch bath is prepared by pouring 2 quarts of boiling water over a cup of cornstarch or laundry starch moistened with cold water and stirring as it thickens. This solution may be added directly to the bath without straining through a mesh bag. Cold uncooked starch also may be used in the same quantity.

Several simple packaged preparations such as

Aveeno (oatmeal-bran extract) are available, although their cost is relatively high. *Sodium bicarbonate,* $1/4$ to $1/2$ cup, may be added to any colloidal bath if ordered by the physician for its drying action on the skin. *Camomile tea* (approximately two handfuls steeped in 2 L. [2 quarts] of water) added to a sitz bath is often prescribed in the treatment of severe pruritus ani.

If the skin lesion is infected, such as might occur in severe neglected eczema, following burns, or in advanced pemphigus, *medicated baths* may be ordered. Potassium permanganate (1:40,000) and antibacterial solutions often are used.

Compresses and dressings

Dressings often are referred to in dermatologic practice as open, closed, or fixed dressings. *Open dressings* are ones for which no outer covering is used. *Closed dressings* have an outer covering such as bandages. *Fixed dressings* may have a covering of collodion starch paste, gelatin paste, or other material.

Compresses may be either sterile or unsterile, depending on the skin condition, but regardless, every effort must be made to prevent new infection of skin lesions by thoroughly washing the hands before any procedure is begun. Hot moist compresses are used to increase circulation and to hasten healing of infection such as a boil. If it is safe to do so, the basin of solution may be kept hot by placing it on an electric plate at the patient's bedside. Cold moist compresses are used to reduce inflammation and to lessen itching. A solution of 3% aluminum acetate (Burow's solution) or 5% magnesium sulfate is often used for cold compresses in the treatment of conditions such as poison ivy dermatitis. Ice may be added to the bowl of solution for unsterile compresses. If it is used, the solution must be changed frequently since it will become diluted. In applying sterile cold moist compresses the basin containing the solution can be placed in a bowl of crushed ice. For either hot or cold sterile compresses, two pairs of forceps with which to wring them are needed. Sterile compresses are discarded after each use.

Equipment for applying compresses may be placed at the patient's bedside so that he may help with the treatment if he is able and wishes to do so. If sterile compresses are used, the patient needs special instruction before participating in his care.

Wet dressings are used to soften crusts, to promote and remove drainage, to combat infection, to allay itching, and to provide constant protection to healing tissue. A few of the many solutions used for wet dressings are potassium permanganate (1:10,000), hydrogen peroxide, and mineral oil in equal parts, acetic acid or vinegar, and physiologic solution of sodium chloride. Sometimes the entire dressing must be changed each time it is moistened because remoistening the original dressing would increase the concentration of the drug used more than is advisable.

If the wet dressing can be safely remoistened without being changed, an Asepto syringe may be used. Care should be taken to avoid contaminating the dressing, however. Care also must be taken to moisten all parts of the inner dressing and yet to prevent fluid from running through outer dressings to other parts of the patient's body or onto the bed. The frequency with which a complete change of dressings is necessary depends on the type of lesion and the amount of drainage. Any skin maceration (softening and withering) should be reported to the physician. Wet dressings may be alternated with either powder dressings or exposure to the air with or without a heat lamp.

Pieces of worn-out linen are best for wet dressings, since they do not stick or hold heat. If linen is not available, gauze is the best substitute. Cotton becomes soggy and uncomfortable and tends to hold heat and cause itching. Several thicknesses of material should be used, and the compress may be covered with waxed paper or oiled silk. Rubberized or plastic materials tend to hold in heat and increase itching but are sometimes used (Fig. 28-2), depending on the nature of the lesion being treated. An outer wrapping sometimes is used. Old Ace bandages that have lost their elasticity make satisfactory outer wrappings.

Either dry or moist dressings may be covered with *boiled starch dressings.* These rather bulky dressings are made of gauze dipped in thick boiled starch and then wrapped about the part and allowed to dry. They provide a firm protection for the healing lesion. Such an outer dressing may be ordered when the physician suspects that the skin lesion may be self-inflicted or that the patient has an active part in preventing its normal healing. This circumstance is most likely to occur in patients with industrially associated skin lesions, in young children, or in patients with strong attention-seeking motives. The adult patient who is suspected of disturbing a lesion purposefully needs close observation to prevent him from doing it. He should be given special consideration since his need for attention is greater than that of the usual patient.

Paste dressings such as an Unna paste boot may be used in the treatment of stubborn eczematous lesions, stasis dermatitis, and ulcerations of the legs. (This dressing is described on p. 395.)

A large variety of *dressing materials* are needed in caring for dermatologic patients. The effectiveness of medications and dressings may depend largely on the imagination and resourcefulness of the nurse. The nurse in a dermatologic unit often becomes a collector. Old linen, table napkins, muslin, binders, stockings, gloves, and the like, which may

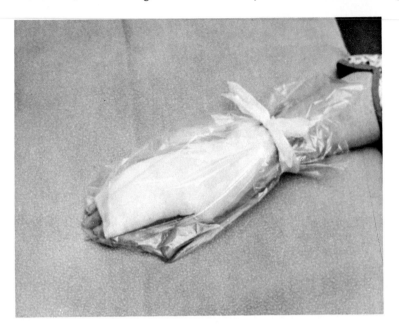

FIG. 28-2. A plastic bag can be used to cover wet dressings and protect the patient's clothes and bed.

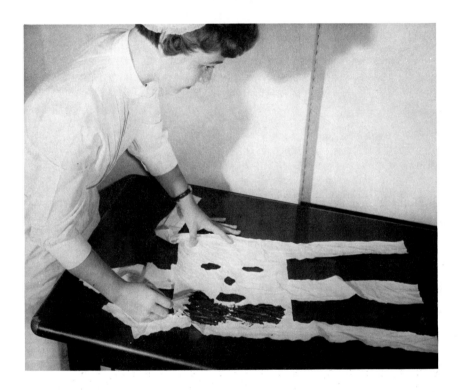

FIG. 28-3. Ointment may be spread on a piece of discarded sheet that is to be used as a mask to cover the face. Note that the ointment is applied to the dressing rather than to the patient's skin. In actual practice the table would be protected from soiling.

be cut up to prepare suitable dressings for every conceivable location on the body, are saved for future use. The cheaper and older the dressings, the better for everyone concerned since they may become lost in the laundry or so soiled and stained that it seems best to destroy them. A white stocking makes an excellent head dressing when shortened and tied with attached chin straps. Old white cotton gloves or mittens are often better than dressings for lesions on the hands, and stockings with the foot cut off make excellent circular dressings for arms or legs. The stock-

inette used in the plaster room may be useful for arm and leg dressings. Suits of long underwear, long stretch stockings, and pajamas may be used when large portions of the body must be treated. Pieces of worn-out sheet may be cut into four- or six-tailed bandages, which are useful in securing dressings under the jaw, on the chin, or on the scalp (Fig. 28-3). Old pillowcases can be used to make a mask to cover the face. The knitted finger dressings used in treating minor surgical wounds are useful in securing dressings on fingers and toes.

External medications and their application

External medications are used in dermatology for many purposes and in many different forms. The list of medications available is endless. The nurse should know the purpose for which a local application is ordered, the drug (or drugs) contained in the preparation, and any toxic signs that may occur from its use. For detailed descriptions, the student is referred to texts on pharmacology and to specialized medical texts on skin diseases and their treatment.[2,35]

Action of external medications. External medications have many actions, and frequently the single preparation ordered has several actions. Preparations used to treat skin disease may be *antiseptic.* Ammoniated mercury ointment, 5%, is one example, and bacitracin and many other antibiotic drugs are used. Penicillin and sulfa preparations are generally not used locally because local use may lead to a sensitivity that would prevent their future value to the patient if severe illness should require their use systemically. Preparations may be *cooling* and thus lessen inflammation and discomfort—cold cream is an example of a cooling preparation—or they may be *astringent,* constricting local blood vessels and thus lessening inflammation, congestion, pruritus, and general discomfort. Burow's solution (aluminum acetate) is widely used for its cooling and astringent effects. Preparations such as calamine lotion or Lassar's paste (zinc oxide ointment) may be *soothing,* thus lessening pruritus or pain and thereby fostering healing. Other preparations such as coal tar ointments may be *stimulating* and even mildly *irritating* and thus may foster healing. Drugs such as salicylic acid in Whitfield's ointment are *keratolytic* in their action and soften outer skin so that it may be removed, thus permitting other drugs to be effective. Some drugs such as coal tar and dibucaine (Nupercaine) are *antipruritic* in their action.

Hydrocortisone and its related preparations are now widely accepted as useful drugs in dermatologic treatment and have proved of great value in the medical management of stubborn pruritus. The fluorinated steroids (Kenalog, Aristocort, Fluonid) have proved especially effective as topical medicaments. There is some danger of systemic absorption when fluorohydrocortisone preparations are used topically, but usually not enough of the drug is used to produce a systemic reaction. Occasionally these preparations may be injected directly *into* the skin lesion.

Forms of external medications. External medications are incorporated into various media so that suitable selection for the particular skin ailment can be made. *Powders* are widely used for their cooling and drying effect and as vehicles for antibacterial or disinfectant drugs. Thymol iodide (Aristol) and sulfanilamide powder are examples. When large areas must be covered, *lotions* or powders suspended in liquids are often used for their cooling, refreshing, and antipruritic effects. One such preparation, calamine lotion, is widely used in the treatment of eczema, hives, and insect bites. It may be used with phenol, 1%, which has an anesthetic effect and allays itching. Care must be taken in using preparations containing phenol, however, since it may burn people with sensitive skins. Infants, old people, and persons with open skin lesions tolerate it poorly. *Liniments* are prepared with a medication and an oily substance emulsified in water. They facilitate the application of medication to large areas when dressings are not desired. Liniments are widely used by the general public for discomfort following vigorous exercise, for massage, and for their counterirritant effect. *Ointments* usually are made with medications added to a base of petrolatum, lanolin, white wax, tallow, or cold cream. Ointments may be protective or antiseptic or have a variety of other uses. They may contain a keratolytic agent (salicylic acid) to soften the outer skin layers and enable other drugs to be effective. Some such as tar ointments are antipruritic. *Pastes* have 50% or more of powder in the ointment base. *Cold cream,* in which water is emulsified into the ointment base, gives a cooling reaction when in contact with the skin.

Application of external medications. The nurse should know exactly how much medication is necessary for therapeutic effects so that waste is avoided and so that excessive amounts may not be left on the skin to cause caking, stickiness, and discomfort. In *some* circumstances it may be necessary to remove old medication before applying new medication. This should be done once or twice daily unless otherwise specified by the physician. Cleanliness and gentleness are important in removing it.

Lotions and *liniments* must be shaken well, and those that do not appear to mix thoroughly with shaking should not be used. Lotions should be applied with clean hands or with gauze. Gauze, not cotton, should be used because cotton holds the powder solute. A paintbrush also may be used. A firm, gentle pressure should be exerted with it so that "tickling" is avoided (Fig. 28-4).

Powders should be used sparingly, as their excessive use on moist surfaces leads to caking and hardening, which may cause trauma on removal. Care should be taken not to spread powder in the air, since sensitivity to inhaled powders is common.

Ointments should be carefully applied in small amounts, using a tongue depressor or clean fingers. On occasion they may be removed at prescribed intervals. Trauma may be avoided in applying ointment by spreading the ointment or paste on a linen, muslin, or gauze dressing and then applying the dressing to the lesion (Fig. 28-5). Care should be taken to estimate correctly the size of dressing need-

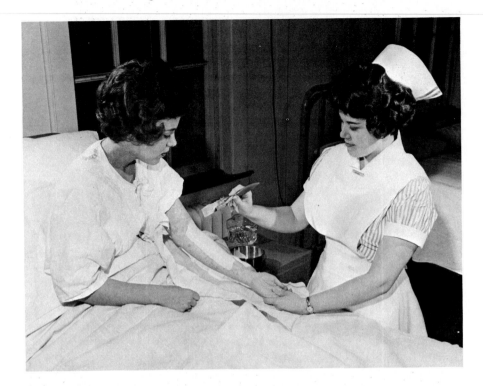

FIG. 28-4. Lotions may be applied to the skin with a paintbrush.

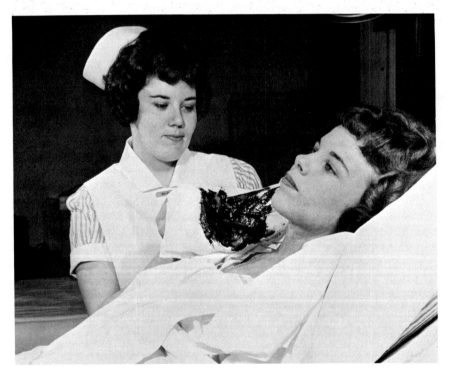

FIG. 28-5. When pruritus is severe, ointments can be applied to the dressing, which is then placed directly on the skin.

ed. Many healing ointments, such as scarlet red, and some liniments contain dyes that stain linen. Therefore the oldest bed linen available should be selected for patients receiving this treatment.

Drugs and other preparations used for skin ailments often are costly. The nurse should know the cost of the preparation used; and if the patient is caring for himself at home, he should be taught to use only enough for therapeutic benefit. In the hospital it is well to have individual jars of ointment for each patient to prevent contamination between patients and to avoid waste of medication kept in large jars. Sometimes it is best to use clean fingers to apply costly ointments. When external medications are used on infants and young children, special care must be taken to ensure that they are not ingested.

Sometimes a bulky external dressing can be used and will prevent the child from getting to the medication. At other times, elbow restraints or even wrist or ankle restraints must be used.

Teaching the patient

Many patients with skin diseases are not hospitalized. In the home and in the clinic the nurse must be specific in her instruction to the patient or to the family member who will be responsible for his care. It is best to write out instructions specifically. A common mistake that patients make when at home is to believe that if some is good, more is better. While a skin ailment may respond to an ointment rubbed on very gently and lightly, trauma from vigorous rubbing may counteract all benefit and may even make the condition worse. The patient, in his eagerness to cure the condition, may not realize how vigorous his own administrations are. The nurse can help the patient to improvise equipment that he needs. He may need to be taught how to apply ointment and how to sterilize linen for dressings by scorching it with an iron and then folding it inward until ready for use. The inside is then applied next to the lesion. Heating the dressing in the oven at 500° F. for 20 minutes also sterilizes it. It should be folded before sterilization.

■ DISEASES OF THE SKIN

Some of the many causes of skin disease are fungal and parasitic infections, response to bacterial organisms and viruses, reactions to ingestion of toxic substances, sensitivity to substances taken internally or encountered externally, and new growths. Some skin diseases are of unknown cause. Others are part of a systemic disease that may or may not be communicable. Only a brief description of a few of the more common skin diseases can be given here, and grouping must be somewhat arbitrary in a book of this kind.

Dermatology is a complex subject with a vocabulary all its own. *Dermatoses* is the term used to designate conditions of the skin that are largely noninflammatory, whereas *dermatitis* is the term used to designate inflammation of the skin whether due to infection, irritation, or any other cause. Considerable time and effort must be spent in learning terminology if the specialty of dermatology is to have meaning for nurses. The following are some of the more common skin lesions.

macule Circumscribed, discolored area, usually small, and not causing skin elevation.

papule Circumscribed area that is elevated, although usually not over 0.5 cm. in diameter.

vesicle Papule that is filled with clear fluid held beneath superficial skin layers.

pustule Circumscribed area containing pus and not usually over 0.5 cm. in diameter.

bulla Large elevation of outer skin layers containing either serous or purulent fluid.

nodule Large elevation of the skin usually involving the deeper skin layers and subcutaneous tissue.

excoriation Break or abrasion in the skin surface.

crust Dry exudate over a lesion.

scar Fibrous tissue covering of a lesion after healing and repair.

ulcer Erosion of skin substance.

scale Outer layer of epithelium as it loosens from the skin surface.

lichenification Leathery thickening of the outer skin layers.

Pruritus is a symptom, not a disease, and the best treatment is to remove its cause. Causes may include systemic disease such as liver disease with jaundice or diabetes mellitus in which sugar is not fully metabolized. Pruritus of the vulva, for example, may herald the onset of diabetes since sugar in the urine causes irritation and itching. Emotional stress is a real factor in the cause and control of pruritus, and even persons who have an average amount of emotional reserve will develop localized areas that itch excessively during periods of emotional strain. Pruritus is present in a very large proportion of all dermatoses and in almost all cases of dermatitis.

Insect infestation

Several kinds of pediculi attack human beings: *Pediculus humanus* (capitis, or *head louse,* and corporis, or *body louse*) and *Phthirus pubis (pubic louse).* Other lice from animals may bite human beings, but they have a short life unless the animal host is nearby. Head and pubic lice attach themselves to the skin and live on the victim's blood. Their eggs are laid along the shafts of the hair, along with a substance that encircles the hair shaft to secure them. The substance is dissolved fairly readily by an alkaline solution or by an acid solution such as vinegar.

The person infested with lice has itching of the area involved. This is caused by the lice biting him to obtain blood. On inspection the skin in the area may appear reddened and bites may be seen. The lice and eggs (nits) also may be seen. *Pediculus humanus* var. *capitis* is grayish in appearance, 0.15 cm. ($^1/_{16}$ inch) long, and often can be found on the nape of the neck, where it is most likely to lay its eggs. Pubic lice are about the same size, brownish, and crab shaped. They may occasionally be found in the axillae and on the eyebrows as well as in the pubic region. Body lice, about 0.3 cm. ($^1/_8$ inch) in length and dark in color, attach themselves to the underwear of the host, usually along the seams. The nits are yellowish and are laid in clumps along the seams of clothing. They are easily removed after they have been killed.

Pediculi are most often found among individuals who have poor personal hygiene habits. They may, however, be easily acquired in city living. Many children get head lice from their classmates or in crowded buses. Pubic lice may be acquired from toilet seats. Pediculi produce much more consternation on the part of the patient or his family than is warranted. They are easily killed. Effective treatment consists of one or more applications of preparations such as benzyl benzoate emulsion (25%) or gamma benzene hexachloride cream or lotion (Kwell) applied to the skin at night and followed by a bath in the morning. Gamma benzene hexachloride may also be used for shampooing the hair. It is left on for 5 minutes and then rinsed off the hair. Underwear and bedclothes should be changed and boiled or autoclaved. Outer clothing that cannot be autoclaved or washed should be dry-cleaned. Pressing the inner surface or lining with a hot iron sometimes suffices for clothing that cannot be washed or cleaned.

Bedbugs are dark brown, oval-shaped insects, about 0.45 cm. ($^3/_{16}$ inch) in length, which have an unpleasant odor. They usually hide in bed frames and mattresses in poor housing units. However, they may also be acquired on crowded city buses.

Bedbugs usually bite at night. The victim awakens with itching bites, and he may notice tiny spots of blood on the bedding. The presence of bedbugs often can be detected if the bedcovers are thrown back at night in a lighted room. They may also be found along the seams of mattresses and in cracks in the bed frame.

Bedbugs are destroyed by the same drugs that are effective in destroying pediculi. Mattresses should be autoclaved. If this is not possible, spraying with benzene hexachloride and extended airing in sunlight are usually sufficient.

Scabies, caused by the itch mite *Sarcoptes scabiei,* usually is found in persons who live in unhygienic surroundings and who bathe infrequently. The female burrows under the skin, leaving a dark trail behind her and causing the skin to itch. It is by the trail that a diagnosis is often made. The mite prefers the delicate skin areas such as the inner surfaces of the forearm and thighs, under the breasts, and between the fingers. Treatment consists of cleansing the skin with warm, soapy water using a brush, followed by local application of preparations such as gamma benzene hexachloride cream or lotion or benzyl benzoate emulsion (25%). After 24 hours the skin should be bathed and clean clothes put on. The patient may be sensitive to the medications used or may have irritation and infection from damage done by the insect pests. Usually mild antiseptic ointments or lotions such as calamine lotion are prescribed for the irritation. Antibiotics may be given systemically if the lesions become infected.

An important problem in treating patients with insect infestations is reinfestation. In crowded living conditions where there may be inadequate facilities for segregation of clothing, every member of the family may be affected and must be treated.

Fungal infections

Fungal infections can be either deep or superficial. Two deep fungal infections, *actinomycosis* and *blastomycosis,* are extremely serious conditions and often lead to death. Fortunately they are quite rare. They usually involve other body tissues besides the skin. Invasion of the lungs and gastrointestinal tract is common. Tissues gradually thicken and then break down and suppurate, sometimes requiring surgical drainage. Penicillin, from 0.1 to 20 million units/day for 6 weeks to 1 year, may be required in the treatment of actinomycosis. Amphotericin B or hydroxystilbamidine, given intravenously, is administered for blastomycosis. A new antifungal agent, the polypeptide X-5079C, is sometimes given.

Barber's itch (tinea barbae) is an extremely unpleasant superficial fungal infection causing lymph gland enlargement and swollen, boggy skin tissue with softening of the hairs of the beard. It is treated with griseofulvin or ammoniated mercury preparations. X-ray therapy may be used to remove the hairs. Barber's itch is entirely preventable by rigorous attention to cleanliness in barber shops.

Tinea of the scalp (tinea capitis), often incorrectly referred to as *ringworm,* is a disease seen most often in children. The condition often starts as a small, reddish papule, although it may begin as a localized area of apparent dandruff with thinning of the hair. Sometimes scaling and pustule formation with matting of the hair and crusting are the first signs. As the roots of the hair become involved, the hairs drop out, leaving bald patches. Since tinea capitis is a disease of children, it is advisable to keep small boys away from barber shops as long as possible, because it is in these establishments that the disease is often spread. The condition is highly infectious among schoolchildren, so that children with tinea capitis are often kept away from school.

It is important to diagnose the condition and begin treatment at once. An important aid to diagnosis and determination of the extent of involvement is the Wood's light, obtained by a special filter from an ultraviolet lamp. The infected hairs fluoresce, or appear luminous, under the light. These hairs are loose and may be removed easily. X-ray therapy may also be used to help remove infected hairs. The area is then treated with a variety of drugs. An antifungal drug, griseofulvin, has been found to be effective in treating tinea capitis. Clothing should be boiled or destroyed and the scalp protected with a stocking cap during treatment. If the treatment has been adequate, hair will eventually return in the affected area.

Tinea pedis (athlete's foot, dermatophytosis) is a superficial fungal infection that is widely spread through the use of showers, swimming pools, and common bath mats and by direct contact with persons who have the infection. It thrives in moist skin areas. Often the first lesion appears as a crack between the fourth and fifth digits of the foot. The disease may spread to the entire foot and cause peeling, cracking, and itching of the skin. The groin, hands, and other parts of the body may become involved. Extensive involvement occurs easily in elderly patients, possibly because of poor circulation in the feet and legs. This condition can incapacitate a person.

The keynote to management of tinea pedis is prevention. It has been said that the fungus cannot thrive on a dry skin. Therefore after a bath the feet should be carefully dried, including between each toe, and then ordinary talcum powder should be dusted between the toes. Medicated powders such as those containing zinc undecylenate (Desenex) are considered even more effective. Persons who exercise vigorously, who stand for long periods at work, and whose feet perspire excessively should have two pairs of shoes, which they wear on alternate days, leaving one pair to air and dry between uses. During hot weather, shoes with straw or nylon mesh insets, which permit ventilation to the feet, are desirable. It is inadvisable ever to walk in public showers with bare feet. Even the foot bath placed before the public shower at swimming pools is not sufficient protection. Paper slippers or one's own shoes should be used. The habit of sharing bath towels even among the closest of friends also should be discouraged. Athlete's foot is common among adolescents, and they should be given instruction in its prevention.

Many agents have been used in the treatment of tinea pedis. At the present time, undecylenic acid preparations are widely used. They are applied generously at night and removed in the morning. Powder is used during the day. Application of ointment may be preceded by soaks in potassium permanganate (1:10,000), which is an old and effective method of treatment. Ammoniated mercury ointment, benzoic and salicylic acid ointment (Whitfield's), and tolnaftate (Tinactin) are also used. Cotton socks or stockings, which absorb perspiration better than rayon or nylon, should be worn during treatment and should be changed and washed daily. Every effort should be made to keep the feet dry. If it can be arranged, direct exposure to the sun is effective treatment. Underclothing of the person with epidermophytosis involving the body should be boiled. Shoes should be destroyed or treated with formaldehyde fumes. Drying and sunning of shoes is not sufficient to kill the fungus. Bath mats and bedclothes should be boiled, and tubs and showers should be scrubbed with 0.1% bichloride of mercury or 0.2% creosol.

Diseases caused by and associated with bacterial infection

Furuncles (boils) are purulent lesions of the skin involving sebaceous glands and hair follicles. They often occur in crops *(furunculosis)* and are caused by the *Staphylococcus* organism in most instances. *Carbuncles* are also caused by the *Staphylococcus* organism and differ from furuncles in that they are much larger and involve not only the skin but also the subcutaneous tissues. Furuncles are likely to occur on the face, neck, forearms, groins, and legs, whereas carbuncles are usually limited to the nape of the neck and the back. They occur most often in poorly nourished, fatigued, or otherwise susceptible persons whose hygiene may be poor, in debilitated elderly people, and in persons who have inadequately treated diabetes mellitus.

A furuncle usually begins as a small pustule at the base of a hair follicle; a carbuncle develops at the base of several hair follicles. Local swelling and redness soon occur, and there is severe local pain, which can be helped by moving the involved part as little as possible. Within 3 to 5 days the lesion becomes elevated, or "points up," the surrounding skin becomes shiny, and the center or "core" turns yellow. A carbuncle has several cores. The boil will usually rupture spontaneously but it may be surgically incised and drained. As drainage occurs, the pain is immediately relieved. The drainage soon changes from a yellow, purulent material to a serosanguineous discharge. All drainage usually subsides within a few hours to a few days, and the redness and swelling gradually subside. As the boil drains, care must be taken to keep the infected drainage off the surrounding skin, because organisms may be harbored in hair follicles and furunculosis may recur.

Hot wet dressings are used to help bring the boil "to a head," but the patient should be warned to discontinue them as soon as drainage starts. They tend to macerate the skin, making it easily infected. The patient also should be cautioned to keep his hands away from the drainage area to prevent spread of the infection.

If the patient is hospitalized, strict isolation procedures are followed until the drainage subsides lest the organism be carried to others. Nurses should be sure to wash their hands thoroughly after caring for the patient, and they should avoid getting the drainage on their own skin. If they do, they should wash the area thoroughly. The patient who is at home must be taught to be scrupulously careful about accidentally passing organisms to others in his family or to persons at work. It is not uncommon for entire families to have some type of staphylococcal infection after one member has had a boil.

Furuncles and carbuncles tend to recur in susceptible individuals, and the staphylococci causing them often are resistant to local treatment and to antibiotics. Sunshine, autogenous vaccine, and pHisoHex to cleanse the skin are used, although their benefits are uncertain. The patient with furuncles must avoid additional infection by washing his hands thoroughly before treating the lesions and by keeping drainage from other skin surfaces. He must be cautioned never to manipulate a lesion about the nose and mouth lest infection be carried to the cranial venous sinus and cause a sinus thrombosis or a brain abscess.

Acne vulgaris is one of the most troublesome and most common skin conditions of adolescence. It is a condition about which the nurse must be informed, since she is often called on in the home, the school, and the community to advise in the total management of young persons with this difficulty. Lack of cleanliness is often blamed for the development of the condition by the patient or his family. In reality, cleanliness plays no part in the initial development of the condition.

Acne vulgaris is definitely known to have a relationship to hormonal activity. It usually makes its appearance at puberty, and in girls its activity can be clearly related to gonadal activity during different parts of the menstrual cycle. Hormonal activity produces hyperkeratosis of follicular orifices, which leads to blocking of the secretions (sebum) and the formation of discolored fatty plugs or blackheads (comedones). After the blackhead forms, there is hypertrophy of the sebaceous glands, and secondary infection occurs. A microorganism called the acne bacillus may contribute to this, and it is known that staphylococci are present in large numbers in the pustules that form. Sometimes cysts and nodules then form, and unsightly scars result despite the best treatment.

Although there is no cure for acne vulgaris, a wide variety of treatments are utilized with varying success. The face should be kept clean by washing with a mild soap or antibacterial solution. A blackhead may be safely removed by applying hot moist compresses for 15 minutes to $1/2$ hour and then removing it with an instrument with a hole in a rounded metal tip that is especially made for this purpose. Pustules should never be squeezed or broken by the patient. He should be taught to avoid touching his face with his hands, since this may cause more infection by grinding dirt and organisms into open pores. It is often difficult for the patient to carry out this instruction, since he may try to hide his face with his hands and may develop the habit of resting his chin in his hands.

Hormones are sometimes given but may cause undesirable systemic effects. The antibiotics are widely used and often produce marked improvement in the secondary infection, but their use must be continued over too long a period to be satisfactory treatment. Staphylococcal toxoid also is sometimes used. Often a quartz lamp is ordered for use in the home, and direct exposure to sunshine is thought to be helpful in destroying infection on the skin and improving its general resistance to organisms.

A variety of diets and other hygienic measures are usually advocated with varying success. Most authorities are in agreement that a diet low in carbohydrates, condiments, and fat is advisable. Rest appears to foster improvement in the condition.

Probably most important is emotional support to the patient in the acute states of the condition and assistance in his adjustment to any scarring that may occur. Unfortunately this condition appears at a time in life when the patient is adjusting to becoming an adult, and disfiguring blemishes sometimes precipitate serious emotional reactions. The greatest understanding on the part of all members of the family is necessary. The pancake makeup used by many adolescent girls in an attempt to hide the affliction often makes it worse. Among adolescent boys there is sometimes the mistaken belief that masturbation leads to acne. Some people believe that acne is aggravated by sexual abstinence and that it will be cured by marriage. This is not so, although acne is largely a self-limiting disease that tends to disappear at the marriageable age. Persons who have residual scars should know that a procedure known as *dermal abrasion*, or *planing*, often helps tremendously in removing scars (p. 241).

Acne rosacea is a skin condition that usually affects people over 25 years of age. The actual cause is unknown. It begins with redness over the cheeks and nose, which is followed by papules, pustules, and enlargement of superficial blood vessels. Many persons who have acne rosacea are of unstable emotional makeup. Achlorhydria has been found in many patients with this condition, and some favorable response has been obtained by giving hydrochloric acid. The treatment for acne rosacea is nonspecific and often not very satisfactory. Some patients respond to ultraviolet light treatment, and preparations containing naphthol and sulfur produce striking results in some. The condition is often accompanied by some pruritus, and the patient must be cautioned against touching the face since this may cause infection and aggravate the condition.

Impetigo contagiosa is a superficial skin disease produced by a form of *Streptococcus* often in association with staphylococci. It is largely a disease of children and may be endemic in nurseries unless special precautions are taken. The disease begins as a vesicle usually in the area of the mouth or nostrils, but it can be anywhere on the body. It becomes pustular and dries to form a honey-colored crust, which comes off as the lesion heals. Scarring does not result unless superimposed infection or trauma occurs. Greatest care must be taken to isolate the patient and to prevent reinfection with fingers and clothing. There is no common agreement as to treatment, but penicillin is now usually ordered either locally as ointment or systemically, or both locally and systemically. Other antibiotics may also be given. Ammoniated mercury ointment and gentian violet are old, reliable methods of treatment.

Erysipelas is caused by the hemolytic streptococcus. It is an acute febrile disease in which there is localized inflammation and swelling of the skin and subcutaneous tissues, usually of the face. A bright, sharp line separates the diseased skin from the normal skin. Elderly people with poor resistance are most often affected. Erysipelas was a serious disease before the advent of antibiotic and sulfonamide drugs, but it responds quickly to these drugs.

Viral diseases

Verrucae (warts) are caused by a virus that may be transmitted from one person to another. Warts should be removed to prevent crops of them from developing. Electrodesiccation (drying by electric current) is one of the better methods of treatment. It is safer than the use of acids such as nitric acid, which may injure normal tissue. Warts sometimes disappear spontaneously, and this unexplained characteristic leads to the many tales of their being charmed by a variety of means. Warts may grow inward on the soles of the feet and cause severe pain and incapacity. These are known as *plantar warts.* They may be treated with x-ray therapy, frozen with liquid hydrogen (the most common), or peeled with salicylic acid, among many modalities available.

Herpes simplex, or the common *cold sore,* is caused by a virus thought to be related to the virus of encephalitis. A cluster of vesicles appears on a reddened, swollen base, usually under the nose or on the lips. The lesion is painful and frequently cracks open. However, a crust gradually forms and the lesion heals in about 10 days. The fever blister of the lip and the herpetic lesion of the genitalia are caused by two *different* subtypes of herpes simplex virus. The canker sore is an aphthous ulcer; its etiology is unknown.

The treatment of herpes simplex is not specific and is not very satisfactory. Hot moist compresses sometimes relieve the discomfort from lesions on the lips and genitalia. Lip lesions sometimes respond to application of spirits of camphor. Small tubes of lip ice containing camphor can be used. Tincture of benzoin also helps to dry the lesions. Pooled human gamma globulin may be helpful to some persons. The drug 5-iodo-2-deoxyuridine (5-IDU) has been used successfully to treat herpes of the eye, but it does not appear to be effective in the treatment of skin lesions.[14] At present, photoinactivation using the vital dyes neutral red and proflavine applied to the opened vesicles in conjunction with light exposure is having some success. Also, either of the two applied to the open vesicles seems to help.

Herpes zoster, or *shingles,* is caused by the same virus (V-Z) that causes varicella (chickenpox). Varicella is believed to be the primary infection in a nonimmune host, while herpes zoster is thought to be the response in a partially immune host. Although herpes zoster is far less communicable than chickenpox, persons who have not had chickenpox may develop it after exposure to the vesicular lesions of patients with herpes zoster. For this reason, susceptible persons should not care for patients with herpes zoster. In herpes zoster, clusters of small blisters usually form in a line. They follow the course of the peripheral sensory nerves and often are unilateral. Since they follow nerve pathways, the lesions never cross the midline of the body. Nerves on both sides, however, can be involved. Itching and severe pain usually precede the development of the blisters by several days and continue throughout the course of the disease. Herpes zoster can be a serious condition in any adult and may even lead to death from exhaustion in elderly debilitated individuals. It is one of the most drawn-out and exasperating conditions found in elderly patients and leads to discouragement and demoralization. One attack of this aggravating condition, however, usually confers immunity. Herpes zoster often occurs in patients with Hodgkin's disease and in those with lymphoid and some bone cancers due to reduced cell-mediated immunity.

Treatment of herpes zoster consists of keeping the blisters dry and using local applications to allay itching. Calamine lotion with phenol is often prescribed. Alcohol injection of the offending nerves may be tried in an attempt to allay pain and itching, and general systemic medications, including sedatives and analgesics, are often necessary. Even after the blisters have crusted and disappeared, there may be severe pain and itching in the surrounding tissue. In extreme cases, death and sloughing of involved tissue occur.

Dermatitis caused by sensitivity to internal and external toxic agents

Dermatitis is inflammation of the skin that usually goes through the stages of redness or erythema, vesicle or blister formation with oozing, and crusting, scaling, and thickening of the skin. *Atopic eczema* is actually the name for a symptom complex designating skin reaction to an irritating factor of endogenous origin and not acquired from the external environment. In the strictest sense of the word, atopic eczema most accurately describes the skin lesions of hypersensitive persons who often also have asthma or hay fever. Infantile eczema, for example, often occurs soon after birth and may be outgrown only to be replaced by asthma or hay fever. The tendency to develop these conditions is inherited. (For a discussion of allergic reactions, see p. 91.)

Contact dermatitis identifies the acute skin inflammations and reactions caused by contact with irritating factors in the environment. Skin conditions caused by industrial products fall into this group. Primary irritants such as acids affect persons who must have their hands and arms in solutions during the larger part of their working hours. Sensitivity to chemical products such as nylon and plastics plagues many workers in the dye and solvent industries. People whose work demands constant wetting of the skin often develop dermatitis. Use of detergents, petroleum products, tars, and resins may cause either direct irritation or sensitivity that may lead to contact dermatitis. Biologic products cause contact dermatitis in some persons. Nurses and physicians have been known to become so sensitive to penicillin and streptomycin that they must wear rubber gloves when handling the drugs. Some people have had to abandon working where the drugs are used. There are many materials in the home that may lead to the development of contact dermatitis. Nail enamel and various cosmetics and related products such as deodorants and depilatories are examples. Some women develop contact dermatitis from contact with metal such as nickel, which may be used in the clips of earrings or in other jewelry. A common form of contact dermatitis is caused by contact with the oil of certain plants. *Poison ivy, poison oak,* and *sumac* are the most common offenders. This condition is known as *dermatitis venenata.*

The symptoms of contact dermatitis vary from redness with itching and burning to blister formation and severe edema followed by secondary infection. Its treatment consists of finding and removing the cause. In the home a large number of household cleaning agents, plastic products, and related materials must be considered. Occasionally the person who develops a sensitivity to materials encountered in his daily work must change his mode of employment permanently.

Dermatitis venenata is largely preventable. Everyone should be taught to recognize the leaves of the poisonous plants that are commonly found in his part of the country. Sensitivity to poisonous resins varies with individuals. Almost all people, however, are sensitive to some extent, and everyone should wear clothing that protects his skin if he is knowingly in contact with poisonous plants. Some persons are so sensitive that minute particles of the irritating oil carried in smoke or borne in the air after someone has crushed the plant are sufficient to cause a severe skin reaction. Pets may carry the irritating resin to their owners. The resin can remain on clothing for several days.

If there has been known contact with the oleoresin of a poisonous plant such as poison ivy, the skin should be washed thoroughly with alkaline laundry soap or detergent and then sponged with alcohol. Preferably this should be done within 10 minutes of exposure. To relieve the symptoms, cool compresses dipped in Burow's solution (aluminum acetate) in a 1:20 dilution are often applied for 10 to 20 minutes every few hours, and a lotion such as calamine may be alternated with the compresses. The greatest care must be taken not to involve new areas by contact with the exudate from active lesions. Although the condition usually does not last over a week, it may persist in some sensitive individuals for weeks and even months. Corticosteroids may be given. They seem to hasten the drying of lesions and limit the progress of the condition. Self-treatment in cases of extensive exposure to poisonous plants is dangerous since secondary infections may occur. The public should be taught this fact.

Neurodermatitis (lichen simplex chronicus) is an inflammation of the skin of neural origin. There usually is no lesion of the skin but only redness. Pruritus often is severe. Thickening and hardening (lichenification) of the skin occurs. The patient is often a tense, nervous person who has developed a neurotic habit of rubbing and scratching his skin. Local applications of corticosteroid creams or ointments usually produce improvement in most persons.

Dermatitis medicamentosa is the name used to designate reactions of the skin to drugs taken internally. Bromides are frequent offenders, and in recent years a large number of patients have suffered severe, prolonged drug reactions as a result of treatment with penicillin and other antibiotics. Iodides, barbiturates, and sulfonamide drugs frequently cause skin eruptions. The skin lesions vary in dermatitis medicamentosa. In some instances they are highly colored and sharply defined, whereas in others they may resemble urticaria, with large, flat wheals covering almost the entire body.

The treatment for drug sensitivity consists of finding and discontinuing the offending medication. Pruritus must be relieved and infection prevented. It is important to reassure the patient since he may become panicky when a generalized eruption is superimposed on the illness for which the drug was prescribed. The skin lesions sometimes disappear as suddenly as they appeared.

Exfoliative dermatitis is usually caused by drugs containing heavy metals such as mercury, bismuth, or arsenic. The condition is seen less often since the antibiotics and the bacteriostatic drugs have largely replaced drugs containing the heavy metals. Signs include redness, edema, and massive desquamation (shedding of epidermal cells). The patient may lose the entire outer layer of skin from the soles of his feet and the palms of his hands. Colloidal baths are often used to allay the itching. Lotions may be used to reduce itching and to make the erythema and desquamation less conspicuous. Patients with exfoliative dermatitis should be reassured that the loss of skin is not harmful and will not cause scarring.

Urticaria, or *hives,* is a disease of the skin characterized by *wheals,* which may vary in size and appearance. The condition can be acute or chronic. When the lesions are very large and are accompanied by large areas of edema that do not pit on pressure and that occur most often about the eyes, mouth, hands, and genitalia, the term *angioneurotic edema* is used. Urticaria is generally conceded to be caused by the body's reaction to some foreign substance to which it is sensitive. In some instances the cause is easily determined. Many people, for example, develop hives immediately after the ingestion of certain foods such as eggs, strawberries, and shellfish and after receiving drugs such as penicillin. In other cases the cause of hives is obscure. Urticaria may disappear spontaneously after a few minutes or may persist for hours or days. Usually there are severe itching, redness, and local heat. Calamine lotion is used for local relief of the pruritus, and the antihistaminic drugs are often given. Epinephrine (Adrenalin) and corticosteroids also may be used. The only real danger from this condition is the possible occurrence of giant hives in a vital area, such as on the mucous membrane of the larynx or glottis. Patients who have repeated attacks of hives that do not respond to an antihistaminic drug are advised to take (and are taught to give themselves) an injection of epinephrine when the hives appear or at the first sign of respiratory difficulty.

Other toxic skin reactions

Erythema multiforme is a skin condition believed to occur secondary to an underlying systemic disease such as an infection. The skin eruption is characterized by red to purple maculae, papules, and blisters. Most often the lesions occur on the wrists, back of the hands, ankles, tops of the feet, knees, elbows, face, palms, and soles of the feet.[1] The entire body may be involved. The skin eruption may be preceded by fever, chest pain, and arthralgia. The treatment is to seek out the underlying cause and eliminate it if possible. Other treatment is supportive and corticosteroids are often used. Local treatment includes baths, soaks, and dressings. Fluids are forced, and the patient is encouraged to take a high-calorie diet. Lesions may appear in the mouth. If so, special care is needed, including frequent mouth irrigations with hot salt solution or alkaline solutions such as Dobell's solution.

Communicable diseases such as measles, chickenpox, smallpox, scarlet fever, and typhoid fever produce skin reactions. Nodes and hemorrhagic spots in the skin also accompany severe acute rheumatic fever.

Dermatoses of unknown cause

Psoriasis is a very common benign skin disease of unknown origin. It causes a dry, scaly eruption on any part of the body but occurs most often on the elbows, back, shins, scalp, and chest. For some un-

known reason, psoriasis is often found in persons suffering from atrophic arthritis. The lesions have a shiny metallic (fish scale) appearance.

A variety of topical modalities are utilized in treating psoriasis. Ultraviolet light exposure is beneficial for some patients. The most widely used regimen today is topical steroids applied several times throughout the day with or without plastic suit occlusion at night. This may be followed by a tar bath in the morning and ultraviolet light exposure. A short course of therapy with an antimetabolite such as methotrexate may be tried. This drug is contraindicated in pregnancy and for anyone with a history of a peptic ulcer. No precautions need to be taken in bathing. In fact, bathing is beneficial in removing the scales.

Lesions may fade with treatment, only to recur eventually in the same area or elsewhere. The disease is not curable and may wax and wane continuously. If the patient does not know these things, he may lose confidence in his physician and may seek a quick cure. Because psoriasis is so common (it comprises about 5% of all skin disease) and so stubborn in response to treatment, manufacturers of patent remedies find a lucrative field for their products among persons who have the disease. Anyone who reads the daily papers or watches television regularly has seen numerous promises of cure. The patient should be warned lest he takes these advertisements seriously and waste his money.

Pemphigus is a skin condition characterized by enormous vesicles called bullae, which appear all over the body and on the mucous membranes. The lesions break and are followed by crusts that heal and leave scars. The cause of pemphigus in unknown. The condition may appear to clear up, and there may be remissions, but lesions eventually appear in such large numbers that a large part of the skin surface is raw and oozing and becomes infected. Prior to the use of systemic corticosteroids, pemphigus was uniformly fatal. Cortisone and ACTH (adrenocorticotropic hormone) cause marked improvement in symptoms and may produce remissions lasting for months or even years.

Nursing care of a patient with pemphigus is very difficult. Bradford frames or Stryker frames may be used in an effort to move the patient as painlessly as possible and prevent weight bearing on raw surfaces. Dakin's solution compresses may be applied to oozing lesions to help control odors and infection. Special mouth care, including frequent gargles with normal saline solution or alkaline mouthwashes, may be necessary if the lesions appear in the mouth. In an attempt to prevent secondary infection, reverse protective isolation may be used (p. 80).

Emotional support and encouragement of both the patient and his family are extremely important. The patient may fear that he is so repulsive that no one will take care of him. He needs constant reassurance that the nursing staff is interested in him and will care for him. The family and friends should be prepared for the patient's appearance before they visit him if they have not seen him recently. The family should be encouraged to visit often and to behave as normally as they possibly can. Fortunately pemphigus is a relatively rare disease.

Degenerative skin diseases

Corns are thickened skin lesions with a center core that thickens inwardly and causes acute pain on pressure. They are often caused by the pressure of ill-fitting shoes and occur on the toes. A corn is best treated by correction of shoes and by placing a small felt pad with a hole in the center over it to relieve pressure. Popular corn remedies seldom produce a cure, since their active ingredient is usually salicylic acid, which only dissolves the outer layer of skin. As soon as the medicated pad is removed, a new layer of skin forms unless pressure is relieved.

Soft corns occur between the toes where the skin is moist. They are extremely painful and difficult to treat. Sometimes x-ray treatment is required to effect a cure.

Calluses, or thickening of circumscribed areas of the horny layer of the skin, often appear on the plantar surface of the foot when the metatarsal arch has fallen and there is constant pressure against the sole of the shoe. They are often successfully treated by relief of the pressure and by regular massage with softening lotions and creams. They must be distinguished from plantar warts.

Stasis dermatitis is a common skin condition of the lower extremities in older persons. It is usually preceded by varicosities and poor circulation. With the reduction in venous return from the legs, substances normally carried away by the circulation remain in the tissues and irritate them. The skin is often reddened and edematous. Pruritus may be quite severe. Breaks in the skin are often caused by scratching, and infection then is introduced by the hands, clothing, and other sources.

The most important treatment for stasis dermatitis is prevention by careful attention to the treatment of peripheral vascular conditions and preventing the constriction of the circulation to the extremities (p. 379). Unna paste boots (Fig. 18-9) are often ordered for this condition.

Seborrheic keratoses occur most often in persons past middle age. The lesions resemble large, darkened, greasy warts and are often found around the trunk, on the back, and under the breasts. They seldom become malignant but should be observed at intervals for any change. They often can be removed easily with dichloracetic acid or carbon dioxide snow.

Angiomas are tufts of blood vessels that may occur spontaneously either as tiny bright red lesions or as purplish vascular lesions. The lesions should be watched closely, for although they do not usually become malignant, they may suddenly develop extensive vascular channels that may be difficult or impossible to remove surgically.

Malignant and premalignant lesions

Malignancies of the skin are more accessible to treatment than are those in any other part of the body. Education of the patient in reporting suspicious lesions and prompt action by nurses and physicians when such lesions are reported should make malignancies of the skin a largely controllable disease. By far the best treatment is early and complete surgical removal of the lesion.

Leukoplakia occurs as raised, even shiny areas of various sizes on the mucous membrane of the mouth and also of the genitalia in women. About 25% of the lesions become cancerous if not removed. Surgical removal is the treatment of choice. However, if the lesions are too extensive to be removed by surgery, radiotherapy or electrodesiccation may be used. In the early stages, leukoplakia of oral mucosa may be controlled by careful mouth hygiene. The patient who smokes should stop smoking. Smoking is definitely known to aggravate the condition. Any loose or jagged teeth are removed, periodontal treatment is given if necessary, and frequent mouth irrigations with an alkaline solution are advised.

Senile keratoses usually begin as scaly raised lesions in exposed parts of the body. The lesion is firm to pressure, and there is usually an elevated surface or border that bleeds easily. Senile keratoses require prompt surgical treatment because they may undergo malignant degeneration and become squamous cell carcinomas.

Basal cell carcinomas involve the lower or basal layer of skin cells. They grow slowly and rarely metastasize, but can be locally invasive. A typical form known as a *rodent ulcer* often develops from senile keratoses. The lesions frequently ulcerate, crust over, and heal, leaving a small scar, and then recur at the same site.

Pigmented moles are often precancerous. These skin lesions may be present at birth or may appear at any time of life. The darker the lesion, the more dangerous it seems to be. The blue or greenish black type (melanotic nevus) is the most dangerous of all. Yellow and brownish moles are less likely to become malignant. Blue or black moles should be removed even if they are not raised above the normal skin surface. Most physicians agree that any mole that shows signs of growth or that is in a part of the body where it is traumatized by clothing should be removed at once. The *malignant melanoma,* deriving its name from the melanin, or pigment, in the basal layer in the skin, is the most dangerous of all cancerous skin lesions. The mortality is extremely high, and often wide metastasis has occurred before the lesion is noticed.

Squamous cell carcinomas originate in the outer prickly or squamous layer of skin cells. Usually the lesion begins as a warty growth with a hard, horny outer layer that breaks down to form an ulcer. The lesions often occur in areas of irritation such as on the bridge of the nose in persons who wear glasses or on the lower lip in those who smoke pipes. If not diagnosed and treated early, squamous cell carcinomas metastasize rapidly.

Sarcoma and *fibrosarcoma* are lesions that may develop quite suddenly from seemingly innocuous nodules somewhere in the skin. Unfortunately metastasis often occurs before the original node shows much change. For this reason any nodule in the skin should be reported to a physician at once.

Mycosis fungoides is one of the most dreaded of all skin diseases. It begins as an itching, thickened lesion in the skin and progresses to a tumor stage,

which finally breaks down and destroys the skin. A large, soft, mushy vegetative lesion develops that destroys all the normal adjacent structures. Lesions may break out in several parts of the body. While the patient lives, all resemblance to his normal self is lost, and the disease, which lasts an average of 7 years from the date of onset of symptoms, is invariably fatal.[1] X-ray therapy is sometimes used to allay itching in the early stages, and nitrogen mustard is sometimes given intravenously. Corticosteroids delay the process somewhat but do not affect the final outcome. The nursing care for mycosis fungoides in late stages is similar to that required for pemphigus. Electron beam irradiation has been helpful because it can be applied to the total skin surface; the rays are adjusted so that deep tissues are not affected.[25]

REFERENCES AND SELECTED READINGS*

1 Beeson, P. B., and McDermott, W., editors: Cecil-Loeb textbook of medicine, ed. 13, Philadelphia, 1971, W. B. Saunders Co.
2 Bergersen, B. S.: Pharmacology in nursing, ed. 12, St. Louis, 1973, The C. V. Mosby Co.
3 *Bowden, L.: Current trends in treating malignant melanoma, A.O.R.N.J. 17:84-91, March 1973.
4 *Carney, R. G.: The aging skin, Am. J. Nurs. 63:110-112, June 1963.
5 Criep, L. H.: Dermatologic allergy: immunology, diagnosis, management, Philadelphia, 1970, W. B. Saunders Co.
6 *Edwards, E.: Mycosis fungoides, Am. J. Nurs. 61:61-63, Feb. 1961.
7 *Goldman, L.: Prevention and treatment of eczema, Am. J. Nurs. 64:114-116, March 1964.
8 *Iverson, P. C., and Staneruck, I. D.: Dermal abrasion, surgical care and nursing care after dermal abrasion, Am. J. Nurs. 57:860-864, July 1957.
9 Jones, F. A.: The skin—a mirror of the gut, Geriatrics 28:75-81, April 1973.
10 *Kimmig, J., and Janner, M.: Frieboes/Schonfeld color atlas of dermatology (American edition translated and revised by Herbert Goldschmidt and Donald M. Pillsbury), Philadelphia, 1966, W. B. Saunders Co.
11 Kinmont, P. D.: Pruritus as a dermatological problem, Practitioner 208:622-632, May 1972.
12 Kligman, A. M., and others: Acne vulgaris: a treatable disease, Postgrad. Med. 55:99-105, Feb. 1974.
13 Korting, G. W.: Diseases of the skin in children and adolescents, Philadelphia, 1970, W. B. Saunders Co.
14 Lewis, G. M., and Clayton, E. W.: Practical dermatology, ed. 3, Philadelphia, 1967, W. B. Saunders Co.
15 Management of common skin problems, Postgrad. Med., J. Appl. Med. 52:63-194, Nov. 1972.
16 Marlow, D. R.: Textbook of pediatric nursing, ed. 4, Philadelphia, 1973, W. B. Saunders Co.
17 Mathews, K. P.: A current view of urticaria, Med. Clin. North Am. 58:185-205, Jan. 1974.
18 Mihm, M. C., Jr., and others: Early detection of primary cuta-

neous malignant melanoma, N. Engl. J. Med. 289:989-996, Nov. 1973.
19 Mitchell, D. M.: Eczema, Practitioner 208:597-606, May 1972.
20 Nahmias, A. J., and others: Infection with herpes-simplex viruses 1 and 2. I. N. Engl. J. Med. 289:667-674, Sept. 1973; II. 289:719-725, Oct. 1973; III. 289:781-789, Oct. 1973.
21 Nelson, W. E., editor: Textbook of pediatrics, ed. 9, Philadelphia, 1969, W. B. Saunders Co.
22 Osment, L. S.: Tinea capitis, Am. J. Nurs. 60:1264-1266, Sept. 1960.
23 Pegum, J. S.: Advances in the treatment of diseases of the skin, Practitioner 209:453-459, Oct. 1972.
24 Piper, W. N.: Poison ivy, poison oak and poison sumac, Am. J. Nurs. 54:814-816, July 1954.
25 Pol, M. L.: Mycosis fungoides and electron beam therapy: the nursing concepts and related care of these patients, Clinical Sessions ANA (1966), New York, 1967, Appleton-Century-Crofts.
26 Reisner, R. M.: Acne vulgaris, Pediatr. Clin. North Am. 20:851-864, Nov. 1973.
27 Robin, M.: How emotions affect skin problems in school children, J. Sch. Health 43:370-373, June 1973.
28 Rodman, M. J.: Some newer drugs for skin diseases, R.N. 31:55-65, March 1968.
29 Rowell, N.: Urticaria, Practitioner 208:614-621, May 1972.
30 *Ruppe, J. P.: Skin infections: their role in health today, J. Sch. Health 43:373-380, June 1973.
31 *Samitz, M. H.: The industrial dermatoses, Am. J. Nurs. 65:79-82, Jan. 1965.
32 Sauer, G. C.: Manual of skin diseases, ed. 3, Philadelphia, 1973, J. B. Lippincott Co.
33 Shecky, W. B.: Consultations in dermatology, Philadelphia, 1972, W. B. Saunders Co.
34 Soter, N. A., and others: Clinical dermatology, I. N. Engl. J. Med. 289:189-195, July 1973; II. 289:242-249, Aug. 1973; III. 289:296-302, Aug. 1973.
35 Sulzberger, M. B., and others: Dermatology, diagnosis and treatment, ed. 2, Chicago, 1961, Year Book Medical Publishers, Inc.
36 *Torrey, F.: Care of the normal skin, Am. J. Nurs. 53:460-463, April 1953.
37 *Wechsler, H. L.: Psoriasis, Am. J. Nurs. 65:85-87, April 1965.
38 Wexler, L.: Gamma benzene hexachloride in treatment of pediculosis and scabies, Am. J. Nurs. 69:565-566, Nov. 1969.

*References preceded by an asterisk are particularly well suited for student reading.

29 The patient with burns

Emergency care
Physiologic changes occurring in severe burns
Management of the patient with burns

■ Burns are wounds caused by excessive exposure of the body to heat. Flame, scalding water, electricity, chemicals, radiation, and x-rays are forms of heat that may cause burns. Scalding water and flame are the two most common causes of burns. This chapter is devoted to nursing care of burned patients. Principles of burn care remain the same regardless of etiology.

Burns are classified as first, second, and third degree, depending on their depth. First- and second-degree burns are classified as *partial-thickness* burns, whereas third-degree burns are *full-thickness* burns (Fig. 29-1). A *first-degree burn* is one in which the outer layer of skin is injured and reddened without blister formation; mild sunburn is a good example. A *second-degree burn* injures all of the epidermis and much of the corium. Blister formation is characteristic and there is usually considerable subcutaneous edema. The deeper layers of the corium are not destroyed and regeneration can occur. First-degree and second-degree burns are likely to be painful because nerve endings have been injured and exposed. A *third-degree burn* is one in which all layers of skin are destroyed, thus making regeneration impossible. Nerves, muscles, bone, and blood supply also may be injured or destroyed in third-degree burns. If the nerves are destroyed, the wound is painless. Victims may experience difficulty with body temperature regulation in relation to the environment. Because epithelialization is impossible, areas that have sustained third-degree burns eventually must be covered either by skin growing from normal skin around the edges of the burned area, by scar tissue, or by skin grafts. Patients experience dryness and itching of burned skin areas due to increased vascularization, destruction of sebaceous glands, and decreased perspiration.

Fire kills 12,000 and scars and injures 300,000 Americans each year, including 50,000 individuals who must be hospitalized for periods from 6 weeks to 2 years. Many of these deaths could have been prevented. Nurses can help prevent accidental burns from occurring by participating in health education programs that stress fire prevention and the consequences of fires such as burns, deformities, and death and by promoting legislation that would control some of man's thoughtless practices and make his working and living environments safer. Public health nurses are in an unusually advantageous position to recognize unsafe practices in the home and to help families develop safe habits of living.

Approximately 80% of accidental burns occur in the home and primarily are caused by ignorance, carelessness, and curiosity of children. Infants and children are the most common victims of fires in and about the home. Young children should be supervised in their play and should never be left at home alone. Children should be taught at an early age about the hazards of fire. Parents must carefully check play areas for all fire hazards such as live extension wires, matches, and unprotected floor heaters and should remove them. Serious burns to children often result from pot handles that project beyond the stove top. A large number of children have been burned to death or permanently disabled and/or disfigured by fireworks. Legislation in many states now prohibits the sale of fireworks, but violations of the law and accidents still occur.

Activities persons were engaged in when they caught on fire in their homes are shown in Table 29-1.

■ STUDY QUESTIONS

1 What are some of the precautionary measures you have already learned that must be observed when applying heat to the skin?
2 From your knowledge of anatomy and physiology, list the harmful effects of loss of a large area of skin.
3 Review the principles and techniques of surgical asepsis.
4 Name some ways of helping a patient increase fluid intake. What kinds of foods are high in protein? What are some ways in which high-protein foods may be given to the critically ill patient?

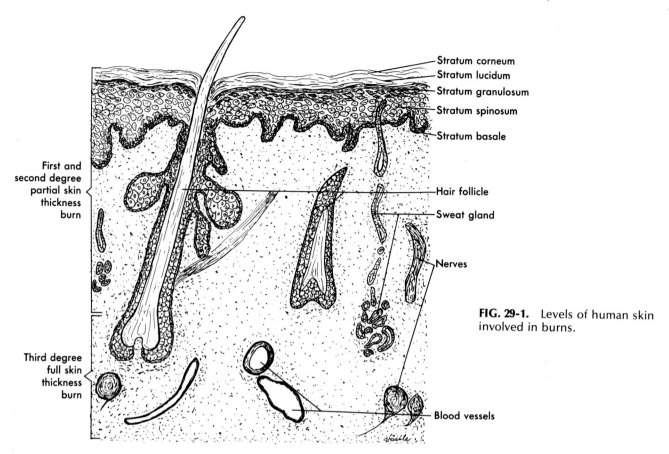

First and second degree partial skin thickness burn

Third degree full skin thickness burn

Stratum corneum
Stratum lucidum
Stratum granulosum
Stratum spinosum
Stratum basale

Hair follicle
Sweat gland

Nerves

FIG. 29-1. Levels of human skin involved in burns.

Blood vessels

Table 29-1   Activity of persons burned by fire*

Playing with matches/lighter	175	11.3†
Smoking	152	10.0
Using matches/lighter	116	7.5
Fell asleep while smoking	100	6.4
Reaching across stove	86	5.5
Sleeping	77	5.0
Standing too close to stove	64	4.1
Leaning against stove	47	3.0

*From Flammable fabric investigations, Washington, D. C., 1973, Department of Health, Education and Welfare, Food and Drug Administration, Bureau of Product Safety, FY66-FY72.
† Percent based on 1,554 cases in which activity is known.

Each year brings increased demand for careful inspection and regulation of places in which the ill and infirm are housed. Aged persons frequently are housed in old and poorly equipped structures and many of them have been burned to death. Attention is being focused on places where large numbers of people congregate. Laws now require that doors in public buildings be hinged to swing outward, that draperies and decorations be fireproof, and that stairways with special fire doors be used in new apartment buildings and hotels. These laws have been passed as a result of serious fires in which many persons have lost their lives. Rigid enforcement of laws requiring that industrial products be labeled when known to be flammable and that new products be tested carefully for their flammable qualities before being placed on the market is further evidence of government effort to protect the public from accident by fire.

Sunburn should be cautioned against, as even a relatively mild first-degree burn of a large part of the body can cause change of fluid distribution and kidney damage. Camp nurses should keep this in mind in their educational programs for children and camp counselors. (For further discussion of sunburn, see p. 271.)

■ EMERGENCY CARE

The nurse may be called on to assist with injuries at the scene of a fire. If flame is involved and the victim's clothing is on fire, his first reaction is to run, which only fans the flame. Rolling the burning person in a blanket on the ground to exclude oxygen, thereby putting out the fire, is one of the best procedures. The person whose clothing is aflame should never stand since this increases the danger of inhalation burns in which heat and smoke are drawn into the lungs. Persons who are burned on the face and neck or those who have inhaled flame, steam, or smoke should be observed closely for signs of laryngeal edema and airway obstruction. Immediate arrangements should be made to transport the patient to a hospital, a burn center if available (see Table 29-2 for list of burn centers), or a physician's office. Often burns are more severe than they may appear to be. Thus all patients with burns, even if the burns appear to be superficial, should be seen by a physician. The hospital or physician should be notified, so that preparations can be made for the arrival of the patient, since a well-prepared and well-equipped team of personnel is needed to care for the severely burned person.

While awaiting transportation to a medical facility, the patient should be kept quiet and lying down. Loss of natural body heat may be prevented in part by covering the victim with blankets, coats, or whatever is available. External heat should not be applied since this may cause dilation of blood vessels and further loss of body heat. If clothing adheres to the burned surface, it should not be removed. Exposed

Table 29-2 Burn units and centers in the United States*

Location	Physician(s) in charge	Hospital(s)	Bed capacity (no.)	Annual admissions (no.)
Chicago, Ill.	John Boswick, M.D.; Nelson Stone, M.D.	Cook County Hospital	35	425
San Antonio, Tex.	Basil Pruitt, Col. M.C.	U. S. Army Surgical Research Unit, Brooke Army Medical Center	60	390
Cincinnati, Ohio	Bruce MacMillan, M.D.; Robert Hummel, M.D.	Shrine Burns Institute, Cincinnati General Hospital	55	325
Los Angeles, Calif.	John Winkley, M.D.	Los Angeles County General Hospital	30	325
Galveston, Tex.	Duane Larson, M.D.; Stephen Lewis, M.D.	Shrine Burns Institute, John Sealey Hospital	30	300
Boston, Mass.	Oliver Cope, M.D.	Shrine Burns Institute, Massachusetts General Hospital	30	225
Milwaukee, Wis.	George Collentine, M.D.	St. Mary's Hospital	30	225
Richmond, Va.	B. W. Haynes, M.D.	Medical College of Virginia Hospital	36	220
Dallas, Tex.	Charles Baxter, M.D.	Parkland Memorial Hospital	12	200
Atlanta, Ga.	H. Harlan Stone, M.D.	Grady Memorial Hospital, Emory University Hospital	25	180
Brooklyn, N. Y.	I. C. Song, M.D.; Bertram Bromberg, M.D.	King's County Hospital	6	175
Ann Arbor, Mich.	Irving Feller, M.D.	University of Michigan Medical Center, St. Joseph Mercy Hospital	14	150
Mobile, Ala.	John Crosby, M.D.; Byron Green, M.D.	Mobile General Hospital	8	150
St. Paul, Minn.	James Lafeve, M.D.	St. Paul Ramsey Hospital	10	150
Akron, Ohio	Clifford Boeckman, M.D.	Children's Hospital of Akron	14	140
Houston, Tex.	Melvin Spira, M.D.	Ben Taub General Hospital	12	140
Columbus, Ohio	E. Thomas Boles, M.D.	Children's Hospital	20	125
Orange, Calif.	Irving Rappaport, M.D.	Orange County Medical Center	8	125
Tulsa, Okla.	Frank Clingan, M.D.	Hillcrest Medical Center	10	125
Albany, N. Y.	Mark Wong, M.D.	Albany Medical Center	10	120
Detroit, Mich.	James Lloyd, M.D.	Children's Hospital	11	120
Cleveland, Ohio	Richard Fratianne, M.D.	Cleveland Metropolitan General Hospital	15	115
New York, N. Y.	Ronald Ollstein, M.D.; George Crikelair, M.D.	Harlem Hospital Center	20	100
Phoenix, Ariz.	William Price, M.D.	Maricopa County General Hospital	9	100

*Modified from Feller, I., and Crane, C. H.: J.A.M.A. **215:**463-464, Jan. 1971.

burned surfaces should be covered with sterile dressings or with the cleanest material available. *Oils, salves, and ointments should not be used on burns* since these materials hamper treatment. Towels soaked in cool water may ease the pain and reduce the edema. Ice should be avoided because the sudden vasoconstriction causes severe shifting of fluid. Pain in extensive burns is best controlled by gentle and minimal handling and by the application of dressings to exclude air from the burned skin surfaces. Occasionally deep, third-degree burns are almost painless, since nerve endings have been destroyed, and for the first few minutes the patient may appear not too badly affected. Usually, however, some part of the body has sustained first-degree and second-degree burns that cause pain.

Since the extent of the burn is extremely difficult to determine, if there is any question, no fluids should be given until a medical estimate can be made. For obviously small burns, fluids may be given with caution. Nothing should be given by mouth if the patient is nauseated or vomiting.

Burns occurring about the eyes should be lavaged with copious amounts of cold, clean water, and if the burn was caused by acids, the procedure should be repeated in 10 to 15 minutes.

■ PHYSIOLOGIC CHANGES OCCURRING IN SEVERE BURNS

The lives of many badly burned patients are now being saved, since in recent years much has been learned about the physiologic changes occurring in patients with severe burns. When tissues are burned, vasodilation, increased capillary permeability, and changes in the permeability of tissue cells in and around the burn area occur. As a result, abnormally large amounts of extracellular fluid, sodium chloride, and protein pass into the burned area to cause blister formation and local edema or escape through the open wound. Visible fluid loss makes up only a small part of the fluid lost from the circulating blood and other essential fluid compartments (see Table 5-6). Most of the fluid loss occurs deep in the wound, where the fluid extravasates into the deeper tissues. Burns of areas such as highly vascular muscle tissue or the face are believed to cause greater fluid shift than comparable burns of other parts of the body. Fully one half of the extracellular fluid of the body can shift from its normal distribution to the site of a severe burn. The extracellular fluid constitutes about 20% of the body weight. Three fourths of it surrounds the cells and one-fourth is found in blood plasma (see Table 5-6). For a person weighing 67.2 kg. (150 pounds), this means that from 10 to 15 pounds or from 5,000 to 7,500 ml. of fluids may be removed from the interstitial spaces and bloodstream. Hypovolemic shock occurs, resulting in a tremendous drop in blood pressure and inadequate blood flow through the kidneys, which in turn leads to further shock, anuria, and death within a short time if treatment is not given promptly or is inadequate.

Dehydration, hypoproteinemia, shock, and electrolyte imbalance develop. Hyperkalemia (excessive amounts of potassium in the blood plasma) occurs as a result of the injury to the epithelial and red blood cells and from diminished urinary output. Increased red blood cells trapped in the burned area are destroyed, and the injured cells continue to hemolyze. Renal damage and hematuria may occur as a result of reduced blood volume and passage of the end products of the hemolyzed cells through the glomeruli. Anemia develops as red blood cells trapped in the burned area are destroyed and the injured cells continue to hemolyze.

Burns increase the production and loss of heat, and water vapor is lost through the open wound; these in turn cause increased metabolism and weight loss. There often is evidence of adrenocortical hyperfunction after a burn due to generalized body stress.

Normal skin function is diminished or eliminated, resulting in physiologic alterations. These include (1) loss of protective barriers against infection, (2) escape of body fluids, (3) lack of temperature control, (4) destroyed sweat and sebaceous glands, and (5) diminished number of sensory receptors. The severity of these alterations will depend on the extent of the burn and the depth to which damage has occurred.

■ MANAGEMENT OF THE PATIENT WITH BURNS

The severely burned patient presents a challenge to the physician and nurse who care for him. Determination of the severity of the burn, its treatment, and the prognosis of the patient is dependent on (1) the presence of preexisting conditions such as cardiac, pulmonary, renal, and hepatic disease and injuries sustained during burn trauma such as fractures or internal injuries; (2) the area of the body that is burned (burns of the hands, feet, face, neck, and most joint surfaces may produce the most serious loss of function and the most conspicuous disfigurement); and (3) the degree and depth of tissue injury.

Immediate treatment

On arrival at the hospital the patient's clothes are carefully removed and the physician evaluates the patient's condition. Respiratory status is evaluated first. An airway should be established if any distress is present. Preventive intubation should be done if any heat inhalation occurred. Endotracheal intubation is preferred over a tracheostomy because edema of the respiratory passages frequently

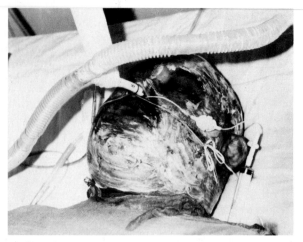

FIG. 29-2.   Patient with severe edema 5 hours after burn occurred. Airway was managed with endotracheal intubation. Edema subsided and patient was extubated 4 days after admission. (Courtesy Burn Center, Cleveland Metropolitan General Hospital, Cleveland, Ohio.)

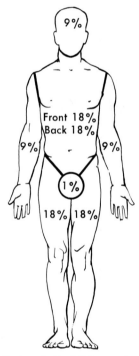

FIG. 29-3.   The "rule of nine's" is used to estimate the amount of skin surface burned.

subsides within a few days and avoidance of surgical trauma is desired (Fig. 29-2). Oral fluids should be withheld and a nasogastric tube is usually inserted as fluids via this method help to prevent paralytic ileus. A Foley catheter is also inserted so that there can be accurate monitoring of urinary output. A central venous line will be required to permit fluid replacement and monitoring of fluid volume. Morphine sulfate or meperidine hydro-

chloride is often given intravenously to the patient with an extensive burn. The intravenous route is used because of inadequate absorption at peripheral sites. Large doses of sedatives and analgesics are avoided because of the danger of respiratory depression and because they may mask other symptoms. *The patient should be weighed. This measurement will be used to determine fluid therapy and to evaluate progress.* Venous and arterial blood samples are taken to determine protein, electrolyte, red blood cell, pH, and blood gas levels.

The severity of the burn is assessed by the percentage of body surface involved and the depth of the burn wound. For adults, the "rule of nine's" is used (Fig. 29-3). These calculations are modified for infants and children under 10 years of age because of their relatively larger heads and smaller extremities. (See pediatric textbooks for these figures.) The age of the patient is important in estimating the severity of the burn. Infants tolerate burns poorly and the mortality in this group is high, even with small burns. In burns involving up to 30% of the body surface in older children and in adults under the age of 50, the mortality rate is quite low. As the age of the patient increases beyond 50, the mortality rate rises even in burns of less than 30%.[3]

Fluid therapy

Replacement of fluids and electrolytes is an essential part of the treatment and is instituted as soon as the extent of the burn and the patient's condition have been determined. Ideally, fluid therapy is started within an hour following a severe burn. A central venous line inserted into a vein permits the rapid administration of fluids and electrolytes.

Three types of fluid are considered in calculating the needs of the patient: (1) colloids, including plasma and plasma expanders such as dextran, (2) electrolytes such as physiologic solution of sodium chloride, Ringer's solution, Hartmann's solution, and Tyrode's solution, and (3) nonelectrolyte fluids such as distilled water with 5% glucose.[4] Medical authorities do not agree as to the proportion of colloid and electrolyte fluids needed. Several formulas are described in the medical literature to guide physicians in determining the type and amount of fluids to be administered, based on the patient's weight and age and the percentage of the body burned.[4,19,31] The present trend is to administer balanced salt solutions (such as Ringer's), water, and plasma and to use whole blood only if a large number of red cells are destroyed or if anemia develops.

Fluid needs for the first 24 hours are calculated from the time of the burn. Usually the patient receives one-half the total amount in the first 8 hours, one-fourth in the second 8 hours, and one-fourth in the third 8 hours. One half of the total amount given on the first day is given in the second 24 hours. If vomiting occurs or if a nasogastric tube is inserted and attached to suction, additional fluids containing electrolytes may be given intravenously. The amount of fluid replacement required during the first 48 hours is determined by assessment of several factors; these include urinary output, serum electrolyte levels, blood gas findings, central venous pressure, body weight, desire to maintain the hematocrit at slightly above normal levels, level of consciousness, and vital signs.

Patients complain of moderate to severe thirst. The nurse should give fluids by mouth only in the amounts ordered and should record them accurately. Unlimited oral intake and failure to measure it may result in too much fluid in the circulating blood and in water intoxication. Monitoring techniques, more sophisticated than central venous pressure recordings, are being used in the management of the burn patient. This includes the insertion of a catheter into the pulmonary artery to monitor sensitive fluid shifts.

Renal function

The rate of urinary output is probably the most reliable measure of determining the adequacy of fluid therapy during the first 48 hours. Hourly checking and measuring of urinary output is one of the most important responsibilities of the nurse. Usually a retention catheter is inserted and drained into a calibrated container. The amount of urine is measured and recorded every hour. The care of the patient with an indwelling catheter is discussed on p. 455. The urine should be observed for color and analyzed for a positive hematocrit level. The physician should be notified if hematuria is present and/or a positive Hemastix reaction. A urine flow of 30 to 50 ml./hour is adequate for an adult.[4] The urine flow should be at least 15 ml./hour for infants and 25 ml./hour for older children.[18] If the urinary output rises above or falls below these figures, the physician should be notified immediately. Fluid therapy will need to be adjusted accordingly. Lack of urinary output may indicate insufficient fluids or acute tubular necrosis. The administration of too much fluid may cause pulmonary edema.

After the first 48 to 72 hours the urinary output is no longer a reliable guide to fluid needs, since water deprivation may occur even when the urinary output for adults is 1,000 ml./day or more. Severely burned patients require a large fluid intake to compensate for the loss of fluid into the tissues and from the wound. Fluid needs then are determined by measuring serum electrolyte levels. Fluids administered during the first 48 hours are given to maintain circulating blood volume. A diuresis phase usually occurs 2 to 5 days after the burn and indicates a shift of fluid back to the intravascular compartment.

Observation

The severely burned patient needs constant nursing observation and care. The nurse must check for changes in the condition of the patient and report any changes promptly. The patient who has been burned by hot air or steam must be closely watched for signs of respiratory complications. Difficulty in breathing, coughing and expectoration of blood, and cyanosis are signs that the trachea and lungs have been burned. These signs must be reported immediately. Depending on the severity of the symptoms, emergency treatment may include oxygen, suctioning, and postural drainage. Establishment of an airway may be necessary if severe edema of the throat develops (Fig. 29-2). Persistent vomiting should be noted and the amount recorded, since this loss must be considered in estimating the total amount of fluid needed. If a sphygmomanometer can be applied, blood pressure should be taken as often as every 15 minutes. Rate and volume of the pulse should be carefully noted. Skin color and level of consciousness are often important in determining whether or not the prognosis is favorable. Restlessness is always significant, and mania is indicative of a poor prognosis. Signs of water intoxication should be watched for, and these include tremor, twitching, nausea, diarrhea, salivation, and disorientation.

Prevention of hospital-acquired infection

Every effort is made to prevent introduction of infection to the burned area. Local and systemic infections (septicemia) are the most common complications of burns and are a major cause of death, particularly in burns covering more than 25% of the body.[28] The primary source of bacteria appears to be the burn wound. The organisms that usually infect burn wounds are *Staphylococcus aureus, Pseudomonas aeruginosa (pyocyanea)* (p. 87), and the coliform bacilli. In the past few years there has been an increasing incidence of *Candida albicans* infections. Antibiotics may be given prophylactically, or they may be withheld until an infection does occur. Cultures of the patient's nose, throat, wound, and unburned skin and a punch biopsy may be taken on admission and at intervals to determine the bacteria present and their sensitivity to antibiotics.

All who attend the patient (as well as visitors) should wear gowns and masks to prevent the introduction of their organisms into the wound. Persons with upper respiratory infections should not be permitted near the patient. Good aseptic surgical techniques should be used in the emergency room. Sterile gloves should be used when applying dressings. Particular care must be taken when bathing groups of patients in hydrotherapy tanks. Sometimes the patient is transferred to the operating room, where sterile surgical techniques can be carried out. The extent of local cleansing depends on the severity of the burn and the judgment of the physician. Detergents and/or antiseptic preparations such as povidone-iodine (Betadine) are effective cleansing agents. A rather extensive debridement may be carried out at the initial cleansing. The wounds then are treated by methods that will be described later in this chapter. If the exposure method is used, strict isolation technique is observed when caring for the patient. Some hospitals use a specially built isolation system (bubble) in order to protect the patient from the hospital environment[24] (p. 80). If silver nitrate dressings are used, the patient is not isolated and clean rather than sterile technique is used.

Tetanus toxoid and/or antitoxin is usually given to the patient who has received extensive burns. The patient may receive both a booster dose of toxoid (0.5 ml.) and 3,000 units of antitoxin if he has not been immunized or has had no booster dose in the previous 4 years.[4]

Local treatment

There are several methods of treating the burned area, depending on the location of the burn, its size and depth, the facilities available, and the patient's response to the therapy. One method may be started and then replaced with another during the course of treatment. Only those commonly used today are described here.

Open or exposure method of treatment. The exposure method of treatment was accidentally discovered to be effective in 1888 when, during a serious steamboat fire on the Mississippi, those in attendance ran out of bandages and later observed that the neglected persons fared better than those who received more intensive local treatment.[16] Today, the exposure method is used most often in the treatment of burns involving the face, neck, perineum, and broad areas of the trunk. The burned area is cleansed and exposed to the air (Fig. 29-4). The exudate of a partial-thickness burn dries in 48 to 72 hours and forms a hard crust that protects the wound. Epithelialization occurs beneath this crust and may be complete in 14 to 21 days.[4] The crust then falls off spontaneously, leaving a healed, unscarred surface. The dead skin of a full-thickness burn is dehydrated and converted to an eschar (black, leathery dead tissue covering) in 48 to 72 hours. Loose eschar may be gradually removed through the use of whirlpool baths or debridement (Figs. 29-5 and 29-6). Uninfected eschar acts as a protective covering. The danger of infection exists as bacteria proliferate beneath the eschar. Spontaneous separation, produced by bacterial action, occurs unless surgical debridement is performed. An escharotomy (linear incision of constricting eschar) may be necessary when con-

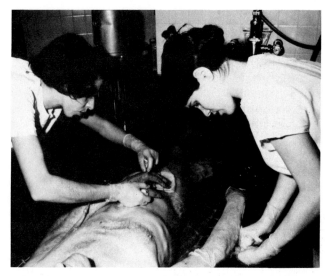

FIG. 29-5. Nurses debriding patient in a hydrotherapy bath. (Courtesy Burn Center, Cleveland Metropolitan General Hospital, Cleveland, Ohio.)

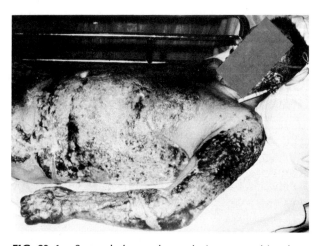

FIG. 29-4. Severely burned man being treated by the open method. (Courtesy Burn Center, Cleveland Metropolitan General Hospital, Cleveland, Ohio.)

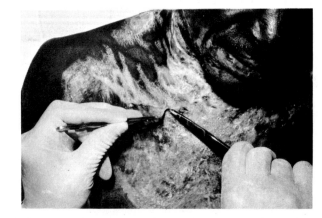

FIG. 29-6. The nurse's role in burn centers may include debridement of patient's eschar. (Courtesy Burn Unit, Cook County Hospital, Chicago, Ill.)

striction of circulation and/or respiration is evident (Figs. 29-7 and 29-8).

To decrease the possibility of infection, the patient with exposed burn wounds should be placed in a unit or room where only "clean" surgical cases are cared for. He usually is placed on sterile linen. A cradle may be used since no clothing or top bedclothes are allowed directly over a burned area. In summer months, screen doors and window screens should be used to keep out flies, which may introduce direct infection or lay eggs in the open wounds.

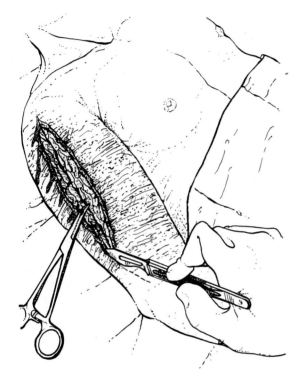

FIG. 29-7. Escharotomy surgically performed for circumferential burn of upper arm.

Sterile cornstarch can be sprinkled on the bed to help prevent sticking caused by drainage from cracks in the crust as the patient moves about. Infants may need to have their hands restrained to prevent them from picking off crusts. Until the wounds are healed, children's toys need to be sterilized to prevent them from causing infection.

The nurse caring for the patient should wear a sterile gown and mask. In most hospitals it is fairly simple to make up a "burn pack" to be autoclaved. This pack can include sheets for the canopy and bed, loin cloth and halter, bath blankets, pillowcases, towels, washcloths, and bedpan covers, as well as gowns and masks for those in attendance.

Patients having exposure treatment complain of pain and chilling. Pain may be controlled by administering morphine sulfate, meperidine hydrochloride (Demerol), barbiturates, or propoxyphene hydrochloride (Darvon) as ordered. Discomfort can be decreased if drafts are avoided and the temperature of the room is kept at 24.4° C. (85° F.). Patients lose more heat from burned surfaces than from the normal skin surfaces, since there is no vascular bed to contract and retain heat in the body. The humidity of the room also should be controlled. A humidity of 40% to 50% usually is considered satisfactory. Portable electric humidifiers and dehumidifiers can be used to achieve and maintain this level.

Many patients prefer to turn themselves, and, if dressings are used to cover small areas, they may wish to help remove the dressings. They should be permitted to help themselves since this is often less painful and more acceptable and promotes independence in self-care. A new nonadherent plastic dressing (Microdon) that does not stick to the wound is now available.

If the burn is extensive, a CircOlectric bed draped with a sheet is an ideal way to care for the patient

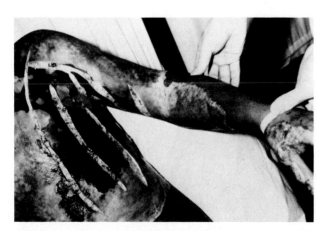

FIG. 29-8. Escharotomy used to alleviate circulatory and pulmonary constriction. (Courtesy Burn Center, Cleveland Metropolitan General Hospital, Cleveland, Ohio.)

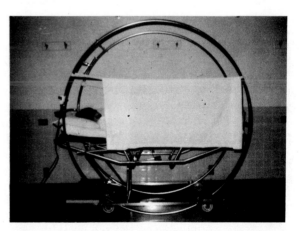

FIG. 29-9. Another exposure method of treating burns. A sheet is draped over the CircOlectric bed so that burned areas are not touched. (Courtesy Burn Unit, Cook County Hospital, Chicago, Ill.)

(Fig. 29-9). However, if a CircOlectric bed is not available, a burn bed may be prepared by draping a Balkan frame with sheets to make a tent. A thermometer should be hung within the canopy, a small section of the canopy should be left open to prevent humidity from rising, and the temperature in the tent should be maintained at about 24.4° C. (85° F.). Portable heating elements may be used at the bedside or small electric light bulbs may be strung up inside the tent to maintain temperature. The bulbs should be enclosed in wire frames for safety and should be placed out of the reach of children. If the lights are used and there are no burns about the face, sometimes patients rest and sleep better when wearing sunglasses. Others find that cloth eyeshades are helpful in keeping the light from their eyes. The burned patient can be kept from embarrassing exposure and can be kept warm in the tent while wearing only a halter and loin cloth. Maximum freedom is provided for him to get on or off the bedpan, move about, and perform exercises for the prevention of contracture and the improvement of circulation.

Topical ointments. Local applications may be ordered to stimulate healing of burned areas. Sterile petrolatum or a local anesthetic cream may be applied to first-degree burns. Ointments, particularly those containing antibiotics, are commonly used in the treatment of severe burns. These include mafenide (Sulfamylon), povidone-iodine (Betadine) ointment, silver sulfadiazine (Silvadine), furazolium, and neomycin.

Mafenide is a white cream containing sulfonamide. A layer of medication 3 to 5 mm. thick is applied directly to the wound once or twice a day. The wound is usually left open to the air. Washing of the wound and reapplication of the cream is necessary when the wound is no longer covered with ointment.

Povidone-iodine ointment is a reddish brown germicidal preparation of 10% povidone-iodine (1% available iodine) with broad-spectrum microbicidal action. It kills gram-positive and gram-negative bacteria, fungi, yeasts, viruses, and protozoa. It is nonirritating and nonsensitizing and permits air to reach the site after application. It is applied at least three times daily. The methods of application are (1) "buttering"—using the gloved hand, a $\frac{1}{4}$-inch thick layer is spread on burned surfaces and (2) the modified closed technique—single-thickness povidone-iodine-impregnated gauze is applied to the affected areas, and additional ointment is spread on top of the gauze layer.

Silver sulfadiazine is an investigational topical agent being tested in some centers. It is applied directly to the wound once or twice daily with a sterile gloved hand or an impregnated gauze roll. It is effective against gram-positive organisms and *Candida albicans*.

Furazolium is a research drug that can be applied either directly to the wound or gauze rolls may be saturated with it. It is a bright saffron-colored cream that is very soluble in water and is heat stable. At high concentrations it is bactericidal to all organisms with the exception of *Proteus* and yeasts.

Neomycin is a bactericidal agent that causes miscoding in the messenger RNA of bacterial cells. It is effective against most organisms but has a serious toxic effect and can cause irreversible hearing loss or kidney failure when used over a long period of time.

In addition to ointments, two other solutions are used frequently in burn care. These are sodium chloride solution and a mixture of equal parts of acetic acid, peroxide, and normal saline solution, commonly referred to as "thirds." Normal or balanced saline solutions are applied to clean granulation tissue or to new grafts to maintain moisture or are used with fine mesh gauze to provide for slight debridement. The "thirds" solution has limited antimicrobial action and is most effective against organisms that are affected by changes in pH. It is also used to clean dirty granulation tissue.

Closed method of treatment. In the closed method of burn treatment the wounds are washed and dressings are changed at least once each day and frequently twice. Commonly the dressing consists of gauze impregnated with one of the topical ointments discussed previously and a gauze wrap. When a dressing is in place, nursing observation should include checking for signs of impaired circulation such as numbness, pain, and tingling and being alert for signs of infection (odor on dressings, elevated temperature and pulse rate). In order to improve venous return the patient is not allowed to stand for more than a short time when the lower limbs are involved, and upper limbs are elevated when the patient is sitting or lying down.

Dressings and soaks. Saline solution dressings may be used to treat small infected areas, and it is important to keep them moist because drying causes the dressing and the exudate to shrink. This shrinkage produces pain and may cause hemorrhage from newly developed superficial blood vessels. Hydrotherapy is a valuable adjunct to therapy and should be used when available.

Tub baths at 37.7° C. (100° F.) may be used to soak off extensive dressings over infected areas as well as to remove eschar. Although the water in the tub cannot be kept sterile, many patients benefit a great deal from its cleansing effects and from the fact that dressings are removed so much more easily and less painfully. The patient must receive careful personal care before being placed in the tub so that fecal contamination is minimal. Those in attendance should wear gowns and gloves until the wounds are healed. The patient should never be left unattended during this procedure because fainting and injury may occur.

Silver nitrate treatment. Although silver nitrate is being used less often than in the past, some physicians still prescribe it. In this treatment, thick gauze dressings are saturated with a 0.5% solution of silver nitrate, and the dressings are kept wet so that the solution remains in constant contact with burned surfaces. The purpose of these dressings is to retain moisture and heat and to reduce evaporation. The proponents of this method of treatment believe that it reduces mortality, lessens pain, eliminates odors, and has a bacteriostatic effect.[31,44] The dressings are removed every 12 or 24 hours and the patient is placed in a bath of salt solution with the temperature carefully maintained at the same level as the body. When skin grafts are applied, silver nitrate dressings are placed over the graft and donor sites on the first postoperative day. Because the silver nitrate solution is hypotonic, electrolytes are lost into the wound. Therefore, throughout treatment, frequent determinations of blood sodium levels are necessary, and sodium that is lost may need to be replaced.

Isolation technique is not required when the burn is treated with silver nitrate dressings, but clean dressings and sterile gloves and instruments are used. Because everything that comes in contact with the silver nitrate solution is stained black, the nurse wears a gown and gloves when applying the solution to protect skin, nails, and clothing. Although linen can be specially treated to remove stains, great care must be taken to prevent splashing the solution on the furniture, walls, and floors.[28]

Skin grafts. Skin grafts are applied to cover the burn wound and speed healing, to prevent contractures from occurring, and to shorten convalescence. Successful grafting reduces the patient's vulnerability to infection and prevents the loss of body heat and water vapor from the open wound or eschar. Most skin grafts are applied between the fifth and twenty-first day after the initial injury, depending on the depth and extent of the burn and the condition of the base. Small areas of third-degree burns such as those that occur on the dorsum of the hand may be excised and skin grafted during the first 24 to 48 hours to hasten healing and to help restore function more quickly. The wound is prepared for the graft as described on p. 235.

Split-thickness grafts usually are used. These grafts include the upper layer of the skin and part of the under layer but are not taken so deep as to prevent regeneration of the skin at the site from which they were taken (donor site). They grow as normal skin on the burned areas (recipient sites). These grafts are removed with a dermatome from almost any unburned part of the body. They may be removed in strips or small squares (postage stamps) (Fig. 29-10). Another type of split-thickness graft is

the *mesh graft,* which is used when few donor sites are available and there are large areas of burned body surface to be covered. The graft is removed with a dermatome and then meshed with a special instrument. The meshing of the graft makes it more distensible and thus it can be used to cover wider areas of the body surface (Fig. 29-11). Grafts may

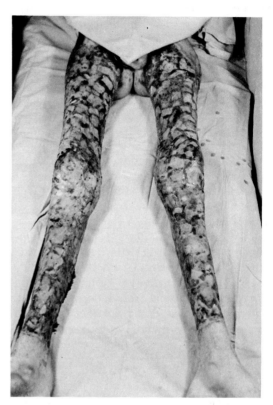

FIG. 29-10. Postage stamp grafts have been cut from split-thickness graft and have been used to partially cover large burned areas on lower limbs. (From Artz, C. P., and Reiss, E.: The treatment of burns, Philadelphia, 1957, W. B. Saunders Co.)

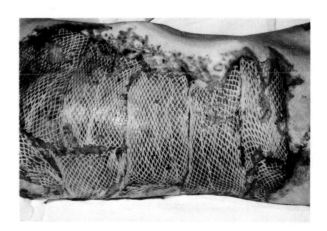

FIG. 29-11. Mesh graft covering a full-thickness burn. (Courtesy Burn Unit, Cook County Hospital, Chicago, Ill.)

be laid on the burn wounds and held in place with dressings or sutured into place and left exposed. Pressure dressings may be applied to secure the graft, provide even compression, and act as a splint. If the loss of skin is so great that life is threatened, the skin of other persons, that of recently deceased persons, or stored postmortem skin is taken to cover burned surfaces (homografts). The use of homografts helps to limit infection and loss of water, electrolytes, and protein and helps to reduce pain in the burn wound. Homografts may survive 4 or 5 weeks before being rejected, but they usually are needed only about 10 days if applied to cover a large granulating wound.[3]

The donor site, which presents an oozing, painful surface, may be covered with sterile gauze and a pressure dressing (Fig. 12-4) or it may be covered with a fine mesh gauze and left exposed to the air. The drainage from the wound dries and serves as a protective covering. The wound usually heals within 2 weeks. Many patients complain of quite severe pain in the donor site, and the nurse should not hesitate to give medications that are ordered for pain. The pain should subside within a day or two. Sometimes an odor develops from dead tissue at either the donor site or the recipient site, which is distressing to the patient, and should be reported to the physician. If infection has developed, antibiotics may be administered and the wound treated with wet dressings.

Heterografts of materials such as pigskin or a synthetic substitute are being used commonly to provide temporary protection to wounds, reduce pain, promote granulation, and reduce surface bacterial count.

Nutrition

To meet the increased metabolic needs, to maintain the patient's nutritional state, and to repair and replace tissue destroyed or injured by the burn, the protein, fluid, and vitamin and mineral intake must be increased as well as the total caloric intake. The actual caloric and protein needs of the burned patient are highly variable, depending on the extent and depth of the injury. A diet containing 1.6 to 4 Gm. of protein/kg. of body weight is required to replace nitrogen losses, and 45 to 85 calories/kg./day is desirable.[2] The caloric requirement for children usually is estimated as follows: for children up to 1 year, 100 calories/kg. of body weight; for children from 1 to 3 years of age, 90 calories/kg. of body weight; and for children between 4 and 12 years of age, 70 calories/kg. of body weight.[37] Supplemental vitamins, particularly ascorbic acid to aid in wound healing and vitamin B complex to meet the increased metabolic needs, also are required as well as iron preparations such as ferrous gluconate. Depending on the extent of the burned area and serum electrolyte levels, sodium chloride, potassium, and calci-

um preparations also may be administered intravenously or orally.

The patient who is burned may have nausea and vomiting to such an extent that nutrition must be provided entirely by the intravenous route. Paralytic ileus also may occur, and peristaltic action may be absent for a few days. Food and fluids are withheld until peristalsis returns. A solution containing 3 to 4 Gm. ($1^1/_2$ teaspoons) of table salt and 1.5 to 2 Gm. ($^1/_2$ teaspoon) of sodium bicarbonate in 1,000 ml. (1 quart) of water (Haldane's solution) flavored with lemon juice and chilled can often be retained when other fluids would be vomited. It supplies electrolytes as well as fluid. Carbonated beverages are also an acceptable means of supplying some necessary electrolytes as well as sugar. Sodium citrate (packaged in envelopes) to be added to water has been stockpiled for use in treating severely burned patients in the event of a major disaster. Salty solutions such as meat broths often are given to help replace sodium chloride that is lost into the tissues and in wound exudate, but broths or fruit juices that contain potassium are withheld for 48 hours or until the serum potassium levels go down.

The diet is advanced as quickly as possible to a regular one but, because of the patient's poor appetite, the utmost imagination and ingenuity on the part of the dietitian and the nurse are needed to motivate the patient to eat what he needs. Sometimes relatives are helpful in suggesting favorite foods, and the patient's knowledge that special preparations are being made in the hospital may encourage him to take more food. If the patient is able to feed himself, his appetite may improve. It is important that painful and disagreeable changes of dressings and other treatments be timed so that they do not immediately precede meals.

The high-protein powdered milk preparations are valuable in increasing the amount of protein taken and often seem to leave the patient with less of a feeling of oversatiation than may result from large servings of meats that are often high in fat. They are also valuable because the very ill patient can take fluids more easily than he can chew and swallow solid foods.

Bulk foods and fruit juices must be stressed in the diet of the severely burned patient because they aid in elimination. Fecal impaction is a common problem for burn patients. Bulk-forming laxatives such as preparations of the psyllium seed (Metamucil) may be given, or a fecal softener such as dioctyl sodium sulfosuccinate (Colace) may be ordered.

Prevention of contractures

Contractures are among the most serious long-term complications of burns. Two major types of contractures occur—those caused by muscle and joint stiffening and those occurring after skin grafting. Many patients must undergo painful reconstructive surgery as a part of rehabilitation, which would not have been necessary if those in attendance had been alert to the prevention of contractures. A large responsibility for the prevention of contractures rests with the nurse, who is with the patient more than anyone else. Nursing care should be planned so that the patient's position is changed regularly during the day and night. Early skin grafting prevents many contractures by mobilizing the patient sometimes months earlier than would otherwise be possible.

Burned patients often have severe pain as healing progresses. They are anemic, debilitated, and very often in a state of depression. The nurse must never let sympathy for the patient interfere with concern for his ultimate good. The patient must be helped to maintain range of joint motion and thus prevent scars from healing in positions that will result in deformity. It is important that he understand why ambulation or motion is necessary even though it may be painful. Since normal skin and normal tissues grow while scar tissue shrinks, children are more likely to develop deformities than adults, and what begins as a minor deformity in childhood may become a major one with increased growth.

For a definite interval of time each day, patients with burns should lie prone and also flat on their backs with no pillow or elevation of the head of the bed. This can be accomplished more easily if the patient is placed on a Stryker frame, a Foster bed, or a CircOlectric bed. Prolonged rest in a semi-Fowler's position or with the pillow pushing the head forward must be avoided. Many patients like this position because it enables them to see about the room better. The resourceful nurse can often turn the bed so that the patient can look about without having to assume positions that may lead to the formation of contractures. It is often advisable to change the bedside table from one side of the bed to the other at intervals. Mirrors help these patients keep in better touch with their environment, provided that viewing disfiguring burns on the face can be avoided.

If burns have been sustained about the neck, chin, and face, the patient should always lie in a position of hyperextension of the neck for most of each day. A pillow may be placed under his shoulders and the bed lowered to a level position. Facial exercises are encouraged to prevent scars from tightening as they form. Chewing gum and blowing balloons provide exercise that helps to prevent facial contractures.

Burns on the hands can easily result in contractures unless the part is kept in a position of hyperextension. If the patient has only one hand burned, he can be taught to exercise it, using his unaffected hand. Tight scarring in the axilla may be prevented by bandaging the arm loosely to the head of the bed

in a position of external rotation. Splints and shell casts may be used to prevent contractures of knees and plantar flexion deformity of the foot. These deformities can result from poor position during sleeping hours.

Exercises for prevention and correction of contractures are begun as soon as the patient's vital signs are stable. Supervision by a physical therapist is desirable. When burns are completely covered (by healing or graft), exercises may be performed more easily in an occupational therapy or physical therapy department where the patient also may benefit from a change in environment. In the department of physical medicine, exercises often are done in water. A Hubbard tank may be used for this purpose (Fig. 29-12). The occupational therapist may help the patient to improve his range of motion in a satisfying and efficient fashion by teaching him functional activities of daily living and crafts suitable for his particular needs such as typing, weaving, or a host of other activities. The nurse must know what the patient is being taught by the physical therapist and the occupational therapist so that progress can be continued when he returns to his room.

The patient who is not hospitalized and the one who returns home early because of skin grafting needs instruction in how to prevent contractures from developing. Contracture clinics are available for burn patients and are associated with some burn centers. If public health nursing services are available, a physical therapist or occupational therapist may be called on to assist the patient at home. If this service is not available, the nurse in the hospital or the public health nurse may have to take responsibility for teaching the patient how he may prevent contractures from developing.

Special beds to facilitate care

Stryker frames, Foster beds, and CircOlectric beds are used in the care of some severely burned patients, since they facilitate the use of the bedpan and urinal, permit change of position with a minimum of handling, and permit larger skin surfaces to remain free from body pressure than is possible when the patient lies in bed. These special beds are particularly useful when both back and front of the trunk, thighs, and legs have been burned. They allow turning of the patient with a minimum of handling and thus help to decrease pain (Fig. 29-13). A regular schedule for turning the patient must be established to prevent thrombophlebitis, emboli, contractures, and decubiti. (For details of use of these beds, see textbooks on orthopedic nursing.)

Emotional aspects of care

The emotional impact of severe burns is enormous and reality based. During the first few days the patient is too ill to fully comprehend what has hap-

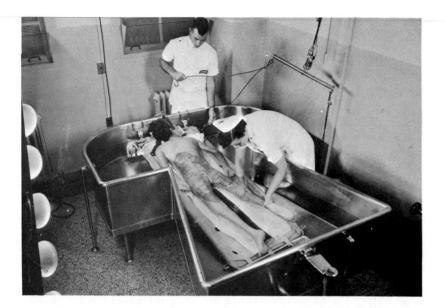

FIG. 29-12. If the burn has healed sufficiently, the patient may be placed in a Hubbard tank, where exercises are done more easily under water. (From Artz, C. P., and Reiss, E.: The treatment of burns, Philadelphia, 1957, W. B. Saunders Co.)

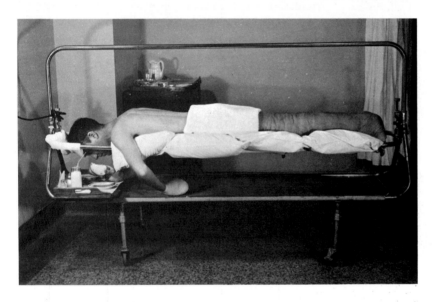

FIG. 29-13. Stryker frames are used in the care of some severely burned patients since they facilitate turning and caring for the patient. (From Artz, C. P., and Reiss, E.: The treatment of burns, Philadelphia, 1957, W. B. Saunders Co.)

pened. He fears he may not survive. Fear of death is a major concern.[21] Then comes the long healing period and the realization of endless implications. The patient's reaction is determined by his own personality makeup, by his degree of total adjustment to life, and by the extent and location of the burns. Burns on the face make adjustment particularly difficult. All kinds of fears arise to harrass the patient. "Will my husband (or wife) still care for me? Can I ever let my children see me?" To the adolescent, the thought of being different or conspicuous may be unbearable. Fears about not being taken back on the job often haunt the wage earner who is badly burned. If possible, the patient should not see facial burns until a good deal of healing has taken place or until skin grafting has been performed. The patient will exhibit readiness by asking to look in the mirror. Interaction with other burned patients who are fur-

ther along in their healing process may help the patient feel that he, too, will recover. In some instances, the recovery is incredible, and although differences in skin pigmentation remain, the redness that accompanies burns and newly healed skin often fades considerably within a few months. Pigmentation problems are more acute for persons with brown or black skin. Their skin may be a different shade, freckled, or whitish in color.

Patients who are severely burned usually are exhausted and often demoralized by the pain, treatment, and frequent dressing changes. Anticipation of painful procedures may frighten the patient. Diazepam (Valium) may be helpful in decreasing anxiety and providing muscle relaxation. The pain can be minimized in many instances by giving medication before the dressings and treatments are scheduled, explaining the necessity of the procedure to the patient and gaining his cooperation, using careful technique, and permitting the patient to participate in the treatment whenever possible. Depending on the age of the patient and the extent of the burn, television, games, puzzles, weaving, and painting may distract him from the pain and also provide occupational therapy.

Clinical observation indicates that the burned individual experiences concern about changes in his appearance and its effect on those about him. Since the skin, peripheral blood vessels, and lymph vessels are damaged, the burned patient's sense of body boundary probably is altered. Patients undergoing debridement following loosening of burn eschar describe sensations of having their skin torn away from them. It has been asserted that persons who perceive their body boundaries as being well-defined tend to be more confident and have higher goal and task completion drives. It is therefore possible that those who lose a part of that sense of definiteness will tend to take a more languid approach to life with less successful interactions with others.[40]

The patient should have an opportunity to talk about his problems and fears. He may discuss these with the nurse when he cannot express them to relatives, and the nurse must be prepared to listen and help him accept necessary changes in his life-style. (See current literature for further discussion.[40,41]) Almost every burned patient needs the help of the social worker for himself and for his family. The nurse should recognize this need and initiate the referral. Visiting hours can be used to talk with relatives who may be able to give information that will clarify the patient's needs and resources. This time also provides opportunity for the nurse to help relatives and friends accept their loved one's change in appearance and to help them plan for his return to the community.

Rehabilitation

Complete recovery and rehabilitation of the severely burned patient is a long and costly process. Many industries have compensation insurance to cover part of the cost, and the patient should be encouraged to discuss his financial problem with his physician and with the social worker if one is available. If the patient is under 21 years of age, he will be eligible for care financed in part by the Office of Child Development (formerly the Children's Bureau) through its aid to states for their programs for crippled children. This care will cover surgical procedures and care, special rehabilitative services, and social service.

Patients who have been burned should have medical checkups at regular intervals indefinitely and should be advised to report any unusual change in the burn scar at once. There is a fairly high frequency of malignant degeneration of scar tissue following burns. This is particularly true when the burn is caused by electricity or by x-rays.

Comprehensive team approach

Comprehensive care of the burn patient can best be provided by a multidisciplinary team approach. This is a desirable method designed to meet the complex and varied needs of the patient. The nurse's role in the team is to coordinate the interactions of the various disciplines and to incorporate the team's suggestions and approaches into an effective plan of care. Because this type of care is most likely to be available in specialized burn units and centers, patients are frequently moved to these units when it is safe to transport them. When such specialized care is not available, the nurse may be able to serve as a catalyst and suggest the active involvement of as many disciplines as are available in the care of the patient.

REFERENCES AND SELECTED READINGS*

1 *Andreasen, N. J. C., and others: Management of emotional reactions in seriously burned adults, N. Engl. J. Med. **286:**65-69, Jan. 1972.
2 *Artz, C. P., editor: The burn patient, Nurs. Forum **4**(3):87-92, 1965.
3 Artz, C. P., and Moncrief, J. A.: The treatment of burns, ed. 2, Philadelphia, 1969, W. B. Saunders Co.
4 Artz, C. P., and Reiss, E.: The treatment of burns, Philadelphia, 1957, W. B. Saunders Co.
5 Artz, C. P., and Yarbourgh, D. R., III: Major body burn, J.A.M.A. **223:**1355-1357, March 1973.
6 Beal, J. M., and Echenhoff, J. E.: Intensive and recovery room care, London, 1969, Macmillan Publishing Co., Inc.
7 Blocker, T. G., Breen, D. B., and Lung, R. G.: Burns. In Meltzer, L. E., Abdellah, F. G., and Kitchell, J. R., editors: Con-

cepts and practices of intensive care for nurse specialists, Philadelphia, 1969, The Charles Press, Publishers.
8 Boswick, J. A.: Symposium on surgery of burns, Surg. Clin. North Am. **50:**1191-1446, Dec. 1970.
9 *Boswick, J. A., and Stone, N. H.: Methods and materials in managing the severely burned patient, Surg. Clin. North Am. **48:**177-190, Feb. 1968.
10 Boswick, J. A., and Stone, N.: The planning of patient care in a hospital burn unit, Surg. Clin. North Am. **50:**275-283, Feb. 1970.
11 Bowden, M. L., and Feller, I.: Family reaction to a severe burn, Am. J. Nurs. **73:**316-319, Feb. 1973.
12 Brentano, L., and others: Bacteriology of large human burns treated with silver nitrate, Arch. Surg. **93:**456-466, Sept. 1966.
13 Burke, J. F.: Treatment of burn infection, Mod. Treat. **3:**1129-1135, Sept. 1966.
14 Burned children, infection, and nursing care, Nurs. Clin. North Am. **5:**131-142, March 1970.

*References preceded by an asterisk are particularly well suited for student reading.

15 Castillo, J.: Treatment of thermal injuries, Surg. Clin. North Am. **53**:627-637, June 1973.

16 Cockshott, W. P.: The history of the treatment of burns, Surg. Gynecol. Obstet. **102**:116-124, Jan. 1956.

17 Current nursing care of the burned patient, Nurs. Clin. North Am. **5**:563-575, Dec. 1970.

18 *Farmer, A. W.: Management of burns in children, Pediatrics **25**:886-895, May 1960.

19 *Feller, I., and Archambeault, C.: Nursing the burned patient, Ann Arbor, Mich., 1973, Institute for Burn Medicine Press.

20 Fox, C. L., and others: Control of Pseudomonas infection in burns by silver sulfadiazine, Surg. Gynecol. Obstet. **128**:1021-1026, May 1969.

21 Hamburg, D., and others: Clinical importance of emotional problems in care of patients with burns, N. Engl. J. Med. **248**:355-359, Feb. 1953.

22 Harper, H.: Nutritional aspects of the burned patient, Plast. Reconstr. Surg. **21**:389-392, May 1958.

23 Hartford, C. E.: The early treatment of burns, Nurs. Clin. North Am. **8**:447-455, Sept. 1973.

24 Haynes, B. W., Jr., and Hench, M. E.: Hospital isolation system for preventing cross-contamination by staphylococcal and Pseudomonas organisms in burn wounds, Ann. Surg. **162**:641-649, Oct. 1965.

25 Hummel, R. P., and others: Topical and systemic antibacterial agents in the treatment of burns, Ann. Surg. **172**:370-383, July-Dec. 1970.

26 Jacoby, F. G.: Nursing care of the patient with burns, St. Louis, 1972, The C. V. Mosby Co.

27 Korlof, B.: Social and economic consequences of deep burns. In Wallace, A. B., and Wilkinson, A. W., editors: Second international congress on research in burns, Edinburgh, 1966, E. & S. Livingstone.

27a *Kunsman, J.: Nursing care after primary excision, R.N. **37**:25-26, Aug. 1974.

28 *Maxwell, P., and others: Routines on the burn ward, Am. J. Nurs. **66**:522-525, March 1966.

29 *Minckley, B. B.: Expert nursing care for burned patients, Am. J. Nurs. **70**:1888-1893, Sept. 1970.

30 *Moncrief, J. A.: Burns, N. Engl. J. Med. **288**:444-454, March 1973.

31 Moyer, C. A., and others: Surgery, principles and practice, ed. 3, Philadelphia, 1965, J. B. Lippincott Co.

32 Nelson, W. E.: Textbook of pediatrics, ed. 9, Philadelphia, 1969, W. B. Saunders Co.

33 Noonan, J., and Noonan, L.: Two burned patients in flotation therapy, Am. J. Nurs. **68**:316-319, Feb. 1968.

34 *Quinly, S., and others: Identity problems and the adaptation of nurses to severely burned children, Am. J. Psychiatry **128**:58-63, July 1971.

35 Rittenbury, M., and others: Probit analysis of burn mortality in 1,831 patients, Ann. Surg. **164**:123-138, July 1966.

36 Sabiston, D. C., editor: Christopher's textbook of surgery, ed. 10, Philadelphia, 1972, W. B. Saunders Co.

36a *Sheehy, E.: Primary excision: innovation in pediatric burn care, R.N. **37**:21-25, Aug. 1974.

37 Silver, H. K., and others: Handbook of pediatrics, ed. 8, Los Altos, Calif., 1969, Lange Medical Publications.

38 Smith, C. A., editor: The critically ill child, Philadelphia, 1972, W. B. Saunders Co.

39 Stone, N. H., editor: Profiles of burn management, Miami, Florida, 1969, Industrial Medicine Publishing Co., Inc. (Reprinted from Industrial Medicine and Surgery, Aug.-Dec. 1968.)

40 Williams, B. P.: The problems and life-style of a severely burned man. In Bergersen, B., and others, editors: Current concepts in clinical nursing, vol. 2, St. Louis, 1969, The C. V. Mosby Co.

41 *Williams, B. P.: Life-styles of severely burned men, Clinical Sessions ANA (1969), New York, 1970, Appleton-Century-Crofts.

42 *Williams, B. P.: The burned patient's need for teaching, Nurs. Clin. North Am. **6**:615-639, Dec. 1971.

43 Williams, S. R.: Nutrition and diet therapy, ed. 2, St. Louis, 1973, The C. V. Mosby Co.

44 *Wood, M., and others: Silver nitrate treatment of burns and nursing care, Am. J. Nurs. **66**:518-527, March 1966.

30 Diseases of the breast

■ The most common diseases of the breast are dysplasia (fibrocystic disease), carcinoma, and fibroadenoma. These conditions occur almost entirely in women. Carcinoma requires the most extensive nursing care and will be discussed in some detail before the other two.

■ CARCINOMA OF THE BREAST

Nurses play a vital role in regard to carcinoma of the breast. Their responsibilities include educating women so that breast cancer may be discovered and treated early, caring for the patient who has had a cancerous breast removed and assisting with physical and emotional rehabilitation, and helping the patient and her family in the home or in the hospital when the lesion is inoperable or when metastasis has occurred.

Incidence, etiology, and prognosis

Carcinoma of the breast is the most common malignancy in women and it is also the leading cause of cancer death in women. In females ages 40 to 44 it is the leading cause of death. There were 29,969 reported deaths from breast cancer in 1971, the majority of the deaths occurring in women between ages 35 and 75.[2] It is estimated that 1 out of 15 women in the United States will develop carcinoma of the breast, with the probability increasing steadily with age. The American Cancer Society estimated that 90,000 new cases will be discovered in 1975 and that 33,000 women will die from the disease.[2] The mortality rate for cancer of the breast in the United States has remained about the same for the past 35 years, with the rate fixed at 24 to 25/100,000.[2] Unfortunately the present 5-year survival rate for all patients with cancer of the breast, whether treated or untreated, is approximately 50%. This low survival rate is due in part to the frequent failure to detect the lesion before regional involvement occurs and failure to seek medical treatment as soon as a lesion is discovered. Studies show that approximately 83% of all women treated when the lesion appears localized have a 5-year life expectancy, compared with 52% for those with obvious regional involvement at the time of treatment.[2] However, survival at the end of 5 years cannot be considered synonymous with cure. Many women who are treated before regional involvement is apparent die of the disease after 5 years, and the 10-year survival rate for these patients is only 33.4%.[47]

Although carcinoma of the breast occurs in young women, it most often immediately precedes or follows the menopause and also develops in those past the climacteric. Most tumors of the breast in women past the menopause are malignant. Benign fibroadenomas occur largely in younger women, and dysplasia (fibrocystic disease) in those between 30 years of age and the menopause.

Causes of carcinoma of the breast are not known. However, some studies have disclosed that it is found more often in women who have never married and in those who have a family history of breast cancer. A recent study indicates that among women with a family history of breast cancer, the risk is greater when there was premenopausal onset and/or bilateral disease than when the lesion developed after the menopause and/or was unilateral.[3] The

■ STUDY QUESTIONS

1 Review the anatomy of the breast and adjacent structures.
2 What are some of the psychologic reactions to be expected when a patient faces the loss of a breast?
3 Review the normal range of motion of the shoulder joint. Make a list of daily activities that involve the full use of this joint.
4 Review the procedure for self-examination of the breasts. Outline how you would teach the procedure to one woman or to a group of women.
5 Review the physiologic processes controlled by the hormones secreted by the ovaries, testicles, adrenal glands, and the anterior and posterior lobes of the pituitary gland. What are the effects of insufficiency or excess of any of these hormones?

mortality rate for women who have never had children is 70% higher than that for women who have had children.

Although it had been thought that hormonal secretions had some relationship to the development of breast cancer, some studies now show that perhaps the estrogenic hormones and progesterone are prophylactic rather than causative factors. Individuals differ as to rate of growth and the probability of metastases, and this "genetic determination" can be an extremely important factor in controlling the outcome for the patient. It is believed that injury does not lead to breast cancer, although a lump in the breast is often discovered after a minor injury has been sustained, perhaps because the woman feels her breast at the time of injury and may note a mass that was already present. There is little evidence that dysplasia (fibrocystic disease) predisposes to the development of carcinoma, although the presence of this condition may make it much more difficult to diagnose an early carcinoma by palpation.

Prognosis in carcinoma of the breast depends to a great extent on early diagnosis, the type of cancer present (slow or fast growing), genetic determination, and complete surgical removal of all tissues containing malignant cells before metastasis occurs. It is estimated that approximately 40% of all patients who seek medical attention for cancer of the breast are incurable at the time of the initial examination. Since the disease develops in a relatively accessible part of the body, it is unfortunate that early diagnosis is not made more often so that more lives might be saved. At the present time the American Cancer Society still recommends removal of the entire breast (radical or modified radical mastectomy) as the surgical treatment for operable breast cancer.[2] They also believe that surgical procedures that remove less than the entire breast have not been scientifically proved to be as effective as mastectomy.

Early diagnosis

Carcinoma may develop anywhere in the breast or on the nipple, although the upper outer quadrant is the most commonly affected area. The early lesion may be discovered by careful inspection and palpation of the entire breast. Mammography is an x-ray technique now used to detect lesions before they are palpable (Fig. 30-1). Early cancers are often easily seen on the developed films as small densities with stippled calcifications within. It is about 80% to 97% accurate in detecting early breast carcinoma. However, mammography has limitations, particularly in the penetration of dense and heavy breasts.[35] Xeroradiography (Fig. 30-2) is a newer technique that is becoming more widely used. In xeroradiography an aluminum plate with an electrically charged selenium layer is used in the place of x-ray film and is exposed in the usual manner using special mammora-

diographic equipment. This technique, which is also known as xeromammography, is recommended for women (1) who have large breasts, (2) who have a family history of breast cancer, (3) who have questionable physical findings, and (4) who have had a mastectomy.[35]

An additional screening device is *thermography.* In this procedure an infrared scanner is used to measure the heat emissions coming from the breast. Abnormal variations in an area due to increased vascularization may indicate the presence of a neoplasm. Early detection of breast masses by using sound waves *(zerography* and *sonography)* is also being explored.

In an attempt to improve early detection the National Cancer Institute and the American Cancer Society have jointly funded the following 27 screening centers that provide free diagnostic services.

East

Guttman Institute, New York, N. Y.
College of Medicine and Dentistry, Newark, N. J.
University of Pittsburgh School of Medicine, Pittsburgh, Pa.
Temple University–Albert Einstein Medical Center, Philadelphia, Pa.
Wilmington General Hospital, Wilmington, Del.
Rhode Island Hospital, Providence, R. I.

South

University of Louisville School of Medicine, Louisville, Ky.
St. Vincent's Medical Center, Jacksonville, Fla.
Duke University Medical Center, Durham, N. C.
Emory University–Georgia Baptist Hospital, Atlanta, Ga.
Georgetown University Medical School, Washington, D. C.
Vanderbilt University School of Medicine, Nashville, Tenn.
St. Joseph's Hospital, Houston, Tex.

Midwest

University of Kansas Medical Center, Kansas City, Kan.
Medical College of Wisconsin, Milwaukee, Wis.
University of Cincinnati Medical Center, Cincinnati, Ohio
Iowa Lutheran Hospital, Des Moines, Ia.
University of Michigan Medical Center, Ann Arbor, Mich.
Cancer Research Center, Columbia, Mo.

West

University of Oklahoma Medical Research Foundation, Oklahoma City, Okla.
Mountain States Tumor Institute, Boise, Idaho
Virginia Mason Research Center, Seattle, Wash.
Samuel Merritt Hospital, Oakland, Calif.
Pacific Health Research Institute, Honolulu, Hawaii
University of Arizona Medical Center, Tucson, Ariz.
Los Angeles County, University of Southern California, Los Angeles, Calif.
Breast Cancer Screening Project, Portland, Ore.

Self-examination of the breasts. For years, physicians have been urging women to learn to examine their own breasts for lesions, since it is not practical to see a physician for these frequent, routine examinations. According to the American Cancer Society, about 95% of patients discover their cancers through

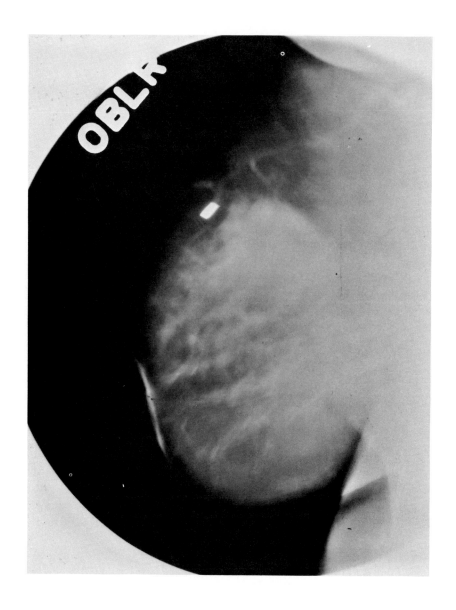

FIG. 30-1. Mammogram of patient with a diagnosis of medullary carcinoma. Main mass of lesion is just below white rectangular mark. "Comet" tails spread to the left and downward from mass. (Courtesy Charles Perlia, M.D., Presbyterian–St. Luke's Hospital, Chicago, Ill.)

breast self-examination. Unfortunately about 60% of these women have cancers that have already spread to the axillary lymph nodes.[2] However, the percentage of women who discover cancer before it has spread has increased since the 1940's and this is attributed, in part, to better education of the public. Authorities believe that a self-examination should be made at least once a month, although women over 30 years of age with a familial history of breast cancer should have a medical examination at least twice a year. All women should have a complete examination that includes palpation of the breasts at least once a year.

The nurse working in the hospital, in industry, in the clinic, in the physician's office, or in the community nursing agency has the responsibility of teaching women how to examine their breasts and of explaining why it is necessary. A movie prepared by the American Cancer Society describing one method of self-examination is available for loan from local chapters of the society. In most large cities the local committee of the American Cancer Society will arrange for showing the film to an audience of 50 or more. In smaller communities the film may sometimes be obtained through the local health department.

Self-examination of the breasts should be done regularly each month. The best time is at the conclusion of, or a few days following, the menstrual period. Some women have engorgement of the breast premenstrually, and the breasts may have a lumpy consistency at that time. This condition usually disappears a few days after the onset of menstruation, although occasionally lumpiness and tenderness may extend throughout the menstrual cycle. Because of this possible change, it is important that the breasts be examined at the same time each month in relation to the menstrual cycle. Women who have passed the menopause should examine their breasts on the same day each month. (See Fig. 30-3.)

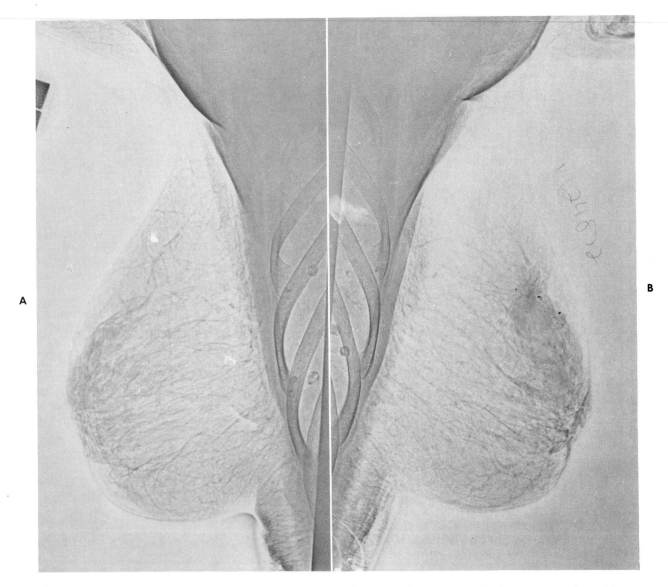

FIG. 30-2. Xeroradiography. **A,** Normal left breast. **B,** Right breast shows a mass in the upper portion with skin thickening and dimpling. The mass has spiculated margins characteristic of neoplasm. An incidental finding is a bone lesion in the right humerus. (Courtesy University Hospitals of Cleveland, Cleveland, Ohio.)

Self-examination of the breasts, as outlined by the American Cancer Society,* should include the following steps:

Step 1. Sit straight before a mirror, arms relaxed at sides. Study the contour of the breasts. Has there been a change since the last examination?

Step 2. Raise the arms high above the head and observe whether there is any deviation from normal in size or shape of the breasts or abnormal puckering or dimpling of the skin.

Step 3. Lie down, place folded towel under shoulder, and raise arm above head on the side being examined. With flat of the fingers, feel gently the inner half of the breast.

Step 4. Bring the arm down to side and feel gently the outer half of the breast, giving special attention to the upper outer section. Examine the other breast in the same way.

Some women need help in learning self-examination; they may, for example, feel a rib when examining the lower half of the breast and become alarmed. However, most women learn quite readily. If a lump of any kind is discovered, it should not be rubbed or touched excessively. It should be left alone, and the advice of a physician should be sought at once.

Nurses who wish further information on how to perform a breast examination are referred to an article written by the American Cancer Society, Inc.[2a]

Signs and symptoms. The only early sign of carcinoma of the breast is a small palpable mass. Pain is

---

*Leaflets on self-examination of the breasts are available free of charge from local chapters of the American Cancer Society, Inc., for distribution to all women.

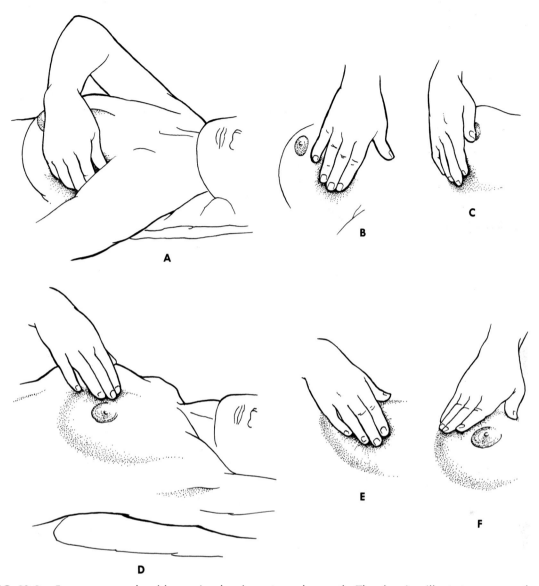

FIG. 30-3. Every woman should examine her breasts each month. The drawing illustrates one method.

seldom a symptom of early cancer. Dimpling of the skin (orange rind appearance) over a hard lump, puckering of the skin, changes in the color of the skin over the lesion, alteration of contour of the breast, distortion of the nipple, serous or bloody discharge from the nipple, and unusual scaling or inversion of the nipple are signs that the lesion is well established and has invaded surrounding tissues. In the advanced phases of neglected cases there may be ulceration of the skin, with subsequent infection of necrotic tissue. Spread to the axillary lymph nodes occurs early. Because of the distribution of the lymph vessels and because there are no lymph nodes between the two breasts to delay spread of malignant cells, these carcinomatous cells may spread rapidly through the lymph vessels with metastasis occurring in the opposite breast and in the mediastinum. Sometimes discovery of enlarged lymph

nodes or pain in the ribs or vertebrae is the first indication to the patient that anything is wrong, particularly when the lesion is deep in the breast tissue and routine palpation of the breast has not been carried out.

Paget's disease of the breast is a condition in which a lesion begins in the duct close to the nipple and rapidly invades the skin of the nipple and areola, progressing to bleeding and ulceration of these areas. Treatment is mastectomy as soon as a diagnosis is established.

Fear of diagnosis. The woman who finds a lump in her breast should not become panicky and decide that she has cancer. Most lumps in the breast are not malignant, and 65% to 80% are found to be benign on biopsy. Women should know that there are other causes for a mass in the breast besides cancer. The lump may be caused by a benign tumor or by a cyst; only the physician can determine this. All women should know that a malignant tumor in the breast does not, as a rule, cause pain. Tenderness in a mass in the breast usually suggests dysplasia (fibrocystic disease).

Women should be taught that the prognosis for cancer of the breast is likely to be much better *if the cancer is discovered early and treatment instituted immediately*. Although 95% of all breast cancers are discovered by self-examination, many are not reported for several months. Fear of mutilation or of death are the two main reasons why some women delay seeking medical advice and treatment and hesitate to risk confirmation of their fears when a tumor is discovered. National statistics on deaths from cancer of the breast are widely publicized, and, as a result, many women fear the disease and delay seeking medical help. Also, some women have had a relative or a friend who died from the disease, which causes the fear to be even more acute. Unfortunately the average woman may tell only her closest friends when a breast has been successfully removed for cancer. As a result, deaths from the disease are much better known than cures by surgery with no recurrence. Some women wish to avoid the expense or embarrassment of an examination, or they rationalize that their trouble would appear trivial to the busy physician. Sometimes they seek the advice of nurses. It then becomes the responsibility of the nurse to stress the urgency of getting medical advice at once.

It will be interesting to see if women will be less reluctant to perform self-examination of their breasts and seek medical advice concerning lumps in the breast now that carcinoma of the breast has received such widespread publicity in the United States.

Management

The only way to determine conclusively whether a tumor is benign or malignant is by microscopic examination of a section of the tumor obtained by biopsy. When axillary lymph nodes can be felt, the diagnosis of malignancy can be made with relative certainty before the operation, and an axillary node may be excised for microscopic study. Most surgeons believe that if there is the slightest possibility of cancer, it is safer to remove the entire mass rather than risk permitting a malignant tumor to remain. Pieces of a tumor are seldom removed surgically because there is danger of releasing malignant cells into the blood and lymphatic systems at the time of the operation.

Emotional preparation. In our culture the breasts have become a primary source of women's identification with femininity. Since much emphasis is placed on the female breast as a symbol of attractiveness, the thought of losing a breast becomes almost intolerable to many women. This is particularly true of those who depend largely on physical attractiveness to hold the esteem of others and to secure gratification of their emotional needs. Psychologists have pointed out that there is a symbolic connection between the breasts and motherhood that is severely threatened when a breast must be removed.[37] All women, including single women and those past the menopause, are seriously threatened emotionally by the loss of a part of the body that is so closely associated with sexual attractiveness and motherliness. Carcinoma of the breast often occurs at the menopause or soon after when some women feel that they have lost much of their sexual attractiveness. Surgical removal of the breast may save a woman's life, but it also may cause her to feel less feminine.

Although she may try to conceal fear, any woman who is hospitalized for removal of a breast tumor is always worried. The surgeon usually discusses the diagnosis and treatment with the patient and sometimes with her family. He frequently talks over the implications of this kind of surgery with the patient's husband, whose attitude and behavior are particularly important to the married woman; the husband can often help her accept surgery and his support is necessary in her future rehabilitation. If it seems that the patient does not fully comprehend the surgeon's explanation, the nurse should report this to the surgeon, who in turn can talk with the patient again and clarify any misconceptions, hopefully alleviating needless anxiety.

The woman who is having breast surgery has a special need to feel understood and accepted by all persons who are giving preoperative care. The nurse can help the patient to express feelings and can help her to understand what breast surgery means to her as a person. Simple explanations may decrease the patient's fear of the unknown. Some patients benefit from a concise discussion of breast prostheses, while the greatest need of others may be for someone to listen as they express feelings about the loss of a breast or the possible loss of life.

The American Cancer Society is sponsoring a volunteer program, "Reach to Recovery," in which the patient has an opportunity to visit with a woman who has had a mastectomy. This encourages the patient, and she will receive practical help from someone who has made a satisfactory adjustment to the same operation.

Preoperative care. The preparation for surgery is similar to that discussed in Chapter 11. If a diagnosis of a malignancy is almost a certainty, x-ray examinations such as a bone survey and liver function studies may be ordered to rule out the possibility of metastases to these areas of the body. Preparing the patient for certain procedures that will take place before and after surgery is of utmost importance in allaying her fears as well as in setting the stage for successful rehabilitation. Should a radical mastectomy be indicated, the patient can be prepared for what she will experience *postoperatively.* She should be told that a dressing may or may not be applied to the incision or that a catheter attached to suction may be used. She should also be told when she will be able to move her arm and whether it will need to be elevated. She should know that she will probably be able to get out of bed the day after the operation. She should know that, if the breast is removed, there will be a tendency for her shoulder to droop on the opposite side because of the inequality of weight and that it can be prevented by close attention to posture. Poor posture may give more evidence that a breast has been removed than will a slight inequality in the breast contours. While padding and prosthetic devices are used to take the place of the breast and restore normal contours to the upper body, stooped, awkward posture cannot be hidden. Exercises that will strengthen muscles and help to improve posture should be discussed with the patient before surgery. Telling the patient about the exercises helps to give her the feeling that there is something in the situation that she can control and contribute to and thus aids in a positive attitude toward rehabilitation.

The operation. At the time of surgery the tumor is removed and a frozen section of the tissue is examined under the microscope. If the tumor is malignant, the first incision is closed. Drapes, instruments, and gloves are changed to help prevent spread of cancer cells, and the more extensive operation is then performed.

If there are no gross signs of extension of the carcinoma, the entire breast, the pectoral muscles, the axillary lymph nodes, and all fat, fascia, and adjacent tissues are removed in one piece. This is a *radical mastectomy.* The judgment of the surgeon regarding the amount of overlying skin that can safely be left to cover the defect determines whether or not a skin graft is to be done. Preoperatively the surgeon may order the skin of the anterior surface of a thigh shaved and prepared surgically in case need for a graft should arise. If the lesion is located in the medial quadrant of the breast, particularly the upper medial quadrant, an *extended radical mastectomy* may be performed to include removal of the parasternal lymph nodes. Lesions in the medial quadrants tend to metastasize to the internal mammary chain of lymph nodes. The nodes may be exposed by splitting the sternum or by dividing the costal cartilages of the second through the fifth ribs. Results of the 5-year survival rate following this procedure are promising but inconclusive at this time. A *modified radical mastectomy* is now often performed for early, well-localized, small lesions of the breast. Removal of the breast and axillary contents, sparing the pectoral muscles, appears to be as curative as the clas-sic radical mastectomy. It cannot, however, remove all lymphatic tissue as well. A *simple mastectomy* (removal of breast tissue without lymph node dissection) sometimes is performed if cancer is believed to be limited to the breast or as a palliative measure to remove an ulcerated carcinoma of the breast in disease that is known to be advanced.

Following removal of the breast and adjacent tissue, a stab wound may be made near the axilla and a catheter inserted and attached to negative suction. Its purpose is to remove blood and serum that may collect under the skin flap, preventing healing and predisposing to infection. There usually is very little drainage from the incision when a catheter is inserted, and a dressing is not always necessary. At one time pressure dressings, rather than a catheter, were commonly used to help prevent the accumulation of fluid under the skin. However, many surgeons now believe that the use of a catheter and a smaller dressing is preferable to the use of a large pressure dressing.

Recently there has been considerable discussion in lay periodicals and in medical journals about the surgical treatment of carcinoma of the breast. In some articles it is suggested that the removal of a lump *(lumpectomy, tylectomy)* is sufficient to treat some carcinomas of the breast and that a mastectomy is not necessary. However, as already mentioned, the American Cancer Society believes that the public should understand that mastectomy is still the recommended treatment and offers the best course of 5-year survival when diagnosis and treatment are made early.[2]

Postoperative care. The operative site should be inspected to determine whether a pressure dressing or a catheter and no dressing is being used. If a catheter is present, it should be attached to negative suction as ordered. Often this is done either in the operating room or in the recovery room. When the patient is returned to the postoperative unit, the catheter and suction should be checked to see that they are working properly. Sometimes a small portable suction unit (Hemovac) is attached to the catheter in the operating room so that constant suction is maintained while the patient is being transported to her room. (See Fig. 23-13.) This unit should be emptied in accordance with specific directions of the manufacturer because the pressure becomes equal to that in the wound if not properly emptied and this prevents further drainage. If the wound is draining properly, fluid will not collect under the skin. The nurse should inspect the wound for swelling if it is not covered with a dressing. Since a dressing may become tight as fluid collects, any swelling should be reported to the surgeon. The catheter usually may be clamped for periods of ambulation and it usually is removed within 3 to 5 days, depending on the amount of drainage. The catheter is commonly left in until the amount of drainage is less than 100 ml. in 24 hours.

The wound or the dressing should be checked often for the first few hours to detect hemorrhage or excessive serous oozing. The bedclothes under the patient must be examined for blood that may flow from the axillary region backward. Any evidence of bleeding should be reported to the surgeon. If the wound is not covered with a dressing, a cradle may be used to protect it from the bed covers. When pressure dressings are used, they should be checked to be certain that they do not hamper circulation. Signs of circulatory obstruction such as swelling and numbness of the lower arm or inability to move the fingers must be reported at once. The nurse, however, should never loosen dressings without specific instruction from the surgeon.

If a graft has been taken from the thigh, this area may be covered with a firm pressure dressing, or fine mesh gauze may be used and the wound exposed to the air. The patient may complain of severe discomfort in this donor site as soon as she reacts from anesthesia.

If dressings are applied over the breast area and the donor site, they usually are not changed for several days after the operation. The skin sutures closing the breast and axillary incision are often removed on the sixth to the eighth postoperative day.

The patient must be encouraged to take deep breaths and to cough deeply at frequent intervals since this helps to prevent congestion in the lungs. The patient may complain of a feeling of constriction over the chest that is painful, causing her to take short, shallow breaths. Supporting the area next to the wound while the patient breathes deeply or coughs may lessen the pain (Fig. 22-16). If the pain is severe, a narcotic will be ordered to reduce the discomfort. Deep breathing and coughing must be done every few hours. Because the patient may be drowsy from sedation, it is best to remain with her to see that she takes deep breaths at specific intervals.

When the patient recovers from the effects of anesthesia, she usually is more comfortable lying on her back with her head elevated. If the arm on the operated side is not elevated, incorporated in the dressing, or supported by a sling, a pillow placed under the lower arm and elbow will help prevent muscle strain and edema. In order to prevent the development of edema of the hand and arm, the pillows should be arranged so that the hand is higher than the arm, and the arm should be above the level of the right atrium. A firm mattress will help to splint the chest wall and lessen pain when the patient moves. The patient may be more comfortable sitting up straight during back care, since turning toward the affected side may be exceedingly painful. A pull sheet or rope attached to the foot of the bed will help the patient to raise herself to a sitting position.

The patient should be encouraged to take fluids by mouth as soon as she has completely reacted from anesthesia. Her time of voiding postoperatively should be noted.

The patient usually is told by the surgeon that the breast was removed when she has recovered from the effects of anesthesia. It usually is her first question and she will try to determine the fact by feeling the dressing. Reactions such as crying, withdrawal, or anger are to be expected, and the nurse should respond with acceptance and understanding. Most patients are helped by a kind yet matter-of-fact attitude toward loss of the breast and by the assumption that there need be no change in their outward appearance or mode of living. After the patient is feeling better, mention of ways by which clothing can be adjusted to preserve normal contours often helps. The patient may be told that bathing suits and low-cut dresses can be worn without the incision being seen if it appears that this information will be of comfort.

Ambulation. The patient usually is allowed out of bed the day after a mastectomy. She needs help when she gets up to use the commode, to sit in a chair, or to walk about for the first time. She must be cautioned not to get out of bed without assistance until she learns to handle herself safely and until narcotics are given less frequently. Assistance should be given even when the patient can walk safely since the nurse should at this time encourage her in her progress and urge her to begin to check her posture regularly. The patient should try to relax the affected side and to use trunk and shoulder muscles to prevent inequality in height of her shoulders.

Arm exercises. Exercises are essential to prevent shortening of muscles and contracture of joints and to preserve muscle tone so that the affected arm can be used without limitations. To prevent additional deformities, exercises should be bilateral ones with the patient using both arms simultaneously. The surgeon decides when specific postoperative exercises should be started. This will depend on the extent of the operation and whether or not skin grafting has been necessary. The nurse should coordinate nursing efforts to help the patient with postoperative exercises with those of the surgeon and physical and occupational therapy departments and with full knowledge of how the mastectomy wound is healing. Usually the patient is encouraged to flex and extend her fingers immediately on return to her room. She should also be encouraged to pronate and supinate her forearm; simply turning the palm up and down will do this. The patient is usually encouraged to brush her hair, brush her teeth, or squeeze a rubber ball with the affected hand and arm on the first postoperative day to help stimulate circulation and restore function.

The nurse should explain to the patient why exercises are necessary and should encourage her to carry them out. It is best for the nurse and the patient to work out a schedule of specific exercises. Everyone finds it easier to follow routines that are well established and that are scheduled for specific times. An exercise routine also helps to keep the patient occupied and thus lessens postoperative depression that usually occurs a few days after surgery. Participation in classes with others who have undergone the same operation usually stimulates the patient to learn the prescribed exercises. As soon as possible, normal activities should take the place of exercises, provided the patient understands how particular exercises can be accomplished by specific tasks. Helpful exercises are suggested in a movie, "After Mastectomy," distributed by the American Cancer Society. The patient must know what motion is intended in each exercise. It is not enough simply to ask her to comb her own hair or to wash her own back. For example, the patient may brush her hair with the arm on the affected side, but she may lower her head and hunch her shoulders in such a way that she does not get normal use of the shoulder joint and attached muscles. The whole intent of the exercise may therefore be lost. A small handbook entitled *Reach to Recovery**is available for use by nurses in teaching patients and for distribution to patients. Smith[45] has outlined exercises for the patient who has had a mastectomy. These should be helpful to nurses in working out appropriate exercises for patients. The following list is only suggestive and is adapted primarily from the two sources just mentioned. All exercises should be done with good, normal standing or sitting posture. The patient should relax as much as possible and should try to develop a smooth rhythmic action. It helps to do as many exercises as possible in front of a mirror.

Care of the hair. This may be done first by resting the elbow on books placed on a small table and brushing only the front part of the hair on the affected side. The exercise should eventually include brushing the hair on the top of the head and doing upward sweeps on the back of the neck. It can include pinning curls in the nape of the neck if this was the patient's practice before surgery.

Climbing the wall (Fig. 30-4). This exercise is usually started while the patient is in the hospital. At home it helps if the patient places a mark on the wall so that each successive day's progress can be noted. (1) Stand with toes as close to the wall as possible and face the wall; (2) bend the elbows and place the palms of both hands against the wall at shoulder level; (3) work both hands parallel to each other up the wall as far as possible (eventually the arms should be completely extended with the elbows straight); (4) work the hands down to the starting position. Housework such

as reaching into high cupboards or closet shelves, hanging out clothes, washing windows, and dusting upper walls will accomplish this exercise.

Arm swinging (Fig. 30-5). This exercise should be started from the standing position with the feet well separated and the body straight. (1) Bend forward from the waist, permitting both arms to relax and fall naturally; (2) swing both arms together sideways, describing an arc as when sweeping (keep elbows straight and arms parallel). Another arm swinging exercise is as follows. (1) Bend forward from the waist, permitting both arms to relax and fall naturally; (2) swing the right arm forward and the left arm backward; (3) swing the left arm forward and the right arm backward.

Attaching a rope (a jump rope is good) to a door knob and twirling it with a rotary motion alternately in one direction and then in the other, using first the affected arm and

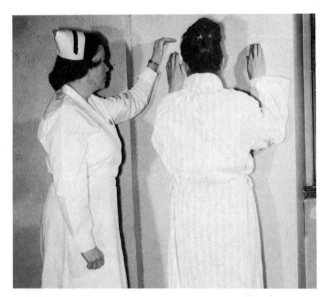

FIG. 30-4. The patient needs help and encouragement in doing postmastectomy exercises.

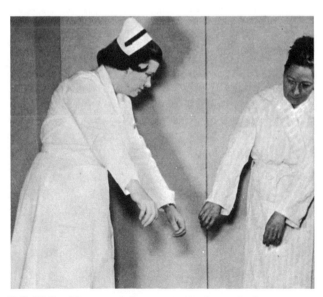

FIG. 30-5. The nurse demonstrates the swinging exercise to a patient who has had a radical mastectomy.

*Published by the American Cancer Society, Inc.; available from local chapters of the society.

then the unaffected arm, gives good exercise to the shoulder. The wrist and elbow must be kept straight. Putting the rope over the shower rod and, grasping each end, alternately lowering and raising the rope until the affected arm is almost directly overhead is another beneficial exercise. It is particularly useful because it gives exercise to both arms at once.

Back buttoning. Stand straight with the feet well apart. Bend the elbow of the arm on the unoperated side and reach back until the fingertips reach the opposite shoulder blade. Repeat, using the operated side. This exercise can be accomplished by fastening a brassiere, washing the back, or massaging or scratching the opposite shoulder blade.

Elbow pull-in. Stand straight with the feet well apart. (1) Clasp the hands at the back of the neck; (2) raise the elbows and bring them forward until they touch; (3) with the hands still clasped behind the neck, bring the upper arms out at right angles to the body.

Elbow elevation. Stand straight with the feet well apart. (1) Place the hand on the affected side on the opposite shoulder; (2) raise the elbow to chin level. Equivalent exercise is obtained in adjusting shoulder straps or pulling a garment over the shoulder and upper arm.

Care of the scar and breast prostheses. The patient should be encouraged to look at the scar before she leaves the hospital. She should be told that the skin will look a little irregular and that sensation may be lessened and may never fully return to the scar tissue. Any signs of redness, infection, or swelling within or outside the scar, however, must be reported at once to the physician. The rate of healing determines when dressings can be completely removed and a prosthesis worn. If a small open area remains and is healing slowly, it may be weeks before a permanent prosthesis can be worn. The patient should be told that the scar will always remain but that in time it will become softer, smaller, and more normal in color. She should be instructed to bathe the area with a soft washcloth as soon as the wound heals. The area should be patted dry because vigorous rubbing may disrupt the newly healed tissue. The scar can be gently massaged with cold cream. Itching of the scar is a fairly common complaint, especially during warm weather; talcum powder or cornstarch often helps to relieve this. If a heavy prosthesis is worn regularly, such as one filled with fluid, it is wise to wear a brassiere padded with lamb's wool for several hours during the day so that there will be free circulation of air over the scar.

While the patient is in the hospital, her daily plan of self-care after discharge should be reviewed with her. The surgeon usually tells the patient how much rest she should have and what she should be able to do at once. The nurse should help the patient to understand the need to exercise her arm regularly in order to prevent any limitation of motion. If the patient is married, she should be encouraged to let her husband see the scar and not try to hide it. Night brassieres can be worn and usually are comfortable and do not interfere with normal sleep. Some patients remain at home, avoid their friends, hesitate to engage in social activities, and thus make life unhappy for themselves and their families. The reasons for withdrawal from social participation include fear of rejection by others because of loss of body intactness.

Healing of the incision so that she is able to wear a fitted brassiere usually reassures the patient and encourages her to participate in home and social activities. It should be pointed out to the patient that she will be able to do everything she normally did before the operation, although total muscle strength in the arm and shoulder may be slightly lessened. Swimming is excellent exercise for the patient who has had a mastectomy, and bathing suits can be fitted so that the loss of a breast is not obvious. Pain in the incision and chest, fatigue, periods of depression, and concern about wound healing are common problems during convalescence. After discharge it may be helpful for the patient to discuss any problems and fears that occur with a public health nurse, a nurse in the hospital clinic, or the surgeon's office nurse.

The nurse in the hospital should help the patient with her immediate preparations to return home. Using needle, thread, and scissors, she can demonstrate to her how to lightly pad brassieres so that they can be used until the scar has completely healed and a prosthesis can be worn (Fig. 30-6). Plain cotton can be covered with gauze and lightly tacked with thread to the inside of the brassiere.

The patient should have help with the selection of an artificial breast before she leaves the hospital. A Reach to Recovery volunteer is often able to be of great assistance in this regard since her recommendations are based on personal experience and the experience of other women who have had a mastectomy.

There are several kinds of artificial breasts, and some hospitals have manufacturers' literature and samples that can be demonstrated before the patient returns home. Sponge rubber prostheses are preferred by many patients since they are light and are easily washed. Other patients prefer the prostheses filled with fluid because their weight more nearly approximates that of the normal breast. Still others prefer the artificial breasts that are filled with air. (See Fig. 30-7.) In large communities the patient can usually be referred to a special corset shop or to the corset department of a department store, where saleswomen are prepared to fit her properly. The artificial breast should fit comfortably and should be covered with a correctly fitted brassiere. The top of the brassiere should touch the skin lightly even when the patient bends forward. If the brassiere tends to slip upward on the operated side, a V-shaped piece of elastic can be attached to the lower edge of the brassiere and to a garter belt or girdle. Lengthen-

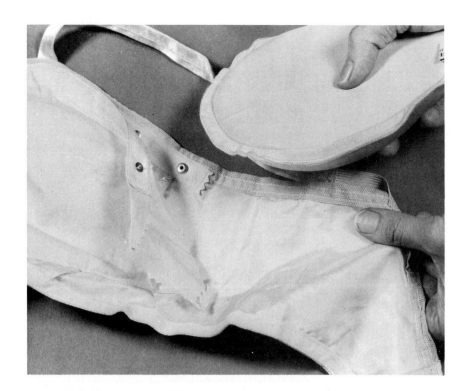

FIG. 30-6. An inner pocket that will hold the padding or prosthesis securely can be made in the patient's own brassiere. Note the snaps that simplify removal of the padding.

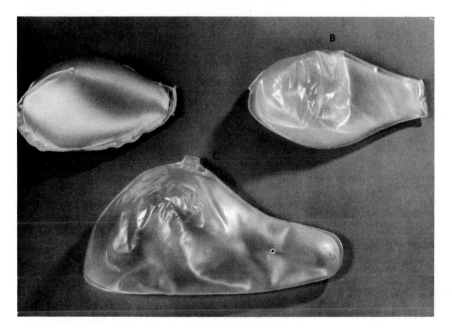

FIG. 30-7. Several types of breast prostheses are available. **A,** Foam rubber prosthesis. **B,** Prosthesis containing fluid. **C,** Prosthesis containing air.

ing the brassiere strap on the operated side helps to prevent discomfort from pressure of the strap. When the patient is seated, erect sitting posture helps keep the prosthesis in the correct position.

Lymphedema. Many patients have swelling of the arm (lymphedema) following a mastectomy. This may follow surgical interruption of lymph channels and infection. Some surgeons feel that lymphedema following mastectomy is decreased when patients are treated with catheter drainage and suction and no dressing.[40] If there is a tendency for edema to

occur, the patient is usually advised to sleep with the affected arm elevated on a pillow. For short periods several times each day, she should sit with the arm elevated on a table or on the arm of a sofa. Regular moderate exercise and use of the arm is believed to help prevent lymphedema from developing. Some surgeons order an elastic sleeve that gives additional support to the vessels in the arm. This should extend from the wrist to the shoulder. It is similar to an elastic stocking (p. 393) and usually may be removed when the patient is in bed. A diuretic such as chlorothiazide (Diuril) may be ordered to help relieve the edema.

Special care must be taken to prevent minor infections of the hands and arms in patients with lymphedema, and if they do occur, medical treatment should be sought at once since the infection spreads quickly because of the improperly functioning lymph system. The patient is advised to use cuticle cream instead of cuticle scissors. She is also advised to wear rubber gloves when using harsh household products and steel wool and to wear canvas gloves when gardening. An electric razor should be used for shaving the axillae. Hangnails or any irritation of the hand or arm should be cared for by a physician.

Therapy used in conjunction with mastectomy

Because carcinoma of the breast seems to be affected by estrogenic hormones, a bilateral oophorectomy is sometimes performed on the premenopausal woman who has had a mastectomy for carcinoma. The closer the woman is to the menopause, the more effective oophorectomy seems to be in tumor suppression. Estrogenic activity may also be reduced by pelvic irradiation. This is most likely to be used in women over 40 who have not entered the menopause. The effectiveness of pelvic irradiation can be determined by examining vaginal smears for loss of estrogenic effect.

Treatment when metastasis occurs

In advanced carcinoma of the breast the treatment is palliative—that is, it affords relief but does not effect a cure. Although some of the procedures may seem radical, they produce temporary regression of the tumor, lessen pain, and permit the patient to remain active. There are several types of treatment. Radiotherapy is often used in conjunction with surgery; it may also be used instead of surgery when the tumor is large, ulcerated, and inoperable. It tends to decrease bleeding, stimulate healing, and may diminish the size of the tumor.

Other treatments are used only when the lesion and symptoms are no longer amenable to surgery or radiation therapy. They are often used in specific sequence and only after recurrence of distressing symptoms of metastasis. The choice of procedure depends on the patient and whether or not she has experienced the menopause. Premenopausal women who do not respond to oophorectomy or pelvic irradiation are usually treated with corticosteroids and chemotherapeutic agents. On the other hand, women who respond to induction of the menopause and who later have a metastasis of their disease are treated with bilateral adrenalectomy or hypophysectomy.

If the patient is more than 1 year past the menopause, she is treated with either estrogens or androgens. At this age, these hormones seem to produce a regression of the tumor in some persons. The reason they do so is not known, although hormonal therapy does prevent physiologic secretion of estrogen from the adrenal gland. If the patient does not respond to estrogenic therapy, corticosteroids and chemotherapeutic agents are used for treatment. Bilateral adrenalectomy or hypophysectomy are only used to treat women who have responded to endocrine therapy and who later develop metastasis. Since adrenalectomy or hypophysectomy are done to curtail the output of the woman's own estrogenic hormones, estrogens or androgens are not given after these procedures.

It is important to remember that not all persons respond to these forms of treatment. The treatment is determined on the basis of the type of lesion, the side effects of the treatment, and the response of the individual patient to previous treatment.

Chemotherapy is ordinarily used for metastatic disease when procedures to curtail endocrine function have failed to slow the progress of the disease. (For details of the drugs given and the nursing care involved, see p. 301.)

Radiotherapy. Radiotherapy may be given if there is suspected or known metastasis. Treatment can be started as soon as the day after surgery and may be continued on an ambulatory basis after the patient leaves the hospital. (For details of care of patients receiving radiation treatment, see p. 295.) Radiotherapy is also used to treat painful metastatic bone lesions, which occur in the spine, ribs, hips, and pelvis of about 30% of all patients who develop metastasis from carcinoma of the breast, and to treat lesions in the brain, which occur in about 10% of all cases of metastasis. If pleural or peritoneal effusions occur, radioactive isotopes such as radioactive gold (^{198}Au) or radioactive phosphorus (^{32}P) may be instilled into the chest or abdominal cavities to attempt to control the formation of fluid. (See p. 300 for discussion of this treatment.)

Hormone therapy. Estrogenic, androgenic, and corticosteroid hormones are used to treat advanced carcinoma of the breast. They seem to be particularly effective in controlling the pain and also the progress of bone metastasis. For example, bone cells may be regenerated in decalcified areas in the spine, and pathologic fractures may heal as a result of hormone treatment. It is estimated that, with hormone treatment, patients with metastases who are responsive to the effects of the hormones have relief of symptoms for 1 year or more. Testosterone propionate is the androgen most often used and may be given in doses of 50 mg. ($^3/_4$ grain) intramuscularly twice a week for an indefinite period. Much larger doses may also be given. Treatment with testosterone will cause secondary changes that are distressing to the patient. These include deepening of the voice, coarsening of the skin, and appearance of hair on the face and the rest of the body. The patient usually gains weight. She should be warned that these changes may occur, and she may need to pay greater attention to details of personal grooming than formerly was necessary.

Diethylstilbestrol (stilbestrol) is the estrogen commonly used. It may be given in oral doses of 15 mg. ($1/4$ grain) daily. The drug is better tolerated if the entire dose is given at bedtime. Occasionally uterine bleeding occurs and is often felt to be a withdrawal effect caused by failure of the patient to take the drug regularly. Increasing the dosage of the estrogen for several days often controls the bleeding. The corticosteroids may produce regression of the tumor in some patients. However, the use of these hormones may cause undesirable side effects (p. 482).

Surgical procedures. Since estrogens are believed to enhance the growth of malignant cells in women who are not past the menopause, several operative procedures are now used to remove the estrogen supply from the body in an attempt to prolong the life of the patient. These include *bilateral oophorectomy* (p. 524) and *bilateral adrenalectomy,* performed when the effect of the oophorectomy has subsided. After an adrenalectomy, the patient needs special nursing care. (See p. 765 for a discussion of this care.) Removal of the pituitary gland, or *hypophysectomy,* suppresses the function of both the ovaries and the adrenal glands. (See p. 767 for a discussion of this procedure and the special nursing needs of the patient undergoing it.)

Psychologic considerations. The patient who has metastasis needs encouragement and help to continue to carry on her normal work either in the home or elsewhere for as long as possible. Some patients who have had to wear a brace because of metastasis to the spine have returned to their jobs for a year or more. Nothing contributes more to the patient's morale than continuing to work and participate in life around her. Appetite improves, and probably the resultant general improvement in health delays complete invalidism for some time. Patients may even continue to work or to carry on normal social activities when they have severe pain that requires regular narcotic or other analgesic treatment.

■ NONMALIGNANT DISEASE OF THE BREAST

Dysplasia and fibroadenoma

Dysplasia (fibrocystic disease). Dysplasia is characterized by thickened nodular areas in the breast that usually become painful during or prior to menstruation. The process is almost always bilateral. A variety of changes take place in the breast tissue, which in some cases includes the formation of cysts. The condition is thought to be caused by hormonal imbalance. There is failure of normal involution following the reaction of the breasts to the cyclic activity of the female sex hormones. The nodules or cysts may be singular or multiple. They may increase in size or remain the same. Usually they are fairly soft and tender on palpation and are movable, sliding under the examining fingers. The woman who discovers such a mass (or masses) in her breast should seek the advice of a physician, who will decide whether or not the lesion should be measured and checked at frequent intervals, whether hormones should be administered, or whether aspiration of the cyst should be considered. There is little evidence that dysplasia predisposes to the development of malignancy, but the presence of nodules in the breast makes the early detection of malignant lesions much more difficult. For this reason, some physicians suggest periodic mammography or xeroradiography of the breast to detect any changes.

Fibroadenoma. Fibroadenomas are tumors of fibroblastic and epithelial origin that are thought to be caused by hyperestrinism. They are usually firm, round, freely movable, nontender, and encapsulated. They occur most often in women under 25 years of age.

The woman who discovers such a mass should not delay in seeking medical consultation. Usually the tumor will be removed under local anesthesia and will be examined microscopically to be sure it is not malignant. Although the hospital stay for excision of an adenoma is short and the patient returns to the surgeon's office or clinic for the sutures to be removed, she needs thoughtful nursing care since she usually is extremely fearful of cancer.

Infections

Infection of the nipple. Infection usually follows cracks in the nipple during lactation. This condition is less common than previously since women are taught to "toughen" the nipple during pregnancy so that cracking during breast-feeding is less likely to occur.

Infection of the breast. An infection can occur in the breast by direct spread from cracked or infected nipples and following congestion or "caking" during lactation when a portion of the breast becomes engorged from blockage of gland ducts. Manual expression of excess milk and hormone treatment for women who are not going to nurse their infants have reduced the incidence of infections of the breast. The microorganisms causing the infection may be transmitted to the mother's breast from the nasopharynx of the newborn infant who has been exposed to infected infants and hospital personnel or from the hands of the patient or those of hospital personnel. Staphylococcal infections are the most common. Infections in the breast can also occur with no specific cause and perhaps follow infections elsewhere in the body. These infections can occur at times other than during pregnancy or lactation.

Infections of the breast cause pain, redness,

swelling, and elevation of temperature. The treatment is usually conservative. Antibiotics are usually given systemically. Sometimes local heat is used, and at other times ice packs may be prescribed. If the condition does not subside with conservative treatment and becomes localized to form an abscess, surgical drainage is necessary. To help prevent infections of the breast from occurring, there is a continued need for strict aseptic technique in nurseries for newborn infants. This includes preventing infected persons (carriers) from coming in contact with mothers and babies.

Gynecomastia. Gynecomastia is a hyperplasia of the stroma and ducts in the mammary glands in the male that occurs during puberty and after the age of 40. It is thought to be due to an abnormally large estrogen secretion. It also frequently is seen following estrogen therapy for carcinoma of the prostate. Gynecomastia is a nonmalignant lesion, but physicians may suggest removal and biopsy of the breast since older men occasionally develop carcinoma of the breast.

REFERENCES AND SELECTED READINGS*

1 Ackerman, L. V., and del Regato, J. A.: Cancer—diagnosis, treatment, and prognosis, ed. 4, St. Louis, 1970, The C. V. Mosby Co.
2 American Cancer Society, Inc.: 1975 cancer facts and figures, New York, 1974, The Society.
2a American Cancer Society, Inc.: Close-up standard breast examination, CA **24:**291-293, Sept.-Oct. 1974.
3 Anderson, D. E.: A high-risk group for breast cancer, Cancer Bull. **25:**23-25, March-April 1973.
4 Bouchard, R., and Owens, N.: Nursing care of the cancer patient, ed. 2, St. Louis, 1972, The C. V. Mosby Co.
5 Cady, B.: Modern management of breast cancer, a point of view, Arch. Surg. **104:**270-275, March 1972.
6 Cancer Advisory Committee: Optimal criteria for care of patients with cancer, J.A.M.A. **227:**57-63, Jan. 1974.
7 Carter, S. K.: Single and combination nonhormonal chemotherapy in breast cancer, Cancer **30:**1543-1555, Dec. 1972.
8 Crile, G., Jr.: Conservative treatment of advanced breast cancer, Am J. Surg. **126:**343-344, Sept. 1973.
9 Crile, G., Jr., and others: Partial mastectomy for carcinoma of the breast, Surg. Gynecol. Obstet. **136:**929-933, June 1973.
10 Dao, T. L.: Ablation therapy for hormone-dependent tumors, Ann. Rev. Med. **23:**1-18, 1972.
11 Donegan, W. L.: Mastectomy in the primary management of invasive mammary carcinoma, Adv. Surg. **6:**1-101, 1972.
12 Egan, R. L.: Contributions of mammography in the detection of early breast cancer, Cancer **28:**1555-1557, Dec. 1971.
13 *Farabee, J. M.: Mammography, chemography offer optimism for breast cancer diagnosis, A.O.R.N.J.**19:**837-842, April 1974.
14 Freundlich, I. M.: Thermography, N. Engl. J. Med. **287:**880-881, Oct. 1972.
15 Gershon-Cohen, J.: Mammography, thermography and zerography, CA **17:**108-112, May-June 1967.
16 *Gribbons, C. A., and Aliapoulios, M. A.: Early carcinoma of the breast, Am. J. Nurs. **69:**1945-1950, Sept. 1969.
17 *Gribbons, C. A., and others: Treatment for advanced breast carcinoma, Am. J. Nurs. **72:**678-682, April 1972.
18 Haagensen, C. D.: Diseases of the breast, ed. 2, Philadelphia, 1971, W. B. Saunders Co.
19 *Harrell, H. C.: To lose a breast, Am. J. Nurs. **72:**676-677, April 1972.
20 *Hartley, I. D., and Brandt, E. M.: Control and prevention of lymphedema following radical mastectomy, Nurs. Res. **67:**333-336, Fall 1967.

21 Healey, J. E., Jr.: Role of rehabilitation medicine in the care of the patient with breast cancer, Cancer **28:**1666-1671, Dec. 1971.
22 *Higginbotham, S.: Arm exercises after mastectomy, Am. J. Nurs. **57:**1573-1574, Dec. 1957.
23 Kaufman, S., and Goldstein, M.: Combination chemotherapy in disseminated carcinoma of the breast, Surg. Gynecol. Obstet. **137:**83-86, July 1973.
24 Kelley, R. M.: Hormones and chemotherapy in breast cancer, Cancer **28:**1686-1691, Dec. 1971.
25 Ketchem, A. S.: Predictable categories of increased risk to breast cancer, A.O.R.N.J. **19:**852-858, April 1974.
26 Lapayowker, M. S., and others: Breast cancer detection by manual surface temperature detector: comparison with results of thermography and mammography, Cancer **31:**377-383, April 1973.
27 Lasser, T., and Clark, W. K.: Reach to recovery, New York, 1972, Simon & Schuster, Inc.
28 Leis, H. P., and Pelnik, S.: Breast cancer, a therapeutic dilemma, A.O.R.N.J. **19:**813-820, April 1974.
28a *Mamaril, A. P.: Preventing complications after radical mastectomy, Am. J. Nurs. **74:**2000-2003, Nov. 1974.
29 Markel, W. M.: The American Cancer Society's program for the rehabilitation of the breast cancer patient, Cancer **28:**1676-1680, Dec. 1971.
30 Mayo, P., and Wilkey, N. L.: Prevention of cancer of the breast and cervix, Nurs. Clin. North Am. **3:**229-241, June 1968.
31 *McCorkle, M. R.: Coping with physical symptoms in metastatic breast cancer, Am. J. Nurs. **73:**1034-1038, June 1973.
32 McLaughlin, C. W., Jr., and others: Cancer of the breast, Am. J. Surg. **125:**734-737, June 1973.
33 *Owen, M. L.: Special care for the patient who has a breast biopsy or mastectomy, Nurs. Clin. North Am. **7:**373-382, June 1973.
34 *Perras, C.: Subcutaneous mastectomy, Am. J. Nurs. **73:**1568-1570, Sept. 1973.
35 *Phillips, C. W., and others: Xeroradiology of the breast, Nurs. Digest **2:**89-92, April 1974.
36 *Quint, J. C.: The impact of mastectomy, Am. J. Nurs. **63:**88-92, Nov. 1963.
37 *Renneker, R., and Cutler, M.: Psychological problems of adjustment to cancer of the breast, J.A.M.A. **148:**833-838, March 1952.
38 Rhoads, J. E., and others: Surgery: principles and practice, ed. 4, Philadelphia, 1970, J. B. Lippincott Co.
39 Rosemond, G. P.: Newer concepts in the management of patients with breast cancer, Cancer **28:**1372-1375, Dec. 1971.

*References preceded by an asterisk are particularly well suited for student reading.

40 Sabiston, D. C., editor: Christopher's textbook of surgery, ed. 10, Philadelphia, 1972, W. B. Saunders Co.

41 *Schmid, W. L., and others: The team approach to rehabilitation after mastectomy, A.O.R.N.J. **19:**821-836, April 1974.

42 Schurman, D. J., and Amstutz, H. C.: Orthopedic management of patients with carcinoma of the breast, Surg. Gynecol. Obstet **137:**831-836, Nov. 1973.

43 Schwartz, G. F.: Evaluation of the patient with a breast tumor, Surg. Clin. North Am. **53:**717-734, June 1973.

44 Segaloff, A.: Hormonal therapy of breast cancer, Cancer **30:**1541-1542, Dec. 1972.

45 *Smith, G. W.: When a breast must be removed, Am. J. Nurs. **50:**335-339, June 1950.

46 Snyderman, R. K.: Symposium on problems of the female breast as related to neoplasm and reconstruction, St. Louis, 1973, The C. V. Mosby Co.

47 Southwick, H. W., Slaughter, D. P., and Humphrey, L. J.: Surgery of the breast, Chicago, 1968, Year Book Medical Publishers, Inc.

48 Strax, P.: New techniques in mass screening for breast cancer, Cancer **28:**1563-1568, Dec. 1971.

49 Zeisller, R. H., and others: Postmastectomy lymphedema: late results of treatment in 385 patients, Arch. Phys. Med. Rehabil. **53:**159-166, April 1972.

31 Diseases of the eye

Health education in care of the eyes
General ophthalmologic management
Disease conditions and related management
Removal of the eye
Blindness

■ Vision is one of man's most priceless possessions. It is essential to most employment and is necessary in countless experiences that make life enjoyable and meaningful. Yet in the United States there are an estimated 475,200 legally blind people today. Approximately 1.7 million Americans cannot read ordinary newsprint even with the aid of glasses.[17] During the next year an additional 35,000 Americans are expected to become blind.[44] The incidence of blindness has increased each decade since 1940.[26]

An apparent reason for the increase in blindness is the longer life span of the American. Although there has been reduction of blindness from infections, certain diseases, and injuries, there has been an increase in blindness resulting from diseases that occur most frequently among older persons. These include diabetic retinopathy, glaucoma, cataract, and retinal degeneration. From 1940 to 1970 there has been a steady growth in the number of persons aged 65 or older in the population, an increase of nearly 45%.[26]

In order to decrease the problem of vision impairment, health workers can focus on (1) prevention of eye disease and injury, (2) early detection of disease and injury, and (3) adequate treatment of disease and injury.

As participants in planning, providing, and evaluating health care, the nurse assumes responsibilities in all these areas. This chapter deals with health education, assessment of persons' needs regarding the eye, medical treatment of certain eye conditions, and specific nursing procedures for a few of the more common eye conditions.

■ HEALTH EDUCATION IN CARE OF THE EYES

Nurses should be able to explain the complex structure of the eye, to teach people to care for their eyesight, and to direct them to the proper specialist. A nurse also should recognize signs suggestive of eye disease and teach them to others. Activities of professional nurses in assisting persons of all ages in regard to vision are outlined below.

1. Protection of sight from impairment or further impairment
   a. Teaching and providing safety measures and first aid
   b. Detecting evidence of disease or impaired acuity
   c. Explaining and administering treatments used to improve sight or prevent further loss (medications, surgery, eye patching)
2. Adjustment of the individual to impaired vision
   a. Identifying basic human needs that have been affected

■ STUDY QUESTIONS

1. Review the anatomy and physiology of the eye. Explain the functions of the three coats of the eyeball. How does the aqueous humor differ from the vitreous humor in location and function? What is the function of the lens?
2. List safety measures that can be taken to prevent accidental damage to the eye. Describe first aid for (a) a foreign body in the eye, (b) irritating chemical in the eye, and (c) a blunt or penetrating blow to the eye.
3. Describe the effect of each of the following drugs on the eye: pilocarpine, atropine, acetazolamide (Diamox), epinephrine, and phenylephrine (Neo-Synephrine). What is the correct procedure for instilling eyedrops and ointments and for applying a sterile eye compress?
4. Have you known anyone with loss of sight? How did impaired vision affect his role in the family, his sense of identity, and his body image?
5. In your community, what services and facilities are available to persons with limited vision? How are these financed?
6. What is the average cost of a pair of reading glasses? A pair of bifocals? Contact lenses? An artificial eye? Does your insurance plan cover these costs?

b. Understanding the effects on adaptation of different degrees of impairment (whether one or two eyes affected, partial or complete loss, acquired or congenital loss)

c. Assisting the newly blinded person through stages of psychologic adaptation to blindness

d. Assisting persons to cope with unmet needs for physical and emotional security, socialization, enhancement of self-esteem, and role identification

e. Using community resources that are available to help persons with impaired vision to cope more successfully (hospital, Lion's Club, school facilities, National Society for the Prevention of Blindness, etc.)

Care of the eyes

Normal healthy eyes do not need special local treatment. The secretions of the conjunctiva are protective and should not be removed by frequent bathing with unprescribed solutions. Boric acid solution and numerous trade preparations recommended to cleanse the eyes are usually unnecessary. Although these preparations are generally harmless, some proprietary solutions contain substances that may cause allergic reactions in sensitive persons.

Many people believe erroneously that eyestrain causes permanent eye damage. Eyestrain actually refers to strain of the ciliary muscles when there is difficulty in accommodation. It causes a sense of fatigue but does not produce serious damage to the eyes. However, a good light should be used when reading and doing work that requires careful visual focus, and extremely fine work should not be done for long periods of time without giving the eye muscles periodic rest. Looking at distant objects for a few minutes helps to rest the eyes after close work. The eyes should be protected by goggles or special dark glasses from prolonged exposure to very bright light such as sunlight over snow. They also need special protection from sudden flashes of light and heat that occur in some industrial occupations. Nurses often are asked the effect of television on the eyes. There is no evidence that prolonged watching of television will damage eyesight.

While adequate nutrition is as important for eye health as it is for maintaining other body functions, persons with nutritionally caused eye disorders are rarely found in the United States. Vitamin deficiencies can cause night blindness (vitamin A), corneal damage (vitamin A), optic neuritis (vitamin B), and other disorders. Although a sufficient vitamin intake is necessary, an excessive amount is wasted and may actually do more harm than good. For example, too much vitamin A can damage the optic nerve.[29]

In the school and home as well as in health agencies the close relationship between diet and good eye health should be taught. Older persons and teenagers are perhaps the worst offenders in this respect. Teenage boys and girls may eat poorly because of poor habits established in early childhood and be-cause of adolescent notions and group preferences; an example is the diet consisting mainly of soft drinks, frankfurters, potato chips, and ice cream. Elderly people may not have the energy or the incentive to prepare and eat proper meals. Persons of all ages should be taught the essentials of good nutrition and should be encouraged and assisted to change their diet patterns when indicated (Chapter 6).

Care should be taken not to irritate the eyes or introduce bacteria into the eyes by rubbing them. Rubbing the eyes may be a natural response of many persons under nervous strain. It may, however, be due to eczematous scaling, infection of the lids, or occasionally to louse attachment on the lashes. Prevention of accidental injury to the eyes should be stressed in child and parent education. Slingshots, BB guns, and even the seemingly harmless rubber bands and paper wads can be dangerous. The nurse can help physical education teachers and others to be alert to hazards to the eyes in gymnasiums and on playgrounds.*

First-aid measures necessary in the event of eye injury should be known by everyone; these measures may be taught in schools and in industry (Chapter 14). The sight of many persons could be saved each year if everyone understood the need for immediate copious flushing of the eye with water when an acid, alkali, or other irritating substance has been accidentally introduced. Much damage is done by the layman's well-intentioned efforts to remove foreign bodies from the eye and by not obeying the important rule of always washing the hands before attempting to examine the eye or to remove a foreign body. Everyone should know that a person who has a foreign object lodged on the cornea must be referred to a physician; the layman should never attempt to remove it. The eye should be closed to prevent further irritation and the lids gently shut and loosely covered with a dressing or patch anchored with a piece of cellophane or adhesive tape. The patient should be advised not to squeeze the eye and should be taken to an ophthalmologist at once.†

The eye is extremely complicated (Fig. 31-1) and seldom is absolutely perfect even when its function appears within normal limits. The eyes should be examined by an ophthalmologist at regular intervals throughout life. Many authorities believe the child should have his eyes examined before starting school, approximately at age 10, and in early adolescence. The young adult should consult an ophthalmologist at least every 5 years. After the age of 40 years the lens becomes firmer and less resilient

---

*Recent articles on eye injuries may be found in the references, especially references 17a, 17b, and 17c.
†"Emergency Eye Care," 1971, Trainex Corp., is a valuable teaching aid.

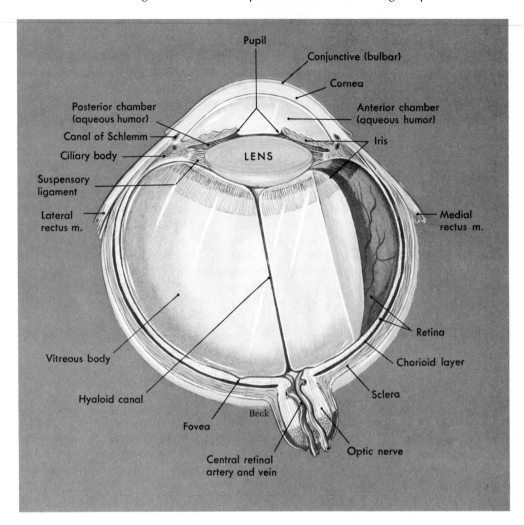

FIG. 31-1. Horizontal section through the left eyeball. (From Anthony, C. P.: Textbook of anatomy and physiology, ed. 8, St. Louis, 1971, The C. V. Mosby Co.)

(presbyopia). The individual begins to hold written material at a distance for better vision, and close vision may become blurred. Medical specialists recommend an eye examination every 2 years after the age of 35.

Since the eyes are often profoundly affected by conditions within the rest of the body, they cannot be considered alone. In fact, nearly all diseases cause some eye change that is diagnostically important. The nurse who is teaching eye health must be aware of total health. When apparently minor disease or abnormality of the eyes occurs, the nurse must be particularly alert for other signs of illness. Many serious medical conditions such as diabetes, renal disease, neurologic disease, and generalized arteriosclerosis may be diagnosed through early recognition of eye symptoms and examination of the eyes by an ophthalmologist.

There is widespread confusion and misunderstanding on the part of the public as to the proper specialist to consult about visual problems. People who demand the best care when other medical and surgical problems arise may fail to seek help from an ophthalmologist when they have eye difficulties.

Many persons do not understand the difference between the *orthoptist,* who directs eye exercises, the *optician,* who grinds and fits lenses, the *optometrist,* who adjusts lenses to changes in refraction and accommodation of the eye, and the *ophthalmologist,* who has had intensive medical training and experience in the diagnosis and treatment of eye diseases. In their search for help a surprisingly large number of people respond to radio advertising and may even purchase glasses from store counters or use glasses originally prescribed for friends or relatives. These people need to understand that eye conditions cannot always be remedied simply by the purchase of a pair of glasses or a change of lenses.

Recognition of eye diseases

Nurses should recognize the signs of eye disease so that they can guide persons with eye problems to appropriate resources. Nurse-teachers and schoolteachers should be alert to changes in the eyes and vision of children during the school year. If changes occur, the child should be referred to an ophthalmologist as soon as possible. If an individual complains of itching or burning of the eyelids after reading or of the sensation of needing to "wash out his eyes," he should consult an ophthalmologist. Frowning, squinting, rubbing the eyes, covering one eye or tilting the head, blinking excessively, headache, fatigue, and irritability on doing close work with the eyes also are signs that medical care may be needed. Constant dull pain in the eyes, blurring of vision, spots before the eyes, rings around lights, and noticeable changes in visual acuity are signs that eye function is affected and should be investigated. Frequent changes of lenses and history of repeated visits to optometrists for lens changes indicate the need for a complete medical examination.

Another detriment to good eye care is the natural human tendency to put things off, to reject any obvious fact that is unpleasant or disturbing, and to assume that an eye condition will "clear up" within a few days. Although the average person thinks of loss of vision as a major catastrophe, he may be careless in giving early attention to eye difficulties that, if neglected, may become serious. The danger of procrastination must be stressed since some eye diseases progress so rapidly that irreparable damage may occur quickly. Neither the patient nor the nurse can know, for example, whether an irritation of the eyes is simple conjunctivitis or incipient acute glaucoma. The patient must never be permitted to postpone treatment and thus risk further infection or progress of disease.

An example of a tragic area of neglect is that of *strabismus* (crossed eyes) in young children. Parents are naturally reluctant to face the fact that something about their child may not be quite normal. They are likely to believe and hope that the child will outgrow the condition or that no accurate medical examination can be done until the child is able to read. However, successful treatment is difficult to obtain after 6 years of age. Delay in treatment of strabismus can result in permanent loss of vision.

People frequently treat eye ailments with proprietary remedies or with eyedrops and other medication that they or others have used at some time in the past. Self-treatment of the eyes is not only dangerous but may also lead to loss of much valuable time for treatment. Many persons fail to realize that there are many disorders that can affect the eyes and that many different drugs are used, each of which has a specific purpose. Two drugs may have completely opposite effects. Since liquids evaporate and drugs deteriorate or become contaminated with bacteria or fungus, use of preparations that a patient or his friends have on hand can contribute to actual damage.

Glasses and special lenses

Eyeglasses are prescribed to improve vision and to relieve discomfort resulting from use of the eyes. Acceptance of glasses seems to be influenced by the improvement in vision that they afford, the personality of the wearer, and the current fashion trends. To some persons, however, glasses may appear as a cosmetic blemish. Because there may be some stigma attached to wearing glasses, the young child will have a period of adjustment after receiving glasses. While the preschool child may reject glasses, he almost always accepts them on entering school when he realizes that without them he cannot see the blackboard. The vogue for attractive frames makes the wearing of glasses more acceptable to teenagers. All persons should be encouraged to wear their glasses as prescribed and to have periodic examinations of their eyes by an ophthalmologist. Instructions for persons who wear glasses should include how to clean their glasses, how to protect them from being scratched or broken, and how to care for them when they are removed.

Federal law now requires that all prescription glasses be made with impact-resistant lenses. Each finished lens must pass an impact test before it is dispensed. *Plastic* lenses weigh less than half of equivalent glass lenses, but cost more and scratch more easily. They are useful for some persons who wear thick lenses that are heavy when made of glass and for those who are active in sports. *Hardened* lenses have been exposed to a tempering process, which makes them extremely hard and resistant to impact and breakage. *Safety* lenses are similar to hardened lenses but are 1 mm. thicker. They are used in goggles worn by workmen whose eyes may be injured by such articles as chips of metal or glass.

Bifocal lenses consists of an upper portion of one focus used for distance and a lower part of another focus used for reading and close work. They make constant changing from distance to reading glasses unnecessary. *Trifocal* lenses are divided into three focuses to give correction for distance, intermediate, and near vision. *Sunglasses* should be carefully ground and should be large enough to exclude bright light around their edges and dark enough to exclude about 30% of the light. The amount of light filtered can be varied according to the needs of the patient.

Contact lenses are thin shells of transparent, ground, plastic material designed to be worn over the cornea (microlenses) or the cornea and sclera (scleral type) to replace eyeglasses. They are inserted after being cleaned thoroughly and immersed in a wetting agent such as methylcellulose. The lenses usually are worn for prescribed periods of time, removed, and then reinserted. Conjunctival secretions provide the lubrication needed for the lenses to be worn in comfort, and the lenses are held in place by capillary attraction and by the upper lid. Although some people wear the lenses continuously, a few can never physiologically or psychologically tolerate the constant presence of a foreign object in the eye. Contact lenses sometimes are prescribed for persons who have a cone-shaped deformity of the cornea (keratoconus), which may prevent satisfactory fitting with conventional glasses. Elderly patients who have lenses removed because of cataracts benefit from wearing contact lenses but may have difficulty adapting to their use.

Recently a hydrophilic contact lens, which absorbs water, has been successfully used for many patients who could not tolerate the hydrophobic hard lens. They are called "soft" lenses because they are flexible while in contact with the cornea. The disadvantages of the soft lens include a higher initial cost and need for more frequent replacement, more difficult cleaning and maintenance, and less acute correction of vision. Current research in this area is being directed toward developing a new material for lenses that is permeable to oxygen, has the comfort of soft lenses, and has the optical qualities of hard lenses. A plastic lens that is permeable to carbon dioxide and oxygen is now on the market. Contact lenses, although expensive, may be used by persons who engage in sports because they do not fog or break easily, or they may be worn for cosmetic reasons. Care must be taken when the lenses are worn that substances such as dirt or dust do not concentrate behind the lens to irritate the cornea. Therefore they are prohibited in some industrial occupations. Occasionally acute, painful corneal abrasions or erosions occur. Persons interested in wearing contact lenses should be encouraged to consult an ophthalmologist and to accept his recommendations regarding their use. The person who dispenses the contact lenses may be an optician, optometrist, or lab technician. Health workers should learn how to check for and remove contact lenses in unconscious persons.

■ GENERAL OPHTHALMOLOGIC MANAGEMENT
Examination of the eyes

Refraction is one of the most common eye examinations. This procedure reveals the degree to which the various light-transmitting portions of the eye bring light rays into correct focus on the retina. Refractive errors account for the largest number of impairments of good vision. The refractive error is tested by means of trial lenses and the Snellen chart. Suitable glasses are then prescribed if needed.

Some specific terminology must be understood before refractive studies can be meaningful. *Emmetropia* refers to a normal eye, whereas *ametropia* indicates that a refractive error is present. *Accommodation* is the ability to adjust vision from far to near objects. This is normally accomplished by the ciliary muscles, which, by means of contraction or relaxation, can cause the lens to flatten or thicken as need arises. *Myopia,* or nearsightedness, is caused by an abnormally long anteroposterior dimension of the eyeball, which causes light rays to focus in front of the retina. *Hyperopia,* or farsightedness, is caused when the anteroposterior dimension is too short, causing light rays to focus behind the retina. *Astigmatism* is a condition caused by asymmetry, or irregular curvature, of the cornea, so that rays in the horizontal and perpendicular planes do not focus at the same point. In *presbyopia,* which occurs in persons past 40 years of age, the lens becomes more firm and responds less to the need for accommodation in viewing near and far objects. Blurring of near objects results, and those who require different lenses for distant and for close vision must obtain bifocal lenses or separate pairs of glasses.

Before refraction is performed, the nurse may be asked to instill a cycloplegic drug into the eyes to dilate the pupil and temporarily paralyze the ciliary muscles. Cyclopentolate (Cyclogyl) usually is used since it is effective in a half hour, and the effect wears off completely by the end of 6 hours. Homatropine occasionally is used for adults and atropine for children, but both of these drugs require longer to take effect, and their effects persist longer. Atropine must be instilled at intervals for 3 days prior to examination and persists in its action for at least 10 days, with some residual effect for up to 3 to 4 weeks. Persons over 40 years of age can be given eye examinations without the use of cycloplegic drugs, because the power of accommodation has become sufficiently weak to permit examination without their use. However, the pupil should be adequately dilated regardless of age for sufficient medical examination of the retina. Small children may not understand the examination and be unable to remain still. They can be wrapped in a sheet to immobilize them.

The nurse who works in a clinic, in an ophthalmologist's office, or in schools must know how to do *vision screening tests* and how to teach others to do them. Distance vision is usually determined by use of a Snellen chart (Fig. 31-2). Examination is done with the patient standing 20 feet from the chart. The chart consists of rows of letters, numbers, or other characters arranged with the large ones at the top and the small ones at the bottom. The uppermost letter on the chart is scaled so that it can be read at 200 feet, and the successive rows are scaled so that they can be read by the normal eye at 100, 70, 50, 40, 30, 20, 15, and 10 feet, respectively. Visual acuity is expressed as a fraction, and a reading of 20/20 is considered normal. The upper figure refers to the distance of the patient from the chart, and the lower figure indicates the distance at which the smallest letters can be read by the person being tested. For example, the person who is able to read, at 20 feet, only the line that should be readable at 70 feet has 20/70 vision in that eye.

The distance from the chart to where the patient stands must be carefully measured. The person

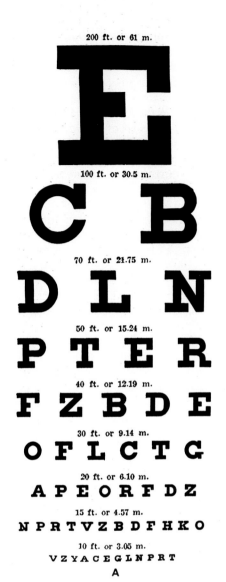

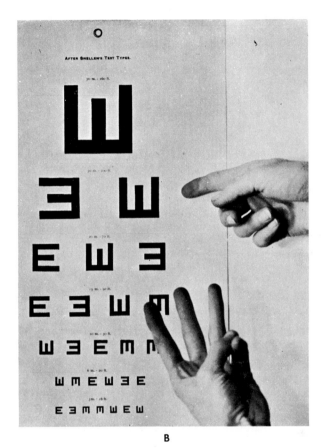

FIG. 31-2. A, Snellen's chart used in testing vision. **B,** Modified Snellen's chart, called the "E" game, for testing vision of small children and persons who are not familiar with the English alphabet. (From Parkinson, R. H.: Eye, ear, nose, and throat manual for nurses, ed. 8, St. Louis, 1959, The C. V. Mosby Co.)

doing the testing usually stands beside the chart and points to the line to be read so that no mistake occurs. Each eye is tested separately, and its performance is carefully recorded. The person is tested with and without glasses. When testing vision, it is best to have the person being examined hold a piece of cardboard over his unused eye rather than have him attempt to read the line with first one and then the other eye closed. The Snellen chart examination is only a basic screening test. Additional detailed procedures must be done to test for nearsightedness, color blindness, and many other abnormalities.

An instrument often used by the ophthalmologist is the *ophthalmoscope.* It magnifies the view of the back of the eye so that the optic nerve, retina, blood vessels, and nerves can be seen through the dilated pupil. The physician may use either the direct (Fig.

31-3) or the indirect (Fig. 31-4) method of ophthalmoscopic examination. The patient may experience a great deal of light sensitivity when examined with the indirect ophthalmoscope. The ophthalmoscope presumably would be damaged by boiling or autoclaving, but it may be wiped clean with alcohol or benzalkonium chloride. If the instrument is contaminated with known infectious organisms, it may be exposed to the sun or air for 24 hours after having been cleaned with a solution such as benzalkonium chloride.

An instrument known as a *tonometer* has been devised for measuring ocular tension and is helpful in detecting early glaucoma. Some ophthalmologists suggest that tonometric readings be taken by the medical internist or the family physician as part of a regular, annual physical examination. The most common indentation tonometer in clinical use is that of Schiøtz. The procedure is performed with the patient lying down and looking upward at some fixed point. The eye may be anesthetized with one or two drops of proparacaine (Ophthaine), 0.5%, after which the tonometer is placed on the cornea. (See Fig. 31-5.) While the weight of the tonometer is supported by the cornea, the amount of indentation that the plunger of the instrument makes in the cornea is measured on the attached scale. This reading is used to determine the pressure within the eye. Readings over 24 mm. Hg (Schiøtz) may suggest glauco-

ma, but tests usually are repeated because temporary increases sometimes may be caused by such things as emotional stress. The applanation tonometer (Goldmann) is more accurate in estimating intraocular pressure (Fig. 31-6). The applanation tonometer is attached to the slit lamp. Instead of indenting the eye, a small area of the cornea is flattened to counterbalance a spring-loaded measuring device, and the pressure is measured directly. Newer means of tonometry currently being investigated include the air tonometer and the scleral and air indentation types.

Although the applanation tonometer cannot be boiled or autoclaved, it is cleansed with soap and water and wiped clean with a solution such as benzalkonium chloride. The Schiøtz tonometer can be dry heat sterilized, and some models can be autoclaved. If alcohol is used for cleansing, it must be removed thoroughly because it is caustic to the cornea.

Areas of opacity within the eye may be detected by means of a fine beam of light projected through the anterior segment of the eye from a *slit lamp.* The limitation of visual field is determined by *perimetry.* The patient is seated in a darkened room at a specific distance from a dark-colored chart on which a dot of light is flashed at consecutive points. Pins are placed on the chart to indicate each dot of light seen by the patient. The placement of the pins describes his field of vision. The tracing can be transferred to the patient's chart for reference. Neither of these two eye examinations requires specific nursing assistance.

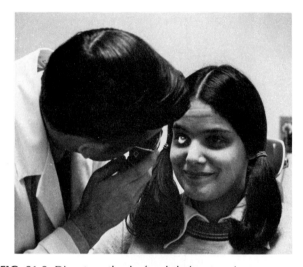

FIG. 31-3. Direct method of ophthalmoscopic examination. The ophthalmoscope is used to examine the optic disc, blood vessels, macula lutea, and fovea centralis of the retina.

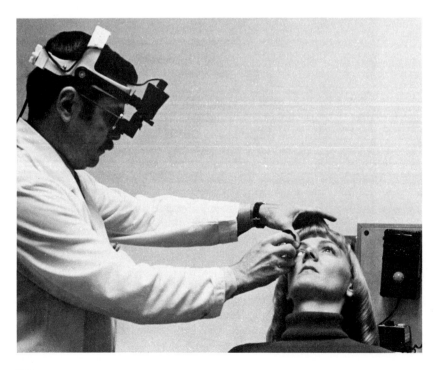

FIG. 31-4. Indirect method of ophthalmoscopic examination. The indirect ophthalmoscope provides a binocular view of the fundus and allows excellent observation of the extreme periphery of the retina.

Gonioscopy is an examination of the angle of the anterior chamber of the eye with a magnifying device. A special contact glass called a gonioscope is placed on the cornea and strong illumination is required for this examination. Gonioscopy is used for patients with suspected glaucoma and diseases of the iris and ciliary body.

The *electroretinogram* (ERG) is a record of the transient, electrical responses produced by the retina following light stimulation. A contact lens electrode is placed on the anesthetized cornea as the stimulus.

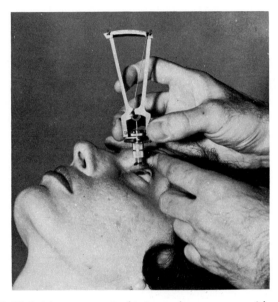

FIG. 31-5. Measurement of intraocular pressure with a Schiøtz tonometer. (From Havener, W. H., and others: Nursing care in eye, ear, nose, and throat disorders, ed. 3, St. Louis, 1974, The C. V. Mosby Co.)

Local treatments

Accuracy in the administration of medications and treatments is essential. Irreparable damage can follow instillation of unprescribed or deteriorated preparations into the eyes. All medication bottles must be checked frequently for smearing or obliteration of labels. Solutions that have changed in color, are cloudy, or contain sediment should not be used. The nurse must know the usual dosage and strength of medications being used. The following is a safe rule: question any dosage that is over 1% in strength unless one is completely familiar with the drug, with the patient, and with ophthalmologic nursing. The nurse who is assigned to care for patients with eye disease should become familiar with the drugs most commonly used, the therapeutic dosages of these drugs, and their toxic signs. In the home the patient should be protected from the use of incorrect drugs from the family medicine cabinet. Medications for the eyes should be placed carefully in a separate part of the cabinet, and dangerous drugs should be removed if the patient is to select and administer his own medications.

The nurse should be aware of the toxic side effects of drugs for ophthalmic use. For example, absorption of atropine instilled into the conjunctival sac may induce flushing of the cheeks, increase in temperature, irritability, and (rarely) convulsions. Osmotic agents that reduce intraocular pressure by increasing plasma osmolarity are contraindicated in patients with poor kidney function. Steroids may cause an exacerbation of an already existing herpes simplex corneal ulcer or increase the intraocular pressure.[25]

Drugs. A large variety of drugs is used for treatment of eye diseases (Tables 31-1 to 31-3). Most of

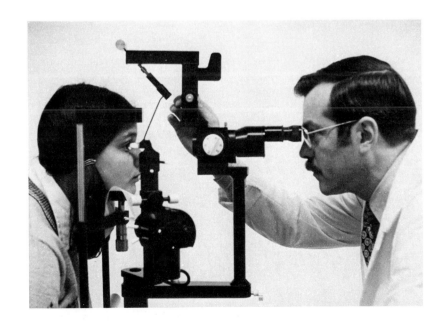

FIG. 31-6. Measurement of ocular tension with the Goldmann applanation tonometer.

them are applied locally as drops, irrigations, or ointments. *Mydriatics* are drugs that dilate the pupil. Mydriasis is necessary for thorough examination of the back of the interior of the eye (fundus). Examples are phenylephrine (Neo-Synephrine) and epinephrine (Epitrate).

Cycloplegics are drugs that not only dilate the pupil but also block accommodation (focusing of the eye) by paralyzing the ciliary muscle. These drugs are used to keep the pupil dilated as part of the treatment for diseases of the cornea and for inflammatory diseases of the iris and ciliary body, after certain operations, and for eye examination. Common cycloplegics are cyclopentolate (Cyclogyl) and tropicamide (Mydriacyl).

Miotics are drugs that contract the pupil, permitting the aqueous humor to flow out more readily and thus reduce intraocular pressure. Miotics such as pilocarpine are most often used in the treatment of glaucoma. *Osmotic agents* may also be used to reduce intraocular pressure. These drugs, for example, urea and mannitol, are given intravenously in the treatment of acute glaucoma or to reduce intraocular pressure during eye surgery.

Secretory inhibitors decrease intraocular pressure by reducing aqueous humor production. Drugs in this classification inactivate the enzyme carbonic anhydrase, which is necessary for the production of aqueous humor. These drugs are given orally and include acetazolamide (Diamox). Local *topical anesthetics* such as tetracaine (Pontocaine) are used frequently for treatments and operations on the eye. Epinephrine (Adrenalin), 1:50,000 or 1:100,000, may be used in combination with local anesthetics to prolong the duration of anesthetics by constricting blood vessels so that the drug remains longer in the injected area and its absorption is delayed. Hyaluronidase (Wydase), which makes cell membranes more per-

Table 31-1 Mydriatic and cycloplegic drugs

Drug	Form and concentration	Duration of effect
Mydriatics		
Phenylephrine (Neo-Synephrine)	Eyedrops, 2.5%-10%	12 hours
Epinephrine (Epitrate)	Eyedrops, 1%-2%	12 hours
Eucatropine (Euphthalmine)	Eyedrops, 5%	6-12 hours
Cycloplegics		
Atropine sulfate	Eyedrops, 1%-3%	2-4 weeks
	Ointment, 1%	
Scopolamine (hyoscine)	Eyedrops, 0.25%-0.5%	1-3 weeks
Homatropine hydrobromide	Eyedrops, 0.5%-3%	1-2 days
	Ointment, 1%-3%	
Cyclopentolate hydrochloride (Cyclogyl)	Eyedrops, 0.5%-1%	4-12 hours
Tropicamide (Mydriacyl)	Eyedrops, 0.5%-1%	2-8 hours

Table 31-2 Drugs used in treatment of glaucoma

Drug	Form	Dose
Cholinergic drugs (miotics)		
Pilocarpine	0.5%-3% solution	1 drop q6h
Carbachol (Carcholin)	0.25%-3% solution	1 drop q6h to q8h
Cholinesterase inhibitors (miotics)		
Physostigmine (Eserine)	0.25%-1% solution	1 drop q6h to q8h
Isoflurophate (DFP) (Floropryl)	0.01%-0.1% solution	1 drop q24h to q48h
Demecarium bromide (Humorsol)	0.125%-0.25% solution	1 drop q12h to q24h
Echothiophate iodide (Phospholine)	0.06%-0.125% solution	1 drop q12h to q24h
Adrenergic agents		
Epinephryl borate (Eppy)	1% solution	1 drop q12h, often used with a miotic such as a cholinesterase inhibitor
Epinephrine hydrochloride (Glaucon)	2% solution	
Epinephrine bitartrate	2% solution	
Carbonic anhydrase inhibitors		
Acetazolamide (Diamox)	250 mg. tablets	1 tablet q6h to q8h
	500 mg. tablets	1 tablet q12h
	500 mg. vials for I.M. or I.V. use	250-500 mg. in 10 ml. diluent
Ethoxzolamide (Cardrase)	125 mg. tablets	1 tablet q6h to q8h
Dichlorphenamide (Daranide)	50 mg. tablets	1 tablet q6h to q8h
Methazolamide (Neptazane)	50 mg. tablets	1 tablet q6h to q8h
Osmotic agents		
Glycerin	Mix with equal amount of orange juice	1-1.5 ml./kg. body wt.
Mannitol (Osmitrol)	10%-20% solution for I.V. use	1-1.5 Gm./kg. body wt.
Urea (Ureaphil)	30% solution for I.V. use	1-1.5 Gm./kg. body wt.

meable, often is mixed with local anesthetic solutions to increase the diffusion of the anesthetic through the tissues.

Physiologic solutions of sodium chloride or mild silver protein (Argyrol) are used as *cleansing agents.* Ophthalmologists may employ uncommonly used *antibiotics* such as bacitracin, polymyxin B, gentamycin, and neomycin for ocular instillation because bacteria are less likely to be resistant to them. Because penicillin causes ocular allergy in about 5% of adult patients, it is not often used.[29]

Table 31-3 Other ophthalmic drugs

Drug	Form	Dose
Antibiotics and antiviral drugs		
Polymyxin B, bacitracin, neomycin, chlorobutanol (Polysporin)	Ointment or eyedrops, 0.1%-1% solution	
Polymyxin B, neomycin, bacitracin (Neosporin)	Eyedrops or ointment	
Bacitracin	Ointment, 500 units/Gm.	
Idoxuridine (IDU) (Herplex, Stoxil)	Eyedrops, 0.1% solution; ointment, 0.5%	
Steroids		
Prednisone	Topical, 0.25%-0.5% suspension; oral, 5-15 mg.	1 tablet q6h
Prednisolone	Topical ointment, 0.1%-0.25%; oral, 5-15 mg.	1 tablet q6h
Methylprednisolone (Depo-Medrol)	Subconjunctival, 0.5 mg.; I.M., 4 mg.	q 2 to 4 weeks
Triamcinolone (Aristocort)	Solution or ointment, 1%	
Dexamethasone (Decadron)	Solution or ointment, 0.1%	
Anesthetics		
Proparacaine (Ophthaine, Ophthetic)	Eyedrops, 0.5% solution	1 drop
Lidocaine (Xylocaine)	Local infiltration, 2%-4% solution	4 ml.
Lubricants and tear substitutes		
Methylcellulose, gonioscopic	Eyedrops, 1% solution	
Methylcellulose (Tearisol)	Eyedrops, 0.1% solution	

A *lubricant* such as methylcellulose may be used for dryness of the cornea and conjunctiva that is caused by deficiency in production of tears or faulty lid closure due to unconsciousness or nerve involvement.

Antiseptic drugs include silver nitrate solution, 1%, and boric acid solution, 2%, administered as drops, and yellow oxide of mercury, 1% to 2%. *Anti-inflammatory drugs* such as cortisone and hydrocortisone as drops and in ointment, 0.1% to 2.5%, are used to control inflammatory and allergic reactions postoperatively as well as for a variety of conditions involving the eyelids, the conjunctiva, and the cornea. Steroids also may be given systemically for the treatment of acute or subacute infections such as those of the iris and choroid.

Astringents such as zinc sulfate preparations are often useful in chronic conjunctivitis. The *dye* fluorescein is used to stain and thereby outline superficial injuries and infections of the external globe of the eye and to check for proper fit of contact lenses.

Techniques. Nursing techniques for giving eye treatments are fully described in texts on fundamentals of nursing, and therefore techniques will not be discussed in detail here. Gentleness is extremely important in performing all treatments. The natural sensitivity of the eye and the reluctance of the normal person to have anything done to his eyes are increased by pain, discomfort, and fear. Nature's powers of repair may be retarded by trauma resulting from pressure on the irritated or inflamed tissues. Hands must be washed thoroughly before giving any eye treatment, and all materials placed in the eyes should be sterile. If the patient is being treated for an active infection, individual medicine bottles, droppers, tubes of ointment, and other equipment should be used. This precaution is also necessary when an infected eye is being treated with an antibacterial drug such as bacitracin and the same medication is ordered prophylactically for the other eye. Many eye medications to be instilled as drops now come in bottles with droppers attached to the stopper. These medications can be used safely to dilate the eyes for examination and to treat noninfectious conditions such as glaucoma since the dropper does not touch the patient when proper technique is used. A good light is necessary when giving treatments, but care must be taken to protect the patient's eyes from direct light.

Eye pads are worn to absorb secretions and blood, to limit movement of the eyes after certain operations or injuries, to protect the eye from light, to eliminate double vision, or to conceal a deformity of the eye. The use of an eye pad is contraindicated in the presence of an eye infection because it enhances bacterial growth. An eye pad is secured with two pieces of tape placed diagonally from cheek to forehead, one on each side of the pad. Cellophane tape and the newer plastic tapes usually are used because they are easy to remove and do not cause allergic irritations. If an eye closes poorly, a drop of a lubricant such as methylcellulose may be ordered to be placed in the eye before it is covered with a dry pad to prevent scratching the cornea. After an operation on the anterior portion of the eye, a metal eye shield may be worn over the dressing to protect the eye from injury until it heals.

Compresses. Warm moist compresses are used in the treatment of surface infections of the cornea, conjunctiva, or eyelid and after many types of eye surgery to help relieve pain, promote healing, and to help cleanse the eye, which is normally cleansed by tears. Compresses may be sterile or unsterile, depending on the eye condition, and should be large enough to cover the entire orbit. If both eyes are involved and the condition is infectious, separate trays must be prepared and the hands carefully washed between treatment of each eye. The temperature of the solution used for compresses should not be over 49° C. (120° F.), and the treatment usually lasts for 10 to 20 minutes and is repeated hourly or several times a day. Great care must be taken not to exert pressure on the eyeball when applying compresses. If there is evidence of irritation of the skin about the eyes from the hot water, a small amount of sterile petrolatum can be used, but it should not be allowed to enter the eyes. Compresses may be heated in a basin placed on an electric plate at the patient's bedside, or they may be heated in a strainer placed in steam and then applied with sterile forceps.

A good compress is made by filling two large, wooden kitchen spoons with gauze or cotton secured with gauze bandage. These can be autoclaved or boiled if a sterile compress is desired. The spoons are then dipped into the warm solution; one is pressed fairly dry with the rounded side of the second spoon and applied to the eye until it cools. The alternate spoon provides for continuous treatment for the prescribed time. The spoon is easy for the patient to hold and obviates handling the compress, thereby lessening the danger of introducing additional infection. Another method of preparing heat applications for the eyes is by means of a *Hydrocolator,* which is an electric water heater with a thermostatic control. It is equipped with special pads to fit the eye that are encased in folds of toweling material for protection from contamination. This convenient piece of equipment can be placed beside the patient's bed.[48] Moist heat also may be applied to the eye by using a clean washcloth soaked in hot water and squeezed free of excess moisture. When the cloth cools, the process is repeated.

Cold moist saline compresses often are ordered to help control bleeding immediately following eye injury, to prevent or control edema in allergic conditions, and to control severe itching. A small basin of sterile solution may be placed in a bowl of chipped ice at the bedside. Sterile forceps are used to wring out and apply the compress. If the compress does not need to be sterile, a washcloth or compresses may be placed on pieces of ice in a basin at the patient's bedside. A rubber glove or small plastic bag packed with finely chipped ice may be adjusted to the eye and necessitates fewer changes of compresses. A piece of plastic material loosely filled and secured with a rubber band is effective also.

Irrigations. Eye irrigations are done to remove secretions, foreign bodies, and chemical irritants and to cleanse the eye preoperatively. Irrigations should be done with the patient lying comfortably toward one side so that fluid cannot flow into the other eye. A plastic squeeze bottle is commonly used unless a very large amount of fluid is needed (Fig. 31-7). If only a small amount of fluid is needed, sterile cotton balls may be used. Physiologic solution of sodium chloride or lactated Ringer's solution is most often used as an irrigating solution. These solutions are isotonic and do not remove from the eye secretions the electrolytes necessary for normal action of the eyes. Irrigating fluid is directed along the conjunctiva and over the eyeball from the inner to the outer canthus. Care is taken to avoid directing a forceful stream onto the eyeball and to avoid touching any eye structures with the irrigating equipment. If there is drainage from the eye, a piece of gauze may be wrapped about the index finger to raise the lid and ensure thorough cleansing.

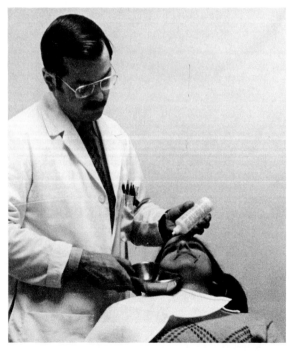

FIG. 31-7. When irrigating the eye, the ophthalmologist directs the fluid along the conjunctiva and over the eyeball from the inner to outer canthus.

Instillation of medications. Eyedrops should be sterile. Each patient should have his own bottle of medication. If the bottle is small, it may be warmed slightly by holding it in the hands for a few moments. Eyedroppers must be sterile. Blunt-edged eyedroppers are available and should be used for children. The dropper is held downward so that medication does not flow into the rubber bulb since foreign material from the bulb can contaminate the solution. When instilling drops, the patient is asked to tilt his head back and look toward the ceiling. The lower lid should be pulled gently outward, and the dropper should approach the patient's eye from the side and not directly (Fig. 31-8, *A*). Drops are placed on the lower conjunctiva. Care must be taken not to touch the eyelids, the conjunctiva, or the eyeball with the dropper. The eyelids should then be closed. The patient should be reminded not to squeeze the eye shut, as this action causes the medication to escape. Absorbent tissue or cotton held against the cheek will prevent the drops from running down the patient's cheek.

To instill ointment, the nurse asks the patient to tilt his head back and to look toward the ceiling. The lower lid is gently pulled down and the ointment is expressed directly onto the exposed conjunctiva from a small, individual tube (Fig. 31-8, *B*). Care is taken not to touch the tissues with the tube. A small, sterile glass spatula may also be used to apply ointment to the eye.

The patient's environment

Most patients with eye conditions are more comfortable when the lighting is dimmed. Screens or curtains can be arranged so that bright light does not enter the room. Bright artificial lighting should be shaded. The patient in the hospital is usually happiest in a room with other patients, especially if both eyes are covered or if he is unable to see. The sound of voices and normal activity around him tends to relieve the feeling of isolation that the blinded person experiences. He benefits from having others around him who may, for example, share newspaper headlines with him. Some patients may prefer to be alone. Radios help the patient to keep up with everyday events. Recordings of entire books are also available.

Accidents present a real hazard when eye disease occurs, especially if an eye is covered or there is loss of vision. It is estimated that 20% of the field of vision is lost if one eye is covered or removed. If the onset of visual loss is slow, the patient and his family may have sufficient time to eliminate common household hazards such as stairs without banisters. The partially blinded person who receives care on an ambulatory basis is taught to have someone accompany him to the physician's office or clinic because he may need additional help for a short time after certain treatments. In the hospital, special measures to prevent accidents are necessary. Side rails may be used, but low beds are safer, particularly for older patients who may forget that they are in a hospital bed. Particular effort should be made to have the space around the patient's bed and chair uncluttered; for example, gooseneck lamps must have short cords that do not fall to the floor. If the patient has serious visual difficulty, hot plates for compresses are not kept at the bedside because the patient may burn himself. Furniture should be firmly anchored with casters locked. Rails along hallways and in bathrooms are also helpful.

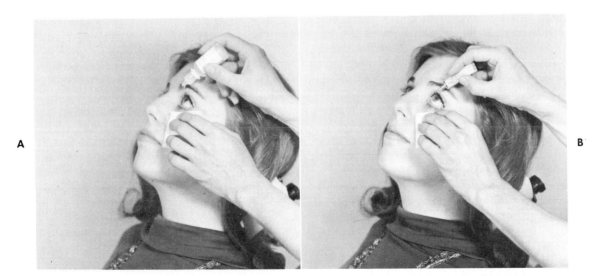

FIG. 31-8. To instill an ophthalmic solution, **A,** or ointment, **B,** tilt the patient's head backward supported by a chairback or a headrest. Use an absorbent tissue pad under forefinger to depress the lower lid to form a conjunctival sac. Introduce medication into sac, never directly at or into the eye. (Courtesy Eye and Ear Infirmary, University of Illinois Hospitals, Chicago, Ill.)

Emotional factors in loss of sight

Emotional reactions to temporary or threatened loss of sight are often severe. Fear of the diagnosis may lead the patient to reject danger signs and delay medical attention. Worries over finances and family support and fear of being conspicuous among others may be added to concern over losing vision. The patient may not act rationally, he may be impatient and demanding, or he may be withdrawn and depressed. While he adjusts to his loss, patience, acceptance, and understanding are necessary from all persons who come in contact with him.

Sudden or jerky movements must be avoided in caring for any patient with eye disease since the natural reaction, blinking, may be painful or impossible. Jerky movements and haste tend to make the patient "on edge" and hamper release of tension and rest. Treatments should be done on time, because delay in treatments may cause anxiety for the patient and/ or delay in healing.

The person who has loss of vision in both eyes depends on sound and tactile sensation to maintain his feeling of security and kinship with those around him. He must be spoken to frequently in a quiet and reassuring voice. This is particularly important when he is in a strange hospital environment and awaiting diagnostic procedures and perhaps surgery. It is upsetting for the patient who cannot see to be touched without first being addressed; such an occurrence can be irritating and humiliating as well as actually dangerous. The nurse must teach all persons who attend the patient the importance of making their nearness known to the patient before touching him. They should introduce themselves and explain why they are there. On leaving the room, they should inform the patient so that he is spared the embarrassment of talking to someone who is not there. A small bell often is given to a patient with visual loss instead of a call signal. It gives the patient who can hear the assurance that his request has been made. The patient who is also deaf presents a real problem. If one cannot direct conversation into his ear and have it heard, there is no alternative but to touch him gently to make one's presence known. If he is to remain in contact with his environment, frequent physical contact must be made with him. Elderly persons who use hearing aids are urged to bring them to the hospital.

Life for the patient who has both eyes covered should be made as normal as possible. If he is used to smoking, he may be permitted to smoke, although someone must be in attendance to prevent a fire. Visitors should be allowed, though sometimes they need assistance in learning how to conduct themselves when they are with the patient who cannot see. They should be as natural as possible; for example, they should not make a conspicuous attempt to avoid such common phrases in speech as "see what I mean." Common sense dictates that gifts should appeal to other senses than vision. Scented colognes and soaps or a small bouquet of highly scented favorite flowers may be brought if the patient is not allergic to these items.

Restraints are sometimes necessary to prevent the patient from disturbing his dressings during sleep. They can be psychologically traumatizing even if carefully explained to the patient. The patient should be told that the restraints are used only to prevent him from accidentally disrupting his dressings. The use of side rails should also be explained. They are primarily to assist the patient in carefully shifting his position and to remind him not to get out of bed. They are not used to keep him in bed forcibly except in the case of patients with delirium tremens or acute brain syndrome.

Preoperative care

In order to formulate a care plan for any patient the nurse gathers information about his ability to meet basic needs such as the need for normal elimination, nutrition, vision, and respiration. Assessment of vision includes inspection of the eye and some measure of visual acuity. In a systematic manner the nurse obtains data by interviewing the patient and/or his family, by physical examination, by reading the patient's records, and by consultation with other health workers. The following are areas to include in the assessment of the eye and vision.*

Facial and ocular expression	Prominence of eyes, alert or dull expression
Eyelids	Symmetry, presence of edema, ptosis, itching, redness, discharges, blinking equality
Iris and pupils	Irregularities in color, shape, or size
Pupillary reflex	Constriction of pupil in response to light in that eye (direct light reaction), equal amount of constriction in the other eye (consensual light reaction)
Lens	Transparent or opaque
Peripheral vision	Ability to see movements and objects well on both sides of field of vision
Acuity with and without glasses	Ability to read newsprint, clocks on wall, and namepins, to recognize faces at bedside and at door
Supportive aids	Glasses, contact lenses, false eye

Routines for preoperative treatment and care vary with the part of the country, the institution, and the

---

*For further information on assessment of the eye see references 1a and 36a.

eye surgeon. If a complete medical examination has not been given before hospitalization, the patient usually spends at least 1 day in the hospital preoperatively. The patient's general condition and his reaction to the anticipated surgery should be observed closely and reported. He should meet the staff in the unit and get to know other patients, particularly if he is to have both eyes covered following surgery. While it is unusual for both eyes to be covered at once, the patient needs to be prepared if this is to be the case. He can become well oriented to his immediate surroundings prior to surgery. Preoperative counseling also includes explaining routines necessary for his care following his return from the operating room. The patient appreciates knowing what he can expect in relation to discomfort, treatments, dressings, tubes, and other equipment. The patient often benefits from meeting and talking to another patient who has successfully recovered from a surgical treatment such as he is to receive. The child should practice having his eyes covered so that he will not be too frightened or restless postoperatively. If possible, the child's mother should be permitted to stay with him before the operation and to sleep in his room.

The preparation of the patient on the evening before surgery is similar to that described on p. 199. If the patient has both eyes covered, it is essential that his call light be available. Since the older patient frequently becomes disoriented with his eyes covered, he should be visited frequently. The child may become frightened and will need to be comforted if his mother is not with him.

The preparation of the eye on the day of surgery consists of the instillation of a combination of drugs such as atropine sulfate, 1%, cyclopentolate (Cyclogyl), 1%, and phenylephrine (Neo-Synephrine), 10%, into the eye at various intervals to dilate the pupil. Topical anesthesia is begun with the instillation of such drugs as tetracaine (Pontocaine), 0.5%, butacaine sulfate (Butyn), 2%, or phenacaine hydrochloride (Holocaine), 1%. These agents are usually instilled in the operating room. Silver protein (Argyrol), 10%, may be instilled also to stain mucous shreds and surface debris so that they can be easily identified and removed during surgery. The medications must be given at the prescribed times so that the eye is prepared at the time of surgery. If anesthetizing drops are instilled before the patient goes to the operating room, the patient is asked to close his eye, and a pad is applied to protect the insensitive eye from injury due to rubbing, dryness, or dirt and dust. If only one eye is to be operated on, a mark may be placed on the forehead over that eye so that it can be identified easily in the operating room. It is vital to carefully check the patient's records so that the surgeon knows which eye is to be operated on.

If a local anesthetic is to be used, chloral hydrate, pentobarbital sodium (Nembutal), or meperidine hydrochloride (Demerol) may be given preoperatively. Atropine sulfate may be included if a general anesthetic is to be administered. When possible, general anesthesia is avoided because the patient may be restless on reacting and disturb the eye dressing, and the strain of vomiting may increase the tension on the suture line. Children, however, require general anesthesia and must be supervised closely until they have reacted fully. The type of anesthesia to be used is decided on by the surgeon and anesthesiologist, depending on the patient's general health.

If the eyelashes are cut, the surgeon uses straight, sharp scissors with fairly short blades that have been lubricated with petrolatum jelly to help prevent the cut lashes from entering the eye. After the skin preparation has been completed and the eye has been irrigated, if local anesthesia is being used, additional anesthetic drugs such as lidocaine (Xylocaine), 2%, may be injected into the operative area at this time. If general anesthesia is given, either intravenous or inhalation agents may be used.

Postoperative care

Specific routines for postoperative care following eye surgery vary in different locations and change rapidly as new techniques are developed. However, general goals of postoperative care are to prevent (1) increased intraocular pressure, (2) stress on the suture line, and (3) hemorrhage into the anterior chamber. A few general principles of postoperative care will be included here.

Immediately after the operation, the patient should keep his head still and try to avoid coughing, vomiting, sneezing, or moving suddenly. He should lie with the unoperated side down to prevent pressure on the operated eye and to prevent possible contamination of the dressing with vomitus. A pillow placed along his back will help keep the patient on his side. During the first 4 to 24 hours the head of the bed usually is elevated gradually; the patient may turn from his back to the unoperated side, but he may not lie on his stomach or on the operated side.

Postoperative confusion is a problem, particularly in elderly persons and in persons who have had both eyes covered. If confusion does occur, the surgeon may decide that the danger of activity due to confusion is worse than activity resulting from having one eye uncovered. For this reason, few surgeons cover the unoperated eye.

Side rails are placed on the bed immediately postoperatively and are kept on while both eyes are covered, if the patient cannot see, or as long as necessary for his protection. The bedside table should be placed on the side of the unoperated eye so that the patient can see it without excessive movement of his head.

Care should be taken that the dressing is not loosened or removed. If the patient is not reliable, he should be attended constantly. Restraints may occasionally need to be applied if the patient does not understand or cannot cooperate and if it is not possible to have him attended constantly. Restraints should be very light in weight and loosely attached to the wrists; usually a 2-inch gauze bandage is used, but a boxing-glove type of hand restraint may be applied. Elbow restraints usually are satisfactory for infants, but if not, the clove-hitch bandage may be used. If the dressings are removed, they should be replaced and the surgeon should be notified. It is usual for some bleeding and serous drainage to occur, but it should be minimal. The lid is edematous, but this condition subsides within 3 or 4 days. Mild pain and pressure can be normal in the postoperative course. However, a sensation of pressure within the eye may suggest hemorrhage; sharp pain is suggestive of infection or hemorrhage. These symptoms should be quickly reported to the surgeon.

Postoperative ambulation depends on the type of operation, the general condition of the patient, and the surgeon's preference. The patient may be up on the first postoperative day, or he may be in bed 5 or 6 days after surgery. Whatever the regimen, supervision and assistance should be given by the nurse to be sure that the patient is able to walk without sustaining injury. Because he cannot see out of the covered eye, he must try to avoid bumping into things and jarring the operative site. To avoid falls, he should not sit down until he has located both arms of the chair with his hands. He usually is advised not to bend or stoop or to lift objects for several weeks after the operation in order to prevent increasing intraocular pressure, which might nullify the surgery. Slippers or shoes that he can slip into without tying or buckling are preferable during this time. Patients who have both eyes covered should be led to their destination (Fig. 31-9). They should be informed of obstacles in their path, alerted when to turn before the turn appears, and told when to move to *their* right or left.

If the patient must remain in bed, he will require the postoperative care discussed on p. 217 to keep him comfortable and to prevent postoperative complications from developing. During this period of inactivity, visits from other patients, family, and friends and listening to the radio or television may help to distract the patient and pass the time. Volunteers may be available to read to patients and to answer their mail. The child will benefit from having his mother with him, listening to stories, and playing with passive games and toys that are familiar to him.

Because increased intraocular pressure may result from the Valsalva maneuver, a stool softener or milk of magnesia often are given postoperatively to

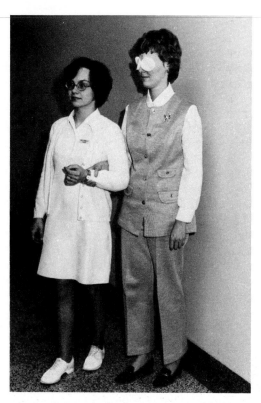

FIG. 31-9. Ambulation of a patient who cannot see. Note that the patient holds onto the nurse's arm and is led to her destination without being held.

lessen difficulty in having bowel movements. Discomfort in the eye usually is relieved by acetylsalicylic acid (aspirin), 0.6 Gm., meperidine (Demerol), 25 to 75 mg., or dextropropoxyphene hydrochloride (Darvon), 32 to 67 mg.

A soft diet may be ordered for a few days postoperatively, although some physicians feel that a diet that permits moderate chewing will decrease abdominal distention and discomfort. The amount of vision he has and his general condition determine whether or not the patient needs assistance in eating. When helping the patient who cannot see, it is important to identify the kind of food he is to receive. The nurse must not allow feeding a patient to become a routine procedure and should not appear hurried. If the patient is to have visual limitation for some time, he must be helped to learn to feed himself. Very exact descriptions of the kind and location of food and equipment and guiding the patient's hands so that he may feel the outline and placement of dishes helps. It is important that, if possible, the bed patient have the bed raised so that he may sit in a somewhat normal position for eating. Having him go through the motions a few times with an empty utensil helps to give him a correct feeling for distance. The patient should have privacy until he learns to handle food in a fairly normal way.

The nurse must help the patient and his family

develop patience. Surgery may not cure the patient's eye condition; it may never be cured but only improved, and the patient should be informed of this possibility by the physician. It should also be explained preoperatively that it may take weeks and even months for him to become accustomed to the type of glasses he may need to wear.

After surgery the patient should follow his surgeon's instructions carefully and keep appointments as scheduled. Many patients must return to the surgeon's office or the clinic periodically for a long time, some indefinitely. The nurse caring for the patient in the hospital has a responsibility to teach him this when he is most receptive to teaching. The nurse working in the community can be invaluable in arranging for clinic care, in helping the patient and his family to avoid discouragement, to administer medications as prescribed, and to report to the physician regularly.

■ DISEASE CONDITIONS AND RELATED MANAGEMENT

Trauma

Trauma may damage the eyelids and adjacent structures, the outer surface of the eyeball, and the deep structures of the eye. (For details of first aid in event of eye injury, see p. 273.) Lacerations of the eyelids should be treated by an eye specialist, because there is danger of scar formation as healing occurs. Any injury to the eyeball should be referred immediately to the specialist.

Patients with *ecchymosis* of the eyelids and surrounding tissues (black eye) should be examined to rule out coexisting skull fractures. Cold compresses will help to control the bleeding, and subsequent hot compresses will speed up the reabsorption of blood from the tissues. The disfigurement will last about 2 weeks and can be covered with cosmetics. *Lacerations* of the eyelid may need to be sutured after the bleeding is controlled and any foreign material is removed. Antitetanus serum usually is given to all patients who sustain eye wounds. *Corneal injuries* are serious since resistance to infection is low in the cornea and scars that form can impair vision. *Injuries to the ciliary body and sclera and injuries involving the orbit* are critical because adjacent tissues usually are also injured and there may be escape of contents of the eyeball and possible infection of the interior of the eye. If these injuries result in wounds that are small and clean, treatment consists of bed rest, antibiotics given systemically and topically, suturing the wound, instilling atropine to put the iris and the ciliary body at rest, and a firm dressing. If the injury is extensive and if sight is lost, enucleation (removal of the eyeball) may be necessary. This is usually not performed before consultation with one or more ophthalmologists.

One of the most dreaded sequelae to eye injury is *sympathetic ophthalmitis*. This complication is a serious inflammation of the uveal tract (ciliary body, iris, and choroid) in the uninjured eye that follows a penetrating injury to the other eye. The cause of this condition is unknown, but it may be due to an allergic reaction to the uveal pigment that is set free in the bloodstream at the time of the injury. Children are especially susceptible, but it may occur at any age. The uninjured eye becomes inflamed and there is photophobia and lacrimation, dimness of vision, and pain in the eye. Sympathetic ophthalmitis may appear 3 to 8 weeks after the eye injury or months or years later, but it never appears if the injured eye is removed within a week of the injury. The decision as to whether or not the involved eye should be removed rests with the surgeon and often depends on the amount of damage to the uveal tract. Before the use of cortisone, sympathetic ophthalmitis usually resulted in total or almost complete loss of vision of both eyes. When cortisone has been given immediately following the injury or at the first sign of involvement of the good eye, it has saved the vision of many patients. Because of increased medical skill in treating perforating wounds and the administration of cortisone at the earliest suggestion of inflammation, sympathetic ophthalmitis has become a rare disease in recent years.

Tumors

Tumors involving the eyelids and structures about the eye as well as the eyeball itself are not unusual. Orbital neoplasms include benign hemangiomas, pseudotumors, lymphomas, mucoceles from the sinuses, malignant melanomas, retinoblastomas, and others. When they are malignant, both vision and life are endangered. Tumors within the eyeball are often silent except for a bloodshot appearance of the eye. Yet, as in all malignant tumors, the prognosis depends on early diagnosis and prompt treatment.

Retinoblastomas are congenital and occur in infants and children under 5 years of age. In about one third of the patients the tumors invade both eyes. In normal parents who have one child with retinoblastoma, there is a likelihood of less than 4% that a subsequent child will have such a tumor. Persons who survive the tumors should have genetic counseling to alert them to the danger of transmission to their offspring.[38] These malignant growths arise from the nuclear layers of the retina, grow rapidly, and spread backward along the optic nerve to invade the brain. Retinoblastomas can also metastasize to distant sites via the bloodstream and lymphatics.

Malignant melanomas occur in the choroid and iris of adults. They grow slowly, but due to the vascularity of the choroid, they metastasize early to the liver and lungs. Medical treatment of tumors of the eye may include enucleation, radiation treatment, use of chemotherapeutic agents, and plastic surgery.

The emotional response to a tumor of the eye is perhaps even greater than to malignancies elsewhere. The surgeon may advise immediate enucleation of the eye in the hope of saving life. If both eyes are affected by retinoblastoma, the most involved eye may be removed and the lesion in the other eye treated more conservatively in the hope of arresting its growth and possibly saving vision. (See p. 841 for a discussion of enucleation.) Both the patient and his family need to be encouraged to talk about their feelings and concerns and helped to readjust their lives in the face of this serious situation.

Infections and inflammation

Infections and inflammation can occur in any of the eye structures and may be caused by organisms, mechanical irritation, or sensitivity to some substance.

Styes. Styes (hordeola) are relatively mild but extremely common infections of the follicle of an eyelash or the small lubricating glands of the lid margins. Staphylococci are often the infecting organisms. Patients should be taught not to squeeze styes because the infection may spread and cause cellulitis of the lids. If warm, moist compresses are used, styes usually open and drain without surgery. These infections tend to occur in crops because the infecting organism spreads from one hair follicle to another. Poor hygiene and excessive use of cosmetics may be contributing causes.

Chalazion. A chalazion is a cyst caused by an obstruction in the ducts of the sebaceous glands (meibomian glands) located in the connective tissue in the free edges of the eyelids. The cysts present a hard, shiny, lumpy appearance as viewed from the inner side of the lid. They may cause pressure on the cornea. Small chalazions need not be removed and may disappear after the application of an antibacterial ointment followed by massage and hot compresses. If they are large or become infected, they usually require a surgical incision and curettage. Chalazions usually are removed in the physician's office or the clinic under local anesthesia. An antibacterial ointment such as neomycin sulfate may be applied to the conjunctiva, and a pad worn for a few days.

Conjunctivitis and blepharitis. Conjunctivitis (inflammation of conjunctiva) and blepharitis (inflammation of the eyelids) are common infections and have a variety of causes. They may result from mechanical trauma such as that caused by sunburn or infection with organisms such as staphylococci, viruses, streptococci, or gonococci. Inflammation is often due to allergic reactions within the body or to outside irritants such as poison ivy or cosmetics. Conjunctivitis caused by the Koch-Weeks bacillus ("pinkeye") is common in schoolchildren and is highly infectious. Conjunctivitis is always accompanied by redness and congestion, which varies in degree and distribution and increased secretions. The secretions may be watery, due largely to an increased secretion of tears, or mucoid, mucopurulent, or purulent, depending on the case.

Treatment for conjunctivitis depends on the cause. Specific antibacterial drugs may be used systemically and locally. Hot moist compresses, irrigations, eyedrops, and ointments often are prescribed. The patient must be cautioned not to touch his eyes since the inflamed tissues are susceptible to new infection, and trauma delays healing. If only one eye is involved, he must be cautioned to leave his uninvolved eye strictly alone. Patients with blepharitis or conjunctivitis rest better in a darkened room than in a well-lighted one. They should be observed carefully for progress of the eye condition. Infections of the conjunctiva can be stubborn and may even lead to involvement of the cornea, with serious consequences to vision. Blepharitis can extend to the conjunctiva.

Corneal ulcer. A corneal ulcer indicates either an abrasion or an infected lesion on the surface of the cornea. Since the cornea has many pain-transmitting fibers, damage to its epithelium is easily recognized because of the pain that is present on blinking. The ulcer may be caused by trauma, by contact lenses, or by infections of the conjunctiva that have spread to the cornea. Persons with a low resistance to infection may develop ulcers from little apparent cause (for example, the individual who has diabetes mellitus). The extent of the ulcer can be outlined by using sterile fluorescein, a green, harmless dye. The ulcer may be self-limiting, it may spread across the cornea, or it may penetrate into its deeper layers.

Nonpenetrating ulcers such as those caused by fingernail scratches heal readily unless infected. Antibiotic drops may be instilled to prevent infection, and a protective dressing may be worn for a few days. Ulcers that penetrate to the deep layers of the cornea may be cleansed with an antiseptic solution, cauterized, treated with antibiotics locally and systemically, and covered with a firm dressing. Atropine sulfate may be instilled to keep the pupil dilated and to put the ciliary body and iris at rest, thus reducing pain. Hot compresses may be applied to help clear the infection, and cortisone may be administered cautiously to control the inflammation. Depending on their location, infected ulcers may destroy corneal tissue, causing partial or total blindness. The corneal ulcer is a form of keratitis.

Keratitis. Inflammation of the cornea is called keratitis. It causes severe pain in the eye, photophobia (sensitivity to light), tearing, and blepharospasm (spasm of the eyelids). Uncontrolled keratitis can result in loss of vision due to impairment of corneal transparency or destruction of the eye by corneal perforation. Keratitis may be acute or chronic and superficial or deep (interstitial). It may be associated with a corneal ulcer or be caused by diseases such as tuberculosis and syphilis. Allergic reactions, vitamin A deficiency, or viral diseases such as mumps, measles, and herpes simplex may contribute to its development in children. If possible, the systemic cause is found and treated. Cortisone may be used cautiously to control the inflammation; antibiotics should be given to treat the infection. Atropine sulfate, which blurs vision for at least 1 week, will keep the iris and ciliary body at rest; hot compresses will help promote healing. Idoxuridine (IDU) applied locally is effective in helping to clear keratitis caused by herpes simplex in 80% of cases. The eyes may be covered to limit eye movements, and the patient may be placed on bed rest.

Corneal grafts (keratoplasty). Loss of vision caused by an opaque or destroyed cornea may be restored by replacing the damaged layers with a corresponding corneal graft obtained from a new cadaver or from an eye freshly removed by operation. For best results, the donor cornea must be removed within 6 hours of death and ideally should be used within 24 hours. Transplants preserved for longer periods may be used for lamellar grafts. The present practice is to keep a waiting list of persons who need grafts, since eye banks are not able to keep up with the demand. Eye Bank for Sight Restoration, Inc.,* is a nonprofit organization that collects and distributes donated eyes throughout the country. Donors or their relatives usually make arrangements for donating the eyes before death.

Corneal transplantation cannot be done if there is any infection. The kind of corneal graft used depends on the depth and size of the damaged part that must be replaced (Fig. 31-10). Corneal transplants, or grafts, may involve the entire thickness of the cornea (total penetrating), only part of the depth of the cornea (lamellar), or a combination of these, in which a small part of the graft involves the entire thickness of the cornea (partial penetrating). Obviously the penetrating graft is the more difficult to establish and requires the more definitive care postoperatively. For the penetrating graft, the eye surgeon seldom uses a donor eye that is over 48 hours old.

Because a large amount of tissue is removed and replaced, the patient who has had a penetrating graft transplant usually remains in bed with both eyes bandaged for 1 to 2 days so as not to disturb the graft. The patient who has had a mixed or partial penetrating graft usually has both eyes bandaged and is kept very quiet for at least 24 hours, whereas the patient who has had a lamellar graft only may

*210 East 64th St., New York, N. Y. 10021.

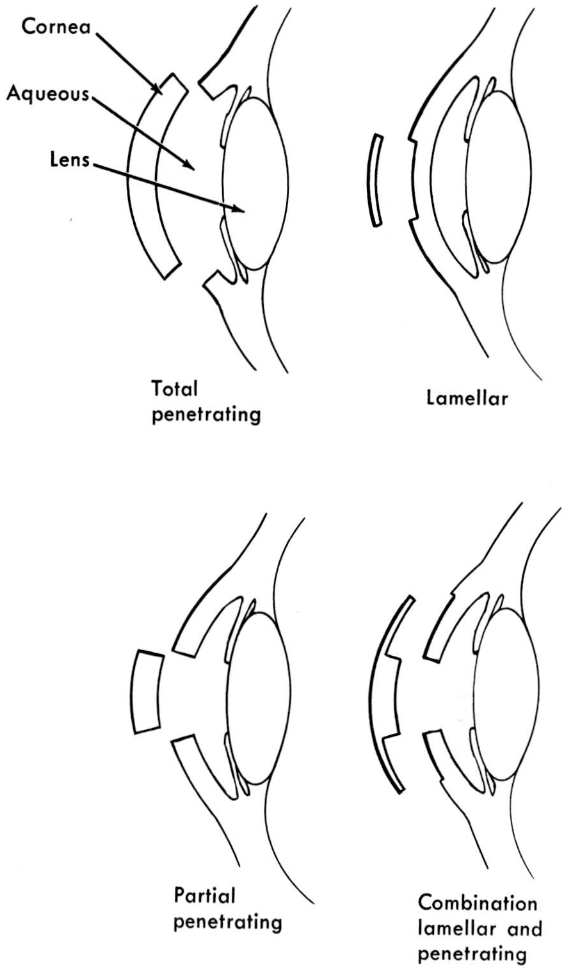

FIG. 31-10. The types of corneal grafts now being used. Note that in the lamellar graft the defect does not penetrate the entire thickness of the cornea.

not have the unaffected eye covered at all and may be out of bed and able to feed himself on the day of the operation. Corneal grafts heal very slowly because of the lack of blood vessels in the cornea and require from 3 weeks to 6 months to heal firmly. The patient is advised to avoid sudden, quick movement, jarring, bending, or lifting during this period in order to avoid disturbing the healing process. Success also depends on the basic disease process.

Complications of corneal transplant operations include the following: blood vessels may grow into the new cornea (compensatory neovascularization) so that clarity may be lost, or the new cornea may become cloudy for no apparent reason. While the operation can usually be repeated, performing a second operation depends on the condition of the patient's eye.

Iritis. Iritis (inflammation of the iris) rarely occurs alone and usually is associated with inflammation of the ciliary body. Then the term *"iridocyclitis"* is used. If the choroid also is involved, the infection is called *uveitis.* These infections produce pain in the eyeball radiating to the forehead and temple, photophobia (sensitivity to light), lacrimation, and interference with vision. There is edema of the upper lid, the iris is swollen because of congestion and exudation of cells and fibrin, and the pupil is contracted and irregular as a result of the formation of adhesions. Iritis and iridocyclitis may be associated with a systemic disease such as syphilis, tuberculosis, toxoplasmosis, or sarcoidosis or it may result from trauma. Usually there is no known cause. The instillation of 1% atropine sulfate or 0.2% scopolamine into the eye puts the iris and ciliary body at rest, relieves pain and photophobia, and diminishes congestion. By keeping the pupil dilated, these cycloplegic drugs prevent adhesions from forming between the anterior capsule of the lens and the iris and tend to cause those already formed to regress. Moist warm compresses may be applied several times each day to help diminish pain and inflammation. The eyes usually are covered, and in the convalescent period, dark glasses are ordered to be worn. The patient is on bed rest during the acute stages. Although acetylsalicylic acid (aspirin) may be helpful for relieving pain, sometimes morphine sulfate is necessary. Cortisone preparations are of great value in controlling the inflammation in many patients, but the inflammation in other patients resists almost all forms of treatment. If a systemic cause cannot be found and treated, the injection of a foreign protein (fever therapy) such as the typhoid H antigen into the body to stimulate its defense mechanism may be used. Complications of these infections of the uvea include the formation of adhesions, keratitis, secondary glaucoma, and the loss of vision.

Strabismus

Strabismus (squint, cross-eye, walleye) is characterized by the inability of the eyes to move together in a coordinated manner. A light source directed straight into normal eyes forms a reflected spot image symmetrically located in each pupil; in strabismus the image is off center in one eye compared to its location in the fellow eye. When the person with strabismus looks straight ahead with one eye, the other deviates. The crossing may be slight or very noticeable. If the eye is turned inward toward the nose, it is called convergent strabismus (esotropia). If the eye is turned outward, it is called divergent strabismus (exotropia).[45] Strabismus may be paralytic or nonparalytic. Paralytic strabismus (inability to move the eye) is caused by loss of function of the ocular muscles resulting from damage to the muscles or the cranial nerves (III, IV, or VI) by tumor, infection, or brain or eye injuries. Its main symptom in addition to the strabismus, unless vision is suppressed in one eye, is double vision (diplopia). Normally, when both eyes look at the same object,

the image of the object is focused by the brain into a single picture. If muscle paralysis causes the eyes to cross, the brain sees two separate pictures. The treatment is directed toward removing the cause of the paralysis, if possible, and straightening the eye.

Nonparalytic strabismus affects 1% of the population and sometimes is caused by an inherited abnormality of the fusion center within the brain.[29] While the eyes of the normal newborn do not focus together, by the age of 6 months he should have developed fusion, or "binocular vision" (the ability to see a separate image with each eye and fuse them into one image). The desire for binocular singular vision keeps the eye straight. Occasionally an infant is born without the ability to acquire fusion, and it can never be acquired. In most cases of strabismus, however, fusion is present but underdeveloped. The child's eyes are crossed, and he may look straight with either the right eye or the left eye but not with both simultaneously. If he fixes (looks straight ahead) with one eye and then the other, he has *alternating strabismus.* If he prefers to use one eye to the exclusion of the other and always uses the preferred eye, he has *monocular strabismus. Suppression* is the ability of the brain to disregard conflicting visual images from the deviating eye. If the child never uses the crossed eye, impaired vision may result. This type of defective vision is called *suppression amblyopia.* It usually can be treated successfully before the child is 6 years of age; thereafter it usually will respond poorly to any therapy. It is the most common cause of partial blindness in children.

Early medical attention is important in strabismus both to save vision and to prevent the emotional trauma that is always associated with crossed eyes. Treatment should begin as soon as the diagnosis is made. During early childhood, occlusion is used to improve vision. The good eye is covered with a patch, bandage, or attachment to the glasses, and the child is forced to use the weaker eye. *Orthoptics* is a nonsurgical treatment of strabismus. Prisms, glasses, and exercises are used to train the child to use the two eyes together. Orthoptics is used as an adjunct to other methods of treating strabismus.

Strabismus in children who are farsighted and who accommodate excessively may be corrected by constantly wearing glasses. Glasses with harness frames can be safely worn by children 5 to 6 months of age. As the child becomes more independent, it is sometimes very difficult to get him to wear glasses consistently. When the glasses are removed, the eyes tend to cross. Long-acting miotics such as isofluorophate (DFP) instilled daily cause constriction of the ciliary muscle and help correct farsightedness. Sometimes the use of glasses and the use of drugs are combined. A recent article on strabismus describes the nature and treatment of the condition.[30a]

Surgery is resorted to if none of the above methods correct the crossed eyes. After the age of 6 years, surgery may achieve only cosmetic improvement and may not correct the already impaired vision. Surgery consists of shortening or lengthening the muscle attachments to straighten the eye. The child may wear a dressing over the eye for a few days and is permitted to move about freely and to be out of bed. Surgery usually is followed by the prescription of corrective glasses and eye exercises, depending on the individual patient. The child's family should understand that the operation may need to be repeated. Parents should be encouraged to continue with medical treatment for as long as recommended. If they believe that the condition is completely cured and neglect medical attention until a conspicuous squint again appears, damage to vision may have occurred. The public health nurse and the school nurse should be particularly alert to children who show signs of strabismus and to direct them to medical care. The establishment of preschool vision screening programs for children in the 3- to 5-year-old age group has been extremely helpful in getting the child with strabismus referred for treatment early enough to be satisfactorily treated.

Glaucoma

Glaucoma is a disease or group of diseases characterized by increased intraocular pressure. The increase in pressure usually is caused by an obstruction to the circulation of aqueous humor through the meshwork at the angle of the anterior chamber of the eye where the peripheral iris and the cornea meet (Fig. 31-11). The blockage may be secondary to an infection or injury or may be caused by a hereditary predisposition to thickening of the meshwork (chronic simple glaucoma). Acute glaucoma is the result of an abnormal displacement of iris against the angle of the anterior chamber. Unless the diagnosis is made early and treatment is effective and continued, increased intraocular pressure leads to destruction of nerve fibers on the optic disc and loss of vision.

The incidence of glaucoma is increasing as the number of older persons in our population rises. While it is seldom seen in persons under 35 years of age, it is the greatest threat to vision in older people. Glaucoma is the second leading identified cause of blindness. It has been estimated that there are about 1 million persons in the United States with glaucoma that has not been diagnosed.

Acute angle closure glaucoma may cause general symptoms of nausea and vomiting in addition to eye pain and dilation of the pupil, as the iris remains dilated. Increased vascularity of the cornea may cause the patient to conclude that he has "pinkeye." There is edema of the ciliary body and the cornea and an increase of tension within the eyeball. Since a marked increase in intraocular pressure for 24 to

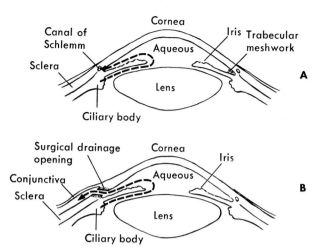

FIG. 31-11. A, Originating from the ciliary processes, the aqueous flows through the pupil into the anterior chamber and normally leaves the eye via the canal of Schlemm. **B,** In glaucoma the normal aqueous outflow is reduced or blocked. The purpose of glaucoma surgery is to create a new channel through which aqueous can leave the eye. (Redrawn from Havener, W. H.: Synopsis of ophthalmology, ed. 3, St. Louis, 1971, The C. V. Mosby Co.)

36 hours may lead to complete and permanent blindness, immediate treatment is necessary. Treatment usually consists of miotics such as pilocarpine drops to constrict the pupil and permit the outflow of aqueous humor, narcotics for pain, and complete rest. If symptoms do not subside within a few hours, an emergency operation such as an iridectomy may be performed to reduce the pressure by providing an outlet for the aqueous humor.

Chronic simple glaucoma may come on slowly, and, at first, symptoms may be absent. Chronic glaucoma gives one characteristic sign that is important: before central vision becomes affected, the peripheral visual fields are impaired so that objects to the side are ignored. Limitation of vision may not be so apparent as in other eye diseases, and much damage can occur before medical aid is sought. The patient may bump into other persons in the street or fail to see passing vehicles, yet not realize that the fault lies in his own vision. A diminished field of vision may cause the driver of an automobile to have an accident. The loss of peripheral vision ("tunnel vision") can progress until the patient is legally blind, yet he may be able to see well straight ahead. The community nurse who recognizes this difficulty may be most helpful in early case finding and in promptly referring patients to an ophthalmologist. Because vision lost due to glaucoma is irreversible, early diagnosis is mandatory.

Chronic glaucoma usually begins in one eye, although if it is left untreated, both eyes often become affected. Symptoms are most apparent in the morning, when a persistent dull eye pain may develop. Frequent changes of glasses, difficulty in adjusting to darkness, failure to detect changes in color accurately, and slight blurring of vision are fairly early signs of angle closure glaucoma. Then follows a steamy appearance of the cornea and further blurring of vision. Tearing, misty vision, blurred appearance of the iris (which becomes fixed and dilated), headache, pain behind the eyeball, nausea, and vomiting can then occur. Halos, resembling street lamps seen through a steamy windshield, may be seen about lights.

All treatment for glaucoma is directed toward reducing intraocular pressure and keeping it at a safe level. Miotics such as pilocarpine are used to constrict the pupil and to draw the smooth muscle of the iris away from the canal of Schlemm to permit aqueous humor to drain out at this point. Acetazolamide (Diamox), a drug that tends to reduce the formation of aqueous humor, is used successfully in some types of chronic glaucoma. Osmotic agents such as urea, mannitol, and glycerol may be used to reduce intraocular pressure in the treatment of acute glaucoma. An effective dose of these drugs will decrease intraocular pressure within $1/2$ hour of administration. Surgical procedures for glaucoma are used to produce a permanent filtration pathway for aqueous fluid. A *cyclodialysis* is performed to form a channel between the anterior chamber and the suprachoroidal space. In an *iridectomy* a portion of the iris is excised to make an opening between the anterior and posterior chambers to permit drainage. If the iris is blocking the angle of the anterior chamber, an iridectomy may be performed to relieve the obstruction. An *anterior sclerectomy* is the removal of a piece of the sclera to permit fluid to escape from the anterior chamber. An *iridencleisis* is a procedure in which a piece of iris is brought into the scleral incision to prevent it from closing, thus providing a permanent fistula for the drainage of fluid. In selected cases the production of aqueous fluid may be decreased by destroying part of the ciliary body. This may be accomplished by diathermy or cryosurgery. Following surgery the patient usually is allowed out of bed at once, although one or both eyes may be bandaged for several days. Postoperative management of patients having eye surgery has already been discussed.

The patient with glaucoma needs assistance in learning to accept his disease. Despite explanation from his physician, he frequently hopes that the operation will cure his condition, that no further treatment will be necessary, and perhaps that the sight he has lost will be restored. It should be explained that the vision lost cannot be restored but that further loss can usually be prevented and his life can be quite normal if he continues under medical care. There usually is no restriction to use of the eyes. Fluid intake generally is not curtailed and exercise is permitted. Bright lights or darkness are not harmful to the eyes of the patient with glaucoma, and there is apparently no relationship between vascular hypertension and ocular hypertension.[29]

The person with glaucoma should be under medical care for the rest of his life, receiving either drug or surgical therapy or both. Following the operation he should return regularly to the physician since one operation does not necessarily mean that drainage will be continued. Any obstruction or closing of the artificial pathway will result in reappearance of symptoms and further visual damage. The patient and his family should know specifically what to do if essential eyedrops are accidentally spilled; for example, they should know what local drugstore is open at night and during holidays. The patient often is advised to have an extra bottle of medication in his home and to carry one with him if he works away from his home. It is advisable also for the patient to carry a card or other identifying information to identify himself as having glaucoma in case an accident occurs.

Cataract

A cataract is a clouding, or opacity, of the lens that leads to blurring of vision and eventual loss of sight. The opacity is due to chemical changes in the protein of the lens caused by slow degenerative changes of age, injury, poison, or intraocular infection. Cataracts can occur at any time of life and may be associated with iritis, uveitis, and other conditions such as diabetes. They may follow the ingestion of injurious substances such as dinitrophenol, which was taken for weight reduction a few decades ago. Cataracts may be congenital, occurring most often in infants whose mothers had German measles during the first trimester of pregnancy.

Cataracts occur so often in the aged that the term "senile cataract" is used. At 80 years of age about 85% of all people have some clouding of the lens. Senile cataracts are listed as the most common cause of blindness in older persons, yet the response of the condition to surgery often is excellent. Patients who are in their nineties can often be operated on with good results.

Operative treatment is the only satisfactory treatment for cataracts. The decision as to when to remove the cataract depends largely on the individual patient and the use he makes of his eyes. If any signs of inflammation are present, surgery is not attempted. It is the nurse's responsibility to refer the patient with a cataract to an ophthalmologist and to encourage him to accept treatment as recommended.

Cataracts usually are removed under local anesthesia. Removal has been simplified in many cases by the use of the enzyme alpha-chymotrypsin, which weakens the zonular fibers that hold the lens in position. Cataracts may be removed within their capsule *(intracapsular technique),* or an opening may be made in the capsule and the lens lifted out without disturbing the membrane *(extracapsular technique).* The lens and its capsule may be frozen with a probe cooled to a temperature of −35° C. (−31° F.) or lower and then lifted from its position in the eye *(cryoextraction).* All these procedures usually are preceded by an iridectomy, which is performed to create an opening for the flow of aqueous humor, which may become blocked postoperatively when the vitreous humor moves forward. Usually only one eye is operated on at a time lest some complication arise or some unexpected behavior of the patient, such as rubbing his operative eye, interferes with healing. If the patient has cataracts in both eyes, both may be removed during one hospitalization. This plan for treatment must be explained to the patient and his family or else he may feel that time is being spent in the hospital unnecessarily.

Following any cataract operation a dressing is applied to the eye and covered with a metal shield to protect it from injury. The unoperated eye also may be covered, but usually it is left free. The patient normally is allowed out of bed the day following surgery. Dressings are changed by the surgeon in 1 to 3 days, and after 1 week to 10 days all dressings are removed. Temporary glasses may be prescribed 1 to 4 weeks after surgery, depending on the rate of healing and the amount of vision in the other eye.

Congenital cataracts respond favorably to a simple operation known as a *discission* procedure. A very small opening is made in the capsule surrounding the lens, and a small, sharp needle knife is passed in pendulumlike manner through the lens. This procedure also is referred to as a "needling" operation. The operation permits aqueous fluid to pass into the cloudy lens, causing the cloudiness to disappear. Congenital cataracts are usually operated on when the child is about 2 years of age or older. A general anesthetic is used, no immobilization in bed is necessary, and the child may be permitted to go home within a day or two of the operation.

A new method of cataract removal is called phacoemulsification. This procedure breaks up the lens and flushes it out in tiny pieces. The phacoemulsification method requires an incision just large enough to insert a needle probe that vibrates 40,000 times/ second to break up the lens. As the lens is broken up, the area is flushed with fluid, and pieces of the lens are carried from the eye by a tiny suction unit. Only one stitch is needed to close the incision. Healing and convalescence are considerably quicker than for patients who have had the cryosurgical removal previously described. The size and shape of the eye are factors in determining if this method is suitable for a particular patient.

The elderly patient sometimes finds it hard to adjust to removal of a cataract. The little remaining ability to accommodate the eye is lost when the lens is removed, and the patient must wear glasses at all times. Cataract glasses magnify, so that everything appears about one-fourth closer than it is and the patient must have perseverance in becoming accustomed to their use. He needs to know that it will take time to learn to judge distance, climb stairs, and do other simple things. He may be surprised to learn that the color of objects seen with the eye from which the lens has been removed is slightly changed, and that if he has had the lens removed from one eye only, he will use only one eye at a time but not both together unless he is fitted with a contact lens for the operated eye. He must wait at least 3 months before permanent glasses can be prescribed. Most younger persons prefer contact lenses after cataract surgery but the older person has difficulty inserting them. There is no restriction of activity once the operative site is healed.

Detachment of the retina

The retina is the part of the eye that perceives light; it coordinates and transmits impulses from its seeing nerve cells to the optic nerve. There are two primitive retinal layers: the outer pigment epithelium and an inner sensory layer. Retinal detachment occurs when (1) a separation of the two primitive layers of the retina occurs due to accumulation of fluid between them or (2) an elevation of both retinal layers away from the choroid occurs due to a tumor. As the detachment extends and becomes complete, blindness results. Myopic degeneration, trauma, and aphakia (absence of the crystalline lens) are the most frequent causes of retinal detachment in children and adults. It may also result from hemorrhage, tumor, or exudates that occur in front of or behind the retina. Detachment of the retina may follow sudden severe physical exertion, especially in persons who are debilitated. However, often there is no apparent cause.

The detachment may occur suddenly or develop slowly. The symptoms include floating spots or opacities before the eyes, flashes of light, and progressive constriction of vision in one area. The floating spots are blood and retinal cells that are freed at the time of the tear and cast shadows on the retina as they seem to drift about the eye. The area of visual loss depends entirely on the location of the detachment. When the detachment is extensive and occurs quickly, the patient may have the sensation that a curtain has been drawn before his eyes or of looking over a fence.

Immediate care for detachment of the retina includes keeping the patient quiet in bed and his eyes covered to try to prevent further detachment. His head is positioned so that the retinal hole is in the lowest part of the eye. Because extended conservative treatment for detachment of the retina has not been successful, early surgery is now the approved method of treatment. Cyclopentolate or phenylephrine is used to keep the pupils widely dilated so that tears in the retina may be identified during the operation. The surgery may be done under either local or general anesthesia. The surgical procedure may include draining the fluid from the subretinal space so that the retina returns to its normal position, thereby closing the opening in the retina. To drain the fluid from the subretinal space, the sclera and choroid are perforated at the time of the operation. The retinal breaks are sealed off by various methods that produce an inflammatory reaction (*chorioretinitis*) in the area of the tear so that the adhesions will form between the edges of the break and the underlying choroid to obliterate the opening. When the tears are small or of recent origin, diathermy may be applied through the sclera with needlepoint electrodes to produce the inflammatory process. An intense beam of visible light directed to the area by means of an elaborate ophthalmoscope may be used to close retinal tears when the retina is not elevated (*photocoagulation*). The *laser* beam is used by some as a source of intense energy to produce the chorioretinitis. Subfreezing temperatures (−40° to −60° C.) may be applied to the surface of the sclera in the area of the hole to produce the inflammatory reaction (*retinal cryopexy*). Nitrous oxide or carbon dioxide under pressure flowing through a tube attached to a delicate instrument is used to produce these low temperatures.

For almost all retinal detachments, including those previously considered inoperable, *scleral buckling* procedures are used. A scleral buckle serves as a splint to hold the retina and choroid together until the choroidal scar can form to permanently seal the hole or tear. The retinal break or tear is closed by the following procedure. The area overlying the treated tear is indented or "buckled" inward toward the vitreous cavity. (See Fig. 31-12.) To create the buckle, a fold is taken in the treated sclera and choroid and sutured into place, or a segment of the sclera is resected and shortened. This procedure may be combined with the implantation of a foreign material such as various-shaped pieces of silicone or with eye-bank sclera to cause further indentation of the choroid. By these procedures, the choroid is pushed into contact with the retinal tear during healing, and vitreous adhesions that have exerted traction, or pull, on the retinal break are relaxed as the size of the scleral shell is decreased.

The patient's postoperative position will depend on the extent and location of his retinal detachment. Because postoperative routines vary a great deal, the nurse must be certain that orders for bed position and for ambulation have been written by the surgeon

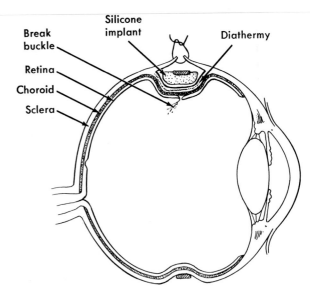

FIG. 31-12. One method of performing a scleral buckling operation.

and that the patient understands exactly how much activity he may have. (See general discussion of the postoperative care of a patient having eye surgery.) Dressings are usually changed daily, but it is about a week before the eye can be fully examined and determination made as to whether or not the operation has been successful. It may be possible to reoperate when surgery has not been successful, although a second operation usually is delayed for at least 1 or 2 weeks. Hemorrhage is a common complication of an operation for detachment of the retina. It may result from cryosurgery, diathermy, or puncture of the choroid to obtain release of subretinal fluids at the time of operation. When dressings are removed, the patient is usually allowed to ambulate progressively over the next several days.

Resumption of sedentary duties may be permitted 3 weeks after surgery, while activities or occupations requiring heavy physical exertion may not be permitted for 6 weeks or more. Restoration of sight will depend on the extent and duration of the detachment prior to surgery as well as the degree of success of the treatment. Some ophthalmologists advise their patients to avoid contact sports for the rest of their lives.

Eye disease resulting from nutritional deficiency

There seems to be a direct relationship between good nutrition and eye health. A lack of vitamin A in the diet can cause changes in the conjunctiva and corneal epithelium. Tears are reduced, and eyes and lid margins become reddened and inflamed. Sensitivity to light is often present, and some loss of visual acuity is noticed at night.

Pathologic changes can occur in the eye as a result of nutritional deficiency, particularly of vitamins A and B. In man, vitamin A deficiency can cause eye defects by damaging the cornea or retina (night blindness). Vitamin B deficiency may cause bilateral optic neuritis, especially in individuals who drink a large amount of alcohol. When damage to the optic nerve has been severe and prolonged, a diet high in vitamin B and other essential nutrients can accomplish only partial recovery.

Eye manifestations of systemic diseases

Diseases and infections that affect other parts of the body also affect the eye. Only a few of the more common conditions will be discussed briefly here. A persistent systemic *hypertension* will eventually produce such changes in the retina as hemorrhage, edema, and exudates, which, if uncontrolled, may result in the loss of sight. If the cause of the elevated blood pressure is eclampsia of pregnancy and is of short duration, the *retinopathy* (any disorder of the retina) usually subsides when the pregnancy is terminated. Retinopathy due to hypertension resulting from renal arteriolar sclerosis or diffuse glomerulonephritis is usually progressive and irreversible. The severity of the hypertension causes narrowing of the retinal arteries, and the blood flow through the retina and choroid is diminished, resulting in degenerative changes in the retina and loss of vision.

Senile degeneration of the macula is a rather common cause of diminished vision in elderly patients. The condition probably results from impaired nutrition of the retina due to changes in the blood vessels caused by senile degeneration of the choroid underneath the macula. The patient occasionally loses central vision and cannot read, sew, or do other activities requiring close and intent vision. He has enough peripheral vision to function independently but requires supervision to prevent accidents. He can be helped with low-vision aids.

Visual loss may follow vascular accidents to vessels anywhere in the eye or in the main blood vessels outside the eye. A cerebral vascular accident may cause hemianopia (blindness for one half of the field of vision in one or both eyes) or total blindness, depending on its location. Arteriosclerosis and atheromatosis, particularly involving the carotid and cranial arteries, may lead to occlusion of the vessels to the optic nerve or of the central vein or artery of the eye. These conditions can cause blindness in one or both eyes.

Diabetes may affect any of the structures of the eye. Senile cataracts occur earlier in persons who have diabetes and progress more rapidly than in most elderly people. *Diabetic retinopathy* produces characteristic changes in the retina (punctate hemorrhages, capillary microaneurysms, and a soapy or waxy exudate) that can cause severe visual damage and eventually result in blindness. Also, diabetes causes the growth of new blood vessels on the surface of the retina and optic disc that later extend out into the vitreous humor (retinitis proliferans). This condition often causes blindness due to recurrent vitreous hemorrhages and retinal detachment. The incidence of diabetic retinopathy seems to depend mostly on the duration of the diabetes. Keeping the blood sugar level under strict control may delay the onset of retinopathy but seems to have little or no effect on the established condition. Photocoagulation of the retina has been used to treat some patients with diabetic retinopathy.[54] Diabetic retinopathy is now the leading cause of blindness in Great Britain and is among the leading causes of blindness in the United States.

Night blindness (nyctalopia) is a condition in which good vision is present in the daytime or with a good light but deficient at night or with a poor light. It may be a symptom of atrophy of rods in the retina, such as in *retinitis pigmentosa,* which may be congenital or may develop in early childhood. Retinitis pigmentosa is a progressive disease in which the pigment epithelium degenerates and its cells migrate and deposit on the retina. Degeneration of the adjacent rod and cone layer causes loss of peripheral vision and then of central vision. There is no treatment for this condition, which leads to poor vision and may cause blindness. Night blindness may also be caused by defective regeneration of the visual purple contained in the outer rods and in the pigment epithelium due to poor ocular nutrition resulting from starvation, anemia, scurvy, vitamin A deficiency, or exposure to a bright light. This condition may respond favorably to the administration of a nutritious diet and vitamin A and iron preparations.

Retrolental fibroplasia

Retrolental fibroplasia, or retinopathy of prematurity, is a disease of premature infants in which a dense, opaque, fibrous membrane forms in the anterior vitreous behind the lens, causing blindness. The cause of the disease is now known to be related to too much oxygen administered to premature infants in the hospital. Because the amount and concentration of oxygen given to premature infants has been curtailed, new cases of retrolental fibroplasia are less common. In premature infants with a birth weight of less than 1,300 grams, retrolental fibroplasia may be unavoidable because of the necessity of administering enough oxygen to keep the infant alive.

■ REMOVAL OF THE EYE

An eye, with or without its supportive structures, may be removed for four reasons: (1) in an attempt to save a life when a malignant tumor has developed, (2) to save sight in the other eye when sympathetic ophthalmia is feared or threatens, (3) to control pain in an eye blinded by disease such as chronic glaucoma or chronic infection, or (4) for cosmetic reasons following blindness from trauma or disease. *Enucleation* is removal of the eyeball, and *evisceration* is the removal of the contents of the eyeball, leaving only the sclera. Occasionally the entire eye with the surrounding structures must be removed *(exenteration)* because of a disease such as cancer. If feasible, the eyeball alone is removed, leaving the surrounding layers of fascia (Tenon's capsule) and the muscle attachments. A silicone, plastic, or tantalum implant is inserted into the eye socket, the cut ends of the muscle attachments are overlapped and sutured around it, and then Tenon's capsule and the conjunctiva are closed. This procedure provides a stump that supplies both support and motion for an artificial eye and therefore gives the patient whose eye has been removed a more normal appearance. The ball-shaped implant is left in place permanently.

Hemorrhage, thrombosis of blood vessels, and infection are possible complications following enucleation, exenteration, or evisceration of an eye. Pressure dressings are used for 1 or 2 days to help control possible hemorrhage. Headache or pain in the operated side of the head should be reported at once since meningitis occasionally occurs as a complication following thrombosis of adjacent veins. The patient is usually allowed out of bed the day following surgery.

An *artificial eye* can be used as soon as healing is complete and edema has disappeared—usually 6 to 8 weeks after operation, although many patients begin to wear an artificial eye after only 3 weeks. Artificial eyes are made of glass or plastic materials. Glass eyes last longer if not broken, but they are heavier. Plastic ones are more expensive and may need to be replaced in a few years because they become more easily scratched or roughened around the edges, causing irritation to the conjunctiva. The plastic prostheses are more popular than the ones made of glass. There are two kinds of artificial eyes: the shell-shaped and the hollow artificial eye. The choice for the individual patient depends on what operation has been done. Artificial eyes may be bought in shades that closely match the normal eye or they may be specially made. Most artificial eyes

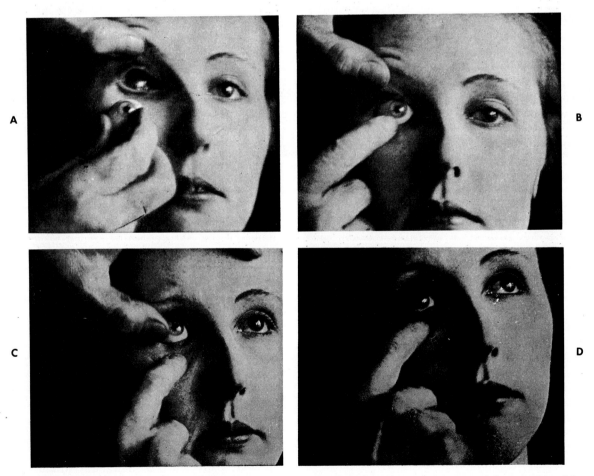

FIG. 31-13. Steps in inserting an artificial eye. (From Parkinson, R. H.: Eye, ear, nose, and throat manual for nurses, ed. 8, St. Louis, 1959, The C. V. Mosby Co.)

are plastic shells fitted and then painted by an artist. The cost varies from $100 to $250 or more. The life expectancy of the prosthesis is as great as 5 years with good care. Despite care taken to match shape and color, the pupil of the artificial eye remains fixed, which is apparent to close observers.

Even young children can be taught to care for their own artificial eye. Usually the eye is removed before retiring and kept either in a clean, dry place after cleansing or in a glass of normal saline solution. The eye should be cleansed immediately after its removal. Care should be taken not to scratch its surface. The eye is removed by gently pressing upward on the lower lid, being certain that the cupped hand is held against the cheek so that the eye does not fall to the floor and break or become lost. It is inserted by gently everting the lower lid, being certain that the narrower end of the eye is placed next to the inner angle of the orifice. Then, by grasping the upper lashes and gently raising the upper lid, the eye is easily slipped into place (Fig. 31-13).

More important than care of the artificial eye is care of the remaining eye. The person who has only one eye is advised to wear protective impact-resistant glasses. The patient should be prepared for the adjustment necessary in learning to carry on normal activities with only one eye and of the accident hazards entailed. Driving a car, for example, is dangerous for the person who suddenly must use only one eye since depth perception is altered. With patience, however, almost all normal activities are possible—surgeons who have had an eye removed have even been able to learn to operate successfully.

■ BLINDNESS

To the ophthalmologist, blindness refers to the condition of being unable to see.[29] Although many nonseeing persons now prefer to be called the "visually handicapped," the term "blindness" is still in common usage. Despite the best efforts of all concerned, some patients will become visually disabled, which is to say that they will become either functionally or legally blind. The National Society for the Prevention of Blindness estimated that there were 475,200 legally blind persons in the United States in 1973. Almost half of our blind population is 65 years of age or over. It is likely that the number will increase in the future since glaucoma, cataracts, diabetic retinopathy, and degenerative diseases associated with arteriosclerosis occur in older people, who as a group are increasing faster than the population as a whole.

The decision as to whether or not the patient should be told of approaching blindness or of certain blindness must rest with the physician. Usually it is considered best for the physician to be completely honest and frank with the patient, provided he is certain that blindness will occur or is irreversible. It then becomes the responsibility of the nurse, working with other members of the health team to help the patient and his family adjust to the condition of blindness.

When the patient has been told that he will become blind, it is to be expected that he will be depressed for a while. This is a normal reaction and is described by psychiatrists as a period of mourning for his dead eyes that the patient must undergo before he can begin to think and plan for his new life.[15] Some patients believe that becoming blind is a symbol of punishment and often need to cope with feelings of inadequacy, guilt, resentment, and loneliness.[29] Family members are extremely important throughout this period, as the patient needs to be sure that they love and accept him in spite of his disability.

Nurses can help the patient during his period of adjustment to partial or complete blindness. They can listen to him talk of what blindness means to him; they can observe exaggerated reactions that might indicate thoughts of self-destruction; they can direct the patient's thinking gradually along positive constructive lines; and they can help to make available to him the resources that he will need.

The child who has never known sight adjusts well and is happy provided that he is treated as a normal child and is neither overprotected nor rejected. It is chiefly the parents who have to adjust to and accept the child's handicap and be willing to use the resources available in the community to develop his independence and enable him to face problems of living. Both the parent and the child may need special consultation and training in order to achieve this end.

Legal blindness

A person is considered legally blind when his central vision in the better eye is reduced to less than 20/200 even with the use of corrective lenses. This means that he is able to see at 20 feet what the normal person can see at 200 feet. In addition, he is legally blind if his visual field is no greater than 20 degrees. Legal blindness entitles a person to certain federal assistance. A 1952 amendment to the Social Security Act made provision for assistance to the blind, and now all 50 states and all territories have approved plans for such aid. Assistance through this program is based on need. The Internal Revenue Act of 1948 permits blinded persons an extra deduction ($750) in reporting income. In 1943 the federal government established a counseling and placement service for the blind in the Vocational Rehabilitation Administration. This agency is now called the Social and Rehabilitation Service (SRS). It shares cost of rehabilitation with the states. The Veterans Administration provides a substantial pension for the single veteran who has enucleation of both eyes.

Rehabilitation

The blind person is handicapped in many aspects of living. Perhaps the greatest loss is in the area of basic skills such as mobility and other activities and techniques of daily living. The blind person may become independent through mobility training, which emphasizes the use of other senses as a means of orienting sightless persons to the environment. Physical therapy exercises in balance, walking, and running are further aids to confident travel. Since two thirds of the persons who are blind lose their vision after the age of 20 years, they must learn a completely new way of life. If the patient has a little time before becoming blind, he may begin learning rehabilitative activities such as learning braille. A device that interprets printed letters as tactile impulses is called the Optacon. This is useful when the material to be read is not available in braille.

Besides loss of basic skills, other losses experienced by the blind include losses in communication skills, losses in appreciation through visual perception of the pleasurable and beautiful, losses of occupation and financial status, and loss of physical integrity and self-esteem.[14]

Important contributions that the nurse can make to rehabilitation are to teach and encourage the patient to carry out the activities of daily living. Members of his family may need assistance to see the importance of letting the patient experience the satisfaction of his own independence. It is imperative that the patient be given an opportunity to preserve self-respect and esteem by caring for his personal needs. He should be urged to feed, clothe, bathe, and otherwise care for himself. The family needs expert counseling and guidance since the natural tendency is to overprotect the patient and possibly render him completely helpless. The nurse can suggest ways in which the home may be arranged to prevent accidents and to permit the blinded person to get about without embarrassment. Many blinded people can learn to be completely independent and may go about in busy city traffic with only a seeing eye dog* to help them or may even go alone with a cane.

The patient will have many questions and many needs. He may, for example, want to go to the occupational therapy department of the hospital to learn to type, or he may want to know how he may arrange to learn braille and what cost is involved. The patient may be anxious to know his chances of learning a new occupation. The participation of nurses in giving direct help will depend on whether they work in a hospital that has a social service department and other good rehabilitation resources or whether they work in a rural public health nursing agency where they may have to seek specific answers for the patient rather than refer his question to others. Nurses who work with patients with eye disease and blindness should familiarize themselves with the local resources in their own community. Voluntary organizations such as the Lions Club, Catholic Charities, the Salvation Army, and others often have programs in local areas. Almost every state has a voluntary organization devoted to this need, and the nurse can learn about it by writing to the state health department. Most state health departments also have a commission that offers various services for the blind. If the patient qualifies, help may also be available through the Veterans Administration.

National voluntary organizations

Two national voluntary health agencies concerned with blindness and the prevention of blindness are the American Foundation for the Blind* and the National Society for the Prevention of Blindness.† Both organizations have literature that is available to nurses and patients on request. The American Foundation for the Blind distributes a free catalog, *Aids and Appliances,* edition 19 (also available to the blind in braille, postage-free and free of charge), which contains a list of devices for the visually handicapped. The catalog includes sewing and kitchen utensils as well as various kinds of tools and instruments (Fig. 31-14). Medical appliances such as special syringes (Fig. 27-9) and aids for the person who must give himself insulin (Fig. 27-9) or other parenteral medication can also be obtained. (See p. 629 for description of aids for the deaf-blind.) Founded in 1908, the National Society for the Prevention of Blindness, Inc., is engaged in the prevention of blindness through a comprehensive program of community services, public and professional education, and research. Publications, films, lectures, charts, and advisory service are available on request. The quarterly publication of this voluntary organization, *The Sight-Saving Review,* covers many aspects of sight conservation and eye health.

Recording for the Blind, Inc.,‡ is a national, nonprofit, voluntary organization that provides recorded educational books free on loan to anyone who cannot read normal printed material because of visual or physical handicaps. "Talking books" produced by this organization are fundamental aids to high school and college students and persons who require educational or specialized material in the pursuit of their occupations. These recordings also may be obtained from many local and state libraries. Talking book machines are loaned free to persons who are legally blind. Information can be obtained from public libraries or organizations for the blind.

---

*The Seeing Eye, Inc., Box 375, Morristown, N. J. 07960.

*15 West 16th St., New York, N. Y. 10011.
†79 Madison Ave., New York, N. Y. 10016.
‡215 East 58th St., New York, N. Y. 10022.

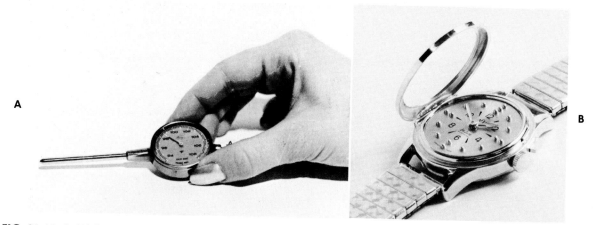

FIG. 31-14. A, Dial-type clinical thermometer with unbreakable stem. Braille (raised) dots mark the scale, one dot at odd numbers and two at even numbers. Raised line is at 98.6° F. A button is pushed to register temperature, which remains set until button is released. Needle then returns to zero. **B,** One of many models of watches available in both braille and inkprint. (Courtesy American Foundation for the Blind, New York, N. Y.)

Schools

Progress has been made in improving educational opportunities for the blind. It is believed now that the blind child, like any other handicapped child, does best when he is accepted and is in as normal an environment as possible. Blind children of school age are being educated in regular public or parochial schools, where special provisions for their individual needs are being met, or they attend special residential schools. Schools emphasize the use of auditory instruction and the development of reading skills through touch perception by the braille system. The child needs to encounter as much of his environment as is practical in order to develop concepts that other children acquire by sight. Many states have legislated funds to provide higher education for the blind and to provide readers for them, and many blind students go on to college and compete successfully with their sighted peers.

REFERENCES AND SELECTED READINGS*

1 Abrams, J. D.: The nature of glaucoma, Nurs. Times **72**:767-770, June 1972.
1a *Alexander, M. M., and others: Physical examination: examining the eye, Nursing '73 **3**:41-46, Dec. 1973.
2 Allen, J. H.: May's manual of diseases of the eye, ed. 24, Baltimore, 1968, The Williams & Wilkins Co.
3 American Foundation for the Blind: Directory of agencies serving the visually handicapped in the United States, ed. 8, New York, 1973, The William Byrd Press.
4 *Ammon, L. L.: Surviving enucleation, Am. J. Nurs. **72**:1817-1821, Oct. 1972.
5 Becker, B., and Burde, R. M.: Current concepts in ophthalmology, vol. II, St. Louis, 1969, The C. V. Mosby Co.
6 Bedford, M. A.: Color atlas of ophthalmological diagnosis, Chicago, 1972, Year Book Medical Publishers, Inc.
7 Bellows, J. G.: Understanding cataracts, A.O.R.N.J. **7**:64-71, May 1968.
8 Blodi, F. C.: Glaucoma, Am. J. Nurs. **63**:78-83, March 1963.
9 *Blodi, F. C., and Honn, R. C.: Tumors of the eye—medical and nursing care, Am. J. Nurs. **56**:1152-1156, Sept. 1956.
10 *Burian, H. M.: Strabismus, Am. J. Nurs. **60**:653-656, May 1960.
11 Buschman, W., and Hauff, D.: Results of diagnostic ultrasonography in ophthalmology, Am. J. Ophthalmol. **63**:926-933, May 1967.
12 Campbell, A.: Tumors of the eye and orbit in childhood, Nurs. Mirror **134**:26-29, May 1972.
13 Carr, R. E., and Gouras, P.: Clinical electroretinography, J.A.M.A. **198**:173-176, Oct. 1966.
14 *Carroll, Rev. F. J.: Blindness, Boston, 1961, Little, Brown & Co.
15 Cholden, L.: Some psychiatric problems in rehabilitation of the blind, Bull. Menninger Clin. **18**:107-112, May 1954.
16 *Condl, E. D., and others: Ophthalmic nursing, Nurs. Clin. North Am. **5**:449-496, Sept. 1970.
17 Editorial, Sight Sav. Rev. **43**:66-67, Summer 1973.
17a *Elkington, A. R.: Intraocular foreign bodies, Nurs. Times **69**:1638-1639, Dec. 1973.
17b *Elkington, A. R.: Non-perforating wounds, Nurs. Times **69**:1562-1563, Nov. 1973.
17c *Elkington, A. R.: Perforating wounds, Nurs. Times **69**:1597-1598, Nov. 1973.
18 *Fulton, M., and others: Helping diabetics adapt to failing vision, Am. J. Nurs. **74**:54-57, Jan. 1974.
19 *Gamble, R. C.: The medical eye examination, Am. J. Nurs. **57**:1590-1592, Dec. 1957.
20 Gellis, S. S., and Kagan, B. M.: Current pediatric therapy, vol. 6, Philadelphia, 1973, W. B. Saunders Co.

*References preceded by an asterisk are particularly well suited for student reading.

21 *Gibbons, H., and Cunningham, F.: Finding and helping the partially seeing child, Nurs. Outlook **7**:524-526, Sept. 1959.

22 Girard, L. J.: Cryotherapy in ophthalmology, Sight Sav. Rev. **35**:87-90, Summer 1965.

23 *Gordon, D. M.: The inflamed eye, Am. J. Nurs. **64**:113-117, Nov. 1964.

24 Gordon, R. D.: Experience with a visually disabled mother, Am. J. Nurs. **68**:1943-1945, Sept. 1968.

25 *Haddad, H. M.: Drugs for ophthalmologic use, Am. J. Nurs. **68**:324-327, Feb. 1968.

26 Hatfield, E. M.: Estimates of blindness in the United States, Sight Sav. Rev. **43**:69-80, Summer 1973.

27 Havener, W. H.: Synopsis of ophthalmology, ed. 4, St. Louis, 1974, The C. V. Mosby Co.

28 Havener, W. H.: Ocular pharmacology, ed. 3, St. Louis, 1974, The C. V. Mosby Co.

29 *Havener, W. H., and others: Nursing care in eye, ear, nose, and throat disorders, ed. 3, St. Louis, 1974, The C. V. Mosby Co.

30 Hewitt, W.: The fate of sensory impulses, Nurs. Times **67**:982-984, Aug. 1971.

30a *Hiles, D. A.: Strabismus, Am. J. Nurs. **74**:1082-1089, June 1974.

31 Judge, R. D., and Zuidema, G. D.: Physical diagnosis: a physiologic approach to the clinical examination, ed. 2, Boston, 1968, Little, Brown & Co.

32 Kelman, C. D.: Phaco-emulsification and aspiration: a new technique of cataract extraction, Am. J. Ophthalmol. **64**:23-35, July 1967.

33 Kelman, C. D.: Phaco-emulsification and aspiration, a report of 500 consecutive cases, Am. J. Ophthalmol. **75**:764-768, May 1973.

34 Koetting, R. A.: Contact lenses and the athlete, J. Sch. Health **41**:75-77, Feb. 1971.

35 Kornzweig, A. L.: The eye in old age, Am. J. Ophthalmol. **60**:835-843, Nov. 1965.

36 McLean, J. M.: Atlas of glaucoma surgery, St. Louis, 1967, The C. V. Mosby Co.

36a *Mechner, F., and Saffiati, L. J.: Patient assessment: examination of the eye. I. Am J. Nurs. 2039-2068, Nov. 1974.

37 Mlynarczyk, R.: How well does your baby see? Parents' Magazine **46**:58-60, Oct. 1971.

38 Newell, F. W., and Ernest, J. T.: Ophthalmology—principles and concepts, ed. 3, St. Louis, 1974, The C. V. Mosby Co.

39 *Nordstrom, W.: Adjusting to cataract glasses, Am. J. Nurs. **66**:1578-1579, July 1966.

40 Oerther, B.: The blind patient need not be helpless, Am. J. Nurs. **66**:2436-2439, Nov. 1966.

41 *Ohno, M. I.: The eye-patched patient, Am. J. Nurs. **71**:271-274, Feb. 1971.

42 *Pereira, P.: Screening for glaucoma, Nurs. Times **68**:771-774, June, 1972.

43 Reinecke, R. D., Stein, H. A., and Slatt, B. J.: Introductory manual for the ophthalmic assistant: a programmed text, St. Louis, 1972, The C. V. Mosby Co.

44 Research to Prevent Blindness, Inc.: Annual report, New York, 1972, Research to Prevent Blindness, Inc.

45 Rubenstein, K.: Ophthalmic cryosurgery, Nurs. Times **63**:1640-1642, Dec. 1967.

46 Rubin, M.: Contact lenses, shells and prosthetics, Nurs. Times **68**:133-136, Feb. 1972.

47 Scheie, H. G., and Albert, D. M.: Adler's textbook of ophthalmology, ed. 8, Philadelphia, 1969, W. B. Saunders Co.

48 *Shepard, M. E.: Nursing care of patients with eye, ear, nose and throat disorders, New York, 1958, Macmillan Publishing Co., Inc.

49 *Smith, J. F., and Machazel, D. P.: Retinal detachment, Am. J. Nurs. **73**:1530-1535, Sept. 1973.

50 *Stocher, F. W., and Bell, R.: Corneal transplantation and nursing the patient with a corneal transplant, Am. J. Nurs. **62**:65-70, May 1962.

51 Stowe, S. M.: Hypophysectomy for diabetic retinopathy, Am. J. Nurs. **73**:632-637, April 1973.

51a The eye in nursing literature 1968-1973: a bibliography, A.O.R.N.J. **18**:1013-1014, Nov. 1973.

52 Uffenorde, T. M.: Nurse's view of eye surgery, A.O.R.N.J. **16**:45-49, Dec. 1972.

53 *Weinstock, F. J.: Emergency treatment of eye injuries, Am. J. Nurs. **71**:1929-1931, Oct. 1971.

54 *Weinstock, F. J.: Tonometry screening, Am. J. Nurs. **73**:656-657, April 1973.

55 Zweng, H. C., and others: Argon laser photocoagulation of diabetic retinopathy, Arch. Ophthalmol. **86**:395-400, Oct. 1971.

32 Neurologic diseases

General management of the patient with
  neurologic disease
Neurologic assessment
Special neurodiagnostic procedures

Neurologic diseases
Common neurologic manifestations
Degenerative diseases
Vascular diseases
Infections
Traumatic lesions
Neoplasms of the central nervous system

■ The specialties of neurology and neurosurgery are complicated and demand special knowledge, skill, and experience. Before the nurse can plan and give competent care to a patient with neurologic disease, assessment of nursing care needs must be made. Basic to all steps of the nursing process is the nurse's knowledge of the patient and his behavior, neuroan-

atomy and physiology, neuropathology, the surgical procedure if one is performed, and the general nursing care needs of neurologic patients. It is suggested that the reader review the relevant neuroanatomy and physiology, pathology, treatment, and the nursing care required by each neurologic patient encountered in nursing practice.

Many neurologic patients have serious emotional and even psychiatric disturbances that may be related in part to their neurologic disease. Psychiatry, however, is concerned largely with functional disorders, whereas neurology is concerned primarily with disorders that have a demonstrable organic or physical cause. There may be neurologic involvement in some medical diseases such as pernicious anemia, diabetes mellitus, and severe infections, but many other diseases are caused by a pathologic process that is primarily in the nervous system. Only a few of the frequently seen neurologic diseases and their management will be considered in this chapter.

■ STUDY QUESTIONS

1 Review basic neuroanatomy and physiology.
2 Review the formation and absorption of cerebrospinal fluid. Trace its circulation within the ventricular system.
3 Identify the structures comprising the upper motor neuron and lower motor neuron. What is meant by the final common path?
4 Distinguish between the pyramidal and extrapyramidal tracts relative to their motor functions. How are motor functions integrated centrally?
5 Review the afferent system. Study the distribution of the spinal dermatomes and compare them with anterior and posterior cutaneous peripheral nerve distributions.
6 Trace a nerve impulse for pain and temperature sensation from the skin on the lateral side of the foot to the cerebral cortex. Start by naming the dermatome.
7 Locate the varied language and speech centers in the cerebrum. Distinguis! between cortical speech and articulation.
8 Locate the neostriatum and the structures comprising it. What alterations in motion occur with lesions in these structures? Review the metabolism of dopamine as to its precursors and metabolic products.
9 Anticipate the general nursing problems that would arise from a neural lesion in each of the following sites: frontal, parietal, temporal, and occipital lobes; cerebellum; thalamus; basal ganglia; and brain stem.
10 What facilities does your community provide for long-term and rehabilitation care of neurologic patients? Is there provision for the delivery of home care from the medical center?
11 Select a patient with a chronic neurologic disease and study how the disease has changed his life-style. How has it affected family life? How has the community been affected?

General management based on common problems arising from neurologic diseases and the resulting dysfunctions, is discussed first. Some of the representative and common clinical neurologic diseases and neurosurgical procedures are described generally in the latter part of this chapter.

■ GENERAL MANAGEMENT OF THE PATIENT WITH NEUROLOGIC DISEASE

Neurologic disease has multiple causes. It may occur in any age group. Pathology or injury may affect the nervous system centrally and/or peripherally. Its onset may occur suddenly as in cerebrovascular accident or traumatic spinal cord injury or it may be slow in onset as in multiple sclerosis or Parkinson's disease. Neurologic disease may be progressive or nonprogressive during its course. Its effects may be reversible when nerve cells regain function; its effects will be irreversible when nerve cell death occurs centrally. Because of the nature of the structure and functions of the nervous system, when pathology or injury occurs at a particular site, the resulting dysfunctions can be related to the site regardless of the pathology producing the dysfunctions. In this way the kind of dysfunction is more relevant to the site than to the disease per se. When dysfunctions are long-standing, as in irreversible and progressive pathology, they produce problems in the daily life of the individual that may necessitate changes in his life-style. The nurse caring for the patient with neurologic disease should be equally knowledgeable about the physical effects of the pathology and how the patient reacts to it emotionally and socially. The following general problems that arise from neurologic dysfunction are the most common and provide a beginning framework for planning nursing care. However, detailed data as pertains to the individual patient should be collected in order to identify his specific problems.

Loss of motor and sensory functions

The loss of some motor and/or sensory function is common in most neurologic diseases. Therefore it will be difficult for the patient to carry out some daily activities that require coordinated movement. The ability to move about at will and control one's actions is precious to every human being. Regardless of the speed of its occurrence, the loss of the ability to function independently or to predict one's movements is psychologically traumatizing. Irritability, defensiveness, fear, and other signs of threat to emotional security are likely to appear and should be met with calmness, patience, and kindness by all who work with the patient. If the patient has a nonprogressive limitation of function due to neurologic damage, he needs reassurance that his condition will not become worse. Unfortunately cure is not possible in many neurologic diseases. The nurse needs to know what

the physician has told both the patient and his family about the prognosis. If assurance of arrest or of improvement of the disease cannot be given, the patient must be helped to live a relatively full life as long as possible, and it is the nurse who often gives much of this help.

The nurse can protect the patient from unwarranted observation and comment by persons who have no part in his care, particularly when he is in a general hospital or in his own home. The peculiarities of gait or mannerisms and the loss of control so common in neurologic disease seem to interest people who otherwise have no concern with them. The unfortunate quality of morbid curiosity in human nature must be faced. The patient should be told how common his particular condition is and that he is not alone with his affliction. The nurse can help him by showing interest in him as a person and not primarily in his physical ailment. Often the patient turns to the nurse as someone with whom he can discuss his reactions to his disease when he cannot discuss them with his family. Listening attentively to the patient's problems is an essential part of neurologic nursing. Knowing when problems are too involved and beyond the nurse's sphere of knowledge is equally essential. A medical social worker can often be of great help to the patient in helping him to think through his feelings about his disease.

It is useless to argue with the patient or to try to talk him out of his fears. Giving a word of encouragement for small achievements, changing the conversation to other topics, and introducing some diversional activity sometimes help. Emotional tension seems to be released by working with one's hands. Making something useful in the occupational therapy department of a hospital or in his own home may be very satisfying to the patient. The patient may receive more satisfaction from weaving a belt or making a wallet than from spending an equivalent amount of time watching television or in a similar passive, time-passing activity. He should not, however, be urged into activities that do not interest him. For example, the patient at home may gain more satisfaction from washing dishes and peeling vegetables than from making some decorative object.

The desire of the patient and his family to shop for a cure is understandable when the diagnosis of a chronic and incurable neurologic disease has been made. The nurse should help prevent the loss of time and financial and emotional resources that this practice usually entails. This is helped by building up the confidence of the patient and his family in the physician and in the clinic or hospital where he is receiving care. The nurse will have to have patience and understanding in answering questions about advertised remedies, news items that may be misleading, and reports from neighbors and friends. At times questions will need to be referred to the physician. Many patients with incurable neurologic disease live out their years in the hope that a cure will be found during their lifetime. They need to feel sure that the persons responsible for their care are alert for new discoveries that may be helpful to them.

The nurse should plan for self-care within the patient's abilities. An assessment of the ability of the patient to carry out personal hygiene, grooming, feeding, toileting, dressing, movement in bed, locomotion, range of joint motion, and speech activities provides the nurse with information necessary to plan nursing care. Physical facilities should be arranged so that the patient can do as much as possible for himself to maintain his self-esteem and to give him some satisfaction. Handrails along hallways, firm locks on bed castors and bedside tables, low beds, and handrails along the sides of the tub and toilet help the patient to handle himself even though his movements are uncertain. It is important to most people to be able to feed themselves. Appetite is better and disposition improves when this is possible. Even a patient with poor coordination may be able to feed himself if food is cut into bite-sized pieces. A special spoon with a large handle may be helpful. If he is clumsy and untidy while eating he will usually want to be protected from the scrutiny of others. The nurse should be calm about failures in attempts to master an activity or else ignore them. Emotional outbursts as a result of frustration should be treated in a matter-of-fact fashion. The nurse needs to know what the patient can do and demonstrate faith in his ability to do these things for himself. Statements such as "You're not trying" or "You couldn't be tired yet" only add to the patient's discouragement and should be avoided. Good judgment is needed in deciding what the patient may safely do without assistance. If any doubt exists, the nurse should consult the physician. Activities that are dangerous for the patient should be known to all nursing personnel. Great frustration may result from attempting activities that are beyond his abilities because they accentuate his limitation. Activities that are stepping-stones to greater accomplishments will result in satisfaction for the patient and will motivate him to further self-help.

It is fortunate that many neurologic diseases progress so slowly that the patient has time to adjust to necessary changes. As difficulty in walking progresses, the patient may benefit from special shoes. Shoes may need to be built up in a variety of ways to provide a stable base of support. They should have low rubber heels, fit well, and provide good support for the arches. As disease progresses, many patients must use a cane; this is a painful step for the patient in his acceptance of the disease, even though built-up shoes and a cane may be less conspicuous than the patient's gait would be without these aids. The nurse can help by suggesting the activities that are safe and possible with the use of a cane. Eventually many patients must resort to a wheelchair. The light

wheelchairs now available make it possible for the quite helpless patient to get about safely in his home and to be taken in a car for trips away from home. Collapsible wheelchairs with removable arms and footrests are available.

The nurse should help the patient and his family to plan the necessary adjustments needed in the home so that he can continue to be partially self-sufficient. Furniture can be arranged to allow the patient to get about more easily in his wheelchair, cupboards and shelves can be lowered, and movable equipment such as lamps and the telephone can be placed on lower tables.

If the patient has difficulty using his fingers and hands for fine movements, the use of shoes with elasticized insteps or elastic laces and the use of Velcro strips or metal grippers on clothing instead of buttons may help him to remain self-sufficient. When the patient is hospitalized, the activities he can perform should be sought in the initial interview and noted on the nursing care plan. If he is at home, the family should know what he can and cannot do so that he is not overprotected.

A decrease, loss, or increase in the sensations of touch, pain, temperature, and proprioception, singly or in combination, result in difficult problems in daily living for the individual. Since these sensations normally help one to be aware of and to discriminate relative to his external and internal environment, any alteration in sensation lessens the ability to be protected completely and accurately. As a consequence, there is a need to adapt to the alteration and plan for safety and comfort. The nurse needs to recognize the specific sensory deficit(s) and assist the individual in planning for self-care to the greatest extent possible. Measures to avoid overstimulation of sensation are necessary in some conditions. The loss of positional and vibratory senses pose difficult problems for some patients.

Aphasia

Aphasia is a disorder of language caused by damage to the speech-controlling areas of the brain. Cerebral hemorrhage and cerebral thrombosis are the most common causes of such damage, but tumors, multiple sclerosis, and trauma may also lead to aphasia. Aphasia caused by cerebral edema following trauma is usually temporary. Occasionally a patient cannot speak following a cerebrovascular accident because motor function of the vocal cords is affected, not because of damage to cortical speech centers. This condition is not a true aphasia.

A variety of abnormalities in speech can occur. The patient may be unable to comprehend the spoken or written word (sensory aphasia), or he may comprehend and yet be unable to use the symbols of speech (motor aphasia). He may also have both disorders at the same time (global). He may be able to write but not to speak; he may be able to speak but

849

may use the wrong words or have a selective loss of words; or he may be able to read but be unable to speak or to write. Sensory aphasia is much more difficult to deal with than motor involvement. Explanations are difficult, and it is hard to reassure the patient, who may become completely confused and undirected in his efforts to speak.

Each patient reacts to language difficulty in a different way, depending on his pattern of adjustment to life's problems. Most patients with aphasia become tense and anxious. They may be irritable and emotionally upset because they are unable to evoke the words they need, and they become discouraged easily in their efforts to speak. Some may quickly refuse to attempt to communicate; others feel ashamed and withdraw from people, including their family and close friends. Yet desire to communicate and persistence in efforts to do so are the essential ingredients in speech rehabilitation.

Nursing care is directed toward decreasing tension and should be started as soon as aphasia occurs in order to help the patient make a satisfactory adjustment to his limitation and in order to make later rehabilitative efforts less difficult. The nurse should anticipate the patient's needs so that he will not have to make repeated attempts to ask for things. The patient should be helped to understand that he may relearn speech and that in the interim there are other means by which he can communicate with others. The most successful approach found to communicate with him will need to be shared with his family and friends and all health workers who interact with him. Other patients can be helped to understand his condition and to make him feel more at ease in a group by not showing amusement or embarrassment at his attempts to communicate. Calmness and patience on the part of the nurse are essential to the patient's acceptance of his difficult program of practicing relearned words and patterns of speech.

The patient's environment should be quiet. Persons who care for him should guard against raising their voices when talking with him as the patient with aphasia is seldom deaf. Although he cannot respond, he should be talked to and have procedures explained in the manner used with any patient. Recreational activities should be soothing and nonstimulating. Music is often relaxing, and the patient may enjoy listening to the radio. If a patient is able to read and comprehend the written captions on television, watching television may be particularly gratifying. Some patients may be made irritable by radio music they do not enjoy or television programs they do not like or cannot follow. Watching the patient's facial expression usually gives the nurse a clue as to the satisfaction derived from these activities.

Gross tests must be performed to determine what specific language abilities have been lost. In some hospitals a trained speech pathologist may be available to make an initial evaluation and to guide members of the nursing staff in making appropriate plans concerning the patient's speech problems. Sometimes, however, this assistance is not available, and the nurse must carry out simple tests that have been ordered by the physician or, more often, devise her own tests. They may be conducted as follows. Spread several familiar objects such as keys, a pencil, a book of matches, a penny, and scissors before the patient: (1) ask him to name each object; (2) as you name each object, ask him to point to it; (3) ask him to write the name of each object as you point to it; (4) ask him to write the name of each object as you say the word; (5) show him a card containing the printed name of each object and ask him to read the word orally and point to the object. It may be too fatiguing for the patient to take all the tests at one time, and they can be phased in gradually. The patient's responses will indicate the best way to communicate with him. If he can only read, one should give him cards with the words and phrases needed in asking for the most common daily necessities. Words needed by most ill persons include yes, no, bedpan, urinal, hot, cold, headache, pain, doctor, nurse, turn, sit up, lie down, bed, pillow, sheet, gown, water, thirst, hunger, comfortable, chair, light, telephone, and wife or husband. If the patient is unable to recognize the written word, he may be able to recognize pictures of objects. If he can write or draw a picture of his needs, he should be given a pad and pencil or magic slate with which to do so.

As the nurse cares for the patient, common objects should be named and the patient encouraged to handle them, to speak their names, and to write or copy their names. The patient should be helped to relearn the names of members of his family and friends. The family can supply these words and others that are particularly important for the patient. Speech retraining should be done for short periods of time because it is exceedingly trying, and fatigue tends to increase difficulty in speaking (dysphasia). Praising the patient for each small improvement and encouraging him to take his mistakes good-naturedly help to make this difficult problem more bearable. The patient's progress in language retraining will depend on his level of intelligence, his age (older patients have more difficulty), the severity of the damage, and whether or not the brain lesion is progressive. Complete language rehabilitation may require months of painstaking work on the part of skilled pathologists.* *A Guide to Clinical Services in Speech Pathology and Audiology*† lists clinics in

---

*Some institutions that specialize in working with patients who have aphasia are ICD Rehabilitation and Research Center, New York, N. Y.; The Institute of Logopedics, Wichita, Kan.; and Vanderbilt University Hospital Clinic, Nashville, Tenn.

†American Speech and Hearing Association, 9030 Old Georgetown Rd., Washington, D. C. 20014.

the United States where speech and hearing services are available. Some of these clinics offer specialized help to persons with aphasia.

Personality and behavioral changes

Personality changes are common in neurologic disease, and occasionally their slow development is the first and only sign of a serious neurologic disorder. These changes should be watched for carefully and reported accurately. Physical changes caused by neurologic disease may affect the personality; reporting these changes may help the physician in his diagnosis and treatment of the patient. Frustrations resulting from restrictions and attempts to get about, anxiety from increasing helplessness, and the fear of helplessness may also cause personality changes.

Changes in judgment and in intellect may become serious. The patient may make poor investments or other unwise decisions in business or family matters. Multiple sclerosis, Parkinson's disease, cerebrovascular arteriosclerosis, and brain tumors are examples of neurologic disorders that may seriously alter judgment. Handling such a situation is extremely difficult because strong emotional reactions may follow curtailment of the patient's freedom in managing his own affairs. The problem is usually dealt with by the physician and the family with the assistance of the social worker. The nurse should not communicate to the patient knowledge of measures taken to prevent the consequence of errors in his judgment.

Unsafe actions resulting from mental, physical, and sensory losses

Judgment defects may lead to behavior that is dangerous both to the patient and to others. It is believed that many automobile accidents are caused by persons with neurologic disease; for example, patients with multiple sclerosis may have blind spots (scotomas), and those with convulsive disorders may lose consciousness for only a few seconds—long enough for an accident to occur. Unfortunately these two diseases appear in young people who feel very keenly the restriction of such activities as driving an automobile. The need to avoid certain other dangerous activities must be stressed; for example, swimming is dangerous for the patient who has uncontrolled convulsive seizures. Emphasis must be positive, however, and it must be placed on the many things that the patient can do. Members of the patient's family should be helped to plan so that the necessary restrictions are not obvious; for example, hiking and camping may be substituted for swimming or horseback riding if the patient has convulsive seizures that cannot be controlled.

The neurologic patient must be protected from accidents in his daily living. Mental and/or physical losses make some activities unsafe. Motor imbalances or incoordination may make locomotion unsafe with or without assistance or supervision. Measures to prevent accidents must be carefully introduced because the patient may resent his limitations so much that he is inclined to reject precautions for his safety. Personality changes and judgment defects again may interfere with his acceptance of measures that would help to ensure his personal safety. Elderly persons with arteriosclerotic brain damage are often great trials to their families; for example, they may decide to paint the outside of the house, when standing on a ladder is obviously dangerous.

The bathroom is a common location of accidents. To prevent falls in the bathtub, handrails should be installed beside the tub, and a rough paint or roughened plastic strips, available at most department stores, should be applied to the floor of the tub to prevent the patient from slipping. It is often helpful to place a rubber or plastic mat in the tub, and many patients at home invest in the type of handrail that clamps to the side of the tub. A low box or a small commercially made seat can be placed in the tub to help the patient get out safely since rising from an elevated seat is less difficult than from the bottom of the tub. One way to prevent accidents in bathtubs is to seat the patient while the tub is empty and dry and to empty it before he gets out. When limitations are severe, it may not be advisable for the patient to take a tub bath without assistance or to take a tub bath at all. Sitting on a shower stool or in a small metal wheelchair in the shower and using a spray device attached to the faucet is safer and is usually satisfactory for the patient.

Bathroom doors should not lock from the inside, since the patient may lock himself in and, in the event of accident, prolong the time needed to reach him. This precaution is particularly important if the patient is elderly or if his sensory perception is impaired. Patients have received severe and even fatal burns from stepping into a tub of water that was too hot or from fainting or suffering a stroke or heart attack as hot water was running into the tub.

Accidents in and about the home may be prevented by special attention to causes of accidents. Scatter rugs should never be used, and any upturned, curled rug edges should be nailed down. Wall-to-wall carpeting with a low pile is best. Floors should not be highly waxed. Toys, lamp cords, or other accident hazards on floors should be removed. The patient should wear firm slippers or shoes. Bathrobes should have buttons instead of long cords or sashes. Good lighting is essential. Nightlights at the bedside, in hallways, and in bathrooms are desirable.

Railings and firm casements on steps and ramps often enable the patient to get about independently for a longer period. It is advisable to caution the family to lock basement doors and even front and back doors when persons who have neurologic disease with judgment defects are in the house. They may open the wrong door and fall down basement steps or go into the street at odd hours and come to harm.

Contractures

Since muscle action is controlled by the nervous system, patients with neurologic disease are likely to develop contractures and deformities. Many changes come on so gradually that they are barely noticed by the patient until they are relatively fixed. In the home as well as in the hospital, much can be done to prevent the progress of deformities. Warm baths often relax tightened muscles enough so that joints can be put through a range of motion. In this way, limitation of joint motion may be prevented, delayed, or maintained status quo. Since muscle and joint stiffness come from prolonged sitting or lying in one position, the patient should be advised to change his position regularly or be assisted to move when limitations are present.

Failure to keep the body in good alignment, both while up and while in bed, may lead to deformity. If the patient is rational and able to help himself, the nurse can teach him to help prevent deformity and preserve his best possible function. A firm mattress and chairs that provide good support are essential. Pillows may be used to support paralyzed parts, and changes of position, both in and out of bed, help to prevent deformities from developing.

Standing for even a few minutes each day will prevent the development of contractures at the hips caused by prolonged sitting. In many communities, walkers may be rented or borrowed from such agencies as the local Red Cross, the public health nursing agency, the local rescue squad offices, or other volunteer groups. Many times the patient can stand safely between two sturdy kitchen chairs, providing he and his family are taught how he may manage himself in this position.

Body parts that are paralyzed must be put through normal range of motion daily so that range will not be further limited if and when the ability to move is restored. The nurse can determine whether or not the patient's range of motion is normal or limited by comparison with her own range of movement. Allowance should be made for individual variations and for changes due to age and to joint disease that the patient may have. Since range of motion for some joints cannot be achieved with the patient in the supine position, it is necessary that he lie prone at least once each day. The nurse should know any special exercises prescribed for the patient so that he can be assisted with them at intervals during the day if this is desirable. Directions for exercises should be in writing and stick drawings will help the patient to understand such details as the angle and arc of motion. (For complete range of joint motion, see Figs. 1-2 to 1-4.)

Pressure areas and skin care

When the nerve supply to a body part is affected by disease, nutrition of that part is impaired because arterial and venous blood flow, which is dependent on normal muscle action, is often decreased as a result of disturbance of nerve impulses. It is well to consider how often the unaffected person normally changes his position during both waking and sleeping hours. Some change is made in distribution of weight on weight-bearing parts of the body, usually every few minutes. When the patient is paralyzed or unable to move, the pressure of body weight further curtails adequate circulation. The skin breaks down easily, and pressure sores may be difficult or impossible to cure. Therefore the patient with a neurologic disorder who is confined to bed or chair must be reminded to change his position frequently if he is able to do so. If he cannot move himself, he must have assistance. When a patient is unconscious, crucial nursing responsibility is to change the patient's position at regular intervals. Light massage of the dependent areas should be given each time the patient is turned. If the patient is completely paralyzed, aged, or particularly debilitated, regular turning and massage may not be adequate to prevent decubiti. An alternating pressure mattress, water flotation mattress, Gelfoam mattress or cushions, sponge rubber, or sheepskin are valuable aids in preventing skin breakdown over bony prominences. Attention should be given to a well-balanced diet, since good nutrition helps to maintain healthy tissues.

Turning patients who are helpless or unconscious involves physical labor. Nursing personnel need to apply the principles of good body mechanics, since that will make the difference between ending the day with a feeling of normal tiredness and satisfaction or ending it with the feeling of discouragement and undue fatigue. (For principles of good body mechanics, see texts on fundamentals of nursing.)

Incontinence is often a problem in the care of the patient with a neurologic disease and this can lead to skin breakdown. Therefore special attention must be given to keeping the skin dry and clean. Care of the incontinent patient is discussed in Chapter 9.

Difficulty in maintaining respiration

When there is dysfunction of respiratory muscles or the nerves innervating these muscles, serious problems in breathing ensue. This often necessitates the use of a respirator to assist or control breathing. Although tank and chest respirators are used infrequently today, when they are used, it is most often in the care of patients with neurologic conditions such as myasthenia gravis, toxic encephalitis, acute infectious polyneuritis, and fracture of the skull. Therefore the nursing care needed is included here. Respirators are mechanical devices used to substitute for normal respiratory action by creating a negative pressure outside the chest wall. This pressure causes air to enter the respiratory passages. A mechanical device is a poor substitute for normal respiration and therefore is usually used as a last resort. For example, the rate of inhalation and rate of exhalation are the same when a respirator is used, whereas in normal respiration the time for inhalation is less than that for exhalation.

Since respirators are used in emergencies, it is essential that they be checked often and kept in working order at all times. If they are kept on a ward or unit of the hospital, a regular day each week should be designated for their routine inspection. There are two main types of respirators and several manufacturers of each. The tank respirator encases the entire body except the head and imposes handicaps on persons who attempt to give nursing care. The chest respirator encloses only the chest. Chest respirators permit the patient much greater freedom and simplify nursing care. They cannot, however, be used for long periods of time since they may not provide adequate aeration of the lungs. Several variations of equipment are available to aid breathing. Some of these respirators employ the use of a mask over the face and do not encase the body, and some can be attached to a tracheostomy tube (p. 612).

Respirators can be dangerous in inexperienced hands. Too much negative pressure can cause inspiration to be too deep and thus traumatize the alveoli of the lungs. The respirator must be tested before the patient is placed in it. This is done in the tank respirator by closing all arm ports and other openings and turning the pressure gauge until approximately the desired pressure is reached. The head opening can be closed by holding a pillow firmly against it. Pressure must again be carefully regulated when the patient is in the machine.

If the patient is conscious, it is imperative that the procedure of placing him into the respirator and the purpose of this treatment be explained to him. Usually he is told that the respirator has been ordered so that he can relax and breathe more easily and thus get necessary rest and sleep. Often the patient is so exhausted from having to remain awake and consciously use his accessory muscles of respiration in an effort to breathe that he welcomes use of the respirator. Occasionally he becomes panicky and "fights" the machine so that adjustment to it is extremely difficult. A nurse must always remain with the patient and help him to breathe with the machine until he becomes accustomed to it.

Before the patient is placed in a respirator, provision must be made for his relative comfort and for care that will be necessary. The mattress should be covered with small sheets in sections that can be easily removed through the arm ports, and the following supplies should be inside the respirator: a piece of plastic material to protect the sheet under the buttocks, bath towels, bath blankets, foot supports, and a thermometer. Soft material such as an old diaper or chamois skin should be used to protect the patient's throat and neck from the rubber collar.

The patient in a respirator must never, under any circumstances, be left unattended. Patients have been known to die because an electric cord was inadvertently disconnected or because some other mechanical failure occurred. Auxiliary nursing personnel, relatives, and volunteers are often asked to stay with the patient when a nurse is unable to do so.

An important concept to remember in care of the patient is that he needs exactly the same care as if he were not in a respirator. He needs to be turned, to have skin care, to have joints flexed and extended, to void, to defecate regularly, and to take fluids and food in normal amounts. Teamwork is essential, and planning should be done so that several essential activities can be carried on at once. For example, when turning the patient to relieve pressure on the sa-

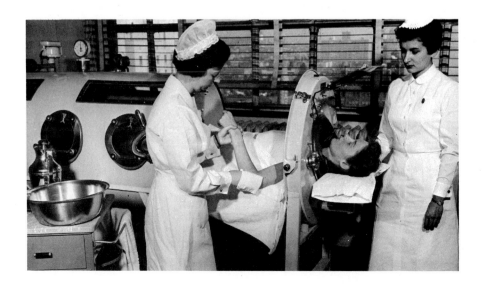

FIG. 32-1. A patient being weaned from a respirator needs encouragement. Short periods out of the respirator are also used to give essential care.

crum, one can also sponge the back, flex the knees, and massage the ankles, provided that equipment for these procedures has been placed in the respirator before the patient has been turned. If the patient can be out of the respirator or can breathe on his own for a short time, this time is used by several nurses and attendants to give essential care (Fig. 32-1).

The greatest care must be taken in helping patients to swallow when in the respirator. It is extremely difficult for anyone to swallow comfortably when lying on his back or in mild hyperextension, much less when breathing cannot be controlled. Swallowing must be done on exhalation. The patient should first try small amounts of liquid or semisolid foods; foods that tend to cause choking (for example, mashed potatoes) must be avoided. A suction machine should always be on hand when a patient first attempts to swallow when in a respirator. If the patient vomits, he must be removed from the respirator at once to prevent aspiration into the lungs.

Although some patients are anxious to be out of the machine, others become dependent on it and must be gradually weaned from the machine. In weaning the patient the respirator is turned off for a few seconds or minutes at periodic intervals, and the patient may be given supplemental oxygen. The nurse stands at the patient's head encouraging him to breathe normally while others in attendance give him physical care. At first the patient is left on the carriage of the machine so that he knows that its use is immediately available. He may then be moved to a bed, where a chest respirator may be used, or to a rocking bed, which tilts at a specified rate and thus assists in breathing. As the head of the bed goes down, the viscera fall against the diaphragm and assist in exhalation, while, as the head goes up, the diaphragm falls toward the abdominal viscera and assists in inhalation. (See Chapter 22 for care of the patient in a respirator.)

Planning with the patient's family

Few illnesses tax the entire physical and emotional resources of the patient's family as do the chronic neurologic diseases. It is imperative that the family participate in long-term plans for the patient. Members of the family may have severe emotional reactions and difficulties in adjustment that may require the assistance of specially trained persons such as a psychiatrist. A social worker or spiritual adviser can be invaluable in listening to members of the family and in helping them to think through their own futures so that they may determine a constructive plan of action for caring for their loved one. Both the patient and his family need time to work through their feelings. Sometimes the enormity of the significance of the diagnosis cannot be grasped

for weeks or even months by either the patient or his family. Toxic polyneuritis in a young husband and father and multiple sclerosis in a young mother are examples of problems of such magnitude that long-term plans cannot be made quickly.

The family may need help in accepting the concept of self-help and independence for the patient. On learning the diagnosis, their first reaction may be to do too much for the patient and thus to hasten his complete dependence on them. Later, when the reality of the burden becomes clearer, they may tire of the restrictions imposed on them and become impatient or needlessly exhausted. Care of the patient may fall too much on one relative who most readily assumes the burden. Sometimes one family member eagerly takes on the greatest responsibility yet resents it. The member may complain that others do not contribute, and yet avoid assistance when it is offered. By reacting in this way the member may be meeting an emotional need. Family crises may sometimes be prevented by careful planning in which each member assumes some specific part of the total responsibility. In the hospital the social worker may be the key person who brings about joint planning by the family. In the patient's home the public health nurse may provide this help.

The relative who is to give nursing care to a chronically ill or terminally ill person should be taught how to give it with a minimum of strain to herself and a minimum of discomfort to the patient. Sometimes the relative may enroll in a home nursing course given by the local chapter of the American National Red Cross. In the hospital, at the bedside of the patient, or in the clinic the relative may learn specific techniques and procedures that will be needed. It should be made known that public health nurses from local agencies are available to give assistance and instruction in the home. If the patient has been in the hospital, it is well for the public health nurse to visit his home to review the plan of care with responsible relatives and to consult with the physician and nurses. Members of the family should be prepared for anticipated changes but should not be given cause for worry about situations that may not arise.

If the patient with neurologic disease has marked personality changes, aphasia, or convulsions, the family may even be afraid of him. Because the family is unaware that the patient may fully understand what is being said, they may make tactless remarks in his presence. When the patient is admitted to the hospital, it is often desirable to have him escorted directly to his room and then to take the family aside to ascertain their insight into the situation. This interview gives the nurse valuable information for beginning a nursing care plan, and it provides the nurse with an opportunity to help interpret the patient's actions and responses so that his family may not inadvertently upset him.

Discharge planning

Planning for discharge of the neurologic patient to his home or other health and welfare agencies is initiated on admission to the hospital, based on all of the considerations previously mentioned. When an actual decision has been made as to disposition of the patient (home, nursing home, extended care facility), the nurse should schedule a discharge planning conference with involved agency members and family to make final plans. Instructions to patient and family are completed and the family is asked to review and demonstrate the necessary care procedures. Equipment is secured for the home as indicated. Referral forms are completed for the appropriate agency that is to be utilized in continuing care. This may, for example, include a request for visiting nurse service in the home, follow-up speech therapy, and/or vocational guidance. A suggested plan for continuing nursing care should, in addition, be forwarded to the agency when the patient is transferred to an extended care facility, nursing home, or visiting nurse service.

■ NEUROLOGIC ASSESSMENT

Complete neurologic assessment of the patient is usually done in phases and is dependent on the condition of the patient and the urgency in collecting the necessary data. It includes a history, neurologic examination, and special neurodiagnostic procedures. Discussion in this section will be directed primarily to description of the components of the neurologic examination. The concept of upper and lower motor neuron signs as related to diagnosis is introduced; reference will be made to these concepts throughout the chapter. The role of the nurse in neurologic assessment is also discussed.

History

As in other specialties, a careful history precedes physical examination of the nervous system. In the course of the history taking the patient's chief complaints are elicited through patient interview. The patient is asked to give a timewise account of his illness in his own words. Special inquiry is made in regard to common neurologic conditions or manifestations such as headache, convulsive seizures, and pain. Later during the course of the neurologic or physical examination, some of the observations made during the history may be confirmed. A skillfully taken history with accurate analysis and interpretation of the chief complaints often hold the key to diagnosis. Some observations made during the history and not confirmed during examination will require further study through special neurodiagnostic procedures.

Neurologic examination

Neurologic examination of the adult conscious patient includes evaluation of the following components by the examiner: cranial nerves; mental status (level of consciousness, orientation, mood and behavior, knowledge, vocabulary, memory); sensory status (touch, pain, temperature, proprioception); language and speech; meninges; and motor status (gait and stance, muscle strength, muscle tonus, coordination, involuntary movements, muscle stretch reflexes). The ongoing discussion of each of these components provides the nurse a framework for the kind of information that should be collected to assist the neurologist and to make decisions about nursing care.

The sequence in performing the neurologic examination varies with the examiner, but it should be one that ensures completeness and thoroughness without exhausting the patient. Throughout the examination the examiner attempts to localize the site of the pathology. Using knowledge of normal neuroanatomy and physiology, abnormal findings with reference to their distribution and symmetry of both sides of the body are noted by the examiner.

Equipment required to perform a neurologic examination (in addition to materials used for a general physical examination) is often assembled for convenience on a neurologic tray. It will include minimally a tongue blade, through which a straight pin with one blunt end and one sharp end is stuck for testing the sensation of pain; a wisp of cotton or a fine brush to test the sensation of touch; a tuning fork to test vibratory and hearing senses; vials containing substances with distinctive odors such as peppermint, tobacco, and coffee to test the sense of smell; test tubes with hot and cold water to test temperature sense; vials containing sugar, salt, vinegar, and quinine to test the varied sense of taste; and a reflex hammer. Other equipment may include a dynamometer to measure hand grip, a colored pencil to directly mark sensory deficits, and a transparent millimeter ruler. A flashlight to test pupillary responses and an ophthalmoscope are necessary for eye examination. A diagram of the anterior and posterior surfaces of the body may be used to record abnormal findings as to specific motor and sensory distribution.

Cranial nerve examination. A general description of cranial nerve testing is included at this point since study of these nerves is essential to a complete study of the nervous system. References on neurologic examination are suggested for more detail as to technique in the testing of each nerve.[24,26,66] It is further suggested in the study of the cranial nerves that the reader recall from anatomy the *number* of the nerve (the sequence of the nerve along the rostrocaudal axis of the brain) and the *name* (explains the function or distribution). More importantly, it is helpful for the nurse to be able to express in a few words the *function(s)* of each cranial nerve so that it has practical meaning.

Cranial nerve I, or the *olfactory nerve,* is tested by occluding each nostril in turn while blindfolded and having the examinee identify variable nonpungent substances through the open nostril. *Anosmia,* or the inability to identify familiar substances, constitutes an abnormal finding. The ability to identify a specific substance, however, has to be differentiated from the ability to name it.

Cranial nerve II, or the *optic nerve,* is tested grossly by having the examinee count the number of fingers the examiner holds up or by reading a section of newsprint. The identification of letters on Snellen's chart (p. 823) provides a more detailed examination. Visual field examination (represented by the entire area of vision of one eye as one stares fixedly ahead) is performed by gross confrontation techniques. The examiner stands approximately 3 feet in front of the examinee and holds his hands about 2 feet apart and has the examinee identify movement of fingers in each quadrant of vision as the finger is moved in toward the center of the eye. All quadrants of each eye are tested separately. Visual field defects fall into patterns of one quarter to one half of the visual field. For example, blindness may be caused by a pituitary tumor compressing the optic chiasm and producing a bitemporal *hemiopia,* or the loss of vision in the temporal halves of each visual field. Lesions between the optic chiasm and the occipital cortex produce homonymous hemiopia, or loss of vision in corresponding halves of both visual fields. Finer tests of the visual fields may be done by perimetry studies following the identification of gross defects. Examination of the fundus of the eye with an ophthalmoscope reveals the condition of the blood vessels in the retina. Congestion of the optic nerve head, or papilledema (choked disc), can be noted. This particularly is indicative of increased intracranial pressure (discussed on p. 884).

Cranial nerve III (oculomotor), cranial nerve IV (trochlear), and *cranial nerve VI (abducens)* are tested at the same time since they generally have to do with extraocular movements in all directions (upward, downward, inward, outward). Ocular movements are tested by having the examinee's eyes follow the examiner's finger in all quadrants of gaze while keeping the head stationary. Double vision *(diplopia),* squint *(strabismus),* and involuntary rhythmic movements of the eyeballs *(nystagmus)* may indicate weakness of some of the extraocular muscles due to deficits of these motor nerves. Lack of conjugate gaze (deviation of both eyes to one side)

is usually due to injury of cranial nerves III and/or VI secondary to increased intracranial pressure. It should be recalled that the muscles that turn the eyeball act in pairs. Consequently, the individual muscles are tested in the field of their greatest efficiency as well as during rotation of both eyes, which is more difficult. Cranial nerve III also controls upper eyelid movement, and weakness of the levator muscle is one cause of *ptosis,* or drooping of the lid. The sphincter, or constrictor muscle of the pupil, is supplied by the parasympathetic fibers of cranial nerve III. The pupil constricts normally when a light is focused on the homolateral retina. As a result of the decussation (crossing) of fibers, both in the optic chiasm and in the *pretectal* area, the homolateral as well as the contralateral pupil responds; this is known as a crossed or *consensual light reflex.* Pupils also normally constrict under the stimulus of accommodation and convergence. In addition to the pupils being tested with a flashlight for direct and consensual light reflexes, the pupils are measured as to equality of size and shape. After a head injury, a dilated and fixed or sluggish pupil may be observed on the side of the cranial injury. *Argyll Robertson* pupils, on the other hand, are small and do not respond to light, although they react to accommodation for near objects; they are associated with syphilis. In this way pupil inequality *(anisocoria)* may assist in diagnosis of some neurologic diseases.

Cranial nerve V, or the *trigeminal nerve,* is tested as to its motor component by asking the examinee to bite a tongue blade and to resist its being removed as the examiner pulls on it and attempts to push it to the opposite side. The masseter, temporalis, and pterygoid muscles are palpated at the same time for size and strength. In weakness the opened jaw tends to deviate to the side of the weakened muscles. The sensory components supplying the face are tested for touch, pain, and temperature and any deficits noted as to distribution. (See discussion of sensory status as to the technique of examination.)

Cranial nerve VII, or the *facial nerve,* which has to do with facial movement, is tested by asking the examinee to perform specific facial movements. The inability to smile, close both eyes tightly, look upward and wrinkle the forehead, show the teeth, purse the lips, and blow out the cheeks constitutes weakness or paralysis of facial muscles innervated by this nerve. Special attention is given to asymmetry. Bell's palsy, caused by compression of this nerve, is a common lower motor neuron type of facial paralysis. Lesions affecting the facial nerve produce paralysis of half of the entire face, including the eyelids, forehead, and lips. Forehead function, by contrast, remains intact in upper motor neuron lesions. The sensation of taste is tested by placing salty, sweet, bitter, and sour substances in turn on the side of the protruded tongue for identification.

Cranial nerve VIII, or the *acoustic nerve,* is tested grossly by having the examinee listen and identify whispered words or the ticking of a watch and the vibrations of a tuning fork at prescribed distances. Bone and air conduction of sound is also compared with a tuning fork. If the vibration is heard longer when placed on the mastoid bone than when placed near the auditory canal, there is a defect of transmission in the acoustic membrane or the auditory ossicles. In the normal ear, air conduction is greater than bone conduction. In *Weber's test* the base of the tuning fork is placed on the vertex of the skull to note if sound is normally heard equally in both ears. If the cochlear nerve is involved on one side, the sound will not be detected on that side; in middle ear disease, or blockage of the external auditory canal, the sound is lateralized and heard on the affected side. To measure hearing sense most accurately, an electric audiometer is used and an audiogram is made.

The vestibular function of cranial nerve VIII is tested by caloric and rotational stimuli. The performance of these tests is complex, and it is not regularly done.

Cranial nerve IX (glossopharyngeal) and *cranial nerve X (vagus)* are tested together. Both nerves supply the posterior pharyngeal wall, and normally when the wall is touched, there is prompt contraction of these muscles on both sides, with or without gagging. This test is thus unreliable in regard to either nerve alone. Since cranial nerve X supplies soft palatal, pharyngeal, and laryngeal muscles, the detection of abnormalities is made through testing of voice sounds and cough sounds. In unilateral involvement of the motor portion of the vagus nerve there is harshness and nasality of the voice. The soft palate deviates to the intact side when tested by having the examinee say "ah." Bilateral involvement produces more severe effects in speech and there is also difficulty in swallowing *(dysphagia),* with regurgitation of fluids through the nose because of palatal and pharyngeal involvement. Sensory function is not usually tested in the vagus nerve.

Cranial nerve XI, or the *spinal accessory nerve,* is tested by having the examinee rotate his head against resistance, while any weakness of the sternocleidomastoid muscle on the opposite side is observed and palpated by the examiner. The ability of the person to elevate and retract his shoulders bilaterally is also tested. Weakness or paralysis of these muscles constitutes abnormality of this nerve.

Cranial nerve XII, or the *hypoglossal nerve,* is tested by having the examinee protrude his tongue in the midline and wiggle it from side to side. When this nerve is involved, there is deviation of the tongue toward the side of the lesion. Atrophy of the tongue is shown through wrinkling and loss of substance on the affected side. In an upper motor neuron lesion there is involvement of the tongue on the opposite side (contralateral) to the lesion.

Mental status. Specific abnormalities of higher cerebral function are particularly significant in the recognition of organic brain disease. Bedside observations of mental function are important.

A determination of the level of consciousness (awareness of self and environment) is necessary. The operational methods for determining the level of consciousness are through inspection of responses to visual and auditory stimuli, loudness of conversation, pain and pressure stimuli, vital signs, and reflex responses. Generally, minimal impairment of depressed consciousness is manifest by excessive drowsiness, with the patient capable of being aroused to a normal level of awareness. With increasing depression of consciousness, there is lethargy or stupor, making it possible to arouse the patient to some degree but with an inability to sustain consciousness; in coma the patient is unresponsive and loses reflex responses as depression increases. Because such grading is subjective to some extent, the actual responses of the patient to specific stimuli are recorded objectively, without making a judgmental grading. (See Chapter 10 for a discussion of the care of the unconscious patient.) Although many metabolic and toxic states produce changes of consciousness, destructive lesions of the brain may directly decrease it. There also may be elevation of consciousness as in insomnia, agitation, mania, and delirium. The latter is the classic clinical example of elevation of consciousness with insomnia, agitation, anxiety, tremulousness, hallucinations, and convulsions (the final outcome of excessive cerebral activity).

The patient is also tested as to his orientation to time (day of month, week), place, and person. Disorientation to place and person indicates a profound cerebral disorder. It is helpful to remember that orientation depends on the ongoing sensory impressions.

The identification of mood and behavior is also necessary in mental examination, since a particular mood may be associated with a particular disease. For example, emotional lability is often seen in bilateral (diffuse) brain disease, where the mood shifts easily and quickly and from one extreme to the other. Euphoria is a superficial elevation of mood accompanied by unconcern even in threatening events. Does the mood swing in a direction appropriate to the subject matter of conversation? Personality change with the appearance of violent temper and aggressive behavior may be present in destructive lesions of the inferior frontal parts of the limbic system.

Knowledge and vocabulary are tested in reference to common knowledge and current events. The ability to think abstractly may be tested by asking the person to explain the meaning of a proverb. Calculation is tested by examining the ability to subtract serially 7 from 100. *Dyscalculia* is the inability to solve simple problems. Recent memory loss is more common in brain disease than is remote memory loss. More definitive tests of mental function may be indicated by the aforementioned gross bedside tests.

Sensory status. General sensory function of the trunk and extremities is tested as to both superficial and deep sensations (the face is omitted since it is tested by examining cranial nerve V). Areas of sensory loss, or abnormality, are mapped out on a body diagram according to the distribution of the *spinal dermatomes* and peripheral nerves (Fig. 32-2). Testing superficial sensation includes light touch, pain, and temperature. Each is tested in turn with appropriate stimuli. The examiner determines the extent to which the patient feels touch (cotton), pain (pinprick), and temperature (hot and cold water) in the sites mentioned. An area in which sensory loss is absent *(anesthesia)* is differentiated from areas in which a sensation is intensified *(hyperesthesia)* or lessened *(hypoesthesia). Paresthesia* is an abnormal sensation that is perceived as burning, prickly, or itching. Deep sensation *(proprioception)* that includes joint and vibratory (deep pressure) and pain perception from deep-lying structures is tested. Passive movement is evaluated, in both the upper and lower extremities, by the examiner passively moving the examinee's digits in different directions and having him identify the direction with his eyes closed. Deep pain sense is determined by compression of deep structures such as the Achilles tendon and calf muscles and noting extremes of response. Vibratory sense is tested by placing the tuning fork on selected bones in the upper and lower parts of the body (sternum, ankle bone, etc.) and asking the person to identify the buzzing sensation felt. The ability to identify and judge the size, weight, and form of an object placed in an outstretched palm while the eyes are

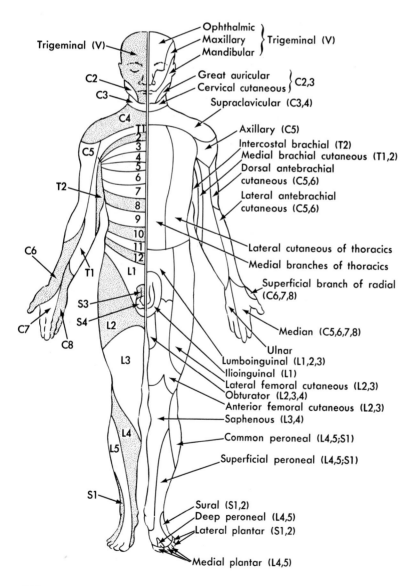

FIG. 32-2. Peripheral distribution of sensory nerve fibers. Anterior view. Right: Distribution of cutaneous nerves. Left: Dermatomes (shaded) or segmental distribution of cutaneous nerves. (Redrawn from House, E. L., and Pansky, B.: A functional approach to neuroanatomy, ed. 2, New York, 1967, McGraw-Hill Book Co.)

closed is also made *(stereognosis).* Since stereognosia is based on normal reception of touch stimuli, it is included at this point; it is also related to the recognition and interpretation of that which is perceived by other cortical senses.

The ability to recognize objects through any of the special senses is known as *gnosia.* Sensations require a high degree of cortical integration or a great degree of knowing or interpretation. The elaboration of sensation as to its ultimate meaning in the individual depends on certain association areas in the cortex. *Agnosia* is not knowing a specific sensation; if the sense of touch is affected, it is called *astereognosia;* if sight and sound are involved, it is termed relative to the sensation deficit. Thus *agraphognosia* means a loss of graphic or writing sense, for example. *Anosognosia* refers to a lack of disease awareness or body parts. Lesions involving a specific association area produce a specific type of agnosia.

Language and speech. These functions are assessed grossly by the examiner while the history is taken. When a problem is apparent, referral may be made to a speech pathologist for a definitive diagnosis and suggestions for treatment approaches. It is important for the nurse to recall from neuroanatomy that language per se is not represented in one area in the cortex but is concentrated in a cortical field that is inclusive of parts of the temporal lobe (superior and lateral), the temporoparietal-occipital junction, and the frontal lobe (opercular region). Also, language is a function of the dominant hemisphere, which is the left one in the majority of individuals. Lesions or injury in any of the language areas will produce some type (or combination) of impairment in the use of language (motor) or in the understanding of language (sensory). This impairment of language is called *aphasia* generally; the specific type has to be diagnosed. Deficits are not usually limited to one area and may be mild or severe. Aphasia with reduced output (motor) may be caused by lesions in Broca's area; aphasia with fluent output but difficulty in reception may be caused by lesions in Wernicke's area. Global aphasia is almost a complete loss of language functions. (See p. 849 for discussion of nursing care of patients with language deficits.)

Speech is tested through the detection of weakness and/or incoordination of muscles used in speech articulation. Limitations are observed during cranial nerve testing and particularly in reference to cranial nerves V, VII, IX, X, and XII. Involvement of the motor component of these nerves, as previously discussed, may produce alterations in phonation, resonance, and articulation. The examiner asks the examinee to produce different speech sounds in order to localize the problem. Disorders of speech *(dysarthria)* may be single or a variety of alterations in speech sounds may be present as characteristics of a particular disease. For example, speech in cerebellar disease is often thick and explosive, with a prolongation of speech sounds occurring at intervals (called scanning); in parkinsonism, speech is referred to as hyperkinetic and is characterized by a decrease in loudness and in vocal emphasis patterns that make sounds appear monotonous to the listener.

Apractic speech is a rare yet interesting disorder in which there is difficulty in the production of speech volitionally in the absence of motor paralysis. It is essentially a problem in motor programming through cortical integration. (Apraxia is a general term and relates to motor acts other than speech.)

Meninges. To test for meningeal irritation, or stiff neck, the head is passively flexed sharply toward the chest while the patient is in a recumbent position. In the presence of meningeal irritation there is marked resistance to the flexion, accompanied by rigidity of the neck (nucha), spasm, and pain. There is also resistance to extension and rotary movements of the neck. *Brudzinski's sign,* indicating meningeal irritation, is also elicited by passive neck flexion. When the neck is flexed, the hips and legs flex involuntarily. *Kernig's sign* is a classic test used in the diagnosis of meningitis. In this test the examiner flexes one of the examinee's thighs to a right angle and then attempts to extend the leg on the thigh (there are many variations of this test). A positive Kernig's sign is present when there is spasm of the hamstring muscles with resistance to extension of the leg and with neck and head pain.

Motor status. Function of the motor system is assessed as to these components: gait and stance, muscle strength, muscle tonus, coordination, and involuntary movements.

Gait and stance should be recognized as a complex activity that requires muscle strength, coordination, balance, proprioception, and vision. Gait, or walking, and associated movements thus give considerable information about motor status. Changes in gait may be characteristic of a specific neurologic disease. In evaluating gait the patient is asked to walk freely and naturally. He may be asked to walk heel to toe in a straight line since this exaggerates abnormalities. In evaluating stance the examinee is asked to stand with his feet close together, first with eyes open and then closed *(Romberg's sign).* Patients with problems of proprioception have difficulty maintaining a stance with their eyes closed; patients with cerebellar disease have difficulty even with their eyes open, and they walk with a wide-base, staggering gait. The hemiparetic gait, as seen in upper motor neuron disease, is characterized by circumduction of the affected leg and inversion of the foot. Patients with Parkinson's disease walk with a slow shuffling gait and, as they start walking, increase the rapidity until almost running (propulsive). They also have difficulty stopping, and deviation in the center of gravity causes retropulsion or lateropulsion. There is, in addition, a loss of associated movement of the arms in walking. *Ataxia* is a general term meaning lack of coordination in performing a planned, purposeful motion, as in walking. It can be caused by disturbance of position sense or by cerebellar or other diseases. It is important to recognize gait disturbances and to interpret cause only after all studies have been completed.

Muscle strength, or power, is assessed systematically, including trunk and extremity muscles. During the test the examinee attempts to resist the examiner in moving his muscles when placed in fixed positions. Weakness of a specific muscle is identified by the examiner as to distribution and degree of muscle weakness. *Akinesia* is loss of muscle power. Evaluation may include all major muscles. At other times testing may be made only through gross tests of the extremities such as hand grip or foot strength and/or the ability to move all extremities. *Hemiplegia* is complete paralysis of one half of the body (linear), whereas *hemiparesis* is weakness or incomplete paralysis in the same distribution. *Paraplegia* is paralysis of the lower extremities, and *quadriplegia* is paralysis of the four extremities. The reader should note the distribution of motor nerves to skeletal muscles. (The distribution varies from that of sensory nerve distributions.)

Muscle tonus is tested by the examiner passively moving the limbs through a full range of motion. An increase *(hypertonia)* or a decrease *(hypotonia)* can be differentiated by the skilled examiner. Overextension and overflexion are found in *hypotonia.* In hypertonia, resistance to passive movement increases rapidly and then suddenly gives way to pyramidal spasticity; this is known as *clasp-knife rigidity.* A steady, passive resistance throughout the full range of motion is characteristic of parkinsonism *rigidity;* the combination of passive resistance and parkinsonism tremor with small regular jerks is called *cogwheel rigidity.* In *decorticate rigidity* the upper limbs are flexed and pronated and the lower limbs are extended. In *decerebrate rigidity,* on the other hand, the upper limbs are extended and pronated and the lower limbs are extended. In hypertonia, extremities tend to stay in fixed positions and feel firm, while in hypotonia the extremities assume a position that is governed by gravity.

Coordination of muscle movements or the ability to perform skilled motor acts may be impaired at any level of the motor system. However, the cerebellum is primarily responsible for control, so that movements take place in a smooth and precise manner. Disturbance in cerebellar function may result in ataxia (as discussed relative to gait), difficulty in controlling the range of muscular movement *(dysmetria),* and an inability to alternate rapid opposite and successive movements *(adiadochokinesia).* Simple motor activities are evaluated on command

of the examiner to perform rapid and rhythmic movements. For example, the nose-finger-nose test requires the examinee to alternately touch his nose and the tip of the examiner's finger with variation in rate and level. Other tests include the knee pat (pronation-supination) and heel-knee or shin test, during which the patient slides his heel over the shin toward the dorsum of the foot. There are many such tests that are often modified by the examiner.

Involuntary movements need to be observed and described during neurologic examination. Description of abnormal movements *(hyperkinesia)* is difficult but necessary. Observation of the presence or absence of the following is helpful: amount and location of muscles involved, amplitude of movement, speed of onset, duration of contraction and relaxation, and rhythmicity. The effects of posture, rest, sleep, diversion of attention, voluntary movements, and emotional stress each need to be questioned and/or tested. Involuntary movements are usually increased by emotional stress and may subside during sleep. Involuntary movements can be the result of organic disease and yet may be psychosomatic in origin. A few of the more common types of involuntary movements are considered generally and as to quantity of movement. *Tremor* consists of rhythmic to-and-fro movements. They are usually of small amplitude and are due to alternate contractions of opposing groups of muscles. They are continuous while the patient is awake and may or may not be present during sleep. *Chorea* consists of short, sharp, rapid movements, usually of small excursion and irregular; movements occur in different parts of the body and persist during sleep. *Hemiballismus* is a variation of chorea in which movement is confined to one side of the body and affects the limbs to a great extent. *Athetosis* consists of slow, sinuous, and more sustained movements that may be of considerable amplitude; movements occur within the neck and trunk as well as the extremities and may be called *torsion spasms. Myoclonus* consists of an irregular, abrupt, and shocklike contraction of a part of a muscle, a muscle, or a group of muscles. Myoclonus may involve the extremities or the trunk and may be consistent in site.

Although all muscles can be made to contract reflexly, only a few reflexes are tested clinically. *Muscle stretch reflexes* (MSR's) (also called myotactic and deep tendon reflexes) that are tested more routinely include the biceps, triceps, brachioradialis, quadriceps, and gastrocnemius-soleus muscles. (Superficial reflexes are omitted in this discussion.) Since the muscle reflexes are simple monosynaptic reflexes, they may be diminished in normal response *(hyporeflexia)* or lost *(areflexia)* completely through interruption of afferent sensory fiber transmission or with extensive destruction of efferent motor fibers or the anterior horn cells. On the other hand, release

Table 32-1 Grading of muscle stretch reflexes (MSR)

Scale	Interpretation
0	Areflexia
±	Hyporeflexia
1 to 3	Normal
3+ to 4+	Hyperreflexia

of the monosynaptic reflex from the influence of suprasegmental fibers (pyramidal and supplementary motor systems) produces an increased muscular response *(hyperreflexia)*. The general method for testing muscle stretch reflexes is through mechanical stimulation of the muscle spindles through stretching and by tapping a tendon or a bone or by flipping a digit (Hoffmann's sign). The degree of response, below or above normal, is noted and graded on a scale. The most important feature of any reflex pattern of a person is not the absolute value on the scale, but asymmetry, or difference between one side and the other. Stick figures are commonly used to record the bilateral values (scale may range from 0 to 4+). See Table 32-1 for one example of how reflex-

es are graded on a scale. Since the threshold for muscle stretch reflexes has a normal range of variability, some individuals with generalized hyporeflexia and hyperreflexia will not have pathologic conditions but will rank at the end of the normal range. Areflexia is usually a pathologic condition.

One reflex often referred to clinically is the plantar reflex. This reflex, when present, results in extention of the great toe (moves toward dorsum) with fanning (abduction) of the other toes when pressure is applied to the plantar surface of the foot laterally from the heel toward the toes. This response is known as *Babinski's sign* and is associated with upper motor neuron disease.

Other reflexes may be classified as pathologic. These are reflexes that are present in infancy for variable periods. They are thought to be released by acquired diseases of the cerebrum. Examples include the sucking, pouting, and grasp reflexes.

A reflex, when positive, may assist in localizing a lesion, as does a positive unilateral Babinski sign. Reflex findings, however, are only used in relation to total assessment data and are not used alone. Refer to neurology texts for techniques on eliciting specific reflexes. Variations of grading scale values used should be noted. It should be recognized that grading is somewhat subjective.

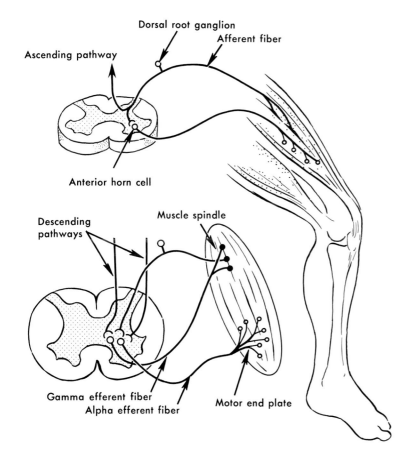

FIG. 32-3. Structures comprising the lower motor neuron, including the motor (efferent) and sensory (afferent) elements. Shown on the right is an anterior horn cell in the anterior gray column of the spinal cord and its axon terminating in a motor end plate as it innervates extrafusal muscle fibers in the quadriceps muscle. Detailed in the enlargement on the left are the sensory and motor elements of the gamma loop system. A gamma efferent fiber is shown innervating the polar or end region of the muscle spindle (sensory receptor of the skeletal muscle). Contraction of the muscle spindle fibers stretch the central portion of the spindle and cause the afferent spindle fiber to transmit an impulse centrally to the cord. The muscle spindle afferent fibers in turn synapse on the anterior horn cell and are transmitted via alpha efferent fibers to skeletal (extrafusal) muscle, causing it to contract. Muscle spindle discharge is interrupted by active contraction of the extrafusal muscle fibers. (Adapted from Truex, R. C., and Carpenter, M. B.: Human neuroanatomy, ed. 6, Baltimore, 1969, The Williams & Wilkins Co.)

Upper and lower motor neuron signs

An important concept in neurologic examination and diagnosis by the neurologist rests on identifying the abnormalities of motor function that result from pathology of or injury to upper and lower motor neurons. The ability to differentiate between upper and lower motor neuron lesions is the first step in the localization of the site of a neural lesion that manifests itself by disturbances in normal motor function. When the site of the neural lesion has been decided, the neurologist can then consider the pathology that may have caused it.

In relation to *lower motor neurons* (LMN's) it is necessary to recall that they consist of the large anterior horn cells in the spinal cord as well as the motor cranial nuclei in the brain stem and all of their respective axons that innervate striated muscle (Fig. 32-3). Although many fiber systems initiate and modify muscular action in some way, it is the LMN that achieves, or effects, the muscle action. This is also known as the *final common pathway,* as shown in Fig. 32-4. When a lesion selectively involves the LMN in some part (cell body, motor root, isolated peripheral nerve), it characteristically results in flaccid muscle weakness or paralysis, loss of reflex activity, loss of muscle tone, and atrophy confined to the involved muscle(s). Each effect will be discussed briefly at this point and compared later with upper motor neuron effects on muscle.

The degree of muscle weakness occurring in the involved muscle(s) in a LMN lesion bears a direct relationship to the extent and severity of the lesion. Since the anterior horn cells and their neurons, which innervate a single muscle, extend longitudinally through several spinal segments, and since several anterior horn cell columns exist at each spinal level, a lesion confined to one spinal segment will thus cause muscle weakness *(paresis)* rather than paralysis of the muscle. Some motor neurons are thus preserved. Complete paralysis occurs in LMN

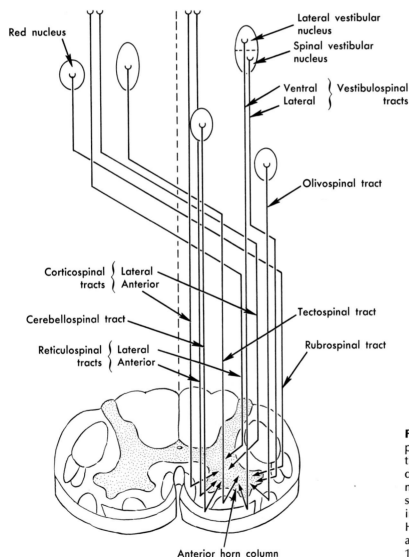

Red nucleus

Lateral vestibular nucleus

Spinal vestibular nucleus

Ventral } Vestibulospinal
Lateral } tracts

Olivospinal tract

Corticospinal { Lateral
tracts { Anterior

Cerebellospinal tract

Tectospinal tract

Reticulospinal { Lateral
tracts { Anterior

Rubrospinal tract

Anterior horn column

FIG. 32-4. The principle of the final common pathway is illustrated. Numerous nuclei and their respective pathways or tracts are shown descending and terminating around the lower motor neuron of the ventral column of the spinal cord where they exert their combined influence on motor activity. (Redrawn from House, E. L., and Pansky, F.: A functional approach to neuroanatomy, ed. 2, New York, 1967, McGraw-Hill Book Co.)

lesions only when the lesion involves the column or anterior horn cells in several spinal segments that innervate a particular muscle or the ventral roots arising from these cells. A lesion in a single motor nerve root will cause varying degrees of muscle weakness in several muscles.

Muscle weakness per se cannot be classified as either lower or upper motor neuron since it is common to both. It is the *distribution* of the muscle weakness that is important to distinguish. In summary, a LMN lesion weakens or paralyzes individual muscles, or sets of muscles, in the root or peripheral nerve distribution (based on knowledge of individual nerve distribution and in segmental distributions as in dermatomes).

The involved muscle(s) is flaccid due to the absence of normal muscle stretch reflexes (areflexia) or reduced reflexes (hyporeflexia) since there has been interruption of the reflex activity at the involved site. Flaccidity of the muscle is further evidenced by hypotonia with reduced or absent electrical impulses to the muscle. Localized muscle atrophy, or wasting, is apparent on inspection and corresponds to the spinal segmental distribution of muscle involvement. This develops more slowly than the other muscle manifestations and is thought to be due to denervation (blocking).

Atrophy also increases with nonuse of the muscle. In some LMN lesions the affected muscle bundle or unit exhibits small localized, spontaneous and involuntary contractions known as *fasciculations.* These are visible through the skin and should not be confused with fibrillation. The fasciculations are thought to represent the discharge of muscle fibers arising from a single lower motor unit. They are coarse in large motor units but may be fine in smaller motor units, as in the hands.

The criteria for a LMN lesion site or disease includes segmental or localized muscle weakness and atrophy in the same distribution, with absent or decreased muscle stretch reflexes in the affected muscles.

The *upper motor neurons* (UMN's) arise from the motor cortex of the cerebrum (precentral gyrus), descend through long projection pathways via the pyramidal system (corticospinal and corticobulbar), and eventually synapse with the LMN's (Fig. 32-5). Some clinicians equate the UMN's only with the descending pyramidal system; other clinicians include in addition the rubrospinal, vestibulospinal, and reticulospinal descending fiber systems that can also influence the LMN's. When neural impulses are transmitted through all descending fiber systems to lower spinal segments, muscle tone, reflex activity, and somatic motor activity are maintained, mediated, or controlled in some way. It is believed that the pyramidal system is primarily responsible for the initiation and stimulation of muscle activity required

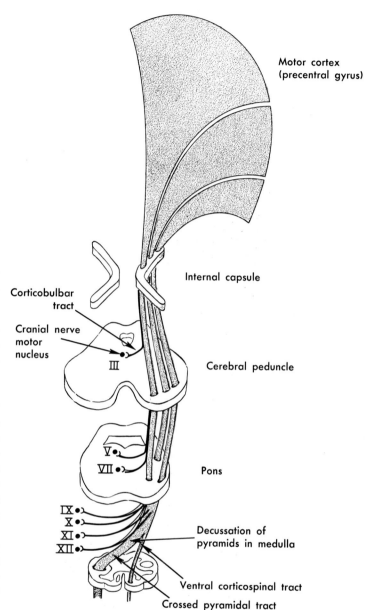

FIG. 32-5. Structures comprising the upper motor neuron, or the pyramidal system, are illustrated. The pyramidal system fibers are shown to originate primarily in cells in the precentral gyrus of the motor cortex; converge at the internal capsule; descend to form the central third of the cerebral peduncle; descend further through the pons, where small fibers are given off to cranial nerve motor nuclei along the way; form pyramids at the medulla, where the majority of the fibers decussate; and then continue to descend in the lateral column of the white matter of the spinal cord, where they synapse with anterior horn cells at all segments of the cord. A few fibers descend without crossing at the medulla level. (Adapted from an original painting by Frank H. Netter, M.D.; from The Ciba Collection of Medical Illustrations, Copyright by Ciba Pharmaceutical Co., Division of Ciba-Geigy Corp. All rights reserved.)

for precise and fine voluntary muscle movements. Thus all descending systems collectively combine their influences on the LMN's so that volitional neural impulses are modified to result in fine, orderly, and smooth movements.

When lesions involve the UMN's at a wide variety of locations, characteristically *after a period of time* there is paresis of muscle movements, increased muscle tonus, and increased reflex activity. Since cerebrovascular accident (stroke) is the most common UMN lesion seen clinically, discussion is directed primarily to it. Trauma, neoplasia, and degenerative disease produce similar findings when located in UMN sites.

The *distribution* of paralysis or paresis is also significant in UMN lesions. The degree of muscle paralysis or paresis, however, does not bear such a direct relationship to the size of the lesion or the extent of involvement of the pyramidal system. It is important to realize that the paralysis is not that of individual muscle distribution, but paralysis of movements in *hemiplegic* (and *paraplegic* and *quadriplegic*) distributions. Hemiplegia, or paralysis of both the upper and lower extremity on the same side, is the common distribution in stroke. Unilateral lesions of the motor cortex and the brain stem always produce paralysis of movement contralateral to the lesion if it is rostral to the decussation of the pyramids; ipsilateral paralysis of movement occurs if the lesion is caudal to the pyramids. The distribution or degree of paralysis is not always equal or the same within the hemiplegic distribution. For example, the face and arm may be weak or the weakness may involve the leg alone, depending on the parts of the motor cortex involved. The following may be considered UMN signs: weakness of the mouth muscle associated with eye muscle weakness (forehead muscle is intact), weakness of forearm and wrist extensors, and weakness of the hip flexors and foot dorsiflexors. These muscle weaknesses result in the characteristic gait and appearance of the patient with a stroke. There is circumduction of the affected leg with inversion of the foot that drags. The arm is held semiflexed at the elbow and wrist. The facial muscles around the eye and mouth droop.

For a variable period of time the muscles on the involved side are usually flaccid, with hypotonia and hyporeflexia. Gradually the muscles become spastic, with hypertonia and exaggerated hyperreflexia. The spasticity is characterized by increased resistance to passive movement, hyperreflexia, clasp-knife phenomenon, and *clonus*. The latter is related to the hyperreflexia, in which the contraction of one muscle group is sufficient to stretch the antagonistic muscles and perpetuate the contractions. A unilateral Babinski sign is present on the hemiparetic side. Atrophy of the muscle results from disuse and occurs late.

UMN lesions within the brain stem also produce the characteristic motor manifestations as just described and, in addition, involvement of the cranial nerve nuclei and sensory pathways that are near the midbrain lesion site.

A complete transection of the spinal cord immediately produces loss of motor function, muscle tone, and reflex activity as well as somatic and visceral sensations below the level of the injury. Usually, when examined after a year, the same motor losses are present along with extensor spasticity and clonus. A bilateral positive Babinski sign is also present. The problem of localizing the site of an UMN brain stem lesion is made more difficult by the close proximity of the descending fiber systems and cranial motor nuclei in the brain stem area. Table 32-2 summarizes and compares the characteristic clinical syndromes as seen in UMN and LMN lesions.

Role of the nurse

The role of the nurse in neurologic assessment includes independent systematic neurologic assessment of the patient and assisting the physician with special neurodiagnostic procedures. It should be made clear that neurologic assessment by the nurse is but one part of nursing assessment, as discussed in Chapter 1. The nurse should understand that patients with neurologic complaints or patients with known neurologic conditions often dread examination and tests more than other patients. They may fear that a procedure such as a lumbar or ventricular

Table 32-2 Clinical syndromes of upper motor neuron (UMN) and lower motor neuron (LMN) lesions

Motor component	UMN characteristics	LMN characteristics
Reflex	Hyperreflexia, extensor toe sign (Babinski's sign)	Hyporeflexia or areflexia
Muscle tonus	Hypertonia, clasp-knife spasticity, clonus	Hypotonia, flaccidity
Muscle movement	Paralysis or paresis of movements in hemiplegic distribution, etc.	Paralysis or paresis of individual muscles in peripheral nerve distribution
Muscle wasting	Late atrophy from disuse	Early atrophy of denervation
Muscle fasciculations	Not present	Present

puncture, for example, will cause further disability; they may be reluctant to have neurologic deficits proved or exposed. A patient may further sense a serious diagnosis and dread its confirmation. The nurse must be able to secure the trust and cooperation of the patient in order to support the patient and secure needed information. The nurse should, in addition, be knowledgeable of the purposes, preparation, and complications of each neurodiagnostic procedure in order to assist intelligently. The nurse must be able to explain the procedure to the individual patient in such a way as to satisfy his concerns.

On admission of the patient to the hospital, the neurologic nurse performs a neurologic examination for the purpose of providing baseline data for planning nursing care. Information collected from the examination should be accurate and recorded clearly so that it is useful to other nurses and health team members. Such primary information is thus both complementary and supplementary to that collected by the neurologist and other paramedical personnel. Secondary data in turn should be collected by the nurse to further assist in planning care of the patient. Neurologic examination is a dynamic process and requires continuing assessment.

The initial neurologic examination, as performed by the nurse, includes the same components of neurologic examination (cranial nerve, mental status, sensory status, language and speech status, motor status) as discussed earlier (p. 855). Techniques used in eliciting responses are the same. The assessment is modified to serve nursing purposes. The examination does not purposefully duplicate the more detailed examination performed by the neurologist for diagnostic purposes. The gross tests, as previously discussed, are usually sufficient to identify the major functional neurologic deficits relative to each component. Once the gross deficits are identified, some will need to be identified more specifically. This is often done in collaboration with the neurologist, occupational therapist, physical therapist, speech pathologist, and psychologist. An abbreviated neurologic examination is described by Truscott,[96] which may be of assistance to beginning nurse practitioners. The routine that he recommends omits unnecessary tests, avoids wasted motions, and yet permits accuracy of information. The sequence of examination selected by the individual nurse should be one that is based on a systematic approach and is comprehensive without tiring the patient. The depth and comprehensiveness of information collected from the examination often corresponds with the knowledge, skill, and experience of the nurse.

From a nursing standpoint it is important to identify neurologic deficits, both grossly and specifically, so that nursing interventions can be decided. It is also important that the nurse assess and identify neurologic deficits and recognize critical changes in status so that these can be accurately reported to the neurologist. The examination should include a detailed appraisal of the functional status of the patient relative to his ability to perform self-care activities (p. 9) that are often limited by motor, mental, and/or sensory deficits.

■ SPECIAL NEURODIAGNOSTIC PROCEDURES

Special neurodiagnostic procedures of the nervous system include examination of the cerebrospinal fluid by lumbar puncture, radioisotope brain scan, neuroradiologic studies of the spinal cord, and brain and electrodiagnostic studies to measure the electrical activity of the brain and muscles. Each is discussed generally as to use, methodology, and nursing care responsibilities. Special tests relating to a specific disease are discussed in the section pertaining to the disease.

Lumbar puncture

This procedure is used to obtain cerebrospinal fluid for examination and to detect spinal subarachnoid block. The cerebrospinal fluid (CSF) is examined for an increase or decrease of its normal constituents; it is also examined for foreign substances such as pathogenic organisms and blood. Cerebrospinal fluid normally is a clear fluid that is formed in the lateral ventricles of the brain. It passes through the third ventricle, the aqueduct of Sylvius, the fourth ventricle, and finally into the cisterna magna at the base of the brain. From this location between the arachnoid and the dura mater, the fluid bathes the entire brain surface and passes down to surround the spinal cord. The main purpose of the spinal fluid is to provide mechanical protection for the brain and spinal cord. The exact manner of its production and absorption is not entirely clear nor is the rate of its production clearly determined. It is thought that approximately 150 to 200 ml. of spinal fluid circulate within the system.

Spinal fluid normally is under slight positive pressure; 80 to 180 mm. of water is considered normal. It is measured on a manometer when a spinal puncture is done. When a brain tumor or other space-occupying lesion is within the cranium, the spinal fluid pressure usually is greatly increased. For this reason a lumbar puncture is not performed in a choked disc or when a brain tumor is suspected lest the quick reduction in pressure produced by removal of spinal fluid cause the brain structures to herniate into the foramen magnum, which would put pressure on vital centers in the medulla and might cause sudden death. The neurologist often writes "No spinal tap" on the patient's chart to be certain that no other medical staff member attempts this procedure.

Normally each milliliter of spinal fluid contains 0 to 5 lymphocytes. An increase in the number of cells may indicate an infection. Tuberculosis and viral infections may cause an increase in lymphocytes, while pyogenic infections may cause increase in polymorphonuclear leukocytes, which may be in large enough numbers to make the fluid cloudy. Bacterial infections such as tuberculous meningitis often lower the blood sugar level from the normal level of 40 to 60 mg./100 ml. (approximately one-half the normal level). They may also reduce the chloride level from the normal 720 to 750 mg./100 ml. In the presence of degenerative diseases and when a brain tumor is present, the spinal fluid protein is usually increased from the normal level of 30 to 50 mg./100 ml. Study of the spinal fluid may occasionally reveal the actual organism causing disease. The serologic test for syphilis may be positive in spinal fluid even when the blood serologic result is negative.

Blood in the spinal fluid indicates hemorrhage from somewhere into the ventricular system. It may be caused by a fracture at the base of the skull that has torn blood vessels, or it may be caused by the rupture of a blood vessel that may occur, for example, with a congenital aneurysm. Occasionally the first specimen of spinal fluid contains blood from slight bleeding at the point of the puncture. For this reason the specimens of fluid are numbered, and the first one is not used to determine the cell count.

Strict aseptic technique is mandatory in all procedures in which the cerebrospinal fluid system is entered. The nurse is responsible for seeing that all equipment is sterile and that safe technique is used throughout the procedure. The nurse always explains the procedure to the patient and sees that a permit for it is signed when hospital policy requires it. If the patient is uncertain about any details of the procedure, the nurse should not hesitate to ask the physician to give him further explanation. The nurse tells the patient what to expect during the procedure and how he may help to make it as uncomplicated as possible.

Details of the lumbar *(spinal) puncture procedure* and a list of the equipment needed are given in texts on fundamentals of nursing.

The physician or nurse will explain to the patient that the needle is inserted below the level of the spinal cord so that there is little danger of injury. (See Fig. 32-6 for the site of insertion of the lumbar puncture needle.) The patient will be positioned with both his knees and his head flexed at an acute angle so that there is maximal lumbar flexion and separation of interspinous spaces. He should have constant nursing attention during the procedure. Even when a local anesthetic is used (usually procaine, 1%), the patient should be prepared to feel slight pain and pressure as the dura is entered. He should be reminded not to move suddenly and may be told that he may experience a sharp shooting pain down one leg. This pain is caused by the needle's coming close

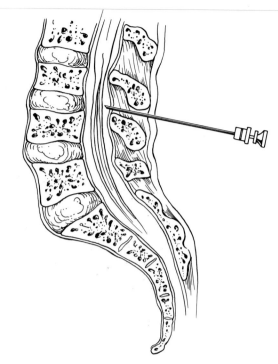

FIG. 32-6. Position and angle of the needle when a lumbar puncture is performed. Note that the needle is in the fourth lumbar interspace below the level of the spinal cord.

to a nerve and is similar to hitting one's "funnybone"; however, the nerve actually is floating in fluid and is safe from injury.

The nurse prepares the equipment, assists the physician, assures sterility, monitors the patient during and immediately following the procedure, and arranges for suitable labeling and disposition of specimens. The manometer must be held above the point where the physician's hands need to come in contact with it (Fig. 32-7). The nurse may be asked to compress the jugular vein first on one side, then on the other side, and finally on both sides at the same time and may be asked to help the physician to recall the spinal pressure under each of these circumstances. The pressure should be exerted with the fingers flat against the patient's neck, avoiding his trachea. This test, known as *Queckenstedt's test,* is simple, but it may alarm the patient if he has not been informed that pressure may be exerted on his neck for a few seconds.

Headache is fairly common following a lumbar puncture. Although its exact cause is unknown, it is thought to be due to loss of spinal fluid through the dura. The sharpness and size of the needle used, the skill of the physician, and the emotional state of the patient are probably the determining factors in whether or not a headache will develop. If one does develop, it is treated with bed rest, an ice cap to the

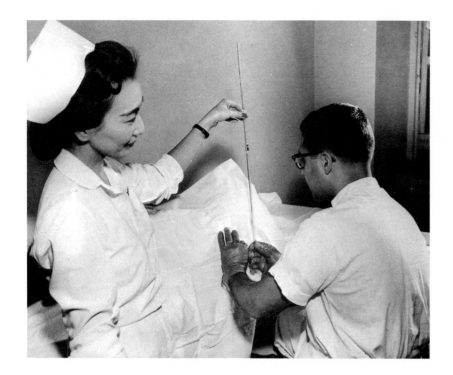

FIG. 32-7. The nurse assisting the physician with a lumbar puncture may support the manometer and record essential readings.

head, and an analgesic. Most headaches from this cause disappear within 24 hours.

Lumbar punctures are often performed on patients who are ambulatory and who go home immediately after the procedure is completed. It has been found that they suffer no more from headaches than do those who are treated more conservatively with bed rest and no elevation of the head.

In a *cisternal puncture* the cerebrospinal fluid system is tapped by inserting a short-beveled needle immediately below the occipital bone into the cisterna magna (Fig. 32-8). This procedure may be more frightening to the patient than a lumbar puncture since the approach is closer to the brain. The patient should have a detailed explanation by the physician before any head preparation is done or before he is placed in the required position. A permit for surgery is usually required. The back of the patient's neck may be shaved, and he is placed on his side at the edge of the bed or on a treatment table, with his head bent forward and held firmly by the nurse or another assistant. The patient is observed immediately following the procedure for dyspnea, apnea, and cyanosis, but these complications seldom occur. A cisternal puncture is often performed on children. In some outpatient departments it is more commonly performed than a lumbar puncture because it is less likely to be followed by headache.

Radioisotope brain scan

Radioactive isotopes are used with a scanner to detect brain lesions. This procedure is particularly successful in the detection of cerebral neoplasia and infarcts. A positive brain scan does not, however,

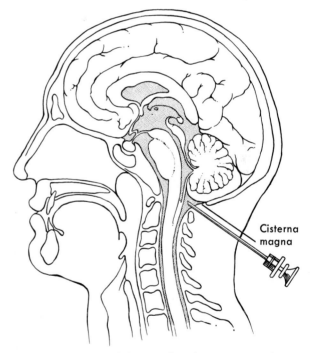

Cisterna magna

FIG. 32-8. Position of the needle when a cisternal puncture is performed. Note the needle length and the short bevel.

provide histologic information about the kind of lesion. In this way a brain scan provides information similar to that provided by other screening procedures such as electroencephalography. It is used adjunctively with neurologic examination and radiologic studies.

It is known that abnormal brain tissue selectively concentrates radioactive isotopes to a greater extent than does the normal brain tissue that is peripheral to a lesion. The procedure for the brain scan is a relatively simple one and consists of no physical preparation other than the intravenous administration of a radioactive isotope indicator such as mercury. This is followed by scanning of the patient's scalp with a special sensing device to pick up the concentrated areas of uptake. Serial scans and the structural features of the isotope uptake may suggest a particular pattern that is indicative of a specific lesion, but this is not reliable for a differential diagnosis. When mercury is used as the isotope indicator, a mercurial diuretic, meralluride (Mercuhydrin), is administered several hours prior to the procedure. This permits a greater concentration of radioactive mercury to be circulated to the brain tissue since meralluride minimizes the uptake of mercury by the kidneys. Areas of concentration show up as very dark areas, as viewed in Fig. 32-9. ^{99m}Technetium pertechenate (^{99m}Tc) is also becoming widely used for brain scans.

Neuroradiologic studies

There are multiple radiologic procedures of the brain and spinal cord that are best carried out and interpreted by a neuroradiologist. These include plain radiographs and special contrast studies of the ventricular system (including the cisternal and subarachnoid space) and cerebral vessels.

Routine or plain radiographs. Routine or plain radiographs of the brain and spinal cord are usually taken first using varied projections to detect any developmental, traumatic, and degenerative bone abnormalities.

Pneumoencephalography.   Pneumoencephalography (air encephalography) is a special contrast study of the ventricular and cisternal systems that permits accurate localization of brain lesions. It is known to provide greater visualization of the posterior fossa than ventriculography. This technically difficult and uncomfortable procedure combines a spinal or a cisternal puncture with an x-ray examination. Air or oxygen, used as a contrast medium, is injected (25 to 30 ml.) and rises to the ventricles, where its presence can be noted on x-ray examination. Abnormal shape, size, or position of the ventricles or failure of the ventricles to fill with the gas is diagnostically significant. (See Fig. 32-10.) The procedure usually is performed under local anesthesia, but a general inhalation, rectal, or intravenous anesthetic may be used for nervous or unstable patients. Headache is usually severe during and following encephalography. Nausea and vomiting are not uncommon. A nurse must be in constant attendance to observe the patient while a second person assists the physician.

The patient who is to have a pneumoencephalogram may be prepared as for surgery—no food or fluids by mouth for 6 hours before the procedure, and a sedative the evening before and $^{1}/_{2}$ hour prior to the procedure. A permit must be signed and dentures removed (p. 201).

The procedure may be started in the patient's room or in the treatment room. The patient is then

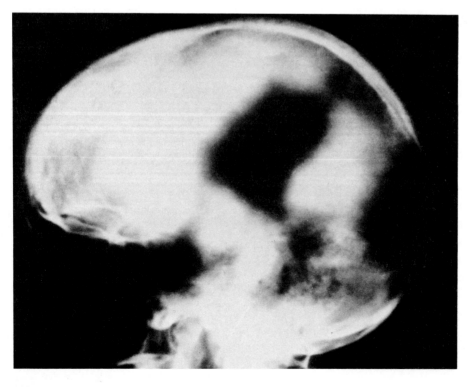

FIG. 32-9. Radioisotope brain scan. An intracranial mass, a brain tumor, is seen in the two dark areas (parietal and occipital) of the scan where an abnormal uptake of ^{197}Hg-tagged chlormerodrin accumulated. (Courtesy Abbas M. Rejali, M.D., Department of Radiology, Case Western Reserve University, Cleveland, Ohio.)

taken to a special room in the x-ray department or operating room. The equipment needed is the same as that for a spinal puncture with the addition of a three-way stopcock, a 20 ml. syringe with which to withdraw spinal fluid and inject air, a calibrated glass to measure any fluid that is removed, and an ampule of caffeine and sodium benzoate and an ampule of epinephrine (Adrenalin) for use in case of respiratory distress. Emergency oxygen equipment is also often requested.

The pressure of the spinal fluid is taken as soon as the needle is inserted into the lumbar spine arachnoid. As the procedure is carried out, the patient is watched carefully for headache, nausea, and vomiting, and his vital signs and color are noted and recorded. The head of the bed or table is gradually

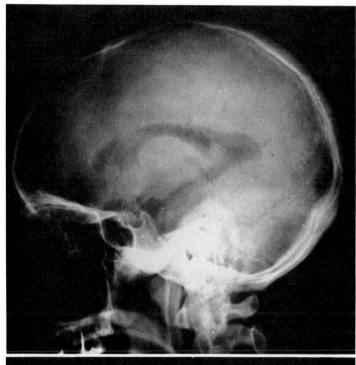

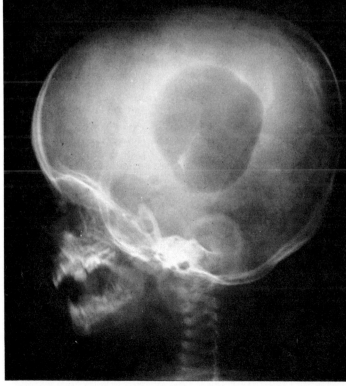

FIG. 32-10. Pneumoencephalogram. **A,** Lateral view showing the outline of a normal ventricle. **B,** Lateral view showing marked distention of the ventricle with cerebrospinal fluid (due to hydrocephalus).

raised, and some physicians like to have the patient's head gently rotated after the air has been injected in the belief that this gives better filling of the lateral ventricles.

On his return from the x-ray department the patient is placed in bed with his head flat. Usually he is more comfortable without a pillow. If a general anesthetic has been administered, he is kept on his side and constantly attended until awake. Vital signs are taken every 15 minutes for the first hour, then every 1/2 hour, and every hour for several hours or until they become stabilized. They are then taken every 4 hours. The level of consciousness is also noted. Any changes should be reported to the physician at once. The patient usually has a severe headache and may benefit from an ice cap applied to the head; he should be given fluids through a straw so that his head is not raised. Acetylsalicylic acid (aspirin), dextropropoxyphene hydrochloride (Darvon), or other nonnarcotic analgesics are given for severe headache. Narcotics may be excluded. If the patient complains of noises in his head, he should be assured that they are temporary, since they are caused by gas in the ventricles and will disappear when the gas is absorbed. If the patient has any history of convulsions or unpredictable behavior, side rails should be placed on the bed and a tongue blade should be at the bedside. Occasionally an emergency tracheotomy set is kept on the unit for 48 hours following this procedure.

Infrequently, reactions to pneumoencephalography are severe and include continued vomiting, convulsions, shock, and signs of increased intracranial pressure with respiratory difficulty. A severe prolonged headache may also follow this diagnostic procedure, although the headache usually disappears in 24 to 48 hours. For the first day or two the patient should be fed and encouraged to be as quiet as possible. He should move about in bed but have assistance in turning from side to side. Usually after 48 hours he can be out of bed gradually. He may find that his headache and nausea increase when he is up, but they will be relieved by lying flat and will gradually subside.

Craniotomy should be performed promptly when a tumor is detected during the procedure to prevent brain stem compression.

Ventriculography. Ventriculography is similar to pneumoencephalography except that air is introduced directly into the lateral ventricles through trephine openings (burr holes) into the skull. This procedure is always performed in the operating room. It may be used when the suspected diagnosis is such that a spinal or lumbar puncture is contraindicated because of the extreme pressure within the skull or because the spinal canal is blocked. The preparation is similar to that for encephalography except that the top or the back of the head must be partially shaved,

depending on the physician's orders. An intravenous or general anesthetic is commonly used, and the patient may go directly from the x-ray department to the operating room for attempted removal of a tumor or for other brain surgery. If the radiograph is normal, the patient is cared for in a manner similar to that following encephalography. Tissue and skin over the burr holes are sutured and the wounds covered with a collodion dressing.

Myelography. In myelography, either gas or a radiopaque liquid is injected into the spinal subarachnoid space via lumbar puncture, and radiographs are taken. It is useful in the identification of lesions in the intradural or extradural compartments of the spinal canal. Observation of the flow of the radiopaque dye fluoroscopically through the subarachnoid space provides valuable information. Lesions in the spinal cord or in the subarachnoid space produce a blocking at some point, as shown in Fig. 32-11.

This procedure is thus similar to that for a spinal puncture except that after the air or the radiopaque substance is injected, the patient's head is elevated on two pillows and he is taken to the x-ray department. After the fluoroscopic examination and radiographs are completed, the dye is removed by lumbar puncture because it can cause serious irritation to the meninges. If some of it remains, care is taken to keep the patient's head elevated, and repeated attempts to remove the dye are made under fluoroscopy. One disadvantage of this test is the irritating quality of the available dyes. Therefore the test is not performed when relatively certain diagnosis can be made by other means, and air is often used in preference to the dye.

Cerebral arteriography. Cerebral arteriography is a method of radiologic visualization of the cerebral arterial system during the injection of radiopaque material. Carotid, vertebral, and brachial arteriography are commonly used. The selection of the puncture site is determined by the clinical problem. For example, a direct left percutaneous brachial injection site is used to visualize the left vertebral artery but not

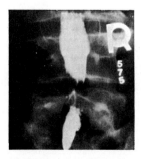

FIG. 32-11. A myelogram showing an almost complete block of the interspace between the fourth and fifth lumbar vertebrae. (From Moseley, H. F., editor: Textbook of surgery, ed. 3, St. Louis, 1959, The C. V. Mosby Co.)

the left carotid artery; if material is injected directly into the left carotid artery, the left anterior circulation can be visualized. Arterial aneurysms, anomalies, or ruptured vessels are often detected. The large blood vessels of the circle of Willis at the base of the brain and the larger vessels penetrating the cerebrum can often be seen by this means (Fig. 32-12). Before the test is performed, a permit is signed by the patient or a responsible relative. Usually a sedative is given the night before, and scopolamine, atropine sulfate and sodium phenobarbital, or meperidine (Demerol) is given ½ hour before the procedure is performed. Occasionally, when the patient is confused or extremely restless, a general anesthetic is given. If this is necessary, the procedure is usually performed in the operating room. If the dye can be injected directly into the carotid vessel without surgical exposure of the artery and if general anesthesia is not necessary, the procedure is usually performed in the x-ray department.

Following the test, the patient is watched for changes in vital signs. Occasionally neurologic deficits result or intensify following this procedure. Decreased hand grip on plantar pressure and facial weakness on the side opposite the injection site are significant. Convulsive seizures or aphasia may occur. Occasionally a delayed allergic reaction to the dye occurs, and this reaction may be serious (p. 94). An ice collar applied to the neck helps to prevent bleeding from the vessel and local edema, which might cause respiratory difficulty because of a carotid artery hematoma. Usually, however, the patient experiences little, if any, discomfort and can resume his usual activities within a few hours.

Electrodiagnostic examination

The electrodiagnostic examinations include electroencephalography and electromyography.

Electroencephalography. An *electroencephalograph* measures the electrical impulses of the brain; the *electroencephalogram* (EEG) is a pictured recording of the electrical activity of the brain amplified many times and recorded in a manner similar to that of the electrocardiogram. Certain characteristic patterns in the record are normal, and by study of the recordings of brain action, areas of abnormal action can sometimes be detected. This test is only an adjunct to other diagnostic tests, but it

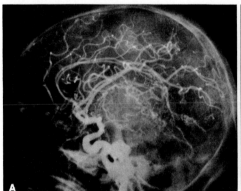
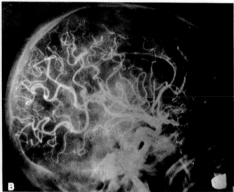

FIG. 32-12. A, Cerebral arteriogram showing elevation of middle cerebral arteries by glioblastoma multiforme containing abnormal vascular network. B, Arteriogram showing the opposite normal side for comparison. (From Moseley, H. F., editor: Textbook of surgery, ed. 3, St. Louis, 1959, The C. V. Mosby Co.)

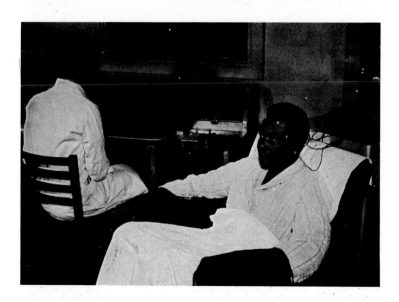

FIG. 32-13. A patient ready to have an electroencephalogram. (From Carini, E., and Owens, G.: Neurological and neurosurgical nursing, ed. 5, St. Louis, 1970, The C. V. Mosby Co.)

may be helpful in locating the site of a lesion. Before the examination the patient should be quiet, and the procedure should be explained to him so that no undue excitement occurs. The scalp should be clean, but no other local preparation is necessary. Approximately 16 tiny electrodes are attached to the scalp with collodion, and the patient should be prepared for this procedure. No hair need be cut, which is often reassuring to the patient. (See Fig. 32-13.) Occasionally the electrodes used are tiny pins that are stuck into the scalp. The patient should know that this procedure will not be painful because there are very few nerve endings in the scalp. The examination is done in a special room where outside electrical activity is eliminated. The patient usually sits in a comfortable chair or lies on a stretcher or table with his eyes closed. The test may last for an hour or more. Recordings may be made during sleep or when deprived of sleep and provide valuable information. Anticonvulsive drugs may be discontinued in the patients with known convulsive disorders prior to the EEG. In general, the EEG is used to provide evidences of focal or diffuse disturbances of increased brain function produced by organic lesions.

Electromyography. The *electromyograph* measures the electrical activity of muscles; the *electromyogram* (EMG) is a recording of the variations of electric potentials (voltage) detected by a needle electrode inserted into skeletal muscle. The electrical activity can be heard over a loud speaker and viewed on an oscilloscope and on a graph at the same time. No electrical activity can be detected in normal muscles at rest, but during volitional movement, action potentials can be detected. However, in motor disease, electrical activity of various types and abnormal patterns appear in resting muscles. An EMG provides direct evidence of motor dysfunction and can be used to some extent to detect a dysfunction located in the motor neuron, the neuromuscular junction, or muscle fibers. Thus it is particularly helpful in the diagnosis of lower motor neuron disease, primary muscle disease, and defects in the transmission of electrical impulses at the neuromuscular junction such as in myasthenia gravis. There is no special preparation for this procedure. The patient may be fearful that electrode needles will electrocute him and should be assured that there is no danger.

Echoencephalography

Echoencephalography is a rapid and simple diagnostic procedure that has become popular. Information provided is supplementary to an EEG and complementary to radiologic studies as to the nature and location of brain lesions.

Ultrasonic pulses (capable of reflection or refraction at cerebrospinal fluid and brain tissue surfaces) are delivered to the head in such a way that the beam intersects the site under study at a perpendicular angle, traverses the area, and is then reflected back. The returning echoes are then converted back to electrical impulses and recorded on a screen. For example, when a transducer is placed on the right temporal bone and directed toward the opposite temporal bone, the sound beams traverses the third ventricle area (which has two parallel walls) and is reflected back. This procedure provides a right, left, and lower trace, or picture, that gives reliable information as to position of the midline of the brain. Shifts from the midline, as caused by right or left hemispheric brain masses, can be inferred. Estimation of ventricular size can also be made from the traces.

Neurologic diseases

Diseases selected for inclusion in this section are classified both from a broad pathologic standpoint and from the standpoint of the anatomic site or localization of the causative neural lesion. The latter classification is viewed as more relevant in planning nursing care. The preceding discussion of upper and lower motor neuron lesions (p. 862) is particularly relevant to classification of diseases and should be reviewed by the reader at this point. Diseases associated with disturbances in motor function are classified in Fig. 32-14 relative to upper and lower motor neuron structures. A discussion of specific medical treatment, surgery, and nursing intervention accompanies each major disease classification. Manifestations that are common to neurologic disease such as headache, convulsive seizures, pain, and increased intracranial pressure are discussed first. Autonomic dysfunctions are not discussed per se.

■ COMMON NEUROLOGIC MANIFESTATIONS
Headache

The complaint of headache is one of the most common manifestations in both neurology and general medical practice. Headache is not a disease but a symptom of disease or of bodily reaction to harmful substances such as drugs or to excessive psychic pressure. The conditions that cause headache are almost infinite in number. Headache may be caused by systemic disease or infection, by hypertension, or

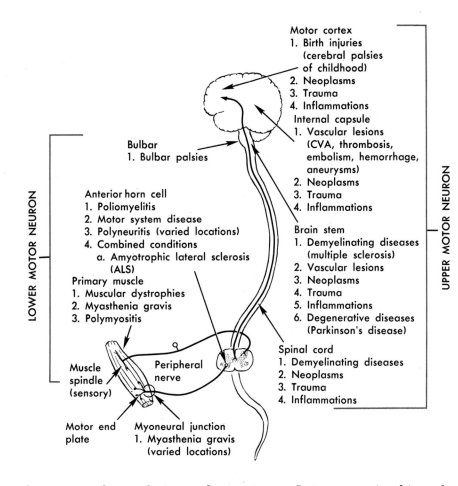

Motor cortex
1. Birth injuries (cerebral palsies of childhood)
2. Neoplasms
3. Trauma
4. Inflammations

Internal capsule
1. Vascular lesions (CVA, thrombosis, embolism, hemorrhage, aneurysms)
2. Neoplasms
3. Trauma
4. Inflammations

Brain stem
1. Demyelinating diseases (multiple sclerosis)
2. Vascular lesions
3. Neoplasms
4. Trauma
5. Inflammations
6. Degenerative diseases (Parkinson's disease)

Spinal cord
1. Demyelinating diseases
2. Neoplasms
3. Trauma
4. Inflammations

Bulbar
1. Bulbar palsies

Anterior horn cell
1. Poliomyelitis
2. Motor system disease
3. Polyneuritis (varied locations)
4. Combined conditions
   a. Amyotrophic lateral sclerosis (ALS)

Primary muscle
1. Muscular dystrophies
2. Myasthenia gravis
3. Polymyositis

Muscle spindle (sensory)

Peripheral nerve

Motor end plate

Myoneural junction
1. Myasthenia gravis (varied locations)

LOWER MOTOR NEURON

UPPER MOTOR NEURON

FIG. 32-14. Disturbances in motor function are classified pathologically along the upper and lower motor neuron structures illustrated. It should be noted that the same pathologic condition occurs at more than one site in the upper motor neuron shown on the right. A few pathologic conditions involve both upper and lower motor neuron structures, as in amyotrophic lateral sclerosis, for example. Other lesion sites include the myoneural junction and primary muscle, making it possible to classify the conditions as neuromuscular and muscular, respectively. (Modified from Chusid, J. G.: Correlative neuroanatomy and functional neurology, ed. 15, Los Altos, Calif., 1970, Lange Medical Publications.)

by pressure from a lesion such as a tumor. It may be caused by drugs, by foreign substances to which the person is hypersensitive, by anoxia, or by the inhalation of poisonous gases. In addition, headache may be caused by congestion in the sinuses, contraction of scalp and neck muscles due to fatigue and tension, and eyestrain. Headache often occurs either before or during the menstrual period.

The nature of headaches varies depending on the cause. For example, frontal headache may be caused by sinusitis and is characteristically relieved if the patient sits up and if local heat is applied to the face overlying the sinuses. Brain tumors often cause a dull, constant headache that increases in severity over time. Headaches caused by emotional tension are usually steady and bandlike. They commonly precede or follow periods of tension and become worse as the day progresses.

Headaches are probably treated by the laity more often than any other condition, including the common cold. However, the public should know that persistent headaches are abnormal and need investigation by a physician. Patients have been known to treat a headache for months in the belief that it was due to a sinus infection, only to learn finally that it was caused by hypertension or a brain tumor. Persistent headaches, even when a physical cause has been ruled out, indicate that the patient should re-

view his mode of living and make some adjustments. The nurse can sometimes help him see the wisdom of this course. She can also advise against the widespread use of the coal-tar analgesics in treatment of headaches. Occasional use of acetylsalicylic acid by the laity for minor indispositions is considered safe by most medical authorities. The use of phenacetin and similar coal-tar preparations is not advisable unless prescribed by a physician. Prolonged and excessive use of these preparations has caused gastric bleeding (from a decreased prothrombin level) and agranulocytosis in some individuals.

Patients with headaches seen by the neurologist include those with vascular headaches of the migraine type, hemiplegic headache, and the cluster headache.

Migraine syndrome. The layman's term for migraine headache is "sick headache." This condition is now believed to be much more common than was previously supposed. Before the acute onset there may be fatigue, chilliness, and irritability. These symptoms occasionally precede the acute attack by as much as a day or more. The acute symptoms are severe but vary in intensity, frequency, and duration. Broadly defined, migraine is a recurring vascular headache. Usually the headache is present on awakening in the morning, and one side of the head is more affected than the other. Pain is usually keenest in the temporal area but may be anywhere in the head, and sometimes the face is also affected. There may be spots before the eyes, partial blindness, dizziness, nausea, and vomiting. The pain is often so intense that the patient is forced to seek isolation in a dark room. The acute attack usually lasts from a few hours to a day, but occasionally may last for a week or even longer. It concludes with a feeling of relaxation and need for sleep. Dull head and neck pain, probably due to tension during the attack, may persist for some time.

The precipitating cause of migraine headache is a constriction and then dilation of cerebral arteries. The initiating cause of this is unknown, but it has been repeatedly demonstrated that nervous tension contributes to the attacks. The person who develops migraine headaches is usually one who works hard and strives for perfection. Migraine headaches often follow a period of overwork and increased stress. After an attack the patient feels better, probably because he has been forced to rest. Hope for a cure of this condition lies in changing the patient's attitudes toward the world and himself, and usually this is not easy.

Specific treatment of migraine includes drugs and psychotherapy. Acetysalicylic acid is seldom effective for classic or common migraine. Ergotamine tartrate is one drug that has been effective. Beneficial effects are probably related to vasoconstrictor action on smooth muscles of the cranial blood vessels. For best results, ergotamine tartrate should be taken early, before the headache is full-blown. The usual dosage is 2 mg. ($\frac{1}{30}$ grain) orally or 0.25 mg. ($\frac{1}{250}$ grain) subcutaneously or intramuscularly. Occasionally it may be administered intravenously for quicker action or in combination with other drugs so that a larger dosage may be tolerated. The disadvantages of this drug are that it can cause nausea and vomiting, tingling sensations, and muscle tightness. Dihydroergotamine is a preparation that is also used since it causes fewer toxic reactions. It may be administered by any parenteral route. Interval treatment between attacks includes efforts to reduce the frequency and severity of the headaches.[105]

Cluster headache. Cluster headache is another type of vascular headache referred to the neurologist. It is abrupt in onset and usually unilateral. It is associated with flushing, sweating, increased lacrimation, and rhinorrhea. Pain episodes are clustered or spaced closely together and there are long remissions.[7]

Convulsive seizures

Convulsions as a sign and symptom are of particular significance in neurologic disease. They occur in many childhood and adult illnesses. Convulsions result from cerebral anoxemia, hypoglycemia, disturbances of calcium balance, electrolyte imbal-

ances, excessive hydration, the ingestion of drugs and poisons with convulsive activity, infections that produce high temperature elevations, and numerous metabolic disorders. In the majority of individuals with convulsions a *localized* organic lesion in the central nervous system serves as the focus for the abnormal neuronal discharges from the damaged brain tissues, such as neoplasms, inflamed areas or abscess, vascular formations or hematoma, congenital formations, trauma, or other space-occupying lesions. Quite often the lesion is microscopic in size and is related to the trauma of birth or scars from infantile and/or childhood infections. Convulsions may also be caused by *generalized* inflammatory and degenerative brain diseases. Convulsions may also be hysterical in origin but are not considered true seizure disorders. Convulsions are seen most frequently in association with epilepsy, which may be considered a disease *sui generis.* Epilepsy, however, is also only a symptom and not a diagnosis.

The word convulsion is frequently used interchangeably with the words "seizure," "attack," and "fits." A convulsion by definition refers to violent or abrupt involuntary contraction of muscles. The word "seizure" connotes the abruptness or spasmlike character of the event or the attack. In this sense, *seizure* and *attack* relate to the whole event. Attack is the best term to use in conversation with the laity; the term "fits" has unpleasant connotations. The terms "seizure" and "convulsions" each label the condition correctly and professionally.

Pathophysiology. Convulsions or seizures are brief and stereotyped "cerebral storms." They result from episodic, excessive, simultaneous, and disorderly ganglionic discharges. The patterns or forms of seizures vary and are dependent on the area of the brain from which the seizure arises. The pattern is stereotyped in the individual, although variations may occur with progression of the cerebral lesion. Seizures can involve essentially all parts of the brain at once or only a minute focal spot. The excessive neuronal discharges are thought to originate in the brain stem portion of the reticular activating system; these then spread throughout the central nervous system, including the cortex and the deeper parts of the brain. This process may last from a few seconds to as long as 3 to 5 minutes; the process may stop immediately as in petit mal. It is not known what stops the seizure at a given time, but it is believed to result from fatigue of the neurons involved in precipitating the seizure and/or inhibition by certain structures within the brain. The excessive neuronal discharges result in *tonic convulsions* with the contraction of all muscles at once or in *clonic convulsions* with alternate contraction and relaxation of opposing muscle groups with characteristic jerking movements of the body. The seizure, regardless of type, is always inappropriate to the immediate situation. The seizure is followed by an inhibition of cerebral function. This period may last longer than the seizure itself. The inhibition of function is often incomplete and is dependent on the area of the brain from which the seizure arises.

Epilepsy. Epilepsy is one of the oldest diseases known to man. It was described in detail by Hippocrates. The term "epilepsy" means seizure or "state." The disease was at one time thought to be of a divine origin and perhaps for this reason has been linked in the public mind with the occult, the strange, and the unmentionable. No disease has been more carefully concealed within families, and many attitudes toward the disease have persisted from early times to the present day. Attitudes may also be affected by the frightening experience of having seen a person during a severe seizure, by the belief that mental deterioration always occurs in epilepsy, and by the fact that the tendency to develop epilepsy may be inherited.

Because of the emotional overtones associated with convulsive disorders, it is often exceedingly difficult for parents to believe that their child might have such a condition. Sometimes they give an inadequate report to their family physician and receive the desired assurance that the child will probably outgrow the disorder. Many children would be spared severely traumatizing experiences at school and elsewhere if parents could only be convinced that the advice of a specialist is needed.

Epilepsy, often called idiopathic epilepsy, is a disease of unknown cause. The disease is not directly inherited, although abnormal brain waves, as shown in the EEG, are found in many relatives of persons having seizures, and it is likely that a predisposition to the disease is inherited. It is believed that some alteration of chemical balance touches off the seizure in susceptible persons. There are no accurate figures available, but it is believed that there are over three fourths of a million persons in the United States who have epilepsy.[70] Epilepsy is largely a disease of younger people; approximately three fourths of the sufferers have seizures before the age of 20 years. The life expectancy of persons with epilepsy is less than for the population as a whole, primarily because the person often dies of an accident incurred during a seizure.

Types of seizures. There are several types of epileptic seizures, including grand mal, petit mal, focal, psychomotor, and combined forms. Seizures are either centrencephalic (generalized) or focal in origin. "Status epilepticus" is the term used when the patient goes from one seizure to another without regaining consciousness; in this sense it is not a distinct type. Each major seizure type is discussed briefly.

The *grand mal seizure* (big sickness) is by far the most common type. It is the most dramatic type and is often the final common event in convulsive disorders. Grand mal is generalized and is characterized by a loss of consciousness for several minutes (variable) and with tonic and clonic convulsions (or motor activity). The clinical sequence is the aura, cry, loss of consciousness, the fall, tonic and clonic convulsions, and incontinence. The symptoms that occur during the prodrome are called an *aura*. Prodromal symptoms occur in about 50% of all patients and usually include a change in sensation or a change in affect. There may be numbness, flashing lights, dizziness, tingling of the arm, smells, or spots before the eyes. The patient may find it difficult to describe the aura precisely, but it gives conclusive warning of an impending seizure. The specific warning serves a useful purpose in that it enables the individual to seek safety and privacy before the onset of the seizure. Occasionally it occurs as much as a day before the seizure so that the individual who works can remain at home and fellow workers may not know of the attacks. Grand mal is heralded by a sharp cry as air is rapidly inhaled. Following this there is a loss of consciousness, which is variable in duration (usually in minutes rather than in seconds). The individual then slumps or falls, depending on his position at the time. This is followed by a tonic contraction of all muscles; the legs are extended and the arms are flexed; jaws are clenched and the tongue is frequently caught between the teeth. The eyes roll upward and the pupils dilate and become fixed. There is cessation of respiration and cyanosis occurs. As the tonic phase stops, it is replaced by a series of clonic contractions with the characteristic jerking movements. Breathing returns and it is shallow and irregular at first. There is often frothing at the mouth and it may be streaked with blood if the tongue and lips have been bitten during the convulsion. There is often fecal and/or urinary incontinence during the clonic phase or earlier. As the clonic phase subsides in a few minutes, there is relaxation of muscles. Partial consciousness is regained and color improves. During the *postictal period* the individual appears groggy and confused. He often complains of headache or muscular pain and usually falls into a deep sleep. During this phase the pupils may remain dilated, and there may be abnormal plantar reflexes. After a variable period of time, the patient awakens and is frequently unaware of the seizure. A dull headache and depression may persist. It is possible that the latter is caused in part by the knowledge that a seizure has occurred. Seizures may occur during sleep in some individuals. In such instances the occurrence of the seizure is known on awakening by the presence of blood on the pillow or the soiled bed from fecal or urinary incontinence.

Petit mal seizure (little sickness) is characterized by an abrupt loss of consciousness that occurs without warning. This loss of consciousness, with arrest of all voluntary activity, is very brief, usually about 10 to 20 seconds. In the classic petit mal seizure there is a sudden vacant facial expression, a stopping of all motor activity except perhaps a slight symmetric twitching of the face and arms, or a loss of muscle tone. Consciousness returns as quickly as it left, and the individual may resume speaking at the point interrupted, unaware that the seizure occurred. The individual may learn to recognize when he has lost a few seconds of time. Petit mal seizures usually occur many times a day and are not accompanied by an aura, falling, or tonic and clonic convulsive phases. In some instances the loss of consciousness may be accompanied by an exaggerated loss of muscle tone so that the patient falls; this is termed *akinetic. Myoclonus* may also occasionally be found in some petit mal seizures with the characteristic sudden, involuntary, jerking contractures of the neck or extremity muscles. Petit mal seizures occur most frequently in children and adolescents, particularly at the time of puberty. Although they do not represent the dramatic and frightening aspects of the grand mal seizure, they are disconcerting to the individual of any age group. Also, since this type of seizure is not preceded by an aura, the momentary loss of consciousness presents problems relative to safety.

Focal motor and/or *sensory seizures* are those that arise initially in the motor and/or sensory areas of the brain adjacent to the rolandic fissure. The clinical manifestations seen in this type of seizure are thus dependent on the site of the focus and differ from the generalized motor seizure (grand mal). If, for example, the abnormal neuronal discharge is initiated in the precentral or motor region of the cortex for the thumb, the individual would experience a tonic contracture of the thumb muscles. If the abnormal neuronal discharge spreads to adjacent parts of the motor strip, there is a progressive involvement of associated musculature with a *march* of movements from thumb to hand, arm, face, etc. The discharge may or may not march. The localized seizure that does march or spread progressively to other muscles following initiation is known as a *jacksonian seizure.* Focal motor seizures commonly begin in the hand, face, and foot but may arise in any part of the motor strip. The seizure may end in a shower of clonic movements, or it may end in a generalized convulsion. When abnormal neuronal discharges arise in the lower part of the motor strip that controls salivation and mastication, seizures are then manifest by chewing, smacking of the lips, and swallowing movements; salivation may be profuse. Other seizures may begin with a forced turning of the head and eyes. Such attacks are termed *aversive* and originate in the eye-turning fields of the brain; the head turns away from the side of the lesion or focus. When the abnormal neuronal discharges, on the other hand, arise in the postcentral or sensory strip of the cortex, the seizure is initiated with complaints of disturbed sensations such as a numbness, tingling, prickling, or crawling feelings. Similar to focal motor seizure, a march of sensations may or may not occur. The neuronal discharge may spread from the sensory area to the motor area.

Psychomotor seizures, variously known as psychic equivalents and automatisms, are characterized by the performance of automatic activities, impairment of consciousness, and psychic symptoms. No apparent convulsions occur. Consciousness may be lost or amnesia occurs. During the attack the individual may appear drowsy, intoxicated, violent, behave abnormally, and engage in antisocial activity. He may continue to carry on activities at an automatic level such as driving a car, typing, eating, and going to the bathroom. The individual is unable to make decisions and is not open to reason during the attack. No concern is given to the usual social amenities. States of furor may occur during attacks, and crimes have been committed. For this reason the diagnosis of this type of seizure is of interest to lawyers and judges as well as physicians. Psychic symptoms may occur with visual and auditory illusions and hallucinations, a sense of unreality, and déjà vu (a sense that a new experience has occurred in all details some time before). Psychomotor seizures may, in addition, include visceral symptoms with autonomic complaints such as chest pain, respiratory arrest, tachycardia, urinary incontinence, gastrointestinal discomforts, and blanching. There may be abnormal sensations of taste and smell (uncinate). This type of seizure is often associated with the temporal lobe.

Medical treatment. The treatment of patients with convulsive seizures should be based on a careful study of the patient to detect any remedial lesion or metabolic cause. When these have been eliminated or treated, care is then directed toward the prevention of seizures. It should be pointed out that only rarely will the elimination of causative factors result in the complete disappearance of seizures. Some authorities believe that the only prevention of epilepsy per se is genetic counseling, since the predisposition to develop the disease appears to be inherited. There is no known cure for idiopathic epilepsy, although seizures can be controlled by anticonvulsive drugs and the regulation of mental and physical hygiene. The period of treatment is years, or a lifetime, for the majority of patients.

From the standpoint of mental hygiene, the individual with convulsive seizures should use all resources to overcome feelings of self-consciousness and inferiority resulting from attacks. Adults should be assisted in obtaining productive work that helps to occupy their time and provides remuneration. Children should be kept in school unless the frequency of attacks disturbs the activities of the classroom and unless mental deficiency requires special facilities. In some instances a continuing schedule of psychotherapy is of benefit. Family members need to be educated in regard to their attitudes toward the individual's illness. Excessive attention and overprotection is to be avoided. The family should understand the problems of convulsive seizures and the prescribed therapy but should not make a chronic invalid of the patient. Commitment to an institution is not preferred unless mental deterioration or violent, intractable attacks make it necessary. Destructive or psychotic individuals, on the other hand, should not remain at home if it negatively affects the lives of other family members.

The physical activity of the person under treatment for convulsive seizures should be regulated so that eating, sleeping, and exercise schedules are at about the same time daily. Exercises should be moderate and should not include competitive sports that are exhausting. Diet should be simple and wholesome with adequate carbohydrate and proteins; alcohol should be avoided. Bowels should be regulated by training, diet, and the judicious use of mild laxatives. The patient should have a regular time for sleep and arising and should not be allowed to stay in bed excessively. Swimming, horseback riding, and other dangerous sports are allowed with the proper safeguards. Activities that endanger the lives of others such as driving dangerous machinery and cars should be prohibited when seizures are *not* under control (despite treatment). Success in prevention of seizures in persons under treatment is to a great extent dependent on the skill of the neurologist in selecting the type of anticonvulsant drug to be used and the regulation of dosage. The choice of medications to be used depends on the type of seizure suffered by the individual. The patient and family must understand the importance of taking the prescribed drugs on schedule and in correct dosage. Anticonvulsant drugs act generally on the cerebral cortex and are not selective in acting on the part of the brain involved in abnormal neuronal discharges.

There are currently many drugs that can be used to prevent the occurrence of grand mal and petit mal seizures and to a lesser extent psychomotor seizures in a high percentage of individuals. Selected commonly used drugs as related to seizure types are listed in Table 32-3 along with the average daily dose and toxic effects. Drugs may be used singly or in combinations, relative to the response of the patient. Highly refractory cases may require several drugs in full therapeutic dosages. Diphenylhydantoin (Dilantin) has the highest therapeutic index and is the drug of choice for grand mal seizures. When the pa-

Table 32-3 Anticonvulsants used to prevent seizures

Drug	Use related to seizure type	Average daily dose	Toxic effects
Diphenylhydantoin (Dilantin)	Grand mal, focal, psychomotor	0.4-0.6 Gm. (divided dose)	Ataxia, vomiting, nystagmus, drowsiness, rash, fever, gum hypertrophy, lymphadenopathy
Phenobarbital (Luminal)	Grand mal, focal, psychomotor (adjunctive)	0.1-0.4 Gm. (divided dose)	Drowsiness, rash
Primidone (Mysoline)	Grand mal, focal, psychomotor	0.5-2.0 Gm.	Drowsiness, ataxia
Mephenytoin (Mesantoin)	Grand mal, focal, psychomotor	0.3-0.5 Gm.	Ataxia, nystagmus, pancytopenia, rash
Ethosuximide (Zarontin)	Petit mal, psychomotor, myoclonic, akinetic	750-1,500 mg.	Drowsiness, nausea, agranulocytosis
Trimethadione (Tridione)	Petit mal	0.3-2.0 Gm. (divided dose)	Rash, photophobia, agranulocytosis, nephrosis
Diazepam (Valium)	Status epilepticus, mixed	8-30 mg.	Drowsiness, ataxia
Carbamazepine (Tegretol)	Grand mal, psychomotor	0.3-2.0 Gm.	Rash, drowsiness, ataxia

tient fails to respond to diphenylhydantoin alone, either phenobarbital, primidone (Mysoline), or related drugs may be added; in refractory individuals all three drugs may be utilized. The same three drugs are also often used in combination in psychomotor seizures, but the seizures are not so readily controlled as in grand mal. Carbamazepine (Tegretol) appears to hold some promise in controlling psychomotor seizures. Ethosuximide (Zarontin) and trimethadione (Tridione) are the drugs of choice in petit mal seizures. The dosages of anticonvulsant drugs are difficult to establish and regulate due to the high incidence of side effects and the toxicity of the drugs. The drug of choice is introduced in average therapeutic dosage and is increased in dosage until control is reached; if toxicity is reached before control of the seizures, the dosage is decreased to the previous nontoxic or tolerated dosage. Additional secondary drugs are usually introduced at this point and increased similarly until control is obtained. It is important that convenient dosage schedules are established for the individual; dosage may be staggered, with a smaller dose given during the day and a larger dose during the evening.

Corticosteroids are used occasionally in myoclonus. Bromides are used less frequently than in the past and have been replaced to a great extent by the above-mentioned anticonvulsant drugs. The ketogenic diet is prescribed infrequently for patients with petit mal. The difficulty in administration of this diet and the effectiveness of ethosuximide has led to decline in its use.

Failure of the patient to take the prescribed drugs and inadequate dosages are frequent causes of failure in treatment. Some medical centers have facilities to determine the blood level of drugs, which provide an accurate check on the therapeutic and toxic levels of the drugs as taken by the patient. Unfortunately most drugs that are helpful in controlling seizures produce toxic effects. It should be recognized that effects on the kidneys and bone marrow can be serious. The individual must remain under medical supervision in order to regulate the drugs and to make changes when toxicity occurs. Patients with convulsive seizures often engage in wishful thinking once control is reached and believe that they have outgrown their disease. They often think that they can get by without taking the drug since they have gone for some time without a seizure.

Nursing intervention. The nurse has responsibilities regarding the diagnostic, therapeutic, and instructional programs of patients with known seizures. The community health nurse and the clinic nurse will need to follow selected patients with seizures for extended periods. The patient and family need to learn what to do during a seizure, to assume responsibility for drug therapy, and seek assistance when toxic or side effects occur.

The primary responsibility of the nurse during the time the patient is having a seizure is to protect him from injury to self and to observe and record the characteristics of the seizure. (The discussion here is related more to a generalized motor seizure.) If the patient is in an upright position, he should be lowered to the floor or bed and adjacent articles and equipment moved away in order to prevent injury during uncontrolled body movements. Constricting clothing should be loosened, especially around the neck area. The head should be supported and turned to the side to allow the tongue to fall forward so that it does not occlude the airway. No effort, however, should be made to restrain the patient either manually or by commercial restraints. Attempting to resist body movements of a patient as in grand mal seizure may result in injury to bones and soft tissues. It is best to permit the patient as much range of motion as possible without injury to himself. Padded side rails are helpful for the patient confined to bed and for the individual who has a pattern of seizures during sleep. Pillows should not be used for padding since there is some danger of suffocation. If the jaws are *not* already clenched at the time when first observed, a padded tongue blade or rubber wedge should be inserted between the back teeth in order to prevent injury to the tongue and mouth tissues. At the same time care must be taken to avoid pushing the tongue back and thus occluding the airway. In many instances the jaws and teeth are already clenched and efforts to insert a tongue blade or any nearby substitute may damage the teeth and gums. The idea that one should pry the mouth open and insert a tongue blade or anything has probably been overemphasized. One needs to make a judgment as to whether it is better to insert something or not relative to the phase of the seizure and the actual condition of the patient. It is the policy of many hospital nursing services that a padded tongue blade be kept at the patient's bedside when seizures are anticipated. It seems best to place it in the drawer of the bedside cabinet rather than taped conspicuously to the bed. A single oral airway may also be kept at the bedside along with other emergency equipment, depending on the severity of seizures and condition of the patient.

Accurate observation of the seizure should be made from the beginning when possible, since it provides needed information that may assist the physician in locating the site of a cerebral lesion or focus. Taking time to fully record the observations made is equally important. It is more important that the nurse fully describe the seizure than to name or classify the seizure. There is a tendency for nurses and others to forget the variations of seizure types and to relate more to the grand mal seizure. Important observations to be made and recorded for any seizure type include the following:

Aura	Presence or absence; nature, if present; ability of patient to describe it (somatic, visceral, psychic)
Cry	Presence or absence
Onset	Site of initial body movements; deviation of head and eyes; chewing and salivation; posture of body; sensory changes
Tonic and clonic phases	Movements of body as to progression; skin color and airway; pupillary changes; incontinence; duration of each phase
Relaxation (sleep)	Duration and behavior
Postictal period	Duration; general behavior; ability to remember anything about the seizure; orientation; pupillary changes; headache; injuries present
Duration of entire seizure	
Level of consciousness	Length of unconsciousness if present

When a patient with known seizure activity is admitted to the hospital, it is important for the nurse to obtain a history of the pattern of seizure activity as to frequency, time of day, whether aura is present or not, any precipitating factors, and any seizure characteristics. In this way nursing actions can be planned more specifically. Admission of a patient with known seizures and under treatment provides the nurse an opportunity to test the patient's understanding of his condition and prescribed therapy. The nurse should follow through on the reason for admission and ascertain if it has relevance to further nursing follow-up.

Management of the patient with status epilepticus. Because of the emergent nature of this condition, it warrants separate discussion in a nursing text. Status epilepticus may be defined as a recurrent generalized seizure activity occurring at such frequency that full consciousness is not regained between seizures; it is prolonged beyond 15 to 20 minutes. Although relatively rare, it can lead to death from exhaustion. It demands emergency medical and nursing care measures.

The patient with status epilepticus is often in a coma for a period of 12 to 24 hours or longer, during which there are recurring seizures. The seizures may cease spontaneously and consciousness returns, or death may result from the repeated attacks. Vigorous therapy is thus directed toward arrest of the seizures. Effort is directed first toward assuring an adequate airway as related to seizure effects on the airway and possible drug complications. Endotracheal tubes, laryngoscope, aspirating equipment, and oxygen should be in the patient unit prior to administration of drugs. This is important, since the large drug dosages and the type of drugs used often lead to pulmonary complications. Drug therapy is via the intravenous route. Medications commonly used include sodium phenobarbital, diazepam, and paraldehyde. Results appear to be best from large or full therapeutic dosage (not divided). Administration is stopped in the event of respiratory depression or if the seizure terminates. At times it may be necessary to give general anesthesia. Oxygen may be used to counter the effects of cerebral hypoxia. Solutions of glucose may be ordered to assist in dehydration and increase the concentration of the prescribed drugs.

The nurse has the responsibility of assisting with the administration of drugs through careful observation and regulation of intravenous flow rate of the prescribed drugs. Constant monitoring of vital signs for respiratory depression and cardiac changes is necessary in response to the drugs and the continuing seizures. The responsibilities pertaining to the observation and recording of seizure activity are the same as those discussed previously (p. 878). It may not be possible to note the separate seizure phases because of the frequency of the attacks. A safe environment must be provided by the nurse, since the patient cannot protect himself. It is also important to provide a quiet and nonstimulating environment. The head of the bed should be lowered, and the patient turned in a side-lying position to lessen the danger of aspiration during seizures; side rails should be padded.

Home care. Members of the family must learn to care for the person during and following a convulsion. They should have a mouth gag on hand at all times and should know how to insert it correctly, and they should be alert for accident hazards. One of the most important things for the family to learn is the need to be calm and accepting in regard to the patient's seizures. They should attempt to keep him from engaging in activity that may be dangerous and from exposure to curious persons during convulsions, but they should not contribute to the patient's feeling that he is different from others. More widespread general knowledge about the disease would help to prevent friends and neighbors from adding to the problems the patient and his family already have.

Public attitudes. One of the most important aspects in epilepsy is changing the public's attitude toward the disease. The patient and the public must be made to look on convulsive seizures not as bizarre catastrophes but as relatively normal events that should be dealt with rationally. Many persons with epilepsy lead normal, productive lives. Indeed, many outstanding figures in world history had seizures, including Julius Caesar, Lord Byron, and Napoleon Bonaparte. Studies do not bear out the popular assumption that there usually is mental deterioration with epilepsy. Nor is there any evidence that personality changes are the result of pathologic progress; they are probably the result of society's attitude toward the person with epilepsy. For example, some people who are found to have epilepsy are automatically and immediately suspended from their work, even when it is such that they are not dangerous to themselves or others. Some employers refuse to hire a person with known epilepsy, and yet at least 80% of all persons with epilepsy are employable. The patient is haunted by fear of being seen during a seizure, fear of being found to have seizures, fear of losing his job, and fear of losing the companionship of others. Children with epilepsy have been segregated in separate schools, and only recently have some major cities passed laws ensuring children with epilepsy the right to attend public schools if they are under adequate medical care. In many schools, children are barred from the classroom according to the inclination of the teacher. Limitation of environment and educational opportunity often limits the patient's knowledge, but this does not mean that his learning capacity is poor.

Interest in epilepsy and in the problems of the epileptic person has been increased by various organizations such as the National Association to Control Epilepsy, Inc.,* and the National Epilepsy League, Inc.† Membership in these organizations is open to health personnel, to persons with epilepsy, and to other interested citizens. The nurse should encourage concerned citizens to support these organizations.

Pain

Types of neurologic pain. Pain, other than headache, is one of the most common neurologic symptoms. It is difficult to distinguish between pain produced by lesions within the nervous system that cause objective sensory abnormality and peripherally produced pain as in incurable cancer. Neurologic pain may arise from lesions involving the peripheral cutaneous nerves, the sensory nerve roots (posterior), the thalamus, and the central sensory pain tracts. As in other types of pain, the quality of the pain and its distribution are important for the nurse to assess.

The quality of neurologic pain and/or *paresthesia* may vary from mild to excruciating pain. The sensation of pain may be increased *(hyperalgesia)*, decreased *(hypalgesia)*, or blocked *(analgesia)*. The nurse may find that it is difficult for the patient to describe his pain accurately. It is perceived variously as "burning," "pins and needles," or "numbness." The constancy of the sensation makes it difficult for the patient to bear.

Peripheral cutaneous nerves are particularly vulnerable to trauma and vascular effects. The pain resulting from peripheral nerve lesions is usually limited to the anatomic area supplied by the affected nerve. Thus the location or distribution of the pain sensation may be compared with charts showing the distribution of peripheral sensory fibers. For example, a lesion involving the lateral cutaneous nerve of the thigh produces pain limited to the area of the skin supplied by this nerve. Pain of this type is often described as a burning or sharp sensation.

Root pain or radicular pain, on the other hand, is limited to the dermatomes supplied by the affected sensory nerve root. (Refer to Fig. 32-2 for distributions.) However, pain from lesions arising from deep somatic and visceral structures may radiate beyond the dermatome. The nurse should understand that radicular pain is often aggravated by anything that causes direct or indirect movement of the spinal cord. Such actions as sneezing, coughing, or straining increase intrathoracic and intra-abdominal pressure and indirectly produce distention of veins in the epidural space, thus affecting the dura that surrounds the nerve roots. It should be recalled that the sensory nerve roots are fixed directly to the spinal cord. Lesions may extend to the motor roots and, in addition, produce motor symptoms and signs. From a nursing standpoint, the patient with root pain should not lie in a horizontal position for long periods. This causes a tensing or traction on the thoracic lumbar and sacral nerve roots. Sitting up may help to relieve this tension on the nerve roots. In moving a patient with root pain, sharp flexion of the neck and leg extension should be avoided, since this intensifies the pain by causing more direct movement of the meninges and roots.

Pain resulting from central lesions within the thalamus is confined to the contralateral side of the body. It should be recalled that the thalamus is concerned with sensory impulses from the opposite side of the body. In massive thalamic lesions the entire contralateral half of the body may be involved; in a less extensive thalamic lesion, contiguous portions of the body may be affected. This type of pain is described by patients as burning, pulling, and swelling. It is often aggravated by emotional stress and fatigue. It is influenced by cutaneous stimulation, and the nurse may find it difficult to care for the patient both physically and emotionally. It is most important that nurses understand the physiologic basis of the discomfort and why the patient has persistent complaints.

Lesions involving the central spinothalamic tract produce pain sensation distributed to the level of the tract involved. Crossed axons of the pain tract ascend the spinal cord in the lateral column within one or two segments of the level of entry. Hemisection of the spinal cord involving the spinothalamic tract thus produces loss of pain and temperature perception on the contralateral side at a level one or two segments below the injury. Tract pain is similar to

---

*22 East 67th St., New York, N. Y. 10021.
†130 North Wells St., Chicago, Ill. 60606.

thalamic pain, but may be less distressing.[66] (See Chapter 8 for a general discussion of pain.)

Intractable pain. Unbearable pain that does not respond to definitive treatment of the causative lesion is classified as intractable. The pain is chronic and often disabling. The individual's degree of disability and suffering (despite the physiologic basis for the pain) must also be related to psychologic and personality factors. It is difficult to objectively evaluate a patient's complaints of pain. The chronic complainer of pain is often stereotyped as a difficult patient. It is possible to alleviate intractable pain surgically through deafferentation at varied sites such as by neurectomy, rhizotomy, and cordotomy. Pain arising from nervous system lesions, as discussed previously, must be differentiated from the pain resulting from incurable cancer. Surgery is more commonly performed for the latter type.

Neurectomy. When pain is localized to one part of the body, it can be relieved by interruption of the peripheral or cranial nerves supplying the area. The nerve fibers to the affected area are severed from the cord (cell body) in an operation known as neurectomy. (See the nerve pathways illustrated in Fig. 32-15.) The nerve may also be effectively destroyed by injecting it with absolute alcohol, but the results are unpredictable. Not only pain fibers are interrupted by these procedures but also fibers controlling movement and position sense. Therefore this type of treatment cannot be used to control pain in the extremities. A neurectomy probably is most often performed to relieve the suffering of patients with trigeminal neuralgia, in which case it is referred to as a *fifth nerve resection.* A neurectomy may also be performed to control incapacitating dysmenorrhea and is called a *presacral neurectomy.*

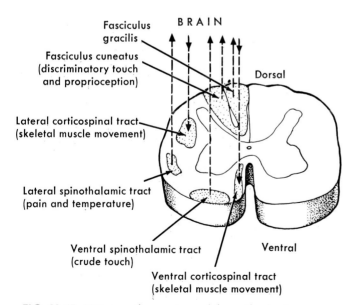

Fasciculus gracilis
Fasciculus cuneatus (discriminatory touch and proprioception)
BRAIN
Dorsal
Lateral corticospinal tract (skeletal muscle movement)
Lateral spinothalamic tract (pain and temperature)
Ventral spinothalamic tract (crude touch)
Ventral corticospinal tract (skeletal muscle movement)
Ventral

FIG. 32-15. Nerve pathways to and from the brain.

Rhizotomy. Resection of a posterior nerve root just before it enters the spinal cord is known as a rhizotomy. This procedure frequently is useful in controlling severe pain in the upper trunk such as that caused by carcinoma of the lung. It is also done to relieve severe spasticity in patients with paraplegia. However, it cannot be used to relieve pain in the extremities, since position sense is lost. The incision is made high in the thoracic or low in the cervical area and involves a laminectomy. The postoperative observation and care are similar to that necessary for any patient who has had a laminectomy, except that the patient who has had a rhizotomy is usually a poorer operative risk and may be suffering from a severe debilitating disease and therefore develops complications such as decubiti more easily. It is important for both the patient and the nurse to realize that this operation will not prevent pain at the level of the incision because the resected nerves affect only the area below the incision.

Cordotomy. A cordotomy is an operation performed to relieve intractable pain in the lower trunk and legs and is most often performed on patients with extensive carcinoma of the pelvis. The incision is made high in the thoracic area, two laminas are removed, and the pain pathways in the spinothalamic tract (anterior and lateral aspect of the cord) on the side opposite the pain are severed (Fig. 32-15). If the pain is in the midline, the interruption must be made bilaterally. However, the two operations must be performed separately to avoid extensive damage to the cord from edema.

Following surgery, nursing care is similar to that given a patient who has had a cervical laminectomy for removal of a protruded nucleus pulposus. Frequently temporary paralysis, or at least leg weakness, and loss of bowel and bladder control follow a cordotomy; it results from edema of the cord and will gradually disappear in about 2 weeks. During the period of paralysis the patient may be helped out of bed by using a hydraulic lift, as demonstrated in Fig. 32-16. Back care, with special attention to pressure points, should be given every 2 or 3 hours since position sense is lessened and the patient is often debilitated. It is advisable to use an alternating air pressure mattress until the patient is allowed out of bed. Sometimes a Foster bed or a Stryker frame enables the nurse to give the patient better care. Because of the decreased position sense, special attention needs to be given to placing the patient in proper body alignment by using foot blocks. If quadriceps-setting exercises are begun in the early postoperative period, retraining in walking will be less difficult for the patient. It usually is easier for the patient to use a walker when he first begins to walk, but he should progress to a cane. Many patients will always feel more secure with a cane. Occupational therapy should be designed to strengthen the leg

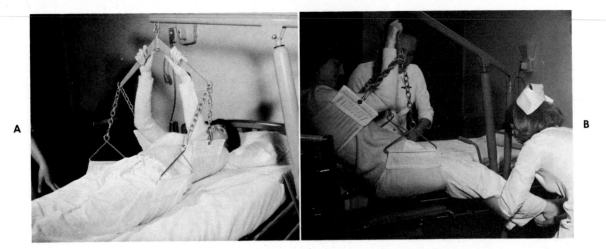

FIG. 32-16. The hydraulic lift can be used to move a paralyzed patient from bed to chair. **A,** Patient lying in canvas slings ready to be moved. **B,** Moving patient to chair. Note that one nurse is guiding the patient's body into the chair while the other nurse is moving the patient's legs. This lift may also be used to move a patient who is unable to grasp the overhead bar. (Courtesy Neuropsychiatric Institute, University of Illinois Hospitals at the Medical Center, Chicago, Ill.)

muscles. The use of a treadle sewing machine or a treadle sander will give exercise to the ankle. A bicycle provides for hip and knee flexion and extension. Therapy can be started as soon as the patient can be out of bed comfortably for at least 2 hours at a time.

Because temperature sensation is permanently lost, the nurse must be careful to avoid burning or otherwise injuring the patient's lower trunk and legs and must teach the patient and his family to avoid injury. The lower portion of the body, especially the feet, should be inspected routinely for any breaks in the skin or unnoticed infection.

Currently percutaneous cordotomy is the preferred surgical technique. It permits more precise control of the size and site of the surgical lesion than does the direct thoracic approach described previously. It is also less traumatic surgically for the debilitated patient who has often been on continuous drug therapy for long periods.

The procedure consists of inserting a spinal lumbar puncture needle laterally between the cervical (C1 and C2) level. A wire electrode is then inserted into the anterior cord and a lesion is made at a designated site, under radiologic and stereotactic control, in order to destroy the ascending pain fibers. The procedure is performed under local anesthesia, and the patient will note a sensation of tingling in the corresponding body area when the electrode is stimulated minimally. This assists the surgeon in locating the exact site for the surgical lesion.

Preoperatively the patient is evaluated carefully as to his candidacy for this type of surgery and to establish baseline data. It is important to identify and exclude the individual whose pain is more functionally based. Cordotomy in this instance would not

be successful in relief of the pain. Pulmonary function is also carefully evaluated. Regional anesthetic blocks (with an epidural catheter) are often evaluated prior to surgery for a 24-hour period or longer in order to test the benefits to the individual. Placebo blocks with normal saline solution are also done and the results compared with the anesthetic block. The patient is carefully monitored regularly by the nurse during the regional blocks as to hypalgesia and analgesia responses.

Postoperatively the patient is observed particularly for postural hypotension when initially ambulated. The sympathetic fibers in the cord controlling blood pressure lie in close proximity to the surgical site, and blood pressure may be affected for a period of time. Temperature sensation is also expected to be lost after this type of surgery. Bladder function and motor function may also be affected and should be observed carefully by the nurse following surgery. Usually such deficits do not increase following unilateral cordotomy but may after bilateral cordotomy. The value of accurate presurgical baseline data of all components is particularly necessary for good postsurgical care of the patient with a cordotomy.

Trigeminal neuralgia. Trigeminal neuralgia (tic douloureux) is characterized by excruciating, burning pain that radiates along one or more of the three divisions of the fifth cranial nerve (Fig. 32-17). The pain typically extends only to the midline of the face and head since this is the extent of the tissue supplied by the offending nerve. There are areas along the course of the nerve known as "trigger points," and the slightest stimulation of these areas may cause pain. Patients with trigeminal neuralgia usually are very unhappy individuals who try desperately to avoid "triggering" the pain. It is not unusual

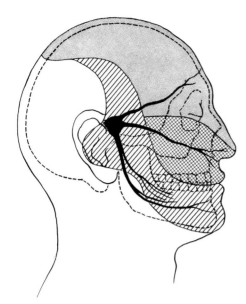

FIG. 32-17. Pathway of the trigeminal nerve and the facial area innervated by each of the three main branches.

to see them lying in bed with the covers over their heads in an effort to avoid drafts. They frequently have been unable to eat properly for some time, since chewing causes pain. They may therefore be undernourished and dehydrated. They may have slept poorly and not washed, shaved, or combed their hair for some time. Oral hygiene must often be neglected because of pain.

The patient is usually treated medically first before attempting surgery. In caring for the patient with trigeminal neuralgia preoperatively or in caring for the patient who is being treated medically, it is important that members of the nursing staff be sympathetic toward the patient's behavior. Every effort should be made to avoid placing the patient in a draft and to avoid walking swiftly to his bed, because the slight motion of air created may be enough to cause pain. The bed should not be jarred or the bedclothes fanned. It is unwise to urge the patient to wash or shave the affected area or to comb his hair, since he may either become upset in feeling that it is required or he may comply and set off another siege of pain. He will probably prefer to do things for himself if touching his face is involved. It is sometimes possible for him to give himself mouth care if applicators and a lukewarm mouthwash are provided. Often pureed foods or lukewarm fluids taken through a straw is the only diet that can be tolerated.

Carbamazepine (Tegretol) currently is the drug of choice for the treatment of pain (also used for convulsions, p. 878).[61] The inhalation of trichloroethylene (10 to 15 drops on cotton) has been tried with variable success for relieving pain. Drugs such as nicotinic acid, thiamine chloride, cobra venom, and

analgesics have all been tried, but usually they offer the patient little, if any, relief. Sedatives are given to help the patient sleep.[16]

The peripheral branches of the trigeminal nerve may be injected with absolute alcohol. This provides relief for weeks or months, and the procedure may be repeated as necessary. Permanent relief can only be obtained by surgery that consists of dividing the sensory root of the trigeminal nerve intracranially. If not all of the nerve is involved, a partial resection will be done.[16]

Postoperatively it is important to know what branches of the nerve have been cut in order to provide the necessary protection. If the upper branch is completely severed, the patient will lose the corneal reflex on that side. Usually an attempt is made to preserve a few of the fibers of the first division of the fifth nerve, since even a few intact fibers seem to preserve this vital function. Until the physician has tested the corneal reflex and verified its presence, an eye shield is used to prevent dust or lint from getting onto the cornea and causing injury.

The patient should be instructed not to touch or rub his eye but to blink it often, since blinking helps to lubricate the eye. If the reflex is completely absent, each eye should be bathed at least every 4 hours and more often if necessary. The best solution for bathing the eye is normal saline solution. A solution of methylcellulose (0.5% to 2%) may be prescribed to help keep the cornea moist. This solution is sometimes referred to as "artificial tears." Some experts recommend that one or two drops of mineral oil be instilled in each eye following the eye irrigation. However, no medication should be instilled in the eye without an order from the physician. The lids should not be dried, since any material such as cotton, gauze, tissue, or toweling may leave lint. The patient should be taught to care for his eye when he returns home. Any contact with the eye should be carefully avoided when washing the face. The eye should be inspected several times a day, and medical attention should be sought if it becomes inflamed. Patients are safer outdoors if they wear glasses, which will protect the eyes from dust and other flying particles. Contact lenses should never be worn by these patients because the lenses are too irritating.

When the lower branch of the fifth cranial nerve is interrupted, the patient needs to avoid hot foods, since he will not be aware if the mucous membrane is burned. He may have some difficulty chewing and swallowing at first and should be instructed to place the food in the unaffected side of the mouth. Since food may be retained in the mouth on the affected side, mouth care should be given immediately following meals. Dental caries on the affected side will not cause pain. Therefore the patient should visit the dentist routinely every 6 months. He should tell the dentist that he has had a fifth nerve resection so that trauma is avoided. Care must be taken in shaving to avoid nicking the insensitive skin.

Within 24 hours after a fifth nerve resection, many patients develop herpes simplex (cold sores) about the lips. Phenol and camphor (Campho-Phenique), applied frequently, seems to give more relief than any other treatment. Usually the lesions heal in about a week.

An operating microscope is used during surgery on the trigeminal nerve. Microsurgery permits greater precision in selective cutting of fibers; also, the sensation of touch and the corneal reflex are preserved.[16] More recently a method to sever the nerve inside the skull is being utilized. A thin electrode needle is inserted through the cheek and into the nerve. This avoids a surgical procedure, yet may provide permanent relief of pain.

Other cranial nerve surgery. Other cranial nerves may be interrupted as necessary. It is sometimes necessary to resect both the fifth and the ninth nerves to relieve severe pain caused by carcinoma of the sinuses. The nursing problems in each instance are related to the areas that have been desensitized and the resulting handicaps. Often there is temporary and sometimes permanent loss or a change of facial expression after resection of these nerves, which may cause severe psychic problems. When any nerve is resected, whether it be peripheral or cranial, the patient must understand that all sensa-

tion in this area is lost and that he will therefore need to avoid injury, especially from heat, cold, and trauma.

Increased intracranial pressure

Increased intracranial pressure (ICP) is a complex manifestation that is the consequence of multiple neurologic conditions and often requires surgical intervention.

The cranial contents, including the brain tissues, vascular tissues, and cerebrospinal fluid, are contained within a bony vault for protection. Any increase in the volume of any of the cranial contents, singly or in combination, results in increased intracranial pressure since the cranial vault is rigid, closed, and nonexpandable. Several neurologic lesions, either by their nature or by inciting cerebral edema, increase the volume of tissue within the cranium. Any lesion that increases tissue volume is known as a space-occupying lesion. Common examples include cerebral contusions, hematomas, infarcts, abscesses, and other inflammations of brain tissues. Intracranial tumors arising from all types of brain tissues increase cell mass and as a consequence increase intracranial pressure. An increase in the production of cerebrospinal fluid, blockage of the ventricular system, or a decreased absorption of cerebrospinal fluid can likewise increase tissue volume. Space-occupying lesions must of necessity displace and distort the brain and vascular tissues as

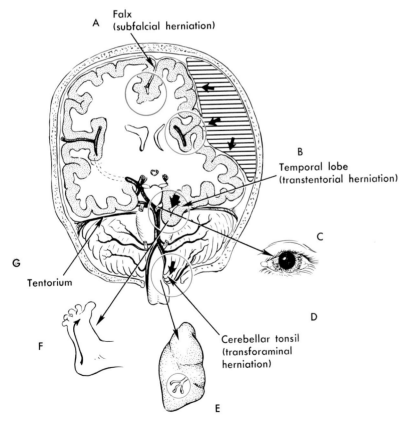

FIG. 32-18. The consequences of increased intracranial pressure are illustrated. An expanding temporoparietal epidural hematoma with medial and downward pressure has produced subfalcial, transtentorial, and transforaminal internal herniations. Note distortion of falx, *A;* bulging of medial temporal lobe at tentorial edge, *B;* and herniation of the cerebellar tonsil with descending pressure on the brain stem, *D.* Also note how major blood vessels are collapsed in the encircled areas. Some consequential effects of continuing and/or expanding pressure on neural structures with alterations in body functions are detailed: *C,* homolateral dilation and fixation of the pupil with ptosis of the eyelid; *E,* life-threatening respiratory arrest through indirect effects on respiratory centers in the brain stem; *F,* contralateral Babinski's sign showing extension of the great toe and fanning of the other toes following plantar stimulation (coronal view of the head, ventral view of brain stem). (Modified from an original painting by Frank H. Netter, M.D.; from Clinical Symposia, Copyright by Ciba Pharmaceutical Co., Division of Ciba-Geigy Corp. All rights reserved.)

pressure increases. Pressure may build up slowly (days/months) or rapidly (minutes/hours), depending on the cause. At first one hemisphere will be more involved, depending on the lesion site, but eventually both hemispheres may become involved if the pressure continues to increase.

As pressure increases within the cranial cavity, it is at first compensated through venous compression and cerebrospinal fluid displacement. When the pressure within the cavity exceeds the compensatory mechanisms in the adult, the only escape for the swollen and displaced brain hemisphere is caudally or by downward herniation. The falx cerebri opposes medial shift of the hemispheres and the tentorium cerebelli opposes downward shift to some extent. Structures that allow internal herniation are the cingulate gyrus, which permits medial subfalcial herniation (under the falx); the uncus, which permits downward transtentorial herniation (across free edge of tentorium); and the cerebellar tonsil, which permits transforaminal herniation (through the foramen magnum). (See Fig. 32-18 for identification of these structures with internal herniations and shifting of the hemisphere.) As a consequence of the herniations, the brain stem is compressed at variable levels, which in turn compresses the vasomotor center, posterior cerebral artery, oculomotor nerve, corticospinal nerve pathways, and fibers of the *ascending reticular activating system* (ARAS). Internal herniation in this way represents the critical state of decompensation. The life-sustaining mechanisms for consciousness, blood pressure, pulse, respiration, and temperature regulation fail.

Nursing intervention. The detection of increased intracranial pressure ideally occurs early, when it is reversible and before the stage of decompensation. The ability of the nurse to make accurate observations, to interpret observations intelligently, and to record observations carefully is without question the most important part of nursing patients with increased intracranial pressure. Timewise, the nurse must know when to notify the physician relative to changes in the patient's condition. The nurse must be capable of implementing nursing, medical, and surgical measures appropriately. Because nurses must understand the neurophysiologic basis of their observations, selected signs relative to increased intracranial pressure are discussed from a nursing standpoint.

Level of consciousness. The mesencephalon and diencephalon that act as way stations to the ascending reticular activating system (ARAS) become compressed following herniation of the brain stem. Nerve impulses are interrupted through the ARAS, which is considered to be the seat of consciousness. A decreasing level of consciousness is an early sign of internal herniation. Any change in the level of consciousness is one of the most important observa-

tions for the nurse to make, report, and record. The patient's response to specific stimuli should be tested. Is the patient oriented to time, place, and person? Does he sleep at inappropriate times but is arousable to a normal level of awareness when shaken or called by his name? How does he respond to simple commands? How does he respond to light or painful stimuli such as pinching or pricking the skin? Are the responses the same on both sides of the body? It is necessary to be objective in recording the stimuli used in testing the specific responses obtained.

Pupillary signs. Pupillary responses are controlled by the oculomotor or third cranial nerve. The oculomotor nerve is compressed by the herniating tissue and specifically by the downward displaced posterior cerebral artery. The pupilloconstrictor fibers of the oculomotor nerve run in a group in the top part of this nerve and are the first to be compressed. As a consequence, the ipsilateral pupil (when the lesion is in one hemisphere) remains dilated and is incapable of constricting. The pupil appears larger than in the other eye and it does not react to light. Eventually, as the cerebral pressure increases and both hemispheres are affected, there is bilateral pupil dilation and fixation. Inequality of the pupil may appear earlier than fixation when the nerve is only stretched; the pupil may respond to light slowly rather than with the usual brisk normal response. The nurse in examining the pupils should note the size and equality first and then test the reaction of pupils to light in a darkened room.

Blood pressure and pulse. The effect of cerebral pressure on blood pressure and pulse is variable. Compensatory changes occur in the cerebral vasculature relative to hypoxia or diminished blood flow. As cerebral pressure rises, the blood pressure rises in response to the hypoxic stimulus in the vasomotor center. The rise in blood pressure may be sudden or gradual. As cerebral pressure rises, the blood pressure rises up to a point or until terminal collapse. Blood pressure readings should be taken in the same arm for comparative purposes. The pulse slows reflexly as the blood pressure rises. Slowing of the pulse rate in conjunction with a rising systolic blood pressure is a significant observation to be made and reported. The pulse should be taken for a full minute and described as to its character.

Respiration. Herniation produces respiratory dysrhythmias that are variable and are related to the level of brain stem compression, or failure. The breathing pattern may be deep and stertorous, Cheyne-Stokes ("periodic"); terminally there is respiratory paralysis. The beginning of periodic breathing is significant. The usual picture is one of slowing of respirations, along with a slow pulse and a rising systolic blood pressure. The nurse should learn to look for variability in vital signs and detect trends as they occur. It is important to remember that the patient with a decreasing level of consciousness will require assistance in keeping his airway clear. Consequently, respiration is further aggravated by this problem.

Temperature regulation. Failure of the thermoregulatory center due to compression occurs late and gives rise to high uncontrolled temperatures. It is important to understand that hyperthermia needs to be controlled, since it increases the metabolic needs of the brain tissues. Temperatures are taken rectally unless otherwise ordered.

Focal motor signs. Compression of upper motor neuron pathways (corticospinal tract) interrupt the transmission of impulses to lower motor neurons and progressive muscle weakness results. For example, a contralateral weakened hand grasp may progress to hemiparesis and hemiplegia. A positive Babinski sign, hyperreflexia, and rigidity are additional motor signs that provide evidence of decreasing motor function from upper motor neuron involvement. Transtentorial herniation of the upper or rostral part of the brain stem produces decerebrate rigidity. The motor inhibitory fibers are blocked, and the patient involuntarily assumes a fixed posture with his arms, legs, and trunk extended and with flexion of the palmar and plantar joints; seizures may also be present. The nurse should use gross tests or more definitive tests to determine motor changes. The worsening in existing motor deficits is significant.

Visual acuity and papilledema. The blind spot of the retina measures the size and shape of the optic papilla or optic disc. As venous congestion and intracranial pressure increase, the resulting pressure is transmitted to the eyes through the cerebrospinal fluid and to the optic disc (choked disc). Since the meninges of the brain reflect out around the eyeball, they permit the direct transmission of pressure along the subarachnoid space through the cerebrospinal fluid. As the optic disc swells, the retina adjacent to it is also compressed. The damaged retina cannot detect light rays. As the size of the blind spot enlarges, visual acuity is lessened. The ability of the nurse to detect papilledema is dependent on her skill in examination of the fundi. Decreasing visual acuity can be detected through the confrontation technique (p. 896). Papilledema is an early sign of increased intracranial pressure; loss of vision is a late sign.

Headache. Headache may occur as an early symptom. It is thought to result from venous congestion and the tension on the intracranial blood vessels as the cerebral pressure rises. The onset of the headache should be noted along with its location and duration. It increases in intensity with cough, straining, and stooping.

Vomiting. The occurrence of vomiting that is projectile is often associated with increased intracranial pressure. Its frequency and character should be noted. The significance of vomiting and headache needs to be associated with other clinical signs such as papilledema and vital signs. In summary, papilledema, headache, nausea, and vomiting are the cardinal signs of increased intracranial pressure.

Observation. The frequency of observation of the patient is often ordered by the physician. However, with significant deteriorating changes in the aforementioned signs, the nurse should make more frequent observations and recordings. Based on the results obtained from observation and the medical history of the patient, the nurse will need to make a decision as to frequency of monitoring. Young[110] reports that alterations in consciousness, blood pressure, pulse, pupillary responses, movement of extremities, temperature, and respiration provide the best guide for the nurse to estimate intracranial pressure. A special craniocerebral nursing record has been developed based on these categories.[110] The patient's condition is regularly compared with an established baseline through continuous monitoring. In some medical centers, electronic monitoring devices are being used to provide a continuous measure of intracranial pressure.

Treatment. The treatment of patients with increased intracranial pressure is planned relative to the underlying cause. When there is a rapidly rising intracranial pressure, it must be relieved by mechanical decompression, such as ventriculotomy or craniotomy. Neurosurgical nursing care is discussed relative to intracranial tumors (p. 925). Drugs such as mannitol and urea may be utilized in order to decrease cerebral edema. They promote osmotic diuresis and make it necessary to plan carefully as to intake and output and electrolyte balance. More recently, corticosteroids have been introduced in the medical management of increased intracranial pressure.

■ DEGENERATIVE DISEASES

The phrase "degenerative diseases" as used here refers to those neurologic diseases in which there is a premature senescence of cells when there is a known or suspected metabolic disturbance and/or when the etiology is unknown.

Multiple sclerosis (disseminated sclerosis)

Multiple sclerosis is a common neurologic disease in northern climates. The exact prevalence of this disease is not known, since in many instances a diagnosis is not made, but probably at least 500,000 persons in the United States are known to have multiple sclerosis. The onset of symptoms usually occurs between 20 and 40 years of age. Symptoms rarely occur before 15 or after 50 years of age. The course of the disease is estimated to be 12 to 25 years.[7] Multiple sclerosis has serious implications for family life, since it affects men and women in the active, productive years, when their responsibilities are greatest. Men and women are affected about equally.

During the past decade there have been major advances in the knowledge of the etiology, pathology, diagnosis, and treatment of multiple sclerosis. The etiology, however, remains unknown despite new findings and the numerous hypotheses that have been advanced as to cause. Mineral deficiency, toxic substances, disturbance of blood clotting mechanism, viruses, and autoimmunity are a few of the causes studied. The latter two are currently the most favored. Experimental allergic encephalomyelitis has been produced in animals by the injection of the basic protein from a homologous neuron sheath.[8] Despite the resemblance to multiple sclerosis, it is not yet clear to what extent this disease represents a human model for multiple sclerosis. The recent discovery of slow viruses (those with a long latent period) in association with the frequent findings of an increase of gamma globulin and immunoglobulin (IgG) in the spinal fluid of patients with multiple sclerosis gives support to these theories. What constitutes an elevation of gamma globulin or of IgG is not clear. Whether the gamma globulin and IgG get into the spinal fluid by transudation or by increased permeability of the blood-brain barrier is still controversial.

Multiple foci of demyelination are distributed randomly in the white matter of the brain stem, spinal cord, optic nerves, and cerebrum. During the demyelination process (primary degeneration) the myelin sheath and the sheath cells are destroyed, but there is early sparing of the axon cylinder. The outer myelin sheath in the spinal cord neuronal pathways is often compared to the insulation on an electric wire. Its destruction causes interruption or distortion of the impulse so that it is slowed or blocked. This type of demyelination differs from that of wallerian degeneration (p. 919) in that damage is always primary to the myelin sheath or sheath cells. There is evidence of partial healing in areas of degeneration, which accounts for the transitory nature of early symptoms. In late stages the degeneration may extend to gray areas of the cord and limit healing.

Because of the wide distribution of areas of degeneration, there is a greater variety of signs and symptoms in multiple sclerosis than in other neurologic diseases. The scarring that occurs at the degenerative lesions as well as the increasing sites provides the name "disseminated sclerosis."

Multiple sclerosis is a chronic, remitting, and relapsing disease. Usually there are acute exacerbations and remissions that may last for a year or more, although eventually exacerbations will recur. There is no record of any patient's having recovered from the disease, although many have lived for 20 years or more and have died from other causes. Exacerbations may be aggravated or precipitated by fatigue, chilling, and emotional disturbances.

Early symptoms are usually transitory and may include double vision (diplopia), spots before the eyes (scotomas), blindness, tremor, weakness or numbness of a part of the body such as the hand, fatigue, susceptibility to upper respiratory infections, and emotional instability. Many patients with early multiple sclerosis may be considered neurotic by their associates and sometimes by their physicians because of the wide variety and temporary nature of symptoms and because of their emotional instability. As the disease progresses, symptoms may include nystagmus, disorders of speech, urinary frequency and urgency, constipation, and changes in muscular coordination and gait. Late symptoms may include urinary incontinence, difficulty in swallowing, and severe muscle spasm and contractures.

Motor signs have upper motor neuron characteristics. Pain is not a common symptom of multiple sclerosis except when there is severe muscle spasm. Death may be caused by infection, usually developing in the respiratory or genitourinary system.

In the hospital the nurse may care for the patient for short periods when he is admitted for diagnosis or for some other condition or when he is terminally ill with advanced disease. Many patients are never hospitalized and will be cared for in their homes by public health nurses.

Diagnosis. The fact that multiple sclerosis involves multiple parts of the nervous system is often characterized by exacerbations and remissions, and frequently includes transient and bizarre signs and symptoms makes it difficult to diagnose with certainty. Because there is no specific diagnostic test, diagnosis is often a clinical judgment. The determination of cerebrospinal fluid gamma globulin by chemical or electrophoretic methods or of cerebrospinal fluid IgG by electroimmunodiffusion, when used with the history and neurologic examination, appears to be the most valuable single laboratory test.[95]

Management. At the present time there is no specific treatment for multiple sclerosis. Many physicians get favorable results from symptomatic treatment and the judicious use of ACTH and the corticosteroids, psychotherapy, social rehabilitation, physical therapy, patient education, and a great deal of compassion. Although ACTH and the steroids are used with increased acceptance, their efficacy remains controversial. These drugs have shown to prevent experimental allergic encephalomyelitis. Currently some clinicians prefer oral prednisone; others prefer intramuscular ACTH; still others prefer intravenous ACTH. Dexamethasone (Decadron), administered intramuscularly or orally, has recently become popular. Its demonstrated antiedema effect may explain the favorable results in acute attacks of multiple sclerosis. The effects of ACTH and the steroids on the demyelinating activity per se are not known.

Symptomatic treatment is often of great benefit. Urinary frequency and urgency, often the source of social disability, may respond to timed doses of propantheline bromide (Pro-Banthine). Prevention of urinary tract infection remains a problem, and such infections are a major cause of death. Cholinergic drugs such as bethanechol (Urecholine) may be of help in the patient with an atonic bladder. Cystometrographic study is important to detect the specific bladder problem. Diplopia can be relieved by an eye patch. Peripheral neurectomies, rhizotomies, and cordotomies are often used for the relief of spasticity, pain, and paresthesias. Many patients get relief from severe spasticity with intrathecal injections of phenol. The mood-elevating drugs are used to relieve depression, which is often present in multiple sclerosis.

Effort is made to keep the patient working for as long as possible, and many men have worked for 5 to 10 years and even longer after the onset of the first symptoms. Women can be helped to plan their shopping, housework, and other duties so that they may continue to function as wives and mothers even when the disease is advanced. The decision as to whether or not the patient is told his diagnosis rests with the physician, and there is not full agreement among physicians as to the proper course of action. Usually the decision is made on an individual basis and depends on the patient's emotional makeup and on his family's ability to cope with the economic, social, and emotional problems that a condition of this kind presents.

The patient with multiple sclerosis should have a daily routine for rest and activity, and he should adhere to it strictly. Rest must be balanced with adequate exercise. The patient is usually advised to exercise regularly but never to the point of extreme fatigue. Because he almost always feels tired, he must look for some special sign that tells him he has exercised enough. If he does more, he may suffer ill effects. For example, a tight feeling in the chest may indicate that the patient must rest or else have severe discomfort. After an exacerbation, it may be difficult for the patient to resume exercises, but it is usually best for him to return to an established schedule as soon as possible.

One side of the body is usually affected more than the other, and the patient may learn to stabilize his gait by leaning toward his uninvolved side. The annoyance of having the foot slap forward in taking a step may sometimes be overcome by the patient if he puts the heel down in a pronounced fashion and rolls the weight forward on the side of the foot.

The patient with multiple sclerosis needs a peaceful, relaxed environment. He should never be hurried and should not be expected to respond quickly either physically or mentally. He may have slowness in speech and slowness in ability to respond, and this difficulty should be ignored by persons around him. Members of the family and friends need help in understanding this problem and in meeting it calmly. The patient may have sudden explosive emotional outbursts of crying or laughing brought on by such simple acts as putting something hot into the mouth. Close members of the family must protect both the patient and visitors from the embarrassment of prolonged emotional outbursts. Reminding the patient of something sad may stop him from laughing and holding the mouth open will sometimes stop the crying.

A sense of optimism and well-being (euphoria) also seems to be characteristic of persons with multiple sclerosis, especially during remissions. It is suspected that this reaction is due largely to the patient's attempts to reassure himself that his condition is not so serious as is supposed. This response is helpful to the patient in many ways, but sometimes it may lead him to overdo and thus increase symptoms.

Good general hygiene is necessary for the patient with multiple sclerosis and includes a well-balanced diet with plenty of high-vitamin foods and fluids. Obesity must be avoided, because it makes it more difficult for the patient to handle himself and detracts from his appearance. The patient should sleep 8 hours each night and should have a rest period after lunch. Fresh air and sunshine are good, but chilling and overheating must be avoided because they may aggravate symptoms or bring on exacerbations. Pressure sores may develop as a result of immobilization and sensory loss. It is essential that the patient and the family understand the importance of checking the skin routinely and of relieving pressure occasionally in order to prevent the development of pressure sores.

Since association with others is good for physical and mental health, the patient with multiple sclerosis must be encouraged and helped to remain an active, participating member of his family and his community for as long as possible. Personal cleanliness adds to a feeling of acceptance and well-being; consequently, these patients should be encouraged to pay careful attention to personal appearance even though they may sometimes feel too tired to put forth the effort. The patient should be encouraged to develop interests and hobbies that will help make up for things he should not do, such as driving a vehicle, and that will help to fill the time when physical activity becomes more difficult. Music, writing, reading, and question games are good hobbies to develop. Interest in politics and in world affairs, which may be followed on the radio if sight is lost, may stand the patient in good stead.

The National Multiple Sclerosis Society* is a na-

*257 Park Ave. South, New York, N. Y. 10010.

tional voluntary organization founded in 1946. Its functions are to encourage and finance research, to gather statistics, and to act as an information center for patients and for the public. Some local chapters also supply equipment to patients. Membership is open to health and welfare workers and to patients and their families. Local organizations are located in many large cities.

Paralysis agitans (Parkinson's disease)

Parkinson's disease is one of the major causes of neurologic disability in the United States, especially in individuals over 60 years of age. Its prevalence is not known for sure. It has variously been estimated to have a prevalence rate of 100 to 150/100,000 population.[13,21] We can expect to see an increasing frequency due to the increased number of older people in our population.

Parkinson's disease is a slowly progressive degenerative disease of unknown cause in which there is destruction of nerve cells in the basal ganglia of the brain. It may follow acute encephalitis and occasionally occurs following carbon monoxide, metallic, or other poisoning. The disease, sometimes termed idiopathic parkinsonism, usually affects older persons. Sometimes it is associated with arteriosclerosis, but in many cases signs of arteriosclerosis are absent.

Advances in knowledge of the regional biochemistry of the brain, particularly of the biogenic amines, have made possible a new understanding of Parkinson's disease and have established a more rational basis for therapy. Parkinson's disease can now be defined as a dopamine deficiency condition with injury or disease of the dopaminergic neuronal system. Most neuropathologists agree that the loss of pigmented neurons occur particularly in the substantia nigra. It has been demonstrated that dopamine, a neurotransmitter substance, is found in high concentrations in the neostriatum (caudate nucleus, putamen, pallidum). In Parkinson's disease it is selectively depleted in these structures. This depletion can be correlated with the degree of degeneration of the substantia nigra in experimental animals. The greater the cell loss in the substantia nigra, the lower the concentration of dopamine in the striatum. The physiologic role of dopamine appears to be the inhibiting modulation of the striatum that it produces by counterbalancing the excitatory cholinergic activity in this area. Acetylcholine, the excitatory neurotransmitter, is in abundant supply in the striatum. Thus there is an imbalance between the depleted dopamine and the acetylcholine. Therapy is now directed toward administering a precursor of dopamine, levodopa, which passes the blood-brain barrier, and/or anticholinergic drugs that act against the acetylcholine.

Parkinson's disease begins with a faint tremor and progresses so slowly that the patient is seldom able to recall its onset. There is not true paralysis and no loss of sensation. Tremor and muscle rigidity are the two outstanding signs of the disease. Parkinson's disease has some characteristics of upper motor neuron signs. It is essentially a problem in motion. Muscle rigidity seems to prevent normal response in commonly performed acts and leads to characteristic changes that make the diagnosis almost unmistakable to persons who have observed patients with the disease. There is a masklike appearance to the face and slowed, monotonous speech. Drooling may occur because of the difficulty of swallowing saliva. This may cause skin irritation that is best prevented or treated by frequent sponging followed by protecting the skin with an emollient such as cold cream. There is a characteristic shuffling gait in which the patient tends to walk on his toes. The trunk is bent forward, and the arms fall rigidly to the sides and do not swing as in normal rhythmic gait. Neuromuscular control may be altered so that the patient is unable to stop his propulsive gait until he meets an obstruction; finally he may become unable to walk at all. The patient usually has a moist, oily skin. Defects in judgment and emotional instability may occur, but intelligence is not impaired. The appetite may be increased and there is heat intolerance. All signs and symptoms increase with fatigue, excitement, and frustration.

Management. Treatment for Parkinson's disease is palliative and symptomatic and depends on the pharmacologic manipulation of the pathophysiologic state. The severity of symptoms and presence of associated disease processes determine the drugs to be used. Anticholinergic alkaloids such as scopolamine hydrobromide and related drugs (hyoscyamine) have been used for more than a century. They act against cholinergic excitatory effects and are more effective in lessening muscle rigidity than in controlling tremor. Many synthetic anticholinergic drugs of varied chemical structure are also available. There is little to recommend one over the other, aside from personal preference, but each has some degree of central nervous system anticholinergic action. However, they are incapable of restoring striatal balance. The preferred anticholinergic agents are trihexyphenidyl (Artane), benztropine mesylate (Cogentin), procyclidine (Kemadrin), and biperiden (Akineton).[10] These drugs have some selectivity of action in that they have greater central than peripheral anticholinergic activity. Optimal results from these drugs depend on a dosage that provides a compromise between the limited symptomatic improvement given by these drugs and the disagreeable symptoms of central and peripheral cholinergic blockade (blurring of vision, dryness of mouth and throat, constipation, urinary urgency and/or retention, ataxia, dysarthria, mental disturbances). Antihistaminic drugs such as diphenhydramine (Benadryl), which are not primarily anticholinergic, exert mild central anticholinergic properties when used alone or in combination with other drugs.

More recently some patients with severe Parkinson's disease have experienced dramatic benefits from levodopa not experienced from anticholinergic drugs. Levodopa assists in restoring striatal dopamine deficiency, since it is a precursor of dopamine. This drug does not affect the underlying process of parkinsonism.[21] In this way, levodopa is more like a replacement drug than a cure. Once benefits are obtained from levodopa, they are likely to be sustained. After prolonged periods of treatment, there may be an increased appearance of side effects. Levodopa is introduced slowly over a period of weeks or months. Usually patients remain on anticholinergic drugs or they may be added as an adjunct. Most individuals experience side effects from levodopa such as nausea and vomiting, orthostatic hypotension, insomnia, agitation, and mental confusion. There have been some cases of kidney and liver damage. Candidates for levodopa should be selected carefully.[21] Amantadine hydrochloride (Symmetrel), an antiviral agent, is known to have antiparkinson activity by blocking the reuptake and storage of catecholamines and allowing the accumulation of dopamine in extracellular or synaptic sites. This drug may not sustain its effectiveness for more than 3 months in some patients. Side effects, although infrequent, include mental confusion, visual disturbances, and seizures.

A surgical procedure has been used with some success in the treatment of selected patients with Parkinson's disease. Descriptions of successful operations in popular magazines have led some patients and their families to believe that a cure for all patients has been found. The nurse should refer those asking questions to a qualified neurologist. Many patients cannot be treated surgically. Results seem to be best in younger patients who have unilateral involvement following other disease and who have marked tremor and rigidity. Treatment consists of destroying portions of the globus pallidus (relieves rigidity) and/or the thalamus (relieves tremor) in the brain by stereotatic methods through use of cautery, removal, or injection of alcohol. Operative techniques involving cooling or freezing with liquid nitrogen (cryogenic surgery) have been attempted with good results in selected cases and with fewer complications than when cautery or alcohol was used. Medications used to control rigidity and tremor are discontinued several days preoperatively so that patients' symptoms will be at their maximum during the operation.[76] Nursing care preoperatively includes seeing that nutrition is adequate as well as other general preoperative care.

Postoperative care includes the most careful attention to the vital signs, use of side rails to prevent accidents in the event of convulsions, disorientation, or temporary hemiplegia, and frequent turning and moving to prevent respiratory and circulatory complications. Excessive salivation and difficulty in blinking the eye on the operated side may be problems requiring nursing attention.

The progress of Parkinson's disease, a condition that often lasts for years, may be slowed by good nutrition, sufficient rest, moderate exercise in fresh air, and other measures that improve general health. Special attention should be paid to posture. Lying on a firm bed without a pillow during rest periods may help to prevent the spine from bending forward, and lying in the prone position also helps. Holding the hands folded behind the back when walking may help to keep the spine erect and prevent the annoyance of the arms falling stiffly at the sides. The tremor often is less apparent when the patient is sitting in an armchair since he can grip the arms of the chair and partially control the tremor in his hands and arms. Unless the patient is well-controlled by medication, drooling can be a real problem and increases with general excitement. A bib can be used to protect the clothing during napping hours. When the patient is dressed, a garment with generous pockets well supplied with soft tissues will help him be less conspicuous and more comfortable.

The patient with Parkinson's disease should continue to work as long as possible. Most physicians advise this unless the occupation is such that continued work is dangerous. The patient should reduce his regular work gradually while developing hobbies and interests in which he may engage when the disease becomes more advanced. Relatives need complete understanding of the circumstances so that they may intelligently assist in the adjustments that will eventually be necessary. Such problems as accidents, personality changes, and progressive helplessness must be anticipated. While drooling and difficulty in swallowing often limit the important social outlet of eating at group gatherings, the patient should have his meals at home with the family as long as possible. Feeding the patient becomes a real problem when the disease is far advanced because of the danger of choking in attempts to swallow; eventually, aspiration pneumonia may terminate the patient's life.

Myasthenia gravis

Myasthenia gravis is a relatively rare disease of unknown cause. It usually occurs in young adults. Nerve impulses fail to pass to muscles at the myoneural junction. It is not known specifically why the motor nerve impulses fail to pass to the muscle and cause it not to contract. It is believed variously to be due to the inability of the motor end plate to secrete adequate acetylcholine, excessive quantities of the cholinesterase enzyme at the nerve ending, or a nonresponse of the muscle fibers to acetylcholine. Relative to the third theory, myasthenia gravis may be considered a primary muscle disease; relative to the first two theories it is a neuromuscular disease with lower motor neuron characteristics. Myasthenia gravis is considered a grave disorder since the respiratory muscles and the bulbar cranial nerves may be involved. During periods of exacerbation or lack of drug control the patient may be cared for in a respiratory intensive care unit. The outstanding symptom is severe generalized fatigue to the point of exhaustion that comes on quickly and, in the early stages of the disease, disappears quickly with rest. Weakness of arm and hand muscles may be first noticed when shaving or combing the hair. Facial muscles innervated by the cranial nerves are often affected, and it may not be possible for the patient to hold his eyelids open, to keep his mouth closed, or to chew and swallow. Occasionally the muscle weakness and fatigue becomes so great that the patient cannot breathe, and a respirator must be used.

There is no known cure for myasthenia gravis. There is, however, a very marked improvement following the use of neostigmine (Prostigmin) or pyridostigmine (Mestinon). These drugs block the action of cholinesterase at the myoneural junction and allow the action of acetylcholine, a chemical necessary for transmission of impulses to the muscles. Treatment is planned so that the patient may be maintained on the amount of drug that he can tolerate without side effects and yet carry out activities essential for normal living. Usually the patient is permitted to adjust his own dosage. The nurse should teach the importance of taking medications at the time prescribed. Patients with myasthenia gravis must often change their method of earning a living. The nurse can help the patient and his family plan so that a minimum of energy is used in activities that are essential to his remaining relatively self-sufficient.

The patient with myasthenia gravis should take particular care of his health. Upper respiratory infections may be serious because he may not have the energy to cough effectively and may develop pneumonia or strangle. The patient who is living at home may feel more secure if there is a tracheal suction apparatus available and a member of his family knows how to use it if an emergency arises.

During acute episodes of the disease a tracheostomy set is kept in the patient's room ready for immediate use. Often it is necessary to suction the patient before he eats. If swallowing is too dangerous, a nasogastric tube is used, and great care must be taken to be certain that the tube is in the stomach before fluid is introduced, since the patient cannot cough to indicate its presence in the trachea. When caring for the patient with severe symptoms of myasthenia gravis, the nurse should remember that he is too weak to do anything for himself. Therefore the patient may not take a drink and may not turn over in bed unless the nurse thinks to help him.

Progressive muscular dystrophy

Progressive muscular dystrophy is a relatively rare disease of unknown cause. The characteristic signs are muscle wasting and weakness. The disease develops most often in children, and boys are affected three times as often as girls. In approximately half of all cases there is a history of at least one other family member who has had the disease, and sometimes several siblings are affected. It is a primary muscle disease.

There are several forms of the disease. One form, *pseudohypertrophic muscular dystrophy,* always develops during childhood and is characterized by enlargement of the muscles of the calf of the leg, accompanied by limitation of muscle function. The child gets from a horizontal to a standing position by turning on his abdomen, getting on his knees, and "climbing up his thighs" with the use of his hands.

There is no effective medical treatment known for progressive muscular dystrophy. Physical therapy is sometimes given, but its benefit is largely psychologic and to help delay contractures. Progressive muscular dystrophy does not have remissions but becomes very slowly but progressively worse. Few children who develop the disease live to adulthood.

Motor system disease

Several motor diseases that in the past were viewed as single disease entities are now recognized as variations of the same disease. Motor system disease includes primary lateral sclerosis, progressive bulbar palsy, spinal muscular atrophy, and amyotrophic lateral sclerosis (ALS). It can be noted that these diseases are named relative to the structures primarily involved—some upper motor neuron, some lower motor neuron, or a combination.

Pathogenesis includes degeneration and loss of motor neurons in the involved structures. Motor cortex cells, bulbar cells, and the corticospinal tract (especially spinal cord) degenerate. Motor nerve roots and nerves show wallerian degeneration; there is a breakdown of axons and myelin in the motor tract. An infantile, hereditary form exists that characteristically affects the anterior horn cells (Werdnig-Hoffmann disease).

Signs and symptoms of motor system disease (also called motor neuron disease) can be associated with upper motor neuron, lower motor neuron, or combined signs relative to the motor system structures affected.

Amyotrophic lateral sclerosis, which is a combined form, is discussed as representative of motor system disease. There is direct involvement of the lateral tracts of the spinal cord with possible eventual involvement of the medulla and the ventral tracts. Myelin sheaths are destroyed and are replaced by scar tissue. The nerve impulses are distorted or blocked. Early symptoms include fatigue, awkwardness of fine finger movements, and muscle wasting. There is progressive muscle weakness, atrophy, and fasciculations. Spasticity of flexor muscles is commonly present. With involvement of the brain stem and medulla, there is dysphagia, dysarthria, jaw clonus, and tongue fasciculations. As the disease progresses, there is disability relative to both upper and lower limbs and one side becomes more involved than the other.

Treatment and nursing care consists of relieving the symptoms with medications, nursing care that includes assistance with activities of daily living as limb deficits increase, and much emotional support. Prostheses are often applied to support the weakening muscles. The patient is always afraid as the disease progresses and respiration is affected. At this time he requires constant nursing attention. Most patients live about 3 years after diagnosis; occasionally there are periods of spontaneous arrest.

■ VASCULAR DISEASES

Cerebrovascular accident

Cerebrovascular accident (CVA) is the most common disease of the nervous system and in 1968 was the third highest cause of death in the United States. The condition is often associated with vascular disease of the heart, the kidneys, other organs, and the peripheral blood vessels. When total deaths due to arteriosclerosis and hypertension are studied, stroke as one subgroup, causes 16.0% of all deaths due to this cause.[99] Usually the vessel involved in a cerebrovascular accident is a relatively large one and affects one side of the brain, which leads to partial or complete paralysis of the opposite side of the body (hemiplegia). *Shock, hemiplegia,* and *stroke* are other terms used in referring to cerebrovascular accidents. The term "stroke" clinically refers to the sudden and dramatic development of focal neurologic deficits. Hemiplegia is one neurologic deficit that commonly occurs. If a small blood vessel is involved, there may be symptoms of short duration or that are less severe as described later in this section. The extent of neurologic deficits is directly related to the specific blood vessels occluded and the area of the brain supplied by the vessels.

The "stroke prone" person often has a history of previous transient cerebral ischemia attacks (TIA) that last for minutes to almost 24 hours. When an attack lasts for several days and resolves, leaving minimal residual evidence, it is known as TIA-IR (incomplete recovery). When the ischemic attack is characterized by a marked and persistent neurologic deficit, the diagnosis of completed stroke (CS) is made.[37]

Vascular lesions of the brain are often categorized as due to embolus, hemorrhage, or thrombosis. Cerebral embolism is usually caused by a mass breaking away from a thrombosed blood vessel elsewhere in the body. This condition has been less frequent since patients with bacterial endocarditis have been treated with antibiotic drugs. Anticoagulant drugs administered in the treatment of coronary artery disease and early ambulation may prevent thrombosis of peripheral blood vessels in hospitalized patients.

Cerebral hemorrhage is caused either by the rupture of a congenital aneurysm or by the rupture of a sclerosed blood vessel in persons who have high blood pressure. Although the symptoms of rupture of an aneurysm and of hemorrhage due to arteriosclerosis and high blood pressure may be similar, the treatment is different. Therefore the nursing care will be considered separately. Cerebral thrombosis is by far the most common cause and accounts for approximately 90% of all cerebrovascular accidents in persons over 65 years of age. It is caused by the formation of a thrombus, or clot, in a blood vessel of the brain. Because the management of patients with cerebral hemorrhage does not differ very much from that for cerebral thrombosis, it will be considered in one discussion.

Cerebral thrombosis and cerebral hemorrhage

Cerebral thrombosis and cerebral hemorrhage may occur at any time, although thrombosis is more likely to occur when the patient is sleeping, and the hemorrhage is more likely to occur when physical or emotional stress is encountered.

Cerebral hemorrhage may be preceded by headache, vertigo, flushing of the face, momentary loss of consciousness, nausea and vomiting, and a foreboding that something is wrong. If a large artery ruptures, a sizable portion of the brain may be deprived of its blood supply and the onset may be sudden. If a smaller vessel ruptures, only a small portion of the brain may be affected, and symptoms may become pronounced only when enough blood has flowed into the brain tissue to produce pressure. Symptoms of cerebral thrombosis are most likely to be obvious on the patient's awakening, but they usually vary in degree. The patient may have only a slight difficulty in speech, in walking, or in recalling events of the day before. The effects of the thrombosis may become progressively worse over a 24-hour period, or the patient may be paralyzed on one side of his body on awakening. If the thrombosis is massive or develops quickly, the patient may die in his sleep without awakening.

Following a cerebral hemorrhage or a cerebral thrombosis, the patient may fall and lapse into total unconsciousness, and convulsions may occur immediately following the accident. Loss of consciousness may come on slowly or quickly and may last for a few minutes or many days until slow recovery occurs, or it may continue until death, which usually does not occur for several days. The pulse is rapid and bounding, the respirations are labored or stertorous, and the blood pressure is elevated; vomiting may also occur. The pupils may not react normally to light, and one side of the body may appear limp. If the paralysis is on the right side of the body, the patient may not be able to speak even if consciousness returns, because the speech center in most right-handed persons is located on the left side of the brain along with the cortical sensory and motor areas for the right side of the body. If the patient is hospitalized, a spinal puncture is usually performed. It may reveal blood in the spinal fluid if hemorrhage has occurred in an intracerebral artery that communicates with the spinal fluid system. As previously discussed, a cerebrovascular accident is the most common lesion involving the upper motor neurons. The vascular lesion often involves variable portions of the corona radiata and internal capsule. Sudden occlusion of a major vessel deprives the local neural tissue of blood and oxygen. Upper motor neuron signs appear as upper motor neuron structures are damaged.

Emergency care. A cerebrovascular accident may occur when the patient is at work or elsewhere outside his home and may be confused with convulsive seizures, diabetic coma, or drunkenness. Emergency care at the scene of the episode consists of turning the patient carefully on his affected side (determined by the puffiness of the cheek on this side) and elevating the head without tilting the neck forward, since tilting may constrict blood vessels and in turn cause congestion of blood within the cerebrum. Turning the patient on his affected side permits saliva to drain out of the mouth and lessens the danger of aspiration into the lungs. Elevation of the head may help to prevent edema of the brain. Clothing should be loosened about the throat to further aid in preventing engorgement of blood vessels in the head, which may lead to cerebral edema. The patient should be kept quiet, moved as little as possible, and protected from chilling. Medical aid should be sought at once.

The prognosis for the patient who has had a cerebrovascular accident is poor, particularly during the first few days. The mortality rate is somewhat higher in cerebral hemorrhage than in cerebral thrombosis. One study showed that of 191 patients sustaining a cerebrovascular accident, 82 survived for 2 days, 43 for 1 month, 28 for 1 year, and only 19 for 3 years.[29]

Nursing intervention. Nursing intervention for the patient who has had a cerebrovascular accident does not differ whether he is in the hospital or in his own home, although oxygen is more likely to be given in the hospital. In an attempt to prevent further thrombosis, bishydroxycoumarin (Dicumarol) and heparin may be given to the patient when he is in the hospi-

tal if it is certain that the cause of the trouble is cerebral thrombosis and not cerebral hemorrhage.

If the patient survives the first few days, he may begin to regain consciousness and some of the paralysis may disappear. It is then that the greatest understanding is needed by persons attending him. He may realize that he cannot talk, that he drools, that he cannot move a hand or a leg, or if he can move the limbs, that the motions are shaky and uncertain. The patient's condition is a terrible shock to him, and it is at this point that the nurse's active part in rehabilitation begins. By quiet assurance a nurse can help the patient feel that his progress toward recovery and self-sufficiency has begun and will continue. The nurse can help by telling him what is going to be done even though he cannot answer. If the patient is right-handed and cannot speak, he has the added difficulty of having to learn to write with his left hand in addition to being partially speechless. The nurse should try to anticipate the patient's needs and should make every effort to understand his indistinct speech, since repeated attempts to make himself understood only augment his misery and frustration. Usually, if partial speech is present at the time of return to consciousness, there is likelihood that speech will improve, and the patient is heartened by the knowledge of this fact. Speech may be affected because of involvement of the tongue, mouth, and throat as well as because of damage to the speech center in the brain. The patient who has sustained a cerebrovascular accident may be overly emotional, and this reaction, combined with his fear and frustration on becoming aware of his condition, is upsetting to his family. He may cry easily, and sometimes family members believe that they are responsible for his sadness when this is usually not true. Family, staff, and other patients need reassurance that they are not the cause of the reaction.

Rest and quiet are important even if the accident has not been serious enough to cause complete loss of consciousness. Some neurologists may prescribe that the head of the bed be kept flat for several days. This is believed to assist cerebral perfusion. No attempt should be made to rouse the patient from coma, although respiratory and circulatory stimulants may be prescribed by the physician. The vital signs should be carefully checked, and the nurse should observe for such things as a rise in temperature within the first day or two, slowing of pulse and respiration, and deepening of the coma, all of which indicate pressure on the vital centers and a poor prognosis.

The patient's eye on the affected side should be protected if the lid remains open and there is no blink reflex. Otherwise damage to the cornea can lead to corneal ulcers and blindness. Irrigations with physiologic solution of sodium chloride, followed by drops of sterile mineral oil, sterile castor oil, sterile petroleum jelly, or artificial tears solution, are sometimes used. After the lid is gently closed, an eye pad may be taped over the affected eye. If a pad is used, it must be changed daily and the eye cleansed and carefully examined for signs of inflammation or drying of the cornea. Eye shields are preferable to pads because they lessen the danger of lint entering the eye.

Mouth care is difficult to give since the patient may be unable to retain fluid and is likely to choke if it is introduced into the mouth. (See p. 189 for details of giving mouth care to the unconscious patient.) Mouth care should be given every 4 hours during the day and night, and special attention must be given to the paralyzed side of the mouth and tongue.

Fluids may be restricted for the first few days after a cerebrovascular accident in an effort to prevent edema of the brain. Then patients will be fed intravenous fluids, or the physician may insert a nasogastric tube and order tube feedings. When the patient is no longer comatose, small amounts of fluid, 5 to 10 ml., can be given several times daily to determine the patient's ability to swallow and to help him regain this function. Returning as soon as possible to a regular diet and a good fluid intake is desirable.

Patience and persistence are necessary in giving food and fluids to the patient. The nurse must make him feel that the problem is not discouraging and that time taken to assist him in eating is well spent. He may encounter so much difficulty in getting food and fluids beyond his partially paralyzed mouth and throat that the effort may not seem worthwhile. Therefore each small step in improvement should be brought to the attention of the patient. Turning him to his back or to the unaffected side may spare him the annoyance and embarrassment of having food spill from the affected side of the mouth. Foods that may cause choking, such as mashed potatoes, stringy meats, and semicooked vegetables, must be avoided. Since food may collect in the affected side of the mouth, it must be irrigated after eating to prevent accumulation of food and subsequent poor mouth hygiene. The patient should assist in feeding himself as soon as possible, since the helplessness of having to be fed by others is detrimental to emotional health. Food such as meats must, of course, be cut up. A covered plastic cup is available with a small center opening through which a straw can be introduced, or one can be improvised by using a straw and a covered plastic food container. This cup is useful for the patient who can draw through a straw but whose hands are unsteady. If the patient can swallow but cannot draw through a straw, an Asepto syringe with a piece of rubber tubing on the end or a pitcher must be used. Turning the patient to his unaffected side before introducing fluids into his mouth often helps him to control the mouthful of fluid and to swallow it successfully. If the patient

with dentures can keep them in his mouth, he should have them placed in his mouth as soon as possible, since wearing dentures also improves his morale and will increase his interest in eating.

Urinary output should be noted carefully and recorded for several days after a cerebrovascular accident. Retention of urine may occur, but it is more likely that the patient will be incontinent. If urinary incontinence occurs, the patient may be told that his control of excretory function probably will improve day by day. Offering a bedpan or a urinal immediately after meals and at other regular intervals helps to overcome incontinence. A retention catheter may be used for the first few days for women patients.

Fecal incontinence is fairly common following a cerebrovascular accident, and again the patient must be reassured that as general improvement occurs, this condition will be overcome. Some patients develop constipation, and impactions develop readily. Elimination must be noted carefully since diarrhea may develop in the presence of an impaction, thus causing it to go unnoticed for several days. Suppositories such as Dulcolax are generally prescribed to be given daily or every other day. However, some physicians order laxatives or enemas. Massage to the abdomen may be helpful in starting peristalsis, but it is done only when ordered by a physician. Warm oil-retention enemas are sometimes given regularly in an attempt to prevent impactions and when impactions occur. Milk of magnesia by mouth is often given, since straining in the act of defecation must be avoided. The patient must be cautioned not to strain and must be assured that the suppositories can easily be repeated if no results are obtained. He usually needs assistance in getting on and off the bedpan. Side rails that he can hold onto in turning himself or a trapeze that he can reach with his unaffected hand is useful if he is permitted this exertion.

The length of time the patient remains in bed depends entirely on the type of cerebrovascular accident suffered and the judgment of the physician in regard to early mobilization. Some physicians prescribe fairly long periods of rest following cerebrovascular accidents, whereas others believe that early mobilization is best. However, the trend is toward early mobilization of the patient with cerebral thrombosis, and mobilization sometimes begins a day or two after the accident has occurred.

While the patient is in bed, he must be moved frequently to avoid the danger of circulatory stasis and hypostatic pneumonia. Care must be taken to see that body weight is not borne on the paralyzed side or on the back for long intervals because pressure sores (ulcers) occur very easily. The patient should not be positioned on the affected side for more than 20 to 30 minutes four times a day. Deep breathing and coughing should be encouraged each time he is turned. Pillows should support the uppermost limbs when the patient lies on his unaffected side to prevent strain on the shoulder and hip joints. The patient can suffer complete dislocation of the hip joint from lack of support to the limb when he is placed on his unaffected side and when the flaccid thigh is allowed to fall forward and downward because the muscles take an active part in holding the head of the femur in its socket. The patient may be turned to a face-lying or partial face-lying position, with pillows again used to maintain good body alignment. This position is good for the patient who is not fully conscious, since it lessens the danger of aspiration of mucus. There should be a regular schedule for turning the patient, and the sequence of desirable positions should be outlined and recorded on the nursing care plan.

Specific rehabilitative measures. The greatest challenge for the nurse in care of the patient who has had a cerebrovascular accident comes after the patient is past the point of danger, for then he must face the long, slow process of learning to use whatever abilities that remain or can be relearned, and he must adjust to his limitations if he and his family are to be reasonably happy for the remainder of his life. If the patient is hospitalized, the physical therapist may make an evaluation of his functional ability before he goes home. If he is referred to a community nursing agency, a physical therapist who is either on the staff of or available to the agency may, with the approval of the physician, assess the patient's limitation in moving about. The therapist may then help the nursing staff in working with the family to set up a regimen of exercises for the patient and to make alterations in and about his home so that the patient can do as much as possible for himself safely and more easily. Simple and relatively inexpensive modifications such as rails on the bathtub and a firm support by the lavatory may make the difference between helplessness and some freedom for the patient. Often, however, no physical therapist is available, and the patient may be cared for at home throughout his illness. If the nurse cares for the patient at home early in his illness, time should be taken to teach the family member who is responsible for his care some of the nursing measures already described under general nursing care. The pamphlet *Strike Back at Stroke,** written for patients and their families, should be familiar to all nurses. It is available to any patient who has his physician's approval for its use. If there is ability to use the arm when consciousness returns, there is reason to believe that the leg function will return sufficiently for the patient to walk. Return of motor impulses and

*Prepared and published by the U. S. Department of Health, Education and Welfare, Public Health Service, Bureau of State Services, Division of Special Health Services, Chronic Disease Program.

subsequent return of function are evidenced by a tightening and spasticity of the affected part. This may appear from the second day to the second week after the cerebrovascular accident. Return of motor impulses is significant for the future use of the affected part but presents new problems for the patient, nurse, and all others who may care for him. Muscles that draw the limbs toward the midline become very active, and the arm may be held tightly adducted against the body. The affected lower limb may be held inward and adducted to, or even beyond, the midline. Muscles that draw the limbs into flexion are also stimulated, with the result that the heel is lifted off the ground, the heel cord shortens, and the knee becomes bent. In the upper limb, flexor muscles draw the elbow into the bent position, the wrist is flexed, and fingers are curled in palmar flexion. This is often seen following a cerebrovascular accident because the adductor and flexor muscles are stronger than the opposing muscles.

Persistent nursing effort must be directed toward keeping any part of the body from remaining in a position of flexion long enough for the occurrence of muscle shortening and joint changes that might interfere with free joint action. If a physical therapist is not available, the total responsibility for preventive measures may rest with the nurse. *Every minute counts in prevention, and the nurse must not miss one opportunity to take a moment from her busy day in the hospital to move the patient's adducted or flexed limbs back to the correct position.* In the home she must teach members of the family who are caring for the patient to exert this same careful attention.

If the patient is lying on his back, a pillow can be placed between the upper arm and body to hold the arm in abduction. A roll made of one or two washcloths serves as a good support to prevent flexion of the fingers, and a splint made from a padded tongue blade may be used to ensure straightening of the thumb or other fingers for periods during the day. A firm box at the foot of the bed holds the foot at right angles and prevents contractures in the dropfoot position.

Range of joint motion should be preserved, and passive exercises are often begun early. The nurse needs no order to put the patient's limbs through complete range of joint motion passively once or twice each day (see Figs. 1-2 to 1-4), but passive exercise in which the limb is to be exercised more than this should be undertaken only when so ordered by the physician. If the nurse does not have a written order, the physician must be consulted as to the amount of passive exercise he wishes the patient to have. A safe rule to follow in caring for any patient with neuromuscular disease is to never force a muscle or a joint past the point of pain. Passive exercise stimulates circulation and may help to reestablish neuromuscular pathways. No difficulty is encountered with these procedures until tightening of the muscles begins to appear, then other physical measures are needed, and the patient's treatment should be under the direction of a physical therapist.

Active exercise of the affected side also may be started early. It is ordered by the physician and, in the hospital, may be directed by the physical therapist. Under the guidance of the physical therapist the nurse checks the exercises while the patient is in the hospital, and the nurse or the physical therapist may teach the exercises to the family in preparation for the patient's return home.

Since the patient will depend a good deal on his unaffected arm and leg when he begins to move about, the unaffected part of the body needs attention to prevent contractures and preserve muscle strength. Even while he is in bed, the patient should exercise his unaffected arm and use it in all normal positions. The unaffected leg should be in a position of slight *internal rotation* most of the time while the patient is in bed, and the knee should be bent several times each day. Exercise to strengthen the quadriceps muscle should be done because the quadriceps is the most important muscle in providing stability to the knee joint needed for walking. Exercise against resistance is obtained by placing two small sandbags that are fastened together saddle fashion over the ankle and having the patient raise his leg. One of the best exercises for strengthening the quadriceps is to have the patient straighten the knee against resistance when he is sitting on the edge of the bed or in a chair; a small bucket of sand hung over the ankle may be used as the resistance, but care should be taken to protect the skin of the ankle from pressure. An ordinary cooking pan with a bucket handle may be used in the home.

When the patient begins to move about and to try to help himself, he may have several problems that can alter his ability to proceed. He may have loss of position sense, so that it is awkward for him to handle his body normally even when he has the muscular coordination to do so. He may have dizziness, spatial-perceptual deficits, diplopia, and altering of skin sensation. He may also have to work harder than other persons to receive a normal amount of air on inhalation, since the involved side of the chest does not expand easily. This difficulty may lead to excessive fatigue unless the nurse and all caring for the patient plan their work so that the patient's effort is not wasted.

Motivation is absolutely essential to rehabilitation. Most patients who have suffered a cerebral thrombosis are motivated and desire deeply to help themselves, even though some are so overcome with the enormity of their limitations that they are very quiet and are misunderstood by those around them. If there is return of hand function in 2 to 3 weeks,

fecal incontinence has disappeared, and no contractures, decubiti, or other complications have developed, there is reason to believe that the patient can learn to care for himself.[79]

The patient needs preparation for each new step in learning to move and care for himself. He must be shown each new activity as it will apply to him, and he then needs practice under supervision and recognition of each accomplishment.

Before standing or walking, the patient may practice raising himself up in bed and may sit on the side of the bed while holding firmly to an overbed table or to a strap with his good hand and pressing his feet on a chair or stool. The patient benefits from wearing shoes, since it is good for his morale and keeps his paralyzed foot in good position.

If preparation for walking has been adequate, the patient usually needs only one crutch when he begins to walk, and then he progresses to the use of a cane. When he first begins to walk, the nurse must remain close to him to allay his fear of falling. He may practice balancing himself by standing between parallel bars or by leaning on the backs of two chairs (provided the chairs are heavy enough to support weight safely). Good walking patterns must be established early, because incorrect patterns are difficult and sometimes impossible to change. A sideward shuffle should be watched for and avoided. The patient should begin by leaning rather heavily on his crutch or cane and lifting his body sufficiently to bring the leg and foot forward so that the toes point straight ahead and not inward. The cane or single crutch is held in the hand opposite the paralyzed or weakened side of the body.

The patient may be taught how to help with his own improvement. Careful and detailed instructions on how to hold and support himself will save him much embarrassment and confusion. By using his unaffected hand, he may, for example, straighten out the flexed fingers on the affected side and move his affected arm to a position where, with the weight of gravity, the elbow will be straightened. Most patients can learn to do activities of daily living (ADL) such as those pertaining to personal hygiene and dressing.

Behavioral changes. Following a stroke, an individual may have difficulty relating to himself and to his environment. After the acute stage, a multibed environment is advocated as it will stimulate him as well as decrease his self-orientation. In the initial stage, bringing familiar articles into the patient's environment can be a very helpful stimulus. Examples are a clock, watch, family pictures, or a Bible. *Hemianopia,* or decreased visual field, occurs rather commonly. Approaching the patient from the side of intact vision and teaching him to scan will not only make him more aware of stimuli but can help prevent injury. Diminished awareness or denial of his affected side (anosognosia) can occur and could be a safety hazard. This possibility should be considered when the patient runs into objects with the wheelchair or allows the affected arm or leg to drag behind him when transferring from chair to bed.[31]

The nurse's observations regarding his mental status are important. The patient may be disoriented and have decreased judgment or poor memory. A constant environment and routine are quite helpful in improving his orientation and his ability to function. Poor judgment and impulsiveness can be major safety hazards. This must be brought to the attention of the physician. The family also will have to be aware of this if they are to care for the patient at home.

Long-range plans. General care and the pattern of living that should be followed after a cerebrovascular accident vary for each patient and are determined by his own circumstances, the amount of recovery he has, and the guidance he received in the early stages of his illness. Despite all effort he may, for example, never be able to negotiate stairs. The medical social worker and the public health nurse are indispensable in helping to arrange the patient's home so that he may live with a moderate amount of self-sufficiency and independence. Members of the family often need help in assisting the patient to accept his limitations, both physical and emotional. They must also make adjustments to actual circumstances. Almost all persons who have cerebrovascular accidents need health supervision for the rest of their lives. Whether or not the patient will be able to return to his own home or must go to a nursing home will depend a great deal on his family's understanding and acceptance of his problems when maximum rehabilitation may have been achieved.

While it is not uncommon for cerebrovascular accidents to recur, the patient may go for years with no further difficulty and eventually die of some other cause. The physician usually explains the prognosis to the patient and to his family. The nurse should know what explanation the physician has given and must sometimes help in interpreting it to the family. Some patients must curtail activity to such a point that they have little enjoyment in living and still have recurrences, whereas others may be active and escape further accidents for many years.

The patient who has sustained a cerebrovascular accident and who has high blood pressure is usually advised by his physician to change his mode of life so that more rest is assured and strain and excitement are avoided. If his work is strenuous, he may be urged to take longer and more frequent vacations. He may be advised to lose weight if obesity is putting an extra strain on his circulatory system and to avoid the use of tobacco because of its constricting effect on blood vessels. Activities of daily living may be modified; for example, the patient may be advised to sit while shaving. If the physician feels that the danger of cerebral hemorrhage is imminent, he may advise against any activities that promote dilation of cerebral blood vessels such as vigorous exercise, hot or cold baths, violent coughing or laughing, straining at defecation, and sexual activity. Occasionally retirement at an early age is necessary. Relocation in a warmer climate or in a more rural area is helpful to some people provided they can afford it and it does not upset the living pattern of the patient and his family too much.

The patient who has continued hypertension usually is given medication such as reserpine or its derivatives. Side effects of these drugs such as stuffiness of the nose, depression and mood changes, and tremor should be explained to the patient if they occur. Anticoagulant drugs such as bishydroxycoumarin (Dicumarol) or warfarin sodium (Coumadin) may be prescribed for an indefinite period following a cerebral thrombosis. The patient and his family should know why blood samples are taken regularly and what signs of overdosage such as epistaxis should be reported to the physician at once.

Cerebral arteriosclerosis and multiple small thrombi. Cerebral arteriosclerosis may lead to deterioration of brain tissue, even though cerebrovascular accidents do not occur. This condition, which usually is associated with high blood pressure, may occur in people in their fifties, although it is usually considered a disease of old age.

Multiple small thrombi may occur in persons whose blood pressure is normal or even below normal if atheromatous changes have occurred in the lining of arteries. This condition causes frequent small and barely perceptible strokes. Both cerebral arteriosclerosis and multiple small strokes from thrombi may produce personality changes. The person who has arteriosclerosis is likely to have a more consistent downward course, whereas the one suffering from multiple small thrombi may have periods of apparently normal physical and mental response between episodes of confusion.

Both cerebral arteriosclerosis and multiple small thrombi cause slowly progressive changes that are particularly distressing to members of the patient's family. Complete brain deterioration may occur. The patient may feel irritable and unhappy with apparently little cause, and no amount of reassurance can make him feel better. The family must be prepared for gradual deterioration of the patient's condition and should make provision for his safety and for the results of the poor judgment he may demonstrate; for example, he may forget to dress appropriately, may give away family possessions, and may enter into unwise business dealings. The family needs help in learning how to treat the patient as an adult and yet deal with his limitations. The physician, the social caseworker, and the nurse can help family members care for the patient in such a way that their own lives are not completely disrupted and yet that they are not plagued by guilt feelings when the patient dies. Institutional care is sometimes necessary, and the family needs encouragement and help in arriving at joint decisions that serve the best interests of all its members.

Cerebral aneurysm

A cerebral aneurysm is a weakening and outpouching of the wall of a cerebral artery and is usually caused by a congenital weakness in the vessel wall. It is caused by an absence of the media or muscle layer of the vessel wall. As a result, the elastic layer develops a berrylike sac that becomes the aneurysm. The aneurysm usually forms where the vessel bifurcates. The most common sites are the internal carotid, the posterior communicating, the middle cerebral, and the vertebral and basilar arterial systems.[94] The internal carotid artery comes from the common carotid artery and branches to form the ophthalmic, the anterior, and the middle cerebral arteries. The posterior communicating artery comes from the posterior cerebral artery. The vertebral and basilar arteries come from the subclavian artery; each of these arteries send communicating branches to the internal carotid branches (anterior and middle cerebral arteries) to form the circle of Willis at the base of the brain. Hemorrhage occurs when the aneurysm ruptures and the blood seeps into the subarachnoid spaces. This condition accounts for the sudden death of young people from "strokes" during strenuous exercise or excitement that causes the blood pressure to rise. The aneurysm commonly ruptures in persons between the ages of 20 and 40 years. Signs and symptoms include sudden explosive headache, photophobia, neck rigidity, nausea and vomiting, loss of consciousness, shock, convulsions, a full, bounding pulse, and noisy, labored respirations.

The following system of grading has been developed to classify the clinical state of the patient by level of consciousness and neurologic deficit.

Grade I Minimal bleeding, alert, no neurologic deficit

Grade II Mild bleeding, alert, minimal neurologic deficit such as third nerve palsy and stiff neck

Grade III Moderate bleeding, drowsy or confused, stiff neck with or without neurologic deficit

Grade IV Moderate or severe bleeding, semicoma with or without neurologic deficit

Grade V Severe bleeding, coma, decerebrate movement

Additional grades are also added for patients over 50 years of age and those with major heart, lung, kidney, and liver conditions that increase risk for procedures.[111]

The immediate treatment for *subarachnoid hemorrhage* is to keep the patient absolutely quiet. He should be very gently moved to bed, and sometimes

it is not advisable to move him to a hospital. He must be kept flat in bed in a darkened room and attended constantly to be sure that he does not raise his head. Blood pressure may be taken as often as every 15 minutes. This procedure is best accomplished and is less disturbing to the patient if the cuff is left (deflated) about the arm. If he is conscious, he is given small amounts of water by mouth, but the water must be given through a straw so that his head is not elevated. Intravenous fluids may be given by slow drip so that blood pressure is not affected, and often an indwelling catheter is inserted to avoid the exertion of voiding. Bowel elimination is usually ignored for several days, and then oil-retention enemas or small doses of bulk laxatives may be given. Under no circumstances should the patient be permitted to strain, cough, sneeze, or otherwise exert himself because these activities increase intracranial pressure. Visitors must be carefully prepared so that they will not upset the patient, and no mail should be given to him unless it is certain that it contains no disturbing information. Hypothermia may be used to lessen the need of the brain for oxygen and thereby decrease the danger of damage to vital brain tissues (p. 209).

About 50% of patients with rupture of an aneurysm recover from the initial episode, but at least 50% of these persons will have recurrences of hemorrhage if untreated. Recurrence may occur within 2 weeks, and the danger of death increases with each recurrence. If the aneurysm is not obliterated by surgery, the patient may die eventually from recurrent hemorrhage.

The only satisfactory treatment for congenital aneurysm is surgery. Before surgery can be performed, however, the location of the aneurysm must be determined by arteriography (angiography), as described on p. 384. The time after the acute rupture when arteriograms are taken and when surgery is performed varies with the patient, his age, the intensity and kind of symptoms he has, and the judgment of the surgeon. Since angiography may increase symptoms, it may be followed by immediate surgery in some instances. Lumbar puncture is also performed initially to verify the presence of blood in the cerebrospinal fluid.

Surgery consists of a craniotomy and location of the aneurysm. When found, the aneurysm may be obliterated by ligation at its neck with the application of a silver clip. If the base of the aneurysm is too large for ligation to be practical, it may be coated with a liquid, adherent, plastic substance that hardens to form a firm support about the weakened vessel wall and thereby prevents rupture. If the aneurysm has not ruptured but has produced symptoms, attempts may be made to produce thrombosis within the aneurysm by use of an electric current and other means.[94]

Both before and after surgery the nurse should

observe for signs of increased intracranial pressure. Common causes of increased intracranial pressure in aneurysm include the local pressure from the aneurysm and the presence of blood or hematoma from the ruptured aneurysm.

Not all aneurysms can be treated surgically at the site of the lesion. If surgery is not feasible, in order to reduce the chances of hemorrhage the common carotid artery in the neck may be completely or partially obliterated to lessen the flow of blood to the site of the aneurysm, *provided* enough blood can be supplied from collateral vessels to preserve vital brain function. The procedure usually is done in stages of several days. A clamp (Silverstone or Salibi clamp) that has a detachable screw stem and can be tightened gradually is used.[94] Usually the surgeon adjusts it each day, and the nurse who attends the patient watches him closely and is instructed to release the clamp at once if there is evidence of inadequate blood supply. Neurologic checks are done regularly by the nurse relative to placement of the clamp in the dominant or nondominant hemisphere. Any signs of muscle weakness in the face or in either extremity on the side opposite the incision or any changes in the level of consciousness, vital signs, or sensory or muscular coordination or control should be reported to the neurosurgeon at once. Immediate removal of the clamps may prevent irreversible complications such as hemiplegia, aphasia, and loss of consciousness. If symptoms of inadequate blood supply appear, further surgical treatment cannot be done safely, although the clamp may be left indefinitely to partially obliterate the vessel. If complete occlusion can be tolerated, the vessel may be permanently ligated. Thrombus formation with resultant cerebral embolism may complicate the patient's postoperative course following any surgery for a cerebral aneurysm. It is a feared and often fatal complication.

Before surgical treatment of an aneurysm is attempted, the surgeon usually explains the hope for cure and the risks involved to the patient's family. The nurse must appreciate how distressing the situation is for the family and should realize that the time spent waiting to know whether or not the outcome will be favorable seems interminable to them. The reasons for details of nursing care should be explained to them if they are with the patient. For example, it is important that both the patient and his family know that blood pressure, pulse rate, respiratory rate, and other pertinent observations will be taken frequently, since these procedures can be most upsetting if they are not explained.

If the surgery is successful, the patient will be cured, although usually he will be advised to avoid strenuous exercise and emotional stress for the rest of his life. Occasionally he may have a severe physical or mental handicap resulting from damage to brain tissue during surgery.

If the aneurysm cannot be successfully treated, however, the family should be aware that there is always the danger of sudden death. The patient must be protected from strenuous activity and excitement.

Carotid endarterectomy. Atherosclerosis of the extracranial carotid system has been considered important in the etiology of some strokes. This atherosclerosis most commonly involves the common carotid artery at or distal to its bifurcation into the internal and external carotid arteries. Narrowing (stenosis) of the internal carotid artery reduces blood flow to the corresponding side of the brain and is thought by many to be the source of small particles of blood clot that dislodge from the area of stenosis and embolize to the smaller blood vessels of the brain to cause strokes. Complete occlusion of the internal carotid may occur from this process with or without stroke manifestations.

Carotid endarterectomy essentially involves the reaming out of these diseased vessels. Postoperative care of these patients should include close attention to neurologic signs (changes in strength, mentation, speech, and level of consciousness). (See p. 366 for a discussion of cardiovascular surgery.)

■ INFECTIONS

The nervous system may be attacked by a variety of organisms and viruses and may suffer from toxic reactions to bacterial and viral disease. Sometimes the infection becomes walled off and causes an abscess; sometimes the meninges, or coverings of the brain and spinal cord, primarily are involved; and sometimes the brain itself is affected most. Organisms and viruses may reach the nervous system by a variety of routes. Untreated chronic otitis media and mastoiditis, chronic sinusitis, and fracture in any bone adjacent to the meninges may be the source of infection. Some organisms such as the tubercle bacillus and probably the pneumococcus reach the nervous system by means of the blood or the lymph system. The exact route by which some infective agents such as the meningococcus in epidemic meningitis and the viruses that cause encephalitis reach the central nervous system is not known.

Meningococcal meningitis (epidemic) and poliomyelitis are reportable communicable diseases. Because they are becoming less common and because they are discussed in specialized texts on communicable disease nursing, they will be mentioned only briefly here.

Meningitis

Meningitis is an acute infection of the meninges usually caused by pneumococci, meningococci (epidemic), staphylococci, streptococci, or aseptic agents (usually viral). Any other pathogenic organism, such as the tubercle bacillus, that gains access to the subarachnoid spaces can cause meningitis. Mild forms of the disease do occur and may be referred to as *meningism.* They may be caused by the specific viruses. A common form of the disease is lymphocytic meningitis, believed in many instances to be associated with a virus.

The incidence of bacterial meningitis is higher in fall and winter when upper respiratory infections are common. Children are more often affected than adults because of frequent colds and ear infections. Disease caused by the enteroviruses is more common in the summer and early fall than in other seasons of the year.

The onset of meningitis (except when due to tubercle bacilli) is usually sudden and characterized by severe headache, stiffness of the neck, irritability, malaise, and restlessness. Nausea, vomiting, delirium, and complete disorientation may develop quickly. Temperature, pulse rate, and respirations are increased. The diagnosis is usually confirmed by doing a lumbar puncture. Usually the offending organism can be isolated from the spinal fluid, and if a pyogenic organism is the cause, the fluid is cloudy. Treatment consists of large doses of the antibiotic most specific for the causative organism. This antibiotic may be administered directly into the spinal canal as well as administered by other routes.

Nursing intervention. Isolation is required for the patient with meningococcal meningitis until the acute illness is over. Particular care should be taken in handling discharges from the nose, mouth, and throat. Nursing care for the patient with meningitis includes the general care given a critically ill patient who may be irritable, confused, and unable to take fluids and yet who is dehydrated because of elevation of temperature. The room should be kept darkened, and noise should be curtailed as much as possible. The patient must be observed very carefully and must be constantly attended if he is disoriented. Padded side rails should be placed on the bed.

Residual damage from meningitis includes deafness, blindness, paralysis, and mental retardation. However, these complications are now rare, because the infection is effectively treated with antibiotics before permanent damage to the nervous system occurs.

Encephalitis

Encephalitis is inflammation of the brain and its coverings. Occasionally the meninges of the spinal cord are also involved. Encephalitis can have a variety of causes. A generalized inflammation of the brain can be caused by syphilis, and encephalitis can follow exogenous poisoning such as that which follows the ingestion of lead or arsenic or the inhalation of carbon monoxide. It can be caused by reaction to toxins produced by infections such as typhoid fever, measles, and chickenpox, and occasionally it follows vaccination.

Encephalitis caused by a virus and occurring in epidemic form was first described by von Economo in Austria, and the name von Economo's disease is still used to identify the widespread epidemic in the United States that followed the influenza epidemic in 1918. This form of the disease has not recurred since 1926. Von Economo's disease was also called encephalitis lethargica and sleeping sickness, a term still used by laymen. The demonstration that viruses can affect the central nervous system after a prolonged incubation period has resulted in considerable search for viral agents in many chronic neurologic diseases.

The death rate from encephalitis varies with epidemics but is generally fairly high. The most common and most serious sequela for patients who do recover from the acute disease is paralysis agitans, which may come on suddenly or develop slowly. Other residual neurologic symptoms may also occur and occasionally incapacitate the patient completely.

Acute viral encephalitis. Viral encephalitis appears to be caused by a number of viruses, some of which may be interrelated. Acute viral encephalitis can be classified as epidemic and sporadic forms. The primary causes of acute epidemic encephalitis are members of the arbovirus (those transferred by a biting arthropod to man) or togavirus group (named after properties of the virus). The sporadic or nonepidemic form in the United States is caused primarily by the herpes simplex virus.[69]

Clinical features of *acute epidemic encephalitis,* caused by the arboviruses that infect man (about 12 cause illness), are similar. The eastern equine form is more severe than the western form. The onset is abrupt with a high fever, headache, nuchal rigidity, and vomiting. Drowsiness or coma and focal or generalized convulsions develop within 24 to 48 hours after the onset. Focal neurologic signs develop, such as hemiplegia and cranial nerve palsies. There are typical findings in the cerebrospinal fluid. It is estimated that about three fourths of the patients die with the eastern equine form. Those who survive have neurologic deficits.

Nursing care consists mainly of symptomatic or supportive care and careful observation. Any change in appearance or behavior must be reported at once since the progress of this disease sometimes is extremely rapid. The patient is kept in bed, and side rails are used if disorientation develops. The patient must be constantly attended to prevent injury. If the temperature is high, sponging or other hypothermia measures may be ordered. Frequent changes of linen may be necessary if perspiration is excessive. There is no specific medical treatment for this disease. No isolation is necessary since encephalitis is not transmitted from man to man. Control of arboviral infection consists of avoiding exposure to the biting arthropod, eradication of the mosquito or tick vector, and immunization.

Acute encephalitis (nonepidemic) caused by the herpes simplex virus, occurs sporadically. It occurs at any age, but over half of the cases are in persons at least 15 years of age. Upper respiratory complaints often precede the onset of neurologic symptoms by at least 24 hours or longer. Headache and focal or major convulsions are the common early signs of cerebral involvement. A persistent high fever and coma are common. Spinal fluid proteins may be moderately elevated and red blood cells are often present when spinal fluid is examined. Herpetic skin lesions are not common. Treatment is supportive with anticonvulsant drugs and steroids to reduce cerebral edema.[71]

Poliomyelitis

Poliomyelitis is an acute febrile disease caused by three different strains of one of the smallest known viruses. With discovery of the Salk vaccine and its wide use since 1956 and the availability of a safe "live virus" vaccine (Sabin vaccine), this disease, which had been a serious crippler of children and young adults, promises to become quite rare. In 1967 there were only 41 cases reported in the United States and nine deaths.[106]

The incubation period for poliomyelitis is from 7 to 21 days. The virus attacks the anterior horn cells of the spinal cord where the motor pathways are located and may cause motor paralysis. Sensory perception is not affected since posterior horn cells are not attacked. Poliomyelitis sometimes takes a somewhat different form and attacks primarily the medulla and basal structures of the brain, including the cranial nerves; the term *"bulbar"* poliomyelitis is used for this form.

An important responsibility of the nurse is to help prevent poliomyelitis by encouraging immunization. Since this dreaded disease is now largely preventable, it is deplorable if all children and young adults do not receive protection. (See p. 311 for the recommended immunization schedule.)

Guillain-Barré syndrome (polyneuritis)

This disease, known variously as acute infectious polyneuritis and Landry-Guillain-Barré syndrome, is often serious because of the extent to which the nervous system may be affected. There is patchy demyelination found in nerve roots, root ganglia, and spinal and peripheral nerves. Axons are generally spared so that recovery may occur early; in severe forms, wallerian degeneration occurs with involvement of the axons, making recovery slow. In the severe forms there is an elevation of the protein in the cerebrospinal fluid. It is probably caused by a virus. The disease is most common in persons 30 to 50 years of age and is seen equally in men and women. If the seventh, ninth, and tenth cranial nerves are involved, the patient may have varying degrees of difficulty in swallowing, speaking, and breathing. The vital centers in the medulla oblongata may be affected, and the patient may die of respiratory failure. A dramatic illustration of the nursing needs of these patients is depicted in the film *Mrs. Reynolds Needs A Nurse.** Patients with less severe involvement may recover fully, although a year or more may transpire before the patient is completely well.

Neurosyphilis

In the late or chronic stage of syphilis, infection may involve the brain and spinal cord. The oculomotor nerves may be involved, causing inability of the pupil to react to light (Argyll Robertson pupil). *Tabes dorsalis* is the name given to the involvement of the posterior columns of the spinal cord and the posterior nerve roots. Since the sensory nerves are primarily involved, sensory symptoms predominate. The patient may have severe paroxysmal pain anywhere in the body, although perhaps the most common location is in the stomach. This condition, known as gastric crisis, may be confused with ruptured peptic ulcer or other acute conditions of the stomach or gallbladder. There may be areas of severe paresthesia on the skin. A common finding in tabes dorsalis is loss of position sense in the feet and legs. The patient is unable to sense where he places his feet, and his resultant slapping gait is highly characteristic of the disease. He has real difficulty walking at night because he depends on sight in placing his feet normally. Visual loss or even total blindness also occurs. Tabes dorsalis can cause trophic changes in the limbs and changes in the joints so that stability is lost (Charcot's joint).

General paresis is the term used to designate another late manifestation of syphilis in which there is degeneration of the brain with deterioration of mental function and varying evidences of other neurologic disease. Since patients with this condition occupy many beds in mental hospitals, the disease is discussed quite fully in texts dealing with nursing care of the mentally ill.

■ TRAUMATIC LESIONS

Parts of the nervous system commonly subjected to trauma include the craniocerebrum, spinal cord, and the peripheral nerves. With the exception of the latter, each is protected by a bony covering. The phrase "traumatic lesions," as used here, includes lesions resulting from direct physical force and injuries that result from sustained compression. Attention is

---

*Produced by Smith, Kline, & French Laboratories, 1500 Spring Garden St., Philadelphia, Penn. 19101.

directed primarily to the former in the following discussion.

Craniocerebral trauma

Craniocerebral trauma, or head injury, causes death and serious disability in people of all ages. Mortality from all types of head injury in the United States was 18,000 in 1967; another 13,000 were permanently disabled.[100] Primary traumatic lesions result from industrial, motor vehicle, and military accidents. It is estimated that 70% of motor accidents result in head injury. Brain injury causes more deaths than does injury to any other organ.

Craniocerebral trauma may result in injury to the scalp, skull, and brain tissues, either singly or collectively. Some of the variables that may modify the extent of the injury to the head include the location and direction of the impact, rate of the energy transfer, the surface area of energy transfer, and the status of the head at the time of the impact. Injuries vary from minor scalp wounds to concussions and open fractures of the skull with severe damage to the brain. The amount of obvious damage is not indicative of the seriousness of the trouble.

Contusions, abrasions, and lacerations of the scalp may occur. Lacerations of the scalp bleed profusely because of its large blood supply. A patient may bleed to death quickly if the external bleeding is not controlled. Most bleeding, however, is minor and controlled readily. An internal hematoma of the scalp may form and resemble a depressed fracture. Infection of the scalp may result from the presence of foreign debris. It should be stressed that the absence of external scalp injury does not preclude serious craniocerebral damage.

The skull indents and deforms when a physical impact occurs. Fractures commonly result, and they are classified as in other parts of the body (p. 956). Skull x-ray films may detect the fractures; a negative x-ray film does not exclude the presence of a fracture such as a hairline fracture. Fractures can occur distant to the point of impact. A compound and depressed fracture causes serious complications. The presence of a skull fracture does not necessarily indicate that brain injury has occurred. There is often a reverse correlation between skull damage and brain damage. Complications of skull damage may include injury to cranial nerves, epidural hemorrhage, and brain contusion.

Types of lesions. Damage to the brain tissues per se may include concussion, contusion, and/or laceration. Each is discussed briefly to differentiate them as to degree of damage and significance. The dura may remain intact in brain damage and is thought of as a *closed injury,* or the dura may be opened from a direct blow or from penetrating objects such as bone fragments or knives and is then classified as an open injury. A *concussion* is characterized by immediate and transitory impairment of neurologic function due to the mechanical force. There is no demonstrable structural alteration. There may be loss of consciousness that is instant or delayed and is usually recovered. The effect of a blow on the cranium to the soft brain tissues contained within the closed cavity is one of sudden and continuing movement. This effect can be likened to what happens as one stops suddenly when moving quickly with an open dish of fluid—some of the fluid spills. The only difference is that instead of spilling in the closed cavity, the brain tissues strike the bony covering forcibly. The sustained damage is variable in degree. There is damage to the brain stem centers. The alteration in consciousness in concussion is due to a lessened blood supply to the tissues, especially to the brain stem. No longer is concussion synonymous with loss of consciousness. Any person exhibiting an alteration in consciousness following a blow on the head should be observed by a physician for a period of time, since damage is not always immediately apparent. A *contusion* is a structural alteration characterized by extravasation of blood cells. It can be likened to bruising without tearing of the tissues. The contusion may be at the site of the impact or on the opposite side. A concussion or contusion site may be classified as a *coup* (at the site), *contrecoup* (opposite the site), or *intermediate.* Contusions often damage the cortex. *Laceration* of the brain tissues and blood vessels is a tearing of the tissues that may be due to a sharp fragment or object or a shearing force. It is obvious that hemorrhage may be a serious complication.

In summary, when the head receives a direct blow or injury, the brain moves in the skull and suffers varying degrees of damage. In addition, the brain swells to a great extent. It is unfortunate that the capacity of the brain to swell far exceeds the capacity of the closed cranial cavity to expand. Most deaths from head injury are from the brain swelling rather than from the actual primary destruction of vital centers. Brain edema is thus a major cause of increased intracranial pressure and its consequences as previously discussed on p. 884. Local and systemic disturbances in circulation occur with resulting anoxia. The brain damage may be minor or severe. There is often a great disparity between functional neurologic derangement and structural damage that can be demonstrated.

Hemorrhage resulting from craniocerebral trauma may occur at the following sites: scalp, epidural, subdural, subarachnoid, intracerebral, and intraventricular. Epidural and subdural hematomas are discussed because of the need for careful and continuing observations by the nurse. An *epidural hematoma* forms as blood collects between the dura and the skull. Since bleeding in this area is commonly due to laceration of the middle meningeal artery, it is capable of producing rapid clot formation. If lethargy or unconsciousness develops after regaining consciousness, an epidural hematoma may be suspected. Bleeding needs to be controlled promptly and the blood evacuated. Common sites for bleeding include basal and temporal skull fractures. The nurse should be alert for potential epidural hematomas when it is known that fractures exist in these sites. A *subdural hematoma* forms as venous blood collects below the dural surface. Since the bleeding is under venous pressure, the hematoma formation is relatively slow. However, the clot formation will cause pressure on the brain surface and may eventually displace brain tissue. If this expanding clot is not evacuated, it can contribute to a rise in intracranial pressure and its sequelae. Thus a subdural hematoma can become serious because of its location and compression of vital areas. If a patient who has been conscious for several weeks or months after a head injury becomes unconscious and develops neurologic symptoms, a subdural hematoma should be suspected. Nurses need be aware of the delayed signs of head injury as well as the immediate and more obvious ones. The focal neurologic signs from clot formation can be related to the site of the clot.

Fractures of the *base of the skull* are usually serious because of their site. When one is sustained, vital centers, cranial nerves, and nerve pathways may be permanently damaged. Trauma and the resulting edema may obstruct cerebrospinal fluid flow directly (or indirectly) with resultant increased intracranial pressure. If the injury has caused a direct communication between the cranial cavity and the middle ear or the sinuses, meningitis or a brain abscess may develop. Bleeding from the nose and the ears is suggestive of a basal fracture. Serosanguineous drainage from these orifices may contain cerebrospinal fluid.

Management. It is likely that most nurses will be called on to care for a patient with craniocerebral trauma several times during their nursing practice. For this reason, nurses need to be knowledgeable about treatment and nursing care. The saving of life and preservation of neurologic function is dependent on understanding the pathophysiology involved. The ability of the nurse to follow through the prescribed therapy and to make nursing decisions based on this understanding is essential. The immediate care is directed toward lifesaving measures and the maintenance of normal body functions until the time when recovery is assured. With appropriate continuing care and rehabilitation, even the severely injured may regain consciousness, recover to some extent, and return to an active life.

Care at the scene of the accident. The patient with an obvious head injury should be kept absolutely quiet. The wound should be covered with the cleanest material available, and pressure should be applied to the bleeding scalp *provided* there is no evidence of a depressed fracture. If it is apparent that a sharp instrument has penetrated the bone or if brain tissue is protruding through the wound, the wound must be left strictly alone, and no attempt should be made to remove the instrument of injury. No matter how serious the injury seems to be, no patient should be regarded as hopeless. Some truly remarkable recoveries have followed injuries in which contents of the cranial cavity were exposed. The patient should be kept warm, and a clear airway should be assured. If there is bleeding into the mouth, he should be turned carefully to one side, provided that several persons are available to help. The patient must be turned "in one piece," with the greatest care taken that the cervical spine is kept absolutely straight. A support must be placed under the head when the patient is on his side. No other moving of the patient should be permitted until an ambulance has arrived and experienced help is available.

Any person who has sustained a blow to the head must be watched closely following the accident. Even if consciousness has been regained almost immediately, the patient should sit quietly and not attempt to help others. Pulse and respiratory rate should be noted and cyanosis watched for. Vomiting may be a sign of increased intracranial pressure following injury, although sometimes it is an emotional response to shock.

Care in the hospital. The patient who has a skull fracture or other serious head injury must be attended constantly. The major aims of medical and nursing management are (1) to be constantly alert for changes in the patient's condition, especially changes that indicate any increase in intracranial pressure; (2) to sustain the patient's vital function until he has recovered sufficiently to resume them on his own; and (3) to minimize complications that will be life-threatening or interfere with full recovery.[75] (See p. 884 for a discussion of the components of increased intracranial pressure.)

Many neurosurgeons feel that alert and intelligent nursing care is often the decisive factor in determining the outcome of the patient. Side rails should always be on the bed, and a padded tongue blade or an airway to protect the tongue should be kept at the bedside since restlessness may come on suddenly and convulsions may occur. Usually the bed is kept flat, although some neurosurgeons believe that the danger of edema to the brain may be reduced by slight elevation of the head of the bed.[86]

REST AND CONTROL OF CONVULSIONS. The patient should be kept absolutely quiet. No vigorous effort should be made to "clean the patient up" during the first few hours after an accident. Rest is much more important. Sudden noises, flashes of light, and the clatter of equipment can increase the patient's restlessness and should be avoided. Portable equipment may be used to take radiographs. The nurse must remain in the room with the patient to help him move and to protect him from exertion. Restlessness may be due to the need for a slight change of position, the relaxation of a limb, or the need to empty the bladder. If nursing measures fail to allay extreme restlessness, the physician may order sodium amytal intramuscularly or paraldehyde. Morphine is not given to relieve pain because it will depress the patient's responsiveness and cause pupillary constriction, thus interfering with the necessary observation of pupillary change. Codeine or other mild analgesics may be necessary, however.

Twitching or convulsive movement of a body part should be recorded in detail and reported at once. In some medical centers, anticonvulsants are given prophylactically when seizures are anticipated; they are always given once seizures occur.[75]

VITAL SIGNS AND TEMPERATURE CONTROL. Usually the blood pressure, pulse, and respiratory rate are taken and recorded every 15 minutes until they become stabilized and remain within safe limits. Leaving the deflated blood pressure cuff on the arm helps to prevent disturbing the patient unduly when the pressure must be taken often. Developing the habit of not forcing the mercury column much above the expected reading also sometimes enables the nurse to take the blood pressure and yet barely disturb the patient. The eyes should be observed for inequality of the pupils and the lips and fingernails for cyanosis. A sudden sharp rise in temperature, which may go to 42° C. (106° F.) or higher, and a sudden drop in blood pressure indicate that the regulatory mechanisms have lost control and the prognosis is poor. When there is elevation in temperature, measures will need to be instituted to reduce the temperature to normal. Although hypothermia has been used in the treatment of patients with severe brain contusions, it is being used less often because of some of the undesirable side effects. Instead, the nursing measures usually employed to reduce temperature such as the administration of aspirin, tepid sponges, ice bags to the groin and axillae, and reduction of the temperature in the patient's room are used. Electrically controlled cooling mattresses are also frequently used.[75]

TREATMENT OF RESPIRATORY INSUFFICIENCY. One of the most common complications of severe head injury is respiratory insufficiency. Cerebral anoxia, which is a sequela of respiratory insufficiency, is a leading cause of death in these patients.[65] The patient who has respiratory insufficiency may have hypoxia, hypercarbia, hypotension, and dyspnea. Most generally these patients will have a tracheostomy performed and will receive respiratory assistance with one of the mechanical respirators (p. 594). Blood oxygen, carbon dioxide levels, and pH will have to be checked frequently to determine whether or not respiratory exchange is adequate. The patient will have to be suctioned as necessary to maintain a patent airway. (See p. 616 for further nursing care of the patient with a tracheostomy.)

DRAINAGE FROM EARS AND NOSE. The patient's ears and nose should be observed carefully for signs of blood and for serous drainage, which may indicate that the meninges have been torn (common in basal skull fractures) and that spinal fluid is escaping. No attempt should be made to clean out these orifices. Loose sterile cotton may be placed in the outer openings only. This procedure must be done with caution so that the cotton does not in any way act as a plug to interfere with free flow of fluid. The cotton should be changed as soon as it becomes moistened. Usually the flow of fluid subsides spontaneously. Antibiotics usually are given when a basal fracture has been sustained. Suction is never used to remove nasal secretions in any patient who has a head injury or who has undergone brain surgery because of the danger of causing further damage. Meningitis is a possible complication when communication to the nose and ears occurs. If there is evidence of drainage of spinal fluid from the nose, the patient should not cough, sneeze, or blow his nose. These activities may, in addition to contributing to the development of meningitis, enable air to enter the cranial cavity, where it may increase symptoms of intracranial pressure.[101]

LUMBAR PUNCTURE. A lumbar puncture is performed with caution following a head injury because of the danger of lowering spinal fluid pressure in the spinal canal, which may cause herniation of the brain stem into the foramen magnum resulting in severe pressure on vital centers. If a spinal puncture is performed, the patient must be watched exceedingly carefully during and following the procedure for such signs of pressure on vital centers as changes in respiratory rate and pulse rate.

CONTROL OF CEREBRAL EDEMA. Cerebral edema and increased intracranial pressure are common problems in patients with head injuries. When the patient's condition is deteriorating because of cerebral edema, dexamethasone is usually administered intravenously. The usual dose is 10 mg. initially, followed by 4 mg. intramuscularly every 6 hours thereafter. The steroids are also useful in combating shock associated with head injury. Usually they are employed only during the acute phase because of their associated side effects (p. 82). Other drugs used to reduce cerebral edema include intravenous mannitol and urea.

Electrolyte balance. Careful monitoring of electrolytes is necessary. Several types of sodium inbalance are known to occur in head injury. *Natriuresis,* or increased urinary excretion of sodium, is common. More recently this has been attributed to the inappropriate ADH syndrome (with an increased plasma level of ADH, serum hyponatremia, and hypotonicity). This aggravates cerebral edema. Hypernatremia, or cerebral salt retention, may also occur. No specific variations in potassium or chlorides have been noted. Plasma cortisol levels are also elevated in acute head injury.[5,9,32]

INTAKE AND OUTPUT. The patient's intake and output should be carefully measured and recorded. Fluid intake may be restricted to 1,500 to 2,500 ml. daily, and it is the nurse's responsibility to see that this is spread over the 24-hour period. Fluids may be given parenterally, by nasogastric tube, or by mouth, depending on the condition of the patient. The nurse must use caution in administering fluids orally, since the patient may have difficulty in swallowing. He may also have difficulty with vomiting and aspiration. The urinary output should be approximately 0.6 to 1 ml./kg. body weight/hour. This means that a man weighing 175 pounds should eliminate between 45 and 80 ml./hour, and if dehydrating drugs have been given, this amount may be greater. If necessary, an indwelling catheter will be inserted.

BOWEL FUNCTION. Bowel function is not encouraged for several days following a head injury. Mild bulk laxatives, bisacodyl (Dulcolax) suppositories, and oil-retention enemas may be prescribed. The patient is cautioned repeatedly not to strain in an effort to defecate since straining increases intracranial pressure.

Complications of head injuries. Patients with severe head injuries are candidates for several complications, some of which will be discussed in this section. As with any other patient who is seriously ill, the patient may develop atelectasis, pneumonia, or a urinary tract infection (secondary to catheter drainage). These infections are treated with a suitable antibiotic. *Stress ulcers* of the stomach and duodenum are also common after a head injury and are apparently caused by autonomic imbalances associated with the injury.[75] The ulcers are usually treated with anticholinergic drugs or with nasogastric tube feedings and antacids. Fluid and electrolyte imbalance may occur as discussed previously, and appropriate laboratory studies such as blood urea nitrogen and serum electrolytes are made frequently. The physician adjusts the intake of fluids and electrolytes in accord with the laboratory findings.

PROLONGED UNCONSCIOUSNESS. General nursing care as described in Chapter 10 is necessary for the patient with a head injury who remains unconscious for some time. Patients may be unconscious for as long as a month or more and yet finally make a satisfactory recovery provided good supportive care has been given.

EXTRADURAL HEMATOMA. Because of the danger of extradural hematoma, as discussed previously, many physicians believe that any patient who has sustained any injury to the head with loss of consciousness should be hospitalized for at least 24 hours. If he is asleep during this time, he should be awakened hourly to determine his state of consciousness. Some physicians believe that fluids should be restricted to 1,000 to 1,500 ml. for the first day or two and that a dehydrating substance should be given. If the patient does remain at home, the family should be told to watch him closely for signs of increased intracranial pressure, to awaken him hourly during the night after injury, and to bring him to a hospital at once if drowsiness, stupor, paralysis, convulsions, or inequality of the pupil size occur. The surgical treatment for extradural hematoma consists of making a burr hole through the temporal bone to relieve the pressure caused by the bleeding and to attempt to control the bleeding; sometimes a craniotomy is performed. Occasionally the patient has so much damage to the soft tissue of the brain that he dies despite relief of pressure caused by the bleeding. Usually such a patient is unconscious after the accident and is taken to a hospital at once.

The patient's family. Often when a person has sustained a serious head injury, members of his family are in a state of shock and need special attention. Occasionally the physician orders sedatives for them. If they are not permitted to see the patient because he is in the operating room or undergoing tests, they should be kept informed of his progress. A quiet, pleasant waiting room and a helpful word as to where such facilities as the telephone are located do a great deal to make them more comfortable.

Convalescence. The length of convalescence will depend entirely on how much damage has been done and how rapid recovery has been. Patients are usually urged to resume normal activity as soon as possible, since this seems to decrease the tendency to develop psychoneurotic responses to the injury. Patients may complain of headache and occasional dizziness for some time following a head injury. These difficulties should disappear within 3 to 4 months. Loss of memory and loss of initiative may also persist for a time. Occasionally convulsions develop due to the formation of scar tissue in injured brain substance or in its coverings. Such scar tissue may often be surgically removed to effect a complete cure. Loss of hearing and strabismus (cross-eye) sometimes complicate basal skull fractures and require a long period of rehabilitation. Sometimes corrective surgery can be performed for the strabismus.

Metabolic disorders and coma. Various metabolic disorders may cause coma *with or without accompanying head injury* and must routinely be excluded in any case of coma. Among the most common metabolic disorders are diabetic acidosis, electrolyte imbalance, hypoglycemia, and hepatic, pulmonary, and renal insufficiency. Other causes of coma include intoxications with alcohol or drugs such as barbiturates. Treatment varies and is determined by the condition causing the coma. Details of treatment and nursing care can be found under the specific condition involved.

Spinal cord trauma

Spinal cord injury (SCI) from accidents is a frequent and increasing cause of serious disability and death in the United States. It has been estimated that there are more than 100,000 individuals with serious spinal cord injury in the United States today.[100] Violent accidents are occurring more frequently and the patients are living longer. Automobile, diving, and other athletic accidents are the major cause in civilian life, and war injuries are a major cause among the military personnel.

Types of lesions. The spinal cord may be damaged by lesions arising outside the cord or by intramedullary lesions. The latter is a less common cause and is usually the result of intramedullary tumors (p. 930). Variable types of lesions arising *outside* the cord eventually cause damage within it. (The word "lesion" as used here is inclusive of both disease and injury.) For example, there may be direct extension of an extramedullary vertebral tumor to the cord, the protrusion of a ruptured intervertebral disc into the spinal canal (p. 918), or a fracture of the spine from direct trauma with resultant tearing of the spinal cord (Fig. 32-19). All such lesions may produce compression of the cord. The anatomy and size of the spi-

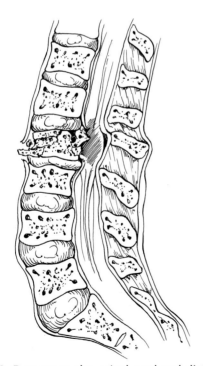

FIG. 32-19. Damage to the spinal cord and distortion of adjacent structures that may occur in traumatic injuries to the spine.

nal cord subjects the cord to compression with even minimal inward encroachment by extramedullary lesions. Edema then forms and contributes even more to cord compression. With damage to any part of the vertebral column, the cord itself becomes more vulnerable to damage. Recognition of the function of the spinal cord as the only conducting system of nerve impulses to and from the brain makes one realize the seriousness of spinal cord damage from any cause.

Severe traumatic lesions of the spinal cord, as from accident, may result in total *transection* of the spinal cord or a tearing of the cord from side to side at a particular level. This represents the most serious damage to the cord. With a complete loss of spinal cord functions, a partial transection or *cross section* is less serious and disabling. Because of the suddenness of a transection and the extensiveness of the tear, this results in a state known as *spinal or neural* shock. It is transitory and refers more to the areflexic state of the body than to cardiogenic shock. Following the injury, afferent impulses are unable to ascend from below the injured site to the brain, and efferent impulses are unable to descend to points below the site. Because transection represents an acute form of spinal cord damage, it is used as an example to relate and discuss the symptoms of spinal cord damage. There is considerable variability in the extent to which signs and symptoms are manifest in the individual patient.

Signs and symptoms of spinal cord injury. The signs and symptoms of cord transection and of lesser cord lesions depend on the level at which the lesion occurs and the degree of the damage. In the immediate stage of a transection there is a complete loss or deficit of motor and sensory functions as well as somatic and visceral sensations below the level of the tear. The individual has flaccid paralysis, areflexia, and hypotonia due to the disruption of nerve impulses as related to the injured level. Within hours, days, or weeks the involved muscles gradually become spastic and hyperreflexic with the characteristic signs of an upper motor neuron lesion. These changes are thought to represent the release of the muscle stretch reflexes from the inhibitory influence of the damaged pyramidal tract, resulting in hyperactive responses. Another theory is that damage of the extrapyramidal descending fibers, in close proximity to the pyramidal fibers, permits unmodified excitatory impulses to reach the lower motor neurons via the muscle spindles. There is thus an increased sensitivity of the lower motor neurons to afferent stimulation from the muscle spindles. Nurses need to be able to explain spinal shock to patients and their families so that the return of involuntary movements are not confused with voluntary movements.

Damage at the cervical cord level is the most critical level for an injury to occur. It causes paralysis of all four extremities and the trunk (quadriplegia). The sparing of any one muscle movement of the shoulder, arms, and fingers is dependent on the specific cervical level of the injury. At the C4 level, for example, there would remain scapular elevation movements only. All other muscle movements in the arms, chest, trunk, and legs are lost. In the immediate stage, muscles of internal organs such as the bladder and bowel are atonic. Perspiration is diminished, as is touch sensation. Since the diaphragm and intercostal muscles are affected, respiratory failure and death may result unless the patient receives adequate respiratory assistance. A pulmotor is sometimes necessary during transportation of the patient to the hospital where equipment to aid respiration is available. Pain is not usually an early problem.

At the thoracic level, injury results in chest, trunk, bowel, bladder, and lower extremity muscle losses. The amount of remaining function varies in this area relative to the specific level. Fortunately the individual has use of his upper extremities; the lower extremities are not functional (paraplegia).

Injury at the lumbar and sacral levels results in paralysis of the lower extremities. The center for micturition is located in the conus medullaris (S2 to S4) and is linked to the detrusor muscle of the bladder by parasympathetic sensory and motor fibers that run in the pelvic nerves; together they form the reflex arc. Sympathetic motor fibers (T11 and L2) control the trigone of the bladder. Somatic lower motor neuron fibers travel through the pudendal nerves to the external urethral sphincter and external anal sphincter and the perineal muscles. Impulses descend via the pyramidal system and synapse with the anterior horn cells at the sacral level and thus provide central control over micturition. Lesions above the conus result in a bladder that is capable of emptying itself reflexly or involuntarily after the spinal shock phase. The bladder is hypertonic and it is variously known as an "upper motor neuron bladder" and "automatic bladder." The emptying occurs spontaneously or automatically. The patient has no control over the act of micturition. Voiding may occur at intervals of 3 or 4 hours; there may be frequency, urgency, and incontinence. The reflex arc of micturition is intact in this type of bladder. When the cord lesion is at, or below, the micturition center, there is destruction of the center and/or the sacral nerve roots; the reflex arc is no longer intact. This type of bladder is known as a "lower motor neuron bladder" or an "autonomous bladder." Any contractions of the bladder muscle are the result of impulses transmitted through an intrinsic nervous mechanism that is within the bladder wall. The contractions, however, are not of sufficient strength or duration to empty the bladder. This can be done only by abdominal straining or by manual compression. Since the bladder musculature is hypotonic or flaccid, re-tention of urine and infection are common complications.

When injury occurs in the lower sacral area and the cauda equina nerve roots, away from the cord, the signs are variable and less severe. Often there is paraparesis and scattered lower motor neuron signs.

Alterations in sexual function occur from injury at different cord levels. Women appear to experience less alteration than do males. Male infertility is common. There is impotence, decreased sensation, and difficulty in erection and ejaculation. There is need for research in this area to identify more fully the extent of alterations.

Diagnosis of spinal cord injury or compression from accidents. Diagnosis is made from the history of the trauma, neurologic examination, and selected studies. It is most important to first detect if there has been any cervical vertebra fracture or displacement and concomitant spinal cord damage. Radiographs are always taken to detect fracture dislocations of the vertebrae or their parts. X-ray films are often taken while the injured patient is still on the stretcher in the emergency room. This lessens movement of the spinal column at a critical period. Myelograms and/or lumbar puncture may be done to detect subarachnoid blockage. Myelography can be carried out with ease and without moving the patient when contrast material is introduced through a lateral puncture at the junction between the first cervical vertebra and the base of the skull. In this way the contrast material flows downward across the site of a cervical fracture dislocation to demonstrate the presence or absence of subarachnoid block. Further diagnostic measures are often delayed until there has been correction of any cervical fractures as established by x-ray films. The thoracic and lumbar spine areas rarely justify priority diagnosis and treatment. There is, however, need to determine the presence of spinal compression in these areas. Both the lumbar and cervical spines are prone to flexion and extension movements that result from severe trauma.

It should be understood by the nurse that there are important variations in the neuroanatomy of the vertebral column at the cervical, thoracic, and lumbar areas as well as important segmental variations in the spinal cord itself. In the cervical area the vertebrae are unstable (to permit movement of the neck) and the cord at this level houses the most important neural structures in a copious dural tube. The anterior horn cells innervating the diaphragm (above C4) and the upper extremities are located in the cervical cord segments as well as the long motor tracts to the remainder of the body. In the thoracic area, by contrast, there is a stable bony column supported by the rib structures. The thoracic spinal cord fills the subarachnoid space almost completely and injuries in this area produce bony malalignments and are often associated with serious neurologic deficits. Finally, in the lumbar area the vertebrae are heavier and are supported by massive lumbar paraspinal muscles. The lumbar vertebrae thus have more stability than the cervical vertebrae but less than the thoracic vertebrae. The lumbar spine is more apt to be injured at the junction between the thoracic and lumbar area. The cauda equina, rather than the spinal cord is housed below L1. The tip of the spinal cord, or the conus, houses the micturition center.

Treatment and rehabilitation measures. The therapeutic and rehabilitative measures are discussed briefly relative to the immediate, intermediate, and late stages of care. It should be made clear that a tremendous variation in therapy is required for the individual patient, as related to variations in levels of injuries and in combinations of injuries to the spine and the cord.

Immediate stage. During the stage immediately following the injury the cervical area is given priority in treatment due to the neuroanatomic and physiologic features of the cervical vertebrae and cord. Therapy is directed first to realignment of the cervical bony column in the presence of demonstrated fractures, dislocations, or other cervical lesions. Any concomitant damage sustained by the cervical cord (or other levels) can be worsened by continuing bony instability. Therapeutic measures necessary to protect the cervical cord may include simple mobilization, skeletal traction, and/or surgery for spinal decompression through varied operative techniques. Stabilization of cervical vertebrae is usually accomplished by skeletal traction through the application of Crutchfield tongs (p. 916) or Vinke tongs. Once skeletal traction for the bony cervical abnormality has been established, further diagnostic and therapeutic measures are considered. The neurologist or neurosurgeon is also guided by the presenting neurologic deficits through continued monitoring of neurologic or spinal cord function. With the introduction of the anterior surgical approach to the cervical spinal column by Cloward,[18] early surgical intervention is now more frequently attempted, since sometimes, despite skeletal traction, extruded cervical disc materials produce continued compression of the cord. The primary advantage of the anterior surgical approach (or anterior laminectomy) is that it provides immediate stabilization of the spinal column by techniques of interbody cervical fusion and the direct removal of any extruded disc materials. Surgery, however, may be delayed by some neurosurgeons for several weeks after the injury, irrespective of the absence or presence of neurologic deficits, and when spontaneous healing of the fracture site provides a more stable cervical area. If evidences of spinal cord compression are demonstrated early, surgery may be warranted by the anterior approach.

Tracheostomy and respiratory assistance is almost always required in the immediate stage following upper cervical cord injury. Careful monitoring of blood gases and regular pulmonary toilet is essential. For this reason the patient may be admitted to a pulmonary intensive care unit. He is placed on a Stryker or a Foster frame with skeletal traction attachments.

Less immediate attention to thoracic fracture immobilization is necessary for the patient *with limited neurologic* deficits. He is often treated later with simple bed rest, hyperextension, and bracing (p. 914). Diagnosis is necessary, however, to determine the presence or absence of spinal cord compression at this level. Patients who show subarachnoid blockage and have associated neurologic deficits are treated through early surgical decompression. The onset of instantaneous paraplegia following direct thoracic trauma is often reversible through spinal decompression.

An early to an intermediate laminectomy may be performed in the presence of even severe lumbar neurologic deficits. Stabilization of the spine is done at the time of the primary surgical intervention or delayed until later in the posttraumatic period. Long delays in lumbar laminectomies or exploration in patients who show early partial recovery are reported to be beneficial for recovery of some neurologic function.[57]

Also threatening to the life of the individual is the extent and effects of paralysis. Immediately, during the areflexic period, medical attention is directed toward the prevention of complications that occur as a result of the loss of motor function. In addition to the more obvious effects apparent in the involved skeletal muscles, there may be loss of vasomotor tone, bladder tone, and bowel peristalsis. The prevention of bladder and bowel distention must be avoided since they may result in mass reflex or autonomic hyperreflexia (p. 912). Pressure sores and contractures that develop when one is unable to move himself and/or to sense the need to do so often result in serious consequences and should be prevented. The establishment of early rehabilitation programs are necessary to prevent such complications and to enhance the return of muscle strength.

There has been increased interest in the early treatment of the spinal cord injury. This interest was stimulated by demonstrations that experimentally produced cord injuries in animals are reversible if treated early. Some forms of early treatment such as localized spinal cord cooling and myelotomy are undergoing experimentation in some university centers.[1,27] It is too early to assess their value at this time. Continued research in the immediate care at the time of injury is crucial to progress in treatment. Also, care received during transportation requires study and control since poor first-aid care negates the effects of optimal care given during the later stages.

The use of adrenal corticosteroids for the prevention and alleviation of spinal cord edema has recently gained more acceptance. The efficacy of steroids in the reestablishment of membrane stability and in the control of central nervous tissue edema has been documented clinically.[11] Methylprednisolone (Solumedrol) at a dosage level of 60 to 80 mg./day (or equivalent dosage of other corticosteroids) may be utilized for the first week or longer following injury.

Intermediate stage. During this stage of treatment, rehabilitation and nursing care measures are focused on mobilization and patient-family education. Quadriplegics and paraplegics need to learn to live with the sequelae of paralysis. The goal of rehabilitation is to minimize the disability and assist the patient toward independence to the extent possible. A psychiatrist may assume responsibility for care at this time.

Early mobilization of the patient is important regardless of the level of injury. At first, mobilization includes active or passive turning movements and range of motion exercises. This helps to prevent pressure sores and contractures and to develop independence in bed activities. Later, mobilization is progressively effected through crutch walking and/or bracing or wheelchair activities. Mat exercises and resistive exercises are initiated to increase muscle strength and endurance.

In addition to instruction about mobilization techniques, the patient is trained to be functional in activities of daily living, with or without equipment and as related to his life-style. Activities included are those self-care activities that one performs during an ordinary day such as bathing, grooming, dressing, eating, elimination, communication, and ambulation. Specific activities related to occupation are often delayed until the late stage. The patient needs to know how to obtain bowel and bladder automaticity, and he needs to know how to prevent bladder infection. It is essential to understand how to prevent pressure sores when one sits in a wheelchair most of the day, and it is important to know how to manage the wheelchair itself. The patient's family is included in instruction since many patients may require some supervision and/or assistance in activities of daily living following discharge from the hospital. The reaction of family members to spinal cord injury is often great. The family as well as patient need help in coping. In addition to medical and physical rehabilitation measures, there is equal need for psychologic, emotional, sociologic, and vocational rehabilitation. The trauma of spinal cord injury also results in numerous interpersonal problems and makes adjustment to one's environment difficult.

Late stage. Education and medical and surgical follow-up are continued through the late stage as related to the rehabilitation goals of the individual patient. There may be need for surgical treatment of spasticity, or mass reflex, with denervation procedures.

Orthotics, or the application of external appliances to support a paralyzed muscle or to promote a specific motion required in activities of daily living, may require further follow-up care. It is of interest that electrostimulation of muscles of the bladder through remote control to regain micturition control in the paraplegic patient is now being tested clinically.[12] Success of this electronic spinal neuroprosthesis will assist in preventing urinary complications that are often a cause of death. Functional intramuscular electrostimulation of paralyzed upper extremities muscles is also currently being tested.[78] Since there is little or no external splinting required in the latter orthosis, it will be cosmetically appealing to the quadriplegic if successful.

In summary, although most of the complications of paralysis are now preventable, it is regretable that complications do occur during and after hospitalization. Under optimal conditions a spinal cord injury patient would be evacuated by a knowledgeable first-aid team from the site of the accident to a regional spinal cord center. At the center a team of specialists would supervise treatment while planning a long-term rehabilitation program. Rehabilitation begun in the center eventually would be carried out consistently until patient discharge. Thereafter the center would provide a continuity in management throughout the residual stages.

General principles of management

The general principles of management common to all types of spinal cord injuries (including transection) are presented in the following discussions. Nursing care specific to fracture of the spine and ruptured cervical intervertebral disc follows (p. 916).

Position and movement. Before moving a patient with acute spinal cord injury onto a bed from the stretcher on which he is admitted, the physician should be consulted about the type of bed he wishes used. The selection will depend on the physician's preference, the type of injury, the size of the patient, and the equipment available. If a regular bed is to be used, a full-length fracture board should be placed on top of the bedspring under the mattress. This board prevents sagging of the mattress and motion of the spine. If the bed is to be gatched, the board must be hinged, or two or more boards with correctly placed breaks can be used. Mattresses containing springs should not be used. Instead of springs and one mattress, some physicians prefer two hair mattresses placed on top of the fracture board. Some use the knee gatch to provide hyperextension to the spine in selected thoracic and lumbar fractures (Fig. 32-20); the bed must then be made

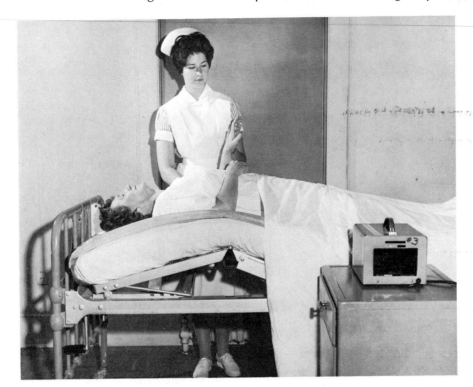

FIG. 32-20. Hyperextension for spinal fracture can be accomplished by gatching the bed with the patient head to foot in the bed. This patient is placed so that the highest point is directly under the fracture. An alternating air-pressure mattress is often used on the bed to prevent pressure sores. The patient must be observed carefully for changes in sensation or use of the extremities.

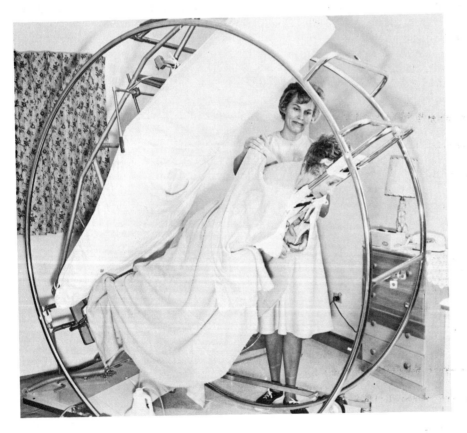

FIG. 32-21. CircOlectric bed used by a paralyzed patient being cared for at home. (Courtesy Stryker Corp., Kalamazoo, Mich.)

up "head to foot." Sponge rubber mattresses are widely recommended and, when available, are commonly used when there is the possibility that for some time the patient will be moved very little and with extreme difficulty. If available, an alternating air-pressure mattress often is used. It alternates the points of pressure at regular intervals. Since it may be dangerous to move the patient for some time and since he may have loss of sensation and paralysis of part of the body, pressure areas develop easily. The

910

mattress and entire bed foundation must be well protected with plastic sheeting so that incontinence will not cause damage.

Before moving the patient, the bed foundation should be completely adjusted, with gatches raised as ordered, bolsters placed in the desired positions, and a turning sheet available so that a minimum of motion will be necessary. Three to five people are needed to move the patient from the stretcher to the bed, depending on his size and the location of injury. The physician should supervise moving the patient. The body should be supported in proper alignment, and if necessary, a manual hyperextension should be applied to the spine as the patient is moved (p. 265).

Many facilities now have CircOlectric beds, and these are especially useful in the care of the patient with a spinal cord injury. The Stryker frame, often used for these patients, can provide for only two positions, prone and supine, and movement must be in a horizontal direction. With the CircOlectric bed, many more position changes such as vertical, horizontal, and sitting are possible. Movement of the bed is vertical and can be stopped at any angle while good body alignment is maintained. Patients on a CircOlectric bed can be placed in sitting or standing positions, thus preventing hypotensive reactions that often occur when patients have been immobilized horizontally over a period of time (Fig. 32-21). CircOlectric beds can also be operated by hand in the event of a power failure or when the use of an electric model is contraindicated.

Observation. The nurse must carefully observe the patient with a spinal fracture, a cord tumor, or a ruptured intervertebral disc for signs of cord compression. The motion, strength, and sensation in the extremities should be tested at least four times a day and more frequently if specifically ordered. Any change in motion or sensation should be reported at once as related to level, since immediate surgery may be needed to relieve pressure on the cord. Some of the laminae may be removed to prevent pressure from edema.

General hygiene. If cord damage has occurred, nursing care will depend on the level of the injury. Patients with cervical lesions, for instance, will be unable to do anything for themselves. Meticulous skin care, maintenance of correct body alignment, preservation of range of joint motion, and attempts to preserve muscle tone are imperative nursing measures in the care of any paralyzed patient. No external heat such as that from a hot-water bottle should be used if the patient has loss of sensation, since he will not feel excessive heat. Care should also be taken to be sure that bathwater is not too hot, and paralyzed areas should be inspected daily for any signs of skin irritation. There will be no perspiration in areas supplied by nerves coming from below the cord injury. At first this may cause the patient to

have an elevated temperature, which may be treated as described on p. 84. Later, there may be excessive perspiration of the unaffected areas, which will need to be bathed frequently.

Skin care. The loss of sensation and paralysis following a spinal cord lesion can result in pressure sores unless attention is immediately given to prevention. Pressure sores are an unnecessary and costly additional disability that can delay rehabilitation for many months. In many instances, surgery is necessary to repair the decubitus.

The keys to prevention are elimination of pressure and promotion of cleanliness. The patient should be turned every 1 to 2 hours, depending on skin tolerance. When physically able, the patient in a wheelchair should do push-ups every hour to relieve pressure on the ischium. Otherwise he must return to bed at planned intervals to prevent pressure sores from developing. Bony prominences such as the sacrum, ischium, trochanters, heels, iliac spines, and pretibial areas are the most frequent sites for breakdown. These areas must be checked each time the patient is turned and must be massaged periodically. If a sore does occur, the patient should not put pressure on the area. Devices to relieve pressure such as gel or water flotation seat pads and mattresses, foam mattresses, and sheepskin are helpful in preventing pressure areas.

Diet. If the patient's arms are paralyzed or if he is not allowed to move them, he will need to be fed or use adaptive devices. The diet for any patient who is immobilized because of spinal injuries should be high in protein to increase the resistance to decubiti. Most fruit juices and foods high in calcium are limited, since urinary calculi tend to form quite easily in patients who are completely immobilized and in those who have fractures. Juices such as cranberry or prune juice are preferred since they aid in promoting acidic urine. (See Table 20-1, p. 440.)

Urinary output. The patient may have urinary retention because of injury to lumbar and sacral spinal nerves. Since he may have no sensation of needing to void, the nurse should check carefully for voiding and for distention of the bladder. A Foley catheter may be inserted into the bladder, or a cystostomy may be performed. Later, if the injury is not in the lumbar area, automatic bladder function may be established (p. 177). The presence of an indwelling catheter makes the patient highly susceptible to urinary infection. The best means of preventing infection is maintenance of fluid intake (3 to 4 L. daily) and meticulous aseptic technique in changing and irrigating catheters. The patient *must* know the signs of infection and *must* have a genitourinary check-up once a year or more frequently.

Gastrointestinal function. Following an acute injury to the spinal cord, the patient often has abdominal distention. A rectal tube may be used, and neostigmine may be administered hypodermically to stimulate peristalsis. A nasogastric tube or a Miller-Abbott or Cantor tube attached to suction may be tried.

Stool softeners, adequate fluids, prune juice, and suppositories are recommended to obtain bowel function. Long-term use of laxatives and enemas is discouraged, although they may be necessary during spinal shock. If it is necessary to give an enema, 200 ml. should be sufficient; no more than 500 ml. should ever be used. The aim of bowel re-education is to get the patient in the habit of defecating every day or every other day at the same hour. It may be difficult to achieve an adequate bowel program with a flaccid bowel. However, good results often are achieved by using the methods described. A permanent loss of bowel control may occur. (See p. 183 for care of and rehabilitation measures for patients with fecal incontinence.)

Pain. Patients with spinal injuries often have a great deal of pain at the level of the injury that radiates along the spinal nerves. A thoracic injury causes chest or back pain, whereas a lumbar injury causes pain in the legs. Analgesics such as acetylsalicylic acid or other nonnarcotic analgesics are ordered. Narcotics may be given for a short time, but are contraindicated for long-term use because the patient's problem may be chronic. Psychologic assistance is often recommended to help the patient learn to cope with pain. If the patient has a high cervical injury, no narcotics should be administered because respirations may be further depressed. Sometimes the paravertebral nerves are injected with 95% alcohol to relieve thoracic pain. This measure may provide relief for several weeks or even months.

Autonomic hyperreflexia. Autonomic hyperreflexia (mass reflex) occurs in patients with cord lesions above the sixth thoracic vertebra; most commonly it occurs in cervical injuries. The clinical signs are bradycardia, paroxysmal hypertension, sweating, and severe headache. The hypertension can be profound and may result in death if not treated immediately.

The most common causes are visceral distention (distended bladder, impacted rectum). If the patient complains of these symptoms, the patency of the catheter should be checked and a new catheter inserted immediately if the catheter is plugged. This should result in reversal of symptoms. In addition, a ganglionic blocking agent such as hexamethonium chloride (Methium chloride), 12.5 mg. intravenously, may be administered.[84] The patient must be made aware of the symptoms of autonomic hyperreflexia and call the nurse or physician immediately if they occur.

Prevention of respiratory complications. Respiratory complications are common following injury of the spinal cord. The patient should be encouraged to take frequent deep breaths, fully expanding the lungs. If he cannot be turned, deep-breathing exercises should be supervised, and he should take 10 to 15 deep breaths at least every 2 hours. Intermittent positive pressure breathing treatments (IPPB) may

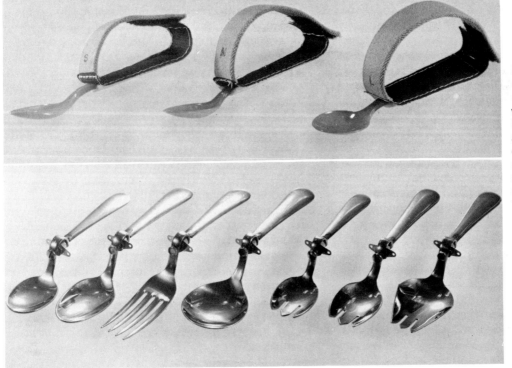

FIG. 32-22. Self-help devices for the quadriplegic. **A,** Spoons with small, medium, and large universal cuff attachments which fit over the hand. **B,** Swivel spoons, forks, and sporks (combination spoon and fork, last 3 to the right), which are used with the universal cuff. (Courtesy Fred Sammons, O.T.R., Chicago, Ill.)

be helpful in promoting deep breathing. Patients who can be turned should have position changes at least every 2 hours and should be encouraged to take deep breaths. If coughing is not contraindicated, it should be encouraged also, but the physician should be consulted before urging the patient to cough. Patients who have injuries of the thoracic spine tend to splint their chests and have shallow breathing. Analgesics may be given to control the pain so that the patient will no longer splint his chest and will breathe more deeply.

Rehabilitation. Anyone who has developed paralysis will undergo a period of emotional adjustment. The disability is a loss the patient will mourn; therefore the nurse can expect the patient to go through

the process of grieving. This means he will move through various stages of shock, denial, and depression to eventual recovery or adjustment.[84] The patient with paraplegia or quadriplegia *must* be knowledgeable about self-care related to diet, hygiene, skin, bowel and bladder function, and fluid intake. The major responsibility for teaching this care to the patient and family rests with the nurse. Many self-help devices are available for these patients (Figs. 32-22 to 32-24).

As the patient recovers, every possible effort should be made to help him do as much as possible for himself. Supplies should be placed within his reach on special trays or on overbed tables, and he must be given time to perform what daily personal

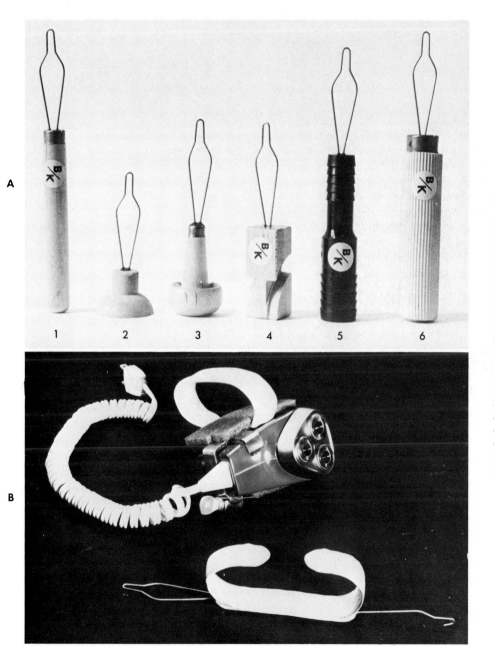

FIG. 32-23. Self-help or assistive devices. **A,** A variety of button hooks are available. From left to right, the hooks are designed to meet the needs of patients with the following disabilities: *1,* hemiplegia or quadriplegia; *2,* hemiplegia (especially CVA) or upper extremity amputation; *3,* hemiplegia; *4,* upper extremity amputation and hook prosthesis (note that handle is cut to be gripped by the hook); *5* and *6,* hemiplegia or quadriplegia. **B,** Electric razor with universal cuff and a combination button hook and zipper pull. These are designed to be used by the quadriplegic patient. (Courtesy Fred Sammons, O.T.R., Chicago, Ill.)

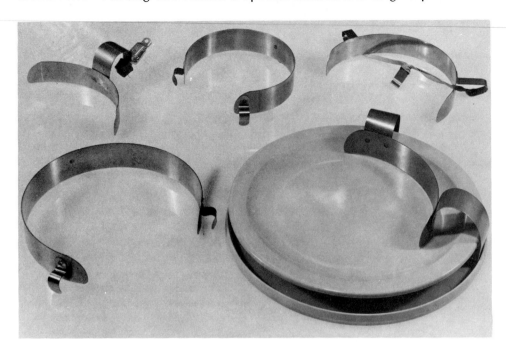

FIG. 32-24. A variety of food guards. Lower right-hand corner shows food guard attached to plate. Food is pushed against guard to help get it onto utensil and to prevent it from being pushed off plate. (Courtesy Fred Sammons, O.T.R., Chicago, Ill.)

care he can manage for himself. Diversional activity should be started to keep him constructively occupied. An occupational therapist can help the nurse in selecting appropriate activities. However, if an occupational therapist is not available, the patient may do any light handiwork that he enjoys and that is feasible, provided he can use his arms. A radio, television set, and reading material may help to pass the time. If the patient's neck is hyperextended, books that can be projected on the ceiling are useful if they do not cause eyestrain. Volunteers are exceedingly helpful in reading to patients. The patient's family and friends should be encouraged to visit often and to keep him up-to-date on activities in his home and community.

Rehabilitation depends on the extent and level of the cord injury, the emotional reactions of the patient, his age, and other factors. Muscle exercises often can be started long before the patient is allowed up, and this practice lessens the period of rehabilitation necessary for returning to activity. The patient should be kept in proper body alignment at all times to prevent shortening of muscles and contracture of joints. The patient who must be kept on his back should have a small, round bolster placed under the knees so that the proximal end of the tibia is supported without any popliteal pressure. Bath towels or a small pillow can be used to fashion such a bolster. A firm, flat pillow should be placed under both calves, and the feet should be firmly dorsiflexed against a footboard. Foot drop and contractures at the hips and knees may take months to overcome, and they may prevent the paralyzed patient from being able to walk even when he uses braces and crutches. Part of the nurse's responsibility is to teach

the patient proper methods of transfer from bed to wheelchair or commode (Figs. 32-25 and 32-26).

Before the patient is permitted to be up following a spinal injury, a brace may be prescribed. A *Taylor back brace,* made of padded and covered metal bars to support the back, is often used. It has sturdy straps that come forward to be fastened over a muslin "apron." All braces and corsets must be custommade and are quite expensive. The cost of a back brace varies according to the materials used in construction. Costs range from $85 to $125, depending on the prescription. The brace or corset should be applied before the patient gets out of bed, and he will need help in getting into it. The patient should wear a thin knitted undershirt next to the skin to keep the brace clean and to protect the skin. Correct use so that the brace fits contours of the buttocks and chest as designed makes a great deal of difference in the patient's comfort. Care should be taken that the apron is smooth and that tapes are not twisted. The patient's emotional reaction to wearing a brace or a corset is important, since it vitally affects ultimate rehabilitation. Attention to small details that help in initial acceptance of this somewhat uncomfortable and unfamiliar piece of "clothing" is important. The patient should practice putting the brace on while he is in the hospital if he must wear it for some time. A close member of his family may visit the hospital and learn to assist him. Patients who live alone and who are unable to care for their braces themselves may need to have a public health nurse help them in the home or teach someone else to assist. The patient wearing a brace should be especially careful in crossing streets and in engaging in activities such as walking down stairs, since he is limited in his ability

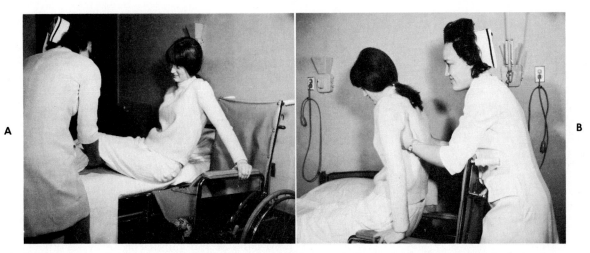

FIG. 32-25. Two methods of transferring the patient with paraplegia from bed to wheelchair. In both methods patient pushes up with her arms to lift buttocks from bed to chair. **A,** Patient is moving sideways into chair as nurse transfers patient's legs. Note that wheelchair is placed next to bed and that the right armrest has been removed. **B,** Patient is moving backwards into wheelchair. The paralyzed legs rest on bed and must be lifted down. Patients with spinal tumors or injuries are often paraplegic. (Courtesy Neuropsychiatric Institute, University of Illinois Hospitals at the Medical Center, Chicago, Ill.)

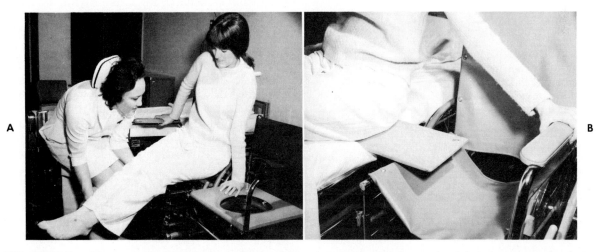

FIG. 32-26. Teaching paraplegic patient methods of transfer. **A,** Moving from wheelchair to commode chair requires the same technique as moving from bed to chair. Note that adjacent arms of both chairs have been removed. **B,** A sliding board may also be used to provide a firm surface on which to move from bed to chair. (Courtesy Neuropsychiatric Institute, University of Illinois Hospitals at the Medical Center, Chicago, Ill.)

to shift his balance quickly to prevent an accident.

Following fracture of a cervical vertebra, a neck brace may be ordered. This brace fits in such a manner that the chin rests on a cup, and the neck is kept in slight hyperextension. Patients who have a ruptured cervical disk may also need to use a neck brace, and the *Thomas collar* is often used (Fig. 32-27). A Thomas collar can be quite cheaply improvised as follows: (1) cut a piece of firm cardboard the width desired; (2) pad it with cotton or dressing pads and secure with bandages; and (3) cover the collar with stockinette and carefully stitch at the top and bottom, avoiding bumps or knots that may irritate

the skin. The collar is usually anchored at the side with wide adhesive tape and must never be removed without specific orders from the surgeon. The collar extends well up under the chin and prevents flexion of the neck. A Thomas collar, as constructed by a specialist in bracing, costs from $18 (plastic and adjustable) to $45 (with chin piece) relative to the kind of support provided. The patient who wears any brace to hyperextend the neck has difficulty in seeing where he is going and must be cautioned about this problem because accidents can occur easily during everyday activities such as crossing streets and going down stairs.

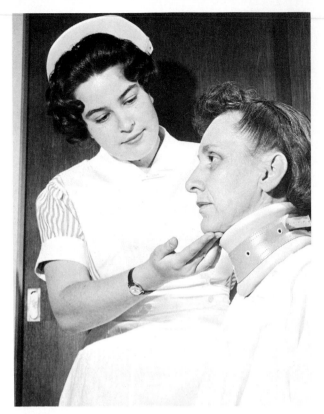

FIG. 32-27. This patient has been fitted with a neck brace following a cervical fracture. As the patient becomes accustomed to the brace, the nurse checks to see that skin irritation does not occur.

All patients who have had spinal injuries should wear shoes with firm lasts and low heels. If the woman patient has always worn moderately high heels, she should continue to wear them rather than to wear flat-heeled shoes. Shoes that tie are preferable. The patient is usually asked to have his family bring his shoes to the hospital so that they may be examined by the physician and so that they may be worn when he first walks about in the hospital.

Nursing care of the patient with a fracture of the spine

Fractures of the spine may cause compression of the bodies of the vertebrae or smashing of the laminae, with or without dislocation of parts, and compression of the spinal cord may result. (The emergency care of patients suffering fracture of the spine is discussed on p. 265.) Nurses should know and be able to teach others what symptoms indicate spinal fracture and how to care for a patient with a spinal fracture so that cord damage is not caused or increased. Spinal fractures should be suspected after automobile accidents, falls, and diving accidents.

Hyperextension. The patient with a spinal fracture may be placed in hyperextension since this position causes the least pressure on the spinal cord. Hyperextension may be accomplished by various means. Skeletal traction may be used. Small burr holes are drilled in the outer portion of the skull over each parietal region. *Tongs* (usually Crutchfield) are then inserted into the holes, the skin around the tongs is sutured, and a collodion dressing is applied. From 10 to 20 pounds of weight are attached to a rope coming from the center of the tongs and extend-

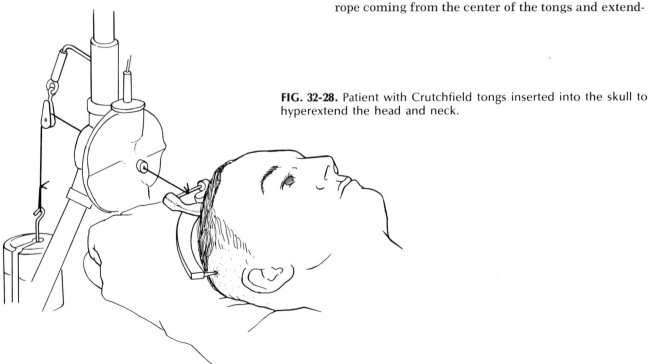

FIG. 32-28. Patient with Crutchfield tongs inserted into the skull to hyperextend the head and neck.

ing over a pulley attached to the head of the bed. If Crutchfield tongs are to be used, the bed should be made up "head to foot." The nurse must be sure that the patient does not slip up in the bed enough for the weights to rest on a rung of the bed or on the floor. The rope should be free of the mattress or any other obstruction that might decrease the amount of pull needed and thus harm the patient (Fig. 32-28). Sandbags are often placed above the patient's shoulders to help prevent his slipping toward the "head" of the bed. Occasionally the "head" of the bed may be elevated by placing the bed on blocks to give countertraction and to prevent the patient from slipping toward the "head" of the bed. Since elevation of the "head" of the bed increases the traction, it must not be done without a specific order.

In order to obtain traction and hyperextension, a leather chin strap (Sayre strap) attached to a pulley and weights, as described for use with tongs, may be employed. The strap fits snugly under the chin and against the occipital protuberances. Leather straps from front and back meet a metal spreader to which the pulley rope is centrally attached. Skin care of the patient's chin is extremely important when this kind of traction is used. The amount of pressure on the skin and soft tissues depends on the amount of weight used. Traction must not be released without an order, but the chin may need to be gently massaged as often as every hour. The nurse can exert gentle pressure on one side of the chin as she massages the other side with her other hand. Alcohol and powder should not be used, and frequent sponging of the skin is necessary to protect the leather from perspiration and to make the patient more comfortable. A small piece of rubber sponge, sheepswool, or chamois is helpful if signs of skin irritation and pressure occur. When feeding the patient, the nurse should take care not to soil or moisten the leather chin strap.

Hyperextension may also be accomplished by gatching the bed with the patient head to foot in the bed and placing him so that the high point is directly under the fracture (Fig. 32-20). If the bed gatch is not at the desired position, a small, firm, round bolster, the width of the mattress, may be placed under the top mattress at the desired level. Several tightly rolled bath blankets may be used to make a bolster of the desired size. Obviously a fracture board must be used to give firm support and it must be hinged to permit use of the gatches. This method of obtaining hyperextension is commonly used following fracture of a thoracic vertebra.

Members of the family should be prepared for seeing the patient in head or neck traction. Tongs are particularly frightening to them. Both the family and the patient should understand that the tongs do not go through the skull but only into the outer layer of bone. Actually, many patients get so much relief from pain from this type of traction that they accept it surprisingly well. An adjustable mirror attached to the head of the bed enables them to see about the room. Usually they are happier and more content when in a unit with other patients around them.

The patient who is placed in hyperextension cannot readily be moved about in bed. He may stay in traction for as long as 6 weeks. Care must be taken to prevent skin breakdown. On the physician's order the patient may be "logrolled" off his back periodically. His head must be held firmly and maintained in proper alignment with the body as the patient is turned.

Patients who are immobilized in head or neck traction or kept in hyperextension develop pneumonia easily. The patient must be instructed to take from 10 to 15 deep breaths regularly each hour when he is awake. The nurse should remain with him to see that it is done at least several times each day. Arms and legs usually may be exercised passively if the patient is paralyzed and unable to move himself, but a physician should be consulted before this is done.

Care of the skin is a major responsibility of the nurse, and the patient must be given back care at least every 2 hours. The nurse's work is made much easier if the patient is on a sponge rubber mattress, since two nurses working together can give the patient back care without moving him. Each nurse depresses the mattress with one hand and massages the patient's skin with the palm of the other. No part of the back should be neglected, although not all the surface of the back must be done at once, since this might tire the patient too much. The use of a bedpan presents a problem, but an orthopedic or a child's bedpan may be placed under the patient without moving him if two nurses work together. The part of the mattress under the buttocks should be depressed with one hand and the bedpan slipped into place with the other. To maintain correct spinal alignment, one of the nurses should insert a small towel roll at the small of the patient's back directly above the bedpan.

Extreme care must be taken in feeding any patient who is in hyperextension and lying on his back, since it is difficult to swallow in this position. Obviously, if the patient chokes, he cannot turn or be raised forward. A suction machine should always be on hand for immediate use in case the patient should aspirate into the trachea. The patient should practice swallowing saliva before he attempts to take fluids or solid foods. Usually he does best when given fairly soft food such as baked custard at first, because liquids tend to flow into the nasopharynx quite easily. Ideally the patient should be fed by the nurse. When it is necessary to delegate this task to others, the nurse should teach them and provide adequate supervision. Since feeding the patient takes time, it must be planned for; he must not be allowed to feel that he is a nursing problem on this account. Adequate food intake is necessary to prevent pressure areas from developing and to preserve general tissue health. Also, since meals are psychologically important to all people, the patient needs the emotional support that attractive meals will give when carefully fed to him.

Stryker frame and Foster bed. If the patient with a spinal injury can be placed flat in bed but cannot be turned in bed, a Stryker frame or a Foster bed may be used (Fig. 29-13). These beds make it possible to change the patient's position from abdomen to back without altering his alignment. Usually the patient on one of these beds is turned every 2 to 4 hours. The bed cannot be used for very obese patients because space between the frames is inadequate and cannot be adjusted sufficiently. The beds have two metal frames to which canvas covers are attached. The canvas used for the back-lying position has an opening under the buttocks to allow for use of a bedpan, and the canvas used for the prone-lying position can be cut out so that the male patient can void. When the patient is in the prone position, the canvas should extend from below the shoulders to the ankles, and a narrow head strap should be used to support the forehead. In the prone position the patient can eat, read, and do light activities with his hands. The canvas may be covered with thin sponge rubber mattresses cut the same size as the canvas and covered with bed linen. To turn the patient, the linen, mattress, and opposite canvas and frame are placed in that order over the patient. The frame is then fastened by bolting it securely in place to the metal attachment at head and foot. Straps are placed around both frames, and then two people release pivot pins at either end of the frame and slowly rotate the patient on the frame from his abdomen to his back or vice versa. The pins are reinserted, and the upper frame, canvas, and mattress are removed. The bed has armboard and footboard attachments to use, if desired, for permissible activity or for good alignment. The patient may be quite apprehensive about being placed on this bed, and, if possible, a demonstration of turning should be given to him before he is moved onto it. Another advantage of these beds is that they wheel easily, so that the patient may be taken to a recreational area for a change of surroundings. This type of bed is unsafe for a very restless or disoriented patient, although the straps may be used to give some security and protection.

Plaster jacket. A plaster jacket that extends from the shoulders to below the hips is sometimes used to treat the patient with a fractured vertebra below the cervical area. A fracture board and a firm mattress should be used. As soon as the patient returns from the plaster room, the nurse should check the cast at the top and bottom for crumbs of plaster, which can usually be removed at first but later are difficult to remove as they work downward or upward. The cast should be examined to be certain it is cut out enough to permit use of a bedpan. If it is not, the nurse must remind the physician, since it must be done before the patient has a bowel movement. The patient can usually urinate safely without soiling the cast. Plastic material may be used to cover the cast edges, and the head of the bed may be raised on blocks so that gravity can help to simplify voiding. The gatch must never be raised without an order, since this may cause the cast to crack. When the cast is dry, its edges should be bound with small petal-shaped pieces of adhesive tape to protect the skin from irritation. This procedure is known as "petaling" the cast.[58] The lower portion should be covered with plastic material fastened on the edge and pushed up under the cast so that it will remain in place when a bedpan is used. This material can easily be removed and changed if it becomes soiled.

If abdominal distention is troublesome, a "window," or opening, may be cut in the cast over the abdomen. The edges of this opening must also be bound. Such a window is useful in checking for distention of the bladder. Skin under the cast should be massaged with alcohol and powder. The nurse should slip her hand palm downward as far as she can reach to feel for crumbs or bits of plaster and any areas of skin tenderness, which may be caused by pressure or irritation. The cast is usually loose enough to permit threading a thin piece of terry cloth toweling from top to bottom under the cast to partially cleanse the patient's skin. This procedure is done by having the patient lie down, which permits the toweling to be pushed along the upper surface of the body, which "falls away" from the cast while he is in this position until it can be reached at the other end of the cast. The patient then turns slowly and supports himself by holding the upper rungs of the bed. Pillows may be needed to support the cast at the hips at this time. The toweling must not be too wet or the lining of the cast will become moist, but soap may be used, and the use of a scented cologne is often gratifying to women patients. (For further details, see orthopedic nursing texts.[58])

Management of the patient with a ruptured cervical intervertebral disc

The patient with a ruptured cervical intervertebral disc usually complains of pain and muscle weakness in the arms. Immediate surgery may be necessary to relieve cord compression, since the compression may cause respiratory failure.

Following surgery for a ruptured cervical disc, the patient should be closely watched for decrease in chest expansion because edema may temporarily paralyze the diaphragm and intercostal muscles. If there is a decrease in chest expansion, the patient may need to be given respiratory assistance at once.

The patient who has had surgery for a ruptured

cervical disc is placed flat in bed postoperatively with only a small pillow at the nape of the neck. The head should not be flexed, because pressure may then be exerted on the cord and cause respiratory failure. The patient may be turned, but the turning sheet should extend above the head. On the third postoperative day he may be placed in a semi-Fowler position, and pillows should be placed well down under the shoulders. Arm movements, even to eat, are prohibited until this time. The patient is allowed up on the fifth postoperative day, and a Thomas collar may be used to prevent forward flexion of the head for several weeks. More specific information on cervical fusion can be found in neurosurgical and orthopedic textbooks.

Peripheral nerve trauma

The peripheral nerves that lie outside the brain and spinal cord include the cranial and spinal nerves and their branches and plexuses. The disorders involving the peripheral nerves are similar to those that affect the central nervous system and are the result of traumatic, degenerative, vascular, inflammatory, neoplastic, and metabolic causes. *Neuropathies,* noninflammatory disorders, may involve one peripheral nerve (mononeuropathy) or involve multiple nerves (polyneuropathies). *Neuritis* refers to an inflammatory disorder, while *neuralgia* means a painful nerve disorder. Although discussion in this section is limited to neuropathies due to trauma, it should be clear that regardless of cause, the resulting nerve dysfunction will be similar and will be related to the site of the lesion. Some of the more common neuropathies (other than trauma) include nutritional, alcoholic, diabetic, lead, arsenic, hereditary, and infectious neuropathies.

Traumatic causes of peripheral nerve injury commonly include gunshot and knife wounds, fragmented fracture wounds, and surgical transections as in denervation surgery and amputations. They variously result in stretching, laceration, and compression of the peripheral nerve; there also is much variation in the degree of injury. Fortunately the axons of peripheral nerves are capable of regeneration under favorable conditions.

Following trauma (or disease), the axon undergoes *secondary* or *wallerian degeneration* distal to the lesion (that is distal to the cells of origin) and for several segments proximal. The axon and the myelin sheath (secondary) degenerate and immediately undergo fragmentation; the fragmented particles are completely ingested within several weeks; the axis cylinder remains. Schwann cells and fibroblasts begin to proliferate along the degenerated fibers. (Myelin in *peripheral fibers* is formed by the Schwann cells.) During the regenerative phase, new axoplasm forms at the proximal edge of the injury and the regenerating fibers now grow distally and enter the empty neurolemma sheath, which has in the meantime proliferated. Myelin then forms around the regenerated axon. When a nerve has been severely damaged and fibrous tissue is abundant, regeneration is interfered with by a tangled mass known as a *traumatic neuroma;* this may have to be removed surgically.

The clinical signs and symptoms resulting from peripheral nerve lesions depend on the exact location of the lesion and the specific function of the involved nerve or nerves. Since peripheral nerves contain both sensory and motor components, there may be deficits in both components distal to the site. There will be alterations in pain, touch, temperature, proprioception, and stereognosis. Motor alterations include lower motor neuron signs such as flaccid paralysis and muscle wasting in those muscles innervated by the affected nerves.

Nursing care is specific to the areas of the body affected by the sensory and motor deficits. Plans for care are based on the nurse's understanding of the distribution and function of the involved peripheral nerves. The flaccid muscles demand attention to prevent deformities. Due to the atonia or hypotonia of the paralyzed muscles, they will be pulled excessively by the muscles that normally oppose them into abnormal or contracted positions. When associated tendons shorten, the contracture is permanent. Positioning of extremities in neutral or counterpositions will help in preventing deformities. Those areas of the body in which there is a loss of sensation need to be protected from injury. The patient needs to be taught protective measures such as not staying in one position too long since he cannot sense that damage is occurring in an area served by a damaged nerve. When positional sense is lost, there is also need to teach the patient to protect himself in walking and in other activities. Pain is usually localized and there may be more paresthesia than pain. The painful areas need to be protected from external stimulation when present. Following surgical intervention, careful positioning of the operative area, as prescribed, is important. Finally, the promotion of general health measures assist in the creation of conditions favorable to nerve regeneration.

■ NEOPLASMS OF THE CENTRAL NERVOUS SYSTEM

Neoplasms of the central nervous system include those arising from cells of structures within the cranium as well as those arising within or outside the spinal cord. Only the more common intracranial and intravertebral tumors will be discussed.

Intracranial tumors

Primary *intracranial* tumors, or *neoplasms,* arise from the intrinsic cells of brain tissues and the pituitary and pineal glands. *Secondary* or *metastatic* tumors are also a contributing type of intracranial tumor. Intracranial tumors are only one example of intracranial lesions. Variable intracranial lesions occur, such as hemorrhage, abscess, and trauma, and cause similar signs and symptoms as a neoplasm dependent on the site of the lesion.

Nurses should be aware that with the development of newer diagnostic techniques, modern surgical and radiologic methods, chemotherapeutic agents, and an increased understanding of functional anatomy of the cerebrum, the prognosis for patients with intracranial tumors is more favorable today than in the past. The prognosis, however, is dependent on early diagnosis and treatment since, as the tumor grows within the cranial cavity, it exerts lethal pressure on vital brain centers and causes irreparable brain damage and death. Although approximately one half of all primary brain tumors are benign, they may cause death by exerting lethal pressure on vital centers of the brain. It is important to remember that although cells of the central nervous system can regain function, even after cerebral edema, dead cells cannot regenerate. Early treatment is thus necessary in order to preserve cerebral functions. Early treatment also becomes important as newer techniques have been developed that improve operative risks and postoperative prospects for patients with intracranial tumors. These techniques include hypothermia (p. 209), the establishment of controlled hypotensive states during surgery by means of sympathetic blocking agents such as trimethaphan camphorsulfonate (Arfonad), and dehydration of cerebral tissues by administering urea compounds and/or mannitol before, during, and after surgery. Because the attitude of the nurse about the treatment of brain tumors cannot help but be communicated to the patient and his family, the nurse should make an effort to communicate a hopeful attitude while stressing the importance of early diagnosis and treatment of intracranial tumors.

Pathology. The symptoms of intracranial tumors result from both local and general effects of the tumor. Locally, the effects are from infiltration, invasion, and destruction of brain tissues at a particular site. There is also direct pressure on nerve structures causing degeneration and interference with local circulation. Local edema develops and, if it is long-standing, it is often sufficient to interfere with the function of nerve tissues. A brain tumor of any type situated anywhere in the cranial cavity may cause an increase in intracranial pressure. The increased intracranial pressure is then transmitted throughout the brain and the ventricular system. Eventually the ventricular system is distorted and displaced sufficiently to cause partial ventricular obstruction at some site, even though the tumor is some distance from the ventricular system. A tumor may directly obstruct a particular ventricle early when it grows adjacent to the ventricle, as shown in Fig. 32-29. Cerebral edema forms even at some distance from the tumor and generally adds to the increasing pressure. Papilledema results from the general effects of the increased intracranial pressure. Death is usually from brain stem compression resulting from herniation. The mechanism for the occasional acute focal symptoms that occur is thought to be due to rapidly increasing cerebral edema, or to functional decompensation of edematous tissues.[108]

Signs and symptoms. Every nurse should recognize the early and progressive symptoms of intracranial tumors. The presenting symptoms and the rapidity of their progression depends on the location of the tumor as well as on the type of brain tissue involved. The onset of symptoms begins either with evidences of neurologic dysfunction, which may be generalized

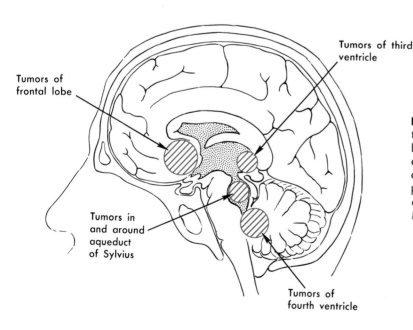

Tumors of third
ventricle

Tumors of
frontal lobe

Tumors in
and around
aqueduct
of Sylvius

Tumors of
fourth ventricle

FIG. 32-29. Sites of brain tumors adjacent to the ventricular system are illustrated. Note how a developing tumor at varied sites with extension distorts, compresses, and obstructs the ventricular system at some point so that increased intracranial pressure occurs early. (From Yahr, M. D.: Hosp. Med. **9**(9):8, 1973; by permission.)

or focal, or with symptoms of increased intracranial pressure. Progressive involvement of the brain occurs in either a stepwise or linear manner regardless of the type of onset. Subsequently, both types of symptoms are present if the tumor is untreated.

Focal and generalized signs and symptoms of neurologic dysfunction as a rule are referable to a specific area of the brain. Occasionally the concomitant occurrence of focalizing signs and symptoms and the symptoms of increased intracranial pressure produce false focalizing signs that are difficult for the neurologist to interpret. Localizing signs usually appear slowly and increase in severity over time. Such signs are rarely abrupt in appearance but their appearance may vary from a few weeks with highly malignant tumors to years with a benign tumor. Some benign tumors may, however, produce acute signs. In many instances, especially if the tumor is infiltrating brain tissue, an alert observer may recognize subtle changes that may suggest the need for neurologic examination before the signs and symptoms of increased pressure appear. The first noticeable symptom may be a change in personality or judgment. If motor areas of the cerebrum are involved, there may be weakness of the eyelid and facial muscles, as illustrated in Figs. 32-30 and 32-31, respectively. Sometimes the patient complains of paresthesia or anesthesia of a part of the body. He may complain of unpleasant odors, a sensation that often accompanies tumors of the temporal lobe. If the speech centers are involved, the patient may be unable to use words correctly or he may be unable to understand the written or spoken word. The patient may complain of loss of visual acuity or of double vision. These signs are indicative of pressure on the optic nerve or on one or both abducent nerves. Unexplained loss of hearing in one ear is suggestive of a brain tumor, although there are other causes to be ruled out. Other localized signs may include a staggering, wide-based gait that is suggestive of a cerebellar tumor. Convulsions occurring for the first time after middle age are suggestive of a brain tumor in the cerebrum or its coverings. Such tumors occurring within the cerebral lobes present disturbances that can be related to the different lobes as visualized in Fig. 32-32. Observation of such disturbances by the nurse assist in the location of brain tumors.

Signs and symptoms of increased intracranial pressure resulting from intracranial tumors usually occur after localized signs and symptoms have been present for varying time periods. However, signs and symptoms of intracranial pressure may occur first when a brain tumor is located within or near a ventricle, as previously shown in Fig. 32-29. The signs of increased intracranial pressure are the same as those discussed on p. 884. Headache at first is transitory and later becomes more constant; it increases in intensity with straining, coughing, stooping, and change of position. Nausea and vomiting usually occur as headache increases. Alteration in mental

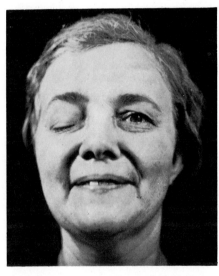

FIG. 32-30. This patient has a marked ptosis of the right eyelid. (From Davis, L.: The principles of neurological surgery, Philadelphia, 1942, Lea & Febiger.)

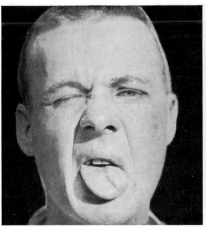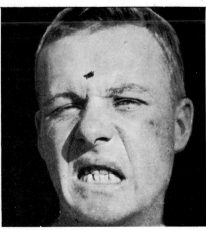

FIG. 32-31. This patient has muscle weakness due to left facial nerve and hypoglossal palsy. Note the deviation of the tongue and drooping of the mouth on the left side when the patient clenches his teeth. (From Davis, L.: The principles of neurological surgery, Philadelphia, 1942, Lea & Febiger.)

921

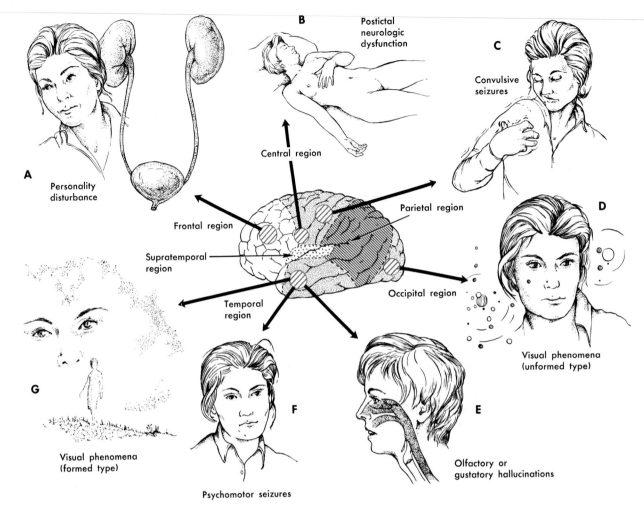

Fig. 32-32. Cerebral lobe tumor sites and examples of their respective localizing manifestations are pictorialized. **A,** Frontal region: specific personality disturbance. Inappropriate affect with lack of concern, facetiousness, and indifference to urinary control. Behavioral changes range from subtle personality patterns to frankly psychotic behavior or intellectual impairment. **B,** Central region: postictal neurologic dysfunction. Transitory period following a convulsive siezure (12 to 24 hours) during which the segment of the body most involved in the attack shows marked neurologic dysfunction. Has same implications as focal features of the attack. **C,** Central region (of motor-sensory strip): convulsive seizures. Jacksonian or focal sensory and motor convulsions in opposite hemisphere. **D,** Occipital region: visual phenomena—unformed type. Flashing lights sensation precede a convulsion. **E,** Temporal region: olfactory or gustatory hallucinations. Olfactory and gustatory hallucinations predominate in a seizure. **F,** Temporal region: psychomotor seizures. Psychomotor seizures during which automatic behavioral patterns are carried out. **G,** Temporal region: visual phenomena—formed type. Visualization of formed objects or revisualization of former events. (From Yahr, M.D.: Hosp. Med. **9**(9):8, 1973; by permission.)

responses also occurs as the tumor grows and the pressure increases.

Types. Brain tumors are named for the tissues from which they arise. The more frequently encountered ones include gliomas, meningiomas, pituitary adenomas, and acoustic neuromas; the brain, in addition, is a frequent site for secondary tumors from other organs.

Gliomas account for about one half of all brain tumors. They arise in any part of the brain connective tissue. As a rule, in adults they infiltrate primarily the cerebral hemisphere tissues and are not so well

outlined that they can be completely excised surgically. The less malignant gliomas are the *astrocytomas* and the *oligodendrogliomas.* The most malignant and rapid growing forms are the *glioblastoma* and *medulloblastoma.* Gliomas not infrequently start as one type and develop into more malignant forms if untreated.

The *meningiomas,* which account for 13% to 18% of all primary tumors in the intracranial cavity, arise from the meningeal coverings of the brain. They occur most frequently in the meninges over the cerebral hemispheres in the parasagittal region along the ridge of the sphenoid bone and in the anterior fossa in relation to the olfactory groove or the sella turcica. When located in the posterior fossa, they arise from the cerebellopontine angle, from the tentorium, or rarely in the region of the foramen magnum. Meningiomas vary widely as to size and histologic findings. They are usually benign but may undergo malignant changes. The neurologic signs and symptoms produced by meningiomas relative to these sites may include anosmia, optic atrophy, extraocular palsies, visual defects, papilledema, pituitary disturbances, and cerebellar dysfunction. Meningiomas frequently cause seizures and involvement of the limbs as related to their presence in the convexity of a cerebral hemisphere.

Pituitary adenomas may arise from eosinophilic, chromophobe, and basophilic cells of the pituitary gland. Each type produces endocrine dysfunction. The first two types, in addition, produce neurologic deficits by compression of adjacent structures such as the optic chiasm. *Eosinophilic adenomas* result in the overproduction of growth hormone, causing acromegaly or gigantism, depending on whether the growth hormone overactivity occurs before or after closure of the epiphyseal lines. *Chromophobe adenomas* similarly produce signs and symptoms of pituitary deficiency related to several target glands. Basophilic adenomas are usually small and do not grow into contiguous structures. They are one cause of Cushing's syndrome. Refer to Chapter 27 for a more complete discussion of the pituitary gland and its functions.

Acoustic neuromas constitute about 8% of all primary intracranial tumors. Neuromas may arise from any cranial nerve. The tumor affecting the acoustic nerve usually arises from its sheath but usually extends to affect the nerve fibers. The signs and symptoms resulting from these slow-growing tumors are related to compression of adjacent cranial nerves (trigeminal and facial), cerebellum, and the brain stem.[108]

Metastatic tumors that arise primarily in the lung, kidney, breast, colon, and other organs account for about one fifth of all intracranial tumors. Primary brain tumors, conversely, rarely metastasize to other organs.

Treatment. The general methods of treatment for intracranial tumors include surgical removal when feasible, radiotherapy, and chemotherapy. Therapy choice is related to the tumor type and the specific site of the tumor.

When gliomas are located in areas that are not critical to vital function, they are usually removed surgically. However, because gliomas infiltrate and some forms are malignant, they are difficult to completely excise and treat. Surgery is often combined with radiotherapy and chemotherapy. When the tumor is located in a more critical area, the tumor is biopsied, if possible, and the patient treated with radiotherapy and/or chemotherapy (with nitrosureas).

Meningiomas are commonly treated by complete excision of the tumor (and overlying bone if infiltrated), since they are usually located in areas that permit removal.

The choice of treatment for pituitary adenomas is made individually relative to each patient and the effects produced from pituitary encroachment and endocrine dysfunction. Treatment often includes radiotherapy or surgery or both.

Acoustic tumors are usually treated surgically with an effort to preserve the facial nerves and their functions.

Nursing intervention. When admitting the patient with a potential or known brain tumor to the hospital, the nurse during the initial assessment should carefully observe him for signs of neurologic dysfunction and/or symptoms of increased intracranial pressure. Thorough and accurate observations and careful recording by the nurse are necessary to establish baseline information for comparative purposes. Even before the neurologist examines the patient, the nurse needs to make specific plans for nursing care based on admission observations and assessment. Decisions as to nursing actions necessary to assist the patient with his personal needs such as bathing, eating, walking, and communication need to be made relative to his neurologic dysfunctions. The mental status of the patient also needs to be assessed carefully, since slowness in mentation and depression of awareness that limit ability to participate in self-care may be present. The patient may demonstrate functional limitations in all activities when tested. Emotional and physical agitation needs to be prevented through control of the environment. If the patient has signs and symptoms of increased intracranial pressure, activities that increase intra-abdominal and intrathoracic pressure need to be prevented.

The nurse may be able to assist the neurologist to locate the site of a brain lesion by accurately reporting and recording observations. For example, noting that the patient has less severe headache when his head is in a certain position may be important because it suggests that the position relieves the pressure. If possible, the exact location of the headache should be determined. Careful description of the course of convulsions may also help to locate a tumor. Any symptoms indicative of early or increasing intracranial pressure should be reported promptly. Any focal or generalized signs of neurologic dysfunction should also be recorded. These observations, in addition to findings from the neurologic examination, provide the neurologist with the data to analyze the patient's problem and to select the best treatment for the patient.

The nurse assists the neurologist with neurodiagnostic procedures selected to determine the site of the tumor. No one diagnostic procedure is entirely diagnostic in brain tumors, and if the patient's condition is stable, electroencephalography, brain scan, and/or echoencephalography will be used to determine the exact site and nature of the tumor. Patients with increased intracranial pressure but with no evidences of specific neurologic deficits are evaluated as rapidly as possible. In emergency situations, arteriography or ventriculography may be used to locate the tumor.

A lumbar puncture may be helpful in assessment of patients with potential brain tumors; it is not carried out in patients with symptoms of increased intracranial pressure except in special circumstances. Immediate surgery known as decompression of the skull may be performed to allow for expansion of brain tissue outside the cranial cavity, thus relieving pressure. Brain scans are particularly useful in screening patients for suspected brain tumors by demonstrating the size and site of the tumor. A negative brain scan does not, however, exclude a tumor since a small tumor may not be visualized. Conversely, a positive scan may be caused by a cranial lesion other than a tumor. Electroencephalography is particularly useful in the detection of abnormal brain waves, generally or focally, within the cerebral hemispheres or their coverings. The echoencephalogram is helpful in identifying displacement of the ventricular system and the pineal gland from their normal midline positions. Displacement to the right of the midline or to the left may be indicative of a tumor within the respective hemisphere. Radiographic studies of the skull are carried out initially and may reveal increased intracranial pressure and abnormal calcifications.

Preoperative care. Written permission for surgery on the brain must be given by the nearest relative unless the patient himself is able to sign a permit. Even then close relatives are usually consulted, and the neurosurgeon obtains their consent before surgery. The patient and his family are usually very threatened by the prospect of brain surgery and should be encouraged to express their fears. The nursing staff should provide time for this as part of essential nursing care of the patient. The patient may also wish to have his spiritual advisor visit him prior to surgery.

Treatments and procedures should be explained to the patient even though he may not seem to understand fully. Enemas may not be given prior to surgery because of the danger of increasing intracranial pressure further by exertion and by the absorption of fluid. Narcotics, excepting codeine, are rarely ordered preoperatively since they may cause further depression of cerebral function. Any order for their use should be carefully verified by the nurse. If the head is to be shaved, the procedure may be delayed until the patient is in the operating room. Long hair should

not be discarded but should be returned to the patient unit because the patient may wish to have it made into a wig. The availability and popularity of synthetic wigs also helps in the solution of the feeling associated with the loss of hair. It is rarely necessary to shave the entire head and some surgeons have only a small area shaved. Hair along the front hairline can often be left so that after the operation it can be drawn backward to cover the scar.

Operative care. Since cranial surgery is commonly performed in the treatment of brain neoplasia when feasible, as well as for other cranial lesions, the following discussion about operative and postoperative care is applicable to cranial surgery generally.

A surgical opening through the skull is known as a craniotomy. It is a basic preparatory procedure for cranial surgery. A series of burr holes (trephine) is made first and then the bone between the holes is cut with a special saw (Gigli) to permit removal of the bone. Bone is then removed in such a way that it can be replaced. The opening depends on the lesion site. Brain surgery may be done under hypothermia to lessen bleeding during the procedure. Drugs for hypotension may be used such as levarterenol bitartrate (Levophed). Fluorescein sodium, a dye, may be administered intravenously 1 hour preoperatively to help localize a tumor during surgery. Tumor tissue tends to retain the dye, which can be seen under ultraviolet light. The dye will cause the skin and the scleras to appear jaundiced for several days. The nursing staff, the patient, and his family should be aware of this.

When the brain lesion is in the *supratentorium* (above the tentorium or in the cerebrum), the incision is usually made behind the hairline (Fig. 32-33). When the incision is into the *infratentorium* (below the tentorium or in the brain stem and cerebellum), it is made slightly above the nape of neck. Neither of these incisions is apparent when the hair has regrown.

Following craniotomy and removal of the bone, an incision is made into the meninges and the tumor is removed or other cranial surgery performed. The removed bone is carefully saved or preserved. Following brain surgery, the bone may be replaced immediately (as in bone flap with muscle attachment) or when there are no evidences of infection or increased intracranial pressure. Not infrequently the bone is left out for variable periods to prevent pressure from cerebral edema postoperatively or to permit expansion of an inoperable tumor. The preserved bone, in this instance, is used as a mold for a bone prosthesis, which is inserted with wire at a later date, or the bone is reinserted. Sterile acrylic is the material presently used to make the bone prosthesis. The acrylic can be molded directly into the skull opening after covering the dura with a thin plastic sheet at the time of

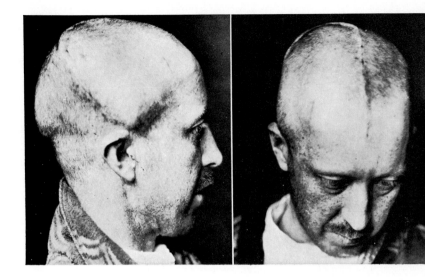

FIG. 32-33. Subtemporal decompression combined with unilateral frontal flap. These photographs were taken 1 week after surgery. The only place the scar might show is in the middle of the forehead. The scar is imperceptible if made accurately in the median line. Note the slight bulging of the right subtemporal decompression. (From Sachs, E.: Diagnosis and treatment of brain tumors and care of the neurosurgical patient, ed. 2, St. Louis, 1949, The C. V. Mosby Co.)

surgery, or it can be molded from the preserved bone at a later time. The removal of part of the skull, without replacement, is called craniectomy. When a tumor cannot be removed because of its location and nature, a subtemporal decompression is made by leaving an opening in the dura and skull.

Limitation of some functions may necessarily follow complete removal of brain tumors occurring in cerebral hemispheres. Portions of the frontal lobe are removed in some instances with little residual damage. Patients with tumors located where they are readily accessible to removal, such as meningiomas and tumors of outer cerebrum, have the best prognosis.

Although neurosurgery is most frequently performed in the treatment of brain tumors, it may be used in the treatment of hematoma or a brain abscess. It may also be employed to repair a cerebral aneurysm. Surgical procedures, in addition, are performed to produce destructive brain lesions in selected sites, as in the treatment of Parkinson's disease and in the control of intractable pain.

Immediate postoperative care. To facilitate change of head dressings and other treatments following surgery, the patient may be placed in bed "head to foot." Whether in the patient unit or in recovery room, the nurse should be certain that the following are readily available: side rails for the bed, suction machine or wall suction with disposable suction catheters, an airway, a padded tongue blade, a lumbar puncture set, and an emergency medication tray (cardiac and respiratory stimulants, amobarbital sodium [Amytal], anticonvulsive drugs), syringes, intravenous and hypodermic needles, and a tourniquet. An emergency tracheostomy tray should also be readily available on the unit.

Immediately after the patient is returned from the operating room, he is placed on his side to provide an adequate airway. If a large brain tumor has been removed, he must not be turned on the affected side, since this position may cause displacement of brain structures by gravity. Otherwise he may be turned to either side. The primary objective is to eliminate pressure at the operative site. Handling of the brain tissues and surgical trauma causes cerebral edema, which contributes to increased intracranial pressure. If there has been supratentorial surgery, the head of the bed is elevated at least 45 degrees, and a large pillow is placed under the patient's head and shoulders. This position should lessen the possibility of hemorrhage, provide for better circulation of the cerebrospinal fluid, and promote venous return. All of these measures assist in decreasing cerebral edema and in preventing increased intracranial pressure. Internal bleeding would also contribute to a rise in intracranial pressure. If an infratentorial tumor has been removed, the head dressing may extend down to the shoulders to support the neck and hold the head in slight hyperextension (massive dressings are used less frequently by some neurosurgeons). The bed should be kept flat with only a small pillow under the nape of the neck. See Fig. 32-34 for one type of infratentorial head dressing. Any flexion of the neck should be avoided, either midline or laterally. Since infratentorial incisions are made adjacent to the medulla and vital centers, there is more danger of respiratory complications and brain stem compression. Suction, if permitted, would produce coughing which, if vigorous, would in turn affect intracranial pressure adversely. Deep breathing needs to be carried out regularly by the nurse to prevent atelectasis, especially in infratentorial surgery.

The head dressing should be inspected regularly by the nurse as to the amount and kind of drainage (Fig. 32-35). Serosanguineous drainage on the dressings should be measured and marked, as is done with other dressings, so that it can be accurately checked for an increase in amount. Yellowish drainage should be reported immediately to the physician because it

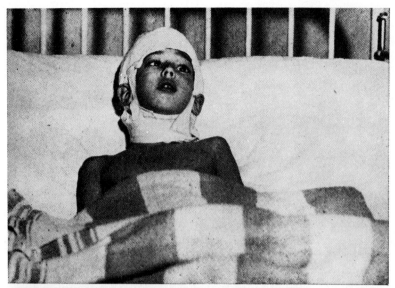

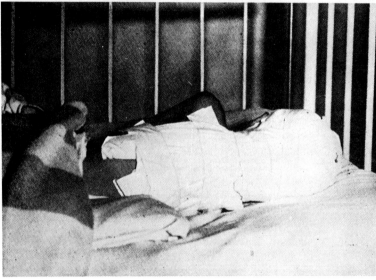

FIG. 32-34. Patient with an infratentorial craniotomy dressing. Note that the adhesive straps extend down the back to prevent the patient from flexing his neck. (From Sachs, E.: Diagnosis and treatment of brain tumors and care of the neurosurgical patient, ed. 2, St. Louis, 1949, The C. V. Mosby Co.)

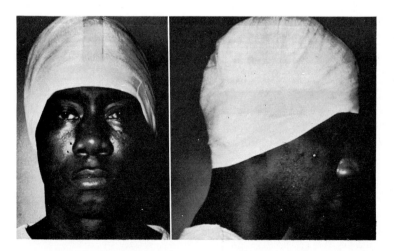

FIG. 32-35. Typical head dressing for the patient who has had a supratentorial craniotomy. (From Carini, E., and Owens, G.: Neurological and neurosurgical nursing, ed. 5, St. Louis, 1970, The C. V. Mosby Co.)

probably indicates loss of spinal fluid. If the head dressing appears to be soaked with any kind of drainage, it should be reinforced with sterile gauze sponges and covered with a sterile towel held in place with adhesive tape. Every half hour the towel should be removed and the dressing checked and reinforced with sterile towels if necessary. An unprotected wet dressing may cause the wound to become infected, which might even lead to meningitis. Sometimes the neurosurgeon may need to change the entire dressing.

The nurse should observe the patient regularly, recording his blood pressure, rectal temperature, pulse rate, respirations, state of consciousness, pupillary responses, and inequality of the size of the pupils, muscle strength (hand grip), and ability to move. If he is unconscious or semiconscious, his response to painful stimuli such as pinching or pricking is noted. Specific observations are usually made and results recorded every 30 minutes for 6 hours, every hour for at least a day, and every 3 to 4 hours until the third or fourth postoperative day. *Frequency of making and recording specific observations depends on the patient's condition.* Temperature is usually taken every hour for 4 hours and then at least every 4 hours for 24 hours. If the lesion was in the infratentorium, the temperature may be taken every 2 hours for 2 or 3 days because edema of the brain stem might occur and upset the temperature control center in the hypothalamus. (The treatment for hyperthermia is discussed on p. 84.) Any change in the patient's vital signs, state of consciousness, or ability to use muscles should be reported at once. If he appears to be restless, he should be watched closely for further signs, since restlessness may forewarn of hemorrhage or of irritation to the brain. Irregular or fixed pupils indicate pressure or disturbance that may be due to hemorrhage. In a patient who has intracranial bleeding the blood pressure rises and the pulse rate drops as the intracranial pressure increases. This process continues until the pressure becomes so great that all regulating control is lost and the blood pressure drops and the pulse rises just before death.

The family during the postoperative period. The family should be prepared to see the patient. They should know that he will return from the recovery room with a helmetlike head dressing and that edema may distort his features. If he is unconscious or has any noticeable limitation such as aphasia, they should be so informed before entering his room. If he is alert, members of the family should be advised to sit quietly at the bedside since talking will tire the patient. If a supratentorial incision has been made, the family should be warned that when they see him on the day following surgery, he may be unable to open one or both eyes, may have generalized facial edema, and may have discoloration of the skin about the eyes (ecchymosis) (Fig. 32-36). Periocular edema is caused by postoperative cerebral edema. It usually improves in 3 or 4 days. Ice compresses to the eyes may make the patient more comfortable.

Fluids and food. Fluid intake and output should be accurately recorded. If there is no special medical order to the contrary, 2,500 to 3,000 ml. of fluid should be given each day. Some neurosurgeons routinely restrict fluids to 1,500 ml./day for the first 3 days after a craniotomy.[86]

Since the gag and swallowing reflexes may be depressed or absent after infratentorial brain surgery, fluids by mouth are usually withheld for at least a day and intravenous fluids are substituted. They should be run very slowly to prevent increased intracranial pressure. The neurosurgeon tests these reflexes. If they are present, water is carefully given by mouth. The patient should be placed on his side or in a semisitting position. Fluid is most easily given by placing the rubber-protected tip of an Asepto syringe into the patient's mouth and allowing him to suck through it. Fluid should not be injected into his mouth. If he coughs or cannot swallow, the fluid should be discontinued.

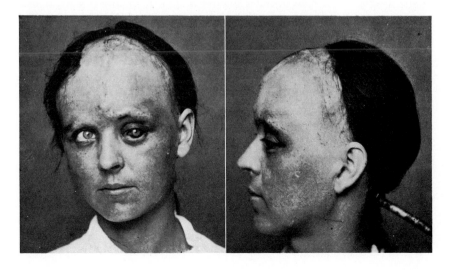

FIG. 32-36. This patient had surgery for a left-sided brain tumor 8 days prior to the taking of these photographs. The conjunctiva of the left eye still shows ecchymosis. Note the area of hair and eyebrow shaved. (From Sachs, E.: Diagnosis and treatment of brain tumors and care of the neurosurgical patient, ed. 2, St. Louis, 1949, The C. V. Mosby Co.)

A regular diet is usually given as soon as it is tolerated. After supratentorial surgery, the regular diet may be given on the second postoperative day. Any patient who has had a craniotomy, however, should be fed for at least 48 hours to prevent undue fatigue. He may need to be fed for a longer time to ensure adequate food and fluid intake. If the patient is unable to take food and fluid by mouth, liquid foods by nasogastric tube are started 48 hours postoperatively.

Urinary output. Care must be taken to see that the patient voids sufficiently. Urinary output must be carefully recorded, and sometimes an indwelling catheter may be used for a few days following surgery. A decrease in output must be reported, since it may indicate the onset of a metabolic disorder of central nervous system origin. If a pituitary tumor has been removed, special attention must be paid to urinary output because surgery on the pituitary gland may alter the control of water balance causing diabetes insipidus. Patients who have had surgery of the pituitary gland usually are given pituitary hormones to control excessive loss of fluid and electrolytes in the urine (p. 767).

Bowel function. Because straining increases intracranial pressure, the patient is urged not to try to have a bowel movement until the third postoperative day. On the second and third postoperative days the patient may be given a laxative or stool softener if indicated. He should be instructed not to strain. Bowel function is monitored by the nurse. If an impaction should develop, feces must be removed manually by the nurse.

Headache. Patients who are conscious after intracranial surgery may complain of severe headache for 24 to 48 hours. Codeine sulfate usually is given hypodermically every 4 hours for this pain, and acetylsalicylic acid may be given by rectum or by mouth if fluids can be swallowed. An ice cap may be placed on the head, and sudden movement and jarring are avoided. The patient should be protected from loud noises and bright lights. Even if the patient is conscious, he should be turned with a turning sheet for the first 48 hours, since the effort needed to move himself may tire him excessively and cause further headache, increased intracranial pressure, or hemorrhage (see Fig. 32-11). The turning sheet should be placed well above the level of the patient's head. General hygienic care for the patient during the first 48 hours is the same whether he is conscious or unconscious.

Ambulation. The patient who has had surgery for a supratentorial lesion usually is allowed out of bed on the third to fifth postoperative day or earlier. Activity should be increased gradually, and he should be watched carefully for signs of increased intracranial pressure. First, the head of the bed should be elevated to a high Fowler position, and then the patient should sit on the edge of the bed with his feet dangling over the side. If he tolerates this position, 4 to 6 hours later, with the help of two persons, he may be assisted to a chair and usually may sit up for a half hour. He then progresses to normal activity as quickly as he desires and is able. The patient who has had surgery for an infratentorial lesion usually may not be permitted up until the tenth postoperative day. The trend is toward getting up earlier, depending on the patient's condition. Initial progress may be slower, since patients who have been kept flat in bed for some time may be dizzy and experience orthostatic hypotension when arising until the circulatory system readjusts to the change in position.

Head dressings. Usually the wound is covered with gauze dressings, and a special head dressing (neurosurgical roll) is then applied in a recurrent fashion from the back to the front of the head and anchored. If a drain has been used, the head dressing is changed in 24 to 48 hours. Otherwise it is not disturbed until the sutures can be removed. They are usually removed on the third postoperative day following a supratentorial incision and on the fifth postoperative day following an infratentorial incision.

When the final dressings are removed, the scalp needs care. It should be gently cleansed with hydrogen peroxide to remove dried blood. Crusts can be

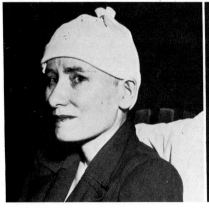
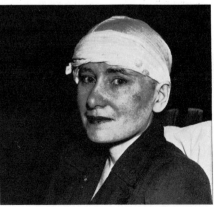

FIG. 32-37. The patient convalescing after brain surgery. In one picture she wears a stockinette cap; in the other, a turban. (From Sachs, E.: Diagnosis and treatment of brain tumors and care of the neurosurgical patient, ed. 2, St. Louis, 1949, The C. V. Mosby Co.)

loosened with mineral oil. The head may then be shampooed, with care taken not to rub the operative area or put traction on the healed suture line. The patient is often given a head covering, which protects the healed wound from dirt and helps to remind the patient not to scratch (an operating room cap may be used). Some neurosurgeons prefer that a stockinette cap be worn at first because it readily reveals any bulging of the wound. A cap may be made by tying one end of a 10-inch piece of tubular stockinette (Fig. 32-37). For women patients, it is psychologically important to cover the operative scar. Some women patients prefer to wear an attractive bandanna. The nurse should inspect the wound at least twice a day. The patient who has had a piece of bone left out will have a depression in the scalp, and he should be warned of the danger of bumping his head in this area. Women patients should be encouraged to have the remaining hair restyled, or they may prefer to wear a wig. Synthetic wigs are relatively inexpensive and should be available to most patients who desire one. If the hospital has a beautician service, restyling may be done before the patient leaves the hospital.

Protective measures. Sometimes the patient must be protected from self-injury after a brain operation. If he pulls at dressings or a catheter or if he scratches or hits himself, he should be attended constantly, and occasionally some kind of hand restraint such as a large mitten made of dressings, bandages, and stockinette fastened at the wrist with adhesive tape may be used. Mittens usually upset the patient less than arm restraints since with mittens he can move his arm freely. The fingers should be separated with gauze to prevent skin irritation and should be curled around a large bandage roll in the palm to prevent hyperextension of the fingers. The hand is then well covered with dressings held in place with a bandage. A piece of stockinette is closed at one end and everted so that the tied end cannot cause injury to the eye. It is then slipped over the bandaged hand and fastened securely at the wrist with adhesive tape. The wrist should be shaved and the skin protected with tincture of benzoin before adhesive is used. At least every other day the mitten must be removed, the hand washed in warm water, and passive exercise given to the fingers before the mitten is reapplied.

Ventricular drainage. Occasionally a catheter is placed in a ventricle of the brain to drain excess spinal fluid and prevent increased intracranial pressure. The catheter is usually attached to a drainage system on a level with the ventricle. The collection bottle is frequently attached to the head of the bed. The tubing and drainage receptacle should be sterile, and care must be taken to prevent kinking of the tubing. If drainage seems to stop, the neurosurgeon should be notified. The catheter is usually left in place for 24 to 48 hours and is then removed by the surgeon.

Complications. Meningitis is a relatively rare complication of brain surgery; it can follow infection during the operation or thereafter. Following supratentorial surgery, the nurse should watch for any clear, watery drainage from the nose. This drainage may be present if there has been a tear in the meninges, which causes subsequent loss of cerebrospinal fluid. The treatment consists of keeping the patient very quiet, avoiding any suctioning or blowing of the nose, and administering antibiotic drugs. The leakage usually subsides spontaneously. Because of the danger of causing damage that might be followed by the drainage of cerebrospinal fluid through the nose, many surgeons request that the nose never be suctioned when supratentorial surgery has been performed. A sign with this caution may be placed at the head of the bed.

Respiratory collapse may follow infratentorial surgery. It is caused by edema of the brain stem or edema above the brain stem that causes herniation of the brain stem into the foramen magnum and pressure on the respiratory center. Any irregularity of respiration, dyspnea, or cyanosis should be reported at once. Equipment should be ready for administering oxygen, doing a ventricular tap, and inserting an endotracheal tube if one is not already present. (For details of nursing care of the patient with an endotracheal tube, see p. 612.) Occasionally a respirator is used (p. 594).

Convulsions are not unusual after a craniotomy, and therefore a padded tongue blade should be at the bedside and side rails should be used even if the patient is unconscious and it is believed that he cannot move. Diphenylhydantoin sodium (Dilantin) may be ordered prophylactically to prevent convulsions. The drug may be given intramuscularly or, infrequently, by rectum until the patient is able to take it orally. If the patient has a history of seizures before the operation or if convulsions occurred in the postoperative period, he may be given this drug for several months.

Loss of the corneal reflex may follow brain tumors or brain surgery. If the eye appears inflamed or if the patient does not seem to blink when objects approach the open eye, the neurosurgeon should be notified. Special eye care such as that given to patients who have had cerebrovascular accidents or who have had surgery for trigeminal neuralgia may be necessary.

The patient may complain of *diplopia* after brain surgery. This condition is often temporary, and the patient should know that it will probably improve. It can be relieved by placing an opaque eye shield over one eye. The eye covered usually is alternated each day to prevent atrophy of eye muscles through disuse.

Radiation therapy is given to many patients following surgery for brain tumors. (See p. 292 for discussion of nursing the patient receiving radiation.)

Long-term care. Some patients who have had cranial surgery will have physical and mental limitations. The patient may have hemiplegia, aphasia, and personality changes, including severe depression. The rehabilitative care and planning both for the patient and for his family are the same as for other patients with chronic and permanent neurologic disease. Specific rehabilitation for patients with hemiplegia and aphasia from this cause is similar to that following a cerebrovascular accident. Preventive exercises should be started as soon as possible postoperatively. Regardless of the eventual prognosis, each patient should be helped to be as independent as possible for as long as possible.

The patient who has had intracranial surgery may need the same protection from injury as do other patients with neurologic disease when judgment defect, disorientation, or locomotor difficulties make it unsafe for him to move about without assistance.

Intravertebral tumors

Primary intravertebral tumors, or neoplasms, occur either as extramedullary (involving tissues outside the cord substance) or intramedullary (involving tissue cells within the cord substance). *Secondary* or metastatic tumors may also involve the spinal cord, its coverings, and the vertebrae.

Types. Extramedullary tumors of the intradural type may at first cause subjective nerve root pain. Subsequently, with tumor growth, this will include motor and sensory deficits relating to the level of root and spinal cord involvement. As the tumor enlarges, it compresses the cord. The nurse can learn to relate the initial signs and symptoms to the segmental level of involvement. A cervical lesion will cause pain and motor and sensory deficits in the arms in relation to segmental level. A thoracic lesion causes pain in the chest, and a lumbar lesion causes pain in the legs. Foot and hand pain are rare, but there may be tingling and numbness in the extremities. Eventually the patient loses all motor and sensory function below the level of the tumor.

An intramedullary tumor, beginning with the spinal cord substance, presents a different clinical picture. A central cord syndrome includes segmental loss of pain and temperature function. In addition, there is often loss of anterior horn cell function, especially in the hands. Most of the central long tracts next to the gray matter become dysfunctional. There is a gradual, progressive, and descending loss of pain and temperature sensations and motor weakness that is pronounced in the arms when the tumor begins in the cervical area. Caudal motor and sensory functions are the last to be lost, including loss of bowel and bladder control.

It is obvious that tumors involving the meninges are more likely to be removed successfully than other types. Even when complete removal is not considered possible, surgery is often performed to remove part of the tumor or to remove part of the bone surrounding the spinal column and thus reduce the obstruction for a time; this is called *spinal decompression.* It can be done at any level of the vertebral column and may include several vertebrae. The operation is sometimes palliative for malignant and nonremovable tumors. Radiation therapy is helpful in the treatment of inoperable intramedullary tumors.

Nursing intervention. Nursing care for a patient with a tumor of the spinal cord is the same as that for a spinal cord injury. The care given after a decompression operation is similar to that given the patient who has had excision of a ruptured nucleus pulposus, except that recovery is much slower (p. 918). The patient who has severe pain requires narcotics.

Convalescent care and rehabilitation depend entirely on the type of tumor and whether or not it has been successfully removed. Even if it cannot be removed, the decompression operation may give relief of symptoms for months and sometimes for years. If the tumor is a slow-growing one, x-ray treatment may be given while the patient is recovering in the hospital and continued after his discharge. The family often needs help in caring for the patient and in meeting his continuing problems. The patient often knows or guesses his prognosis (if little can be done for him medically) because he does not have the mental dulling that so often accompanies brain tumors.

In summary, intravertebral tumors, depending on the site, can produce both upper and lower motor neuron signs as well as sensory deficits. This is also true of other intravertebral lesions such as disc herniation and syringomyelia (cavitation of the spinal medulla) and ependymoma (growths involving the central canal of the cord and ventricles).

REFERENCES AND SELECTED READINGS*

1 Albin, M. S., and others: Effects of localized cooling on spinal cord trauma, J. Trauma **9:**1000-1008, 1969.

*References preceded by an asterisk are particularly well suited for student reading.

2 Alpers, B. J.: Essentials of the neurological examination, Philadelphia, 1971, F. A. Davis Co.
3 American Medical Association drug evaluation, ed. 2, chap. 31, Acton, Mass., 1973, Publishing Sciences Group.
4 Ballinger, W. F., and others: Alexander's care of the patient in surgery, ed. 5, St. Louis, 1972, The C. V. Mosby Co.

5 Barttler, F. C., and Schwartz, W. B.: The syndrome of inappropriate antidiuretic hormone, Am. J. Med. **42:**790-806, 1967.

6 Bassett, C. A. L., editor: National Research Council, Committee on the Skeletal System: the current status of the care of the spinal-cord injured patient, October 1967.

7 Beeson, P. B., and McDermott, W., editors: Cecil-Loeb textbook of medicine, ed. 13, Philadelphia, 1971, W. B. Saunders Co.

8 Bellanti, J. A.: Immunology, Philadelphia, 1971, W. B. Saunders Co.

9 Benson, V. M., McLaurin, R. L., and Foulkes, E. C.: Traumatic cerebral edema, Arch. Neurol. **23:**179-186, 1970.

10 Bergersen, B. S.: Pharmacology in nursing, ed. 12, St. Louis, 1973, The C. V. Mosby Co.

11 Blinderman, E. E., Graf, C. J., and Fitzpatrick, T.: Basic studies in cerebral edema, J. Neurosurg. **19:**319-324, 1962.

11a *Blount, M., and Kinney, A. B., guest editors: Neurologic and neurosurgical nursing, Nurs. Clin. North Am. **9:**591-772, Dec. 1974.

12 Boone, E. T., and Self, L. H.: Nursing care of the paraplegic using an experimental electronic spinal neuroprosthesis to activate voiding, J. Neurosurg. Nurs. **4:**61-74, July 1972.

13 Brain, L., and Walton, J.: Brain's diseases of the nervous system, ed. 7, London, 1969, Oxford University Press.

14 Brunnstrom, S.: Clinical kinesiology, Philadelphia, 1972, F. A. Davis Co.

15 Burt, M. M.: Perceptual deficits in hemiplegia, Am. J. Nurs. **70:**1026-1029, May 1970.

16 Carini, E., and Owens, G.: Neurological and neurosurgical nursing, ed. 6, St. Louis, 1974, The C. V. Mosby Co.

17 *Chusid, J. G., and McDonald, J. J.: Correlative neuroanatomy and functional neurology, ed. 15, Los Angeles, 1973, Lange Medical Publications.

18 Cloward, R. B.: Treatment of acute fractures and fracture dislocations of cervical spine by vertebral body fusion: a report of eleven cases, J. Neurosurg. **18:**201-209, 1961.

19 Conn, H. F., editor: Current therapy, Philadelphia, 1973, W. B. Saunders Co.

20 Cooper, I. S.: Cryogenic surgery, N. Engl. J. Med. **268:**743-749, April 1963.

21 *Cotzias, G. C., and McDowell, F. H., editors: Developments in treatment for Parkinson's disease, New York, 1973, Medam Press.

22 Covalt, D. A.: Rehabilitation of the patient with hemiplegia, Mod. Treat. **2:**84-92, Jan. 1965.

23 *Culp, P.: Nursing care of the patient with spinal cord injury, Nurs. Clin. North Am. **2:**447-457, Sept. 1967.

23a Dalessiso, D. J., editor: Wolff's headache and other head pain, ed. 3, New York, 1972, Oxford University Press.

24 *DeGowin, E., and DeGowin, R.: Bedside diagnostic examination, ed. 2, New York, 1969, Macmillan Publishing Co., Inc.

25 *Delehanty, L., and Stravino, V.: Achieving bladder control, Am. J. Nurs. **70:**312-316, Feb. 1970.

26 *Denny-Brown, D. E.: Handbook of neurologic examinations and case recording, Cambridge, Mass., 1957, Harvard University Press.

27 *Dohrmann, G. J., and Wick, K. M.: Research in experimental spinal cord trauma: past and present a brief review, J. Neurol. Nurs. **4:**115-124, Dec. 1972.

28 Ducker, T. B., and Hamit, H. F.: Experimental treatment of acute spinal cord injury, J. Neurosurg. **30:**693-697, 1969.

29 Eisenberg, H., and others: Cerebrovascular accidents, J.A.M.A. **189:**883-888, Sept. 1964.

30 Fangman, A., and O'Malley, W. E.: L-Dopa and the patient with Parkinson's disease, Am. J. Nurs. **69:**1455-1457, July 1969.

31 Fowler, R. S., and Fordyce, W. J.: Adapting care for the brain damaged patient: Am. J. Nurs. Part I. **72:**1832-1835, Oct. 1972; Part II. **72:**2056-2059, Nov. 1972.

32 Fox, J. L.: Neurosurgical hyponatremia: the role of inappropriate antidiuresis, J. Neurosurg. **34:**506-514, 1971.

33 *Gatz, A. J.: Manter's essentials of clinical neuroanatomy and neurophysiology, Philadelphia, 1970, F. A. Davis Co.

34 *Goda, S.: Communicating with the aphasic or dysarthric patient, Am. J. Nurs. **63:**80-84, July 1963.

35 Gordon, J. E., editor: Control of communicable disease in man, ed. 10, New York, 1965, American Public Health Association.

36 *Guyton, A. C.: Structure and function of the nervous system, Philadelphia, 1972, W. B. Saunders Co.

37 Haas, W. K.: Occlusive cerebrovascular disease, Med. Clin. North Am. **56:**1281-1295, Nov. 1972.

38 Hanes, W. J.: Tic douloureux—a new theory of etiology and treatment, J. Oral Surg. **20:**222-232, May 1962.

39 Hawken, P.: Hypophysectomy with yttrium-90, Am. J. Nurs. **65:**122-125, Oct. 1965.

40 Highland View Hospital, Cleveland, Ohio: Facing spinal cord injury, 1971.

41 *Hinkhouse, A.: Craniocerebral trauma, Am. J. Nurs. **73:**1719-1722, Oct. 1973.

42 *Hodgins, E.: Episode; report on the accident inside my skull, New York, 1963, Atheneum Publishers.

43 *Hohmann, G. W.: Considerations in management of psychosexual readjustment in the cord injured male, Rehabil. Psychol. **19:**50-59, Feb. 1972.

44 Holquin, A. H., Reeves, J. S., and Gelfand, H. M.: Immunization of infants with the Sabin oral poliovirus vaccine, Am. J. Public Health **52:**600-610, April 1962.

45 *Hughes, M. T.: Neuroradiology, a sub-specialty, J. Neurosurg. Nurs. **4:**83-91, July 1972.

46 *Hunkele, E., and Lozier, R.: A patient with fractured cervical vertebrae, Am. J. Nurs. **65:**82-84, Sept. 1965.

47 *Hurd, G. G.: Teaching the hemiplegic self-care, Am. J. Nurs. **62:**64-68, Sept. 1965.

48 Jackson, F. E.: The treatment of head injuries, Ciba Found. Symp. **19:**4-34, Jan.-March 1967.

49 Jasper, H. H., and others: Basic mechanisms of the epilepsies, Boston, 1969, Little, Brown & Co.

50 Jeffreys, W. H., and Hood, H.: The supportive management of acute closed head injuries, Med. Clin. North Am. **46:**1599-1604, Nov. 1964.

51 Kahn, E., and others: Correlative neurosurgery, ed. 2, Springfield, Ill., 1969, Charles C Thomas, Publisher.

52 King, I. M., guest editor: Symposium on neurologic and neurosurgical nursing, Nurs. Clin. North Am. **4:**199-283, June 1969.

53 *Kingdon-Ward, W.: Helping the stroke patient speak, London, 1969, J. & A. Churchill Co.

54 *Kintzel, K. C., editor: Nursing interventions for the patient with CNS dysfunction. In Advanced concepts in clinical nursing, Philadelphia, 1971, J. B. Lippincott Co.

55 Klocke, J.: The role of nursing management in behavioral changes of hemiplegia, J. Rehabil. **35:**24-27, July-Aug. 1969.

56 *Kottke, F. J., and Anderson, E. M.: Deterioration of the bedfast patient—causes and effects, and nursing care, Public Health Rep. **80:**437-451, May 1965.

57 Landau, B.: Late surgery for incomplete traumatic lesions of conus medullaris and cauda equina, J. Neurosurg. **28:**257-261, 1968.

58 Larson, C. B., and Gould, M.: Orthopedic nursing, ed. 8, St. Louis, 1974, The C. V. Mosby Co.

59 *Leavens, M. E., and others: Brain tumors and nursing care of patients with brain tumors, Am. J. Nurs. **64:**78-83, March 1964.

60 *Livingston, S., and others: Petit mal epilepsy, J.A.M.A. **194:**227-232, Oct. 1965.

61 Lutz, E. H.: Treatment of tic douloureux with carbamazepine, Dis. Nerv. Syst. **27:**600-603, Sept. 1966.

62 *Magee, K. R., and Moser, D.: Myasthenia gravis and nursing care of myasthenic patient, Am. J. Nurs. **60:**336-343, March 1960.

63 *Martin, M. A.: Nursing care in cervical cord injury, Am. J. Nurs. **63:**60-66, March 1963.

64 *Matthews, W. D.: Diseases of the nervous system, Oxford, 1972, Blackwell Scientific Publications.

65 Mayfield, F. H., and McBride, B. H.: Craniocerebral trauma. In Meirowsky, A. M., editor: Neurological surgery of trauma, Office of the Surgeon General, Department of the Army, Washington, D. C., 1965, U. S. Government Printing Office.

66 *Mayo Clinic and Foundation: Clinical examinations in neurology, ed. 3, Philadelphia, 1971, W. B. Saunders Co.

67 McAlpine, D., Lumsden, C. E., and Acheson, E. D.: Multiple sclerosis: a reappraisal, ed. 2, Baltimore, 1972, The Williams & Wilkins Co.

68 Medical Research Council: Aids to investigation of peripheral nerve injury, London, 1967, Her Majesty's Stationery Office.

69 Melnick, J. L.: Classification and nomenclature of viruses, Prog. Med. Virol. **14:**321-332, 1972.

70 Merritt, H. H.: A textbook of neurology, ed. 4, Philadelphia, 1973, Lea & Febiger.

71 *Miller, J. D., and Ross, C. A. C.: Encephalitis: a four year survey, Lancet **1:**1121-1126, 1968.

72 Mortimer, J. L., and Peckham, P. H.: Intramuscular electrical stimulation. In Fields, W. S., editor: Neural organization and its relevance to prosthetics, New York, 1973, Intercontinental Medical Book Corp.

73 *Mullan, J. F., and Van Schoick, M. R.: Intractable pain, Am. J. Nurs. **58:**228-230, Feb. 1958.

74 *Musick, D. T., and MacKenzie, M.: Nursing care of the patient with a laminectomy, Nurs. Clin. North Am. **2:**437-445, Sept. 1967.

75 *Nulsen, F. E., Bell, M., and Karb, V.: Head injuries. In Meltzer, L. E., Abdellah, F. G., and Kitchell, J. R., editors: Concepts and practices of intensive care, ed. 2, Philadelphia, 1975, The Charles Press, Publishers.

76 *Olson, C. K., and Tollefsrud, V. E.: Chemosurgery for parkinsonism and when the patient has chemosurgery, Am. J. Nurs. **59:**1411-1416, Oct. 1959.

77 *Olson, E. V., and others: The hazards of immobility, Am. J. Nurs. **67:**779-797, April 1967.

78 Peckham, P. H., Marsalais, E. B., and Mortimer, J. L.: Intramuscular stimulation; applications to upper extremity orthotics. In Proceedings of the fourth annual meeting of the Biomedical Engineering Society, Los Angeles, Calif., 1973.

79 *Peszczynski, M.: The rehabilitation potential of the late adult hemiplegic, Am. J. Nurs. **63:**111-114, April 1963.

80 *Pfaudler, M.: Flotation therapy: flotation, displacement, and decubitus ulcers, Am. J. Nurs. **68:**2351-2355, Nov. 1968.

81 *Quesenbury, J. N: Nursing action—not reaction—for a stroke patient's rehabilitation. In Bergersen, B. S., and others, editors: Current concepts in clinical nursing, vol. 2, St. Louis, 1969, The C. V. Mosby, Co.

82 Reaves, L. E., III: Considerations in rehabilitation of patients with cerebrovascular disease, J. Am. Geriatr. Soc. **12:**996-1001, Oct. 1964.

83 Rocklin, R.: The Guillain-Barré syndrome and multiple sclerosis, N. Engl. J. Med. **284:**803-808, April 1971.

84 Ruge, D., editor: Spinal cord injuries, Springfield, Ill., 1969, Charles C Thomas, Publisher.

85 Russell, D. S., and Rubinstein, L. J.: Pathology of tumors of the nervous system, London, 1971, E. Arnold.

86 Sabiston, D. E., editor: Davis-Christopher textbook of surgery, ed. 10, Philadelphia, 1972, W. B. Saunders Co.

87 Sarno, J., and Sarno, M. T.: Stroke: the condition and the patient, New York, 1969, McGraw-Hill Book Co.

88 *Schlesinger, E. B., and Haber, M. E.: Trigeminal neuralgia and nursing care of the patient with trigeminal neuralgia, Am. J. Nurs. **58:**853-858, June 1958.

89 Schmidt, R. P., and Wilder, J.: Epilepsy: a clinical textbook, Philadelphia, 1968, F. A. Davis Co.

90 Shaternick, J.: Living with myasthenia gravis, Am. J. Nurs. **63:**73-75, Feb. 1963.

91 *Shaw, B. L.: Revolution in stroke care, R.N. **33:**56-61, Jan. 1970.

92 Silverstein, A.: Arteriography of stroke, Arch. Neurol. **12:**387-389, April 1965.

93 *Stryker, R. P.: Rehabilitation aspects of acute and chronic nursing care, Philadelphia, 1972, W. B. Saunders Co.

94 *Taren, J. A., and Martin, M. A.: Cerebral aneurysm and care of the patient with a cerebral aneurysm, Am. J. Nurs. **65:**90-95, April 1965.

95 *Tourtelotte, W. W.: Cerebrospinal fluid in multiple sclerosis. In Vinken, P. J., and Bruyn, G. W., editors: Handbook of clinical neurology, Amsterdam, 1970, North Holland Publishing Co.

96 Truscott, B. L.: An abbreviated neurological examination, Psychiatr. Forum pp. 21-25, Winter 1969.

97 Tweed, G. G., Coyle, N. R., and Miller, B.: Guillain-Barré syndrome, Am. J. Nurs. **66:**2222-2226, Oct. 1966.

98 *Ullman, M.: Disorders of body image after stroke, Am. J. Nurs. **64:**89-91, Oct. 1964.

99 U. S. Department of Health, Education and Welfare, National Center for Health Statistics: Monthly vital statistics report, annual summary for the United States, 1968, vol. 17, Aug. 1969.

100 U. S. National Center for Health Statistics: Types of injuries, incidence and associated disability, Public Health Service Publication no. 1000, July 1965–June 1967, series 10, no. 57, p. 3.

101 Warren, R., and others: Surgery, ed. 2, Philadelphia, 1972, W. B. Saunders Co.

102 *Whitehouse, F. A.: Stroke—some psychological problems and causes, Am. J. Nurs. **63:**81-87, Oct. 1963.

103 Williams, S. R.: Nutrition and diet therapy, ed. 2, St. Louis, 1973, The C. V. Mosby Co.

104 Wintrobe, M. M., editor: Harrison's principles of internal medicine, ed. 7, New York, 1974, McGraw-Hill Book Co.

105 Wolff, H. G.: Headache and other head pain, New York, 1963, Oxford University Press.

106 World almanac and book of facts, 1970 edition, New York, 1969, Newspaper Enterprise Association, Inc.

107 *Yahr, M. D., guest editor: Symposium on clinical neurology, Med. Clin. North Am. **56:**1225-1418, Nov. 1972.

108 *Yahr, M. D.: Brain tumors, Hosp. Med. **9:**8-35, Sept. 1973.

109 Yase, Y.: Amyotrophic lateral sclerosis, Arch. Neurol. **27:**118-128, Aug. 1972.

110 *Young, J. F.: Recognition, significance and recording of the signs of increased intracranial pressure, Nurs. Clin. North Am. **4:**223-236, June 1969.

111 Young, J. F., and Reid, M.: Care in the surgical management of intracranial aneurysms, J. Neurosurg. Nurs. **4:**21-31, July 1972.

112 Zankel, H. T.: Stroke rehabilitation, Springfield, Ill., 1971, Charles C Thomas, Publisher.

33 Musculoskeletal injuries and disorders

■ Among the characteristics that distinguish man as a species are his ability to maintain an erect posture and his bipedal means of locomotion. These preceded the specialization of his thumb and hand and the development of his brain, which enabled him to become a tool-making creature. Thus he is the only animal with the ability to adapt the environment to meet his needs. However, this ability depends on an intact neuromusculoskeletal system.

Consider, then, the consequences for an individual who has an alteration in his ability to stand erect, to walk using only his lower extremities, or to use his upper extremities in a normal fashion. The essence of orthopedic nursing is the nursing care needed to assist an individual to make the physiologic and psychosocial adaptations necessary to minimize these temporary or permanent disabilities.

■ NURSING ASSESSMENT

A plan of care for the patient must be based on a systematic assessment of his needs. In previous chapters, assessment of patients with various pathologic conditions was discussed. Assessment of many of these same areas will be applicable to the patient

■ STUDY QUESTIONS

1 Describe the anatomic structures of bones. What are the functions or purposes of the skeletal system?
2 What part of the joint is the synovial membrane? What tissue constitutes the remainder of the joint?
3 What are the main types of joints in the body?
4 Review the range of motion for the hip, shoulder, knee, elbow, ankle, wrist, and finger joints and give examples of daily activities for which these joints are used.
5 What are the harmful effects of immobilization of a joint?
6 What are some of the exercises to preserve muscle tone in the legs and arms that you might teach the patient?
7 Describe the blood supply to the head, neck, and shaft of the femur.
8 What is the therapeutic action of acetylsalicylic acid? What are the toxic effects?
9 What are the therapeutic effects of heat and cold? What are some of the measures used to provide heat and the related nursing care?
10 Select a patient from your ward, a member of your family, or an acquaintance who has arthritis. How does this person earn his living? What financial problems has the disease presented? What major modifications in the patient's life have been necessary because of the disease? How has his need for recreation been affected?
11 What substances constitute connective tissue? What is the difference between elastic and fibrous connective tissue? What organs would be affected by a disease of the connective tissue? In each case, what specific nursing measures would be important?
12 Review the methods of assisting a patient in and out of bed and to and from bed to a wheelchair.
13 What are some of the changes that might be observed in the skin if circulation is impaired?
14 What determines the strength of a cast?

with an orthopedic problem. For example, the older orthopedic patient may also have cardiovascular or respiratory impairment. As the number of elderly persons increases and medical advances sustain persons with chronic diseases, the percentage of patients with multiple medical and nursing care problems can be expected to rise.

An individual's posture and movements depend on the proper functioning of the neuromuscular and skeletal systems. Neurologic assessment was discussed in Chapter 32. The orthopedic segment of assessment is basically concerned with posture and the ability to ambulate. This information is obtained through careful observation, history taking, and examination. Although others may contribute, a thorough history and physical examination, including testing for muscle strength and range of motion in all joints, will be done by the orthopedist. The nurse's admission interview should include questions concerning the patient's functional ability prior to admission. Some patients may have had no prior disability, such as a skier with a fracture, while others such as a person with severe rheumatoid arthritis may have coped with disability for an extended period of time. For those persons who have been disabled prior to admission, the nurse will want to know what adaptations, if any, the patient has already made in his activities of daily living. The nursing care plan should be designed to allow the patient to maintain his maximum ability. If the patient has a history of pain, the nurse should find out what positions and activity precipitate or aggravate the pain and what measures, including medications, have relieved the pain in the past.

As soon as possible, the nurse should find out the living circumstances of the patient. What will be the physical environment to which he is returning? What human resources are available to him? Discharge planning should begin on admission of the patient. This allows other members of the patient care team, such as the social worker, adequate time to make extensive plans with the patient should it be necessary.

Having obtained data regarding the patient's status prior to the current episode, the nurse must consider the present disorder or injury. To do this the nurse must know the nature of the present problem, the proposed medical plan, the possible complications, and the expected outcomes. A tentative time schedule is helpful in planning long-term goals. Interdisciplinary conferences with personnel from nursing, medicine, physical therapy, social service, occupational therapy, and other departments participating in the patient's care offer the opportunity to view the patient's needs from different vantage points. They also provide an opportunity for each member of the team to describe and suggest those services that he can best offer the patient.

■ PLANNING FOR CARE

Once the health team has identified and discussed the patient's needs and has evaluated services that seem appropriate, the patient and his significant others should be consulted. During the consultation the needs as identified by the health team and alternative courses of intervention are explained to the patient. Suggestions and consent are sought from the patient and his family. A plan of care can be successful only if the providers and recipient of care have compatible goals.

The disorders and injuries of the musculoskeletal system are vast in scope. They range from those that cause the patient only minor discomfort and inconvenience to those that are life threatening. The purpose of this chapter is to discuss those musculoskeletal conditions that commonly necessitate the adult individual's hospitalization and need for specific nursing care. Some clinical conditions present localized signs and symptoms, while others show systemic involvement. A brief review of the nature of the musculoskeletal system will serve as a basis for the discussion of specific conditions.

■ THE MUSCULOSKELETAL SYSTEM

The tissue of the musculoskeletal system is derived from the mesoderm of the embryo. It is capable of differentiating into any one of several types of connective tissue such as bone, cartilage, ligament, muscle, tendon, and fascia.

Each bone consists of an outer layer of dense, compact bone and an inner substance of spongy-looking trabecular bone. The periosteum that covers adult bone is thin and adherent to the cortex. As structures, bones provide a rigid framework for the body, serve as levers for skeletal muscles, and offer protection to vital organs. As an organ, bone contains hematopoietic tissue and is the storage area for calcium, phosphorus, magnesium, and sodium. Any disorder or injury to bone will affect at least one of these functions.

Joints (junctions between two or more bones) allow for some motion of the rigid skeleton as well as for growth. The following discussion will be primarily concerned with synovial joints. The capsule of the joint consists of tough, fibrous, modified connective tissue, which encases the epiphyseal cartilages, and the potential joint space, which contains synovial fluid. The synovial fluid provides lubrication to decrease friction in the movement of the joint. It also provides nutrients to the cartilage, which has no blood supply. The tendons that insert into the capsule as well as the ligaments and muscle tone add stability to the normal joint. Synovial joints are supplied with myelinated and nonmyelinated nerve fibers that terminate in the capsule. The myelinated fibers are very sensitive to twisting, stretching, and increased fluid pressure within the joint.

The basic property of skeletal muscle is its ability to contract. When pulling against a light load, the muscle shortens and provides movement. This is an *isotonic contraction*. An *isometric contraction* occurs when the muscle pulls against an immovable object and therefore no shortening of the muscle occurs. These two types of contractions allow the maintenance of posture as well as locomotion. (In studying disorders that are primarily neuromuscular, the reader should consult a specialized text for the complex physiology of skeletal muscle.)

Tendons and ligaments are comprised chiefly of collagen fibers. Both tendons and ligaments have firm attachment to bone via a continuation of their collagen fibers deep into cortical bone at the site of insertion.

Reactions of the musculoskeletal system to disorders and injuries will be discussed with the specific conditions.

■ CATEGORIES OF RHEUMATIC DISEASES

The category of "rheumatic disease" includes a wide range of clinical conditions that cause pain and stiffness in the musculoskeletal system. The American Rheumatism Society has classified rheumatic diseases into the following 13 categories:

1. Polyarthritis of unknown etiology
2. "Connective tissue" disorders (acquired)
3. Rheumatic fever
4. Degenerative joint disease (osteoarthritis, osteoarthrosis)
5. Nonarticular rheumatism
6. Diseases with which arthritis is frequently associated
7. Disorders associated with known infectious agents
8. Traumatic and/or neurogenic disorders
9. Disorders associated with known or strongly suspected biochemical or endocrine abnormalities
10. Neoplasms
11. Allergy and drug reactions
12. Inherited and congenital disorders
13. Miscellaneous disorders

Several of the more common diseases in these categories will be considered next. It is estimated that 16 million people in the United States have what they describe as "arthritis." Arthritis means inflammation of a joint. However, like the term "rheumatism," it is often used by the public to apply to any pain or stiffness of the musculoskeletal system whether or not the cause is an inflammatory process. Degenerative joint disease (also known as osteoarthritis) is a noninflammatory condition that in-creases in frequency with age. Epidemiologic studies suggest that both host and environmental factors contribute to increased susceptibility to osteoarthritis. Osteoarthritis affects men and women nearly equally except for degenerative disc disease, which more frequently affects men. Rheumatoid arthritis is three times more prevalent in women than in men.

■ NURSING INTERVENTION FOR THE PATIENT WITH A RHEUMATIC CONDITION

Regardless of the specific clinical condition that affects the patient, common general nursing care goals for the patient with a musculoskeletal problem apply.

1. Relief of pain and promotion of comfort
2. Maintenance of maximal functioning and independence
3. Prevention of complications or additional deformities
4. Improvement of function and correction of deformity
5. Education of the patient and his significant others
6. Participation with the patient and other team members in long-range planning

Relief of pain

Pain accompanies all musculoskeletal diseases. It may be exquisite in acute stages of diseases such as rheumatic fever, atrophic arthritis, gout, and diseases of the muscles and tendons. The patient requires the greatest care and gentleness when he must be moved. Fear of pain often makes him irritable and can lead to muscular resistance, which makes the pain worse. Care must be taken not to jar the bed. Heavy bedclothes may cause added pain. If cradles are used, caution must be taken not to accidentally bump an involved part of the body when adjusting or removing the cradle. Footboards help to relieve the pressure of covers, provided the patient can be kept warm during their use. Patients with rheumatic arthritis must be encouraged to change position frequently since their general nutrition is often poor and pressure sores and contractures develop easily. Sometimes a very painful joint such as a wrist, elbow, or ankle can be placed on a pillow, and the pillow and the limb can be moved together when the patient must turn over or otherwise adjust his position (Fig. 33-1).

Medications often are used to help control the pain. Salicylates such as acetylsalicylic acid (aspirin) are widely used for patients with arthritis and have been found to be effective in combating pain and discomfort in almost all types of rheumatic diseases. Since large doses of salicylates may cause local irritation to the stomach mucosa (gastritis),

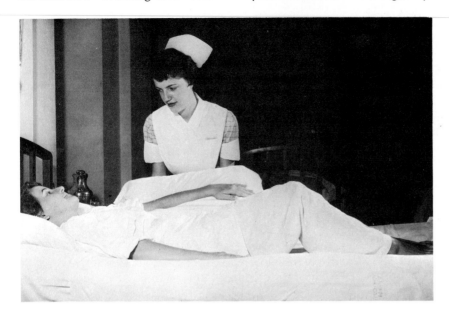

FIG. 33-1. Supporting the painful part on a pillow lessens discomfort when the patient must be moved.

these drugs are given with large quantities of water. They also are given frequently with milk or antacids. The signs of salicylate poisoning—ringing in the ears, nausea, vomiting, and tachycardia—should be watched for, although aspirin usually can be taken over a long period of time without the occurrence of toxicity or the acquisition of tolerance. Liver damage from salicylates seldom occurs. Because salicylates are widely used in the treatment of rheumatic diseases, it is essential that the nurse know how much acetylsalicylic acid, if any, the patient was taking prior to admission. Acetylsalicylic acid is known to prolong bleeding time. This is thought to be due to its effect on the platelets. Because of this tendency to bleed, patients scheduled for elective surgery are usually instructed to refrain from taking any medications containing acetylsalicylic acid for 2 weeks prior to surgery. In the event of trauma or emergency surgery it is imperative that the wounds be checked frequently for evidence of bleeding or a hematoma.

Corticosteroids are frequently given to patients with a rheumatoid disease for their antipyretic and anti-inflammatory effects. They are usually not prescribed until after conservative therapy has failed to relieve symptoms. Oral or parenteral administration is most common, although intra-articular injection of hydrocortisone is also used. It should be emphasized that the corticosteroids relieve symptoms but do not alter the underlying pathology. When corticosteroids are withdrawn, the symptoms will reappear. These drugs are especially useful when the patient is in the stage of exacerbation of a disorder. However, every effort is made to maintain the patient on the smallest possible dose. The side effects of the corticosteroids have been discussed on p. 82. Of particular orthopedic concern is the problem of os-

teoporosis and avascular necrosis, which will be discussed later in this chapter.

Although it is important to find out what medications have been taken by any patient who is admitted, it is especially crucial for patients who may have been receiving steroids. The nurse should seek this information in the initial interview. The physician will also inquire, but an anxious patient may not accurately give his history the first time. The nurse should remember that in periods of stress such as surgery the adrenal cortex of the patient who has been receiving exogenous steroids will be unable to respond with increased production of corticosteroids. Therefore increased doses of steroids will be prescribed, and the patient should be watched closely for signs of adrenal insufficiency.

Determining a program of rest and activity

In the acute phase of the disorder the patient may be placed on bed rest until the inflammatory process decreases, the muscle spasms subside, or the patient generally has an improved clinical picture. As gradual increase in activity is permitted, the nurse and the patient together should develop a plan for his daily activities that provides for adequate rest periods. The patient should be encouraged to do as much as he is able to do without becoming overly tired.

Maintenance of personal hygiene

Despite acute pain, personal hygiene must not be neglected. The patient with acute rheumatic fever often has profuse, sour-smelling perspiration and needs refreshing, warm sponge baths at least daily, as does the patient with an acute attack of gout. The patient with rheumatoid arthritis is often too tired and discouraged to keep himself as well groomed as he should, but few things contribute so much to gen-

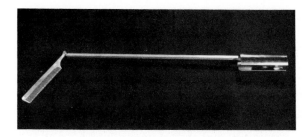

FIG. 33-2. A long-handled comb for use by persons with limited shoulder motion. (Courtesy Fred Sammons, O.T.R., Chicago, Ill.)

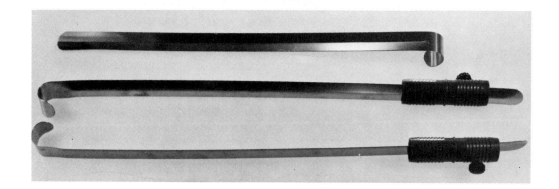

FIG. 33-3. A long-handled shoe horn and dressing aids. (Courtesy Fred Sammons, O.T.R., Chicago, Ill.)

eral morale as attention to personal hygiene. The nurse should give time to cutting fingernails and should assist women patients in setting and arranging their hair. The man with rheumatoid arthritis should be encouraged to shave regularly, and nursing personnel can help by having equipment conveniently placed and by providing time for this activity. If the patient is having much pain, the nurse should see that medications for pain are given about $\frac{1}{2}$ hour before personal hygiene measures are begun.

Every effort should be made to help the patient with a rheumatic disease to become and to remain self-sufficient in caring for his daily needs. Many self-help devices for patients with permanent musculoskeletal limitations are now available for purchase, and many others can be improvised by the resourceful person (Figs. 33-2 and 33-3). For example, the patient who has limited shoulder and elbow movements can sometimes comb his hair using a long-handled comb; eating utensils can be equipped with built-up handles that can be grasped more easily by persons who have a deformity of the fingers; and special buttons, zippers, and hooks can be used to make dressing easier for the person with a limited range of joint motion. The Arthritis Foundation and some of its regional offices in large cities have self-help device centers from which suggestions can be obtained.

Maintenance of posture

Although maintenance of good posture is important for all patients, it is especially important for the patient with a chronic arthritic disease. Poor posture exerts further strain on already damaged joints and

not only may cause pain and fatigue but predisposes to increased deformity.

The patient's bed. A firm bed lessens pain by preventing motion and consequent pull on painful joints and helps to keep the spine in good alignment. In the home or in the hospital the bed should have a firm mattress, and often bed boards are needed. Boards should be long enough and wide enough to rest firmly on the main side and end rails of the bed, not on the bedsprings. The person with arthritis should either use no pillow or should use one small pillow that fits well down under the shoulders so that forward bending of the cervical spine is not encouraged. Knees should not be flexed on pillows, and all patients who must be confined to bed most of the day should lie flat on the abdomen for a part of each day to relieve supine pressure areas.

Sitting posture. Furniture should be such that good posture can be maintained during working and recreational hours with a minimum of drain on vital energy resources. There are five criteria for a good chair: the seat should be deep enough to support the thighs but not so deep that circulation in the popliteal spaces is hampered; the seat should be high enough so that the feet rest firmly on the floor and do not dangle and put strain on the knee joints; the seat should be level or tilted slightly forward so that flexion of the knees and hips is at a minimum and not at more than a right angle; the chair should have arms so that arm and shoulder muscles can provide leverage to help in moving from the chair; the rungs must be such that one foot can be placed partially under the seat in preparation for rising so that the patient is better able to stabilize his center of gravity when he assumes an erect position. Chairs seats a little higher than is usually considered comfortable provide better leverage when arising. Sometimes adding an inch or two to the height of the patient's favorite chair will increase his comfort when sitting and on arising. Occasionally, too, it is necessary to build up the toilet seat. Devices to be placed over the seat to provide height can be improvised or they can be purchased from hospital supply stores. A rail beside the toilet seat is as necessary as arms on any chair the patient uses, since he must use his arms to arise from the seat safely.

If the patient with arthritis has been sitting for some time and finds his knees stiff on attempting to move, he should remember to flex and extend his knees several times before attempting to rise from the chair. By eliminating some of the stiffness before trying to bear weight, he will find that he is much steadier on his feet. Many patients who otherwise find an evening at the movies intolerable are able to enjoy such recreation by remembering this simple practice.

Shoes. The patient with arthritis should always wear properly fitted shoes that give support to the feet. Frequent changes of shoes also are helpful. Sometimes the physician may prescribe corrective shoes or shoes modified to provide special support. For example, a metatarsal bar may be placed on the outside of the sole of the shoe. The patient is usually gratified at the difference such changes make in how he feels after several hours on his feet. Shoes, not soft bedroom slippers, should be worn about the house.

Splints. Splints may be ordered for use during sleeping or waking hours to help prevent deformity caused by muscle spasm. Splints should be well padded and should be removed frequently. The skin should be carefully checked for signs of pressure, particularly over bony prominences. In the home, splints may be made from chicken wire that has been carefully covered and padded.

Exercise. Activities for all patients with arthritic diseases in the chronic stage should be planned to keep joints limber. Most patients with rheumatoid arthritis must do special exercises that are prescribed for them by the physiatrist and taught to them by the physical therapist. The nurse should know what these exercises are and should not only encourage the patient to do his exercises regularly but also should occasionally watch him do them. Some patients are so eager to get well that they are too vigorous in exercising and may cause aggravation of the disease and damage to the involved joints. Others who are tired and resigned to their fate may sit passively, not moving their limbs sufficiently because of slight pain and thus negating the whole purpose of the exercises.

Exercises are often prescribed to be done two or three times a day. To be beneficial, all exercises must involve steady, prolonged contraction before relaxation—not merely "wiggling" the part. Pain experienced during the exercise and disappearing soon afterward is not significant. Pain persisting throughout the rest of the day or into the night probably is an indication that the exercise has been too strenuous and should be decreased. The physician or the physical therapist should be consulted.

The patient and his family need to know why activity is necessary, why exercises are ordered, why it is so important to do them regularly, and what changes take place in muscles and joints when motion is not maintained. They should be told that muscles are very important in holding joints in good position and that without muscle action, joints themselves cannot produce motion. Exercises are necessary to preserve range of joint motion, to strengthen muscles, and to prevent shortening of muscles.

The patient needs to understand the normal range of motion for every joint in his body and should be helped to appreciate why the daily efforts demanded to prevent limitation of any involved joints are so important in his long-term outlook. Drawings and pictures help in this explanation, which is usually given by the physician and augmented by the nurse and the physical therapist. Members of the patient's family also should be taught the positions and exercises so that they may help the patient as necessary. However, they should encourage the patient to do without help the exercises that he is capable of performing alone.

It may be helpful for the patient to take acetylsalicylic acid about $\frac{1}{2}$ hour before doing exercises. Use of heat before beginning the exercises is of great help in making them easier for the patient. The patient may prefer a heating pad, a heat lamp equipped with a 25-watt bulb and placed at least 12 inches from the skin, or warm, moist packs applied for short periods. Bath towels wrung out in hot water and applied directly to the skin are often used because moist heat seems more effective than dry heat in promoting muscle relaxation and alleviating pain. Warm baths rather than moist packs may be preferred by the patient who is caring for himself and who may have difficulty in wringing out the towels. The patient may prefer to do his exercises while lying in a tub of warm water or standing under the shower. If bath oils and bath salts can be afforded, their use makes this routine more enjoyable.

Nutrition

There are no special diets that will cure or even materially alter the course of any type of arthritis except possibly gout. Yet thousands of patients follow special and expensive diets in the hope of cure. More patients with arthritis than with any other disease are the victims of advertising and diet fads.

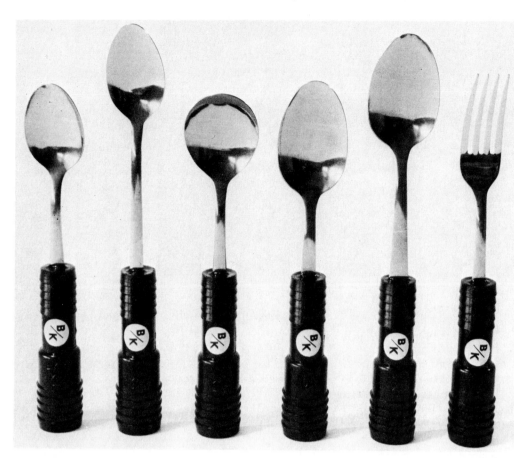

FIG. 33-4. Several different utensils with built-up handles are available. They are used to improve the grasp of the hand. (Courtesy Fred Sammons, O.T.R., Chicago, Ill.)

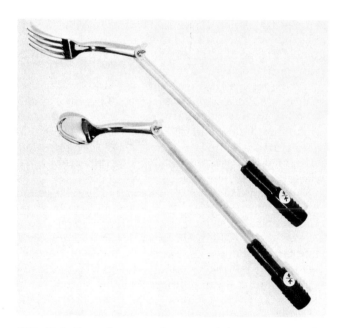

FIG. 33-5. Extension utensils are useful to persons with limited range of motion at the elbow or shoulder. (Courtesy Fred Sammons, O.T.R., Chicago, Ill.)

The essentials of good nutrition, which include fruits, vegetables, protein, and vitamins, are recommended for most patients with arthritis. If the arthritis is metabolic in origin, as is gout, or if the patient is overweight, a special diet may be ordered. Otherwise the patient should be permitted to indulge his food likes and dislikes within the range of the essentials of good nutrition.

The patient should be urged to eat regular meals and should be given plenty of time for meals. Even the patient with marked limitation of movement should be urged to feed himself, although food may sometimes have to be cut up or otherwise prepared beforehand. Built-up handles on eating equipment or specially constructed utensils may enable the patient with severe limitations to feed himself (Figs. 33-4 to 33-6). Other self-help devices for patients with physical disabilities can be found in Chapter 32.

Psychosocial aspects of rheumatoid disease

In general, the patient with a rheumatic disease suffers from some degree of chronic disability. As discussed in the introduction to this chapter, a musculoskeletal disability alters, both literally and figuratively, the individual's place in his world. The entire health team must assist the patient to make the necessary adaptations. Of particular importance in this aspect of care is the social worker. The social

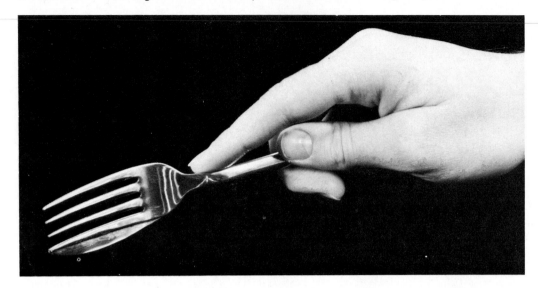

FIG. 33-6. A side-cutter fork for use by a person with one functioning hand. (Courtesy Fred Sammons, O.T.R., Chicago, Ill.)

worker's skill in interviewing and counseling as well as his familiarity with community agencies can greatly assist the patient and family in making necessary adjustments.

Patients vary greatly in their ability to adapt to changing circumstances. Varying degrees of disability have been observed in patients who have approximately the same degree of pathology. The willingness to tolerate pain in the present in order to gain more independence in the future is thought to be a key factor in the person's rehabilitation potential.

Progress is often very slow. Depending on the disease condition, the patient's disability may increase in spite of all efforts, including his own. Therefore patients and their families often become very discouraged. The person who is discouraged and in pain is very vulnerable to promises of a "cure." Millions of dollars are spent each year, by persons who can ill afford the expense, on programs, gadgets, and "medicines" that allegedly are able to "cure." While the ultimate decision to try or not to try a program rests with the individual, the nurse can provide guidance to the patient and his family. Working with the physician and other team members, the nurse has the opportunity to teach the patient about his care and to see that he is referred to reputable resources for additional assistance and information. The local chapter of the Arthritis Foundation can be of great assistance to the individual and his family and is also keenly aware of the relative merits or lack of merits in resources available in the community.

The Arthritis Foundation* has prepared the following material, all of which is helpful to the nurse working with persons who have arthritis. *Arthritis: the Basic Facts; Home Care Programs in Arthritis; Arthritis and Related Disorders: Manual for Nurses, Physical Therapists, and Social Workers;*

*1212 Avenue of the Americas, New York, N. Y. 10036.

and Rheumatoid Arthritis, Osteoarthritis, and Gout.

The American Rheumatism Society suggests a paperback book available at bookstores, for use by the patient and his family.*

■ SPECIFIC DISORDERS

Rheumatoid arthritis

Rheumatoid arthritis is also known as atrophic arthritis and arthritis deformans. It attacks young adults most often and affects women more often than men. Usually it appears during the productive years of life, when career and family responsibilities are greatest. The cause of rheumatoid arthritis is unknown. There are various theories of causation under investigation. Areas of study are infection, metabolism, and the role of the autoimmune response. General debility, fatigue, endocrine imbalance, emotional instability, and psychic trauma all apparently play a part in the development of rheumatoid arthritis. Because the collagen substance of the connective tissue is involved, rheumatoid arthritis is now considered to be a collagen disease. It is a systemic disease characterized by fatigue, poor appetite, low-grade fever, anemia, mild leukocytosis, and increased blood sedimentation rate. The serum of most patients with the disease contains the antibody known as the rheumatoid factor.

The course of rheumatoid arthritis varies greatly from patient to patient. It is marked by periods of remission and exacerbation. The pathology begins with inflammation of the synovium with increased exudate. This eventually leads to thickening of the synovium. The fibrous capsule and ligaments may

*Bland, J. H.: Arthritis, medical treatment and home care, a book for family use, rev. ed., New York, 1963, Collier Books.

become softened and stretched. If this occurs, the joint may subluxate or dislocate. This is frequently seen at the wrist. As the amount of granulation tissue resulting from the inflammation increases, it interferes with the normal nutrition of the articular cartilage and the cartilage becomes necrotic. The invading tissue extends to subchondral bone, causing eventual regional osteoporosis. If the process continues unchecked, it leads to bony ankylosis or fusion with resultant loss of motion in the joint. The inflammatory process includes the synovial membrane covering tendons, and the parts of the muscle that control the joint become fibrosed. This process causes contracture and adds to the deformity. Often the proximal interphalangeal joints of the hands are affected early. The fingers develop a characteristic tapering appearance with a classic ulnar deviation of the hand.

Several joints may be involved at the same time, and if the disease is not arrested, it may progress steadily to other joints. There is spasm of the muscles attached to the involved joints, and wasting of these muscles is greater than would normally be expected from their lessened activity. Subcutaneous nodules may develop. They are usually near joints, over bony prominences, or along extensor surfaces.

The public should be taught that the outlook for rheumatoid arthritis is not hopeless. If the disease is intensively treated, some patients recover from the first attack and, with careful attention to their general health, never suffer a recurrence. If not treated early, the disease has a tendency to relapse and to recur in more severe form. The nurse may be helpful in supporting the patient to seek and continue competent medical care. Approximately 10% to 15% of the patients with rheumatoid arthritis, however, progress to a crippling state despite any kind of treatment.

The basic principles of management of rheumatoid arthritis are (1) rest, (2) relief of pain, (3) maintenance of joint function, (4) prevention and correction of deformities by application of orthopedic principles, and (5) correction of other health factors.[55]

Whenever possible, the patient should rest for 10 to 12 hours out of each 24. This is accomplished by a longer sleeping period at night and an afternoon nap. The nurse should be alert to the physical comfort of the patient and to factors that could interfere with him obtaining the prescribed amount of rest. Rest of weight-bearing joints is especially important during the inflammatory stage. The patient should lie flat in bed on a firm mattress with only one pillow.

As mentioned earlier, salicylates are still the initial drug of choice in the treatment of rheumatoid arthritis. Adults should start with a minimal dose of 3.6 Gm./day in divided doses after each meal and before bedtime. There is considerable variation in the plasma level of salicylates produced by a given dose of aspirin, and the dosage is individually decided and based on desired plasma levels.

Corticosteroids given over extended periods of time and in high dosages may cause cataracts or elevate intraocular pressure and cause glaucoma. Any complaints about vision should be reported at once. These drugs should not be discontinued suddenly because adrenal insufficiency may result. Peptic ulcer may also result from steroid administration and therefore these drugs should be given with meals or with milk or antacids.

Gold salts seem to control the symptoms of rheumatoid arthritis in some persons. However, gold salts may cause serious reactions. They have been known to cause severe renal and hepatic damage,[55] and gold may be deposited on the cornea of the eye.[29] Dermatitis and inflammation of the eyelids and the conjunctivae are rather common side effects.[29] If the patient receiving gold has a sore mouth, excessive salivation, nausea, vomiting, diarrhea, or irritated eyes, the drug usually is stopped. Signs of jaundice should be watched for and reported. The urine usually is tested frequently for albumin.

Aurothioglucose (Solganal) and gold sodium thiomalate (Myochrysine) are the two forms of gold most frequently used. The dosage is usually 10 mg. ($\frac{1}{6}$ grain) intramuscularly as a first test dose. If no ill effects are encountered, a second dose of 25 mg. ($\frac{3}{8}$ grain) is given and then 50 mg. ($\frac{3}{4}$ grain) is given at weekly or biweekly intervals until 750 to 1,000 mg. (12 to 15 grains) has been given.[7] Usually a rest period of at least 4 weeks is planned before another series of injections is started. In some clinics a maintenance dose of 25 to 50 mg. is given every 4 weeks for months and sometimes years. Dimercaprol (BAL) and vitamin B_{12} may be given with gold preparations to reduce the danger of untoward reactions.

Antimalarial drugs such as chloroquine phosphate (Aralen) also seem to relieve symptoms of rheumatoid arthritis and are being prescribed by some physicians. However, they have been found to cause changes in the retina, and blindness may result from their use. Early symptoms are blurred vision, halos around lights, difficulty in adjusting to sun or glare, and diplopia. Therefore vision should be assessed carefully, and the physician should be notified at once if these symptoms occur.

The measures described previously to promote joint function are discussed in the section on the management of the patient with rheumatoid arthritis. Most effective is the use of heat (particularly moist heat) followed immediately by range of motion and muscle strengthening exercises.

Other methods used to prevent or correct deformities include good body alignment with the use of a footboard as necessary and prevention of flexion contractures. No pillow should be placed under swollen and painful knees. Dynamic splints or half-shell molds may be employed to prevent joint deformities. Splints or molds should be removed at least twice daily for the application of heat and for exercise.

Surgical intervention may be necessary to relieve pain and correct deformity. Synovectomies in the early stages of the disease have proved very useful. In later stages, osteotomies to alter the weight-bearing surface, joint replacement, or fusion of the joint may be done. These will be discussed later under types of orthopedic surgery.

Correction of other health factors includes attention to the general health of the patient, with special attention to diet and to the treatment of anemia, if present. Many persons with chronic discomfort and disability become undernourished and underweight. A well-balanced diet and vitamin supplements may improve nutritional status and promote a feeling of improvement. Patients often need to be encouraged in maintaining this kind of diet. In severe anemia, blood transfusion may be necessary because iron therapy, folic acid, and vitamin B$_{12}$ are usually ineffective in the anemia associated with rheumatoid arthritis.[55]

Marie-Strümpell disease

Marie-Strümpell disease affects the spine and is seen primarily in young men. The sacroiliac joint usually is involved first. The patient complains of intermittent low back pain that does not radiate into the buttocks or legs and stiffness. Later the symptoms become constant. The disease progresses upward in the spine and, unless arrested, causes a severe forward-bending deformity. Marie-Strümpell disease sometimes responds to x-ray therapy, and sometimes fusion of the spine is done to prevent further progressive deformity.

Still's disease

Atrophic arthritis that affects children is called Still's disease. It occurs before puberty. There may be slowly progressive joint inflammation, or an acute febrile illness with joint involvement may herald the onset of the disease. The clinical findings and the progress of the disease are almost identical to that in adults except that there may be premature cessation of the growth of bones, and the vertebrae in the cervical spine may become fused. The percentage of patients who develop severe deformities is fairly high.[53a] The nursing needs are no different from those of adults except that the technique for accomplishing care must be adapted to the age of the child. (Adaptations needed by children of various ages are described in Chapter 2.)

Degenerative joint disease

Degenerative joint disease is also known as hypertrophic arthritis and osteoarthritis. The term "degenerative joint disease" is preferred because it most accurately describes the pathologic process involved. Unlike rheumatoid arthritis there is no inflammatory process involved. Degenerative joint disease may be either primary (a normal part of aging) or secondary (degeneration following trauma, infection, or a metabolic disorder). Almost everyone past 40 years of age has hypertrophic changes in the joints. These changes may become symptomatic, depending on their severity and on such mechanical factors as poor posture, obesity, and occupational strain. Weight-bearing joints such as the knees, hips, and spine are most often affected. The patient with osteoarthritis can be given reassurance that pronounced deformity will not occur. Changes within the joint consist of thinning of the articular cartilages and deposition of calcium on the bone surfaces and in the joint spaces. Some enlargement of the joint occurs, but there is no swelling. There is some discomfort, and motion may be limited. Pain is often intermittent, tending to follow chilling, and is possibly due to muscle tension from the cold. Small fragments of bone or cartilage, known as joint mice, occasionally break off, causing severe pain on movement. It may be necessary to remove them surgically. Bony tumors (exostoses) may develop. They are benign growths, but if they develop on weight-bearing areas such as the heel, they can be removed surgically.

The patient with degenerative joint disease is often overweight, and general weight reduction is advised. Pain and discomfort in the joints usually are relieved by aspirin. Activity rarely needs to be limited. In fact, activity alleviates the accompanying stiffness. Care must be taken, however, in placing patients with osteoarthritis in unusual positions such as the lithotomy position, since movement of the hip may be limited. Severe pain and even trauma can be caused by forcing the legs apart or by failure to move both legs in unison.

Although hypertrophic changes in the joints cannot be prevented, their attendant discomforts can be controlled to some extent. This is true particularly if prevention is considered early in life. Obesity should be controlled because it places considerable strain on all weight-bearing joints.

Trauma and excessive use of certain joints can lead to degenerative joint disease. Examples of professions and occupations that seem to be associated with hypertrophic involvement of the upper spine and shoulder joints are dentistry, barbering, and dishwashing. It seems likely that the position assumed during working hours is a contributing factor. Public education and industrial practices that consider the dangers of prolonged work in a position of strain may help to prevent the development of symptoms in some people. The orthopedic principle of alternate rest and activity to prevent strain on particular joints and muscles has real application in the prevention of hypertrophic arthritis. Poor posture throughout life contributes to hypertrophic arthritis. The child should be taught to stand correctly so that strain due to prolonged hyperextension does not occur in joints such as the knee joints. Holding the pelvis correctly with a forward tilt will prevent increased curvature of the lower back with its resultant strain on muscles and joints. Correct mechanical use of the body, such as stooping with knees and hips flexed rather than bending, prevents muscle strain that may pull the joint out of alignment just enough for osteoarthritic changes to develop or to cause symptoms. Holding the head up and back takes a great deal of strain from the joints of the upper spine. It is surprising how many older patients can benefit from posture improvement even though the damage may date from childhood. (For more complete discussion of posture, see specialized texts.[38])

Gout, although it actually is a disease related to faulty metabolism, frequently is classified as an arthritic disease because of the joint symptoms. The Arthritis Foundation also classifies acromegaly (a disorder arising from excessive secretion of the growth hormone) and the blood disorders hemophilia and sickle cell anemia as arthritic diseases. In each of these diseases joint symptoms may be predominant. Only gout, however, is discussed as this form of arthritis in this book.

Gout, or gouty arthritis, is arthritis caused by the deposit of sodium urate crystals in the joints as a result of excessive uric acid in the blood. Eighty-five percent of all patients with gout show a familial tendency to develop the disease, and 95% of all patients with gout are men.

Gout is a chronic disease, although acute exacerbations occur, causing high temperature, malaise, and headache. Attacks are characterized by acute pain, swelling, and tenderness of joints such as those of the great toe, ankle, instep, knee, and elbow. Renal stones form from the uric acid as it is filtered from the blood. Renal damage may occur when acute attacks are repeated over an extended period of time. Subcutaneous deposits of urates (tophi) in locations such as the outer ear occur in about one third of all patients who have gouty arthritis.

Treatment of gout is directed toward control of acute attacks, since permanent joint damage and deformity as well as renal failure can follow repeated attacks. In an acute attack, treatment consists of pain relief and rest of the affected limb. Medications such as colchicine, phenylbutazone, and corticotropin are used to reduce pain. Prevention of recurrences and complications depends mainly on medications (colchicine, uricosuric agents such as Probenecid [Benemid]), dietary regulation, and increased fluid intake (3 to 4 L./day).

Colchicine is the standard drug used in the treatment of acute gout. When an acute attack of gout is imminent, the usual treatment is administration of 0.5 mg. ($^1/_{120}$ grain) of the drug each hour by mouth until nausea, vomiting, diarrhea, or abdominal pain develops, or until joint pain is relieved. Other drugs, including probenecid and sulfinpyrazone (Anturan), are used for their uricosuric action and allopurinol (Zyloprim) for its metabolic effect. Camphorated tincture of opium (paregoric) is then sometimes given as treatment for the gastrointestinal irritation. The usual maintenance dose of colchicine (0.5 mg.) is administered daily or two or three times/week. Some patients may require medication two or three times each day. The usual dosage of probenecid is 0.5 Gm. (7½ grains) daily by mouth for 1 week, followed by 1 Gm. daily for months. The drug may cause gastric distress and is best tolerated if taken with meals. Large amounts of fluid must be given to minimize formation of stones in the kidneys. Since the drug works best in an alkaline medium, sodium bicarbonate, 5 to 7.5 Gm. (75 to 110 grains) daily, is often ordered. However, this dosage may disturb the acid-base balance of the body if continued for too long. Therefore an alkaline-ash diet may be prescribed. The nurse may be asked to check the acidity of the patient's urine with litmus paper each time he voids or to teach him to do so and to record the results. One limitation in the use of probenecid is that salicylates cannot be given at the same time, since this combination diminishes the benefit derived from both drugs.[7] Sulfinpyrazone is similar to probenecid in action and effects. The usual dosage is 50 mg. four times a day. Allopurinol blocks the formation of uric acid. The dosage varies but is usually 200 to 300 mg. (3 to 4½ grains) daily in divided doses.[7]

Patients with gout who are able to maintain normal uric acid blood levels with prescribed medication do not need to be on a restricted diet unless they have other health problems. If overweight, the patient is advised to lose weight, which aggravates the joint symptoms. On the other hand, an alkaline-ash diet may be prescribed to increase the alkalinity of the urine, to decrease the possibility of urate crystal formation, and to enhance the effect of the medication. (See Table 20-1.) This type of diet is high in fruits and vegetables with lower amounts of meat proteins. In either case, a high fluid intake is advisable to minimize uric acid precipitation. The daily urine output for the patient should be 2,000 to 3,000 ml./day.

Early treatment of gout prevents serious complications. However, people often fail to recognize the significance of early symptoms. The most prominent early symptom is pain in the foot during the night. The nurse has a responsibility for being aware of the possible cause of this complaint. Persons who complain of foot pain should be encouraged to seek medical attention.

Degenerative joint disease of the spine

The spine has 23 intervertebral disc joints and 46 posterior facet joints, all of which are subjected to stresses and strains in holding man upright and moving him about. The vertebrae in the spinal column are articulated in a series of "couplets" that are able to move through an intervertebral disc joint and two posterior facet joints. Each disc has an outer layer called the anulus fibrosus and an inner core called the nucleus pulposus. The disc normally functions as a shock absorber. With degeneration, the disc loses its resiliency. Under pressure the nucleus sometimes ruptures and protrudes through the anulus (usually posteriorly or laterally), causing pressure on a spinal nerve root (Fig. 33-7). The facet joints that stabilize the spine are synovial joints and also can be affected by degenerative joint disease (Fig. 33-8.) The most common sites of lumbar herniation are L4-5, L5-S1, and L3-4. A myelogram may be ordered to confirm a suspected protruded disc or to rule out a cord lesion.

Prevention. Injury to an intervertebral disc usually is caused by stress on the back while it is in acute flexion. The injury may be due to one severe episode of loading the disc or it may result from a cumulative effect of years of wear. Many back injuries of this type could be prevented if persons doing extensive lifting and pulling were taught to observe principles of good body mechanics. When a person is lifting heavy objects, the knees should be flexed and the back kept straight. In this position the weight is carried by the large muscles of the thighs and the buttocks, not the back muscles, which give support to the spine. It is always better to pull than to push, and the body should be kept in correct alignment and not twisted to one side whenever one bends, lifts, or carries heavy objects. If one is lifting objects from a high shelf, both hands should be used. This will place the weight of the object on the shoulder muscles rather than on those of the cervical spine.

The nurse must frequently move patients and heavy objects. Therefore the principles of good body mechanics must be learned and practiced. The incidence of back strain and ruptured intervertebral discs is high among nursing personnel. The nurse should be responsible for teaching the principles of good body mechanics to members of the nursing staff. The industrial nurse may have many opportunities to help workers improve their body mechanics and avoid back injury. (For a complete discussion of body mechanics in nursing, see texts on fundamentals of nursing.)

The common complaint of low back pain may result from many causes, among which may be pelvic disease, vascular disorders, neurologic disease, or degenerative joint disease. Although bed rest usually is the initial management for patients with low back pain regardless of etiology, the following relates to the treatment of a patient with a ruptured intervertebral disc. While the patient is on bed rest it is essential

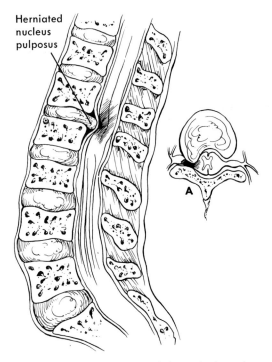

FIG. 33-7. Note compression of the spinal cord caused by herniation of nucleus pulposus into the spinal canal. **A,** Pressure on nerves as they leave the spinal cord.

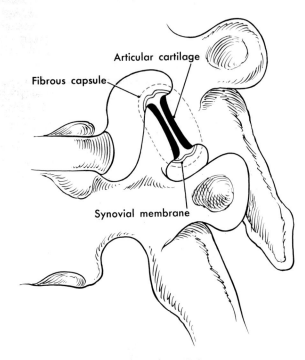

FIG. 33-8. Normal posterior facet joint.

that there be accurate observation and recording of the patient's pain and positions that aggravate or alleviate the pain.

Diagnostic measures. The diagnosis of a herniated disc is usually made on the basis of the history and physical examination. The history of low back pain that is relieved by recumbency and aggravated by flexion of the trunk, coughing, or sneezing is typical. The patient will often complain of sciatic pain radiating down his leg. Some patients, after the initial injury, will have sciatic pain but no pain in their back. Deep pressure over the interspace usually elicits pain. Straight leg raising with the hip flexed and the knee extended (a positive Lasègue sign) will produce the sciatic pain. Neurologic signs and symptoms help in determining the level of the disc involved. The sensory and motor changes depend on the nerve root involved. A patient with fifth lumbar root involvement is usually unable to walk on his heels. If the fifth lumbar disc is causing pressure on the first sacral root, the patient will be unable to walk on his toes. If the back problem has been long-standing, the patient may have some muscle atrophy in the affected leg. Radiographs of the spine are taken. Myelography may be done if needed to confirm the physical

findings or to differentiate a herniated disc from an intervertebral tumor.

Conservative management. Unless there are major neurologic deficits indicating a need for immediate surgery, the patient is usually managed conservatively. (This course of treatment may have been attempted at home prior to admission.) The patient is placed on bed rest. The bed should have a firm mattress with bed boards. The patient with a herniated disc is usually most comfortable when supine with his head elevated a few degrees and his knees flexed. This decreases the lordosis of the lumbar spine and relieves the pressure on the nerve roots. The bed should be flat when the patient is on his side, and he will probably be most comfortable with pillows between his legs. The pillows should support the upper leg and therefore lessen the pull on the back. The patient should be taught to turn himself in a logrolling fashion: to cross his arms over his chest, bend the uppermost knee to the side to which he wishes to turn, and then to roll over (Fig. 33-9). This position helps him to maintain good spinal alignment. If there is any motor nerve loss, a footboard should be used to prevent foot drop. The patient may complain of a burning sensation in his feet because of paresthesia, and a footboard helps by keeping the bedclothes off the feet. If the patient has a sensory nerve loss, hot-water bottles or heating pads should not be used on the feet or legs, and other precautions should be taken to prevent further injury. A small bedpan should be used with a small towel roll placed directly behind it to support the arch of the lower back. The patient should roll onto the bedpan instead of lifting his hips. He should be advised not to strain to defecate since straining will increase pain. Constipation is frequent. The patient is urged to increase the amount of roughage eaten; fresh fruits are helpful. At least 3,000 ml. of fluid should be taken each day, and a regular time for defecation should be established. A mild laxative such as one of the bulk laxatives may be ordered.

Many patients with a ruptured lumbar intervertebral disc suffer from severe muscle spasm in the lower back. A heating pad may relieve it, although codeine or other analgesic drugs are often necessary. Physical therapy in the form of infrared heat, massage, and active and passive muscle exercise carried out in warm water may also be ordered to help relieve the muscle spasm. Exercises are more easily performed in water, and the heat helps to relax muscles. The patient should be transferred to the physical therapy department by stretcher, and extra covers such as a towel to wrap around the head if the hair becomes wet should be sent with him to avoid chilling after the treatment.

The patient with a ruptured disc may be discouraged by the prospects of a long period of bed rest and possible surgery. If he has motor or sensory losses,

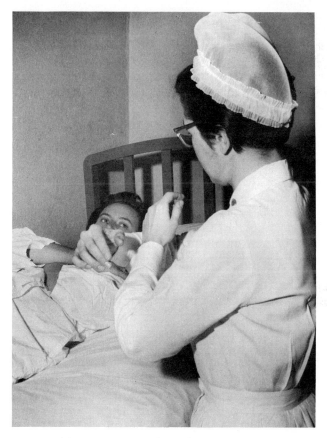

FIG. 33-9. The nurse is teaching the patient with a ruptured disc how to fold her arms preparatory to "logrolling."

he worries lest he become unable to walk. To some people, spinal surgery is synonymous with paralysis. The patient may worry about his family, his finances, his job, and about collecting compensation if the injury was sustained at work. Physicians, nurses, other professional team members, and the patient's spiritual adviser may need to help alleviate his fears and anxieties.

The physician may order traction to relieve muscle spasm. This is usually accomplished by bilateral Buck's extension or pelvic traction. The patient may begin with short periods in traction and gradually increase his tolerance until he remains in traction most of the time.

If the patient shows improvement on bed rest, as do 90% of the patients for whom this is the first occurrence, the physician may order a brace or place the patient in a plaster flexion jacket to provide external support for the spine. This support may be needed for several months until the patient is asymptomatic. The external supports are discarded as soon as possible since prolonged use fosters muscle weakness, which then increases the load on the vertebral column. Before the patient is discharged, he will need assistance in adapting his activities of daily living to protect his back. The occupational therapist can assist in teaching the patient and recommending devices to assist in dressing. The patient who will wear a corset or brace must learn to put this on while lying flat and before getting out of bed. Since straight leg raising and bending at the waist should be avoided, the patient may need assistance in putting on shoes and stockings. However, it is permissible to bend the knees to bring the foot up, and most patients learn to dress themselves.

The nurse should teach and demonstrate principles of body mechanics to the patient since he will need to be particularly careful in lifting. Some patients may be encouraged by the physician to change their type of work. Movement and positions that cause poor alignment of the spinal column and put a strain on the injured nerves should be avoided. A firm, straight chair should be used instead of an overstuffed one. The knees should not be crossed or the feet or legs elevated on a footstool. It is inadvisable for the patient to drive a car since this activity would necessitate stretching the legs. Stairs should be climbed as infrequently as possible, and great care should be taken in walking over rough ground or in stepping off curbs to avoid sudden twisting of the back. If a tub bath must be taken, the knees should be kept flexed. However, getting in and out of the tub may aggravate the symptoms, and showers are preferable. A warm shower before bed and on arising often helps to reduce discomfort. In picking things up off the floor, the patient should assume a squatting posture with the knees bent and the back held straight (Fig. 33-10). Weights heavier than 5 pounds should not be carried.

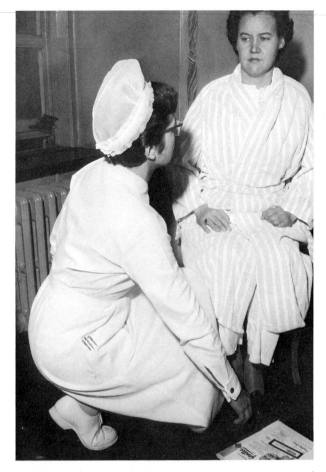

FIG. 33-10. The nurse is demonstrating to a patient with a ruptured disc how to stoop to pick something up from the floor. Note that her back is held straight and that her knees and hips are flexed sharply.

When the acute episode has subsided, the physician may prescribe exercises designed to strengthen the back and abdominal muscles to decrease the load carried by the vertebral column.

Surgical management. When the patient's symptoms fail to respond to conservative management, when there is progressive neurologic impairment, or when the patient has repeated episodes when he resumes activity, surgical intervention is usually indicated. The pressure on the nerve root is relieved by removing the disc (discectomy). This is most often done through a posterior approach in which a portion of the lamina is removed (laminectomy).

Postoperative nursing care of a patient who has had a laminectomy is similar to that needed in conservative management. In addition, the patient needs the nursing care indicated for any postanesthesia patient. The patient should be told preoperatively that he may have much the same pain in the initial postoperative period. Although the pressure from the disc has been removed, there is pressure from edema at the operative site. Postoperatively the patient's motion and sensation in the lower extremities should be

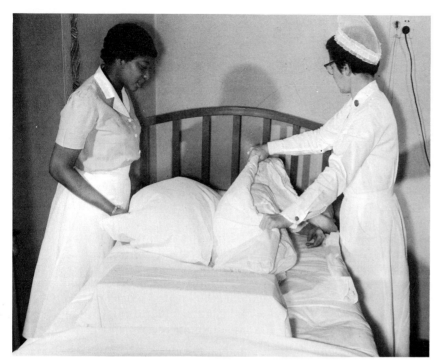

FIG. 33-11. The nurse and the aide are turning the patient who has had surgery for the excision of a ruptured disc. Note that the nurse holds the turning sheet taut with one hand at the level of the patient's shoulder and the other below his buttocks.

checked routinely along with his vital signs. He may continue to have muscle spasms. The patient should be encouraged to move his legs and continue plantar flexion and dorsiflexion of his feet. The patient may have bowel and bladder dysfunction for several days. This should be carefully observed. These complications are treated in the usual manner—with a Foley catheter, rectal tube, or a suppository or enema as needed. As soon as the patient is able to take oral medications, it is very beneficial if the physician prescribes a stool softener.

Physicians vary in their postoperative management of a patient who has had a laminectomy. Generally the patient is allowed a position of comfort in bed. The dressing should be inspected frequently for signs of bleeding or leakage of spinal fluid. Any evidence of either should be reported at once. If the patient is having increased drainage, he may be placed on his back to put pressure on the operative site. As with any dressings, they should be kept dry to prevent contamination.

Following a laminectomy, the patient may be ambulated anytime from the first postoperative day. Orders to ambulate depend largely on the patient's general postoperative condition and the surgeon's preference.

Removal of a disc causes increased stress on the posterior articulations of the spine, which then may develop degenerative changes. Therefore, depending on the extent of the pathology and the type of activities the patient usually engages in, the surgeon may elect to do a spinal fusion. A spinal fusion may also be done when a prior laminectomy has failed to provide relief of symptoms or the symptoms have reappeared. There are numerous techniques for spinal

fusion, details of which may be found in orthopedic texts. Most commonly, lumbar fusion is done through a posterior incision, with the bone for the graft being taken from the iliac crest. The postoperative nursing management is aimed toward preventing any movement at the graft site. The basic nursing care is similar to that for a patient who has had a laminectomy with the exception that more stringent limitations of movement are placed on the patient who has had a fusion.

For the patient who has had a lumbar fusion through a posterior approach, the bed is kept absolutely flat. Raising the head of the bed would increase the lordosis in the lumbar spine, putting strain on and possibly dislodging the graft. The patient usually is kept flat for 10 days to 2 weeks.

Any twisting motion of the trunk must be avoided. The patient should be log-rolled from side to side (Fig. 33-9). He should be taught this preoperatively but should not be expected to assist with this for several days postoperatively. Patients anticipate pain with turning and tend to be very tense. Giving medications for pain before turning the patient is beneficial. Having the patient fold his arms across his chest lessens the possibility of his reaching out and twisting as he is turned. Some surgeons prefer that patients who have had fusions remain flat on their backs for several hours. This is to provide additional pressure on the operative site and increase hemostatis. The patient who has had a spinal fusion is more likely to develop a hematoma than is the person who has had a laminectomy. A pressure dressing is applied and should be checked frequently for drainage. Also, the nurse should note the contour of the area around the dressing as the patient is turned. A change in contour may indicate that a hematoma is developing. The patient may also complain of a feeling of pressure at the site. When the bone graft is taken from the iliac crest, the patient may be very uncomfortable when positioned on that side. It is not unusual for the patient to complain of intense discomfort at the graft site.

A turning sheet, although not essential, makes it easier to turn the patient while keeping his trunk in good alignment (Fig. 33-11). When the patient is on his side, pillows between the legs are needed to maintain proper alignment, as described earlier. Multiple small adjustments are usually necessary to get the patient in a position of comfort. Although for several days the patient will have a great deal of discomfort for which he will need to receive medication, positioning is often the key factor in providing comfort. When the patient is on his side, a pillow behind his back will lend support. If the patient must be transferred from bed to cart, a sheet or roller board should be used along with adequate personnel to maintain proper alignment of the patient during the transfer (Fig. 33-12).

When the patient is allowed to ambulate, he should be gotten out of bed without being placed in a sitting position. Depending on the type of fusion that was done and the preference of the surgeon, the patient may have to wear a brace. This is put on while he is still in bed. He may be instructed to wear this for several months after he goes home. The patient may be gotten out of bed from a side-lying position. At least two people should be present the first time that this is done. Having been horizontal for an extended period of time, the patient may very likely have postural hypotension on assuming an upright position. The patient is moved to the very edge of the bed and then turned on his side. The patient can be instructed to push up with his elbow as one person lifts his shoulders and the other person guides his legs

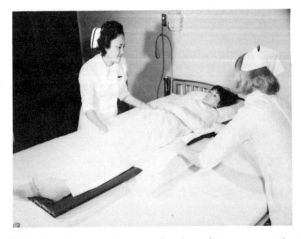

FIG. 33-12. Nurses using a roller board to move patient from bed to cart. (Courtesy Neuropsychiatric Institute, University of Illinois Hospitals at the Medical Center, Chicago, Ill.)

to the floor. The weight of the lower extremities moving to the floor assists in pivoting the trunk upwards when the patient is on his side. After several days of getting out of bed in this manner, the patient will need the assistance of only one person. As his postoperative pain decreases, he will be able to do this by himself. A walker will be a useful source of support when the patient begins to ambulate. When the patient is able to ambulate without problems, he may be allowed bathroom privileges for bowel movements. A raised toilet seat allows the patient to use the toilet with less discomfort. He may not be permitted to actually sit for several weeks. When he is permitted to sit, he should have a firm, straight-backed chair with arms so that he sits bolt upright. Sitting will be his least comfortable position because of the load that this places on the lumbar spine. Although surgery may have corrected the initial disorder, the patient who has had a back problem is very vulnerable to further trauma. He must be taught good body mechanics to avoid putting unnecessary stress on his back.

Other types of arthritis

Almost any organism can affect the joints. The typhoid bacillus, tubercle bacillus, gonococcus, and staphylococcus were common causes of arthritis before the discovery of the specific antibiotic drugs and the control of communicable diseases. Arthritis can also result from trauma to the joint, or it may be associated with new growths within or about the joint or with neurogenic changes. See Table 33-1 for a summary of characteristics of various types of arthritis.

Rheumatic fever

Rheumatic fever is a systemic disease that is believed to be a sequela of infection with group A hemolytic streptococcus. Most commonly the attack of rheumatic fever occurs several weeks following a streptococcal infection. The patient often does not remember having had a previous infection, but careful questioning may reveal a history of a sore throat a few weeks previously. The symptoms of rheumatic fever—elevation in temperature, inflamed and painful joints, and in some cases cardiac and other symptoms—are felt to be due to antibodies produced in response to the streptococcus organism.

The disease varies in its severity, but most commonly the patient has migratory joint pains accompanied by heat, redness, and swelling. In addition, he may have the usual systemic symptoms found in most infections: anorexia, fatigue, and loss of weight. Rheumatic fever is most common in children between the ages of 5 and 15, although it can occur at any age. The incidence is highest among those members of the population who are most susceptible to any infection. Thus the incidence is highest among the lower economic groups who live in

Table 33-1 Summary of characteristics of various types of arthritis

Characteristics	Rheumatic fever	Rheumatoid arthritis	Degenerative Joint disease	Gout
Synonyms	—	Atrophic arthritis Arthritis deformans	Hypertrophic arthritis Osteoarthritis Degenerative arthritis	—
Average age of onset	5-11 yr.	30-50 yr.	50-70 yr.	20-40 yr.
Sex (ratio)	—	Women 3:1	Women 5:1	Men 19:1
Build and weight	—	Asthenic—underweight	Stocky—overweight	Overweight
Joints involved	Any; moves from joint to joint	Any, often fingers and other joints; progressive	Weight-bearing joints—joints—knees, hips, spine, fingers; localized	Terminal joint of great toe of foot—spreading to any joint, tarsal and metatarsal joints
Subcutaneous lesion	Rheumatic nodules over tendon surfaces; indicate poor prognosis	Nodules over bony prominences, painful on injury, no prognostic significance	Heberden's nodes on fingers, painful at times, no prognostic significance	Tophi, prognostic of difficulty in control of blood urates
X-ray findings	None	Clouding of fluid space, fraying of inner joint margins, lessening of joint space	Lipping of bony margins, lessening of joint space	Clouding of joint spaces
Outward appearance of joints	Swollen, tender, reddened, painful	Swollen, painful, reddened, shiny	Enlarged, no swelling	Swollen, painful, reddened, shiny
Termination	No joint damage or limitation of motion	Ankylosis, deformity	Some limitation of motion, deformity, some ankylosis	Limitation of motion, deformity, possible renal calculi

substandard, overcrowded housing and who are poorly nourished.

There seems to be some evidence that the incidence of rheumatic fever in the United States is declining. One possible explanation for this decline is the widespread use of antimicrobial agents to treat childhood infections. This is supported by the fact that when outbreaks of rheumatic fever have threatened a military base, the use of prophylactic antimicrobial therapy has reduced the incidence of the disease.

The joint manifestations of rheumatic fever are not permanent and no deformity occurs. A serious complication of rheumatic fever is rheumatic heart disease (p. 332), and one of the aims of medical therapy is to prevent its occurrence. To this end adequate treatment with penicillin during the acute phase of rheumatic fever and its prophylactic use for years afterwards are advocated.

Although not all medical authorities would agree on the need for absolute bed rest, it is generally accepted that the patient should be on bed rest until the acute symptoms subside and longer if there is evidence of cardiac involvement.

Penicillin is usually ordered once or twice daily for 10 days or a long-acting form of the drug may be given. Oral penicillin may also be prescribed and it is the form most often used for long-term prophylactic follow-up of the patient. If there is any doubt that the patient will adhere to the regimen of a daily prophylactic dose of penicillin, a long-acting parenteral form will be given. Sulfonamides (sulfadiazine, sulfisoxazole) are also used for continuous prophylaxis. They are most commonly prescribed for individuals who are allergic to penicillin.

During the acute phase of the disease, the patient commonly receives salicylates in large doses to relieve joint pain and fever. It is usually necessary to attain blood levels of at least 25 mg./100 ml. to obtain full therapeutic effect.[35a] Thus the dosage of salicylates will be adjusted in accordance with the serum level of the drug. The nurse should expect the patient to develop toxic manifestations of salicylate therapy and should be alert for their occurrence. At one time sodium bicarbonate was commonly administered with the salicylates to reduce gastric irritation; this is no longer recommended, however, since it also increases the excretion of salicylate and interferes with the maintenance of an adequate blood level.

Corticosteroids may be given either alone or in combination with salicylates. If combined therapy is used, the steroid is usually discontinued as soon as the signs of inflammation subside and the salicylates are continued alone. There seems to be no medical agreement on whether or not the corticosteroids should be used in the treatment of rheumatic fever; however, there is agreement that they should be used to treat the patient with symptoms of cardiac involvement. Since both the salicylates and corticosteroids suppress symptoms of inflammation without altering the underlying disease process, the symptoms may recur once the therapy is discontinued.

Because there are several different strains of group A hemolytic streptococci and they do not confer cross-immunity, it is possible for an individual to have more than one attack of rheumatic fever. Each succeeding attack is usually more severe and more likely to result in cardiac involvement.

Since the incidence of rheumatic fever is especially high in the poverty areas of large cities, some cities have begun rheumatic fever case registries to aid them in administering long-term prophylactic penicillin therapy and medical follow-up. This is necessary because in most states rheumatic fever is not a reportable disease as are the communicable diseases of childhood.

The nursing care of the patient with rheumatic fever will be determined by his symptoms and his medical therapy. As in any febrile condition, fluids are usually ordered in large amounts (3 to 4 L. daily). Relief of joint pain can be minimized by proper positioning and support of the affected joints. These patients often become very bored and restless, especially when confined to bed for long periods of time; thus the nurse may be taxed to develop diversional activities for the patient in accord with his physical limitations. The American Heart Association publishes many booklets that are helpful in understanding rheumatic fever. One of the most useful is *Home Care of the Child with Rheumatic Fever.*

Nonarticular rheumatic disease

Bursitis, or inflammation of the connective tissue sac about a joint, may be acute or chronic. It usually is caused by trauma, strain, and overuse of the joint, but pathogenic organisms and toxins may cause it also. The shoulder bursa is the most often affected and may be exceedingly troublesome. Severe pain occurs, especially on movement of the joint.

The main treatment of bursitis consists of controlling the pain and preserving joint motion. Treatment and the response of individual patients vary widely. During the acute attack treatment includes the local application of heat, diathermy, medications to control pain, and temporary immobilization of the part. Medications used include salicylates and phenylbutazone as well as other analgesics such as meperidine (Demerol) or codeine. X-ray treatment is sometimes given in an attempt to dissolve the calcium

deposits that form within the bursa, causing pain. Sometimes the bursa may be aspirated to remove some of the irritating deposits. Sterile normal saline solution with procaine (Novocain) may be used. Hydrocortisone may be injected into the bursa or used systemically for its anti-inflammatory effects. If there are large particles of calcium, surgery may be necessary for their removal. In bursitis of the shoulder, attention should be given to preserving the range of joint motion in the shoulder. Pendulum exercises are almost always ordered, and the nurse may demonstrate them and stress their importance to the patient.

In some cases, recurrence of bursitis may be prevented by avoiding excessive use of the joint. The patient with chronic bursitis should continue physical therapy and exercises are prescribed by the physiatrist.

There are many other forms of nonarticular rheumatism. Lumbago, stiff neck, fibrositis, tendinitis, and tenosynovitis are examples. These conditions can be very painful and may cause distress out of all proportion to their seriousness. So far, unfortunately, there seems to be no specific cure for any of them, and the greatest comfort comes from the use of local heat and mild analgesic agents such as acetylsalicylic acid. Constant pain is demoralizing to the patient, and one of his greatest needs is a sympathetic person to listen to his problems and to give encouragement.

Collagen diseases

The collagen or connective tissue diseases are a group of clinical entities in which there is derangement of collagen substance; they are not well understood. Because of the occurrence of immunologic abnormalities in these diseases, it is thought that they may represent an autoimmune reaction. Collagen and elastic substances are the fibrous constituents of connective tissue. Connective tissue makes up the extracellular framework around which cells develop and organs and other essential structures are formed and carry out their function. The collagen substance may respond with inflammation and degeneration. Because of its extremely wide distribution in the body, disease involvement is widespread also. There are several collagen diseases, including polyarteritis, systemic lupus erythematosus, scleroderma, and dermatomyositis. As can be seen in Table 33-2, both the characteristics and clinical manifestations of these diseases vary. Diagnosis is often difficult and elusive. Serologic tests are being used increasingly and are often fruitful in their results. Because of multiple-organ involvement, nursing care must be directed toward the individual patient's needs and the medical regimen being followed. Two of the diseases, systemic lupus erythematosus and scleroderma, are described in more detail. (For more informa-

Table 33-2 Summary of characteristics of some collagen diseases

Characteristics	Systemic lupus erythematosus (SLE)	Dermatomyositis (polymyositis)	Polyarteritis nodosa	Progressive systemic sclerosis (scleroderma)
Occurrence	20-40 yr. Females 4:1	30-50 yr. Females 2:1	20-50 yr. Males 4:1	30-50 yr. Females 3:1
Symptoms	Skin rash, Raynaud's phenomena, joint pains, photosensitivity	Edema, dermatitis, profound symmetric muscle weakness	Respiratory disease, abdominal illness, fever, hypertension	Skin changes, Raynaud's phenomena, calcium nodules, edema
Organs involved	Any organs in body (commonly multiple organs) skin, joints, kidney (75% of cases), liver, heart, central nervous system	Skin, muscle (pelvic girdle, shoulder girdle, neck muscles), diaphragm	Kidneys, heart, gastrointestinal tract, liver, lungs, brain, peripheral nerves	Skin, lungs, esophagus, kidney
Primary process	Inflammation → fibrosis	Fiber necrosis, inflammation → fibrosis	Inflammation of small arteries	Fibrinoid degeneration
Diagnosis	Blood serology (often false positive), LE prep, antinuclear factors (ANF), serum proteins, renal biopsy, history of symptoms	Muscle biopsy, electromyogram, elevated SGOT, blood serology (often false positive), history of symptoms	Peripheral neuritis, muscle biopsy, infarcted bowel, bronchospasm (may present as asthma), history of symptoms	Skin changes, x-ray studies (bowel, lung, barium swallow), "birdlike facies," history of symptoms
Treatment	Symptomatic relief: salicylates for joint pain, steroids, immunosuppressives, antimalarials	Symptomatic relief: complete rest, analgesics, steroids, treatment of underlying malignancy if present	Symptomatic relief: analgesics, steroids	Symptomatic relief: steroids not very effective
Prognosis	Some die within a few weeks, others live many years with remissions and exacerbations, slow debilitating process	May have remissions, guarded prognosis, die of respiratory insufficiency or cardiac failure	Poor often die within 6 months	May live 30-50 years or die within a few months

tion, the student is referred to specialized texts.[48])

Systemic lupus erythematosus is a serious disease involving the collagen substance of connective tissue in the skin, blood vessels, and serous and synovial membranes. It is now known to be fairly common, and young women are most often affected. The cause of systemic lupus erythematosus is unknown. It may be acute or chronic and usually runs a long course with exacerbations and remissions. About half the patients have skin lesions. Pleuritis, pericarditis, peritonitis, neuritis, and anemia are common.

The initial manifestation of systemic lupus erythematosus is often arthritis. In most instances the joint symptoms are transient and respond to treatment. Avascular necrosis, particularly of the femoral heads, is not uncommon. The necrosis is thought to be associated with the use of corticosteroids.

Erythema (redness), usually in a butterfly pattern, appears over the cheeks and bridge of the nose. The margins of the lesions are usually bright red, and the lesions may extend beyond the hairline, with partial alopecia (loss of hair) above the ears. Lesions also occur on the exposed part of the neck. Chronic discoid (round) lesions are also fairly common and may undergo vascularization, degeneration, and subsequent atrophy. Lesions slowly spread to the mucous membranes and other tissues of the body, or they may originate there. The lesions do not ulcerate but cause degeneration and atrophy of tissues.

No specific treatment for systemic lupus erythematosus is available. Adrenocorticosteroid therapy is used to control active manifestations. With this treatment and supportive treatment of systems involved, many patients live for years. Bed rest and salicylates are used during exacerbations, and antimalarial drugs such as chloroquine are sometimes surprisingly helpful. If the patient has skin lesions, rest in a darkened room during the acute stages and permanent avoidance of sunshine are usually prescribed.

Scleroderma (progressive systemic sclerosis) is a generalized systemic disease involving the collagen substance throughout the body. The cause of this relatively rare condition is unknown. Middle-aged persons are most often affected, and women are affected more frequently than men.

The word "scleroderma" means "hard skin" and accurately describes the skin manifestations that are predominant in this disease. Usually local areas such as the face and fingers are first affected, and sometimes the condition is confused with rheumatoid arthritis and with Raynaud's disease in the early stages. Usually there is pain on joint motion because the skin and muscle contractures produce a deformity of the joint. The skin may first appear slightly edematous, then turn pale, become steadily more firm, and finally become fixed to underlying tissues and mildly pigmented. The face becomes masklike, chewing may be impossible, and the patient may have difficulty swallowing. Finally, all body motion becomes so restricted that the patient has the appearance of a living mummy. Tissues of essential organs such as the heart, kidneys, and liver may be affected in a similar manner, and fatal impairment of their function may result. Chest expansion may be impaired by firming of the skin so that respiratory failure threatens.

There is no cure and no specific treatment for scleroderma, and the disease is fatal within a period of months or years. Death usually is caused by failure of involved organs or systems such as the liver or the circulatory system. Intensive treatment with corticosteroids in the early stages has proved helpful in some cases. Salicylates and mild analgesics are used for joint pain, and physical therapy is ordered to slow the development of contractures and deformity.

In advanced stages of the disease, meticulous nursing care is imperative. It includes mouth care, care in assisting the patient while eating to prevent choking, skin care and prevention of decubiti, and attention to the emotional support of the patient, who is becoming more helpless daily.

Avascular necrosis of bone

Unlike some other forms of connective tissue, bone has a highly developed vascular system and will die without an adequate blood supply. There is a well-developed collateral blood supply to most bone so that infarction due to vascular interruption is infrequent. Several areas of bone, however, have a rather precarious blood supply. One such area is the femoral head. Hence avascular necrosis of the femoral head is a common late complication of a fracture of the femoral neck since the blood supply to the head comes up through the neck and has been interrupted by the trauma. Avascular necrosis of the femoral head is also seen in patients with systemic diseases such as alcoholism, sickle cell disease, and lupus erythematosus. Patients who have had prolonged corticosteroid therapy have an increased incidence of avascular necrosis.

The patient usually has a history of gradually increasing hip pain with increasing deformity. Flexion contractures may develop. Joint replacement is the treatment usually chosen when there has been complete destruction of the head.

■ OPERATIVE PROCEDURES

Surgery is being increasingly used to correct deformity and improve function of the musculoskeletal system. Surgery is indicated when other measures are ineffective. Advances in other fields such as bioengineering have made possible reconstructive surgery in patients for whom there were formerly very limited means of treatment available. These advances are most notable in the area of joint replacement.

The patient having orthopedic surgery has many of the same needs of any other surgical patient. He, too, needs preoperative teaching regarding postanesthesia care. Since he is very likely to be relatively immobile, he especially needs to understand the importance of good pulmonary toilet. Because the integrity of the locomotor system will be altered in some way during surgery, there are three major questions to be answered in anticipating patient care requirement: (1) What is the operative procedure? (2) What limitations in positioning and/or ambulation will this necessitate and for how long? (3) What are the consequences of these limitations for this particular person?

The following discussion will be limited to commonly used operative orthopedic procedures of bone and joints.

Arthrotomy

An arthrotomy is an opening of a joint. This is usually done for explorations, drainage, or removal of damaged tissue within the joint. The knee is very frequently the joint involved and often the arthrotomy is done to remove a torn meniscus. After an arthrotomy, the joint must be protected until healing takes place. Following an arthrotomy of the knee the patient is often placed in a Robert-Jones dressing. This is a large bulky compressive dressing sometimes referred to as a "soft cast." Circulation and sensation to the distal part of the extremity must be checked frequently. The dressing also acts as a protective splint, preventing flexion of the knee.

Depending on the procedure, the surgeon may order straight leg raising exercises to be done postoperatively. The patient will have limited weight bearing on that leg and most probably will use crutches for a prescribed amount of time.

Arthrodesis

An arthrodesis (fusion) is done to permanently immobilize a joint, to provide relief of pain, or to stabilize a joint. Spinal fusions are a type of arthrodesis and have been discussed on p. 947. A triple arthrodesis of the foot is often done to stabilize the foot when there is inadequate or absent neuromuscular control. The three joints involved are the subastragalar, the astragaloscaphoid, and the calcaneocuboid joint. A joint that has been fused must be immobilized until bony healing has occurred. For a triple arthrodesis this means that the patient will be held in a short leg cast with no weight bearing for 8 to 12 weeks.

Arthroplasty

An arthroplasty is the reconstruction of a joint. A common interposition arthroplasty is the "cup" or "mold" arthroplasty of the hip joint. The usual indication for this procedure is osteoarthritis of the hip. In this procedure both the acetabulum and the femoral head are reshaped. A Vitallium cup is interposed between the head of the femur and the acetabulum. In the immediate postoperative period the patient is placed in some form of traction with an apparatus to allow him to begin prescribed exercises. The period of hospitalization is usually 5 to 6 weeks during which the patient will undergo an extensive program of physical therapy. The patient will not be permitted full weight bearing for at least 6 months and therefore will be on crutches for at least that length of time. An exercise program to be done at home will be prescribed and followed for several years. The cup arthroplasty provides relief of pain, increase in motion of the hip, and decrease in deformity. To achieve these results a patient must be highly motivated and committed to the long-term exercise program.

Replacement arthroplasty. The replacement arthroplasty is one of the most rapidly expanding areas of orthopedic surgery. The results are quickly apparent and very dramatic. Partially for these reasons this type of surgery has received wide coverage in the lay press. Many patients with diseased joints seek out an orthopedic surgeon with the expressed hope that they might benefit from joint replacement. However, not all persons with diseased joints are candidates for joint replacement. Joint replacement is still a relatively new procedure and is usually considered when there is no other operative procedure that would be effective for the individual. A major factor in the use of joint replacements is wear. All artificial joints have a finite life and therefore are used most frequently in the older individual.

The hip is a joint that is commonly replaced. As discussed previously, the hip joint may be involved with osteoarthritis, rheumatoid arthritis, and numerous other systemic diseases. When the patient has far-advanced destruction of both the femoral head and the acetabulum with resultant pain and deformity, a hip replacement may be considered.

The prosthesis consists of an acetabular portion (cup) and a femoral component. There are numerous types of total hip replacements in use (Fig. 33-13). Some prostheses (McKee-Farrar, Ring) are made entirely of metal (Vitallium or stainless steel). Other prostheses (Charnley, Charnley-Müller, Trapezoidal-

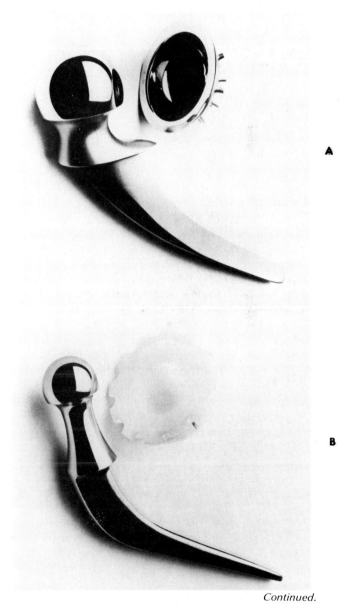

Continued.

FIG. 33-13. A, McKee-Farrar prosthesis. **B,** Charnley prosthesis. **C,** Charnley-Müller prosthesis. **D,** Trapezoidal-28 prosthesis. (Courtesy Zimmer USA, Warsaw, Ind.)

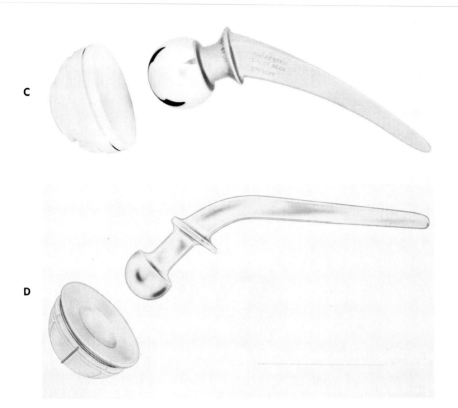

FIG. 33-13, cont'd. For legend see p. 953.

28) have a metal femoral component and a high-density polyethylene acetabular component. The metal component moving within a polyethylene cup is expected to cause less friction and therefore it should wear at a slower rate. The designs of the different prostheses vary in size of the femoral head, shape and length of the femoral neck, and shape of the acetabular component. Each type of prosthesis has its own mechanical advantages and disadvantages of design, and each prosthesis is inserted by a particular operative technique. The relative merits of the design and operative techniques are discussed at great length in the orthopedic literature. As in any new and expanding field, changes are constantly being made. For this reason it is essential that the nurse caring for a patient with a total hip replacement become familiar with the literature pertaining to the prosthesis and procedure being used for each patient.

A discussion of the general nursing care requirements of a patient with a total hip replacement follows. Many of the total hip prostheses that are in current use are held in place by polymethylmethacrylate. This material is a filling agent that gives off heat as it solidifies. The temperature is high enough to cause some minimal local tissue necrosis. Because necrotic tissue is a good culture medium for bacterial growth, there is an increased risk of infection. Although any bone infection is serious, it has especially grave consequences for a patient having a joint replacement. *Infection at the prosthesis site causes total failure of the surgery.* The prosthesis must be removed and cannot be replaced. The patient is then left after healing with a pain-free but unstable hip. For this reason, the utmost care must be taken in preparing the operative site to guard against infection. Each hospital will have its own procedure for preoperative preparation, but the goal is the same. Nursing care is directed at keeping the patient and his environment as free as possible from potential sources of contamination. Once the joint is replaced and the wound closed the patient has no more risk of infection than any other surgical patient.

The postoperative positioning of the total hip patient is directly dependent on the design of the prosthesis and the method of insertion. Positioning is generally directed at keeping the patient's operative leg in *abduction* and in limiting flexion of that hip. To plan care for the patient the nurse must have the following information:

1. What degree of flexion in the operative hip is permitted and for how long?
2. In what rotation is the leg to be held?
3. How much weight bearing is allowed on the operative leg?
4. What exercises, if any, are to be done?

Nursing care of the patient with a Charnley total

hip replacement will serve as an example of a partial care plan regarding positioning and ambulating. The Charnley prosthesis has a small (22.5 mm.) head that, once healing has taken place, can be flexed to 90 degrees without dislocating it. In the Charnley procedure the greater trochanter is detached with all its muscles still in place. After placement of the prosthesis, the trochanter is wired back into place. Until bony union takes place (6 to 8 weeks) pull on the abductor muscles attached to the trochanter must be avoided. However, weight bearing on the operative leg is permitted.

During surgery a drain or drains are usually placed in the wound to prevent formation of a hematoma. The drains are connected to constant suction and are usually the self-contained vacuum type such as the Porto-Vac (Fig. 11-11). It is imperative that the system remain closed and that sterility be maintained. Because the drains are inserted deep in the wound, contamination of the tubing would provide a portal of entry for bacteria. The drains are usually removed in 48 hours.

Since the patient remains in bed for 3 postoperative days, nursing care is directed at keeping him as active as possible within the specified restrictions. His head may be elevated for comfort (usually about 60 degrees) for short periods of time. He is encouraged to spend some time flat with his hip in full extension. He is instructed in the use of the overbed trapeze and taught how to shift his weight using his unoperated leg and the trapeze. His leg is maintained in abduction with an abduction block and he is turned only slightly side to side. The patient is encouraged to do plantar flexion and dorsiflexion of the feet as well as quadriceps and gluteal-setting exercises to promote venous return and prevent thrombi. These exercises are taught preoperatively.

Because of the increased risk of thromboembolic phenomena in hip surgery, prophylactic anticoagulant treatment is often prescribed. The various methods of treatment are debated in the literature. While there is not general agreement on which method is preferable, three types of treatment are most common: (1) the patient is maintained on acetylsalicylic acid, usually 600 mg. four times a day; (2) the patient receives low molecular weight dextran, which increases microcirculation and decreases platelet cohesiveness; and (3) the patient receives small dosages of heparin. Each method has its particular advantages and hazards with which the nurse must be familiar. (Refer to specialized texts for further details.)

Ambulation begins on the third to fourth postoperative day. Nursing personnel and physical therapy assist the patient to stand without flexing his operative hip more than 60 degrees. The amount of walking, using a walker for support, that the patient is allowed is variable and depends on his progress. The patient is usually discharged 3 weeks after surgery. He must use crutches and limit his hip flexion to 90 degrees for 2 months.

To assist him in making the necessary adaptations the nurse, physical therapist, and occupational therapist evaluate his ability to carry out activities of daily living throughout his postoperative course. Necessary equipment is secured for him. A raised toilet seat extension must be used for 2 months to protect against the extreme hip flexion needed to rise from a standard toilet seat. Long-handled shoe horns and devices to pick up dropped items (reachers) are also needed by these patients.

Some surgeons, depending on the prosthesis used and their personal preference, will place the patient in various slings or traction to facilitate motion of the hip while maintaining the desired position. It is important for the nurse as well as the entire health team to understand what will be required of the patient in the postoperative period so that the necessary preoperative teaching can be done.

A replacement arthroplasty of the knee is also in common use. Once again there are numerous prosthetic designs, each with its distinct mechanical advantage. Nursing care of the patient with a total knee replacement is not usually nearly as complex as that for a patient with a total hip replacement. Postoperatively the patient will have a bulky compression dressing on his leg. The leg must be elevated to prevent edema and the usual neurocirculatory checks of the extremity are required. Active straight leg raising exercises are begun as soon as the patient reacts from anesthesia. The patient may be out of bed in a chair with the leg elevated. On approximately the fifth postoperative day the large dressing is removed and the patient begins active flexion and extension exercises. The exercises may increase his discomfort greatly. He will need considerable encouragement as well as prescribed medication and other nursing comfort measures. Once the patient is able to do straight leg raising he begins to ambulate with crutches. He will remain on crutches for approximately 8 weeks.

Total replacement arthroplasty of the elbow has also been done, although not as frequently as that of the hip and knee. Following surgery the patient is placed in a cylinder cast for 1 week, while only a sling is worn during the second postoperative week. The patient is encouraged to try to flex his arm as well as extend it while still in the cast. He continues these exercises and excellent function is usually achieved by 3 weeks.

Various implants have been used on the finger joints of persons with severe rheumatoid arthritis. Silastic implants are used in the metacarpophalangeal joint and the proximal interphalangeal joint. Dynamic splinting is used to guide motion as the patient begins his exercises on approximately the third postoperative day. The period of rehabilitation is approximately 3 months.

Osteotomy

An osteotomy is a frequently used orthopedic procedure that involves cutting a bone to change alignment. It is sometimes used to change position of the femoral head and thus alter the weight-bearing surface in a diseased joint. It may also be used to correct angulation or rotational deformities. Postoperatively the extremity involved is immobilized in some manner. The nursing care of the patient is the same as that of a patient who has a fracture in the area. An osteotomy may be thought of as an intentional fracture.

Synovectomy

Synovectomy (removal of the synovial membrane) is often performed in the early stages of rheumatoid arthritis when the destruction is still confined to the synovium and has not progressed to affect the surface of the joint. It is frequently performed on the knee. The patient is placed in a bulky compressive dressing for approximately 48 hours postoperatively. While still in the dressing, the patient usually begins isometric quadriceps exercises prescribed by the physician. As his pain decreases, the patient is encouraged to exercise more actively. Ambulation begins on the parallel bars and progresses to crutches. The patient may usually bear weight on his operative leg when he is able to demonstrate active straight leg raising.

Rheumatic nodules may sometimes be removed surgically if they have become irritated by trauma or pressure or if they are particularly unsightly. Hospitalization for this treatment is usually of only 1 day's duration. In a similar fashion, the tophi of gout may be excised, particularly if they have opened and are draining or are causing pain.

Patients with hypertrophic arthritis may be operated on when bony tumors, or exostoses, develop and cause pain, particularly on weight-bearing areas such as the heel. Pain-causing calcium deposits within the joint also may be removed surgically in the patient with hypertrophic arthritis or bursitis.

■ TRAUMA

The patient who has suffered trauma to his musculoskeletal system, like the postoperative patient, has had an interruption in the integrity of the locomotor system. The same basic data are needed to plan his care. Only trauma as seen in fractures will be considered here. When sufficient force is applied to bone it breaks. As it breaks, the original force is dissipated through the soft tissue. Small fragments of bone may become embedded in the soft tissue such as muscle, blood vessels, and nerves. It is because of the potential injury to soft tissue that an extremity that has sustained a fracture must be carefully checked for neurocirculatory impairment.

Definitions and terminology

A bone is said to be fractured or broken when there is an interruption in its continuity. This is usually caused by a blow or injury sustained in a fall or other accident. A fracture may also occur during normal activity or following a minimal injury when the bone is weakened by disease such as cancer or *osteoporosis.* This is called a *pathologic fracture* and causes collapse of the bone. A bone may fracture when the muscles involved are unable to absorb energy as they usually do. This type of fracture, a *fatigue fracture,* has been seen in persons who have been on long foot marches and the muscles have become fatigued.

There are several types of fractures. A fracture is *complete* when there is complete separation of the bone, producing two fragments. It is *incomplete* when only part of the bone is broken. The part of the bone nearest to the body is referred to as a proximal fragment, whereas the one most distant from the body is called the distal fragment. The proximal is also called the uncontrollable fragment since its location and muscle attachments prevent it from being moved or manipulated when attempting to bring the separate fragments into correct alignment. The distal is referred to as the controllable fragment since it can usually be moved and manipulated to bring it into the correct relationship to the proximal fragment. Fractures in long bones are designated as being in the proximal, middle, or distal third of the bone.

If the skin is intact, the fracture is classified as simple or closed. A fracture is classified as *compound* when there is a direct communication between the skin wound and the fracture site.[1] An open or compound fracture has a high risk of contamination and this is an important factor in its treatment. When the two bone fragments are in good alignment with no change from their normal position despite the break in continuity of bone, the fracture is referred to as a *fracture without displacement.* If the bone fragments have separated at the point of fracture, it is referred to as a *fracture with displacement.* This may be slight, moderate, or marked.

The line of fracture as revealed by x-ray examination or fluoroscopy is usually classified as to type. It may be *greenstick,* with splintering on one side of the bone (this occurs most often in young children with soft bones); *transverse,* with a break straight across the bone; *oblique,* with the line of fracture at an oblique angle to the bone shaft; or *spiral,* with the fracture lines partially encircling the bone. The fracture may be referred to as *telescoped* if a bone

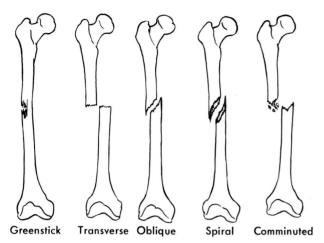

Greenstick　Transverse　Oblique　Spiral　Comminuted

FIG. 33-14. Types of fractures.

fragment is forcibly pushed against and into the adjacent fragment. If there are several fragments, the fracture is referred to as *comminuted*. (See Fig. 33-14.)

Symptoms of fracture and related injury

The signs and symptoms of fracture vary according to the location and function of the involved bone, the strength of its muscle attachments, the type of fracture sustained, and the amount of related damage.

Pain is usually immediate and severe following a fracture. It may continue and is aggravated by attempted motion of any kind and by pressure at the site of injury. Loss of function is another characteristic sign. If the person attempts to use the injured part, he may be unable to do so. If there has been marked displacement of fragments, there will be obvious gross deformity, and there may be motion where motion does not usually occur. When the fractured limb is moved gently, there may be a characteristic grating sound (crepitus) as the bone fragments come in contact with each other. The nurse should never under any circumstances attempt to elicit this sign since it may cause further damage and increase pain. It is possible, though unusual, for a fracture to occur with no displacement of fragments, little or no swelling, and pain only when direct pressure is applied to the site of fracture or on use of the limb or body part. Fractures of this kind might be missed if x-ray examinations were not routinely ordered when there was reason to suspect that a fracture may have occurred.

Since the bones are firmer than their surrounding structures, any injury severe enough to cause bone fracture will also cause injury to muscles, nerves, connective tissue, and blood vessels that may be evident by hemorrhage externally or into surrounding tissues. Bleeding may not be fully apparent for several hours, and discoloration of the skin (ecchymosis) may not be apparent until several days after injury. Edema may follow extravasation of blood into the tissues and localization of serous fluid at the site of injury, and paralysis or other evidence of nerve injury may develop. Occasionally a large nerve becomes locked between two bone fragments, causing immediate paralysis. The patient who has a fracture usually has signs and symptoms of injury of both bone and surrounding tissues. He may go quickly into shock from severe tissue injury or intense pain.

Immediate management

Perhaps the most important basic principle in the care of a patient with any fracture is to provide some kind of splint before moving him. This is constantly emphasized in the emergency care of patients at the scene of accidents (p. 264). It is equally important for the nurse to remember to preserve body alignment when caring for patients who are in traction or some other mechanical apparatus.

When a patient with a known or a suspected fracture is to be admitted to the hospital, his bed should be provided with a fracture board. This is a good practice regardless of the part fractured because the patient with a known fracture of the ankle, for example, may be found also to have a fracture of the pelvis or of the spine on further examination.

Since it is known that edema will occur following a fracture, the injured part usually is elevated routinely. One or more protected pillows should be used, and these can support the extremity if moving must be done. If a temporary splint has been applied, this should not be removed without orders from the physician no matter how crude or soiled it may be. The limb encased in the splint can be elevated.

The injured part should be observed at frequent intervals for local changes in color, sensation, or temperature. Care should be taken that emergency splinting bandages do not cause constriction as edema develops. Tingling, numbness, or burning pain may indicate nerve injury. Coldness, blanching, or cyanosis usually indicates interference with circulation. Increased warmth and swelling may indicate infection. Gas bacillus infection is a dreaded complication in grossly contaminated compound fractures. Sudden increase in edema and pain associated with darkening of the tissues should be reported to the physician at once. Tetanus immunization usually is given when a compound fracture has been sustained (p. 311).

The nurse should be alert for early signs of shock, especially if the injury is severe. Vital signs should be taken every 15 minutes until the patient's condition has stabilized.

The nurse should anticipate that the physician may order local cold applications during the first 24 hours following a fracture, since these help to reduce hemorrhage and edema and contribute to the patient's comfort. Ice bags are often used and must be covered and moved at regular intervals to prevent skin damage.

Pain is usually relieved in the first few hours by giving acetylsalicylic acid or narcotics. Adjustment to sudden immobilization is difficult for the patient, and the nurse must appreciate what it means to him to be unable to move about freely. Even a fracture of an arm bone may make the patient quite helpless at first. He may be unable to move or use the rest of his body without severe pain. Sometimes treatment of the fractured bone makes it physically impossible for him to care for some of his most basic physical needs. The patient usually needs a sedative such as secobarbital (Seconal) to help him sleep the first few nights after he has sustained a fracture.

Complications

Fat embolism is a serious complication that may follow a fracture, especially a comminuted fracture of a long bone. One source of the emboli is thought to be the fat of the bone marrow. There is evidence of a change in lipid metabolism after a fracture and the metabolic influence on the development of fat emboli is also under investigation. The signs of a fat embolus are similar to the signs of other kinds of emboli and consist of sudden severe pain in the chest, pallor, dyspnea, prostration, and collapse. The development of these signs and symptoms constitutes a medical emergency and the physician should be called at once.

Petechial hemorrhages of the skin and conjunctivae are a classic sign of systemic fat embolism. These usually appear on the second or third day after injury and are commonly found in the conjunctivae, skin of the neck, shoulders, and axillary folds.

There is no specific treatment for systemic fat embolism. Treatment is geared to supportive measures. The patient can usually breathe best in high Fowler's position and will require oxygen therapy. Oxygen will be given to lower the surface tension of the fat globules and reduce local anoxia. Intravenous fluid may be given for its emulsifying effect. Intravenous alcohol is also being tried. Blood transfusion may be necessary to relieve shock and maintain an adequate hemoglobin level. If the patient has heart failure, he will be digitalized. He should be kept as quiet as possible and subjected to no unnecessary movement. Some experts feel that proper immobilization and careful handling of patients with bone injuries may help prevent the occurrence of fat emboli.

Ischemic paralysis (contracture) is a somewhat rare complication of a fracture and develops when an artery is injured by trauma or pressure so that arterial spasm occurs. *Volkmann's contracture* is a complication of fractures about the elbow caused by

circulatory impairment due to pressure from a cast, constricting bandages, or injury to the radial artery. The muscles of the forearm atrophy and the fingers and forearm are permanently flexed (clawhand). Signs of coldness, pallor, cyanosis, pain, and swelling of the part below the cast must be watched for and reported promptly so that pressure may be relieved by either loosening the bandage or removing the cast in order that circulation may be restored before contracture can develop.

Common methods of treatment and related care

Objectives in the treatment and care of fractures include reduction of the fracture, maintenance of the fragments in the correct position while healing takes place, prevention of excessive loss of joint mobility and muscle tone, prevention of complications, and maintenance of good general health so that, with healing of the fractured bone, the patient can continue as before his accident or injury.

Reduction of fractures. "Reduction" is the term used for the return of bone fragments to their normal position. This may be accomplished by closed manipulation, traction, or surgery.

Closed manipulation. When closed manipulation is used to reduce a fracture, the patient is often given a general anesthetic. The physician then reduces the fracture by pulling on the distal fragment (manual traction) while he (or someone else) applies countertraction to the proximal fragment until the bone fragments engage or fall into their normal alignment. The physician may also apply direct pressure over the site of the fracture to correct angulation or lateral displacement of a fragment. Usually when this type of reduction is used, a cast is applied to hold the fragments in the desired position while healing occurs.

Traction. Continuous traction (pull on the affected extremity) for a period of days or even weeks may be necessary to reduce fractures of the femur because the large muscles draw the bone fragments out of normal alignment so that immediate reduction by manual traction is impossible. Continuous traction may also be used to reduce fractures when there has been very extensive tissue damage and when the physical condition of the patient is such that anesthetics cannot be given. Therefore traction may be used for immobilizing the limb while soft tissue healing takes place, reducing the fracture, and maintaining correct position of fragments during bone healing.

Open reduction. Open reduction may be necessary if closed manipulation or traction is unsuccessful. Open reduction has the advantage of allowing visualization of the fracture and surrounding tissues. The fragments can be arranged and held by internal fixation if necessary. This method is indicated when there is soft tissue caught between bone fragments or when there is known damage to nerves or blood vessels. The disadvantages of open reduction are the need for anesthesia and, primarily, the possibility of introducing organisms into the fracture site at time of surgery. In certain specific fractures, open reduction may be the treatment of choice. However, it is usually not used if closed reduction or traction will do.

Healing of fractures. When a bone is broken, bleeding occurs and a hematoma forms around the damaged bone ends. The hematoma is not absorbed during healing, as are hematomas that occur elsewhere in the body, but becomes changed into granulation tissue. From the sixth to the tenth day after injury the granulation tissue changes into a tissue called the *callus*. Callus is different from other granulation tissue in that it contains cartilage, calcium and phosphate ions, and osteoblasts. The callus temporarily holds the bone fragments together, but will not support weight or withstand much strain. It eventually is replaced by true bone that grows from beneath the periosteum of each fragment to meet and fuse across the defect. The length of time required for a bone to heal depends on its location, blood circulation to the part, and age and general physical condition of the patient. Fractures in young children unite much more quickly than do those in older persons. Fractures of the humerus usually heal within 10 to 12 weeks; of the forearm, within 8 to 10 weeks; of the femur, in 6 months; of the lower leg, in 3 months; and of the spine, within 6 to 12 months. The larger the bone, the longer it usually takes to heal.

Delayed healing or *delayed union* is said to occur when the fracture has not healed within the usual time for the particular bone involved. Delayed healing will occur if the space between the two bones is such that neither the callus nor bone cells can bridge the gap, if the callus is broken or torn apart by too much activity, if muscle or fascia is caught between the fragments, if an infection develops, or if there is poor blood supply to the part or marked dietary deficiency. Occasionally delayed union occurs with no obvious cause. Open reduction and more complete immobilization may be necessary.

"Nonunion" is the term used when healing does not take place even in a much longer time than is usually needed. Congenital conditions and obscure medical disease occasionally account for this, and nonunion may occur in the aged. When this occurs, the patient may have to wear a brace to support the limb. If the fracture is in the lower extremity, crutches may have to be used indefinitely. Surgery may be performed and an attempt made to unite the fragments with a bone graft. Nonunion occurs most often in the middle of the humerus, the neck of the femur in older people, the lower third of the tibia, and the carpal bones.

Treatment by immobilization of the reduced fracture. The purpose of immobilization is to hold the bone fragments in contact with each other until healing takes place. All activity of the part that might cause separation of the fragments is restricted, and the fractured bone is kept in position by immobilizing the entire limb. Usually immobilization includes the joints immediately proximal to and distal to the fractured bone. Bandages, adhesive tape, plaster-of-Paris casts, splints, traction, internal fixation, and bed rest are methods of securing immobilization. Metal pins, screws, plates, and nails, all made of stainless steel or Vitallium, are used to hold the fragments together when an open reduction is done; a plaster-of-Paris cast is often used to provide extra protection when internal fixation is used. This is especially true in treatment of compound fractures of the leg.

Plaster casts. Plaster-of-Paris casts have been used for many years and are still widely used in the treatment of fractures. Unless a cast has been applied to the entire trunk, the patient who is treated with a plaster-of-Paris cast can usually move about and carry on most of the activities of daily living. Often he may, for example, return to school or to work and participate in many activities without damage to the site of injury. Use of casts shortens hospitalization, and many patients with simple fractures can be treated in a physician's office or the outpatient department of a hospital. After a short period of observation, they can be discharged and treatment continued under close medical or nursing supervision.

Plaster-of-Paris casts do, however, restrict activities because of their weight and their inflexibility. A cast can cause complications due to interference with normal physiologic functions and can cause actual physical injury if incorrectly applied and improperly cared for. A cast applied to the arm or shoulder may limit the kind of clothing worn and may interfere with eating, writing, or other uses of the arm. If applied to the leg, a cast may change body alignment, put strain on certain muscle groups, and limit locomotion.

The nurse must not only know how to maintain the effectiveness of the cast, but must understand how the patient is affected by it. The patient must be helped to be as independent as possible. The nurse should help to prevent development of complications and be alert for early signs of complications, which must be reported to the physician promptly.

Application of the cast. Most hospitals have a room set aside for the application of casts that provides the necessary space and contains all the equipment required for this procedure. Some hospitals also have a cart equipped with plaster and other cast materials that can be taken to the bedside for use. Plaster-of-Paris bandages come in various widths

(2 to 8 inches). Each roll is wrapped in waxed paper to prevent sifting of the plaster from the bandage and to prevent deterioration from exposure to moisture. The bandage itself is made of crinoline into which plaster of Paris (gypsum or calcium sulfate dihydrate) has been rubbed. When water is added, the gypsum assumes its crystalline state and the wet plaster bandage can be molded to fit the shape of a body part or wrapped about a limb. When the water evaporates, the cast becomes firm and is able to withstand considerable stress and strain. The number of layers of plaster used determines the strength of the cast.

After reduction has been accomplished and before the cast is applied, the skin is usually protected with sheet wadding (a thick, nonabsorbent cotton web covered with starch to hold it together), and felt or sponge rubber is used over bony prominences to protect them from pressure. Tubular stockinette, from 2 to 18 inches wide, is used as lining for the cast and is applied so that it will extend over the edge to cover the round edges of the plaster. The excess stockinette and sheet wadding are usually folded back over the cast after it has been applied and bound down with a final roll of plaster.

If the cast is applied elsewhere than in a special plaster room, the floor and table should be protected from wet plaster. When the physician is ready to apply the cast, the bandage is placed in a bucket of water at 21° to 24° C. (70° to 75° F.) for 5 seconds. The bandage should be carefully removed from the water so that none of the plaster is lost. It should be held horizontally with an end in the palm of each hand and gently compressed to remove excess water. It should then be quickly handed to the physician so that it can be used before it begins to set. Only a few bandages should be placed in the water at a time. The bucket containing the water should be lined with a cloth or paper to collect waste plaster. When the procedure has been completed, the cloth or paper containing waste plaster can be removed and discarded into a garbage can and the water emptied into the sink, if there is no loose plaster. Plaster of Paris will clog ordinary plumbing and should never be emptied into ordinary drains.

Care of the cast. Plaster bandages are fast setting (3 to 7 minutes). Thin casts may dry completely in several hours, but thick casts may require several days to become completely dry. The cast can be cracked or broken by inadequate support or by unwise handling before it is dry. A wrinkle in the plaster and indentations caused by the fingertips from continuous pressure can alter the inner shape of the cast and cause pressure on the body part encased in the plaster.

A fracture board should always be used to provide a firm mattress and prevent uneven weight on the fresh plaster cast. To protect the new cast and ensure its efficiency, the patient should be carefully transferred from the stretcher onto his bed. If he is conscious, he can move onto the bed with the assistance of one nurse while another supports the wet cast at the areas of greatest strain—usually at the joints. If the patient is asleep or is in a body cast, three or four people should lift him onto the bed. The entire cast and the patient's head and his extremities must be fully supported.

The wet cast should not lie unsupported on the hard bed because it may become flattened over bony prominences and weight-bearing areas such as the back of the heel, buttocks, and shoulders, and this can cause pressure. The wet cast should always be fully supported on a pillow or pillows that are protected with waterproof material to prevent their becoming damp. Although the pillows must be protected with a waterproof material, they should also be covered with cloth so that the waterproof material is not directly in contact with the cast. Some heat is given off as the cast hardens. If the cast is completely surrounded with a waterproof material, not only will it not dry but a burn may result. The patient should be in proper body alignment, and there should not be any break in the support provided by the pillows to cause weakening of the cast. If the patient has a cast on the leg, the foot should extend over the edge of the pillow or the bed to avoid pressure on the heel.

In order for the cast to dry, there must be provision for evaporation by exposure to circulating air. A hair dryer can be used to provide warm moving air; this is particularly helpful when wet, humid weather delays drying. Heat from radiant lamps is not advocated because it can cause severe burns beneath the cast. Cradles equipped with electric bulbs are not recommended unless there is also provision for free circulation of air; moisture-laden air becomes trapped under the cradle and delays the drying process. The cast should not be covered with bed linen until it is dry. Therefore the bed must be made in such a way that the cast is exposed but the patient kept warm and free from drafts. Blankets may be used to protect body parts not encased in plaster.

The patient in a body cast should be turned to ensure uniform drying of the cast, to prevent continuous pressure on any one area while the cast is drying, and to make him more comfortable. Sufficient personnel should be used in turning the patient to ensure support of the patient and the cast. The patient should be turned every 2 hours. Patients are usually more comfortable turned toward the uninjured side. Whether or not the patient in a cast may be turned toward the affected side depends on the type of injury sustained.

To protect body and long leg casts from becoming soiled or wet, waterproof material should be applied around the perineal area. Continuous dampening will soften the cast and impair its effectiveness, and a soiled cast lining will irritate the patient's skin and cause an offensive odor. The area can be covered with plastic material, oiled silk, or waxed paper, which can be anchored with adhesive or cellophane tape and changed as necessary.

Patients often like to decorate their casts. However, casts should never be covered with paint, varnish, or shellac. Plaster of Paris is porous and allows circulation and air to the skin. When the plaster cast is covered with a substance that decreases the porosity, the skin underneath the cast may become macerated.

If the cast becomes soiled, scouring powder on a damp cloth will usually remove surface stains. The area must be allowed to thoroughly dry again. There is no way to clean a badly soiled cast; therefore it is essential that preventive measures be used to keep it clean.

Care of the patient in the cast. Care of the patient in a cast depends on the patient's general condition, with the cast presenting one more factor to deal with. After the patient has been carefully transferred into bed and the cast is supported on pillows, the nurse should check the patient's general condition. If he has had an anesthetic, he must be watched carefully until vital signs are normal (p. 217). After reduction and immobilization, he should be observed for signs of delayed shock such as sudden faintness, dizziness, pallor, diaphoresis, or change in pulse rate. Medication as ordered should be given for general pain. Complaints of pressure may be relieved by elevating the extremity or changing the patient's position. However, continuous pressure or pain that is unrelieved by change in position must be reported to the physician at once.

Areas of pressure are usually over the instep, lateral border of the foot, heel, malleoli, iliac crests, and sacrum. Changes in skin color should also be observed carefully since they, too, indicate that pressure may be restricting circulation.

The skin below the cast should be inspected frequently and routinely for signs of circulatory impairment. There may be swelling and slow return of color after pressure has been applied to the fingers or the toes below the cast. The skin also may be cold or cyanotic. The patient may complain of tightness of the cast and of numbness or tingling of the fingers or toes. These signs and symptoms should be reported immediately so that the cast can be divided to relieve constriction if necessary. Most swelling occurs within the first 24 to 48 hours. Interference with circulation is usually caused by a tight cast or by edema. Occasionally it is caused by bruising of a blood vessel during manipulation or surgery.

Compression of a nerve can also occur. The nerve most often affected is the peroneal nerve, which is located below the head of the fibula on the lateral side of the leg. Continuous pressure on this superficial nerve by a leg cast results in paralysis with a loss of the ability to dorsiflex the foot or to extend the toes. Any complaint of pressure on the lateral side of the leg, numbness or tingling of the foot, or burning pain in the area covered by or distal to the cast must be reported at once. These indicate pressure on a nerve. When there is pressure on the nerve or circulatory impairment, the pressure must be relieved at once. Failure to do so can result in nerve paralysis and/or lack of circulation to the part with resultant necrosis. The ultimate consequence can be loss of the extremity. Pressure is relieved by cutting the cast and the padding underneath it. The cast is bivalved or sometimes wedged. The cast that has been split in two can be held in place by bandages. This will provide adequate temporary immobilization for the part while relieving the pressure on the nerve or that caused by edema. Signs of nerve compression and/or circulatory embarrassment constitute an emergency that must be reported to the physician, and action must be taken immediately. A cast cutter should be readily available and the nurse must know how to bivalve a cast should it be necessary to do so. Plaster on the skin should be removed with plain water. The skin around and directly under the cast edges should be washed and then massaged with alcohol to prevent skin irritation. Creams and lotions may be used with due caution. They tend to soften the skin under the cast and also may cause the skin to stick against the cast lining. In addition, continuous use of excessive lotions dampens the inside of the cast. The skin should also be inspected for pressure areas and signs of irritation from rough plaster edges. As the patient remains in the cast, his elbows may become irritated from bracing himself to move about in bed. Frequent massage and protective pads help to prevent this. An orthopedic frame with a trapeze will assist the patient to move about in bed.

If the patient is in a body cast or a long leg cast, the head of the bed should be elevated when a bedpan is used. If the cast is new and still damp, it is better to elevate the head of the bed on shock blocks instead of using the gatch, which will put a strain on the cast and may cause it to crack. A pillow should be placed against the small of the back, and a cotton pad protected with plastic material may be tucked under the sacral area to protect the cast from soiling. The leg in the cast should be supported with pillows so that the patient does not feel insecure in this position. An overhanging trapeze will permit him to help lift himself as the nurse places the bedpan under him. Side rails also assist the patient to turn and give him protection from falling out of bed.

Many patients are discharged after the cast is dry if there is no evidence of circulatory or nerve impairment. If a cast is applied to the arm, the patient should wear a sling to support the full weight of the cast, and the hand should be supported to prevent wristdrop from developing. The ends of the sling should be secured with two pins instead of being tied at the back of the neck. If the sling is to be worn for some time, sling ties may be lengthened with bandage or muslin so that they can be crossed in the back and brought around and tied in the front of the body. This helps to prevent forward and downward pull on the neck, which may cause a postural defect and fatigue. A member of the patient's family should be taught how to apply the sling correctly.

Depending on the injury, the patient may or may not be permitted to bear weight on his cast. If weight bearing is permitted, the cast is usually fitted with a rubber heel or walking iron that prevents wear on the plaster. Weight bearing is never permitted until the cast is completely dry.

Cast removal. The cast is usually removed when radiographs show that union is sufficient to allow safe removal. This is often done in the physician's office or in the hospital outpatient or emergency department. The cast is bivalved with manual or electric plaster cutters. While the procedure is not painful, the patient may feel some pressure or vibration. The skin is usually dry and scaly and should be washed with mild soap and water and lubricated with mineral oil. Since there is usually some

stiffness of the joints, the limb should be moved very gently (Fig. 33-15). The patient is usually encouraged to move the limb as much as he is able within limits of pain or stiffness. Exercises for the stiff joint are usually started. After a leg cast is removed, swelling and edema occur for some time when the leg is placed in a dependent position. The patient should be advised to sleep with the limb elevated and to elevate it at intervals during the day. Elastic bandages or stockings may be prescribed to help prevent dependent edema.

Traction

Continuous traction, or pull, is used to reduce and immobilize fractures, to overcome muscle spasm, and to stretch adhesions and correct certain deformities.

Skin traction. Skin traction is achieved by applying wide bands of moleskin or adhesive directly to the skin and attaching weights to these. The pull of the weights is transmitted indirectly to the involved bone. *Buck's extension, Bryant's traction,* and *Russell traction* are the three most common forms of skin traction used for injury to the lower extremities.

Buck's extension is the simplest and provides for straight pull on the affected extremity (Fig. 33-16). It is often used to relieve muscle spasm and to immobilize a limb temporarily, such as the leg when a hip fracture has been sustained by an elderly person and internal fixation is to be done within a short time. The skin of the leg is usually shaved, and tincture of benzoin is applied to protect it. Because physicians disagree about the advantages of shaving and

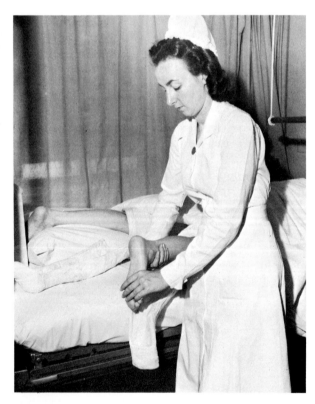

FIG. 33-15. Use of a bivalved cast permits removal of the extremity to give care and exercise. (From Anderson, H. C.: Newton's geriatric nursing, ed. 5, St. Louis, 1971, The C. V. Mosby Co.)

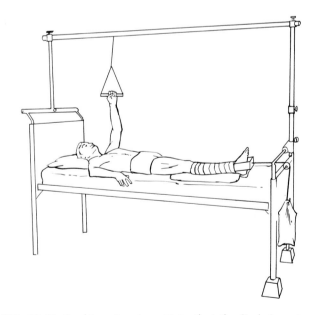

FIG. 33-16. Buck's extension. Note that the limb is not raised but lies parallel with the bed. Note also the blocks to raise the foot of the bed to provide countertraction and to help keep the patient from moving to the foot of the bed.

applying tincture of benzoin to the skin, the nurse should check before proceeding with these measures. Adhesive tape or moleskin is placed on the lateral and medial aspects of the leg and secured with a circular gauze or elastic bandage. The tape should not cover the malleoli, as skin breakdown is certain to occur over these bony prominences. The tapes are attached to a spreader bar. The spreader bar should be sufficiently wide to pull the tapes away from the malleoli. Rope is attached to the spreader, passed through a pulley on a crossbar at the foot of the bed, and suspended with weights. The maximum weight that should be applied by skin traction is 8 pounds. Greater amounts of weight will cause skin damage. Removable foam boots for Buck's extension are commercially available. These have the advantage of not being fastened to the skin. The foam, held in place by Velcro straps, provides enough friction to stay in place. Regardless of the method of skin traction that is used, the skin must be thoroughly inspected for signs of breakdown.

There are other methods of applying Buck's extension although the principles are the same. Some orthopedists prefer to use foam rubber strips in place of adhesive or moleskin on the lateral and medial aspects of the leg. Others paint the leg with Ace adherent and then cover the leg with stockinette before attaching the moleskin strips to the stockinette.

Not everyone will be able to be placed in Buck's extension; contraindications include stasis dermatitis, arteriosclerosis, allergy to adhesive tape, severe varicosities or varicose ulcers, diabetic gangrene, and marked overriding of bone fragments that would require 10 pounds or more of weight to reduce the deformity.

Russell traction is widely used because it permits the patient to move about in bed somewhat freely and permits bending of the knee joint. This is skin traction in which four pulleys are used. A Balkan frame must be attached to the bed before the procedure is started. Moleskin or adhesive is then applied to the leg as in Buck's extension. The knee is suspended in a hammock or sling to which a rope is attached. This rope is directed upward to a pulley that has been placed on the Balkan frame at a point located over the tubercle of the tibia of the affected extremity. The rope is then passed downward through a pulley on a crossbar at the foot of the bed, back through a pulley on the footplate, back again to another pulley on the crossbar, and then suspended with weights. Because there is double pull from the crossbar to the footplate, the traction is equal to approximately double the weight used (Fig. 33-17). Since there is upward pull from the hammock, skin under the popliteal space should be protected with a piece of felt or sponge rubber and should be inspected regularly. The patient's heel should just clear the bed so that there is no weight or pressure on the heel. Usually a pillow is placed lengthwise under the thigh, and a second pillow is placed under the leg. This traction results in slight flexion of the hip. The angle between the thigh and the bed should be approximately 20 degrees. Usually the foot of the bed is elevated on blocks to provide counteraction. Any complaints of pain or discomfort should be reported to the physician at once. Occasionally thrombophlebitis develops from inactivity and from pressure on the popliteal vessels. Often the patient is permitted to have the head of the bed elevated slightly, but as elevation of the head of the bed

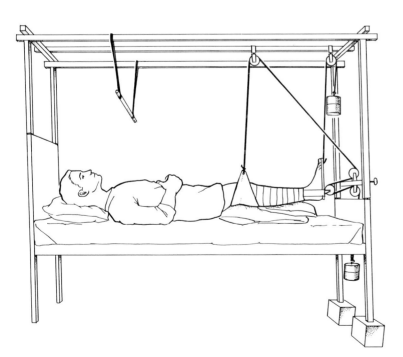

FIG. 33-17. Russell traction. Note that the Balkan frame is attached to the bed, that the leg is supported on pillows, and that the heel extends beyond the pillow.

does reduce the amount of the traction, the nurse should check with the physician about the amount of elevation permitted. Russell traction is used in the treatment of intertrochanteric fracture of the femur when surgery is contraindicated, especially in the aged. Bilateral Russell traction may be used to treat back pain since it immobilizes the patient and reduces muscle spasm.

Skeletal traction. Skeletal traction is traction applied directly to bone. Under general or local anesthesia a *Kirschner wire* or *Steinmann pin* is inserted distal to the fracture (the site of insertion varies with type of fracture). For a fractured femur the pin is often inserted through the tibia. The pin protrudes through the skin on both sides and the ends are covered with corks or metal protectors. Small sterile dressings are usually placed over the entry and exit sites of the pin. The utmost care must be taken to guard against infection at the pin site. Infection on the surface can proceed to the bone along the pin tract. This results in osteomyelitis. A metal U-shaped spreader or bow is attached to the pin. The rope for the traction is attached to the spreader. Skeletal traction can be used for fractures of the tibia, femur, humerus, and neck or cervical spine. Skeletal traction to the cervical spine is achieved by use of *Crutchfield tongs* applied to the skull (p. 916).

Balanced traction. When a balanced or suspension apparatus is used in conjunction with skin or skeletal traction, the patient is able to move about in bed more freely without disturbing the line of traction. The extremity is balanced with countertraction, and any slack in the traction caused by the patient's movement is taken up by the suspension apparatus. The use of balanced traction also facilitates nursing measures such as bathing the patient, caring for his skin, and placing the bedpan correctly.

A full or half-ring *Thomas* or *Hodgen splint* is used for balanced traction. Straps of canvas or muslin are placed over the splint and secured to provide a support for the leg. The areas under the popliteal space and heel are left open to prevent pressure on these parts. If it is desirable to have the knee flexed and to permit movement of the lower leg, a *Pearson attachment* is clamped or fixed at the level of the knee to the Thomas splint. It is also covered with muslin or canvas to support the lower leg. The leg is put through the ring and placed on the canvas support. The ring is placed firmly against the ischium. When a half-ring splint is used, the ring is placed on the anterior aspect of the thigh. Rope is attached to the ring or to the frame on either side of the ring and to the end of the Thomas splint, directed upward to pulleys on the frame, and then suspended with weights. Rope is also attached to the end of the Pearson attachment, directed upward to a pulley on the overbed frame, and suspended with weights. (See Fig. 33-18.) A foot support may be fastened to the Pearson attachment to prevent foot drop, or the foot is left free so that the patient can exercise it more fully. Skin or skeletal traction is applied as described earlier.

The ring is made of smooth, soft, moisture-resistant plastic material or of leather. It is not necessary to wrap the ring with padding. The padding cannot be changed after it is applied and inevitably gets damp from perspiration, bedpan accidents, and bathing the skin. The padding holds moisture against the skin and causes skin irritations. When the patient is bathed, the skin beneath the ring must be moved

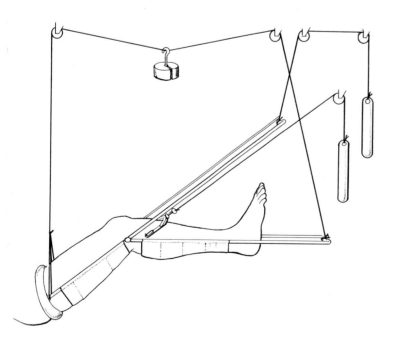

FIG. 33-18. Balanced traction used in conjunction with skeletal traction.

back and forth so that all areas are washed, dried thoroughly, and powdered. The patient may be turned toward the leg in the splint.

Nursing intervention for the patient in traction. Before the nurse attempts to give care to a patient in traction, the patient's difficulty and what is to be achieved by the use of traction must be clearly understood. Any deviation from the basic rules for care of a patient in traction must be approved by the physician. For example, the patient with arthritis may be permitted to partially release traction by sitting upright for a few moments, whereas the patient with a fresh fracture of the femur would harm himself by doing this.

In order for traction to be effective, the patient must lie on his back. Turning onto the side or sitting up changes body alignment, and the pull (traction) is lost or becomes less effective. Patients in traction can usually be turned slightly from side to side to relieve skin pressure. The motion allowed depends on the injury and kind of traction used. The nurse must ask the physician what the limitations of motion are so that appropriate nursing care can be planned. The patient will be extremely limited in activity. The nurse should explain this to the patient and help him to be as comfortable as possible while remaining in the correct position. The patient who must lie flat often feels handicapped and helpless because he cannot readily see what is going on about him. Ceiling mirrors and prism glasses may be used to help the patient feel less isolated. Television sets are sometimes placed on high wall shelves or suspended from the ceiling so that they can be seen by patients who must lie flat in bed.

The nurse must be certain that the *weights hang free* with no obstruction to interfere with straight, even, continuous pull. Traction should be inspected frequently. For example, when traction is being applied to the lower limb, bedclothes must not press on the rope or against the footplate. The footplate must never push against the foot of the bed or the pulley, since this will completely negate traction. There should be no knots in the rope, since these may become caught in the pulley and interfere with traction. The rope should be long enough so that weight will not be hampered by the pulley as the patient pulls himself up in bed, yet not long enough to rest on the floor if he slips to the foot of the bed. The rope must be strong enough so that it will not break if more weights are added. The weights must be securely fastened so that they will not drop off if they are disturbed accidentally, and the equipment should be visible so that it is not jarred or swung inadvertently. Sandbags are often used for weights and are tied to the rope. When regular scale weights are used, they should be fastened with adhesive tape so that they will not slip off. Jarring the bed and swinging the weights may cause pain and upset the

patient. Any extremity in traction must be checked frequently for adequate circulation. Patients in *Buck's extension* or *Russell traction* should be checked for inversion of the foot or foot drop on the affected side. These signs would be indicative of peroneal nerve damage.

An important concept in the care of the patient in traction is that the patient should not suffer from lack of any kind of nursing care because of his immobilization. At first glance it might sometimes appear that good back care, for example, is impossible. This is not true. The patient in traction should be on a firm bed and should have an orthopedic frame or overhead attachment so that he can help to lift himself and take some weight off his back for short periods. Usually he can be moved enough for good back care to be given and for linen to be changed. This is accomplished by having the patient raise himself straight up in bed with the help of the trapeze while care is given and the bed linen slid under him. Depending on the site and the extent of the fracture, the physician may permit the patient to turn toward the side of the fracture enough for back care to be given (Fig. 33-19). It is a good practice for a second nurse or an attendant to steady the traction and even increase the pull slightly as the patient carefully and steadily turns or raises himself. The same principles are followed when the patient has the bedpan placed under him. A very small, flat bedpan should be used, and the back above the pan should be supported by a small pillow or a bath blanket folded to the height of the pan.

The patient who is in traction needs the same attention to nutrition, elimination, exercise of noninvolved extremities, prevention of postural defects, and skin care as any other patient who is immobilized. Particular attention must be given to the skin that comes into contact with any traction apparatus. For example, the skin over bony hip prominences may become reddened and painful if a pelvic band is being used, adhesive tape may work downward so that straps may rub against the ankle malleolus when skin traction is used on the lower limb, and a *Thomas splint* may cause injury to the skin of the groin. Skin irritation of this kind must be reported to the physician, who may alter the amount of weight used or take other action. Nursing measures to relieve skin irritation should be taken.

Nursing intervention for a patient immobilized with a fracture. Nursing intervention during the time of immobilization includes prevention of complications and maintenance of general health. The patient whose activity is limited by a fracture usually has digestive and elimination problems. Appetite may be poor, yet increased body requirements must be met if bone repair is to progress normally. The diet should be high in protein, iron, calcium, and vitamins. It should also be high in roughage since

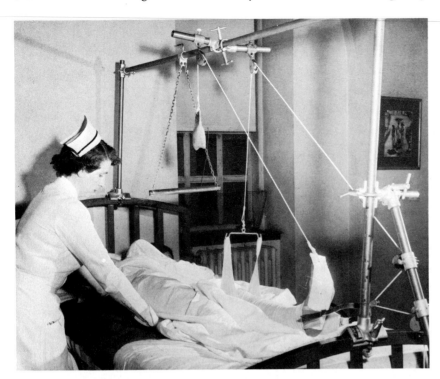

FIG. 33-19. The patient may turn slightly when Russell traction is used. Note the hammock under the knee, the placement of the four pulleys, and the apparatus used to prevent foot drop.

constipation is often a real problem that causes inconvenience and discomfort and may interfere with appetite.

During immobility, catabolic activity is accelerated, producing a rapid breakdown of cellular materials. This leads to protein deficiency and negative nitrogen balance. Decalcification and demineralization of bones also take place during immobility regardless of the quantity of calcium intake. Increasing calcium in the diet is not recommended because it cannot be used by the immobile patient. A diet high in protein is indicated, however, in order to overcome protein deficiency and return the body to a state of *positive nitrogen balance.* Sometimes 150 to 300 Gm. of protein is required daily to achieve this.

The patient who is ambulatory and being cared for at home should be encouraged to eat plenty of uncooked green vegetables and fresh fruits. The patient in the hospital may be permitted to have relatives bring such foods to him if the hospital menu is somewhat limited in uncooked vegetables and fresh fruits.

Thrombosis, embolism, and muscle and joint changes with resultant deformity or limitation of function are possible complications when a patient is immobilized in the treatment of a fracture. It is a nursing responsibility to see that the patient does deep-breathing exercises and exercises his good limbs by means of muscle-setting, resistive, or other exercises, depending on his particular circumstances. Because of the complex arrangement of muscle attachments and because of muscle action,

the nurse needs specific orders from the physician before assisting or encouraging the patient to exercise the involved limb. A safe rule is never under any circumstances to have the patient move or use the joint either immediately distal to or immediately proximal to the fracture unless there is an order permitting this. For example, if the fracture is in the radius, the wrist and elbow joints should not be moved without an order. However, the shoulder can and should be protected from muscle weakness, muscle shortening, and joint changes by regular motion and exercise. The legs, trunk, and unaffected upper limb should be checked regularly (at least daily) to be certain that the patient is doing some systematic routine exercises.

The patient who must remain in bed for a long period of time in traction or in a cast should be in a bed with a firm mattress, and a fracture board should be placed under the mattress. The patient should pay particular attention to his posture from the beginning of his confinement. The lumbar curve in the back can be supported by small pillows, a bath towel, or a rolled bath blanket. The unaffected foot (or feet) should rest against a footboard at least part of the day. This helps to maintain the foot in the normal walking position, prevents the weight of bedclothes from contributing to foot drop, and provides a firm surface against which the patient can do resistive foot exercises. The patient should be taught to check the position of his lower limb when at rest. He should "toe in" to prevent external rotation of the hip and pronation of the foot, which cause serious difficulty when walking is resumed.

The patient's skin should be inspected for pressure areas or signs of other irritation. In caring for patients who are immobilized for a long time, there should be a regular schedule for cutting nails, for giving special attention to the skin, for turning and massage, and for cleansing areas such as the perineum. Urinary output should be measured and observed at intervals since the patient who is immobilized for a time may develop urinary retention and renal calculi.

The patient with a fracture who is confined to bed should do full range-of-joint exercises for all unaffected joints daily (Figs. 1-2 to 1-4). If he is to eventually use crutches, he should practice push-up exercises or other resistive exercises to strengthen the triceps muscle. These can be done, for example, when the patient in a body cast is turned on his abdomen; the patient in traction and in a back-lying position can straighten his elbows while holding weights on his palms.

Patients who have been on bed rest for some time should be mobilized gradually. The change of position from a flat to an upright one causes weakness and dizziness. The patient should be prepared for this and should be closely supervised until he can be safely left alone. A tilt table is useful since it allows the patient to become accustomed to an upright position before actual standing is attempted. The walker is extremely helpful, particularly for elderly patients, since the seat provides a resting place if they become too tired from standing. Often the walker is useful in preparing the patient to use crutches. With increasing frequency, walkerettes, which can be moved by the patient at his own speed, are being used instead of walkers.

Before leaving the hospital, the patient should be relatively self-sufficient in getting in and out of bed and in and out of a chair. If he lives alone, he must be able to manage stairs. When he practices getting out of bed in the hospital, the casters should be removed from the hospital bed to lower it and to make it more stable. A Hi-Lo bed should be kept in the low position to simulate the height of an ordinary bed. A visiting nurse can usually help the patient in his home to adjust to his immediate environment and to supervise his progress. A nursing referral should be sent to the public health nursing agency, so that the visiting nurse will know exactly what the patient may or may not do and what his progress was during hospitalization and at discharge.

Internal fixation

Depending on the location and type of fracture, *open reduction with internal fixation* may be necessary. Open reduction with internal fixation is used only when other methods of reduction are not suitable. Although this method allows direct visualization of the injury, it also carries the possibility of

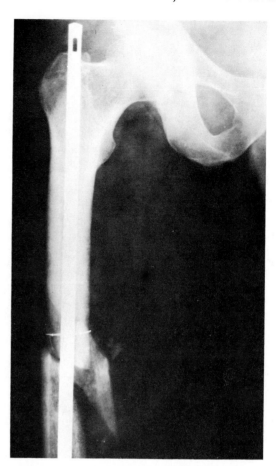

FIG. 33-20. Internal fixation of fracture of middle third of femur by means of an intramedullary nail (Kirschner nail).

infection. Open reduction with internal fixation must be done under the most vigorous aseptic conditions.

Internal fixation is achieved by using a metal device (Fig. 33-20). There are a wide variety of metal pins, wires, intramedullary rods, compression plates, nails, etc. available. Each has its particular advantage and indications for use. The care of the patient who has internal fixation of a fracture depends on the site of the fracture and the device used for stabilization. One general aim, however, does apply to all fractures treated by internal fixation. The part must be protected until healing takes place. Metal will fatigue and break. It cannot be expected to substitute for intact bone. Therefore, depending on the fracture, a cast may be used or the patient may be placed on limited weight bearing until healing occurs.

Immediate postoperative care. Immediately following the patient's return from the operating room, he should be watched carefully for signs of shock and hemorrhage. If a cast has been applied, it may be impossible to detect external signs of bleeding for some time, and the vital signs should be checked at frequent intervals until they have become stabilized. Extensive bleeding under a cast will eventually become apparent either as oozing around the edge of the cast or as staining of the cast as blood saturates the damp plaster. The nurse should also be alert to the patient's complaints of wetness or warmth under the cast that may indicate bleeding that is not yet visible. The surgeon usually requests that the extremity in a cast be elevated on a pillow and that an ice bag be placed on the cast over the fracture site. The nurse should check the circulation of the area below the cast and report any signs of coldness, pallor, cyanosis, or swelling. Other care required is the same as that of any postoperative patient.

Fractures of the hip

Patients with fractured hips are frequently seen in the hospital, so these fractures will be discussed in more detail. The hip joint is a ball-and-socket joint and is formed by the acetabulum, a deep round cavity in the innominate bone, and the upper portion of the femur. The upper part of the femur is composed of a head, neck, greater and lesser trochanter, and shaft. The distal part of the femur ends in two condyles. The head of the femur fits into the acetabulum. The hip joint is surrounded by a capsule, ligaments, and muscles. The greater trochanter serves as a point of insertion for the abductor and short rotator muscles of the hip, whereas the lesser trochanter serves as a point of insertion for the iliopsoas muscle.

The blood supply to the femoral head is of paramount importance in fractures in or about the hip joint. The blood supply to the femoral head varies with age. The chief source of blood supply to the femoral head in adults is the posterior retinacular arteries (Fig. 33-21). The nutrient and periosteal vessels of the femoral shaft extend into the trochanteric region and lower part of the neck.

Fractured hips occur more frequently in women than in men. Some factors explaining this are (1)

women have a wider pelvis with a tendency to coxa vara; (2) usually women are less active and are more prone to senile osteoporosis; and (3) women's life expectancy is greater than that of men.

Fractures of the hip may be classified in two general categories: intracapsular and extracapsular fractures. The patient with a fractured hip will present with pain in the hip. The affected leg will be shorter and externally rotated.

Intracapsular fractures of the hip include those occurring within the hip joint and capsule. These include *capital, subcapital,* and *transcervical* fractures. *Extracapsular* fractures occur outside of the capsule to an area 2 inches below the lesser trochanter (Fig. 33-22).

Impacted intracapsular fractures may be treated by bed rest without internal fixation. Intracapsular fractures of the hip may be treated by the use of nails or pins. The choice of device depends on the location of the fracture and the personal preference of the surgeon. Since the blood supply to the head of the femur comes up through the neck, it is often disrupted in an intracapsular fracture (Fig. 33-22). When the blood supply is interrupted, there will be eventual avascular necrosis of the femoral head (p. 952). This complication occurs in a significant percentage of patients following internal fixation of an intracapsular fracture. For this reason, particularly in the elderly patient, the physician may elect to remove the head of the femur and insert a prosthesis such as the Austin-Moore type (Fig. 33-23).

The care of the patient following insertion of a hip prosthesis is directed toward preventing dislocation. The patient may be placed in a spica cast, in traction, or left free in bed. The type of traction and length of immobilization may vary from 10 days to 3 weeks, depending on the wishes of the orthopedic surgeon. Types of traction used include Buck's extension (Fig. 33-16) and Russell traction (Fig. 33-17). The postoperative position is dependent on the surgical approach. With a posterior approach, the incision is similar to the one used for the neck of the femur, and one end of the incision is carried upward from the trochanteric area toward the posterosuperior iliac spine. When the capsule of the hip is opened posteriorly and the prosthesis is inserted, the leg must be placed in slight external rotation with slight abduction. The head of the bed must be relatively flat. Acute flexion of the hip, adduction, and internal rotation must be avoided to prevent dislocation of the hip prosthesis before complete healing has occurred. With an anterior approach, the upper end of the incision is carried forward to the anterior spine of the ilium. The position of the operated leg is abducted or neutral with internal rotation.

The patient usually may have the head of the bed elevated to 45 degrees. Extreme flexion of the hip is avoided to prevent dislocation.

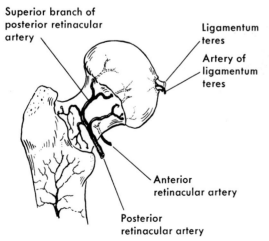

Superior branch of posterior retinacular artery

Ligamentum teres

Artery of ligamentum teres

Anterior retinacular artery

Posterior retinacular artery

FIG. 33-21. Posterior view of the blood supply to the head of the femur.

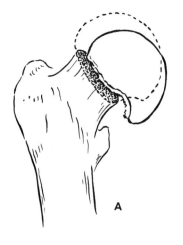
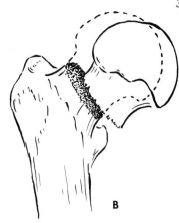
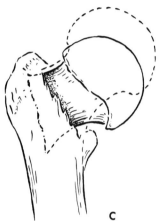
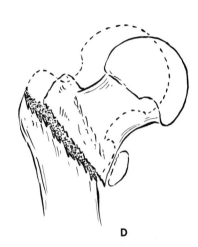

FIG. 33-22. Fractures of the hip. **A,** Subcapital fracture. **B,** Transcervical fracture. **C,** Impacted fracture of base of neck. **D,** Intertrochanteric fracture.

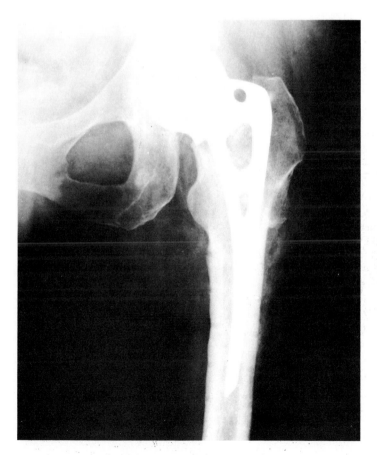

FIG. 33-23. Radiograph showing Austin-Moore prosthesis in place. Tracts of nails and screws of recently removed Smith-Petersen nail and plate are still visible in the remaining bone. (Courtesy The University Hospitals of Cleveland, Cleveland, Ohio.)

Adduction and external rotation must be avoided. If the patient does not have traction or a cast, turning to the unaffected side may be done only on the physician's order. The nurse supports the leg in abduction while the patient turns the rest of his body (Fig. 33-24). Several pillows are placed between the thighs and staggered forward to the foot to avoid adduction. The leg must not slip off the pillows (Fig. 33-25). Sandbags may be used to help maintain this position. Careful instructions must be given to the patient.

Complete healing occurs within 3 weeks and partial weight bearing may be ordered at this time. The management of a patient with a hip prosthesis will be dependent on the surgical approach used and the type of immobilization used. The physician's orders should be checked carefully for the amount of movement and position in bed. Movement of all uninvolved extremities should be encouraged in order to maintain muscle tone and prevent circulatory stasis. Plantar flexion and dorsiflexion of the affected foot are started the first postoperative day. They are done three times a day and later increased to about eight times a day. Quadriceps-setting and gluteal-setting exercises are usually started on the first postoperative day. In the quadriceps-setting exercise the patient is instructed to press the popliteal space against the bed and lift the heel; the patient will feel the kneecap move. This exercise is done five times every hour and later increased until it is done 20 times every hour. The gluteal-setting exercises are done by pinching the buttocks together and attempting to move the leg to the side of the bed. This is done five times every hour; it tightens the abductor muscles.

Abduction exercises may be started 2 to 3 weeks following surgery or when the patient has been taken out of traction. This may be accomplished by the use of roller skating board exercises (Fig. 33-26). The shoe with a skate is placed on the patient's foot. A board with a slight elevation is used with an attached pulley and rope. The patient pulls the rope to abduct the operated extremity. The patient returns the affected leg to the midline. The nurse holds the opposite hip to prevent compensatory adduction when the affected hip is pulled into abduction.[16]

The patient will be taught to crutch walk about 2 to 4 weeks postoperatively. He starts out walking between parallel bars, progressing to a walker and then to crutches with a three-point, partial weight-bearing gait. Before total weight bearing is resumed, the patient may progress to using canes.

Extracapsular fractures are usually caused by direct violence, by a fall directly onto the trochanter, or when the leg is twisted. The leg will be externally rotated. The shaft fragment tends to shorten, producing an acute angle between the shaft and the neck of the femur. Shortening occurs because of the fracture itself and the angulation. Such fractures may be *comminuted*. If the fracture is not treated, the leg will be externally rotated and adducted. The

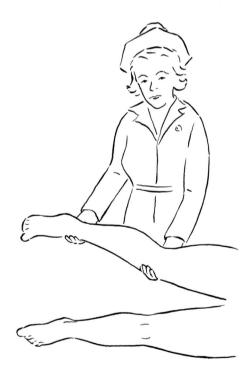

FIG. 33-24. Maintaining abduction position while turning the patient. (Redrawn from Wiebe, A.: Orthopedics in nursing, Philadelphia, 1961, W. B. Saunders Co.)

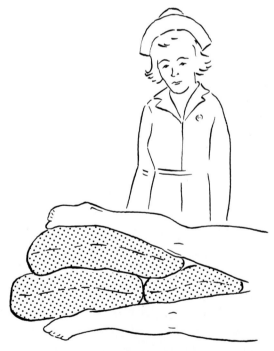

FIG. 33-25. Staggering pillows to avoid adduction of leg. Pillows must be placed so that the leg does not slip off of them. (Redrawn from Wiebe, A.: Orthopedics in nursing, Philadelphia, 1961, W. B. Saunders Co.)

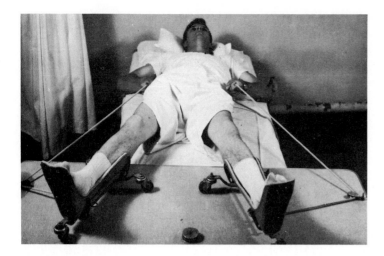

FIG. 33-26. Skates and board used to facilitate abduction exercise of the lower extremity. With the rope arrangement, the patient can passively increase the amount of abduction obtained. (From Larson, C. B., and Gould M.: Orthopedic nursing, ed. 8, St. Louis, 1974, The C. V. Mosby Co.)

intertrochanteric region has a rich blood supply and union usually occurs without difficulty. A common complication is the *varus deformity.* A varus deformity occurs when the angle of the femoral shaft to the neck is less than the normal 120 degrees. An *intertrochanteric* fracture (Fig. 33-22) may be treated by closed reduction and application of a hip spica cast. Russell traction may be used as a temporary measure or if surgery is contraindicated. Reduction by *Russell traction* takes from 6 to 12 weeks. The preferred method of treatment is surgery.

Fractures of the hip are reduced under general or spinal anesthesia. The objectives of treatment include (1) overcoming the shortening by traction or pull; (2) correcting the external rotation so that the leg is rotated while forward pressure is applied to lift the greater trochanter out of the buttock; (3) swinging the leg in abduction; and (4) maintaining the reduction by pinning or support. A lateral incision is made from the greater trochanter down along the outer side of the thigh for 6 or 7 inches. The incision is placed toward the posterior surface of the shaft of the femur to produce easier access to the femur's lateral surface. After reduction, the fracture may be immobilized by a *three-flanged Smith-Petersen nail,* the *Neufeld angled nail,* the *apparatus of Austin-Moore,* or the *multiple pin technique of Roger Anderson* and others (Fig. 33-27). Internal fixation permits more mobility for the patient, thereby reducing systemic complications common in the aged. Complications associated with some methods of internal fixation include displacement of fragments, causing deformities that may require further and more extensive surgery including bone grafts.

Nursing intervention following a hip pinning. Because the nurse will have many occasions to care for patients who have had a fractured hip pinned, the nursing care of these patients will be discussed in some detail. Casts are not usually applied after the pinning of a hip, and the dressing should be inspected frequently for bleeding. The linen under the pa-

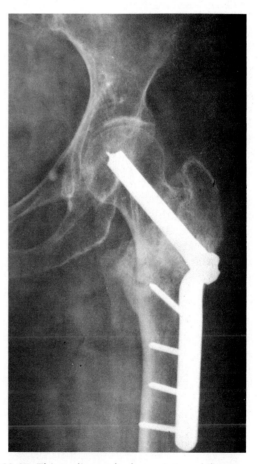

FIG. 33-27. This radiograph shows internal fixation of an intertrochanteric fracture with McLaughlin plate and pins.

tient should also be inspected to be sure that blood has not oozed from under the dressing and down the side of the thigh. Pain usually is severe postoperatively and the patient generally requires narcotics for pain and sedatives for sleep. As these patients are frequently aged women, the nurse should give drugs discriminately to prevent too much depression

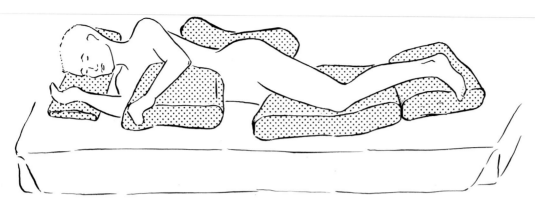

FIG. 33-28. In the side-lying position the top leg should be supported with pillows to prevent adduction of the leg as well as pressure on the lower leg. A small pillow under the head will maintain alignment of the cervical spine. (Redrawn from Wiebe, A.: Orthopedics in nursing, Philadelphia, 1961, W. B. Saunders Co.)

of respirations and activity. The older patient may become confused, particularly when barbiturates have been given. Precautions such as the use of side rails should be taken to prevent falls and further injuries. Side rails also are a help to the patient in moving about in the bed.

A patient who has had his hip pinned may be turned for back care the evening of the operation. The patient may be turned to either side. This will vary according to the physician's wishes. The patient should be turned every 2 hours. If the patient is to be turned to the operative side, the nurse should stand on the side of the bed, reach across the patient, place her hands on the opposite hip and shoulder, and gently roll him toward her. When the patient is turned to the unaffected side, the fractured limb should be kept at the same level as the trunk, supported along its entire length with pillows (Fig. 33-28). To prevent the affected hip from rotating externally when the patient is lying on his back, a *trochanter roll* should be placed gently but firmly against the outer aspect of the hip and upper thigh.

If there are no contraindications, the patient is usually permitted to be up in a chair the morning following surgery. As there can be no weight bearing on the affected extremity for several months, the patient is lifted or assisted in pivoting to the chair. When he is sitting in the chair, the patient's hips and knees should be flexed with the feet resting on the floor. The leg should *not* be elevated in extension because extension fosters external rotation and this puts a detrimental load on the nailplate.

Exercise of the affected extremity should be initiated as early as possible. The nurse should consult with the surgeon regarding desirable exercises for the affected limb as well as the exercises necessary to prepare the patient for crutch walking (p. 401). Often the physical therapist is needed to assist with this. As most patients with hip fracture are in the older age group, progress with crutch walking may be slow, and the ability to use crutches may be hampered by poor vision and physical limitations. Each patient will need to be observed carefully, and plans for discharge to the family or a nursing home will depend on the help and facilities needed and available.

Osteomyelitis

Osteomyelitis refers to an infection of bone by pyogenic bacteria. The infection involves the marrow spaces, the haversian canals, and the subperiosteal space. The bone is involved secondarily. It is destroyed by proteolytic enzymes, and interference with the blood supply causes necrosis. *Acute osteomyelitis* may be caused by introduction of bacteria through a wound, but the most common route of infection is *hematogenous spread* from a preexisting focus such as a boil.

There is initially a small focus of inflammation with hyperemia and edema. Since bone is a rigid material, this edema causes increased pressure and pain. The pus that forms further increases the pressure, which compromises local circulation and results in necrosis of the bone.

The initial treatment of acute osteomyelitis involves rest and large doses of appropriate antibiotics prescribed following culture and sensitivity testing. If dramatic improvement is not seen within 24 hours, the involved bone is usually surgically decomposed to relieve the pressure and provide for drainage. Inadequate treatment leads to *chronic osteomyelitis,* which is extremely difficult to eradicate. After a relatively long period of being symptom free the patient may again present with an acute episode. The infected dead bone separates from the living bone and becomes a *sequestrum.* The infection cannot be permanently cleared until the sequestrum is removed. This is usually done surgically, although it will sometimes happen by a natural process.

Osteomyelitis is extremely difficult to treat and often means years of recurrent episodes of disability for a patient. It can result in failure of surgical procedures such as arthroplasty. A major nursing role in osteomyelitis is in its prevention. Aseptic technique is always indicated when caring for an open wound and the nurse working with the orthopedic patient must be acutely aware that this is one means by which osteomyelitis can be prevented.

REFERENCES AND SELECTED READINGS*

1 Adams, J. C.: Outline of fractures, London, 1969, E & S Livingstone, Ltd.

2 Alba, I. M., and Papeika, J.: The nurse's role in preventing circulatory complications in the patient with a fractured hip, Nurs. Clin. North Am. **1:**57-61, March 1966.

3 American Heart Association: Prevention of rheumatic fever, New York, 1968, The Association.

4 Ansell, B. M., and Bywaters, E. G. L.: Rheumatoid arthritis (Still's disease), Pediatr. Clin. North Am. **10:**921-939, Nov. 1963.

5 Barnes, R.: Salvage procedures, failed treatment of fractured neck of the femur. In Anderson, W. F., editor: Current achievement in geriatrics, London, 1964, Cassell & Co.

6 *Beetham, W. P., Jr.: The management of the collagen diseases, GP **31:**113-123, Feb. 1965.

7 Bergersen, B. S.: Pharmacology in nursing, ed. 12, St. Louis, 1973, The C. V. Mosby Co.

8 Braidwood, R. J.: Prehistoric man, no. 37, Chicago, 1966, Chicago Natural History Museum Popular Series Anthropology.

9 *Bray, A. P., and Thomas, J. R.: Severe fat embolism syndrome following multiple fractures, Nurs. Times **65**(4):109-110, Jan. 1969.

10 *Brewer, E. J., Jr.: Rheumatoid arthritis in childhood, Am. J. Nurs. **65:**66-71, June 1965.

11 Browse, N. L.: Physiology and pathology of bed rest, Springfield, Ill., 1965, Charles C Thomas, Publisher.

12 *Brunner, N. A.: Orthopedic nursing: a programmed approach, St. Louis, 1970, The C. V. Mosby Co.

12a Brunnstrom, S.: Clinical kinesiology, ed. 3, Philadelphia, 1972, F. A. Davis Co.

13 Bryan, R. S., and Lowell, F. A. P.: The quest for the replacement knee, Orthop. Clin. North Am. **2:**715-728, Nov. 1971.

14 *Buck, B. I.: Hip replacement, Supervisor Nurse **3:**75-78, May 1972.

15 *Campbell, E. B., Hogsed, C. M., and Bogdonoff, M.: Lupus erythematosus, Am. J. Nurs. **62:**74-77, June 1962.

16 Clark, W. E. L.: The fossil evidence for human evolution, ed. 2, Chicago, 1964, The University of Chicago Press.

17 *Clissold, G. K.: The body's response to trauma: fractures, New York, 1973, Springer Publishing Co., Inc.

18 Cockin, J.: Osteotomy of the hip, Orthop. Clin. North Am. **2:**59-74, March 1974.

19 Committee on Trauma of The American College of Surgeons: An outline of the treatment of fractures, ed. 8, Philadelphia, 1965, W. B. Saunders Co.

20 Covalt, N. K.: Bed exercises for convalescent patients, Springfield, Ill., 1968, Charles C Thomas, Publisher.

21 Crenshaw, A. H., editor: Campbell's operative orthopaedics, vol. 2, ed. 5, St. Louis, 1971, The C. V. Mosby Co.

22 Dee, R.: Total replacement arthroplasty of the elbow for rheumatoid arthritis, J. Bone Joint Surg. **54B:**88-95, Feb. 1972.

23 Eaton, P., and Heller, F.: Therapeutic nursing care of orthopedic patients, Nurs. Clin. North Am. **2:**429-435, Sept. 1967.

24 Evarts, C. M., and Kendrick, J. I.: Cup arthroplasty, Orthop. Clin. North Am. **2:**93-111, March 1971.

25 *Francis, Sister Maria: Nursing the patient with internal hip fixation, Am. J. Nurs. **64:**111-112, May 1964.

26 Freyberg, R.: Rheumatoid arthritis, the natural history, diagnosis, prognosis and management, Med. Times **95:**742-752, July 1967.

27 Goldner, J. L., and others: Anterior disc excision and interbody spine fusion for chronic low back pain. In American Academy of Orthopedic Surgeons: Symposium on the spine, St. Louis, 1969, The C. V. Mosby Co.

28 Harvey, A. M.: Diseases of the connective tissue (the "collagen" diseases). In Beeson, P. D., and McDermott, W., editors: Cecil-Loeb textbook of medicine, ed. 12, Philadelphia, 1967, W. B. Saunders Co.

29 Henkind, P.: Iatrogenic eye manifestations in rheumatic disease, Geriatrics **20:**12-19, Jan. 1965.

30 Herbert, J. J., and Alain, H.: A new total knee prosthesis, Clin. Orthop. **94:**202-210, July-Aug. 1973.

31 Hoaglund, F. T.: Osteoarthritis, Orthop. Clin. North Am. **2:**3-18, March 1971.

32 Hollander, J. L., editor: Arthritis and allied conditions, ed. 7, Philadelphia, 1966, Lea & Febiger.

32a Hubbard, M. J. S.: One treatment of femoral shaft fractures on the elderly, J. Bone Joint Surg. **56B:**96-101, Feb. 1974.

33 *Kelly, M. M.: Exercises for bedfast patients, Am. J. Nurs. **66:**2209-2213, Oct. 1966.

34 Kirk, J. A., and Kersley, G. D.: Heat and cold in the physical treatment of rheumatoid arthritis of the knee, Ann. Phys. Med. **9:**270-274, Aug. 1968.

35 *Knocke, L.: Crutch walking, Am. J. Nurs. **61:**70-73, Oct. 1961.

35a Krause, R. M.: Rheumatic fever. In Beeson, P. D., and McDermott, W., editors: Cecil-Loeb textbook of medicine, ed. 13, Philadelphia, 1971, W. B. Saunders Co.

36 *Lamont-Havers, R. W.: Arthritis quackery, Am. J. Nurs. **63:**92-95, March 1963.

37 *Larson, C. B., and Gould, M. L.: Fractures of the hip and nursing care of the patient with a fractured hip, Am. J. Nurs. **58:**1558-1563, Nov. 1958.

38 *Larson, C. B., and Gould, M.: Orthopedic nursing, ed. 8, St. Louis, 1974, The C. V. Mosby Co.

39 Lonergan, R. C.: Osteoporosis of the spine, Am. J. Nurs. **61:**79-81, Jan. 1961.

40 Lowman, E. W.: Rehabilitation of the patient with chronic rheumatoid arthritis, J. Chronic Dis. **1:**628-637, June 1955.

41 Lowman, E.: Clinical management of disability due to rheumatoid arthritis, Arch. Phys. Med. Rehabil. **48:**136-141, March 1967.

42 Lutwak, L.: Calcium and nitrogen balance studies during Gemini VII flight, Lectures in aerospace medicine, Brooks Air Force Base, Texas, 1967.

43 *MacGinniss, O.: Rheumatoid arthritis—my tutor, Am. J. Nurs. **68:**1699-1701, Aug. 1968.

44 *Madden, B. W., and Affeldt, J. E.: To prevent helplessness and deformities, Am. J. Nurs. **62:**59-61, Dec. 1962.

45 Martin, D. S.: The necessity for combined modalities in cancer therapy, Hosp. Practice **8:**129-136, Jan. 1973.

46 *Mayer, J.: Nutrition and gout, Postgrad. Med. **45:**277-278, May 1969.

47 *Mayo, R. A., and Hughes, J. M.: Intramedullary nailing of long bone fractures and nursing care after intramedullary nailing, Am. J. Nurs. **59:**236-240, Feb. 1959.

48 *Miescher, P. A., and Mueller Eberhard, E. H. J.: Textbook of immunopathology (2 vols.), New York, 1969, Grune & Stratton, Inc.

49 *Monteirio, L. A.: Hip fracture—a sociologist's viewpoint, Am. J. Nurs. **67:**1207-1210, June 1967.

50 Morris, J. M.: Biomechanical aspects of the hip joint, Orthop. Clin. North Am. **2:**33-54, March 1971.

50a Murray, D. G., and Racz, G. B.: Fat embolism, the role of respiratory failure and its treatment, J. Bone Joint Surg. **56A:**1327-1337, Jan. 1974.

51 *Neufeld, A.: Surgical treatment of hip injuries, Am. J. Nurs. **65:**80-83, March 1965.

52 *Olsen, E. V.: Hazards of immobility, Am. J. Nurs. **67:**779-797, April 1967.

*References preceded by an asterisk are particularly well suited for student reading.

53 Peers, J.: The care and handling of orthopedic implants, RN **28:**66-71, Oct. 1965.

53a Pendleton, T., and Grassman, B. J.: Rehabilitating children with inflammatory joint disease, Am. J. Nurs. **74:**2223-2225, Dec. 1974.

54 *Peszczynski, M.: Why old people fall, Am. J. Nurs. **65:**86-88, May 1965.

54a Rabb, S.: Bunion surgery, Am. J. Nurs. **74:**2185-2187, Dec. 1974.

55 Robinson, W. D.: Diseases of joints. In Beeson, P. B., and McDermott, W., editors: Textbook of medicine, ed. 13, Philadelphia, 1971, W. B. Saunders Co.

56 *Roaf, R., and Hodkinson, L. J.: Textbook of orthopaedic nursing, Oxford, 1971, Blackwell Scientific Publications.

56a Ryan, J.: Compression in bone healing, Am. J. Nurs. **74:**1998-1999, Nov. 1974.

57 *Salter, R. B.: Textbook of disorders and injuries of the musculoskeletal system: an introduction to orthopaedics, rheumatology, metabolic bone disease, rehabilitation and fracture, Baltimore, 1970, The Williams & Wilkins Co.

58 *Schneider, F. R.: Handbook for the orthopaedic assistant, St. Louis, 1972, The C. V. Mosby Co.

59 Schmeisser, G. J.: A clinical manual of orthopedic traction techniques, Philadelphia, 1963, W. B. Saunders Co.

60 *Seegmiller, J. E.: Goals in gout, Postgrad. Med. **45:**99-103, Jan. 1969.

61 Shaw, B. L.: The nursing challenge of lupus: the uncertain killer, RN **31:**32-35, Sept. 1968.

62 Siegel, M., and Seelentreuna, M.: Racial and social factors in systemic lupus erythematosus, J.A.M.A. **191:**77-80, Jan. 1965.

63 Stiles, P. J.: Internal fixation of fractures in patients with diffuse malignant disease, Nurs. Mirror **125:**i-iv, Oct. 1967.

63a Synnestvedt, N.: The do's and dont's of traction care, Nursing '74 **3:**35-41, Nov. 1974.

64 *Talbott, J. H.: Gout and gouty arthritis, Nurs. Outlook **2:**540-543, Oct. 1954.

65 Talbott, J. H.: Gout, ed. 3, New York, 1967, Grune & Stratton, Inc.

66 Thomas, J. E., and Ayyar, D. R.: Systemic fat embolism, Arch. Neurol. **26:**517-523, June 1972.

67 Thomas, S.: Fat embolism—a hazard of trauma, Nurs. Times **65**(4)**:**105-108, Jan. 1969.

67a Townley, C., and Hill, L.: Total knee replacement, Am. J. Nurs. **74:**1612-1617, Sept. 1974.

68 Turek, S. L.: Orthopaedics: principles and their application, ed. 2, Philadelphia, 1967, J. B. Lippincott Co.

69 *Walike, B. C., and others: Rheumatoid arthritis, Am. J. Nurs. **67:**1420-1433, July 1967.

69a Webb, K. J.: Early assessment of orthopedic injuries, Am. J. Nurs. **74:**1048-1052, June 1972.

70 Wiebe, A. N.: Orthopedics in nursing, Philadelphia, 1961, W. B. Saunders Co.

71 Wilde, A. H.: Synovectomy of the knee, Orthop. Clin. North Am. **2:**191-205, March 1971.

72 Williams, J. M.: Fractured neck of femur and subsequent gas gangrene, Nurs. Mirror **124:**63-64, April 1967.

73 Williams, S. R.: Nutrition and diet therapy, ed. 2, St. Louis, 1973, The C. V. Mosby Co.

Index

A

Boldface type indicates major discussion.

Index